Rhinology

Diseases of the Nose, Sinuses, and Skull Base

Thieme

Rhinology

Diseases of the Nose, Sinuses, and Skull Base

David W. Kennedy, MD
Rhinology Professor
Department of Otorhinolaryngology—Head and Neck Surgery
Perelman School of Medicine
University of Pennsylvania
Philadelphia, Pennsylvania

Peter H. Hwang, MD
Professor and Chief
Division of Rhinology and Endoscopic Skull Base Surgery
Department of Otolaryngology—Head and Neck Surgery
Stanford University School of Medicine
Stanford, California

Foreword by

Heinz R. Stammberger, MD, Hon. FRCS (Ed.), Hon. FRCS (Eng), Hon. FACS
Professor and Head
Department of General ENT–Head and Neck Surgery
Medical University Graz
Graz, Austria

Christine Gralapp, MA, CMI
Medical Illustrator

Thieme
New York • Stuttgart

Thieme Medical Publishers, Inc.
333 Seventh Ave.
New York, NY 10001

Executive Editor: Timothy Y. Hiscock
Managing Editor: J. Owen Zurhellen IV
Editorial Assistant: Elizabeth Berg
Editorial Director: Michael Wachinger
Production Editor: Heidi Grauel, Maryland Composition
Medical Illustrator: Christine Gralapp
Front Cover Illustration: © 2012 Department of Otolaryngology-Head & Neck Surgery, Stanford University and Christine Gralapp
International Production Director: Andreas Schabert
Senior Vice President, International Marketing and Sales: Cornelia Schulze
Vice President, Finance and Accounts: Sarah Vanderbilt
President: Brian D. Scanlan
Compositor: Maryland Composition
Printer: Everbest Printing Co.

Library of Congress Cataloging-in-Publication Data

Rhinology : diseases of the nose, sinuses, and skull base / edited by David W. Kennedy, Peter H. Hwang. — 1st ed.
p. ; cm.
Includes bibliographical references and index.
ISBN 978-1-60406-060-7
I. Kennedy, David W., 1948- II. Hwang, Peter H.
[DNLM: 1. Nose Diseases—physiopathology. 2. Nose Diseases—surgery. 3. Otorhinolaryngologic Surgical Procedures. 4. Skull Base—surgery. WV 300]
617.5'1—dc23

2011046233

Important note: Medical knowledge is ever-changing. As new research and clinical experience broaden our knowledge, changes in treatment and drug therapy may be required. The authors and editors of the material herein have consulted sources believed to be reliable in their efforts to provide information that is complete and in accord with the standards accepted at the time of publication. However, in view of the possibility of human error by the authors, editors, or publisher of the work herein or changes in medical knowledge, neither the authors, editors, nor publisher, nor any other party who has been involved in the preparation of this work, warrants that the information contained herein is in every respect accurate or complete, and they are not responsible for any errors or omissions or for the results obtained from use of such information. Readers are encouraged to confirm the information contained herein with other sources. For example, readers are advised to check the product information sheet included in the package of each drug they plan to administer to be certain that the information contained in this publication is accurate and that changes have not been made in the recommended dose or in the contraindications for administration. This recommendation is of particular importance in connection with new or infrequently used drugs.

Printed in China

ISBN 978-1-60406-060-7
eISBN 978-1-60406-705-7

I dedicate this book to my teachers during my student years, residency, and academic career, some of whom were international leaders, some of whom were residents, and some of whom were patients who helped refine our thinking and techniques. I sincerely appreciate your insights and advice. We have learned much, but still have a long way to go. I also dedicate this to my students, for their patience and understanding when I have fallen short on answers because of either inadequate knowledge or the pressures of academic clinical practice and administrative duties. I hope that *Rhinology: Diseases of the Nose, Sinuses, and Skull Base* will help to provide more complete answers to many of the issues and questions that you have raised, and I truly appreciate the contributions you have made.

—DWK

I dedicate this book to my parents, whose enduring love and support have been my wellspring of inspiration.

—PHH

Contents

IV. Surgical Aspects of Skull Base Disease

MENU FOR THE ACCOMPANYING DVD

Foreword

It is rare in the history of medicine that a new diagnostic and surgical concept has had such a decisive and ongoing impact on a specialty as the advent of the endoscope and endoscopic sinus surgery has had on rhinology. The ability to look into the most remote corners and niches of the nose and sinuses has led to improved understanding of pathophysiology, which in turn triggered the curiosity of many clinicians and scientists to further explore the infective, inflammatory, allergic, and immunologic backgrounds of many of the diseases encountered. Transnasal endoscopic surgery developed from its humble beginnings in the early 1970s to a degree of sophistication unimaginable 20 or even 10 years ago. In interdisciplinary cooperation, rhinologists and neurosurgeons have started to go for and through the skull base, toward the pituitary, clivus, petrous apex, and well beyond toward intracranial lesions. Rhinology, over the last few decades, has developed from a field of interest only for idiosyncratic researchers into one of the most exciting and attractive rapidly developing and expanding topics of modern medicine.

This fascinating development and its achievements are documented in a masterly fashion in this book and DVD, for which David W. Kennedy and Peter H. Hwang have to be congratulated. Its plain title *Rhinology: Diseases of the Nose, Sinuses, and Skull Base* does not at first glance reveal the true treasures hidden inside: David and Peter have managed to bring together many of the best experts in their respective fields to contribute chapters—the contributors' names read like the "who's who" of the opinion leaders globally. This book reflects the developments of the last 30 years, and the interdisciplinary nature of rhinology brings together anatomists, physiologists, allergologists, immunologists, radiologists, endocrinologists, basic researchers, rhino- and neurosurgeons, and more. Whereas normally books and their chapters lag behind the latest advances and journal publications, with this book it is different. Here, the contemporary experience of the world's top experts is one of the book's core values; one can clearly "feel" the editors' work throughout the chapters, highlighting work and research in progress whenever appropriate—there is no dogmatic approach anywhere in this book! That Thieme Medical Publishers has taken extra effort by providing the great medical illustrator Christine Gralapp, who has created unique and clear color drawings throughout the volume, adds to the overall outstanding quality of this book. The accompanying DVD is of high quality, illustrative, and very educational. The fact that though the videos are by various experts David Kennedy personally narrates all of them provides a welcome consistency for the viewer.

There has never been a book on rhinology that is as complete and up-to-date as this one—it will be a benchmark for the decades to come!

Heinz R. Stammberger, MD, Hon. FRCS (Ed.),
Hon. FRCS (Eng), Hon. FACS
Professor and Head,
Department of General ENT–
Head and Neck Surgery
Medical University Graz
Graz, Austria

Preface

Rhinology: Diseases of the Nose, Sinuses, and Skull Base is intended to provide a comprehensive multimedia resource for otorhinolaryngologists, head and neck surgeons, and residents and students with a significant interest in rhinology or skull base surgery. Appropriate chapters are also a resource for skull base neurosurgeons who wish to better understand the otolaryngologic aspects of the team approach to skull base lesions.

Since the book *Diseases of the Sinuses: Diagnosis and Management* by David W. Kennedy, William E. Bolger, and S. James Zinreich was published in 2000, much has changed within this rapidly expanding field. Although still far from providing all the answers, our clinical research since then has significantly improved our understanding of the pathogenesis of these common disorders, our sinus surgery has been considerably refined, and endoscopic skull base surgery has become mainstream and widely practiced internationally. This new book provides a broad but detailed compendium of current knowledge and practice within the field.

This book is divided into four sections: Sinonasal Anatomy and Physiology, Medical Aspects of Sinonasal Disease, Surgical Aspects of Sinonasal Disease, and Surgical Aspects of Skull Base Disease. We were able to illustrate the chapters with a large number of excellent color illustrations from artist Christine Gralapp. Additionally, we have included a DVD, also authored by leading surgeons within the specialty, to illustrate the key pearls and pitfalls of the surgical aspects of the majority of the procedures discussed within the chapters. In each instance, we were very fortunate to be able to recruit the leading surgeons within each of their areas of interest and expertise. We hope and expect that this will be an important reference for surgeons looking to improve their surgical expertise or to develop a broader armamentarium of techniques.

The 2000 book became an important resource for otorhinolaryngologists and otorhinolaryngology residents internationally, in terms of the broader aspects of understanding both the underlying disorders and their medical and surgical management. We sincerely hope that you will find this new and more comprehensive book of equal importance to the field. Most importantly we hope that this resource will help you improve the quality of management of patients with sinonasal and skull base disorders. The book encompasses a common area of patient symptomatology where for too long our management has been suboptimal or not based upon current academic research. We hope and expect that you, the reader, will find this a significant contribution in this regard.

Acknowledgments

For the creation of this resource, first and foremost we must thank the contributors, the list of whom includes the vast majority of luminaries within this rapidly expanding field nationally and internationally. We truly appreciate how much of your time you have expended on this work, and we hope you will feel proud of the results. Secondly, we would like to thank the staff of Thieme Medical Publishers for their encouragement and patience as we endeavored to develop this comprehensive resource.

We thank KARL STORZ Endoscopy-America Inc., especially Ali Amiri, Yvonne Bernschneider, and Susan Jaffy Marx, for their kind support of the DVD production. We also thank VCSvideo of Cinnaminson, New Jersey (especially David Fox), for the production work, and we thank artist Christine Gralapp for her superb illustrations.

Contributors

Reza Alizadehfar, MD, FRCPC
Professor of Pediatrics
Department of Allergy and Immunology
McGill University/Montreal Children's Hospital
Montreal General Hospital
Montreal, Québec, Canada

Vijay K. Anand, MD, FACS
Clinical Professor of Otolaryngology
Otolaryngology, Head and Neck Surgery
Weill Cornell Medical College
Presbyterian Hospital
New York, New York

Claus Bachert, MD, PhD
Professor of Medicine
Ear, Nose, and Throat Department
Ghent University
Ghent University Hospital
Ghent, Belgium

Leonardo Balsalobre, MD, MPH
Department of Otolaryngology—Head and Neck
Federal University of Sao Paulo
São Paulo ENT Center, Hospital Professor Edmundo Vasconcelos
São Paulo, Brazil

Fuad M. Baroody, MD
Professor of Surgery
Section of Otolaryngology—Head and Neck Surgery
The University of Chicago
Chicago, Illinois

Pete S. Batra, MD, FACS
Associate Professor of Otolaryngology—Head and Neck Surgery
UT Southwestern Medical Center
Dallas, Texas

Karen Anne Bednarski, MD
Allergy and Asthma Associates
Houston, Texas

Gerald J. Berry, MD
Professor of Pathology
Co-Director of Surgical Pathology
Stanford University Medical Center
Stanford, California

Rajiv K. Bhalla, BSc (Hons), MBChB, FRCS (ORL-HNS), MD
Consultant ENT Surgeon and Rhinologist
Honorary Senior Lecturer
University Department of Otolaryngology—Head and Neck Surgery
Manchester Royal Infirmary
Manchester, United Kingdom

Robson Capasso, MD
Clinical Assistant Professor of Otolaryngology—Head and Neck Surgery
Chief of Sleep Surgery Division
Stanford University
Stanford, California

Paolo Cappabianca, MD
Professor of Neurosurgery
Department of Neurological Sciences, Division of Neurosurgery
Università degli Studi di Napoli Federico II
Naples, Italy

Ricardo L. Carrau, MD, FACS
Professor of Otolaryngology—Head and Neck Surgery
Director of Comprehensive Skull Base Surgery Program
The Ohio State University Medical Center
Columbia, Ohio

Oscar Carrillo, RPSGT
Research Collaborator
Sleep Research
Stanford University
Stanford, California

Roy R. Casiano, MD
Professor of Otolaryngology
Miller School of Medicine
University of Miami
Miami, Florida

Paolo Castelnuovo, MD, PhD
Professor of Otorhinolaryngology—Head and Neck Surgery
University of Insurbia, Varese
Chairman of Otorhinolaryngology—Head and Neck Surgery
Varese, Italy

Luigi Maria Cavallo, MD, PhD
Assistant Professor of Neurosurgery
Department of Neurological Sciences, Division of Neurosurgery
Università degli Studi di Napoli Federico II
Naples, Italy

Yvonne Chan, MD, FRCS(C), MSc, HBSc
Assistant Professor of Otolaryngology—Head and Neck Surgery
University of Toronto
Ontario, Canada

Rakesh K. Chandra, MD
Associate Professor of Otolaryngology—Head and Neck Surgery
Clinical Practice Director of Otolaryngology—Head and Neck Surgery
Northwestern University Feinberg School of Medicine
Chicago, Illinois

Alexander G. Chiu, MD
Professor and Chief of Otolaryngology
University of Arizona
Tucson, Arizona

Deborah J. Chute, MD
Assistant Professor of Pathology
Department of Anatomic Pathology
Cleveland Clinic
Cleveland, Ohio

Martin J. Citardi, MD, FACS
Professor and Chair of Otorhinolaryngology–Head and Neck Surgery
University of Texas Medical School at Houston
Texas Sinus Insititute
Texas Skull Base Physicians
Houston, Texas

Noam A. Cohen, MD, PhD
Assistant Professor of Otorhinolaryngology
University of Pennsylvania
Philadelphia, Pennsylvania

David B. Conley, MD
Associate Professor of Otolaryngology
Northwestern University Feinberg School of Medicine
Chicago, Illinois

Marie-Noëlle Corriveau, MD
Clinical Professor of Otolaryngology—Head and Neck Surgery
Université Laval, Centre Hospitalier Universitaire de Québec
Montreal, Québec, Canada

John M. DelGaudio, MD
Professor of Otolaryngology—Head and Neck Surgery
Emory University
Atlanta, Georgia

Martin Y. Desrosiers, MD, FRCSC
Professor of Otolaryngology—Head and Neck Surgery
Université de Montréal/Centre Hospitalier Universitaire de Montréal
Hôpitale Hôtel-Dieu de Montréal
Québec, Canada

Vikram D. Durairaj, MD, FACS
Professor of Ophthalmology and Otolaryngology—Head and Neck Surgery
Director of Oculoplastic and Orbital Surgery
University of Colorado
Denver, Colorado

Jean Anderson Eloy, MD, FACS
Assistant Professor of Otolaryngology—Head and Neck Surgery
Assistant Professor of Neurological Surgery
University of Medicine and Dentistry of New Jersey
Vice Chairman and Director of Rhinology, Sinus, and Endoscopic Skull Base Surgery
Neurological Institute of New Jersey
Newark, New Jersey

Janaki Emani, MD
Weiss Memorial Hospital
Chicago, Illinois

Victoria A. Epstein, MD
Rhinologist and Skull Base Surgeon
The Permanente Medical Group
San Francisco, California

Felice Esposito, MD, PhD, FACS
Assistant Professor of Neurosurgery
Department of Neurological Sciences, Division of Neurosurgery
Università degli Studi di Napoli Federico II
Naples, Italy

Isabella Esposito, MD
Neurosurgery Instructor
Department of Neurological Sciences, Division of Neurosurgery
Università degli Studi di Napoli Federico II
Naples, Italy

Berrylin J. Ferguson, MD, FACS
Professor of Otolaryngology
University of Pittsburgh School of Medicine
Pittsburgh, Pennsylvania

Juan C. Fernandez-Miranda, MD
Assistant Professor of Neurological Surgery
Director, Surgical Neuroanatomy Lab
University of Pittsburgh
Pittsburgh, Pennsylvania

Nancy J. Fischbein, MD
Professor of Radiology, Otolaryngology—Head and Neck Surgery, Neurology, and Neurosurgery
Standford University Medical Center
Stanford, California

Andrew J. Fishman, MD
Associate Professor of Otolaryngology and Neurosurgery
Northwestern University Feinberg School of Medicine
Chicago, Illinois

Karen J. Fong, MD
Adjunct Clinical Assistant Professor of Otolaryngology–Head and Neck Surgery
Stanford University
Physician and Surgeon
California Sinus Centers
Walnut Creek, California

Giorgio Frank, MD
Director
Center of Surgery for Pituitary Tumors
Neurosurgeon
Bellaria Hospital
Bologna, Italy

Paul A. Gardner, MD
Assistant Professor of Neurological Surgery
Co-Director, Center for Skull Base Surgery
University of Pittsburgh Medical Center
Pittsburgh, Pennsylvania

Anne E. Getz, MD
Assistant Professor of Otolaryngology
Washington University
St. Louis, Missouri

Andrew N. Goldberg, MD, MSCE, FACS
Professor of Otolaryngology—Head and Neck Surgery
Director, Division of Rhinology and Sinus Surgery
University of California, San Francisco
San Francisco, California

Parul Goyal, MD
Assistant Professor of Otolaryngology
Director of Rhinology and Sinus Surgery
SUNY Upstate Medical University
Syracuse, New York

David A. Gudis, MD
Resident of Otorhinolaryngology—Head and Neck Surgery
University of Pennsylvania
Philadelphia, Pennsylvania

Jose G. Gurrola II, MD
Resident of Otolaryngology—Head and Neck Surgery
University of Iowa Hospitals and Clinics
Iowa City, Iowa

Daniel L. Hamilos, MD
Associate Professor of Internal Medicine
Division of Rheumatology, Allergy and Immunology
Massachusetts General Hospital
Boston, Massachusetts

Joseph K. Han, MD
Associate Professor of Otolaryngology—Head and Neck Surgery
Eastern Virginia Medical School
Norfolk, Virginia

Griffith R. Harsh IV, MD, MA, MBA
Professor of Neurosurgery
Stanford University
Stanford, California

Richard J. Harvey, MBBS, FRACS
Associate Professor of Otolaryngology and Skull Base Surgery
Program Head, Rhinology and Skull Base Surgery
St. Vincent's Hospital, University of New South Wales, and Macquarie University
Sydney, Australia

Eric H. Holbrook, MD
Assistant Professor of Otology and Laryngology
Harvard Medical School
Massachusetts Eye and Ear Infirmary
Boston, Massachusetts

Peter H. Hwang, MD
Professor and Chief
Division of Rhinology and Endoscopic Skull Base Surgery
Department of Otolaryngology—Head and Neck Surgery
Stanford University School of Medicine
Stanford, California

Amin R. Javer, MD, FRCSC
Associate Professor of Surgery
St. Paul's Hospital, University of British Columbia
Director, St. Paul's Sinus Centre
Vancouver, British Columbia, Canada

Ben-Zion Joshua, MD
Otolaryngology—Head and Neck Surgery
Soroka University Medical Center
Beer Sheva, Israel

Larry Hilton Kalish, MBBS (Hons I), MMed (Clin Epi), MS, FRACS
Senior Lecturer at University of Sydney
Head of Ear, Nose, Throat Department
Concord Hospital
Sydney Sinus and Allergy Centre
New South Wales, Australia

Michael J. Kaplan, MD
Professor of Otolaryngology
Stanford University School of Medicine
Stanford, California

Amin B. Kassam, MD
Professor of Surgery, Neurological Surgery
Department of Surgery
Chief, Division of Neurosurgery
Director, Minimally Invasive Neurosurgery Center
Co-director, Center for Cranial Base and Cerebrovascular Surgery
The Ottawa Hospital
University of Ottawa

David W. Kennedy, MD
Rhinology Professor
Department of Otorhinolaryngology—Head and Neck Surgery
Perelman School of Medicine
University of Pennsylvania
Philadelphia, Pennsylvania

Robert C. Kern, MD
Chairman and Professor of Otolaryngology—Head and Neck Surgery
Northwestern University Feinberg School of Medicine
Chicago, Ilinois

Manish Khanna, MD
Sinus Institute of Northern Virginia
Alexandria, Virginia

Shaun J. Kilty, BSc, MD, FRCSC
Assistant Professor of Otolaryngology—Head and Neck Surgery
The University of Ottawa
The Ottawa Hospital
Ontario, Canada

Todd T. Kingdom, MD
Professor and Vice Chair of Clinical Affairs
Department of Otolaryngology—Head and Neck Surgery
University of Colorado
Aurora, Colorado

Peter J. Koltai, MD, FACS, FAAP
Professor of Otolaryngology and Pediatrics
Stanford University School of Medicine
Vice President, Medical Staff
Lucile Packard Children's Hospital
Palo Alto, California

Stilianos E. Kountakis, MD, PhD
Professor of Otolaryngology
Chief, Division of Rhinology
Georgia Health Sciences University
Augusta, Georgia

Paul R. Krakovitz, BS, MD
Assistant Professor of Surgery
Section Head of Pediatric Otolaryngology
Head and Neck Institute
Cleveland Clinic Foundation
Cleveland, Ohio

Frederick A. Kuhn, MD, FACS, FARS
Adjunct Professor of Otolaryngology
University of North Carolina
Fellowship and Medical Director
The Georgia Nasal and Sinus Institute
Savannah, Georgia

Andrew P. Lane, MD
Professor of Otolaryngology—Head and Neck Surgery
Director, Johns Hopkins Sinus Center
The Johns Hopkins University School of Medicine
Baltimore, Maryland

Donald C. Lanza, MD, MS
Program Director of Rhinology/Skull Base Fellowship
Sinus and Nasal Institute of Florida, PA
Sinus and Nasal Institute of Florida Foundation
St. Petersburg, Florida

Edward R. Laws, MD, FACS
Professor of Surgery
Director, Pituitary/Neuroendocrine Center
Harvard Medical School
Brigham and Women's Hospital
Bristol, Massachusetts

John M. Lee, MD, FRCSC
Lecturer of Otolaryngology—Head and Neck Surgery
University of Toronto
St. Michael's Hospital
Toronto, Ontario, Canada

Donald A. Leopold, MD, MBA
Professor of Otolaryngology
University of Vermont
Burlington, Vermont

Man-Kit Leung, MD
Adjunct Clinical Instructor of Otolaryngology—Head and Neck Surgery
Stanford University School of Medicine
Palo Alto, California

Francis T.K. Ling, BSc, MD, FRCSC
Adjunct Professor of Otolaryngology—Head and Neck Surgery
Schulich School of Medicine and Dentistry
University of Windsor
Dr. Francis T.K. Ling Medicine Professional Corporation
Windsor, Ontario, Canada

Laurie A. Loevner, MD
Professor of Radiology, Otorhinolaryngology and Neck Surgery, and Neurosurgery
University of Pennsylvania School of Medicine
Director, Head and Neck Imaging
Hospital of the University of Pennsylvania
Philadelphia, Pennsylvania

Valerie J. Lund, MB, BSMS, FRCS, FRCSEd
Professor of Rhinology
Royal National Throat, Nose and Ear Hospital, University College
London, United Kingdom

Bradley F. Marple, MD
Professor and Vice Chairman
Associate Dean for Graduate Medical Education
Department of Otolaryngology—Head and Neck Surgery
UT Southwestern Medical Center at Dallas
Dallas, Texas

Christopher T. Melroy, MD, FARS
Georgia Nasal and Sinus Institute
Savannah, Georgia

Ralph B. Metson, MD
Clinical Professor of Otology and Laryngology
Harvard Medical School
Department of Otolaryngology
Massachusetts Eye and Ear Infirmary
Boston, Massachusetts

Igor Mikityansky, MD, MPH
Radiologist
Windsong Radiology Group
Williamsville, New York

Stefan A. Mindea, MD
Assistant Professor of Neurosurgery
Stanford University School of Medicine
Director, Minimally Invasive Spinal Surgery
Stanford Medical Center
Stanford, California

Howard S. Moskowitz, MD, PhD
Department of Otolaryngology
University of Pittsburgh School of Medicine
The Eye and Ear Institute Building
Pittsburgh, Pennsylvania

Sam P. Most, MD, FACS
Professor of Otolaryngology—Head and Neck Surgery
Chief, Division of Facial Plastic Surgery and Reconstructive Surgery
Stanford University School of Medicine
Stanford, California

Andrew H. Murr, MD, FACS
Professor and Vice Chairman, Otolaryngology—Head and Neck Surgery
University of California, San Francisco
San Francisco, California

Robert M. Naclerio, MD
Professor of Otolaryngology—Head and Neck Surgery
The University of Chicago
Chicago, Illinois

Jayakar V. Nayak, MD, PhD
Assistant Professor
Division of Rhinology and Endoscopic Skull Base Surgery
Department of Otolaryngology—Head and Neck Surgery
Stanford University School of Medicine
Stanford, California

Piero Nicolai, MD
Professor of Otorhinolaryngology
Otorhinolaryngology
University of Brescia—Spedali Civili Brescia
Brescia, Italy

João F. Nogueira, MD
Otolaryngologist
Sinus Centro
Hospital Geral de Fortaleza
Fortaleza, Brazil

Erin K. O'Brien, MD
Senior Associate Consultant
Department of Otorhinolaryngology
Mayo Clinic
Rochester, Minnesota

Richard R. Orlandi, MD
Professor of Otolaryngology—Head and Neck Surgery
University of Utah
Salt Lake City, Utah

John F. Pallanch, MD, MS
Division Chair of Rhinology
Ear, Nose, and Throat Department
Mayo Clinic
Rochester, Minnesota

James N. Palmer, MD
Associate Professor of Otorhinolaryngology—Head and Neck Surgery
Director of Rhinology
University of Pennsylvania
Philadelphia, Pennsylvania

Ernesto Pasquini, MD
Adjunct Professor
Ear, Nose, and Throat Department
Sant'orsola-Malpighi Hospital
Bologna, Italy

Mihir R. Patel, MD
Resident of Otolaryngology—Head and Neck Surgery
University of North Carolina at Chapel Hill
Chapel Hill, North Carolina

Carl Philpott, MD, MB ChB, FRCS
Senior Lecturer in Otorhinolaryngology
Norwich Medical School
University of East Anglia
Honorary Consultant ENT Surgeon and Rhinologist
Director of the Smell and Taste Clinic
James Paget University Hospital NHS Foundation Trust
Norwich, Norfolk, United Kingdom

Jayant M. Pinto, MD
Assistant Professor of Otolaryngology—Head and Neck Surgery
The University of Chicago
Chicago, Illinois

Andrea Pistochini, MD
Assistant Professor of Otorhinolaryngology
Ospedale di Circolo—Varese
Varese, Italy

Michael P. Platt, MD
Assistant Professor of Otolaryngology—Head and Neck Surgery
Boston University School of Medicine
Boston, Massachusetts

Daniel M. Prevedello, MD
Assistant Professor of Neurological Surgery
Director of The Minimally Invasive Cranial Surgery Program
The Ohio State University Medical Center
Columbus, Ohio

Vijay R. Ramakrishnan, MD
Assistant Professor of Otolaryngology
Director of Skull Base Program
University of Colorado
Aurora, Colorado

Matthew W. Ryan, MD
Assistant Professor of Otolaryngology
University of Texas Southwestern Medical Center
Dallas, Texas

Nathan B. Sautter, MD
Assistant Professor of Otolaryngology—Head and Neck Surgery
Oregon Health and Science University
Portland, Oregon

Rodney J. Schlosser, MD
Professor of Otolaryngology
Director of Rhinology
Medical University of South Carolina
Charleston, South Carolina

Theodore H. Schwartz, MD, FACS
Professor of Neurosurgery, Otolaryngology, Neurology, and Neuroscience
Weill Cornell Medical College,
New York Presbyterian Hospital
New York, New York

Kristin A. Seiberling, MD
Associate Professor of Otolaryngology
Loma Linda University
Loma Linda, California

Brent A. Senior, MD, FACS, FARS
Vice Chair of Academic Affairs
Nathaniel and Sheila Harries Professor of Otolaryngology
Chief, Division of Rhinology, Allergy, and Endoscopic Skull Base Surgery
Division of Rhinology, Allergy, and Endoscopic Skull Base Surgery
University of North Carolina
Chapel Hill, North Carolina

Dharmbir S. Sethi, MD, FRCSEd
Department of Otorhinolaryngology
Singapore General Hospital
Singapore

Ameet Singh, MD
Assistant Professor of Surgery (Otolaryngology) and Neurosurgery
Co-Director, Endoscopic Pituitary and Skull Base Surgery
George Washington University Medical Center
Washington, DC

Timothy L. Smith, MD, MPH
Professor of Otolaryngology—Head and Neck Surgery
Oregon Health and Science University
Portland, Oregon

Carl H. Snyderman, MD, MBA
Professor of Otolaryngology and Neurological Surgery
University of Pittsburgh School of Medicine
Co-Director, Center for Cranial Base Surgery
University of Pittsburgh Medical Center
Pittsburgh, Pennsylvania

Domenico Solari, MD
Assistant Professor of Neurosurgery
Department of Neurological Sciences, Division of Neurosurgery
Università degli Studi di Napoli Federico II
Naples, Italy

Aldo C. Stamm, MD, PhD
Affiliate Professor of Otorhinolaryngology—Head and Neck Surgery
São Paulo Federal University
Director, São Paulo ENT Center
Hospital Professor Edmundo Vasconcelos
São Paulo, Brazil

James A. Stankiewicz, MD
Professor and Chair
Department of Otolaryngology—Head and Neck Surgery
Loyola University Medical Center
Maywood, Illinois

Michael G. Stewart, MD, MPH
Professor and Chairman of Otolaryngology—Head and Neck Surgery
E. Darracott Vaughan MD Senior Associate Dean for Clinical Affairs
Weill Cornell Medical College
New York, New York

E. Bradley Strong, MD
Professor of Otolaryngology
Vice Chair, Clinical Director
University of California, Davis Medical Center
Sacramento, California

Shannon S. Sullivan, MD
Assistant Professor of Psychiatry
Stanford University School of Medicine
Faculty Physician
Stanford Sleep Disorders Clinic
Redwood City, California

Dana L. Suskind, MD
Associate Professor of Otolaryngology
Medical Director of Pediatric Cochlear Implant Program
University of Chicago Medical Center
Chicago, Illinois

Hin Ngan Tay, MBBS, MMed(ORL), MRCSEd
Adjunct Assistant Professor of Otolaryngology
Singapore General Hospital, Duke-NUS Graduate Medical School
Singapore

Belachew Tessema, MD
Assistant Clinical Professor of Otolaryngology
University of Connecticut
Farmington, Connecticut

Roy F. Thomas, MD
Rhinologist
Department of Surgery
Otolaryngology Service
Madigan Healthcare System
Tacoma, Washington

Travis T. Tollefson, MD, FACS
Associate Professor of Facial Plastic and Reconstructive Surgery
University of California, Davis Medical Center
Sacramento, California

Elina M. Toskala, MD, PhD
Professor of Otorhinolaryngology and Allergy
Center for Applied Genomics, Children's Hospital of Philadelphia
Philadelphia, Pennsylvania
Department of Otorhinolaryngology, Finnish Institute of Occupational Health
Helsinki, Finland

Manfred Tschabitscher, MD, PhD
Professor of Anatomy
Department of Systematic Anatomy
University of Vienna
Vienna, Austria

Justin H. Turner, MD, PhD
Clinical Instructor of Otolaryngology—Head and Neck Surgery
Stanford University
Stanford, California

Winston C. Vaughan, MD
Director, California Sinus Center
Stanford Hospital
Atherton, California

Allan D. Vescan, MD, FRCSC
Lecturer of Otolaryngology—Head and Neck Surgery
Staff Surgeon
Mount Sinai Hospital/ University of Toronto
Ontario, Canada

Kevin C. Welch, MD
Assistant Professor of Otolaryngology—Head and Neck Surgery
Loyola University Medical Center
Maywood, Illinois

Sarah K. Wise, MD
Assistant Professor of Otolaryngology—Head and Neck Surgery
Emory University
Atlanta, Georgia

Ian J. Witterick, MD, MSc, FRCSC
Professor and Vice Chair
Department of Otolaryngology—Head and Neck Surgery
University of Toronto
Ontario, Canada

Stephen M. Wold, MD
Alpine Ears, Nose, and Throat, PC
Fort Collins, Colorado

Troy D. Woodard, MD
Professional Staff
Otolaryngology—Head and Neck Institute
Cleveland Clinic Foundation
Cleveland, Ohio

Bradford A. Woodworth, MD
James J. Hicks Associate Professor of Surgery
Gregory Fleming James Cystic Fibrosis Research Center
University of Alabama at Birmingham
Birmingham, Alabama

Peter-John Wormald, MD, FRACS, FRCS, FCS (SA), MBChB
Professor and Chairman
Department of Otolaryngology—Head and Neck Surgery
University of Adelaide
South Australia, Australia

Erin D. Wright, MDCM, MEd, FRCSC
Associate Professor of Surgery
Division of Otolaryngology—Head and Neck Surgery, Department of Surgery
University of Alberta
Edmonton, Alberta, Canada

Adam M. Zanation, MD
Assistant Professor of Otolaryngology—Head and Neck Surgery
University of North Carolina
Chapel Hill, North Carolina

1 Sinonasal Development and Anatomy

Sarah K. Wise, Richard R. Orlandi, and John M. DelGaudio

Sinonasal Development

Understanding the anatomy of the paranasal sinuses and surrounding structures is integral to performing safe and appropriate sinus surgery through endoscopic and open techniques. In addition, knowledge of the embryologic development of the paranasal sinuses allows for better comprehension of the spatial involvement of disease processes affecting the sinuses. Because the nasal and paranasal sinus structures develop from multiple bones, rather than a single bone, understanding the developmental relationship between these bones allows the surgeon to better evaluate and treat certain disease processes that affect the sinonasal cavities.

The primary bones from which the paranasal sinuses develop are the maxillary, ethmoid, sphenoid, and frontal bones. There are also lesser contributions to paranasal sinus development from the lacrimal and zygomatic bones. Development of the four sets of paired paranasal sinuses is discussed in detail here. The nasal septum develops from four sources: the perpendicular plate of the ethmoid bone, the maxillary bone (crest), the vomer, and the quadrangular cartilage.

Nasal Cavity Development

Early development of the sinonasal cavity begins during the 8th week of fetal life. At this time, the nasal septum can be seen dividing the right and left sides of the future nasal cavity. At 8 weeks' gestation, the nasal septum is a mesenchymal structure that is partially differentiated into cartilage.[1] Also beginning at 8 weeks, several ridges begin to develop along the lateral nasal wall.[2] These lateral nasal wall ridges are the earliest signs of the developing turbinates. Surrounding the embryologic nasal cavity a cartilaginous capsule forms, and at 9 to 10 weeks the cartilaginous capsule contributes finger-like projections to the developing turbinates.[2] Also between 9 and 12 weeks' gestation, a separate cartilaginous and soft tissue bud forms between the developing middle and inferior turbinates.[1,2] This bud will become the uncinate process (**Fig. 1.1**).

The ridges along the lateral nasal wall, which will ultimately develop into the turbinates, have been reported to be of different origin by various authors throughout history. In 1895, Killian described the inferior turbinate as originating from the maxillary process and termed this developing structure the maxilloturbinal.[3] Killian further described the more superiorly located ethmoturbinals as

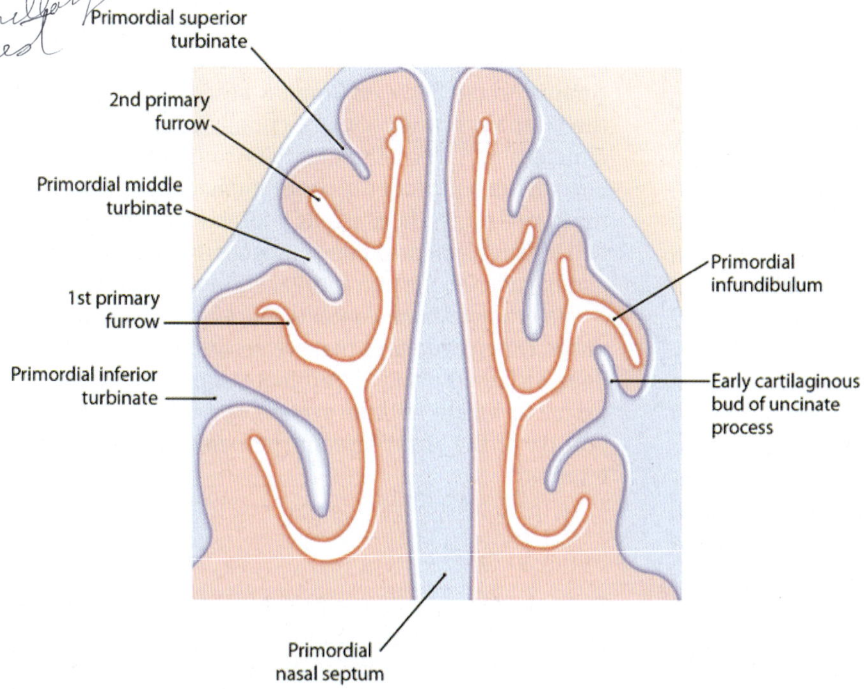

Fig. 1.1 Illustration of cartilaginous nasal capsule at ~9 to 12 weeks of fetal development.

forming the middle and superior turbinates, with a small nasoturbinal forming the agger nasi region. Stammberger supports the maxilloturbinal origin of the inferior turbinate, but notes some subtle differences in the ultimate development of the five described ethmoturbinals, with approximately four of the ethmoturbinals remaining throughout development and eventually forming the agger nasi region (superior portion of first ethmoturbinal or nasoturbinal), middle turbinate (second ethmoturbinal), superior turbinate (third ethmoturbinal), and supreme turbinate (fourth and fifth ethmoturbinals).[4] In contrast to Killian and Stammberger, Bingham et al. have described the inferior turbinate as arising from the cartilaginous nasal capsule along with the middle and superior turbinates and they do not support separate maxilloturbinal terminology.[2]

At 15 to 16 weeks' gestation, the inferior, middle, and superior turbinates are clearly formed and easily visible in embryologic sections.[2] As seen from developmental histologic sections, the middle and superior turbinates arise from precursors of the ethmoid bone, whereas the inferior turbinate bone is independent, receiving contributions of its final adult structure from the cartilaginous nasal capsule and the bone of the maxilla.[2]

Between the ethmoturbinal ridges are primary furrows, which will form the recesses and meatuses that separate the adult turbinates.[4–6] The first and second ethmoturbinals are separated by the first primary furrow, which becomes the middle meatus, ethmoid infundibulum, hiatus semilunaris, and part of the frontal recess in the adult. The superior and supreme meatuses are derived from the second and third primary furrows, respectively. The extent of adult paranasal sinus pneumatization and development differs greatly from person to person. This is thought to result from the extent of invagination and evagination between the developing turbinates and their intervening furrows.[5]

Sinonasal Mucosa and Olfactory Development

In a histologic study of human fetal heads, Wake et al.[1] have elegantly described the development of the sinonasal mucosa. In summary, as the nasal cavity begins to develop at 8 weeks' gestation, a hypercellular mesenchymal capsule forms around the developing nasal structures. Although the majority of the nasal cavity contains undifferentiated cells or stratified cuboidal cells, the nasal septum is partially differentiated into cartilage at this time, and olfactory epithelium can be seen in the superior aspect of the nasal cavity. By 9 to 10 weeks, the cartilaginous nasal capsule has fully differentiated, ciliated pseudostratified columnar or cuboidal epithelium is seen on the septum and inferior turbinate, and primitive blood vessels are present. At 11 to 12 weeks, the septal epithelium has differentiated into characteristic ciliated respiratory epithelium and secretory goblet cells are present, but the lateral nasal wall mucosa continues to be less differentiated. The cribriform plate is present in cartilaginous form at 14 to 16 weeks, with neurovascular bundles penetrating it, and olfactory epithelium is present throughout the superior portion of the nasal cavity. Also at 14 to 16 weeks, stratified squamous epithelium with hair follicles can be seen in the nasal vestibule. The mucosal lining of the developing paranasal sinuses remains spherical or cuboidal with few cilia and glands. By 17 to 18 weeks, the lateral nasal wall and ethmoid sinus mucosa has matured to respiratory epithelium, with higher concentrations of goblet cells anteriorly and ciliated cells posteriorly. At 20 to 24 weeks, secretory cells are more evenly distributed and vascular structures are present throughout the lamina propria, resembling postnasal development. Postnatally, there is partial regression of the olfactory epithelium such that it occupies only the area of the cribriform plate and superior turbinate.

Ethmoid Sinuses

The ethmoid sinus is the first to develop into detectable pneumatized cells in the fetus. Early anterior ethmoid cells, including the cartilaginous beginnings of the ethmoid bulla, form as a result of budding from the middle meatus around 11 to 12 weeks of fetal life.[1,7] At 14 to 16 weeks some anterior ethmoid cells are well formed.[1] Wake et al.[1] report that, by 17 to 18 weeks, the posterior ethmoid buds begin to develop from the superior meatus. Ossification of the ethmoid sinuses and lamina papyracea has occurred by 20 to 24 weeks' gestation.[1,7]

At birth the ethmoid sinuses are the most mature of the paranasal sinuses, being completely developed in the number of cells but not in size.[8] In the newborn, the ethmoid complex is 8 to 12 mm long, 1 to 3 mm wide, and 1 to 5 mm in height. The ethmoid sinuses undergo significant growth during the first decade of life. Wolf et al.[8] note the most rapid expansion of the ethmoid complex between 1 and 4 years of age, whereas Shah et al.[9] have demonstrated the most rapid anteroposterior expansion of the ethmoid sinuses occurs between 3 and 8 years of age. By age 12, the ethmoid sinuses have essentially reached their adult dimensions.[8,9] The ethmoid cells can, however, expand beyond the boundaries of the ethmoid bone to extend into the frontal recess (frontal cells, suprabullar cells, and frontal bullar cells), sphenoid bone (sphenoethmoid [Onodi] cell), and maxillary bone (infraorbital ethmoid [Haller] cell).

The ethmoid bone contains more than the ethmoid sinuses. Other structures that are derived from the ethmoid bone include the middle turbinate, superior turbinate, supreme turbinate, cribriform plate, and the posterosuperior portion of the nasal septum (perpendicular plate of the ethmoid).

Maxillary Sinus

The maxilla begins to ossify at 11 to 12 weeks' gestation, as the early anterior ethmoid sinuses are developing.[1] The maxillary infundibulum becomes evident at week 14 to 16 of fetal life as an invagination of the maxillary bone, found lateral to the uncinate ridge. At this point there is still no true maxillary sinus cavity. By 17 to 18 weeks' gestation, an air space is clearly seen lateral to the developing uncinate process, protruding toward the woven bone of the maxilla.[2] The developing maxillary sinus can be differentiated from the nasolacrimal duct at this stage as well.[2] Thereafter, as the cartilaginous capsule resorbs or ossifies, dependent on location, the maxillary sinus grows larger.[2,5,7,10] Over the second and third trimesters the maxillary sinus continues to enlarge from the maxillary infundibulum.

At birth the maxillary sinus measures ~10 mm long, 4 mm wide, and 3 mm in height.[8] By age 4 the maxillary sinus has expanded laterally to the level of the infraorbital nerve and inferiorly to the level of the inferior turbinate attachment. At 8 years old, growth of the maxillary sinus typically extends laterally past the infraorbital canal and inferiorly to the middle of the inferior meatus. By age 12 the maxillary sinus extends laterally into the zygomatic recess, medially to the nasolacrimal duct, and inferiorly to the level of the floor of the nasal cavity (**Fig. 1.2**). Shah et al.[9] have noted that the transverse diameter of the maxillary sinus expands most rapidly between 1 and 8 years of age, and the maxillary sinus vertical height increases rapidly between 1 and 5 years of age.

The infant's midface is very small, which results in significant differences in the maxillary sinus between the infant and the adult. In the infant and young child, the roof of the maxillary sinus slopes inferolaterally, as the orbit occupies a large portion of the midface. At this stage, the floor of the maxillary sinus lies at a level above the level of the nasal floor due to the presence of unerupted teeth. With midfacial growth and eruption of permanent teeth in childhood, the sinus continues to aerate, resulting in a more horizontal orientation of the orbital floor and inferior growth of the maxillary sinus floor to a level at or below the nasal floor.

The development and ultimate size of the maxillary sinus can be influenced by many factors. Rarely, the maxillary sinus fails to develop, with cancellous bone ultimately filling the maxilla. Early childhood trauma can result in hypoplasia, possibly due to inadequate aeration of the sinus to permit expansion. Failure of eruption of the permanent dentition can result in shortening of the inferior vertical growth of the sinus. Hypoplasia of the maxillary sinus can also occur in the absence of any other factors such as unerupted teeth or trauma. Patients with cystic fibrosis frequently have hypoplastic

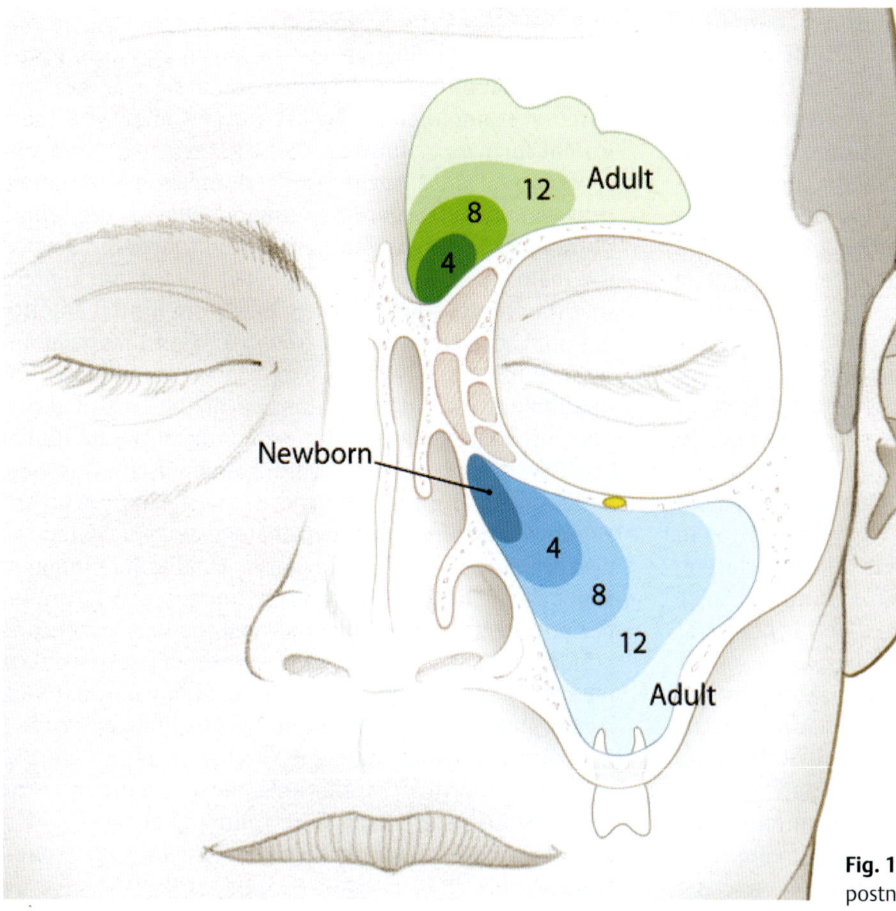

Fig. 1.2 Illustration of maxillary and frontal sinus postnasal development.

maxillary sinuses, possibly related to physiologic obstruction of the ostium, reduced aeration, and impaired pneumatization of the maxilla.[11]

Sphenoid Sinus

Development of the sphenoid sinus begins in the third to fourth month of fetal life as an invagination of the nasal cavity mucosa into the cartilaginous nasal capsule, termed the cartilaginous cupolar recess of the nasal cavity.[12] At this time the nasal cavity invagination that will become the sphenoid sinus is not actually in contact with the sphenoid bone, but rather comes from the area of the posterior ethmoid via the ossiculum Bertini or "Bertini bone."[5,8] At this stage, the sphenoid bone has two ossification centers, separated by the canalis pharyngeus.[8] Over the first few years of life, the cartilage that separates the ossiculum Bertini from the sphenoid bone will be resorbed and pneumatization of the sphenoid sinus will progress into the sphenoid bone itself.

Although Shah et al.[9] were able to identify minimally developed sphenoid sinuses in 33% of newborns radiographically, in most instances only the sphenoid ostium can be identified at birth. Pneumatization of the sphenoid sinus begins at age 1, with the most rapid growth reported between age 3 months and 5 years.[9] Various authors have noted that by approximately age 12, adult size of the sphenoid sinus is reached.[8,12] Wolf et al.[8] have commented that beyond age 12 the sinus may continue to change shape, although the size remains fairly constant. Interestingly, in a study of sphenoid sinus aeration over the lifespan, Yonetsu et al.[13] report that pneumatization of the sphenoid sinus does not reach its maximum until the end of the third decade of life. Following the third decade, these authors note that sphenoid aeration may actually decrease, with possible causes being loss of small vessels, hypoxia, and mucosal atrophy leading to bone deposition.[13]

Surrounding the sphenoid sinus are multiple important neurovascular structures, including the pituitary gland and optic chiasm in the superior medial position, internal carotid arteries and cavernous sinuses in the superior lateral position, and vidian nerves inferolaterally. The degree of sphenoid pneumatization with respect to the sella is often described by visualization in the sagittal plane. Vidic reported that sellar (including postsellar) pneumatization was most common (83.6%), defined as sphenoid pneumatization extending posterior to a vertical line drawn through the tuberculum sella.[12] Further delineating sphenoid pneumatization in the sagittal plane, Batra et al. note that postsellar pneumatization (extending beyond the posterior wall of the sella) is actually found in 65% of cases.[14] Pneumatization of the sphenoid sinus may also occur in surrounding bony processes, such as the pterygoid process, greater and lesser sphenoid wings, anterior clinoid processes, and palatine bone, among others. The greater the aeration, the greater the likelihood that the neurovascular structures that are adjacent to the sphenoid sinus will appear in bony relief on the lateral wall or roof of the lateral extensions (**Fig. 1.3**). In addition, arachnoid granulations often occur in the proximity of the second branch of the trigeminal nerve in the pterygoid recess of well aerated sphenoid sinuses.[15] These areas may ultimately result in spontaneous cerebrospinal fluid leaks or meningoencephaloceles in patients with benign intracranial hypertension.

The degree of postnatal development of the sphenoid sinus may be affected by chronic disease or possibly genetic factors. For example, patients with cystic fibrosis (CF) tend to have hypoplastic sphenoid sinuses (**Fig. 1.4A**). Furthermore, CF patients homozygous for the delta-F508 mutation have a greater incidence of sphenoid hypoplasia than those with other CF genotypes.[11] Whether this is related to the effect of genetic factors on sinus development or postnatal mucosal pathophysiology is unclear.

Frontal Sinus

The frontal sinuses are the last paranasal sinuses to begin developing and the last to complete development. There are various potential interpretations of the exact development of the frontal sinus, with some common themes. In 1916, Schaeffer described several (one to four) frontal furrows or pits being present during embryologic development that ultimately form the frontal sinus and various anterior ethmoid cells.[6] Kasper further delineated these frontal furrows as forming the agger nasi cell (first furrow), frontal sinus (second furrow), and anterior ethmoid cells as they aerate into the ethmoid bone or the orbital portion of the frontal bone (third and fourth furrows) in the majority of specimens dissected.[16] Kasper also notes that the frontal sinus may originate from frontal anterior ethmoid cells and frontal furrows (57%), infundibular anterior ethmoid cells (34%), extension of the ethmoid infundibulum (4%), direct extension of the frontal recess (3%), or least commonly by expansion of a suprabullar cell (2%).[16] Both Schaeffer and Kasper discuss multiple variations of frontal sinus and frontal recess pneumatization, confirming that early anatomists appreciated the distinct variability of this region.[6,16] Finally, Stammberger supports the development of the frontal recess at the superior aspect of the groove between the first and second ethmoturbinals.[4] As endorsed by Bolger, it is easy to imagine that, given the highly complex anatomy of the frontal recess and frontal sinus, these invaginations or furrows may ultimately pneumatize to varying degrees.[5] Contributing to the intricacy of this area, the actual origin of the frontal sinus proper may form from any of the furrows, and multiple furrows may ultimately aerate the frontal bone as well.[5,16]

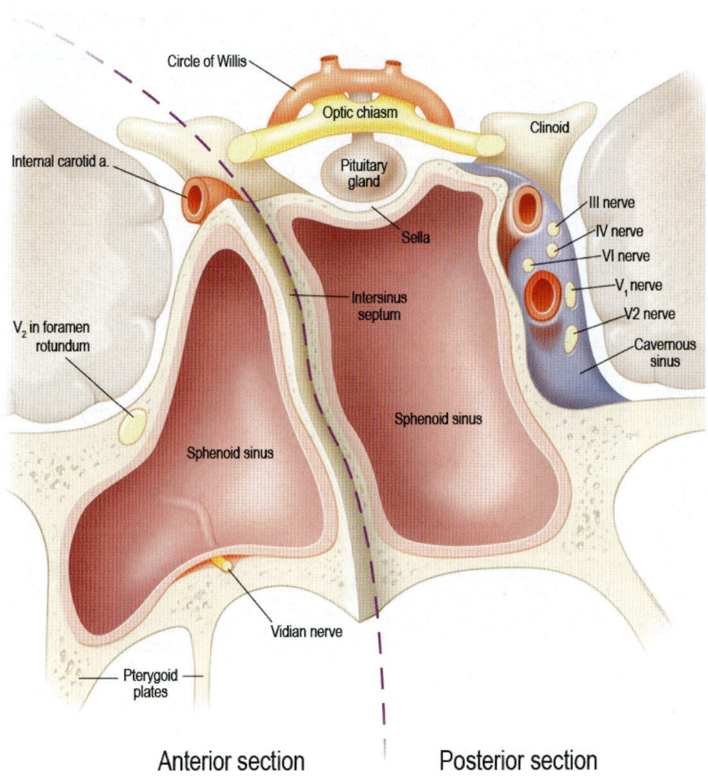

Fig. 1.3 Illustration of adult sphenoid sinus anatomy. The drawing is in an oblique plane, with the left side of the drawing demonstrating structures present more anteriorly, such as the vidian nerve and foramen rotundum, whereas the right side of the drawing shows more posterior structures, such as the cavernous sinus.

At birth the frontal sinus is not visible in most individuals, with only 12% of newborn computed tomography (CT) scans demonstrating minimally developed frontal sinuses.[9] The frontal sinus is present by the age of 4, at 4 to 8 mm in length, 6 to 9 mm in height, and 11 to 19 mm in width.[8] By age 12, the frontal sinus has achieved tetrahedral shape and continues to aerate until early adulthood (**Fig. 1.2**).[8]

As in the sphenoid sinus, the frontal sinus develops mostly in the postnatal period. Because of this, the frontal sinus is also subject to the same developmental issues, such as hypoplasia in cystic fibrosis patients (**Fig. 1.4B**).

Clinical Implications of Paranasal Sinus Development

An example of the importance of understanding sinonasal developmental anatomy as it relates to disease processes can be seen with monostotic fibrous dysplasia. The abnormal bone formation and expansion seen in monostotic fibrous dysplasia does not cross bony suture lines. Therefore, analysis of bony areas involved in this type of fibrous dysplasia can provide information about the embryologic derivation of various parts of the sinonasal cavities, such as the ethmoid and sphenoid bones (**Fig. 1.5**).

In addition, mucoceles that obstruct the frontal recess can originate from multiple sources. Mucoceles involving the frontal recess may derive from agger nasi cells, frontal cells, suprabullar cells, and frontal bullar cells, or from the frontal sinus itself. Understanding the developmental origins of these various frontal recess cells may aid the otorhinolaryngologist and radiologist in evaluating imaging studies to determine the boundaries of the expanded bony walls and planning the location and extent of surgery necessary to adequately treat the pathology.

As a final example, diseases such as CF often result in incomplete development of the sinuses. The maxillary and ethmoid sinuses are present at birth, whereas the sphenoid and frontal sinuses develop after birth. In many patients with CF, the sphenoid and frontal sinuses are rudimentary or absent.[11] This paranasal sinus underdevelopment in CF patients may result from the underlying pathophysiological process in CF, in which thick secretions obstruct the sinuses and inhibit aeration, resulting in possible stunting of the development of the sphenoid and frontal sinuses (**Fig. 1.4A,B**).

Sinonasal Anatomy

Introduction

This section focuses on sinonasal anatomy, beginning with schematic construction of the ethmoid complex. For many paranasal sinus surgeons, initial understanding

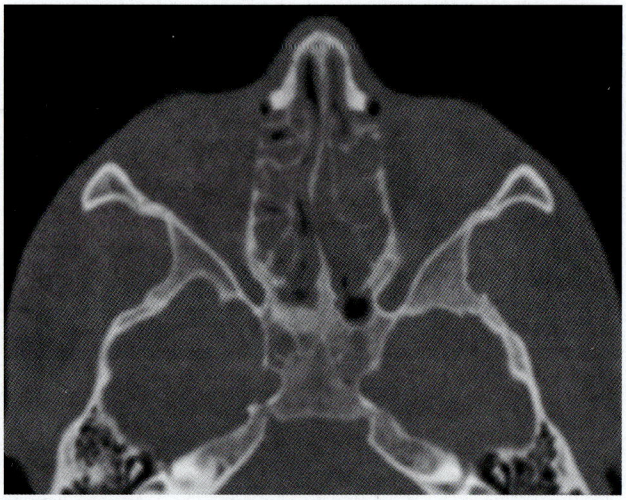

A

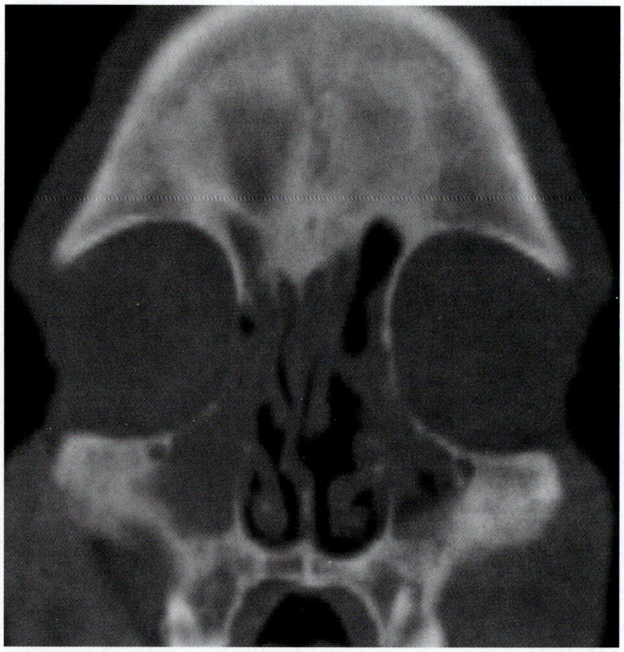

B

Fig. 1.4 **(A)** Axial computed tomography (CT) scan in bone window algorithm of an adult cystic fibrosis (CF) patient. The ethmoid sinuses are relatively well developed, whereas the sphenoid sinuses are underdeveloped. **(B)** Coronal CT scan in bone window algorithm of an adult CF patient with rudimentary frontal sinuses bilaterally.

of the ethmoid sinuses proves challenging. Simplified methodological construction of the ethmoid sinuses and surrounding structures will provide the framework for understanding the anatomy of the maxillary, frontal, and sphenoid sinuses as well.

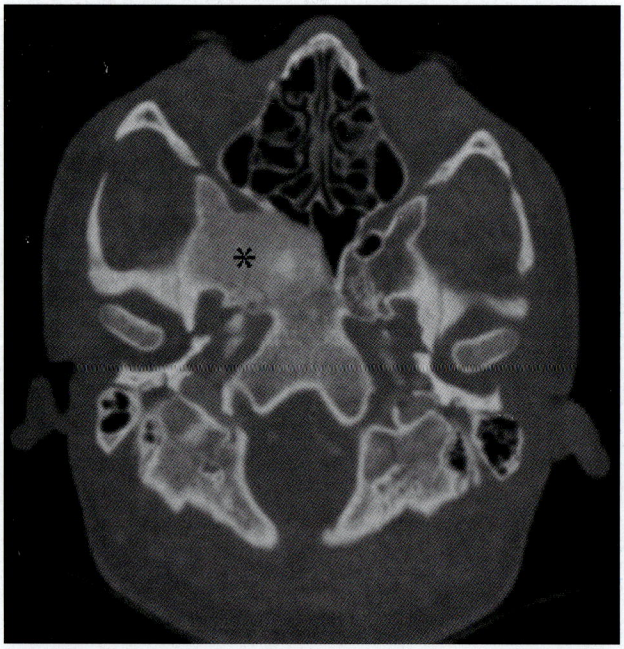

Fig. 1.5 Axial computed tomography scan in bone window algorithm demonstrating monostotic fibrous dysplasia of the right sphenoid bone (*asterisk*). Note that the abnormal bone formation is confined to the right sphenoid bone.

Ethmoid Sinus

The ethmoid complex is just that—complex. Yet a thorough understanding of its anatomy and inherent variations is the key to safe and thorough surgery. Although the anatomy of the ethmoid sinuses can be as individual as a fingerprint, common landmarks and relationships guide its effective dissection. Stepwise construction of complex structures often aids in understanding them. For that reason, the construction of a simplified ethmoid sinus complex follows, along with anatomic descriptions and highlights.

Ethmoid Bulla

Schematic construction of the anterior ethmoid sinuses starts with a sphere. This sphere is then sectioned by a plane, and the smaller portion of the sphere is discarded. The thin sectioning plane or layer represents the *lamina papyracea*. The partial sphere attached to the lamina papyracea represents the *ethmoid bulla* (**Fig. 1.6A**). As implied from our basic construction of the ethmoid complex, the ethmoid bulla is typically a rather large anterior ethmoid air cell that takes origin from the lamina papyracea along the medial wall of the orbit. Although ethmoid anatomy is often quite complicated, the ethmoid bulla is the most consistent and recognizable of the ethmoid cells. As the remainder of the ethmoid anatomy is added to the diagram, the relationship of the ethmoid bulla to surrounding structures will become evident: medial to the lamina papyracea, posterior to the uncinate process, anterior to the vertical basal lamella of the middle turbinate, and posteroinferior to the frontal recess. Stammberger describes minimal ethmoid bulla pneumatization or absence of ethmoid bulla occurring in ~8% of patients, referred to as a torus lateralis.[4]

Uncinate Process, Ethmoid Infundibulum, and Hiatus Semilunaris

A crescent-shaped line is added anterior to the ethmoid bulla and parallel to it. From this line, an outgrowth is then extended posteriorly and slightly away from the lamina papyracea and lateral nasal wall. This hook-shaped outgrowth thus forms a trough with a vertical plane that parallels the anterior surface of the sphere (or ethmoid bulla). The term for this hook-shaped outgrowth is the *uncinate process.* As seen in **Fig. 1.6B**, the uncinate process conforms to the anterior and inferior aspects of the ethmoid bulla, and has a free edge without bony attachments posteriorly. At its anterior superior aspect, the uncinate process attaches to the ethmoidal crest of the maxilla and the posterior portion of the lacrimal bone, near the agger nasi region.[5] At its posterior inferior aspect, the uncinate process fuses to the ethmoidal process of the inferior turbinate bone.

The superior and posterior attachment of the uncinate process deserves special attention, as this attachment can have implications for the configuration of the frontal recess and frontal sinus outflow tract. Publications in the early 20th century, based on frontal recess anatomic dissections by Schaeffer[6] and Kasper,[16] indicate that the developmental origins of the frontal sinus and surrounding frontal recess structures are varied. Due to such variations, the frontal sinus outflow tract may drain directly into the superior aspect of the ethmoid infundibulum (less common), or into the middle meatus without a direct connection to the superior aspect of the ethmoid infundibulum (more common).[6,16] The uncinate process most commonly inserts laterally onto the lamina papyracea, resulting in frontal sinus drainage that occurs medial to the uncinate process insertion and directly into the middle meatus between the superior aspect of the uncinate process and the middle turbinate attachment to the skull base.[5,17] Less frequently, the uncinate process may insert onto the superior aspect of the middle turbinate or directly onto the skull base. In both of these cases, the frontal sinus drainage pathway will be lateral to the uncinate process and into the ethmoid infundibulum, which is described later. Finally, the posterior superior aspect of the uncinate process may have multiple attachments to the lamina papyracea, skull base, and

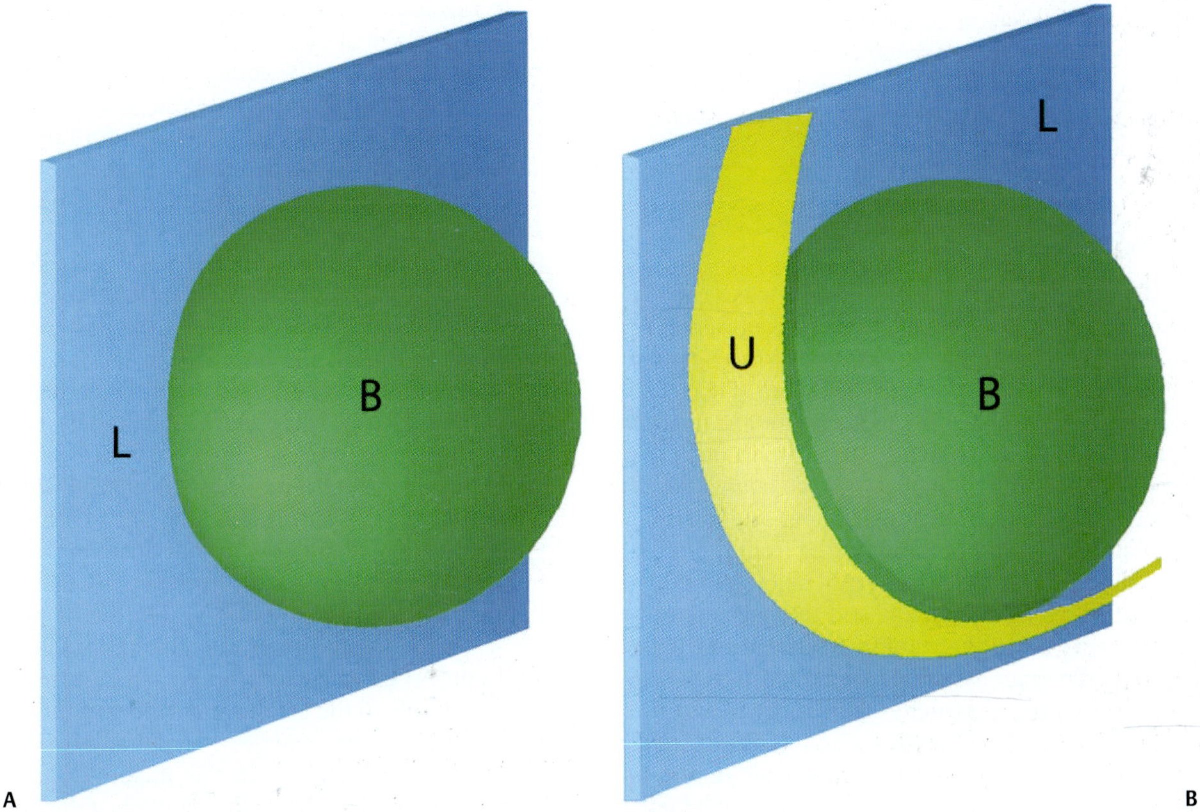

Fig. 1.6 (A) Construction schematic of a lamina papyracea and ethmoid bulla. **(B)** Schematic of the anterior ethmoid complex with an uncinate process added. *B*, ethmoid bulla; *L*, lamina papyracea; *U*, uncinate process.

middle turbinate.[17] It is important to recognize that, due to the extreme variability of pneumatization of the frontal recess, these descriptions of the frontal sinus outflow tract are quite simplified and serve only as a framework for a basic understanding of this region.

The trough that is formed lateral to the uncinate process, within the anterior ethmoid complex, is called the *ethmoid infundibulum*. The ethmoid infundibulum is bounded medially by the lateral aspect of the uncinate process, laterally by the lamina papyracea, and posterosuperiorly by the ethmoid bulla.[5,17] In addition, the frontal process of the maxilla and the lacrimal bone may also contribute to the anterior and superior boundaries of the ethmoid infundibulum.[5,17] The importance of the superior attachment of the uncinate process and its relationship to the frontal sinus outflow tract have already been described. Of note, in the most common scenario of uncinate attachment to the lamina papyracea, the superior aspect of the infundibulum that is formed by the uncinate process attaching laterally to the lamina papyracea is a blind-ended configuration called the *recessus terminalis*.[17]

Access to the three-dimensional ethmoid infundibulum is through a two-dimensional semilunar-shaped gap or opening between the free margin of the uncinate process and the ethmoid bulla, called the *hiatus semilunaris*. Although commonly referred to simply as the hiatus semilunaris, Grunwald further classified this entrance to the ethmoid infundibulum as the hiatus semilunaris inferior.[18] The hiatus semilunaris superior is then defined as the two-dimensional entrance to the sinus lateralis (described later) that is formed by the space between the posterior aspect of the ethmoid bulla and the anterior aspect of the middle turbinate basal lamella.

Agger Nasi Region

Within the anterior portion of the lateral nasal wall, a mound of bone that is often pneumatized is present. The term for this nasal mound is the *agger nasi*. When this area is pneumatized, it is called an *agger nasi cell* (**Fig. 1.7A**). The agger nasi region or cell is found anterior and inferior to the frontal sinus and frequently forms a portion of the anteromedial floor of the frontal sinus. The boundaries of the agger nasi cell are the frontal sinus superiorly and frontal recess superiorly and posteriorly, the frontal process of the maxilla anterolaterally, the nasal bones anteriorly, the lacrimal bones inferolaterally, and the uncinate process inferomedially.[5] In the surgical treatment of frontal sinus disease, the agger nasi cell is important to recognize and remove, as it may contribute significantly to narrowing of the frontal recess and frontal sinus outflow tract. In cases of revision frontal sinus surgery, retained remnants of unopened agger nasi cells may also be identified narrowing outflow from the frontal sinus.[19]

Middle Turbinate

The addition of the *middle turbinate* completes the construction of the *anterior ethmoid* complex (**Fig. 1.7A**). The middle turbinate provides a medial and posterior boundary to the anterior ethmoid complex. The middle turbinate is a complex, three-dimensional structure, whose shape may not be intuitive initially. The portion of the middle turbinate that is initially visible on anterior rhinoscopy or nasal endoscopy is oriented in the parasagittal plane, with a free mucosal edge anteriorly and inferiorly. This portion of the middle turbinate may be pneumatized, forming a *concha bullosa* air cell. Bony attachment of the parasagittal portion of the middle turbinate occurs anterosuperiorly at the crista ethmoidalis of the maxilla, in the region of the agger nasi cell.[4,17] The middle turbinate attachment to the skull base in the parasagittal plane occurs adjacent to the lateral lamella of the cribriform plate of the ethmoid bone.

The portion of the middle turbinate that runs in the coronal plane and attaches to the skull base superiorly and the lamina papyracea laterally is called the *vertical portion of the middle turbinate basal lamella* (**Fig. 1.7A–D**). The basal lamella of the middle turbinate separates the anterior and posterior ethmoid complexes. Although the concept of the vertical portion of the middle turbinate basal lamella may now be easy to grasp via simplified diagrams (**Fig. 1.7A**), in reality the middle turbinate basal lamella is rarely a smooth structure. The middle turbinate basal lamella is frequently indented from both anterior and posterior aspects by the ethmoid complexes on either side, adding to the intricacy of its shape.[4,17] The vertical portion of the middle turbinate basal lamella may also be pneumatized, forming an *interlamellar cell*.[4,5,18] Pneumatization of an interlamellar cell has been described as originating from the superior meatus.[4]

Posteriorly, the middle turbinate basal lamella is oriented in a more axial plane, forming the *horizontal portion of the middle turbinate basal lamella*. The posterior bony attachment of the middle turbinate to the lateral nasal wall occurs at the crista ethmoidalis of the perpendicular process of the palatine bone, which is often used as an anatomic marker anterior to the sphenopalatine foramen.[5,17]

With the middle turbinate now visualized, the term *ostiomeatal complex* or *ostiomeatal unit* may be addressed. A functional rather than truly anatomic term, the ostiomeatal unit refers to the conglomerate of structures and sinuses that surround or drain into the middle meatus.[20] Included are the anterior ethmoid, maxillary, and frontal sinuses; the uncinate process; and the ethmoid infundibulum. Due to the confluent anatomy of this region, and potentially narrow middle meatus drainage pathway, a relatively minor blockage in this important area may lead to obstruction of the frontal, anterior ethmoid, and maxillary sinuses.

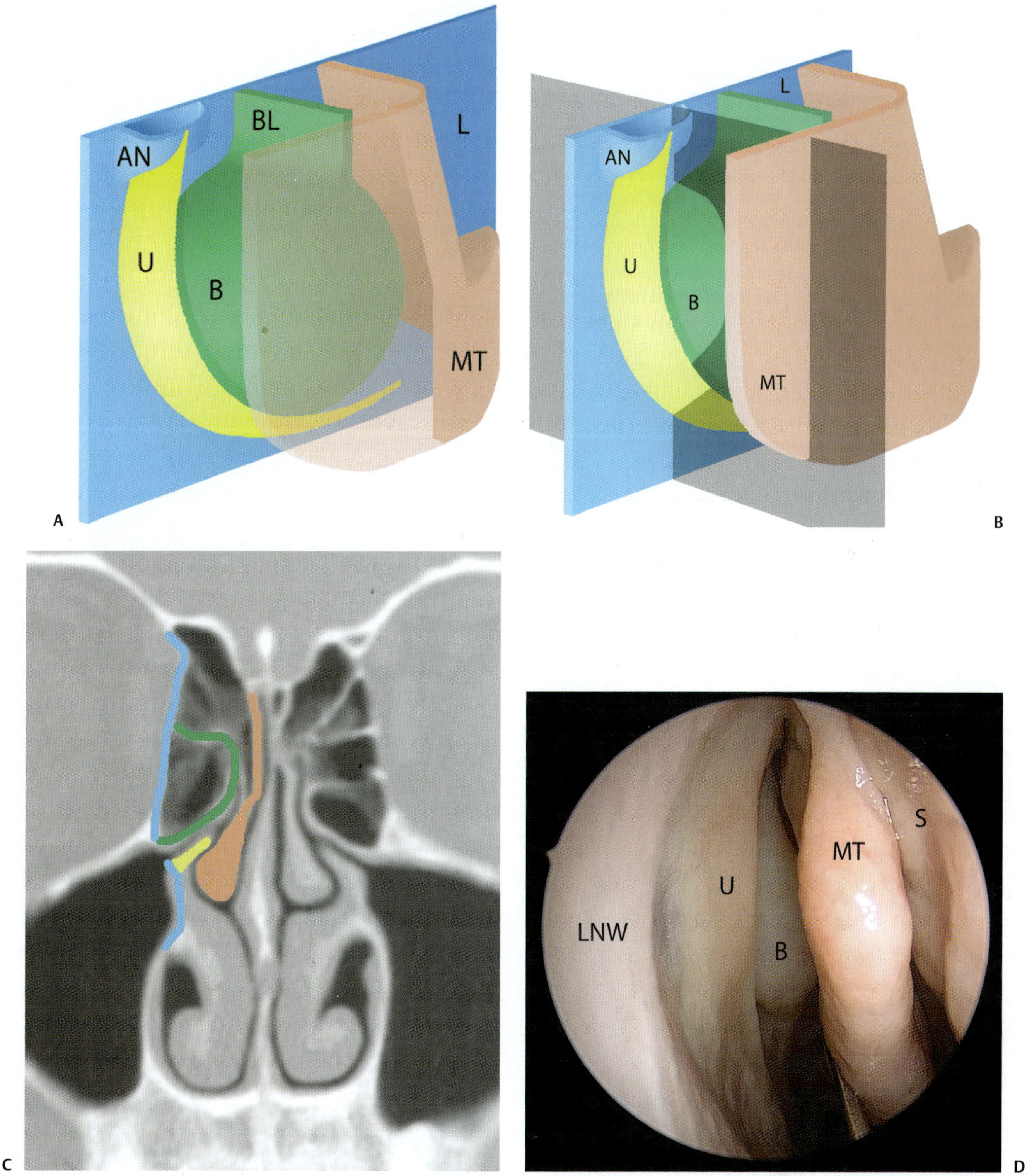

Fig. 1.7 (A) Schematic of the anterior ethmoid complex demonstrating the middle turbinate position, the agger nasi cell, and the bulla lamella. **(B)** A gray slice is placed through the anterior ethmoid complex in the coronal plane to demonstrate the position of structures in the following computed tomography (CT) scan. **(C)** Coronal CT scan in a bone window algorithm showing the ethmoid bulla and surrounding structures. **(D)** Initial endoscopic view of the anterior ethmoid complex from the nasal cavity. *B*, ethmoid bulla (green); *L*, lamina papyracea (blue); *U*, uncinate process (yellow); *MT*, middle turbinate (pink); *AN*, agger nasi cell; *BL*, bulla lamella; *LNW*, lateral nasal wall (blue); *S*, nasal septum.

Retrobullar and Suprabullar Recesses (Sinus Lateralis)

Situated between the bulla ethmoidalis and the middle turbinate basal lamella are the *retrobullar* and *suprabullar recesses*, which lie posterior and superior to the bulla ethmoidalis, respectively (**Fig. 1.8**). Sometimes referred to collectively as the *sinus lateralis*, these spaces are not actually sinuses but instead are potential spaces, or recesses, that are bounded by the ethmoid complex structures. The two-dimensional entrance to the sinus lateralis from the middle meatus is the hiatus semilunaris superior, situated between the posterior aspect of the ethmoid bulla and the anterior aspect of the middle turbinate basal lamella, as described previously.

The sinus lateralis may be pneumatized to varying degrees, and at times, bony partitions may divide the suprabullar and retrobullar recesses. The sinus lateralis is bounded by the lamina papyracea laterally, the ethmoid bulla anteriorly, the middle turbinate basal lamella posteriorly, and the skull base superiorly.

Frontal Recess

Typically there is a superior projection from the bulla toward the roof of the ethmoid cavity which attaches to the skull base. This attachment is called the *bulla lamella* (**Fig. 1.7A**). The space anterior to the bulla lamella, which is bounded by the agger nasi cell anteriorly, the lamina papyracea laterally, and the middle turbinate medially, leads toward the frontal sinus ostium. This space is the *frontal recess* (**Fig. 1.8**). If a bulla lamella is not present connecting the ethmoid bulla to the skull base, the frontal recess may communicate with the suprabullar recess posterior to the ethmoid bulla.[4,17] The frontal recess is described in more detail in the Frontal Sinus section of this chapter and in other chapters in this text specifically devoted to the anatomy and surgery of the frontal sinus.

Posterior Ethmoid Complex

The *posterior ethmoid* complex is now added (**Fig. 1.9A–C**). The posterior ethmoid sinus has as its boundaries: the parasagittal portions of the superior and supreme turbinates medially, the anterior face of the sphenoid sinus posteriorly, the lamina papyracea laterally, the middle turbinate basal lamella anteriorly, and the skull base superiorly. There are approximately one to five air cells that occupy this posterior ethmoid space.[5]

It is important to recognize the critical structures that may be encountered around the posterior ethmoid sinuses. A highly pneumatized posterior ethmoid cell can aerate posteriorly over the superolateral aspect of the true sphenoid sinus[21]; this anatomic variant is commonly referred to as an Onodi cell. The term *sphenoethmoid cell* is now preferred over Onodi cell, as it is more illustrative of the anatomy in this area.[17] When a sphenoethmoid cell is present, the posterior aspect of the lamina papyracea,

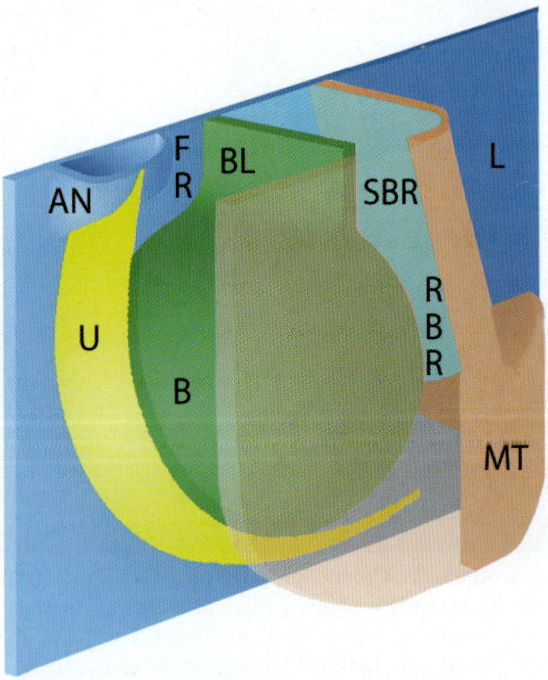

Fig. 1.8 Schematic of the anterior ethmoid complex highlighting the suprabullar and retrobullar recesses. Frontal recess is also demonstrated. *B*, ethmoid bulla; *L*, lamina papyracea; *U*, uncinate process; *MT*, middle turbinate; *AN*, agger nasi cell; *BL*, bulla lamella; *SBR*, suprabullar recess; *RBR*, retrobullar recess; *FR*, frontal recess.

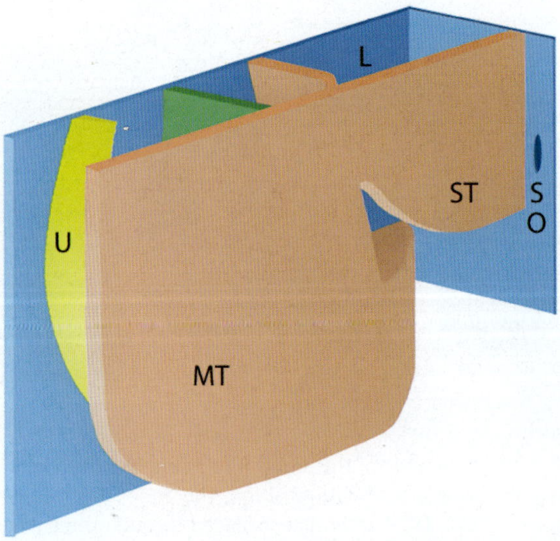

Fig. 1.9 **(A)** Ethmoid complex schematic with the superior turbinate (ST), the posterior ethmoid area, and the sphenoid sinus ostium (SO) shown. The anterior ethmoid is bounded medially by the middle turbinate, whereas the posterior ethmoid is bounded medially by the superior turbinate. The vertical basal lamella of the middle turbinate separates the anterior and posterior ethmoid complexes. (*continued*)

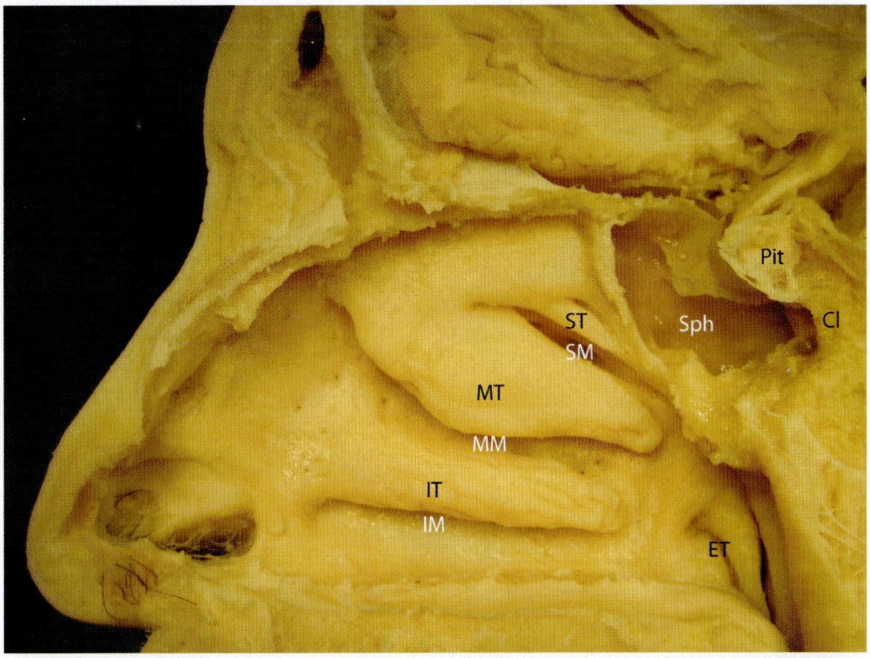

B

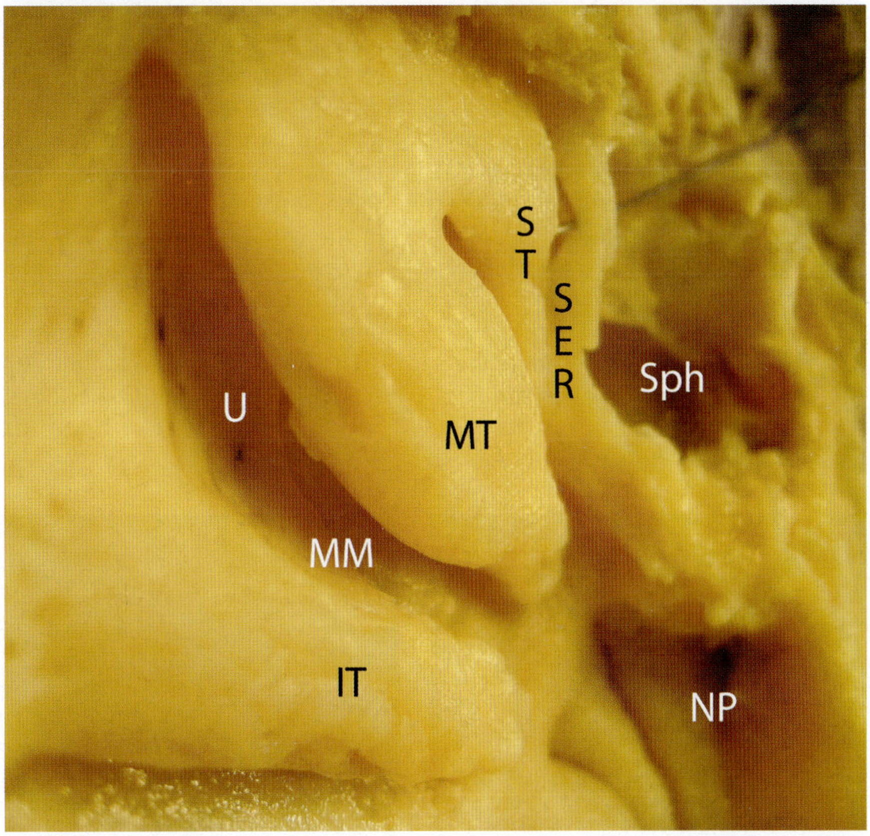

C

Fig. 1.9 (*continued*) **(B)** Sagittal cadaver dissection demonstrating the position of superior, middle, and inferior turbinates and their respective meatuses with respect to the sphenoid sinus and skull base. **(C)** Oblique orientation of a sagittal cadaver dissection revealing a turbinate position with respect to the sphenoethmoid recess, the sphenoid sinus ostium (metal probe), and the nasopharynx. *U*, uncinate process; *L*, lamina papyracea; *ST*, superior turbinate; *SM*, superior meatus; *MT*, middle turbinate; *MM*, middle meatus; *ST*, superior turbinate; *IT*, inferior turbinate; *IM*, inferior meatus; *SO*, sphenoid sinus ostium; *Sph*, sphenoid sinus; *Pit*, pituitary gland; *Cl*, clivus; *ET*, eustachian tube orifice; *SER*, sphenoethmoid recess; *NP*, nasopharynx.

optic nerve, and occasionally carotid artery may be seen as bony reliefs on the superolateral aspect of the posterior ethmoid wall, rather than in the sphenoid sinus. The prevalence of sphenoethmoid cells on imaging has been reported to be 28.1%.[22] A sphenoethmoid cell may often be recognized on CT scan imaging by its position in the superolateral aspect of what initially appears to be a septated sphenoid sinus on a coronal CT scan (**Fig. 1.10A,B**). By tracing this cell in axial, coronal, and sagittal images, the surgeon will often realize the true origin of the cell is from the posterior ethmoid, rather than the sphenoid sinus. In such images, the true sphenoid sinus is most commonly located in the medial inferior position on coronal imaging.

Paranasal Sinus Drainage Patterns

The anterior ethmoid complex is bounded medially by the middle turbinate. Likewise, the superior turbinate forms the medial boundary of the posterior ethmoid cells. Note that the middle and superior turbinates share a common skull base attachment and run in the same parasagittal plane. The vertical portion of the middle turbinate basal lamella is oriented in the coronal plane, dividing the anterior from the posterior ethmoid cells. Following the addition of the middle and superior turbinates, the middle and superior meatuses may be visualized as well. The superior, middle, and inferior meatuses lie in the space inferior and lateral to their respective turbinates (**Fig. 1.9B**). A supreme turbinate may be present in some patients as well, with its meatus inferior and lateral to the turbinate. Due to their developmental origin from the precursors of the middle meatus, the anterior ethmoid, frontal, and maxillary sinuses drain into the middle meatus. The posterior ethmoid sinuses drain into the superior meatus and the supreme meatus, if present.

In examining a partial sagittal dissection of the ethmoid complex, one may appreciate multiple lamellae that lie in an oblique, roughly parallel plane (**Fig. 1.11**).[5,23] From anterior to posterior, the first lamella visualized is the uncinate process, followed by the ethmoid bulla. The third and fourth lamellae are the basal lamellae of the middle turbinate and superior turbinate, respectively. These lamellae may also be seen during endoscopic surgical dissections as work progresses in an anterior to posterior direction.

Addition of the *nasal septum* completes the construction (**Fig. 1.12A,B**). The sphenoid sinus drains into the *sphenoethmoid recess*, which lies medial to the superior and supreme turbinates, lateral to the posterior nasal septum, inferior to the skull base, and superior to the nasopharynx.

Ethmoid Roof and Skull Base

The roof of the ethmoid sinuses is formed by the orbital plate of the frontal bone laterally and the lateral lamella of the cribriform plate of the ethmoid bone medially.[5] Whereas the lateral aspect of the ethmoid roof is thicker (0.5 mm), the medial aspect of the ethmoid roof at the cribriform plate lateral lamella is only 0.2 mm thick. The thinnest point in the ethmoid roof is found along a groove in the cribriform plate lateral lamella at the site of the anterior ethmoid artery (0.05 mm thick), representing the most common site for iatrogenic cerebrospinal fluid leak during sinus surgery.[24]

The thin medial aspect of the ethmoid roof must be observed during any endoscopic sinus surgery. However, Keros

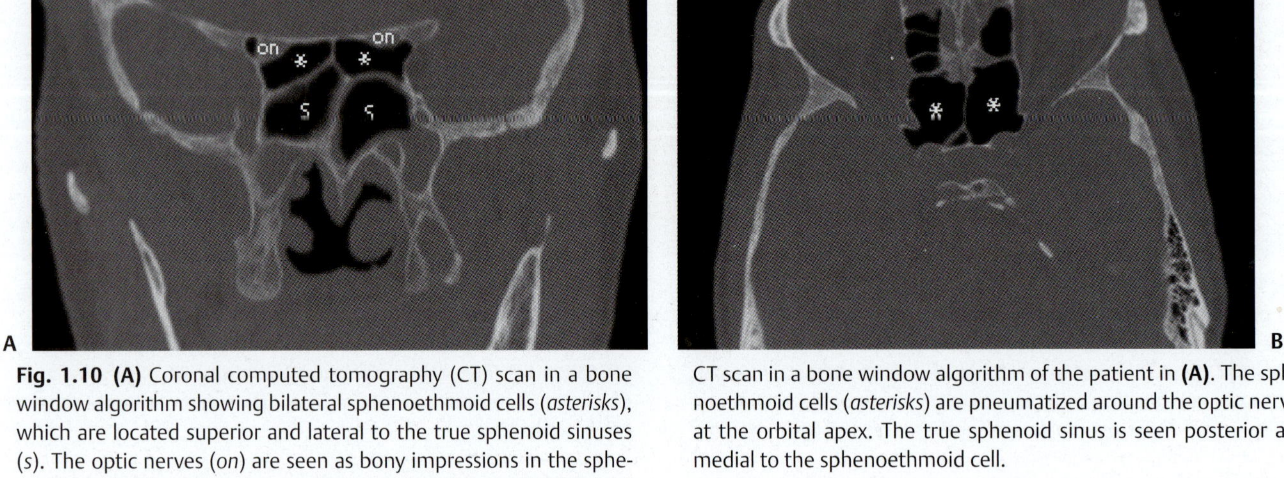

Fig. 1.10 **(A)** Coronal computed tomography (CT) scan in a bone window algorithm showing bilateral sphenoethmoid cells (*asterisks*), which are located superior and lateral to the true sphenoid sinuses (*s*). The optic nerves (*on*) are seen as bony impressions in the sphenoethmoid cells, rather than in the true sphenoid sinuses. **(B)** Axial CT scan in a bone window algorithm of the patient in **(A)**. The sphenoethmoid cells (*asterisks*) are pneumatized around the optic nerves at the orbital apex. The true sphenoid sinus is seen posterior and medial to the sphenoethmoid cell.

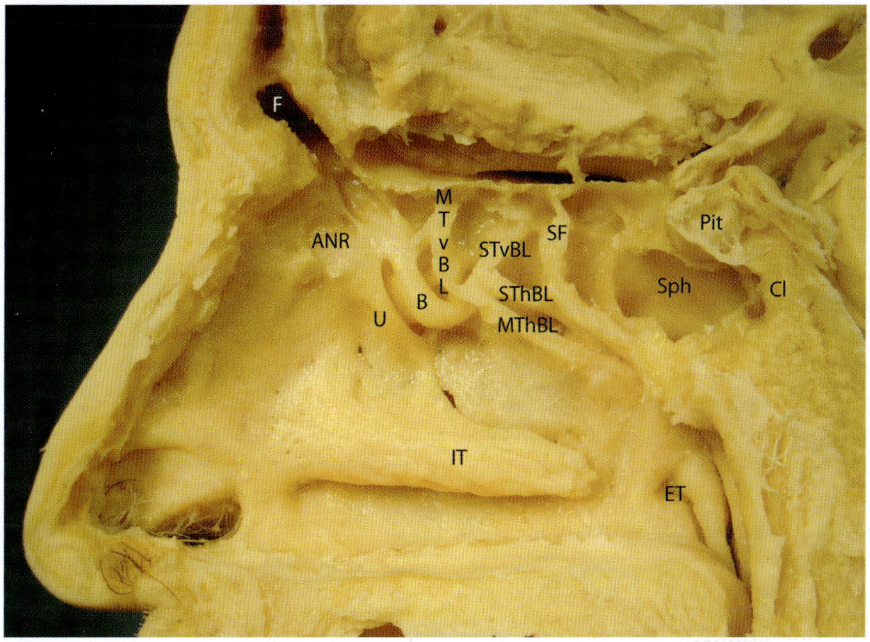

Fig. 1.11 Cadaveric dissection showing obliquely oriented parallel lamellae within the anterior and posterior ethmoid sinuses. *F*, frontal sinus; *ANR*, agger nasi region; *U*, uncinate process; *B*, ethmoid bulla; *MTvBL*, middle turbinate vertical portion of basal lamella; *MThBL*, middle turbinate horizontal portion of basal lamella; *STvBL*, superior turbinate vertical portion of basal lamella; *SThBL*, superior turbinate horizontal portion of basal lamella; *IT*, inferior turbinate; *SF*, face of sphenoid sinus; *Sph*, sphenoid sinus; *Pit*, pituitary gland; *Cl*, clivus; *ET*, eustachian tube orifice.

further delineated olfactory sulcus depth classifications that can highlight the potential for iatrogenic injury to the cribriform plate lateral lamella.[25] Keros type 1 is defined as an olfactory sulcus depth of 1 to 3 mm, and Keros type 2 is an olfactory sulcus depth of 4 to 7 mm. Finally, Keros type 3 represents an olfactory sulcus depth of 8 to 16 mm, and leaves a significant amount of thin cribriform plate lateral lamella along the medial aspect of the ethmoid roof. With increasing Keros type, there is lesser contribution from the thick frontal bone forming the ethmoid roof, with more of the ethmoid roof being formed by the thin cribriform plate lateral lamella. Therefore, as Keros type increases, there is an increased risk of cerebrospinal fluid leak during sinus surgery.[5] Recent radiologic analysis of cribriform plate

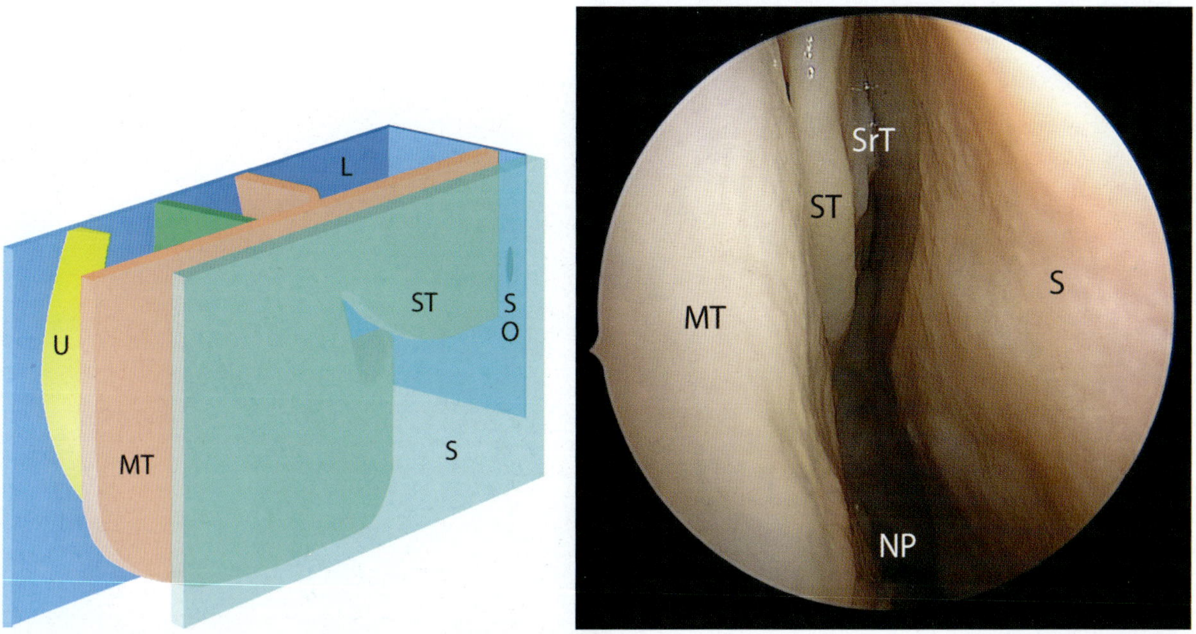

Fig. 1.12 **(A)** Shadowed nasal septum added to the schematic ethmoid complex diagram. **(B)** Endoscopic view of the nasal cavity and the sphenoethmoid recess medial to the middle turbinate. *U*, uncinate process; *MT*, middle turbinate; *ST*, superior turbinate; *SrT*, supreme turbinate; *L*, lamina papyracea; *S*, nasal septum; *SO*, sphenoid sinus ostium; *NP*, nasopharynx.

lateral lamella dimensions performed by Solares et al.[26] has revealed that Keros type 1 was the most common type identified (83%), which differs from Keros' original report of type 2 being the most common (70%).[25]

When studying the anatomy of the ethmoid roof preoperatively, the surgeon must also recognize asymmetries between sides. Due to differences in development, ethmoid roof height may be considerably lower on one side of a patient in comparison to the other, and Keros classifications may also differ between sides. Finally, the vertical orientation of the cribriform plate lateral lamella should also be assessed, as this area may range from truly vertical to obliquely oriented. In more oblique orientations of the cribriform plate lateral lamella, the medial aspect of the ethmoid roof will be quite thin and great care should be exercised in this area.

The anterior ethmoid artery is another important surgical landmark associated with the ethmoid skull base. The anterior ethmoid artery runs in an anteromedial direction from the orbit to enter the skull base at the ethmoidal sulcus in the lateral lamella of the cribriform plate.[24] The anterior ethmoid artery often runs along the skull base, but in well pneumatized ethmoid sinuses, it may be found 1 to 3 mm below the ethmoid roof in a mesentery. On coronal CT scan imaging, the anterior ethmoid artery may be seen leaving the orbit as a projection medially. This anterior ethmoid artery projection can be identified on coronal imaging at the approximate location where the medial rectus and superior oblique muscles are in closest proximity within the orbit, or near the most anterior visualization of the optic nerve just posterior to the globe.

Maxillary Sinus

Within the ethmoid infundibulum trough is the opening into the maxillary sinus or *maxillary ostium* (**Fig. 1.13A–C**). In anatomic descriptions of the maxillary sinus ostium, Van Alyea described the natural ostium of the maxillary sinus as lying in the posterior one-third of the infundibulum in 71.8% of cases.[10] On the anterior and posterior aspects of the uncinate process attachment to the inferior turbinate bone lie the anterior and posterior fontanelles.[5] Representing bony dehiscences of the medial wall of the maxillary sinus, the anterior and posterior fontanelles are made up of only mucosa of the middle meatus, connective tissue, and mucosa of the maxillary sinus. According to Van Alyea, ~23% of patients have defects in the mucosal covering of the medial wall of the maxillary sinus in the posterior fontanelle, resulting in accessory ostia.[10]

In the adult with normal maxillary sinus pneumatization, the boundaries of the maxillary sinus cavity are the alveolar portion of the maxilla inferiorly, the zygoma laterally, the orbital floor superiorly, the pterygopalatine fossa and infratemporal fossa posteriorly, and the inferior

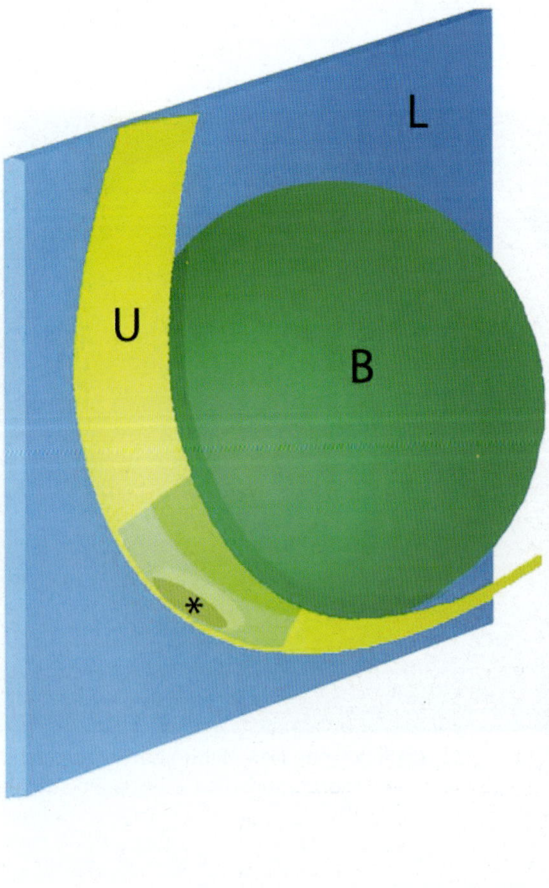

A

Fig. 1.13 **(A)** Schematic demonstrating the position of the maxillary sinus ostium with respect to the uncinate process and ethmoid bulla. **(B)** Endoscopic view of the right maxillary sinus natural ostium with respect to the uncinate process (partially removed), the ethmoid bulla, and the lamina papyracea. (*continued*)

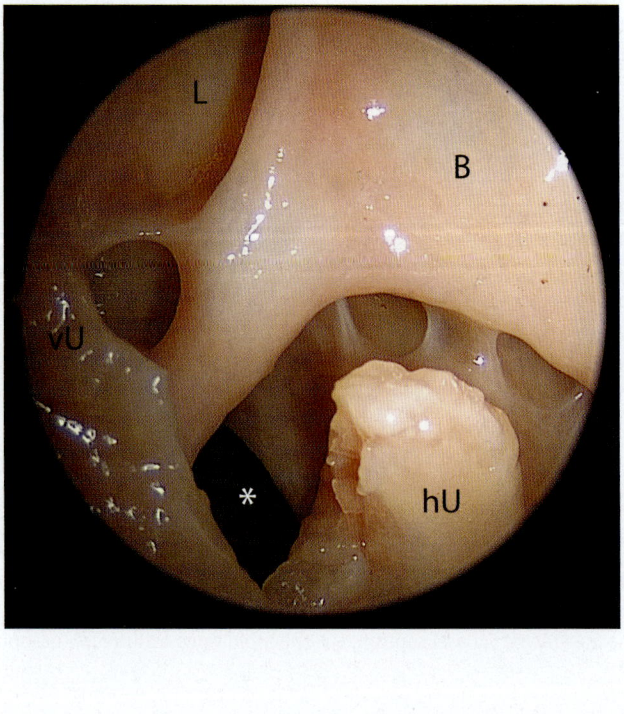

B

C

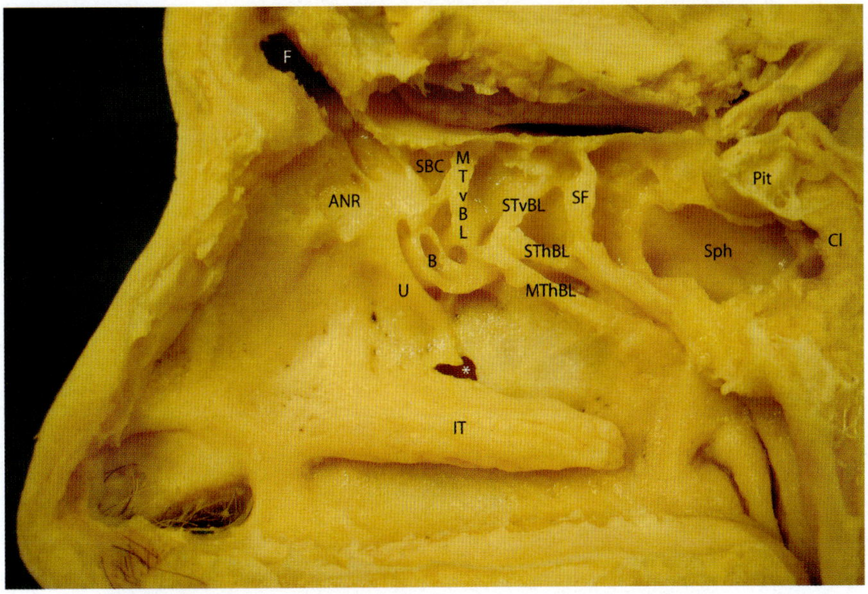

Fig. 1.13 (*continued*) **(C)** Sagittally split cadaveric dissection demonstrating the position of the maxillary sinus ostium with respect to the uncinate process (partially removed). *B*, ethmoid bulla; *L*, lamina papyracea; *U*, uncinate process; *vU*, vertical portion of uncinate process; *hU*, horizontal portion of uncinate process; *, maxillary sinus ostium; *F*, frontal sinus; *ANR*, agger nasi region; *SBC*, suprabullar cell; *IT*, inferior turbinate; *MTvBL*, middle turbinate vertical portion of basal lamella; *MThBL*, middle turbinate horizontal portion of basal lamella; *STvBL*, superior turbinate vertical portion of basal lamella; *SThBL*, superior turbinate horizontal portion of basal lamella; *IT*, inferior turbinate; *SF*, face of sphenoid sinus; *Sph*, sphenoid sinus; *Pit*, pituitary gland; *Cl*, clivus.

turbinate, uncinate process, and anterior and posterior fontanelles medially.[5] As with the other paranasal sinuses, the maxillary sinus may exhibit varying degrees of pneumatization, and in some cases, may be hypoplastic. According to Eggesbo et al., five criteria have been proposed for deeming a maxillary sinus hypoplastic in CF, a common setting of hypoplastic sinuses.[27] These criteria for maxillary hypoplasia include four of the following five: an oval-shaped sinus, an enlarged oval-shaped orbit, a lack of pneumatization of the maxillary sinus below the level of the nasal floor, the medial maxillary sinus wall lateral to a vertical line drawn tangential to the medial orbit, and the lateral extent of the maxillary sinus medial to a vertical line through the middle of the orbit at the level of the infundibulum in the coronal plane. Due to the increased ratio of orbital volume to maxillary sinus volume in cases of maxillary sinus hypoplasia, the paranasal sinus surgeon must exercise caution when operating in and around a hypoplastic maxillary sinus. In these cases, the uncinate process is typically displaced inferolaterally and lies in close proximity to the orbital wall. In addition, owing to the common developmental origins of the uncinate process, the ethmoid infundibulum, and the maxillary sinus, underdevelopment of the uncinate process may be associated with more significant degrees of maxillary sinus hypoplasia.[28]

Originally described in 1765, the Haller cell is the most frequent anatomic variation seen in the maxillary sinus.[17] Now termed an infraorbital ethmoid cell to precisely describe its anatomic location, this cell is thought to pneumatize from the anterior ethmoid (88%) or posterior ethmoid (12%) sinuses.[17,29] By virtue of its location along the inferomedial orbit contiguous with the natural drainage pathway of the maxillary sinus, the infraorbital ethmoid or Haller cell may narrow the maxillary sinus ostium and ethmoid infundibulum and may contribute to obstruction in this area (**Fig. 1.14**).

Frontal Sinus

The most anterosuperior portion of the ethmoid region that connects with the frontal sinus defines the frontal recess.[17] Although the anatomy of the frontal recess may

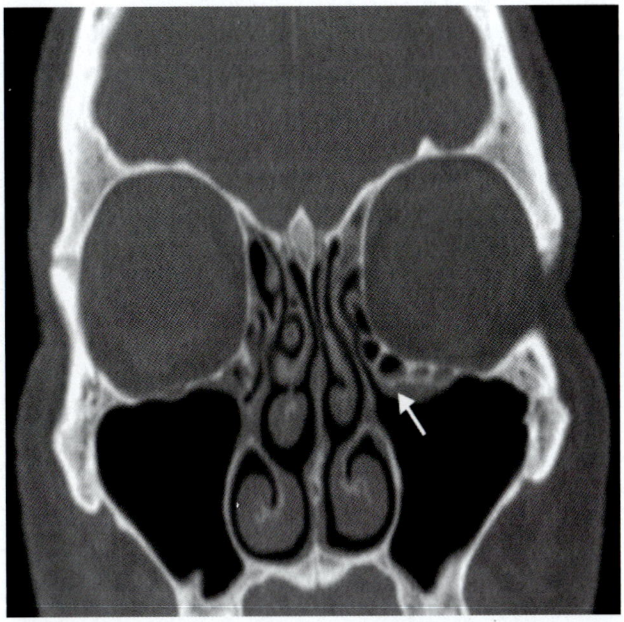

Fig. 1.14 Coronal computed tomography scan image in a bone window algorithm showing a series of infraorbital ethmoid (Haller) cells along the left maxillary sinus ostium and the infundibulum (*arrow*).

vary greatly, the general boundaries of the frontal recess include the posterosuperior aspect of the agger nasi cell, the superior lateral aspect of the middle turbinate within the middle meatus, the anterior wall of the ethmoid bulla and bulla lamella, and the lamina papyracea (**Fig. 1.15A–C**).[5,17] As stated previously, if a bulla lamella is not present, the frontal recess may communicate directly with the sinus lateralis and the suprabullar recess.[17]

Previously termed the nasofrontal duct, the frontal sinus outflow tract does not form a true duct. Rather, the *frontal recess* forms an hourglass shape that is best appreciated in the parasagittal orientation, with the narrowest portion being the internal frontal sinus ostium (**Fig. 1.16**).[17] Superior to the internal frontal sinus ostium, the frontal sinus aerates into the frontal bone. On parasagittal view, the anterior and posterior tables of the frontal sinus can be

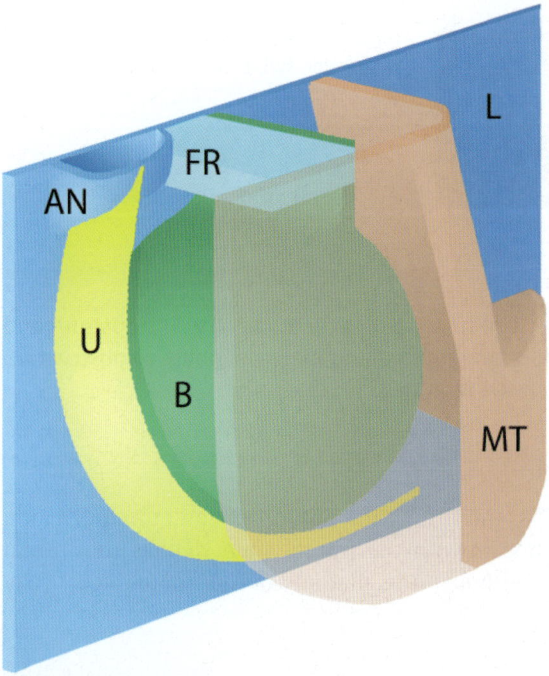

A

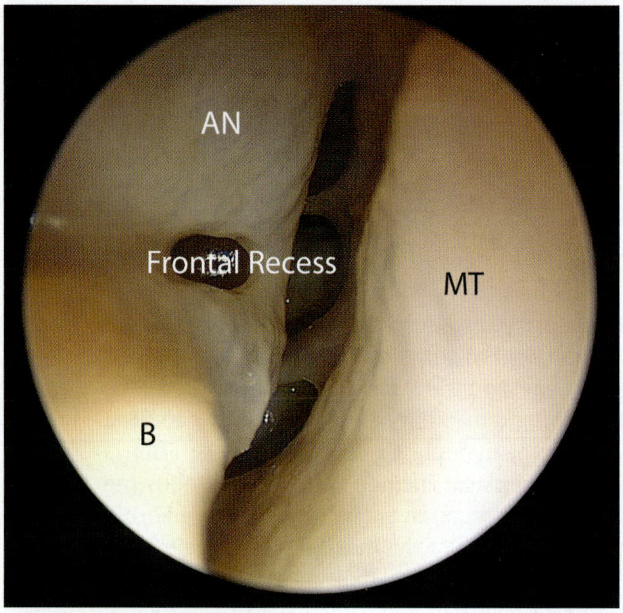

B

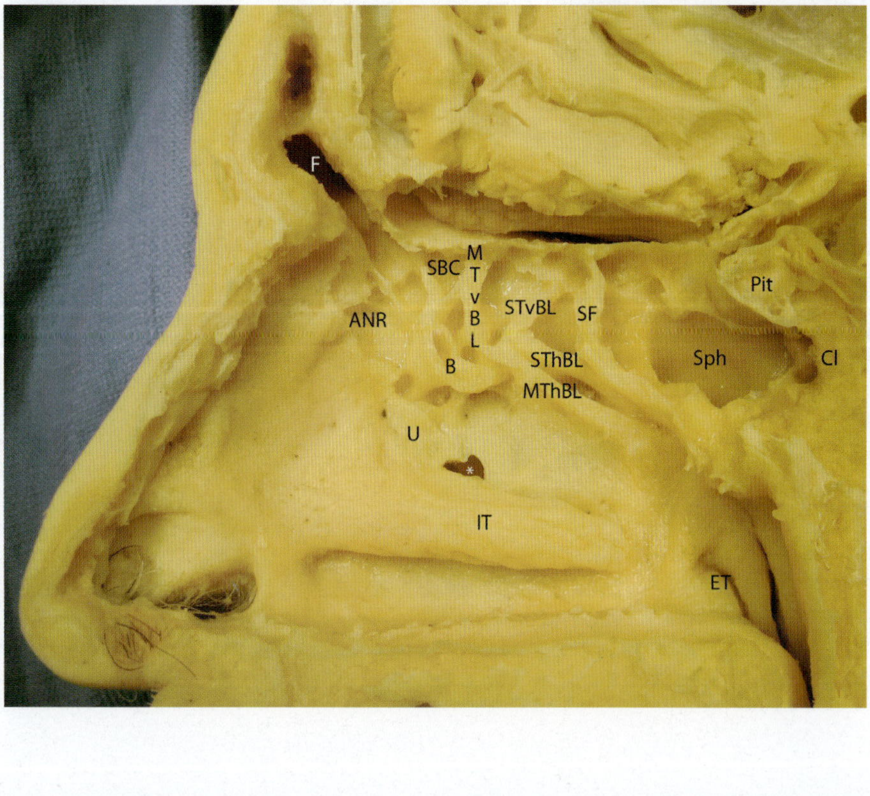

C

Fig. 1.15 (A) Schematic diagram demonstrating the position of a frontal recess with respect to the anterior ethmoid cells and surrounding structures. **(B)** Endoscopic view of the frontal recess, as seen from the inferior aspect of the middle meatus. **(C)** Sagittally split cadaveric dissection demonstrating the frontal sinus outflow tract in relation to the agger nasi region and the ethmoid structures. *B*, ethmoid bulla; *L*, lamina papyracea; *U*, uncinate process; *F*, frontal sinus; *AN(R)*, agger nasi (region); *FR*, frontal recess; *MT*, middle turbinate; *SBC*, suprabullar cell; *IT*, inferior turbinate; *, maxillary sinus ostium; *MTvBL*, middle turbinate vertical portion of basal lamella; *MThBL*, middle turbinate horizontal portion of basal lamella; *STvBL*, superior turbinate vertical portion of basal lamella; *SThBL*, superior turbinate horizontal portion of basal lamella; *IT*, inferior turbinate; *SF*, sphenoid face; *Sph*, sphenoid sinus; *Pit*, pituitary gland; *Cl*, clivus; *ET*, eustachian tube orifice.

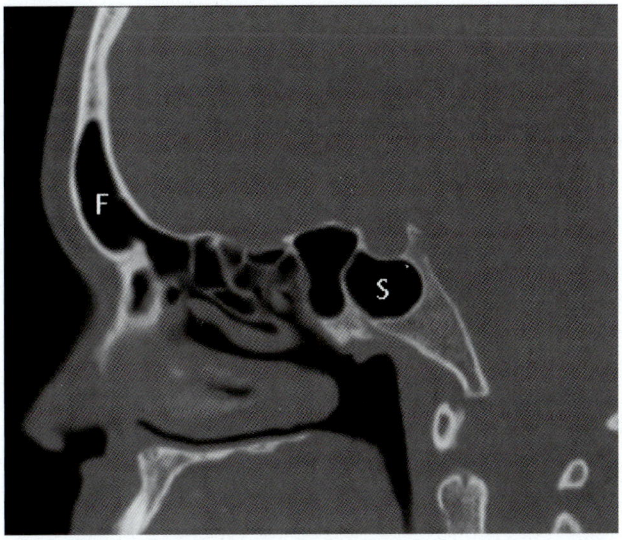

Fig. 1.16 Sagittal computed tomography scan in a bone window algorithm demonstrating the hourglass shape of the frontal recess. *F*, frontal sinus; *S*, sphenoid sinus.

visualized, and their differing thicknesses may be appreciated. The frontal sinus anterior table (4–12 mm) is considerably thicker than the posterior table (0.1–4.8 mm).[30]

There is significant variation in frontal recess and frontal sinus anatomy. The anatomy of this region is covered in detail in later chapters in this text. However, a few common anatomic variations of the frontal recess and frontal sinus deserve mention (**Fig. 1.17**). The *agger nasi cell* frequently forms the anteromedial aspect of the floor of the frontal sinus. Agger nasi cells are quite common and are demonstrated on imaging in ~89% of patients.[31] With significant pneumatization of the agger nasi cell, the frontal sinus outflow tract may be narrowed.[5]

On coronal CT scan imaging, an air cell may periodically be seen extending laterally over the superior orbital rim, at times giving the appearance of a septation in the lateral aspect of the frontal sinus.[31,32] This cell, pneumatizing superolaterally over the orbit, is a *supraorbital ethmoid cell*. It is formed by ethmoid air cell pneumatization of the orbital plate of the frontal bone, and has been reported to occur in up to 62% of cases.[5,23,31] Descriptions of the origins of the frontal sinus by Kasper attributed the derivation of supraorbital ethmoid cells to the third and fourth frontal furrows.[16] Stammberger described the supraorbital ethmoid cell as originating from the sinus lateralis or suprabullar recess and pneumatizing over the roof of the orbit.[4] On endoscopic visualization of the frontal recess, the ostium of the supraorbital ethmoid cell is located posterior and lateral to the internal frontal sinus ostium.[32]

Although significant anatomic variation may occur in the region of the frontal sinuses, the right and left frontal

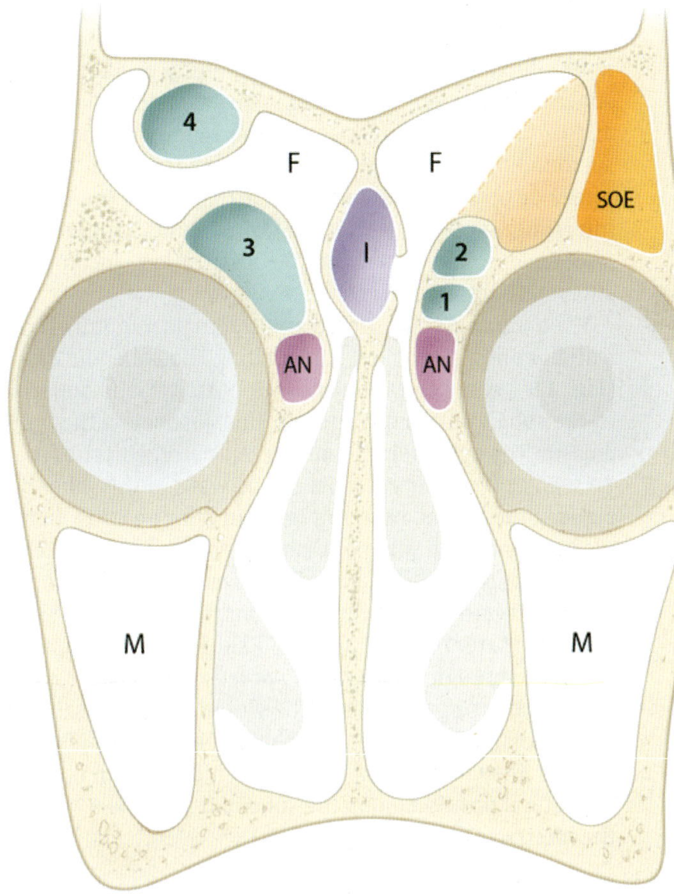

Fig. 1.17 Illustration of the frontal sinus and frontal recess anatomic variations. Coronal representation of various frontal sinus and frontal recess variations. *M*, maxillary sinus; *F*, frontal sinus; *AN*, agger nasi cell; *1–4*, type 1–4 frontal cells; *SOE*, supraorbital ethmoid cell; *I*, frontal intersinus septal cell.

Type I => 1 superior to AN
Type II => mult sup to AN
Type III => 1 large into frontal sinus
Type IV => all in frontal

sinuses are typically separated by a thin bony partition called the *frontal intersinus septum*. Frequently, the right and left frontal sinuses are asymmetric in size, with the frontal intersinus septum oriented toward one side. At times, the frontal intersinus septum may be pneumatized, forming an *intersinus septal cell*.[31,33] By carefully tracing the drainage path of a frontal intersinus septal cell on preoperative imaging, the sinus surgeon will often be able to determine that these cells drain unilaterally into the right or left frontal sinus but occasionally may have a separate ostium that drains directly into the frontal recess.[31]

Frontal cells were broadly described in 1941 by Van Alyea as cells that impinged on the frontal recess and frontal sinus ostium.[34] Currently, the most widely accepted classification of frontal cells was delineated by Bent et al.[35] According to this classification, a type 1 frontal cell is a single anterior ethmoid air cell located superior to the agger nasi cell, which does not pneumatize into the frontal sinus. Type 2 frontal cells are multiple tiered anterior ethmoid cells superior to the agger nasi cell, and a type 3 frontal cell is a single large anterior ethmoid cell superior to the agger nasi cell, which extends into the frontal sinus and has a connection to the frontal recess. Finally, a type 4 frontal cell is an anterior ethmoid cell that appears to be completely contained within the frontal sinus and attached to the anterior table of the frontal sinus. By definition, types 1 to 4 frontal cells have bony connections with the anterior frontal recess or anterior table of the frontal sinus; there are no bony connections to the posterior table of the frontal sinus or the skull base.[31,35]

The frontal recess and frontal sinus present some of the greatest challenges to the sinus surgeon. This chapter presents some of the basic anatomy and anatomic variations present in this intricate area. Knowledge of the frontal recess, agger nasi and supraorbital ethmoid cells, frontal intersinus septal cells, and frontal cells form the basis for understanding this complicated area. However, the varied pneumatization and complexity of the frontal recess and frontal sinus cannot be overstated and often remains challenging, even for the most experienced sinus surgeons. We direct the reader to later chapters in this text devoted to surgery of the frontal sinus for additional discussion of the complex anatomy of the frontal recess and frontal sinus.

Sphenoid Sinus

Positioned in the most posterior medial location of all the paranasal sinuses, the sphenoid sinuses sit at the central skull base. The sphenoid sinus drains through its natural ostium into the sphenoethmoid recess. The sphenoid ostium is located on the face of the sphenoid sinus in an anterior superior location with respect to the sinus itself, and is traditionally taught to be 7 cm at a 30-degree angle from the nasal spine in the adult. On visualization of the face of the adult sphenoid sinus, the sphenoid ostium is typically located ~1.0 to 1.5 cm above the superior aspect of the posterior choana and sphenoid sinus floor, and lies between the nasal septum and the posterior insertion of the superior or supreme turbinate.[36]

The roof of the sphenoid sinus, comprising the sphenoid skull base, is termed the *planum sphenoidale*. In the posterior superior aspect of the sphenoid cavity, a rounded bony projection may be seen when the sphenoid sinus is well pneumatized. This area is the bony covering over the pituitary gland, called the *sella turcica*. Inferior to the sella turcica is the thick bone of the *clivus* that forms the posterior inferior wall of the sphenoid sinuses. The *sphenoid rostrum* forms the face and the floor of the sphenoid sinuses and articulates anteriorly with the vomer bone. In some cases, the inferior lateral aspects of the sphenoid sinuses will be pneumatized, forming lateral pterygoid recesses. In cases of spontaneous cerebrospinal fluid leak, skull base defects are often found in these pneumatized lateral recesses of the sphenoid sinus and specialized trans-pterygopalatine fossa surgical approaches may be needed to address cerebrospinal fluid leaks in this location.[37]

As seen in the frontal sinuses, a *sphenoid intersinus septum* divides the right and left sphenoid sinuses. It is quite common for the right and left sphenoid sinuses to develop asymmetrically and exhibit different size and pneumatization patterns in the adult. In planning and undertaking surgery of the sphenoid sinuses, the sphenoid intersinus septum must be carefully evaluated. The sphenoid intersinus septum may be deviated unilaterally, and in such cases, may insert in the vicinity of one of the surrounding vital structures, such as the internal carotid artery or optic nerve.[5] In a similar manner to the frontal intersinus septum, the sphenoid intersinus septum may also have some degree of pneumatization. Incomplete sphenoid septations may be noted as well.

The paranasal sinus surgeon must remain mindful of critical anatomic structures surrounding the sphenoid sinus (**Fig. 1.3**). The pituitary gland lies posterior and superior to the sphenoid cavity at the midline, just below the optic chiasm. The optic nerves and internal carotid arteries may be seen as bony impressions on the walls of the sphenoid sinus in the lateral, posterior, and superior position. In the well pneumatized sphenoid, a bony indentation representing the *opticocarotid recess* may be seen between the optic nerve and carotid artery impressions. The cavernous sinus is located lateral to the sphenoid sinus lateral wall, with the third through sixth cranial nerves and internal carotid artery traversing through it. The vidian nerve is located in an inferolateral position. In highly pneumatized sphenoid sinuses, the vidian canal may be seen running in an inferior lateral position along the sphenoid sinus floor toward the internal carotid artery.

In radiologic analysis of the intrasphenoid optic canal, Batra et al. determined that the sphenoid most commonly pneumatized to the level of the optic canal (39.8%), with the optic nerve creating an indentation on the lateral wall of the sphenoid sinus.[22] However, in up to 15.6% of sphenoid sinuses and 8.3% of sphenoethmoid cells, the optic nerve was seen freely traversing these air cells. In addition, in 30.5% of cases, the intersinus septum inserted directly onto the optic nerve canal, and in 12.5% of cases, optic nerves were frankly dehiscent of bony covering. In a similar study of the carotid canal, the retrosellar internal carotid artery segment was found to have 90 to 180 degrees of adjacent sphenoid sinus pneumatization in 50% of cases.[14] Furthermore, in 37.5% of cases, the sphenoid intersinus septum inserted directly onto the bony carotid canal, and in 19.5% of cases, the internal carotid arteries were dehiscent. These findings highlight the importance of careful preoperative planning and analysis of imaging studies, due to the proximity of critical structures surrounding the sphenoid sinus.

Conclusion

This chapter presents an overview of the prenatal and postnatal development of the paranasal sinuses, followed by a summary of sinonasal anatomy. Although an understanding of the anatomic principles and relationships outlined in this chapter will assist the sinus surgeon in approaching sinonasal pathology, sinus surgeons should bear in mind that paranasal sinus pneumatization patterns may vary significantly. There is great potential for significant differences in sinonasal anatomy from patient to patient, and even between the right and left sides within the same patient. Therefore, close study of preoperative imaging and knowledge of individual patient anatomy is imperative to prevent complications during paranasal sinus surgery.

References

1. Wake M, Takeno S, Hawke M. The early development of sinonasal mucosa. Laryngoscope 1994;104(7):850–855
2. Bingham B, Wang RG, Hawke M, Kwok P. The embryonic development of the lateral nasal wall from 8 to 24 weeks. Laryngoscope 1991;101(9):992–997
3. Killian G. Zur anatomie der nase menschlicher embryonen. Arch Laryngol Rhin (Berl) 1895;3:17–47
4. Stammberger H. Functional Endoscopic Sinus Surgery: the Messerklinger Technique. Philadelphia: B.C. Decker; 1991
5. Bolger W. Anatomy of the paranasal sinuses. In: Kennedy D, Bolger W, Zinreich S, eds. Diseases of the Sinuses: Diagnosis and Management. Hamilton, Ontario: B.C. Decker, Inc.; 2001: 1–11
6. Schaeffer J. The genesis, development and adult anatomy of the nasofrontal duct region in man. Am J Anat 1916;20:125–145
7. Wang RG, Jiang SC, Gu R. The cartilaginous nasal capsule and embryonic development of human paranasal sinuses. J Otolaryngol 1994;23(4):239–243
8. Wolf G, Anderhuber W, Kuhn F. Development of the paranasal sinuses in children: implications for paranasal sinus surgery. Ann Otol Rhinol Laryngol 1993;102(9):705–711
9. Shah RK, Dhingra JK, Carter BL, Rebeiz EE. Paranasal sinus development: a radiographic study. Laryngoscope 2003;113(2):205–209
10. Van Alyea O. The ostium maxillare: anatomic study of its surgical accessibility. Arch Otolaryngol 1936;24:553–569
11. Woodworth BA, Ahn C, Flume PA, Schlosser RJ. The delta F508 mutation in cystic fibrosis and impact on sinus development. Am J Rhinol 2007;21(1):122–127
12. Vidić B. The postnatal development of the sphenoidal sinus and its spread into the dorsum sellae and posterior clinoid processes. Am J Roentgenol Radium Ther Nucl Med 1968;104(1):177–183
13. Yonetsu K, Watanabe M, Nakamura T. Age-related expansion and reduction in aeration of the sphenoid sinus: volume assessment by helical CT scanning. AJNR Am J Neuroradiol 2000;21(1):179–182
14. Batra PS, Citardi MJ, Gallivan RP, Roh HJ, Lanza DC. Software-enabled computed tomography analysis of the carotid artery and sphenoid sinus pneumatization patterns. Am J Rhinol 2004;18(4):203–208
15. Shetty PG, Shroff MM, Fatterpekar GM, Sahani DV, Kirtane MV. A retrospective analysis of spontaneous sphenoid sinus fistula: MR and CT findings. AJNR Am J Neuroradiol 2000;21(2):337–342
16. Kasper K. Nasofrontal connections: a study based on one hundred consecutive dissections. Arch Otolaryngol 1936;24:322–343
17. Stammberger HR, Kennedy DW; The Anatomic Terminology Group. Paranasal sinuses: anatomic terminology and nomenclature. Ann Otol Rhinol Laryngol Suppl 1995;167:7–16
18. Grunwald L. Deskriptive und topographische anatomie der nase und iher nebenhohlen. In: Denker A, Kahler O, eds. Handbuch der Hals-Nasen-Ohrenheilkunde. Berlin: Springer-Bergmann; 1925: 1–95
19. Kuhn F, Bolger W, Tisdal R. The agger nasi cell in frontal recess obstruction: an anatomic, radiologic, and clinical correlation. Oper Tech Otolaryngol—Head Neck Surg 1991;2:226–231
20. Naumann H. Patholische anatomic der chronischen rhinitisund sinusitis Proceedings VIII International Congress of Oto-rhino-laryngology. Amsterdam: Excerpt Medica; 1965: 12
21. Onodi A. The optic nerve and the accessory cavities of the nose: contribution of the study of cannicular neuritis and optic nerve atrophy. Ann Otol Rhinol Laryngol 1908;17:1–116
22. Batra PS, Citardi MJ, Gallivan RP, Roh HJ, Lanza DC. Software-enabled CT analysis of optic nerve position and paranasal sinus pneumatization patterns. Otolaryngol Head Neck Surg 2004;131(6):940–945
23. Van Alyea O. Ethmoid labyrinth: anatomic study, with consideration of the clinical significance of its structural characteristics. Arch Otolaryngol 1939;29:881–902
24. Kainz J, Stammberger H. The roof of the anterior ethmoid: a place of least resistance in the skull base. Am J Rhinol 1989;3:191–199
25. Keros P. On the practical value of differences in the level of the lamina cribrosa of the ethmoid. Z Laryngol Rhinol Otol 1962;41:809–813
26. Solares CA, Lee WT, Batra PS, Citardi MJ. Lateral lamella of the cribriform plate: software-enabled computed tomographic analysis and its clinical relevance in skull base surgery. Arch Otolaryngol Head Neck Surg 2008;134(3):285–289

27. Eggesbø HB, Søvik S, Dølvik S, Eiklid K, Kolmannskog F. CT characterization of developmental variations of the paranasal sinuses in cystic fibrosis. Acta Radiol 2001;42(5):482–493
28. Bolger WE, Woodruff WW Jr, Morehead J, Parsons DS. Maxillary sinus hypoplasia: classification and description of associated uncinate process hypoplasia. Otolaryngol Head Neck Surg 1990;103(5 (Pt 1)):759–765
29. Kainz J, Braun H, Genser P. Haller's cells: morphologic evaluation and clinico-surgical relevance. Laryngorhinootologie 1993; 72(12):599–604
30. Strong EB, Pahlavan N, Saito D. Frontal sinus fractures: a 28-year retrospective review. Otolaryngol Head Neck Surg 2006;135:774–779
31. Lee WT, Kuhn FA, Citardi MJ. 3D computed tomographic analysis of frontal recess anatomy in patients without frontal sinusitis. Otolaryngol Head Neck Surg 2004;131(3):164–173
32. Owen RG Jr, Kuhn FA. Supraorbital ethmoid cell. Otolaryngol Head Neck Surg 1997;116(2):254–261
33. Merritt R, Bent J, Kuhn F. The intersinus septal cell. Am J Rhinol 1996;10:299–302
34. Van Alyea O. Frontal cells: an anatomic study of these cells with consideration of their clinical significance. Arch Otolaryngol 1941;34:11–23
35. Bent J, Cuilty-Siller C, Kuhn F. The frontal cell as a cause of frontal sinus obstruction. Am J Rhinol 1994;8:185–191
36. Yanagisawa E, Yanagisawa K, Christmas DA. Endoscopic localization of the sphenoid sinus ostium. Ear Nose Throat J 1998; 77(2):88–89
37. Bolger WE, Osenbach R. Endoscopic transpterygoid approach to the lateral sphenoid recess. Ear Nose Throat J 1999; 78:37–46

2 Sinonasal Physiology

David A. Gudis, Bradford A. Woodworth, and Noam A. Cohen

The external nose and nasal cavity represent a critical unit whose function is to cleanse and humidify inspired air, as well as sample it for olfaction. The function of the surrounding paranasal sinuses is less clearly understood, but hypothesized to lighten the skull and generate a "crumple zone" for protection of the brain and eyes from facial trauma. Additionally, the sinonasal unit is the initial contact point for many environmental insults ranging from simple pollution to complex infectious agents. Thus, each structure and region within the sinonasal cavity represents a tier of defense and protection against the external environment.

■ Protection of the Upper Airway

The Nose

As air is inspired through the nose, it immediately encounters the first of many protective features of the sinonasal cavity: the vibrissae. The vibrissae are coarse hairs whose follicles are located just within the nasal meatus. They filter large aerosolized particulate matter from inspired air, and they are aided in expelling the debris by the sweat and sebaceous glands in the stratified squamous epithelium of the anterior nares, the only squamous epithelium of the sinonasal cavity. Vibrissae are present in most mammals, but their innervation and role in sensory function appears to be less pronounced in humans.

Just beyond the meatus of the anterior nares and vibrissae, inspired airflow is regulated by the nasal valves, the next tier of sinonasal defense. The external nasal valve is defined by the angle between the lateral crus and the medial crus of the lower lateral cartilage, the columella, and the nasal sill. The internal nasal valve—the narrowest segment of the upper airway—is defined by the angle between the caudal upper lateral cartilage, the septum, the anterior face of the inferior turbinate, and the nasal floor. Both valves are dynamic such that they limit airflow at variable rates. When the velocity of inspired air increases with forceful inspiration, the pressure of the air passing through the nasal valves decreases relative to the ambient air outside the nasal valve in accordance with the Bernoulli principle of fluid dynamics. This pressure differential causes the nasal valve to decrease in aperture, varying with respect to the individual size, shape, and soft tissue compliance of a particular nose. During times of labored breathing or exercise, the alar muscles contract to dilate the nares to oppose the effect of this air pressure differential. This mechanism allows the nasal valves to ensure that air is not inspired faster than it can be warmed, humidified, and cleaned.

The Turbinates

Inspired air then encounters the turbinates of the nasal cavity. The three shelflike structures project from the lateral wall of the nasal cavity toward the septum and provide a crucial protective function of the sinonasal cavity. The superior and middle turbinates are extensions of the ethmoid bone, whereas the inferior turbinate is an independent osseous structure. Most air passes between the middle and inferior turbinates, with a maximum velocity just posterior to the internal nasal valve.[1] By increasing the total surface area of the nasal cavity, the turbinates significantly contribute to warming and humidifying inspired air. At respiratory rates of up to 7 L per minute, the nasal airway can warm air to 37°C from ambient temperatures as low as 25°C and maintain the humidity of inspired air at ~85% within a wide range of ambient environmental humidity.[2] This controlled temperature and humidity of air entering the lungs facilitates pulmonary alveolar gas exchange.

The orientation and shape of the turbinates streamlines inspired air posteriorly toward the nasopharynx while providing sufficient obstructive resistance to change the airflow from a laminar to a transitional pattern. Additionally, the cross-sectional area of the nasal airway increases substantially just past the nasal valves, leading to a drop in airflow velocity just before the air reaches the turbinates; this too contributes to the loss of laminar airflow.[2] Transitional airflow is neither completely laminar nor completely turbulent, and its dynamics are protective in several ways. The element of turbulence causes much of the aerosolized debris, including pathogens and dust, to precipitate from inspired air and land in the mucus layer of the epithelium. The change in airflow pattern also exposes more air molecules to the warm and moist mucosa of the large turbinates, whereas a laminar flow would shield a central column of air from the mucosa. However, a completely turbulent flow with no laminar component would be undesirable because it would generate higher resistance and lower velocity of the airflow in the nasal passage. Such turbulence becomes useful only during the sniff, the mechanism of olfactory detection whereby quick high-flow (>300 mL/s per nostril) inhalation generates enough turbulence to expose more odorants to the olfactory mucosa, tucked posterosuperior to the superior turbinate.[3] Therefore, the transitional airflow pattern of normal breathing balances the protective features of turbulent flow with the lower resistance of laminar flow.

When nasal resistance is too low, however, patients may paradoxically report subjective complaints of obstruction or difficulty breathing, known as "empty nose syndrome." The turbinates may provide up to 50% of total airway resistance when one breathes nasally. Thus, after excessive surgical turbinectomy, the altered velocity differentials and resistance patterns throughout the upper airway may result in a paradoxical nasal obstruction, with patients reporting shortness of breath and unsatisfying breathing.[4] These clinical sequelae demonstrate the functional importance of turbinates to effectively create a unique transitional airflow pattern that is necessary to protect the upper airway while allowing for normal and comfortable breathing.

Nasal air filtration proves to be remarkably efficient. Humans inspire between 10,000 and 20,000 L of air per day. About 80% of particles 3 to 5 μm in diameter and 60% of particles 2 μm in diameter are filtered by nasal filtration, with the vast majority of this filtration process occurring anteriorly. Studies with radiolabeled water have found that ~95% of pollen-sized particles are trapped in the anterior nasal cavity.[5] However, despite this powerful filtration system, countless contaminants including particulate debris and infectious pathogens pass through to the upper airway and become trapped in the mucus layer of the sinonasal epithelium, generally allowing only particles less than 1 μm to pass into the lungs. Mucociliary clearance is the process by which the mucus layer containing such debris is transported to the gastrointestinal tract for elimination, and it is the definitive mode of defense for both the upper and lower airways.

The Nasal Cycle

In the anatomically normal nasal airway, most people experience asymmetric airflow through the nose. At any time, one nasal passage is typically more widely patent to airflow and has increased secretions from both serous and mucus glands, whereas the other passage is more congested with reduced secretions.[2] This feature of the nasal airway, known as the "nasal cycle," is tightly regulated by a combination of neural control and vasomotor input that results in alternating engorgement and constriction of the arterioles, precapillary sphincters, and most significantly, the venous sinusoids within the erectile mucosa of the nasal passage. The mechanisms governing these vascular changes are not completely understood, but vascular tone is influenced by factors including local metabolic and vasoactive substances, neurotransmitters, and neuropeptides (**Table 2.1**).

This erectile tissue is most fully developed along the anterior nasal septum and on the inferior turbinates, but is distributed throughout much of the nasal airway. At peak congestion, the mucosal edge of the inferior turbinate may protrude anteriorly as far as 5 mm beyond its baseline decongested position.[6] Sympathetic adrenergic input leads to constriction of the vasculature and a patent nasal passage, which plays an additional role in increasing systemic oxygenation in the fight-or-flight response. Parasympathetic input may contribute to vasodilatation and engorgement of the distensible mucosa but appears to play a much smaller role in this process. Rather, parasympathetic input to the sinonasal cavity functions largely to stimulate glandular secretions.[7]

Table 2.1 Endogenous Vasoactive Substances on Nasal Mucosa

Vasodilators	Vasoconstrictors
Histamine	Epinephrine
Vasoactive intestinal peptide	Norepinephrine
Substance P	
Prostaglandin E_2	
Bradykinin	
Nitric oxide	
Estrogen	

The nasal cycle has been described as far back as 1895, when Kayser found that patients had varying airway resistance in each nasal passage, yet a constant total resistance of the whole nasal airway.[8] Some investigators have found using rhinomanometry that ~80% of normal people undergo this recurring process, and that the patent and congested sides alternate every 2 to 7 hours on average.[7] However, the term "nasal cycle" has been called into question, as there is little data to confirm that a consistent rhythmic periodicity exists that predicts the alternating patency and congestion of a nasal passage. Rather, it is now commonly accepted that most people exhibit an irregularly alternating patency and congestion governed by many factors including posture, infection, mucosal irritants, hormones, temperature, and drugs. Kayser was still correct in his original estimation that, despite changing resistance of individual nasal passages, the total resistance of the combined nasal cavities remains largely unchanged,[8] and because there is often no sensation of obstruction from the congested side, the cycle goes unnoticed by most people.

The functions of the nasal cycle are not entirely understood, but it most likely serves both mechanical and immunologic roles. The cycle's mechanical functions include augmenting the efficacy of the turbinates to humidify and warm inspired air. During inspiration of cold or dry air, the blood is directed through the capillaries and venous sinusoids leading to engorgement of the erectile tissue and swelling of the nasal lining. Additionally, the nasal cycle may play a role in controlling nasal secretions, whereby the alternating congestion and decongestion creates a pump-like mechanism for plasma transudate, an important component of these secretions. During the period of decongestion, the increased sympathetic tone that constricts the venous sinusoids of the erectile tissue may raise their intravascular hydrostatic pressure, resulting in increased plasma filtration through the endothelium of the distensible venous sinusoids in the nasal lining.[9] This plasma transudate, as a component of nasal secretions, has been suggested to play a major role in the first line of defense against pathogenic organisms that enter the nose as the primary site of infection. Indeed, studies have confirmed that the amplitude of the nasal cycle as measured in unilateral nasal resistance is increased during acute viral upper respiratory infections,[8] supporting the immunological role of the nasal cycle.

The system of neural and humoral factors that control the nasal mucosa is complex and includes adrenergic and cholinergic fibers as well as vasoactive intestinal peptide and nitric oxide, where parasympathetic input causes engorgement and congestion and sympathetic input causes constriction and patency (**Table 2.1**). Most nasal decongestants are selective alpha agonists that cause precapillary vasoconstriction with selective shunting of blood through the arteriovenous anastomoses, leading to decreased nasal edema.

The Sneeze Reflex

The sneeze reflex is a protective mechanism that causes a forceful nasal expulsion of air and secretions in response to an irritating or noxious stimulus. It protects the upper airway in a manner analogous to the cough reflex of the lower airway. The function of this reflex is to expel the offending irritant from the nasal cavity. The velocity of exhaled air associated with a sneeze may reach in excess of 100 miles per hour.[10] Thus, the sneeze is a highly effective neuromuscular response involving both cranial and spinal nerves. Although the exact neural arcs are unknown, certain neurological deficits have been described that lead to an impaired sneeze reflex.

While the olfactory nerve conveys the specialty olfactory senses (and is discussed in detail in Chapter 4), the trigeminal nerve conveys thermal, noxious, and mechanical stimuli from the nasal cavity. When an irritant is present in the nose, the sneeze reflex is initiated through activation of the afferent fibers of the trigeminal nerve (V_1 and V_2). The efferent parasympathetic fibers, carried from the pterygopalatine ganglion, then stimulate the corresponding mucosa to increase local secretions, the initial effort to flush or dislodge the irritant. Simultaneously, the phrenic nerve stimulates the diaphragm to activate inspiration. Then, the anterior abdominal wall muscles are stimulated to contract, generating a powerful exhalation. Concurrently, the glossopharyngeal and vagus nerves elevate the palate and contract the superior pharyngeal constrictor, causing a brief Valsalva maneuver, before forcing the pressurized exhalation through the nasal cavity.

In cats, a "sneeze center" has been localized to the lateral medulla, the brainstem region containing the glossopharyngeal and vagus nerve nuclei.[11] It has been suggested that an analogous region exists in humans. Wallenberg syndrome is a relatively common manifestation of ischemic insult to the lateral medulla caused by vertebral or posterior inferior cerebellar artery occlusion. Indeed, there have been several case reports of patients with Wallenberg syndrome who have an impaired sneeze reflex.[12] Such patients describe the sensation of the urge to sneeze, but no spontaneous forced nasal expulsion ensues. This complaint corresponds to their neurological deficit of impaired motor function from the glossopharyngeal and vagus nerve nuclei despite intact sensory function of the trigeminal nerve and nucleus, providing evidence that humans may have a localized brainstem center for the sneeze reflex as well.

The Mucosa, Mucus, Cilia, and Mucociliary Clearance

The Mucosa

When aerosolized pathogens and debris pass through the initial tiers of nasal defense and are greater than 0.5 to 1 μm, they become trapped in the mucus layer of the sinonasal mucosa. The sinonasal mucosa protects the cavities and upper airway from inhaled pathogens, toxins, and debris by mucociliary clearance, a specialized function of the unique protective epithelium of the airway. Mucociliary clearance, which comprises mucus production and mucus transport, removes both healthy secretions and pathological debris from the sinonasal airway. Although the cough and sneeze mechanisms may supplement mucus clearance from the lung and nose respectively, mucociliary clearance remains the principal mode of defense of the respiratory system, especially of the paranasal sinuses.

The mucosa consists of a superficial layer of epithelium with variable numbers of goblet cells, an acellular basement membrane, a thick lamina propria containing vascular and glandular layers, and the periosteum (**Fig. 2.1**). The epithelium of each part of the nasal cavity is specialized to suit its particular region. The anterior margin of the nasal vestibule is composed of stratified squamous epithelium. Containing sebaceous glands, sweat glands, vibrissae, and finer hair, the stratified squamous epithelium provides a protective barrier much like the skin of the rest of the face. Around the area of the nasal valves, the stratified squamous epithelium transitions to the pseudostratified columnar ciliated epithelium found throughout the rest of the nasal cavity (with the exception of the olfactory epithelium). This region of epithelial transition, which is 1 to 2 mm in thickness, overlies dense arterial anastomoses. The anastomoses lead to a plexus of capillaries derived from the anterior ethmoid, greater palatine, sphenopalatine, and superior labial arteries. This plexus, known as Kiesselbach's or Little's area, is believed to be the source of 80% of epistaxis, owing to its rich blood supply and anterior location.[13]

The transitional area between stratified squamous epithelium and pseudostratified columnar ciliated epithelium enlarges as a person ages. As the most anteroinferior

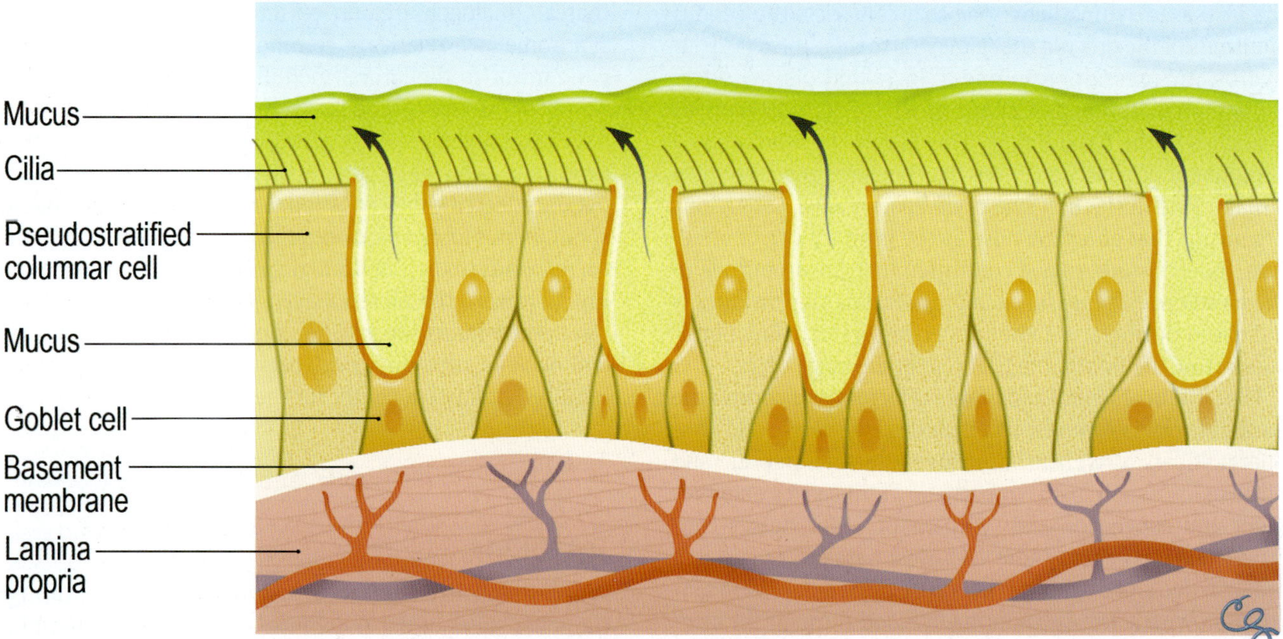

Fig. 2.1 The sinonasal mucosa consists of a superficial layer of epithelium, which is composed predominately of ciliated cells and, to a lesser degree, goblet cells, which rest on an acellular basement membrane overlying a thick lamina propria containing vascular and glandular layers. This mucosa is the primary barrier against inhaled microbes and particulate matter.

columnar epithelium is exposed to years of desiccation from inspired airflow, it may undergo squamous metaplasia, a common adaptive mechanism of stressed epithelium. The total surface area of intranasal squamous epithelium thus often increases over the course of one's life.

The respiratory mucosa of the remainder of the sinonasal cavity and turbinates consists of columnar epithelium (~80%), goblet cells (~20%), and basal cells (less than 5%). Although the nasal columnar epithelium is predominantly pseudostratified, including both ciliated and nonciliated cells, the paranasal sinus columnar epithelium is predominantly simple ciliated columnar cells.[1] Both ciliated and nonciliated columnar cells have hundreds of immotile microvilli along their surface, tiny hairlike projections of actin filaments 1 to 2 μm in length covered by the cell membrane. The microvilli tremendously increase the total surface area of the columnar cells, which likely aids the sinonasal mucosa in mucus production, secretion, and sensation.[14]

The goblet cells, interspersed throughout the columnar cells, contribute to mucus production via secretory granules that contain mucin—a glycoprotein essential to the viscosity and elasticity of mucus. The apical surface of a goblet cell is also covered with microvilli and has a small duct through which it releases its secretions into the nasal cavity (**Fig. 2.2**). Basal cells, attached to the basement membrane by hemidesmosomes, are shielded from the abrasive and contaminated environment of the nasal cavity and paranasal sinuses. In addition to serving as a progenitor cell that can differentiate into goblet or ciliated columnar cells, basal cells may also aid in anchoring the overlying columnar cells to the basement membrane.[15]

The epithelium of the sinonasal mucosa is constructed with three types of intercellular junctions. Adherens junctions, comprised of actinlike filaments, bind epithelial cells to their basement membrane with protein structures

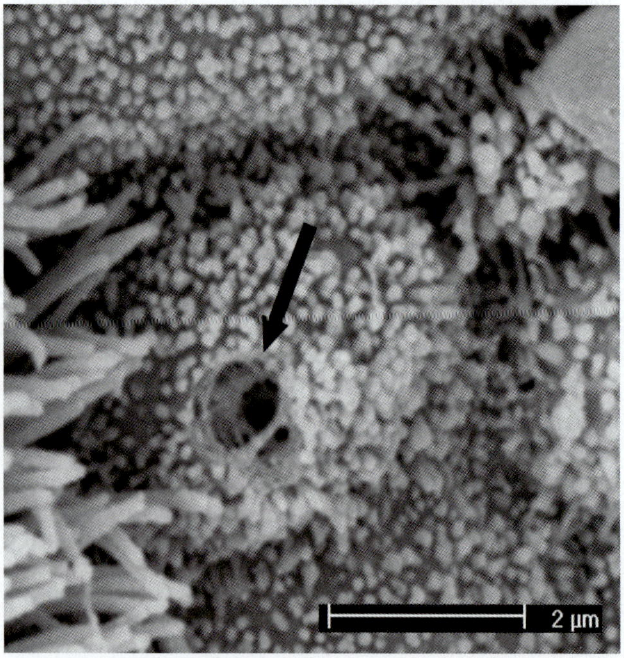

Fig. 2.2 Scanning electron microscopy of a goblet cell. Note the fine microvilli on the surface of the cell and the glandular duct (*arrow*).

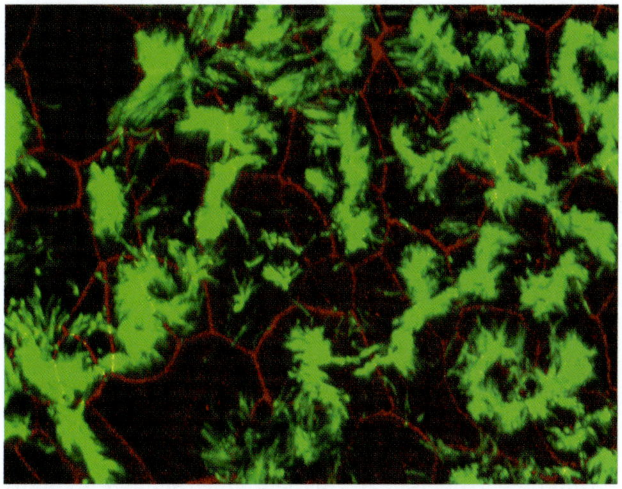

Fig. 2.3 Confocal laser scanning microscopy of sinonasal mucosa stained with immunofluorescence for zona occludens (tight junctions, *red*) and type IV beta-tubulin (cilia, *green*).

including hemidesmosomes, macula adherents, and zonula adherents (**Fig. 2.3**). Tight junctions surround each epithelial cell and ensure that the epithelial layer remains impermeable to water molecules, ions, and potential pathogens. Finally, gap junctions provide small windows connecting the cytoplasm of adjacent epithelial cells. They allow certain ions and charges to pass through and likely play an important role in ciliary coordination.[16]

Beneath the thin basement membrane lies the lamina propria, the layer containing the glands, vasculature, and nerves supplying the sinonasal mucosa. The lamina propria has a superficial glandular layer, a vascular layer, and a deep glandular layer. Anterior serous glands, present on the anterior septum and lateral nasal wall, produce a watery secretion that contributes to the moisture of the nasal cavity. Seromucinous glands are found throughout the cavity and contribute a combination of serous and mucinous secretions. Intraepithelial glands consist of several goblet cells arranged around a lumen and contribute a small amount of mucus to nasal secretions. The parasympathetic fibers that course throughout the lamina propria originate in the superior salivatory nucleus of the brainstem and are carried by the nervus intermedius branch of the facial nerve to the greater superficial petrosal nerve. The sympathetic fibers of the nasal mucosa originate in the sympathetic trunk, synapse in the superior cervical ganglion, and are carried by the deep petrosal nerve. The greater superficial petrosal and deep petrosal nerves then join to form the vidian nerve, which carries the autonomic nervous supply through the pterygopalatine ganglion, where parasympathetic fibers synapse, and the autonomic fibers are then carried to the mucosa by the trigeminal nerve (V_2). The parasympathetic fibers of the lamina propria directly stimulate glandular secretions and can be blocked by atropine or other anticholinergics. The sympathetic fibers of the lamina propria, as mentioned, appear to play a more significant role in mucosal vasoconstriction and decongestion than in regulating nasal secretions.[15]

The Mucus

The epithelium is covered in a mucus blanket that traps cellular debris, pathogens, and particulate matter that precipitates from inspired air. Mucus consists of two layers: the *gel phase* is a discontinuous outer viscous layer that rides along the tips of extended cilia; and the *sol phase* surrounds the shafts of cilia as a continuous inner layer of lower viscosity composed of water and electrolytes (Na^+, K^+, Ca^{2+}, Cl^-). Mucus is an immunologically active substance composed of water (~95%), proteins and peptides (2–3%), salts (1%), and debris (1%), with a slightly acidic pH of 5.5 to 6.5.[17] Its fluid content includes varying concentrations of plasma exudate, submucosal and goblet cell secretions, tears and lacrimal gland secretions, and serous secretions from the olfactory glands of Bowman. Approximately 600 to 1,800 mL of mucus is produced by the sinonasal mucosa per day.[17]

Mucin proteins, secreted by goblet cells, are a group of large threadlike glycoproteins that contain peptide backbones and oligosaccharide side chains. They are an essential component of mucus that give the gel phase its characteristic rheologic properties of viscosity and elasticity. They are secreted in condensed form and undergo hydration to form a gel, which facilitates mucociliary clearance by creating a unique fluid structure that can retain trapped debris while maintaining a pliable and easily transported medium. The mucin proteins themselves may also play an important role in host defense. Their carbohydrate side chains appear to bind surface adhesins on microorganisms, and recognition sites on side chains have been described for adhesins of *Mycoplasma pneumoniae, Streptococcus pneumoniae, Pseudomonas aeruginosa*, influenza virus, and *Escherichia coli*.[18] Therefore, mucin-associated carbohydrates may serve an additional protective mechanism by strongly binding and effectively clearing microorganisms that frequently colonize the upper airways. Mucins may also bind other endogenous proteins within the mucus, including lysozyme and lactoferrin, to protect and structurally support these molecules and facilitate their role in host defense.[19] Furthermore, activated neutrophils, which are central to the acute inflammatory response, stimulate mucin secretion by goblet cells.

Mucus contains many proteins that aid in the local immune defense of the mucosal layer, including the innate immunity proteins lysozyme, lactoferrin, antitrypsin, and surfactant proteins. Lysozyme is a protective enzyme that catalyzes the hydrolysis of bacterial cell walls, and is more effective against Gram-positive bacteria. Lactoferrin is a multifunctional protein with a very high iron affinity that has antimicrobial and immune modulatory activities. By strongly binding iron, lactoferrin deprives local bacteria and fungi of this essential growth nutrient. Lactoferrin may also directly damage the cell wall of Gram-negative bacteria by causing the release of lipopolysaccharides, which are essential to the structural integrity and protective membrane of bacteria.[15] Collectin (collagen-lectin) proteins, such as surfactant proteins (SP-A and SP-D) and mannose-binding protein, exhibit antimicrobial properties and interact with numerous bacteria such as *Staphylococcus* species, *Streptococcus* species, *Klebsiella pneumoniae, P. aeruginosa, E. coli, Aspergillus, Mycobacterium tuberculosis,* and *Salmonella* species.[20] These bacteria have related molecular structures called pathogen-associated molecular patterns (PAMP) that consist of polysaccharides and polynucleotides, such as lipopolysaccharide (LPS). PAMPs differ little from one pathogen to another, but are not found in the host. Collectins bind PAMPs located on microbial membranes via their calcium-dependent carbohydrate-binding domains that promote bacterial clearance.[21–23]

Immunoglobulin A (IgA) and IgG, produced mostly in the mucosa-associated lymphoid tissue (MALT) of the inferior and middle turbinates, are protective antibodies that further augment the defensive barrier of mucus. IgE, which plays a central role in the allergic response (discussed later in text), and IgM are also present in nasal secretions but in lower concentrations. IgA is the major antibody of secretions and mucosal defense, and selective IgA deficiency may result in recurrent sinopulmonary infections. Indeed, IgA deficiency is the most common Ig deficiency responsible for recurrent sinonasal infections.[24] IgA opsonizes pathogens to facilitate their phagocytosis by macrophages and neutrophils, and the aggregation of IgA activates the complement pathway of defense. In concert with lysozyme and complement, IgA also has more specific bactericidal effects against certain pathogens like *S. pneumoniae.*[25] IgG is also very effective at opsonizing pathogens for phagocytosis and activating the complement pathway but plays a less significant role in mucosal secretions. Dendritic cells support the innate immunity of the sinonasal mucosa by processing mucosal antigens and presenting them to T cells, which then engage B cells, in the MALT.[26]

The composition of mucus, while variable, is essential to normal respiratory health, and disorders of mucus production can be debilitating. Cystic fibrosis (CF), an autosomal recessive disease resulting from a mutation in a single gene, involves several organ systems and is considered to be a disease of abnormal mucus production secondary to defective electrolyte transport. The genetic defect is found in the CF transmembrane conductance regulator gene product (CFTR), a cyclic adenosine monophosphate (cAMP)-mediated membrane glycoprotein that forms a chloride channel but also intimately regulates the open probability of the sodium channel, ENaC. The movement of intracellular water from the endothelium into the extracellular mucus layer is an osmotic process that follows electrolyte concentrations, so these patients with defective sodium chloride transport develop abnormally viscous mucus. The goblet cells in such patients subsequently become very engorged and distended. These patients have severely impaired mucociliary clearance and frequently develop severe recurrent sinopulmonary infections.[22]

The Ciliary Structure and Function

Respiratory cilia clear the mucus blanket containing pathogens and debris from both the upper and lower respiratory passages by beating in a coordinated and rhythmic manner. Cilia are cylindrical organelles protruding from the apical surface of epithelial cells and are anchored by intracellular basal bodies derived from centrioles. There are ~50 to 200 cilia per epithelial cell, each measuring 5 to 7 μm in length and 0.2 to 0.3 μm in diameter.[17] Each cilium is composed of a bundle of interconnected microtubules, termed the axoneme, and an overlying membrane that is part of the cell plasma membrane. Microtubules are made of protofilaments, which in turn are composed of alpha- and beta-tubulin dimers. The major beta-tubulin in cilia is the type IV isotype,[27] which is much more abundant in the cilia than elsewhere in the cell and makes for an ideal marker for respiratory cilia in the research setting (**Fig. 2.3**).

The axonemes of motile cilia contain two central singlet microtubules surrounded by nine doublet microtubules (**Fig. 2.4**). Each doublet consists of one alpha-tubule, a complete circle of 13 protofilaments, and one beta-tubule—an incomplete circle of 10 protofilaments. This axoneme

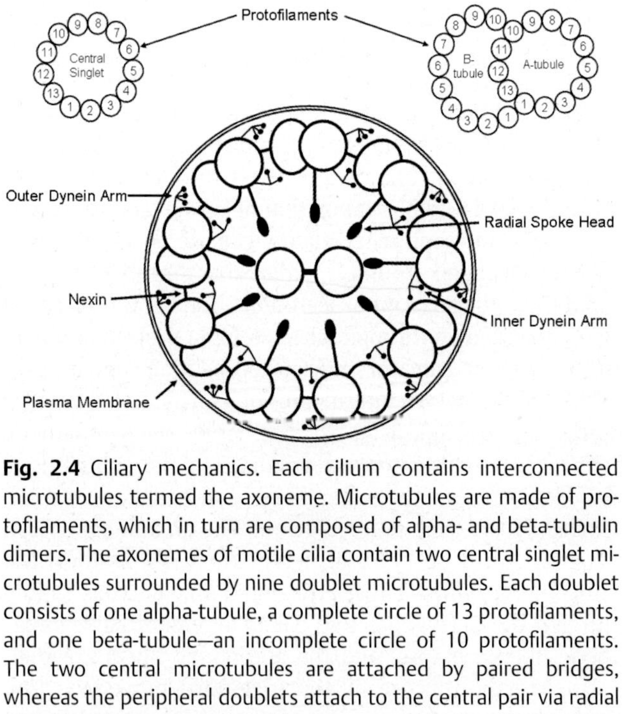

Fig. 2.4 Ciliary mechanics. Each cilium contains interconnected microtubules termed the axoneme. Microtubules are made of protofilaments, which in turn are composed of alpha- and beta-tubulin dimers. The axonemes of motile cilia contain two central singlet microtubules surrounded by nine doublet microtubules. Each doublet consists of one alpha-tubule, a complete circle of 13 protofilaments, and one beta-tubule—an incomplete circle of 10 protofilaments. The two central microtubules are attached by paired bridges, whereas the peripheral doublets attach to the central pair via radial spoke heads. Each outer doublet interacts with the adjacent outer doublets via inner dynein arms (IDAs), outer dynein arms (ODAs), and nexin. Activation of the dynein arms generates a sliding motion of one microtubule doublet against the adjacent doublet.

structure is preserved across the motile cilia of the respiratory epithelium, the oviduct, and the ventricular ependymal cells. The two central microtubules are attached by paired bridges, whereas the peripheral doublets attach to the central pair via radial spoke heads. Each outer doublet interacts with the adjacent outer doublets via inner dynein arms (IDA), outer dynein arms (ODA), and nexin, each having a distinct role in the dynamic motion of cilia bending.[28] Activation of the dynein arms generates a sliding motion of one microtubule doublet against the adjacent doublet. In the *Chlamydomonas*, phosphorylation of the ODAs regulates cilia beat frequency while phosphorylation of the IDAs regulates the wave form pattern of beating.[29] Although the function of the radial spoke heads is not entirely understood, it seems they are involved in regionally limiting the sliding between the microtubules during the ciliary stroke, thus converting the sliding motion generated by the dynein arms into a bending motion of the axoneme.[30]

Each cilium has a forward power stroke followed by a recovery stroke. During the power stroke, the cilium is fully extended, and at the apogee of the arc, the distal tip makes contact with the viscous outer mucus layer (gel phase), thereby transmitting directional force to the overlying mucus blanket. During the recovery stroke, the cilium bends 90 degrees and sweeps back to its starting point within the thinner periciliary fluid layer (the sol phase). The mechanism of ciliary motion depends on a series of ATP-dependent molecular motors that cause the outer doublets of the axoneme to slide relative to each other, producing a vectorial force. The central pair of microtubule singlets divides the axoneme into two opposing halves. As proposed by the "switch point" hypothesis, the dynein motors on one side of the axoneme are predominantly active during the effective stroke, whereas the motors on the other side are mainly active during the recovery stroke. If the microtubules are numbered in a clockwise fashion from 1 to 9, the effective stroke would involve the ODAs on the 9–1–2–3–4 microtubules, and the recovery stroke would involve activity of the dynein in the 5–6–7–8 microtubules.[31] The dynamic force of each power stroke is directly proportional to the number of dynein-microtubule interactions,[32] and there is usually a physiologic reserve available to increase the force of the stroke when necessary.[33] The orientation of the stroke is determined by the orientation of the anchoring basal body of the axoneme (**Fig. 2.5**).[34]

Although it is well established that cilia beat in a coordinated fashion, referred to as a metachronous wave, the mechanism of coordination is not entirely understood. One theory to explain the coordinated wavelike motion of cilia is that gap junctions connecting adjacent epithelial cells may allow a directional propagation of intracellular calcium waves driving the microtubule interactions and, ultimately, the entire metachronous wave.[35] Another possible mechanism relies on the close relationship between the cilia and the hydrodynamic forces surrounding them in their partly liquid environment, where only a relatively small number of coordinated cilia would be necessary to generate a hydrodynamic wave

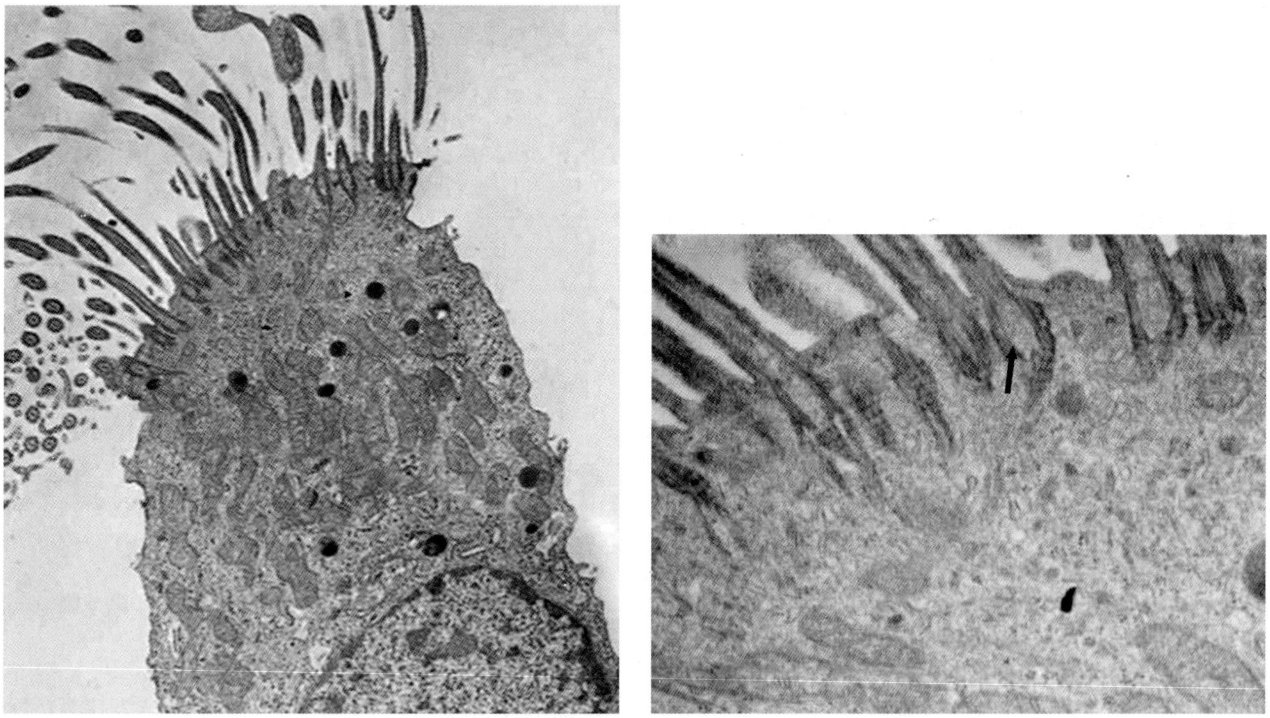

A B

Fig. 2.5 A basal body. Transmission electron micrograph of a ciliated sinonasal epithelial cell. **(A)** The basal bodies anchor the cilia in the cytoplasmic membrane and do not have singlet central microtubules. **(B)** They determine orientation of the ciliary beat and also regenerate the axoneme and new cilia if sheared by external forces (*arrow* indicates basal body).

that, in turn, forces the timed coordinating beating of nearby cilia.[36] Once a metachronous wave is established, spontaneous beating can range from ~9 to 15 Hz in humans, and the cilia tip reaches a velocity of 600 to 1,000 μm/s. The resultant dynamic range of mucus velocity is ~50 to 450 μm/s, or 3 to 25 mm/min. The power and speed of the cilia results in a highly efficient mechanism that can clear the mucus blanket of the entire nose or sinus in 10 minutes.[37]

Ciliary beat frequency (CBF) changes in response to several chemical,[38,39] thermal,[40,41] mechanical,[42] and hormonal[43–45] stimuli. Small changes in both extracellular and intracellular pH can have a profound impact on CBF. An increase in intracellular pH produces an increase in CBF, whereas a decrease in pH produces a decrease in CBF.[46] However, it is not known whether this effect is due to modulation of kinase activity, even though an acidic pH has been demonstrated to inhibit PKA function,[47] or by directly regulating the outer dynein arms of the axoneme.[48] Ciliary beat frequency has also been shown to vary directly with respect to temperature, with the ideal temperature for CBF to be from 32° to 37°C.[40,41,49] Furthermore, direct mechanical stimulation of the cilia promotes an increase in CBF, which coincides with an increase in intracellular Ca^{2+}.[42] This mechanical stimulation is then propagated to the neighboring cells by diffusion of IP_3 through gap junctions, which then activates a release of calcium from the intracellular pools. The end result is an increase in CBF in the entire region surrounding the site of mechanical stimulation.[50]

Extracellular nucleotides (adenosine and uridine) are especially potent regulators of epithelial functions and can stimulate mucociliary clearance in several ways. These nucleotides are released by local epithelium in response to mechanical and osmotic stimuli and act in a paracrine fashion.[51] Through both metabotropic and ionotropic receptors, the nucleotides increase mucus secretion, increase CBF, and gate ion channels involved in maintaining epithelial surface liquid volume.[52] This capability generates a tremendous reserve for dynamic regulation of mucociliary clearance when the respiratory system is environmentally challenged.

Furthermore, adrenergic,[45,53,54] cholinergic,[55,56] and peptidergic[57,58] stimulation have also been demonstrated to stimulate ciliary motility. These environmental and host stimuli are transmitted via surface receptors and channels to trigger activation of second messenger cascades that regulate phosphorylation status of ciliary proteins, thereby modulating the kinetics of microtubules sliding relative to each other. Inositol triphosphate (IP3)-mediated calcium transients have been correlated with increased CBF.[59–61] Additionally, protein kinase A (PKA),[56,62] protein kinase G (PKG),[63,64] and nitric oxide (NO)–dependent mechanisms of CBF stimulation have been proposed.[39,65,66] In contrast, activation of protein kinase C (PKC) appears to decrease CBF.[58,67] Kinase anchoring proteins (AKAPs), kinases, and phosphatases have been demonstrated to be tightly associated with the axoneme, which may allow rapid control of ciliary activity.[68–70]

The Sinonasal Mucociliary Clearance Patterns

The remarkable ability of cilia to create coordinated, microscopic wave movements is equaled by their ability to macroscopically propel mucus in a directional, oriented fashion. The mucus of the paranasal sinuses is directed toward the nasal cavity, where it then travels to the posterior nasopharynx and is eventually ingested into the immunologically active gastrointestinal tract. Appreciation of the natural clearance patterns of the sinuses is critical for successful surgical intervention, especially the frontal sinus, as scarring of confluence regions may lead to mucus stasis.

In the maxillary sinus, mucus must flow superomedially, against gravity, from the most inferior portion of the cavity. Propelled by cilia, the mucus courses upward along the walls of the antrum and medially across the sinus roof toward the natural ostium in the superior medial wall of the sinus, which drains into the ethmoidal infundibulum. The anterior ethmoid cells direct their mucus toward their individual ostia, then into the middle meatus, whereas the posterior ethmoid cells direct their mucus toward the superior meatus and eventually into the sphenoethmoidal recess. The sphenoid sinus also drains through its natural ostium into the sphenoethmoidal recess. The mucus flow pattern in the frontal sinus appears to be unique in that it demonstrates both retrograde and anterograde motion. Mucus along the medial portion of the sinus is carried superiorly, away from the frontal ostium, and then laterally along the roof of the sinus. The mucus along the floor and the inferior portions of the anterior and posterior walls is then carried medially toward the frontal ostium, where it then drains into the frontal recess and the ethmoid infundibulum.

The mucociliary flow from the anterior sinuses (frontal, anterior ethmoid, maxillary) converges at the ostiomeatal complex. From here, the mucus is carried along the uncinate process and inferior turbinate to the posterior nasopharynx, generally passing anteriorly and inferiorly to the eustachian tube orifice (**Fig. 2.6**). The mucociliary flow from the posterior sinuses (posterior ethmoid, sphenoid), however, tends to travel posterior and superior to the eustachian tube orifice toward the posterior nasopharynx. From the posterior nasopharynx, further ciliary motion and swallowing direct the mucus blanket into the gastrointestinal tract, where infectious pathogens are far less likely to survive and create infection. Upper respiratory infections, inflammation, mucosal swelling, and anatomical anomalies may disrupt the normal mucus composition or mucociliary clearance flow pattern. In such cases where obstruction occurs in key areas like the ostiomeatal complex or eustachian tube orifice, associated

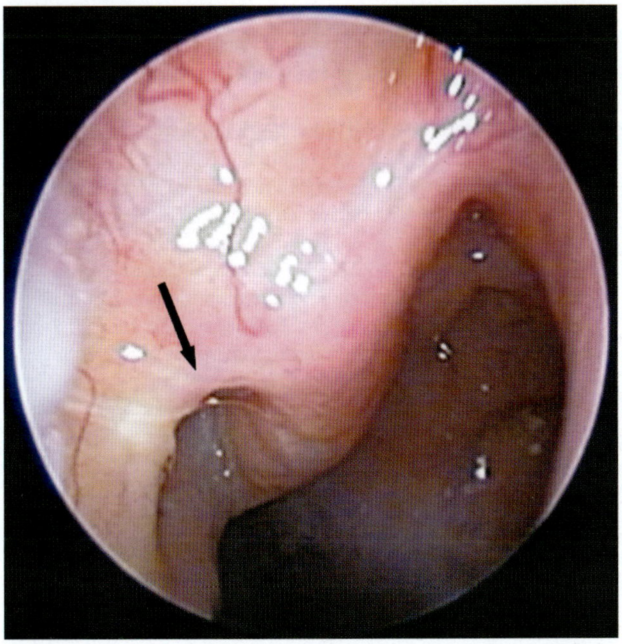

Fig. 2.6 Transnasal endoscopic view of mucus (*arrow*) streaming from the middle meatus and extending over the eustachian tube.

symptomatology commonly results. (Rhinitis and sinusitis will be discussed in detail later in the text.) However, ciliary motion can adapt to a dynamic landscape. For instance, cilia will transport the mucus blanket around irregularities such as septal spurs.

The Ciliary Dysfunction

Mucociliary clearance is dependent on normal cilia function and mucus composition. Thus, disease states that compromise these essential modes of defense tend to result in impaired clearance of infectious pathogens and, ultimately, recurrent sinopulmonary infections. Primary ciliary dyskinesia (PCD), or immotile cilia syndrome, is an inherited disorder of dysfunctional cilia that manifests as severely impaired mucociliary clearance. PCD patients typically present with chronic airway and recurrent middle ear infections. Because embryonic nodal cilia, which are essential for the normal left-right asymmetry of visceral development, are likewise defective, ~50% of PCD patients have situs inversus.[71] Many patients, both male and female, also suffer from infertility because both sperm motility and fallopian tube transport of ova depend on functional cilia. Kartagener syndrome is a subgroup of PCD marked by the triad of chronic sinusitis, situs inversus, and bronchiectasis. The inherited defect of Kartagener syndrome is in the dynein arms of axonemal microtubules, which may result in the absence of the ODAs, the IDAs, or both. Other subsets of PCD patients may demonstrate normal ciliary structure, but random ciliary orientation. Thus, despite normal motility, cilia function is ineffective and results in impaired mucociliary clearance.[72]

In addition to inherited pathologies, exposure to various environmental pathogens can also alter the normal mucociliary clearance system. Infectious organisms that can interfere with their host's mucociliary defense have a survival advantage, and several have indeed adapted such mechanisms. Common bacterial pathogens such as *Haemophilus influenzae*, *S. pneumoniae*, *Staphylococcus aureus*, and *Pseudomonas* produce specific toxins to impair ciliary motion and coordination.[73] Viruses responsible for common upper respiratory infections disrupt the microtubule function of ciliated columnar cells and change the viscosity of the surrounding mucus. Impairing the local defense system facilitates the infectious pathogens' upper airway colonization.

Chronic rhinosinusitis (CRS), affecting more than 35 million Americans of all ages,[74] represents several distinct entities that are clinically indistinguishable. Although the mortality of the disease is low, the morbidity is high with CRS patients, demonstrating worse quality-of-life scores (for physical pain and social functioning) than those suffering from chronic obstructive pulmonary disease, congestive heart failure, or angina.[75] Multiple etiologies contribute to the development of CRS, but a common pathophysiologic sequela is ineffective sinonasal mucociliary clearance, resulting in stasis of sinonasal secretions and subsequent chronic infection and/or persistent inflammation. Although the literature is contradictory regarding mucus viscosity[76,77] and basal ciliary beat frequency[76,78] in CRS, recent work has suggested that a subset of patients with CRS have a blunted ciliary response to environmental stimuli.[79] Additionally, air-liquid interface cultures of respiratory epithelium from patients with CRS have demonstrated an increased transepithelial ion transport compared with normal cultures, thereby altering mucus viscosity and potentially contributing to the pathophysiology of the disease.[80]

■ Conclusion

The respiratory system is regularly exposed to altered environmental conditions as well as constantly bombarded by environmental pollutants, respiratory pathogens, and aerosolized toxins. Thus, the system has evolved multiple physiologic strategies to regulate inspired air flow resistance, temperature, and humidification, as well as tightly modulate its ability to protect and defend itself. Disruption of these physiologic processes secondary to host or environmental factors such as anatomic variations, genetic mutations, overwhelming environmental pollution, or frequent infections contribute to the development of chronic rhinosinusitis. Other chapters of this book address issues in the management of CRS, with each strategy aimed at restoring a disrupted sinonasal physiologic process.

References

1. Wagenmann M, Naclerio RM. Anatomic and physiologic considerations in sinusitis. J Allergy Clin Immunol 1992;90(3 Pt 2): 419–423
2. Mirza N, Lanza DC. The nasal airway and obstructed breathing during sleep. Otolaryngol Clin North Am 1999;32(2):243–262
3. Zhao K, Dalton P, Yang GC, Scherer PW. Numerical modeling of turbulent and laminar airflow and odorant transport during sniffing in the human and rat nose. Chem Senses 2006;31(2):107–118
4. Houser SM. Surgical treatment for empty nose syndrome. Arch Otolaryngol Head Neck Surg 2007;133(9):858–863
5. Heyder J. Deposition of inhaled particles in the human respiratory tract and consequences for regional targeting in respiratory drug delivery. Proc Am Thorac Soc 2004;1(4):315–320
6. Haight JS, Cole P. Nasal responses to local unilateral stimuli in man. Rhinology 1983;21(1):67–72
7. Hanif J, Jawad SS, Eccles R. The nasal cycle in health and disease. Clin Otolaryngol Allied Sci 2000;25(6):461–467
8. Eccles R. A role for the nasal cycle in respiratory defence. Eur Respir J 1996;9(2):371–376
9. Grevers G. The role of fenestrated vessels for the secretory process in the nasal mucosa: a histological and transmission electron microscopic study in the rabbit. Laryngoscope 1993;103(11 Pt 1): 1255–1258
10. Guinness World Records. Guinness Book of World Records. New York: Guinness World Records Limited; 2004
11. Nonaka S, Unno T, Ohta Y, Mori S. Sneeze-evoking region within the brainstem. Brain Res 1990;511(2):265–270
12. Hersch M. Loss of ability to sneeze in lateral medullary syndrome. Neurology 2000;54(2):520–521
13. Doyle DE. Anterior epistaxis: a new nasal tampon for fast, effective control. Laryngoscope 1986;96(3):279–281
14. Busse WW. Mechanisms and advances in allergic diseases. J Allergy Clin Immunol 2000;105(6 Pt 2):S593–S598
15. Naclerio R. Clinical manifestations of the release of histamine and other inflammatory mediators. J Allergy Clin Immunol 1999;103(3 Pt 2):S382–S385
16. Bhargave G, Woodworth BA, Xiong G, Wolfe SG, Antunes MB, Cohen NA. Transient receptor potential vanilloid type 4 channel expression in chronic rhinosinusitis. Am J Rhinol 2008;22(1):7–12
17. Houtmeyers E, Gosselink R, Gayan-Ramirez G, Decramer M. Regulation of mucociliary clearance in health and disease. Eur Respir J 1999;13(5):1177–1188
18. Prince A. Adhesins and receptors of Pseudomonas aeruginosa associated with infection of the respiratory tract. Microb Pathog 1992;13(4):251–260
19. Lamblin G, Lhermitte M, Klein A, et al. The carbohydrate diversity of human respiratory mucins: a protection of the underlying mucosa? Am Rev Respir Dis 1991;144(3 Pt 2):S19–S24
20. Woodworth BA, Lathers D, Neal JG, et al. Immunolocalization of surfactant protein A and D in sinonasal mucosa. Am J Rhinol 2006;20(4):461–465
21. Woodworth BA, Neal JG, Newton D, et al. Surfactant protein A and D in human sinus mucosa: a preliminary report. ORL J Otorhinolaryngol Relat Spec 2007;69(1):57–60
22. Woodworth BA, Wood R, Baatz JE, Schlosser RJ. Sinonasal surfactant protein A1, A2, and D gene expression in cystic fibrosis: a preliminary report. Otolaryngol Head Neck Surg 2007;137(1): 34–38
23. Woodworth BA, Wood R, Bhargave G, Cohen NA, Baatz JE, Schlosser RJ. Surfactant protein B detection and gene expression in chronic rhinosinusitis. Laryngoscope 2007;117(7):1296–1301
24. Sethi DS, Winkelstein JA, Lederman H, Loury MC. Immunologic defects in patients with chronic recurrent sinusitis: diagnosis and management. Otolaryngol Head Neck Surg 1995;112(2):242–247
25. Pilette C, Ouadrhiri Y, Godding V, Vaerman JP, Sibille Y. Lung mucosal immunity: immunoglobulin-A revisited. Eur Respir J 2001;18(3):571–588
26. Rampey AM, Lathers DM, Woodworth BA, Schlosser RJ. Immunolocalization of dendritic cells and pattern recognition receptors in chronic rhinosinusitis. Am J Rhinol 2007;21(1):117–121
27. Antunes MB, Woodworth BA, Bhargave G, et al. Murine nasal septa for respiratory epithelial air-liquid interface cultures. Biotechniques 2007;43(2):195–196, 198, 200 passim
28. Hard R, Blaustein K, Scarcello L. Reactivation of outer-arm-depleted lung axonemes: evidence for functional differences between inner and outer dynein arms in situ. Cell Motil Cytoskeleton 1992; 21(3):199–209
29. Brokaw CJ. Control of flagellar bending: a new agenda based on dynein diversity. Cell Motil Cytoskeleton 1994;28(3):199–204
30. Satir P, Christensen ST. Overview of structure and function of mammalian cilia. Annu Rev Physiol 2007;69:377–400
31. Sanderson MJ, Sleigh MA. Ciliary activity of cultured rabbit tracheal epithelium: beat pattern and metachrony. J Cell Sci 1981;47:331–347
32. Holwill ME, Foster GF, Hamasaki T, Satir P. Biophysical aspects and modelling of ciliary motility. Cell Motil Cytoskeleton 1995;32(2): 114–120
33. Johnson NT, Villalón M, Royce FH, Hard R, Verdugo P. Autoregulation of beat frequency in respiratory ciliated cells. Demonstration by viscous loading. Am Rev Respir Dis 1991;144(5):1091–1094
34. Lee CH, Lee SS, Mo JH, et al. Comparison of ciliary wave disorders measured by image analysis and electron microscopy. Acta Otolaryngol 2005;125(5):571–576
35. Yeh TH, Su MC, Hsu CJ, Chen YH, Lee SY. Epithelial cells of nasal mucosa express functional gap junctions of connexin 43. Acta Otolaryngol 2003;123(2):314–320
36. Gheber L, Priel Z. Synchronization between beating cilia. Biophys J 1989;55(1):183–191
37. Hilding A. The physiology of drainage of nasal mucus: III experimental work on the accessory sinuses. Am J Physiol 1932;100:664–670
38. Wong LB, Miller IF, Yeates DB. Stimulation of tracheal ciliary beat frequency by capsaicin. J Appl Physiol 1990;68(6):2574–2580
39. Jain B, Rubinstein I, Robbins RA, Leise KL, Sisson JH. Modulation of airway epithelial cell ciliary beat frequency by nitric oxide. Biochem Biophys Res Commun 1993;191(1):83–88
40. Mwimbi XK, Muimo R, Green MW, Mehta A. Making human nasal cilia beat in the cold: a real time assay for cell signalling. Cell Signal 2003;15(4):395–402
41. Schipor I, Palmer JN, Cohen AS, Cohen NA. Quantification of ciliary beat frequency in sinonasal epithelial cells using differential interference contrast microscopy and high-speed digital video imaging. Am J Rhinol 2006;20(1):124–127
42. Sanderson MJ, Dirksen ER. Mechanosensitivity of cultured ciliated cells from the mammalian respiratory tract: implications for the regulation of mucociliary transport. Proc Natl Acad Sci U S A 1986;83(19):7302–7306
43. Jain B, Rubinstein I, Robbins RA, Sisson JH. TNF-alpha and IL-1 beta upregulate nitric oxide-dependent ciliary motility in bovine airway epithelium. Am J Physiol 1995;268(6 Pt 1):L911–L917
44. Korngreen A, Ma W, Priel Z, Silberberg SD. Extracellular ATP directly gates a cation-selective channel in rabbit airway ciliated epithelial cells. J Physiol 1998;508(Pt 3):703–720
45. Sanderson MJ, Dirksen ER. Mechanosensitive and beta-adrenergic control of the ciliary beat frequency of mammalian respiratory tract cells in culture. Am Rev Respir Dis 1989;139(2):432–440
46. Sutto Z, Conner GE, Salathe M. Regulation of human airway ciliary beat frequency by intracellular pH. J Physiol 2004;560 (Pt 2):519–532

47. Reddy MM, Kopito RR, Quinton PM. Cytosolic pH regulates GCl through control of phosphorylation states of CFTR. Am J Physiol 1998;275(4 Pt 1):C1040–C1047
48. Keskes L, Giroux-Widemann V, Serres C, Pignot-Paintrand I, Jouannet P, Feneux D. The reactivation of demembranated human spermatozoa lacking outer dynein arms is independent of pH. Mol Reprod Dev 1998;49(4):416–425
49. Green A, Smallman LA, Logan AC, Drake-Lee AB. The effect of temperature on nasal ciliary beat frequency. Clin Otolaryngol Allied Sci 1995;20(2):178–180
50. Dirksen ER, Sanderson MJ. Regulation of ciliary activity in the mammalian respiratory tract. Biorheology 1990;27(3-4):533–545
51. Winters SL, Davis CW, Boucher RC. Mechanosensitivity of mouse tracheal ciliary beat frequency: roles for Ca2+, purinergic signaling, tonicity, and viscosity. Am J Physiol Lung Cell Mol Physiol 2007;292(3):L614–L624
52. Picher M, Boucher RC. Human airway ecto-adenylate kinase. A mechanism to propagate ATP signaling on airway surfaces. J Biol Chem 2003;278(13):11256–11264
53. Wyatt TA, Sisson JH. Chronic ethanol downregulates PKA activation and ciliary beating in bovine bronchial epithelial cells. Am J Physiol Lung Cell Mol Physiol 2001;281(3):L575–L581
54. Yang B, Schlosser RJ, McCaffrey TV. Dual signal transduction mechanisms modulate ciliary beat frequency in upper airway epithelium. Am J Physiol 1996;270(5 Pt 1):L745–L751
55. Salathe M, Lipson EJ, Ivonnet PI, Bookman RJ. Muscarinic signaling in ciliated tracheal epithelial cells: dual effects on Ca2+ and ciliary beating. Am J Physiol 1997;272(2 Pt 1):L301–L310
56. Zagoory O, Braiman A, Priel Z. The mechanism of ciliary stimulation by acetylcholine: roles of calcium, PKA, and PKG. J Gen Physiol 2002;119(4):329–339
57. Wong LB, Miller IF, Yeates DB. Pathways of substance P stimulation of canine tracheal ciliary beat frequency. J Appl Physiol 1991;70(1):267–273
58. Wong LB, Park CL, Yeates DB. Neuropeptide Y inhibits ciliary beat frequency in human ciliated cells via nPKC, independently of PKA. Am J Physiol 1998;275(2 Pt 1):C440–C448
59. Salathe M, Bookman RJ. Coupling of [Ca2+]i and ciliary beating in cultured tracheal epithelial cells. J Cell Sci 1995;108(Pt 2):431–440
60. Korngreen A, Priel Z. Simultaneous measurement of ciliary beating and intracellular calcium. Biophys J 1994;67(1):377–380
61. Lansley AB, Sanderson MJ. Regulation of airway ciliary activity by Ca2+: simultaneous measurement of beat frequency and intracellular Ca2+. Biophys J 1999;77(1):629–638
62. Braiman A, Zagoory O, Priel Z. PKA induces Ca2+ release and enhances ciliary beat frequency in a Ca2+-dependent and -independent manner. Am J Physiol 1998;275(3 Pt 1):C790–C797
63. Zhang L, Sanderson MJ. The role of cGMP in the regulation of rabbit airway ciliary beat frequency. J Physiol 2003;551(Pt 3):765–776
64. Wyatt TA, Spurzem JR, May K, Sisson JH. Regulation of ciliary beat frequency by both PKA and PKG in bovine airway epithelial cells. Am J Physiol 1998;275(4 Pt 1):L827–L835
65. Yang B, Schlosser RJ, McCaffrey TV. Signal transduction pathways in modulation of ciliary beat frequency by methacholine. Ann Otol Rhinol Laryngol 1997;106(3):230–236
66. Uzlaner N, Priel Z. Interplay between the NO pathway and elevated [Ca2+]i enhances ciliary activity in rabbit trachea. J Physiol 1999;516(Pt 1):179–190
67. Mwimbi XK, Muimo R, Green M, Mehta A. Protein kinase C regulates the flow rate-dependent decline in human nasal ciliary beat frequency in vitro. J Aerosol Med 2000;13(3):273–279
68. Porter ME, Sale WS. The 9 + 2 axoneme anchors multiple inner arm dyneins and a network of kinases and phosphatases that control motility. J Cell Biol 2000;151(5):F37–F42
69. Kamiya R. Functional diversity of axonemal dyneins as studied in Chlamydomonas mutants. Int Rev Cytol 2002;219:115–155
70. Smith EF. Regulation of flagellar dynein by the axonemal central apparatus. Cell Motil Cytoskeleton 2002;52(1):33–42
71. Noone PG, Leigh MW, Sannuti A, et al. Primary ciliary dyskinesia: diagnostic and phenotypic features. Am J Respir Crit Care Med 2004;169(4):459–467
72. Rutland J, de Iongh RU. Random ciliary orientation. A cause of respiratory tract disease. N Engl J Med 1990;323(24):1681–1684
73. Ferguson JL, McCaffrey TV, Kern EB, Martin WJ II. The effects of sinus bacteria on human ciliated nasal epithelium in vitro. Otolaryngol Head Neck Surg 1988;98(4):299–304
74. Murphy MP, Fishman P, Short SO, Sullivan SD, Yueh B, Weymuller EA Jr. Health care utilization and cost among adults with chronic rhinosinusitis enrolled in a health maintenance organization. Otolaryngol Head Neck Surg 2002;127(5):367–376
75. Gliklich RE, Metson R. The health impact of chronic sinusitis in patients seeking otolaryngologic care. Otolaryngol Head Neck Surg 1995;113(1):104–109
76. Majima Y, Sakakura Y, Matsubara T, Miyoshi Y. Possible mechanisms of reduction of nasal mucociliary clearance in chronic sinusitis. Clin Otolaryngol Allied Sci 1986;11(2):55–60
77. Atsuta S, Majima Y. Nasal mucociliary clearance of chronic sinusitis in relation to rheological properties of nasal mucus. Ann Otol Rhinol Laryngol 1998;107(1):47–51
78. Braverman I, Wright ED, Wang CG, Eidelman D, Frenkiel S. Human nasal ciliary-beat frequency in normal and chronic sinusitis subjects. J Otolaryngol 1998;27(3):145–152
79. Chen B, Shaari J, Claire SE, et al. Altered sinonasal ciliary dynamics in chronic rhinosinusitis. Am J Rhinol 2006;20(3):325–329
80. Dejima K, Randell SH, Stutts MJ, Senior BA, Boucher RC. Potential role of abnormal ion transport in the pathogenesis of chronic sinusitis. Arch Otolaryngol Head Neck Surg 2006;132(12):1352–1362

3 Radiologic Imaging of the Paranasal Sinuses and Skull Base

Laurie A. Loevner and Igor Mikityansky

This chapter addresses imaging modalities available to assess disease processes of the sinonasal cavity, and provides some direction on when and how to use each imaging modality. We specifically emphasize inflammatory disease and neoplasia. To understand the pathogenesis and imaging appearances of sinusitis and other pathologic processes that affect the paranasal sinuses, a brief review of sinus anatomy as it pertains to mucociliary clearance is essential. Subsequently, focused imaging assessment of disease processes including sinusitis and neoplasms is covered. An understanding of the natural history of sinus carcinomas is also paramount in assessing imaging patterns of tumor spread and in determining surgical and irradiation management.

Anatomy

For a detailed discussion of sinonasal development, see Chapter 1 of this book. The paranasal sinuses and nasal cavity are lined by the ciliated columnar epithelium, which contains both mucinous and serous glands. The common drainage pathway for the frontal sinuses, maxillary sinuses, and anterior ethmoid air cells is through the ostiomeatal complex.[1,2] The ostiomeatal unit consists of the maxillary sinus ostium, the infundibulum, the hiatus semilunaris, and the middle meatus (**Fig. 3.1A,B**). This drainage conduit is centered around the uncinate process, an osseous extension of the lateral nasal wall. Secretions that accumulate within the maxillary sinuses circulate toward the maxillary sinus ostium propelled by ciliated mucosa.[1,3] From the maxillary ostium, mucus passes through the infundibulum, located lateral to the uncinate process. Secretions progress through the hiatus semilunaris, the air space between the posterior edge of the uncinate process and the anterior and inferior surface of the ethmoidal bulla (the largest ethmoid air cell), and then pass into the middle meatus, the nasal cavity, and ultimately into the nasopharynx where they are swallowed.[1,3]

The frontal sinuses drain inferiorly via the frontal ethmoidal recess into the middle meatus, which is the common drainage site also for the anterior ethmoid air cells.[1] The anteriormost of the ethmoid air cells is the agger nasi, but other variants of ethmoid pneumatization may be present, including frontal cells, supraorbital ethmoid cells, and suprabullar cells.[4] Infraorbital ethmoid cells (also known as Haller cells or maxilloethmoidal cells) are located along the anterosuperior maxillary surface just inferior to the orbital floor, typically in close proximity to the maxillary sinus ostium. Present in less than 10 to 18% of imaged patients, infraorbital ethmoid cells are important because they may encroach or obstruct mucociliary clearance from the maxillary sinus and may contribute to sinonasal inflammatory disease.[4]

The posterior ethmoid air cells are located posterior to the basal lamella of the middle turbinate, and secretions originating from the posterior ethmoid sinus drain through the superior meatus and/or the supreme meatus into the sphenoethmoidal recess, the nasal cavity, and finally, into the nasopharynx (**Fig. 3.1C,D**). The sphenoid ostium is located medial to the superior turbinate and drains directly into the sphenoethmoid recess. Cilia are necessary for drainage of the sphenoid sinuses as secretions must be propelled to the sphenoid ostia located superior to the sinus floor.

The anterior and inferior nasal septum is made up of cartilage. The posterior portion of the nasal septum is osseous. The superior posterior osseous portion is the perpendicular plate of the ethmoid bone, whereas the inferior posterior osseous portion is the vomer. The nasolacrimal duct runs from the lacrimal sac at the medial canthus, along the anterior and lateral nasal wall, and drains into the inferior meatus. The three sets of turbinates in the nasal cavity include the superior, middle, and inferior turbinates. Occasionally, there may be a supreme turbinate located posterior and superior to the superior turbinate. Concha bullosae (aerated middle turbinates) are present in up to 50% of patients.[5,6] A large or opacified concha bullosa may obstruct the ostiomeatal complex. In most individuals, there is normal cyclical passive congestion and decongestion that alternates between each side of the nasal cavity, as dictated by the nasal cycle. These periodic fluctuations in blood flow may result in apparent relative hypertrophy of intranasal structures.

Blood supply to the sinonasal structures comes from the internal and external carotid arteries. The arterial supply to the frontal sinuses is from supraorbital and supratrochlear branches of the ophthalmic artery, whereas venous drainage is through the superior ophthalmic veins. The ethmoid air cells and sphenoid sinus also receive blood supply from branches of the sphenopalatine artery (arising from the external carotid circulation) as well as ethmoidal branches of the ophthalmic artery (arising from the internal carotid circulation). Branches of the internal maxillary artery that arise from the external carotid artery predominantly supply the maxillary sinuses.

The venous drainage pattern of the paranasal sinuses (ultimately communicating with the cavernous sinus and

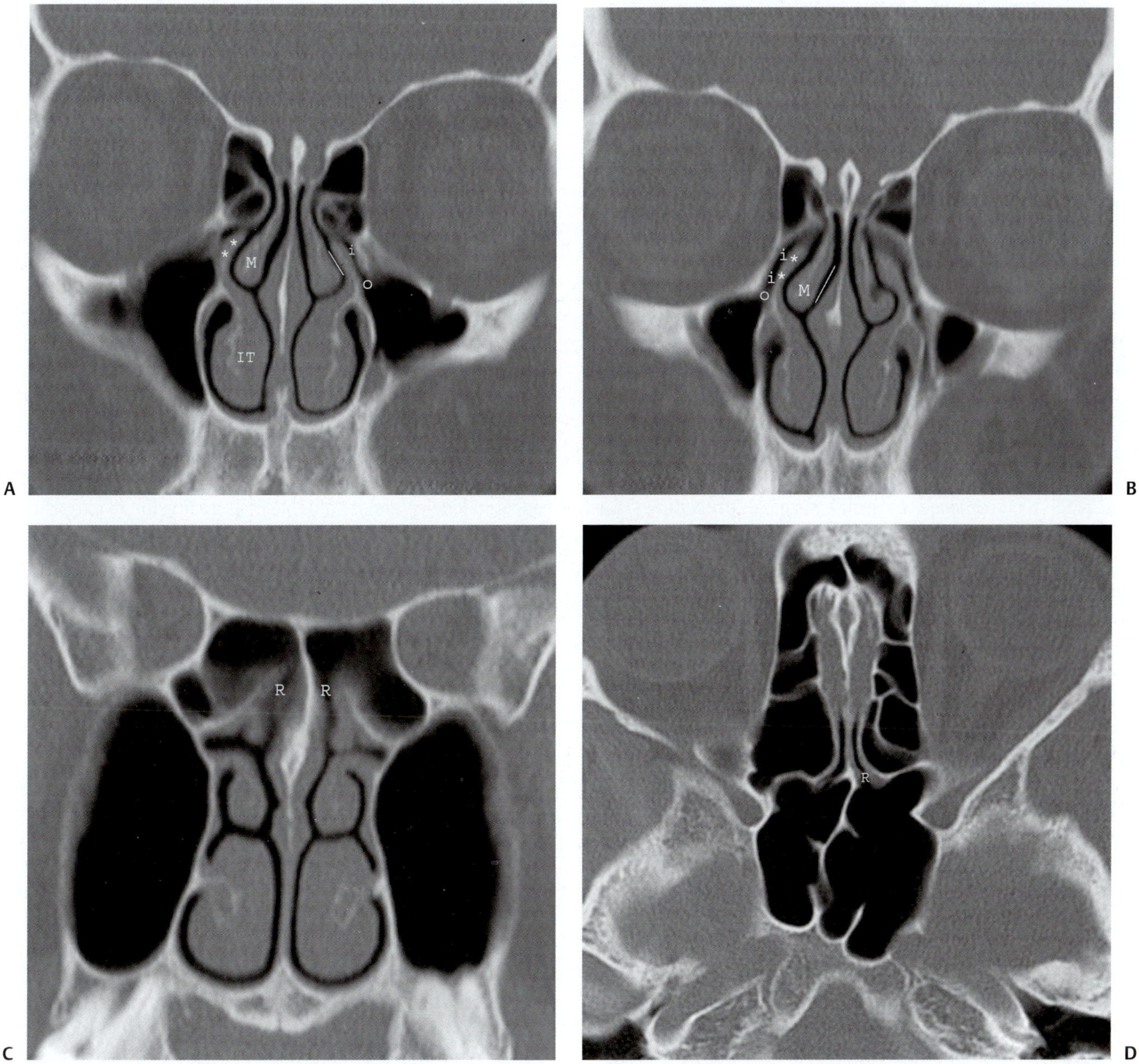

Fig. 3.1 Normal anatomy of mucociliary drainage of the paranasal sinuses. **(A,B)** Direct coronal computed tomography (CT) images in a bone algorithm show the normal drainage pathway of the maxillary sinus, anterior ethmoid air cells, and frontal sinus via the ostiomeatal complex (*OMC*). *, uncinate process; *O*, maxillary sinus ostium; *i*, infundibulum; *white line*, middle meatus; *m*, middle turbinate; *IT*, inferior turbinate. **(C,D)** Coronal and axial CT images in bone algorithm show the normal drainage of the posterior ethmoid air cells and the sphenoid sinus via the sphenoethmoidal recess into the nasal cavity (*R*).

pterygoid venous plexus) is responsible for the potential intracranial complications of sinusitis, including meningitis, subdural empyema, and venous thrombosis. The venous drainage is through nasal veins and/or ethmoidal veins that drain into the ophthalmic veins, which subsequently drain into the cavernous sinus. The maxillary sinuses drain through facial and maxillary veins, the latter communicating with the pterygoid venous plexus.

Imaging Sinonasal Disease: The Radiologist's Arsenal

Plain Film Radiographs

Computed tomography (CT) has replaced plain film radiographs as the primary modality in evaluating sinonasal disease. Functional endoscopic sinonasal surgery (FESS) has supplanted external procedures like the Caldwell-Luc and maxillary antrostomy for the treatment of sinusitis. This has required much better and precise anatomic delineation, which is not provided by plain film radiographs. Overlapping structures on plain film radiographs limit evaluation of the ostiomeatal complex, as well as the individual paranasal sinuses. There is also insufficient detail regarding the osseous framework of the sinonasal cavity. There are a few limited applications for radiographs. They are sometimes obtained in intensive care unit settings when sinusitis is suspected or needs to be excluded and the patient is too sick to come to the radiology department for CT imaging. However, the increasing availability of portable CT units has resulted in progressive decrease in the use of radiographs for this purpose.

Computed Tomography

As FESS has replaced external surgical procedures for treating sinusitis, CT imaging has become necessary to provide the surgeon with precise anatomic information as seen by the endoscopist. Surgery is directed toward removing blockages to mucociliary clearance at the ostiomeatal complex. For the surgeon performing FESS, coronal CT is ideal as it simulates the appearance of the sinonasal cavity from an endoscopic view (**Fig. 3.1A–D**).

Direct coronal thin section imaging (1 to 3 mm) is frequently obtained through the paranasal sinuses.[7] Using the newer helical CT scanners, high quality axial reformatted images may be created from these coronal images. Alternatively, direct axial CT imaging may be performed with subsequent creation of coronal reformatted images. The recent literature suggests the use of low-dose CTs to decrease radiation exposure to the lenses.[8–13] Many computer software programs allow instant three plane reconstructions (coronal and sagittal reconstructions from axial images). Intravenous contrast material is usually not necessary for imaging sinonasal inflammatory disease. Should CT imaging show findings such as bone destruction or an extension of disease outside the sinonasal cavity concerning for a more aggressive process like a neoplasm or invasive sinusitis, magnetic resonance imaging (MRI) should be obtained with and without intravenous contrast (gadolinium) administration, which is a more sensitive study.[7,14,15] If the patient has a contraindication to MRI (i.e., pacemaker) and an enhanced study is indicated, then contrast-enhanced CT is the appropriate alternative study.

Magnetic Resonance Imaging

MRI has become increasingly important in assessing patients with neoplasms of the sinonasal cavity, aggressive infections, and developmental lesions, such as meningoencephaloceles.[7,15–20] A combination of sagittal, axial, and coronal imaging provides excellent anatomic information regarding the extent of sinonasal pathology. Multiple different image sequences are obtained, including T1-weighted, T2-weighted, as well as contrast-enhanced multiplanar imaging. Excellent anatomic resolution may be acquired from an MRI examination performed in a standard head coil. On occasion, imaging of the sinonasal cavity may be performed with a surface coil positioned over the face.[21]

MRI of sinonasal tumors and aggressive infections must include high-resolution unenhanced and enhanced thin section (3 mm) images not only of the sinonasal cavity, but also the orbits, skull base, and the adjacent intracranial compartment.[22–26] Tumor extension into these structures is frequently not evident on clinical assessment/endoscopy. Images should be acquired in both axial and coronal planes. Contrast-enhanced imaging is essential to assess the extent of local disease, as well as the presence of perineural spread and intracranial extension. MRI allows discrimination of inflammation and inspissated secretions from neoplasms (**Fig. 3.2A,B**) and other nonneoplastic masses (i.e., encephalocele), and is valuable in assessing for an extension of disease outside the sinonasal cavity into the intracranial compartment, the eye, and the base of the skull.[22,23,25,26]

Imaging Disease Processes of the Paranasal Sinuses

Inflammatory Disease/Sinusitis

Sinusitis is among the most common ailments in the United States, with over 30 million Americans affected by sinusitis each year.[27] Over 15 million visits to family physicians each year are related to sinus inflammation. Most cases of acute sinusitis are related to an antecedent viral upper respiratory tract infection. There is resultant swelling that results in apposition of the mucosal surfaces within the paranasal sinuses leading to obstruction of the normal drainage pathways. Inadequate drainage of secretions results in bacterial overgrowth and sinus infection. Although literature suggests that use of CT in uncomplicated community-acquired bacterial sinusitis is not cost-effective,[28] unenhanced coronal CT imaging may be obtained in patients with suspected acute sinusitis to assess mucosal disease and/or blockage of the drainage passageways that support this clinically suspected diagnosis (**Fig. 3.3A,B**).[29–31] Although the empiric antibiotic therapy or treatment according to clinical guidelines are considered the cost-effective pathways,[28,32] the imaging still could be used for those patients refractory to medications and antibiotics. If imaging is contemplated to follow-up a patient treated for sinusitis, it is best to obtain imaging 4 to 6 weeks following therapy as the resolution of the radiological findings may lag behind the clinical response.

In patients being assessed with CT imaging for chronic sinusitis, it is important for the radiologist to report the areas of mucosal thickening within the paranasal sinuses as well as the drainage passageways of the ostiomeatal complex and

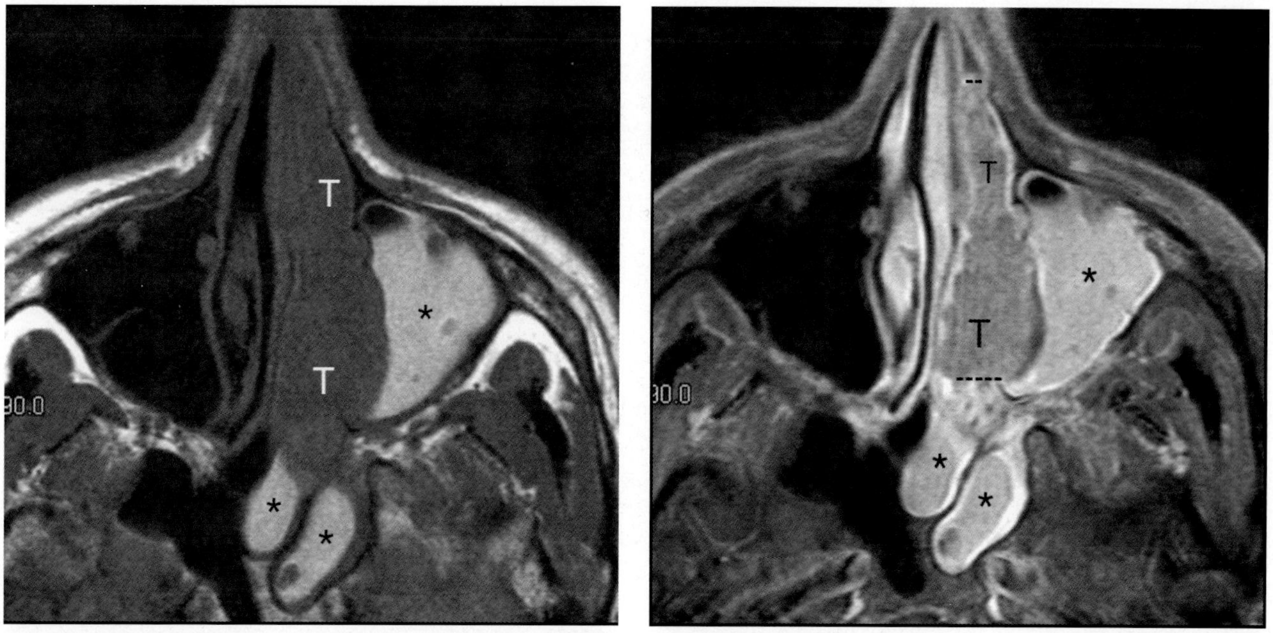

A B

Fig. 3.2 The value of magnetic resonance imaging (MRI) in delineating a tumor from sinus secretions. **(A)** Axial unenhanced T1-weighted MRI shows complete opacification of the left maxillary and sphenoid sinuses with central material that is hyperintense (*bright*) consistent with proteinaceous, inspissated secretions (*asterisk*). There is complete opacification of the left nasal cavity with hypointense tissue (*T*). **(B)** Corresponding enhanced fat-suppressed T1-weighted MRI shows persistent hyperintensity of the central material (*asterisk*) in the left maxillary and sphenoid sinuses. Note that this is not enhancement as these areas are hyperintense on the unenhanced T1-weighted image **(A)** corresponding to proteinaceous secretions. Note the enhancing mass, which represented squamous cell carcinoma in the left nasal cavity (*T*) (compare with unenhanced image **A**). Note how magnetic resonance nicely delineates the margins of the tumor (—).

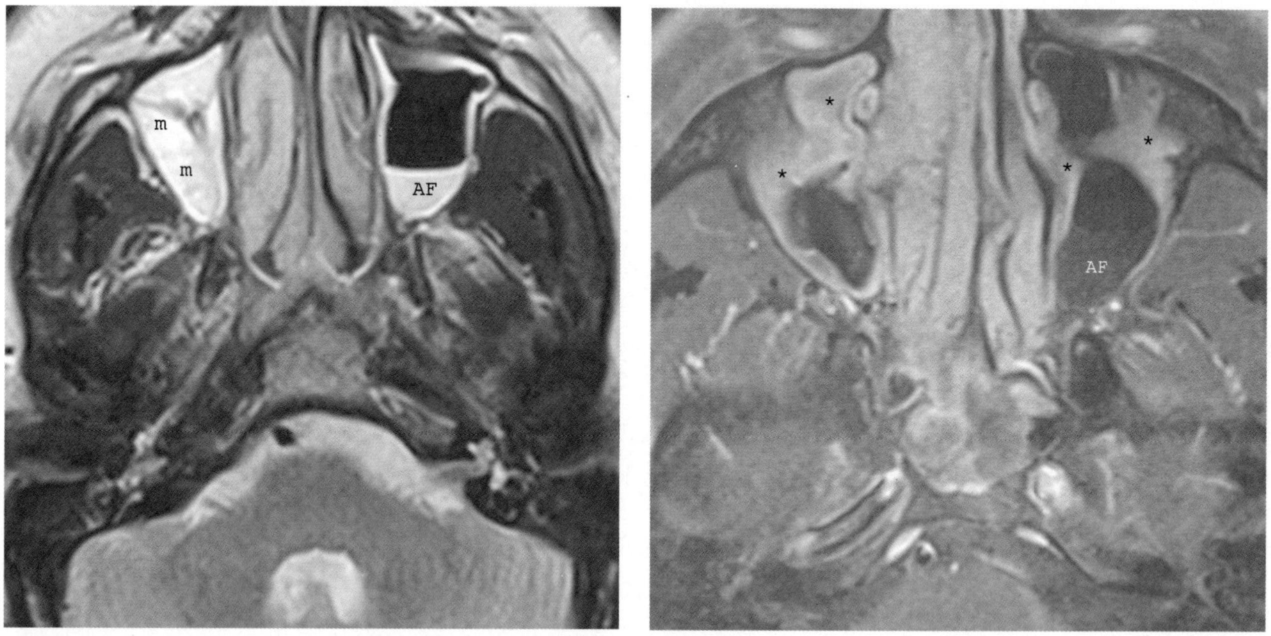

A B

Fig. 3.3 Acute sinusitis in a patient with left facial pain and nasal congestion. Axial T2-weighted **(A)** and contrast-enhanced T1-weighted **(B)** magnetic resonance images show mucosal disease in the bilateral maxillary sinuses (*) and an air-fluid level in the left maxillary sinus.

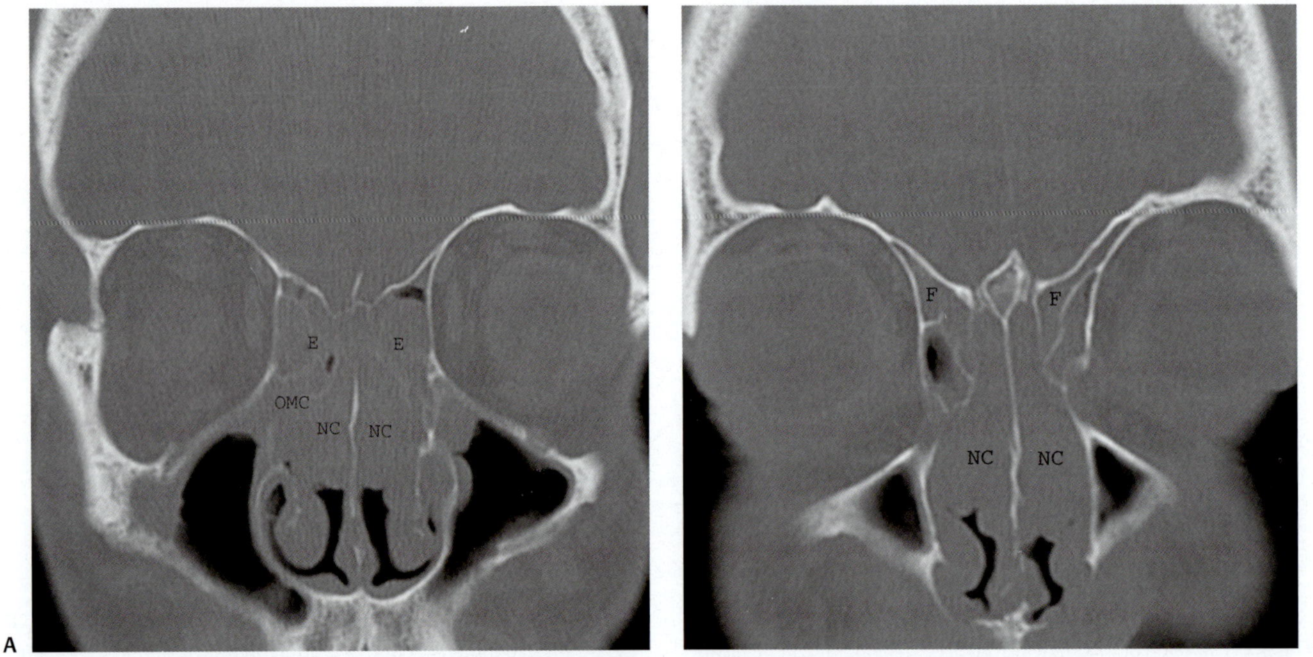

Fig. 3.4 Computed tomography imaging of chronic sinusitis prior to functional endoscopic sinonasal surgery. Coronal images, **(B)** is anterior to **(A)**, show mucosal disease in the bilateral maxillary sinuses, opacification of the ethmoid air cells (*E*), and opacification of the frontal sinuses (*F*). The ostiomeatal complexes (*OMC*) are obstructed. Opacification of the nasal cavity (*NC*) represented numerous polyps.

sphenoethmoidal recess (**Fig. 3.4A,B**).[33,34] The location of sinusitis is as important as the extent of disease in producing symptoms. An evaluation of the nasal cavity and osseous confines (medial orbital walls, cribriform plate, sphenoid sinus roof), and identification of anatomic variants is essential in the assessment of sinonasal pathology. The presence of air-fluid levels or bubbly mucoid material should be reported. Hyperdense sinus contents may reflect the presence of inspissated secretions and/or fungal elements, and is an important finding in diagnosing allergic fungal sinusitis (**Fig. 3.5A,B**). Hemorrhage usually in the setting of trauma or instrumentation is also hyperdense.

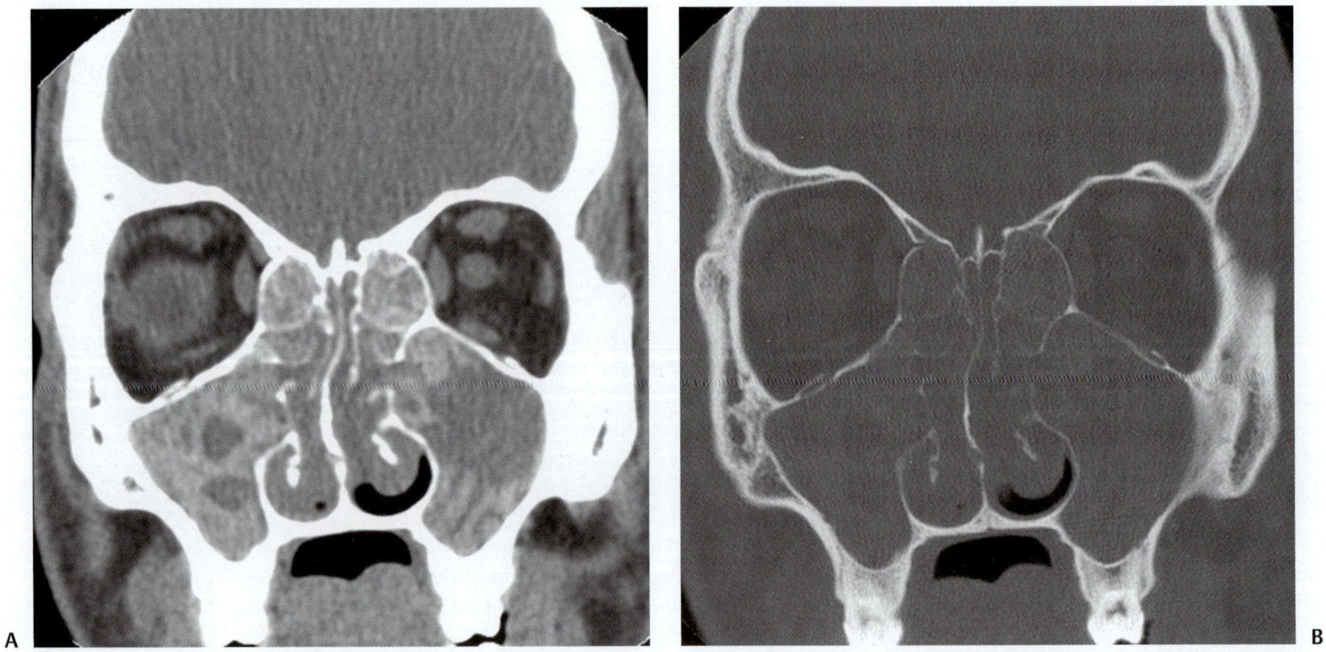

Fig. 3.5 Classic imaging appearance of allergic fungal sinusitis with polyposis. Coronal unenhanced computed tomography scan in soft tissue detail **(A)**, and a bone algorithm **(B)** shows complete opacification of the bilateral maxillary sinuses, ethmoid air cells, and nasal cavity. Note the laminated appearance of the material in the sinuses with areas of hyperdensity (representing fungal elements and proteinaceous material) alternating with low density (inflammatory tissue and mucosal disease). Tissue opacifying the bilateral nasal cavity represents inflammation and numerous small polyps. Note the preservation of the osseous confines of the sinonasal cavity.

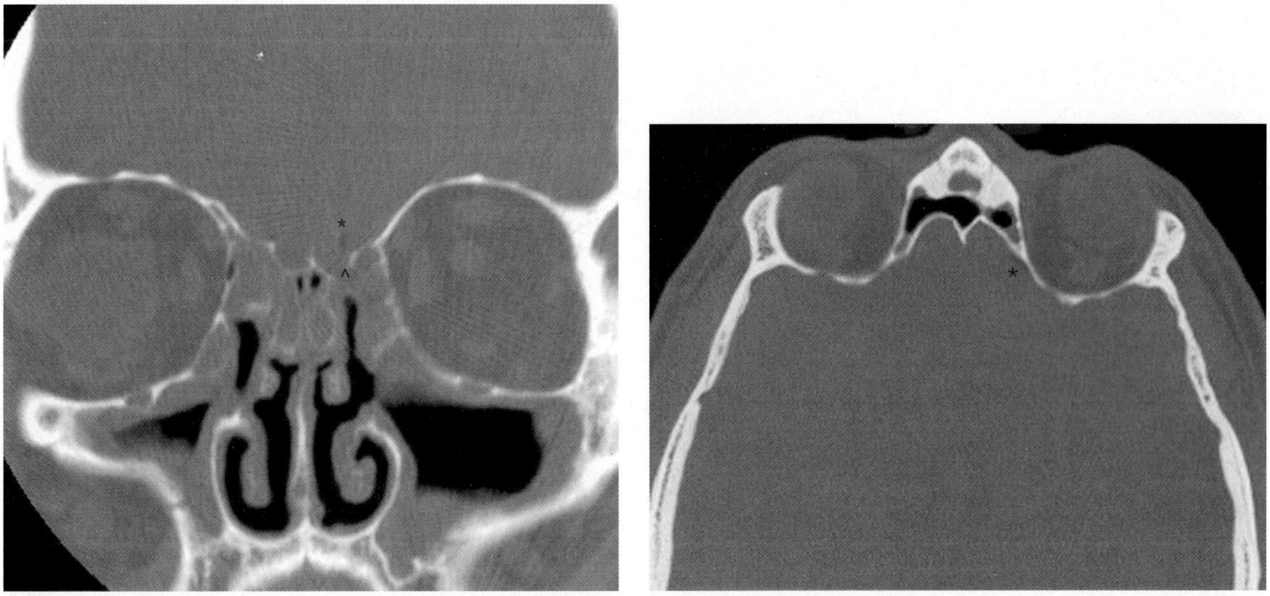

A B

Fig. 3.6 Cerebrospinal fluid leak and meningitis presenting ~10 days following functional endoscopic sinonasal surgery. Coronal **(A)** and axial **(B)** computed tomography scans show intracranial air (*) seen as hypodense or dark areas. There is a surgically created defect in the left ethmoid fovealis (^).

When evaluating patients with chronic sinusitis for potential FESS, it is important to evaluate certain anatomic landmarks on high quality, thin section unenhanced CT images. Direct coronal images may be obtained, or direct thin section axial images may be obtained and coronal reformations created from these. The medial orbital walls, the cribriform plate, and the roof and lateral walls of the sphenoid sinus should be evaluated for osseous deficiencies. An unrecognized defect in the lamina papyracea may result in orbital penetration and hematoma formation, whereas a dehiscence in the cribriform plate or sphenoid sinus could result in a cerebrospinal (CSF) leak (**Fig. 3.6A,B**), intracranial complications (meningitis, encephalocele) (**Fig. 3.7**), or carotid artery complications (perforation, acute subarachnoid hemorrhage; pseudoaneurysm formation).[35–39] The radiologist and clinician must also assess for anatomic variants or secondary changes of the drainage passageways that may impact surgery. For instance, if the uncinate process and/or middle turbinate are opposed to the orbital floor (**Fig. 3.8A,B**) and the endoscopist is unaware, vigorous removal may result in orbital penetration (**Fig. 3.9**).

Post-FESS scanning is not accurate in distinguishing inflammation, granulation, and fibrous tissue. The absence of disease on a postoperative study is reliable, but the converse is not true. False-positive studies are common. In cases of suspected complications following FESS, CT scan is the study of choice. Many of these complications are evident within 24 to 48 hours following instrumentation. CT is accurate in identifying orbital hematomas, optic nerve injury in the orbit, as well as other orbital injuries.[36,39] A CSF leak due to inadvertent injury to the cribriform plate or overly vigorous removal of the attachment of the middle turbinate to the ethmoid fovealis may be immediately evident in the operating room, or may present days to weeks after surgery with rhinorrhea or symptoms of meningitis (**Fig. 3.6A,B**).[35,40]

Complications of acute sinusitis include periorbital cellulitis and abscess formation, meningitis, thrombophlebitis (including cavernous sinus thrombosis),

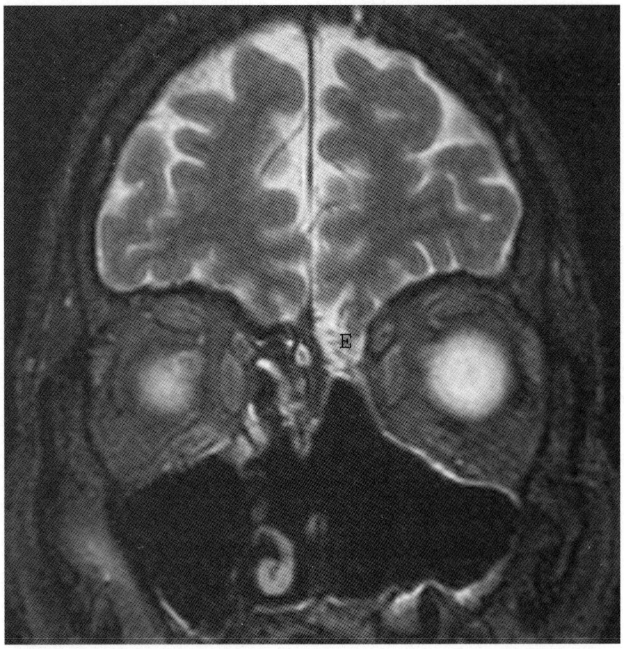

Fig. 3.7 Postfunctional endoscopic sinus surgery meningoencephalocele. Coronal T2-weighted magnetic resonance image shows findings consistent with extensive bilateral functional endoscopic sinonasal surgery. A left frontal encephalocele is noted through a left cribriform plate defect (*E*).

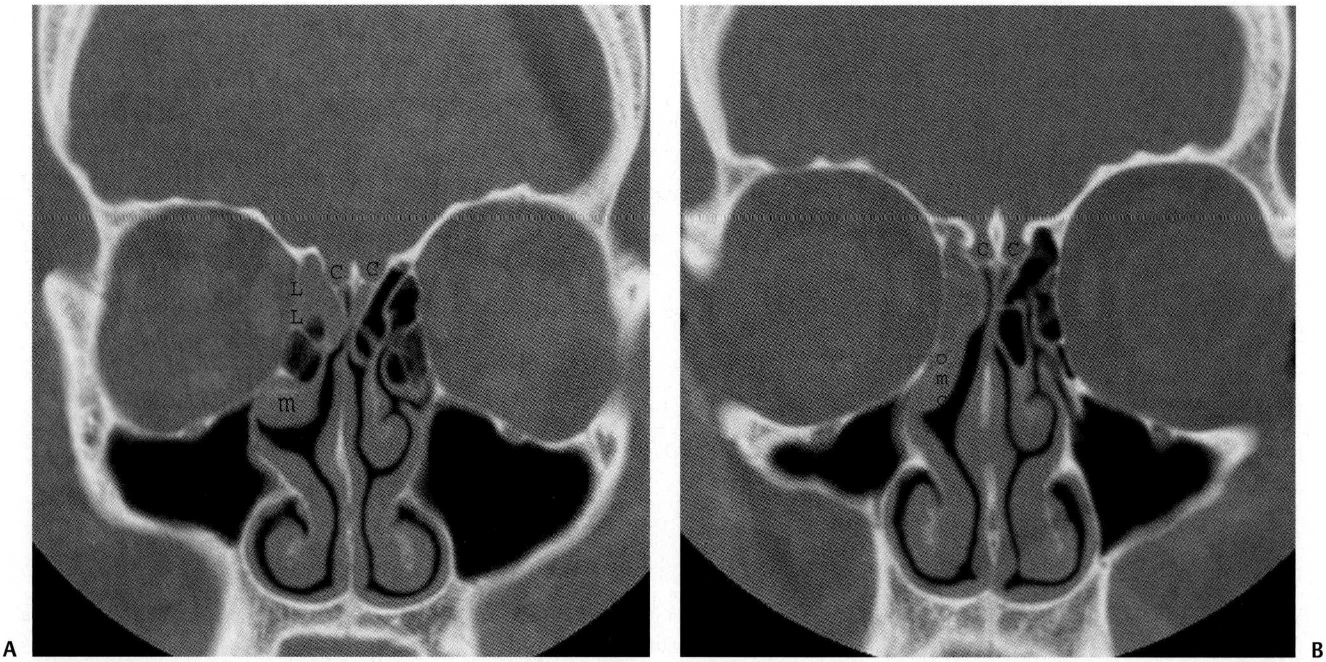

Fig. 3.8 (A,B) Atelectatic right maxillary sinus (silent sinus) identified in a patient prior to functional endoscopic sinonasal surgery for chronic sinusitis. Contiguous direct coronal computed tomography images showing the right ostiomeatal complex (uncinate process and middle turbinate) are apposed to the orbital wall. The cribriform plate (*C*) and lamina papyracea (*L*) are intact. The right ethmoid air cells are opacified.

subdural empyema, brain abscess, and perineural and perivascular spread of infection (especially in invasive fungal disease).[41–44] These acute intracranial complications are most accurately assessed with a combined brain and orbital MRI, including contrast-enhanced imaging (**Fig. 3.10A,B**). Contrast-enhanced CT is reliable in assessing orbital and periorbital infection as long as there is not concern for extension to the orbital apex or intracranial compartment (in which case MRI should be obtained).[7,14,45]

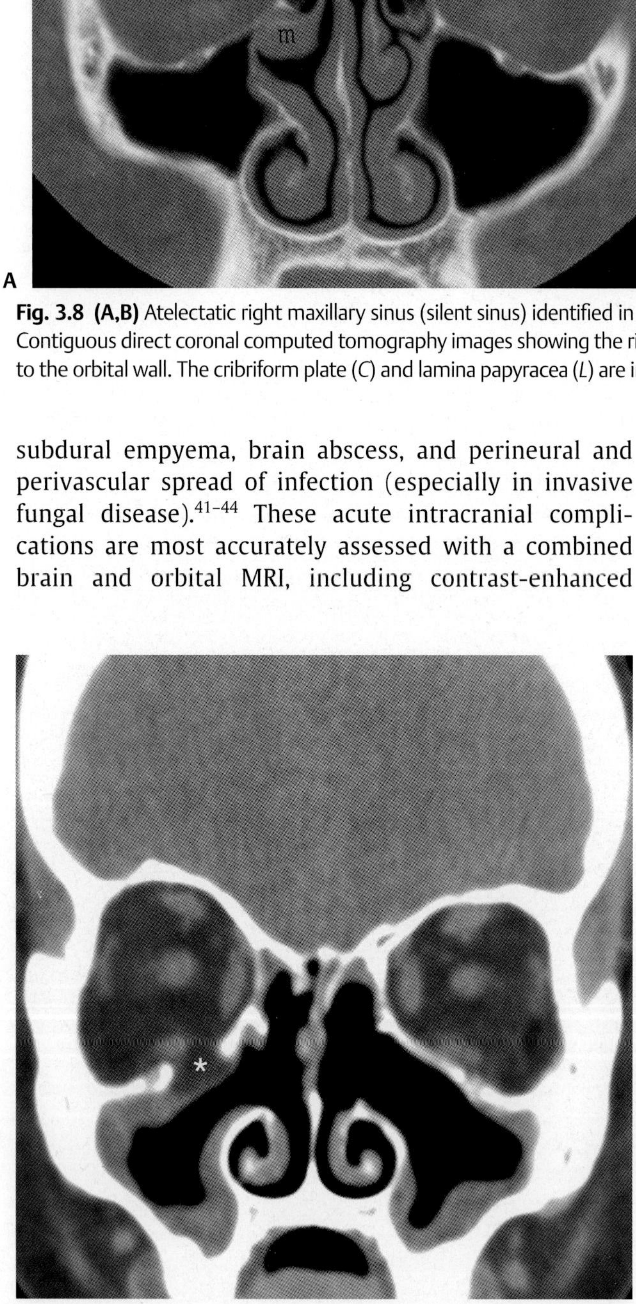

Fig. 3.9 Defect in the orbital floor following functional endoscopic sinonasal surgery. The asterisk shows a defect in the floor of the right orbit with herniation of orbital fat into the defect. The patient had intermittent diplopia.

Mucoceles may complicate chronic sinusitis, facial trauma, or sinus surgical instrumentation. Mucoceles develop from obstruction of sinus ostia or septated compartments of a sinus and represent mucoid secretions encased by mucus-secreting epithelium (sinus mucosa). In over 90% of cases, mucoceles occur in the frontal sinuses or the ethmoid air cells.[46–48] Signs and symptoms of mucoceles are related to a mass effect such as frontal swelling, headache, and orbital pain. Orbital extension may result in proptosis or diplopia.[49] A secondary infection (mucopyocele) or a direct extension into the anterior cranial fossa is not infrequent.[50–54] Advances in endoscopic sinus surgery have led to simple drainage procedures, even for some seemingly very complicated mucoceles.

In the radiologic evaluation of mucoceles, CT best shows the osseous changes of the sinus walls, which may be expanded and thinned. With large mucoceles, the adjacent bones may have frank defects (**Fig. 3.11A**). MRI may better assess the interface of a mucocele with intraorbital and intracranial structures. Enhanced MRI is useful in distinguishing a mucocele, which demonstrates peripheral enhancement, from a neoplasm, which typically demonstrates solid enhancement (**Fig. 3.11B**).[14,55] Mucoceles have a spectrum of signal characteristics on MRI depending on their protein content relative to free water.[56,57]

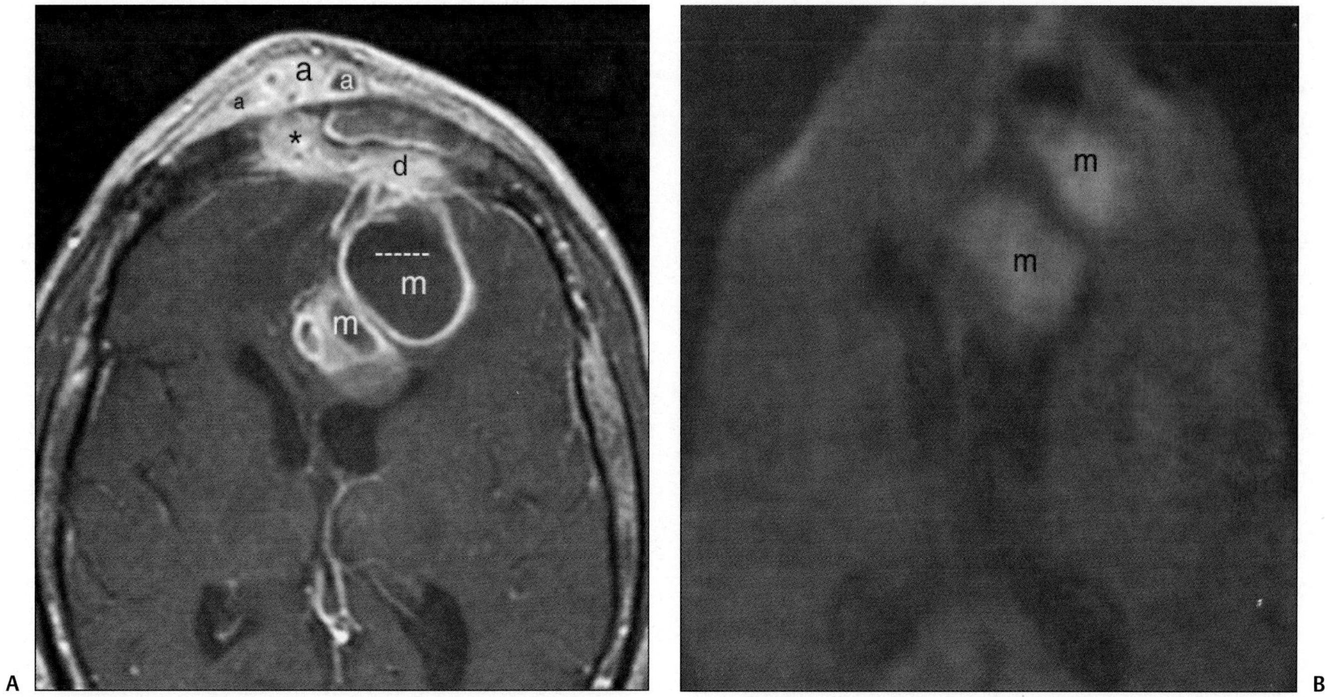

Fig. 3.10 Intracerebral abscess (Pott's puffy tumor) complicating frontal sinusitis. **(A)** Axial enhanced T1-weighted magnetic resonance image (MRI) shows a multiloculated intracerebral mass in the left frontal lobe (*m*). The mass has peripheral enhancement and a fluid-debris level (—). Note enhancement in the frontal sinus (*), dural enhancement (*d*), and an associated subperiosteal abscess overlying the frontal bone (*a*). **(B)** Axial diffusion-weighted MRI shows that the left frontal lobe intracerebral mass is high in signal intensity (*bright*; *m*), consistent with an infection/abscess.

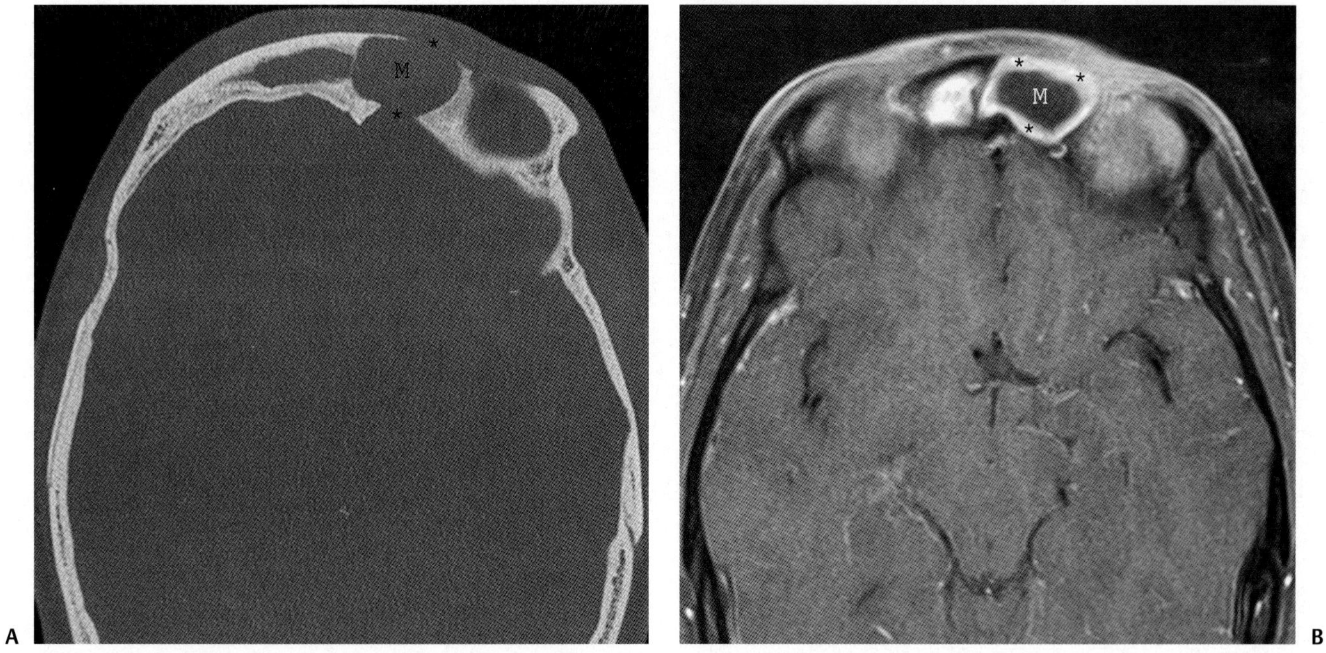

Fig. 3.11 Mucopyocele of the left frontal sinus. **(A)** Axial unenhanced computed tomography image in a bone algorithm shows an expansile lesion of the left frontal sinus (*M*), with remodeling and thinning of the anterior and posterior cortical tables (*). **(B)** Axial contrast-enhanced fat-suppressed T1-weighted MR image shows the mucopyocele (*M*) with no central solid enhancement. Thick circumferential mucosal enhancement is noted (*).

Developmental Lesions

Meningo(encephalo)cele refers to herniation of the meninges, CSF, and/or brain through an osseous defect in the cranium. Meningoencephaloceles are more common than meningoceles. Congenital encephaloceles are due to an abnormality in the process of invagination of the neural plate.[58,59] During embryogenesis, the dura around the brain contacts the dermis in the facial/nasion region as the neural plate regresses. Failure of dermal regression may lead to an encephalocele, dermoid cyst, sinus tract, or nasal glioma. "Nasal glioma" is a misnomer, as it is not a true neoplasm. With nasal gliomas, there is a fibrous connection with the intracranial compartment. Dermoid sinus tracts may have an intracranial connection in up to 25% of cases, and may be complicated by infection (osteomyelitis, meningitis, and abscess). Nasofrontal and sphenoethmoidal encephaloceles are frequently clinically occult, and the differential diagnosis is broad when seen through the endoscope. Anterior basal encephaloceles have an association with other developmental anomalies (**Fig. 3.12**), including migrational abnormalities, agenesis of the corpus callosum, and cleft lip and palate.[60–63]

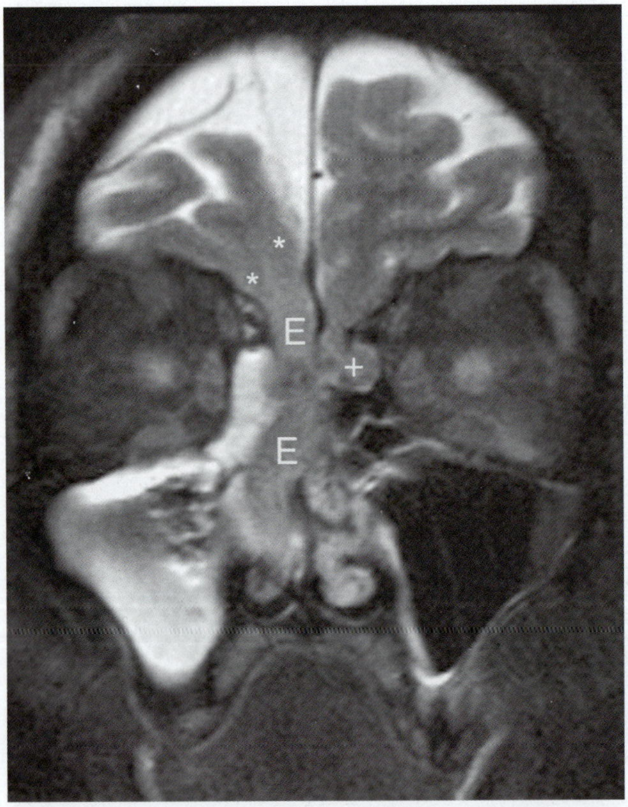

Fig. 3.12 Large congenital basal encephalocele associated with bilateral frontal lobe cortical dysplasia. Coronal T2-weighted magnetic resonance image shows tissue similar in signal characteristics to the brain and contiguous with the brain extending into the right sinonasal cavity through a defect in the cribriform plate consistent with an encephalocele (*E*). Notice the small left encephalocele (+). There is cortical thickening (*) consistent with dysplasia.

In the setting of trauma or surgery, most acquired meningoencephaloceles involve the sinonasal cavity or the temporal bone. Patients may present with rhinorrhea.

A combination of imaging modalities, including nuclear scintigraphy, CT, and/or MRI, can be used to assess CSF leaks and meningoencephaloceles. It is important to determine whether the CSF leak is due to a dural laceration or a meningo(encephalo)cele. Following the placement of pledgets in the nasal cavity, intrathecal instillation of indium-diethylene triamine pentaacetic acid (DTPA) may be used to confirm the CSF leak. Once a leak is established, coronal CT may be performed for anatomic localization. In the hands of skilled otolaryngologists and radiologists, iodinated contrast CT cisternography is rarely necessary. If an encephalocele is suspected, multiplanar MRI easily establishes the diagnosis by showing direct continuity of the tissue in the sinonasal cavity with the intracranial brain (**Fig. 3.7**). Although imaging may be useful in detecting CSF leaks, fluorescein injected intrathecally followed by an endoscopic evaluation may allow for direct visualization of an active leak.

Sinonasal Neoplasms

Evaluation and staging of sinus neoplasms is achieved through a combination of clinical assessment and pretreatment imaging with close scrutiny of the sinonasal cavity, orbits, nasopharynx, oral cavity, cranial nerves, and the intracranial compartment. Imaging is especially important in assessing the skull base and the intracranial compartment, and in distinguishing the tumor from coexistent inflammatory changes. CT and MRI play complementary roles in evaluating sinonasal neoplasms.[2,7,16,24–26,64–73] Both are usually obtained in the evaluation of patients with sinonasal masses. CT is more sensitive and accurate in assessing the osseous margins of the sinonasal cavity, the osseous floor of the anterior cranial fossa, as well as the walls of the orbit.[7,15,18,25,69,74–76] MRI offers improved soft tissue resolution, contrast, and multiplanar capabilities allowing better evaluation of disease extension outside the sinonasal cavity. An extension of the neoplasm outside of the sinonasal cavity into the adjacent anatomic locations significantly impacts upon the patient's operability, the type of resection that will occur, the surgical approach, the necessity for radiation therapy, the placement of radiation portals, and the prognosis.

Benign neoplasms, when large enough, expand the paranasal sinus that they affect and secondarily remodel the adjacent bone. Osseous destruction from benign lesions is less common than with malignancies. However, it is not unusual for contained malignant tumors to have benign imaging features and, conversely, benign tumors to have an aggressive appearance. Papillomas arise from

A

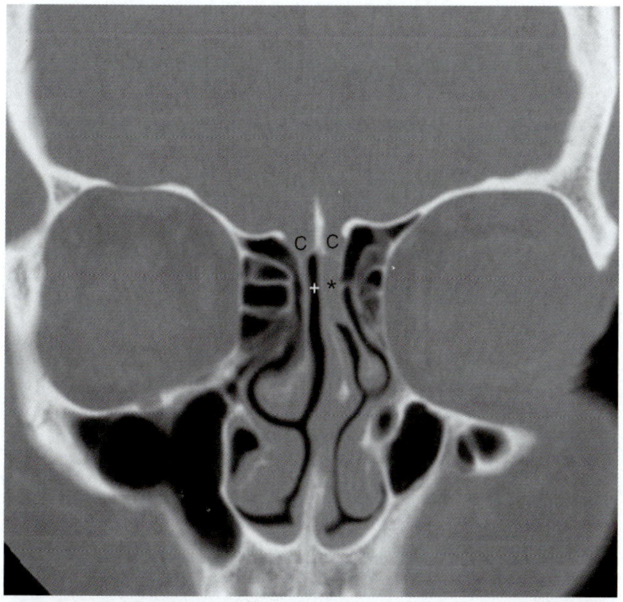

B

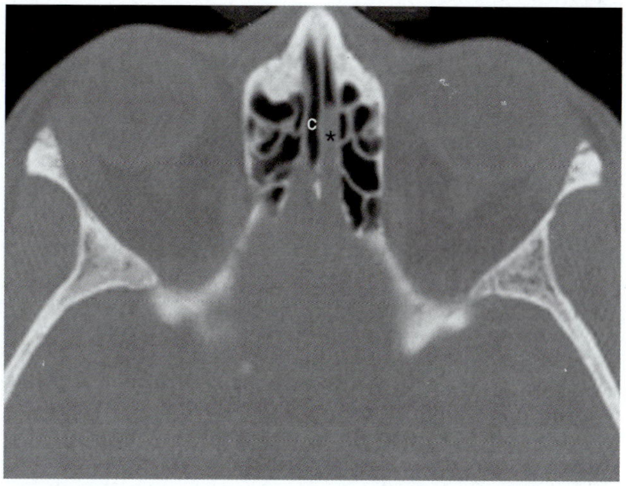

C

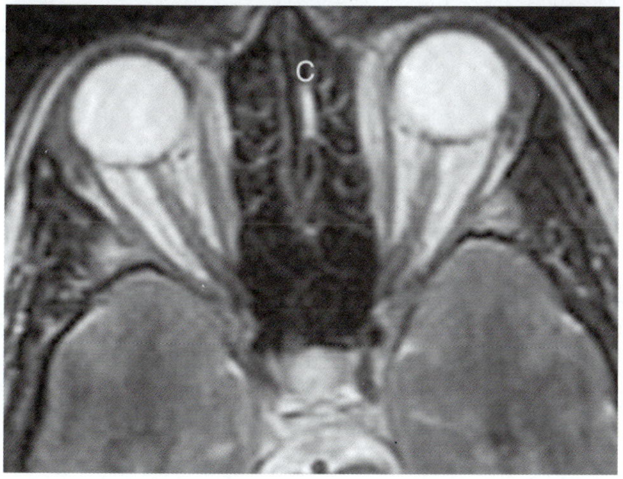

Fig. 3.13 Unilateral opacification of the left olfactory strut representing a cerebrospinal fluid leak. Coronal **(A)** and axial **(B)** computed tomography images show opacification of the left olfactory strut (*). Axial T2-weighted magnetic resonance image **(C)** shows that the material in the left olfactory strut (*) is similar to cerebrospinal fluid (like the vitreous in the orbital globes). *C*, cribriform plate; +, clear olfactory strut.

the columnar epithelium and include inverted, cylindric, and fungiform subtypes. Typically, papillomas occur unilaterally in the sinonasal cavity.[77,78] Inverted papillomas are most common and are benign; however, squamous cell carcinoma may be present in 5 to 15% of cases.[77,78] Papillomas typically arise from the lateral nasal wall at the level of the middle turbinate or, less commonly, within the maxillary sinus. Although a convoluted cerebriform pattern is thought to be associated with an inverted papilloma, it may be seen with other malignancies.[79] Location is usually a tip-off to the diagnosis.[80,81] A focal ostetis on CT imaging may indicate the site of attachment of an inverted papilloma. Inverted papillomas may show a rather aggressive appearance with bony destruction, and occasionally they may erode the skull base (as may benign polyps), simulating a malignant tumor.[82]

Unilateral opacification of the olfactory strut in the absence of other findings in the paranasal sinuses usually represents a CSF leak, a meningoencephalocele, or a neoplasm such as an esthesioneuroblastoma (**Fig. 3.13A–C**). Caution is always required when evaluating masses within the paranasal sinuses. Fibro-osseous lesions such as osteomas, fibrous dysplasia, ossifying or nonossifying fibromas, and chondroid lesions may mimic a malignant mass on MRI. However, these lesions usually have characteristic radiologic appearances on CT imaging (**Figs. 3.14A,B and 3.15A–C**).

Malignant Neoplasms

Carcinomas of the sinonasal cavity constitute 3 to 4% of all head and neck neoplasms.[2,65,83,84] In general, they have a relatively poor prognosis because many present at advanced stages. Squamous cell cancer accounts for ~80% of sinonasal carcinomas. Approximately 25 to 60% of squamous carcinomas involve the maxillary antrum; however, the maxillary sinus is secondarily involved by direct extension in 80% of patients. Approximately 30%

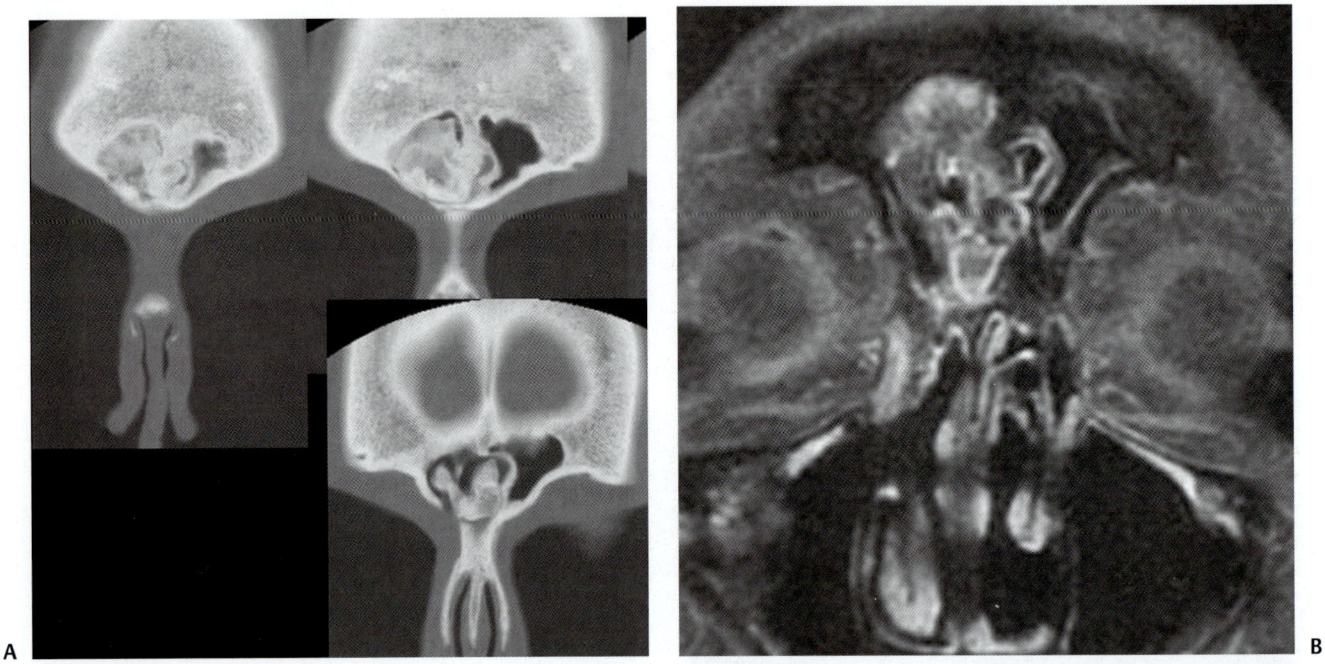

Fig. 3.14 Frontal sinus osteoma. **(A)** Contiguous computed tomography (CT) scans in bone algorithm show the typical appearance of an intrasinus osteoma in the right frontal sinus. There is a mild expansion of the sinus, and a mild extension across the midline septum into the medial left frontal sinus. **(B)** Coronal enhanced T1-weighted magnetic resonance image looks like mucosal disease in the frontal sinuses. This case illustrates the significance of CT imaging in identifying and diagnosing fibro-osseous lesions of the sinonasal cavity.

of squamous carcinomas arise in the nasal cavity, and 10% in the ethmoid air cells. Occupation exposures include nickel, chromium pigment, Bantu snuff, Thorotrast, mustard gas, polycyclic hydrocarbons, cigarettes, and isopropyl alcohol.[2,85] Approximately 10% of sinonasal tumors arise from minor salivary glands.[2,65,83,86] There is a spectrum of histologic types, including adenoid cystic, mucoepidermoid, undifferentiated, and adenocarcinoma. Adenoid cystic carcinomas are most common, accounting for one-third of minor salivary gland neoplasms.[87] Adenocarcinomas may represent minor salivary gland tumors or intestinal-type adenocarcinomas, and have a predilection for the ethmoid air cells.[88–90] These may be more common in wood and leather workers.[38] They are frequently advanced at presentation, with cribriform plate erosion present in up to 50% of cases. Dural invasion is not uncommon.[90]

Delayed presentation is typical of sinonasal malignancies as there is a relative paucity of pain associated with these neoplasms. Because there is frequently coexistent inflammatory disease in the paranasal sinuses that may elicit mild pain, a tumor may initially be overlooked as the patient is treated for presumed infection. Although pain in the early stages of sinonasal malignancies is uncommon, the presence of pain is usually an indication of advanced disease. Pain may indicate perineural tumor spread, skull base extension, or spread to the infratemporal fossa. Other clinical presentations include nasal congestion and epistaxis.

The treatment of choice for sinonasal carcinomas usually includes combined surgery and irradiation.[91–96] Orbital exenteration is often necessary when a tumor involves the orbital contents, usually confirmed during intraoperative assessment.[97,98] In the setting of extension into the central skull base, curative surgery is usually not attempted. The main cause of treatment failure is local recurrence.[83,99]

Findings on CT scans that should raise one's index of suspicion for something other than inflammatory disease include unilateral nasal mass/tissue, unilateral opacification of the olfactory strut, bone destruction, and extension of disease outside the sinonasal cavity. In these cases, MRI often provides important additional information and should be obtained. In suspected sinonasal malignancies, CT and MRI should be completed when possible prior to surgical intervention, including biopsy.[64,100] Advances in pretherapeutic imaging have contributed significantly to the management of sinonasal tumors. Imaging may provide important information regarding the origin of the neoplasm, the extent of the neoplasm, as well as the presence of tumor vascularity. Preoperative imaging may allow optimal localization for tissue biopsy, and may be extremely useful in preparing the surgical approach and minimizing complications.

MRI plays a critical role in distinguishing sinus opacification related to a tumor from that related to inspissated secretions.[7,14,15] Most neoplasms have a more solid enhancement pattern[101,102] following intravenous contrast administration, compared with peripheral enhancement

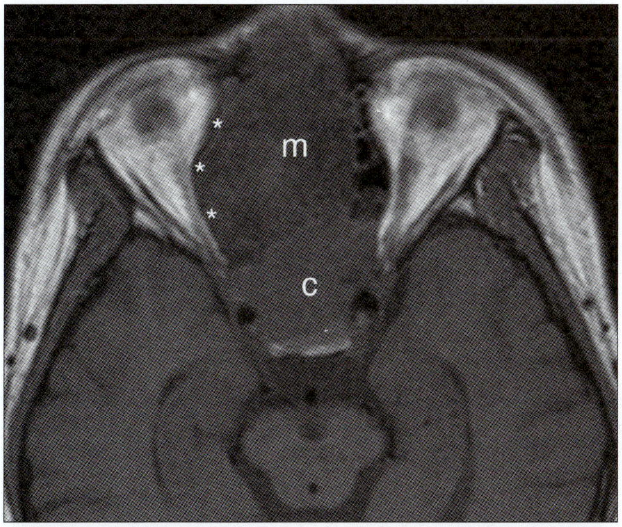

A

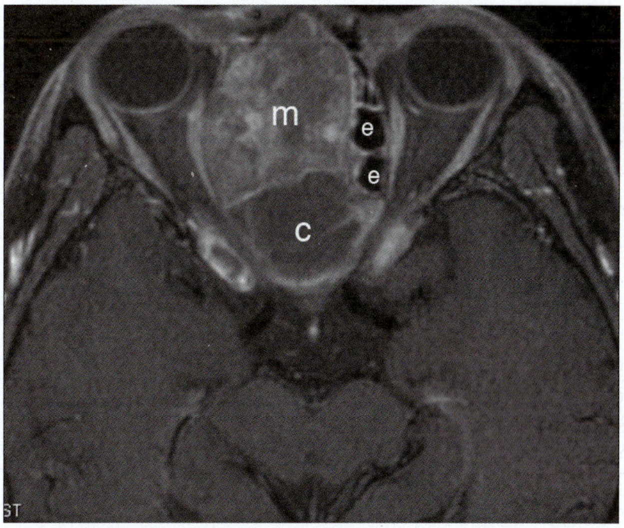

B

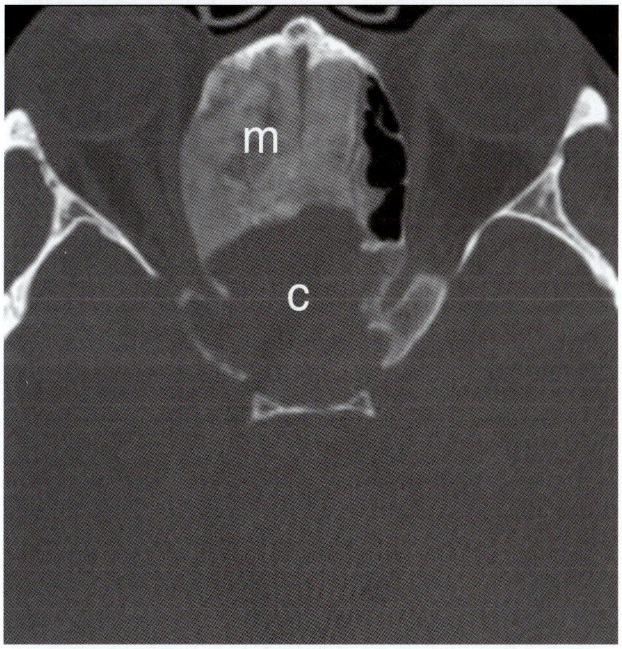

C

Fig. 3.15 Fibrous dysplasia involving the paranasal sinuses. **(A)** Axial unenhanced T1-weighted magnetic resonance image (MRI) shows a demarcated, expansile mass (*m*) at the ventral skull base involving the right greater than the left ethmoid air cells, the sphenoid sinus, and the planum sphenoidale. The portion involving the sphenoid sinus and planum sphenoidale is more cystic in appearance (*c*). Note the smooth, lateral bowing of the right lamina papyracea (*). **(B)** Axial contrast-enhanced T1-weighted MRI shows no solid enhancement of the cystic component (*c*), but avid enhancement of the more fibroosseous component (*m*). On the left, pneumatized ethmoid air cells (*e*) are present. **(C)** Axial computed tomography scan in bone detail shows the characteristic ground glass appearance of fibrous dysplasia (m). The cystic component posteriorly is lucent in appearance (*C*). It is not uncommon to have cystic components in fibrous dysplasia involving the skull base.

seen in benign inflammatory conditions. However, benign masses, such as polyps, may also demonstrate peripheral enhancement. In addition, T2-weighted imaging may be helpful as most histologic types of sinonasal tumors are highly cellular, resulting in intermediate-to-low signal intensity of these tumors on T2-weighted images (similar to the brainstem) compared with inflammatory secretions that tend to be hyperintense (bright).

Patterns of Tumor Spread

Sinonasal malignancies frequently spread by direct (**Fig. 3.16**) or perineural (**Fig. 3.17A,B**) extension outside the sinonasal cavity.[64,69,70] This significantly impacts upon prognosis, operability, the type of resection, and the necessity for chemo-irradiation.[103] Therefore, an understanding of the anatomic boundaries of the individual paranasal sinuses and their contiguous structures is important in mapping tumor extent and in planning the extent of surgery.

The superior and posterior boundaries of the maxillary sinuses are important prognostically, as well as in designing the surgical management.[98,104] The maxillary sinuses are bounded superiorly by the orbit and ethmoid air cells, and posteriorly by the pterygoid plates and the pterygopalatine fossa. Direct extension into the orbit or spread to the intracranial compartment via the ethmoid air cells makes obtaining tumor-free surgical margins more difficult. Extension posteriorly by direct extension or perineural spread may result in neoplastic invasion of the masticator space, the orbit, and/or the intracranial compartment. The medial and inferior margins, the nasal cavity, and the alveolus, respectively, are more readily resected en bloc and are less problematic.

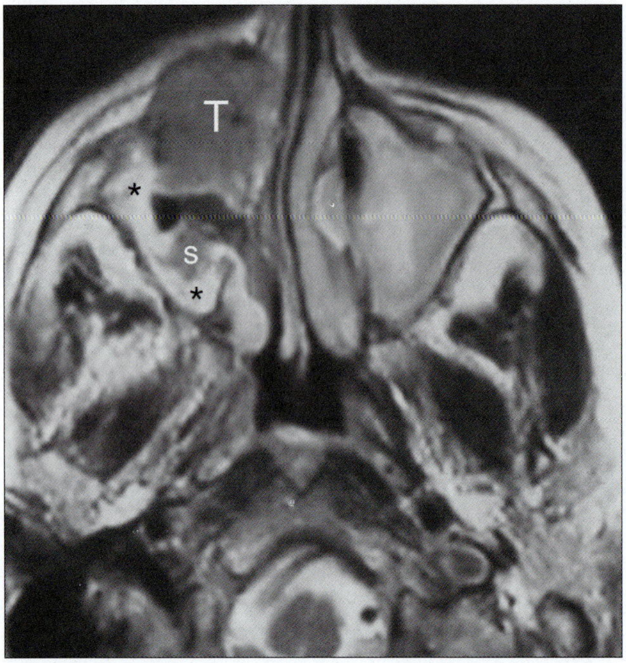

Fig. 3.16 Squamous cell carcinoma of the maxillary sinus with direct extension outside the sinus. Axial T2-weighted magnetic resonance image shows a tumor isointense to the brain (*T*) with extension outside the ventral wall of the sinus into the premaxillary soft tissues. There is mucosal disease (*) and inspissated secretions (*s*). The left maxillary sinus is opacified with inspissated secretions.

Important landmarks of the ethmoid air cells include the fovea ethmoidalis and the cribriform plate superiorly, which provide only a moderately resilient barrier to intracranial spread.[98] Intracranial spread may necessitate an open or endoscopic craniofacial resection.[91] The lateral wall of the ethmoid air cells (lamina papyracea), when violated, may result in intraorbital spread that may require an orbital exenteration.[105–110] Although rare, cancer arising in the sphenoid sinus is difficult to resect because of its central location in the skull base where it is surrounded by numerous vital structures. The sphenoid sinus is bounded superiorly by the pituitary sella and visual tracts, laterally by the carotid arteries and cavernous sinuses, anteriorly by the posterior ethmoid air cells, and inferiorly by the vidian canal and the nasopharynx.

Image Analysis of Sinonasal Neoplasms

It is often difficult for the radiologist to hone down on a particular histologic diagnosis because of the marked overlap of the imaging appearance of different tumors on CT and MRI.[111] The major contribution by the radiologist is an accurate mapping of the tumor extent in the context of an understanding of the anatomic sites that will influence or alter surgical resection, treatment planning, and prognosis. In the setting of sinonasal malignancies, a combination of CT and MRI is usually acquired.[69,70,73,74,112] Potential areas of tumor extension that must be assessed in all patients with sinonasal malignancies include intracranial spread

A

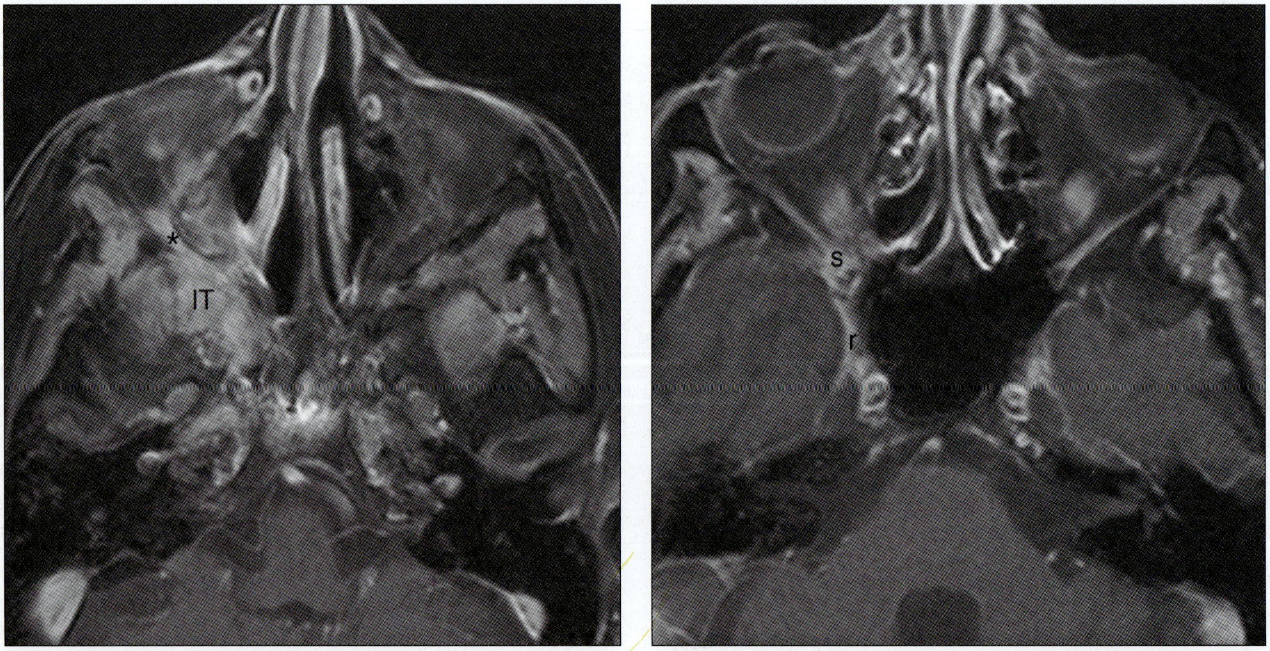

B

Fig. 3.17 Recurrent perineural spread of adenoid cystic carcinoma status post-partial maxillectomy and radiation therapy. **(A)** Axial contrast-enhanced T1-weighted magnetic resonance image (MRI) with fat-suppression shows enhancing tissue in the right inferior orbital fissure (*), and the infratemporal fossa (*IT*). **(B)** Axial contrast-enhanced T1-weighted MRI shows an enhancing perineural spread of the tumor in the foramen rotundum (*r*) and the superior orbital fissure (*s*). The perineural spread of a tumor biopsy is proven.

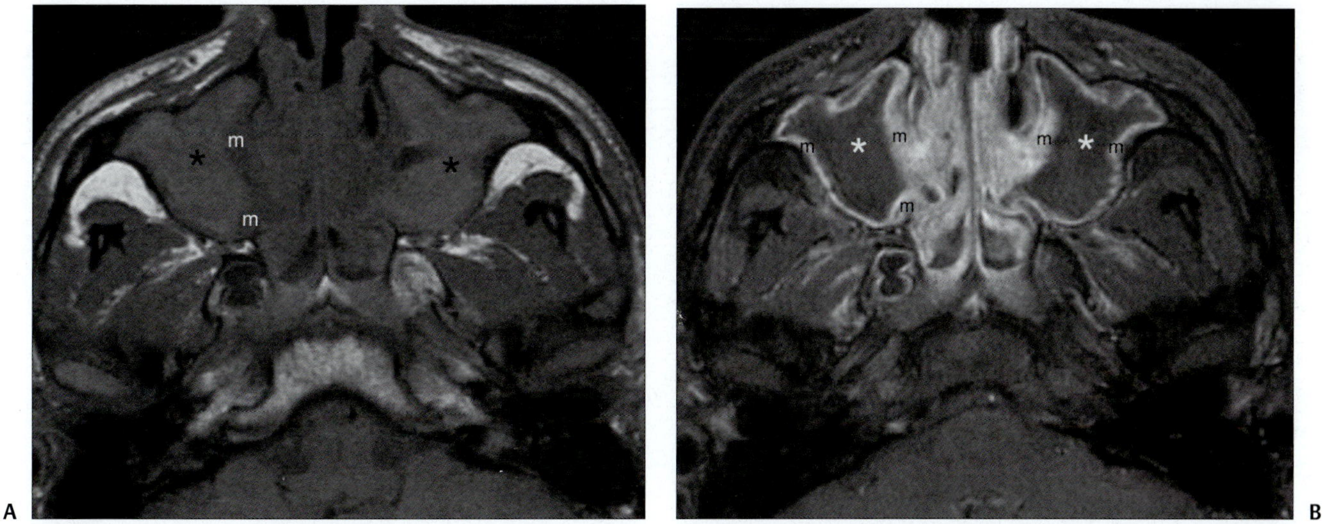

Fig. 3.18 Proteinaceous secretions in the paranasal sinuses on magnetic resonance imaging (MRI). **(A)** Axial T1-weighted MRI shows complete opacification of the bilateral maxillary sinuses with central material that is hyperintense (*bright*) relative to water consistent with proteinaceous material (*). Surrounding mucosal disease is low signal intensity (*m*). **(B)** Corresponding axial contrast-enhanced fat-suppressed T1-weighted MRI shows peripheral enhancement of the mucosa (*m*), with low signal intensity (*dark*) central inspissated secretions without central enhancement (*).

(the anterior and middle cranial fossa), the palate, the orbits, the pterygopalatine fossa, and the skull base.[22–24,111,113]

Histologic specificity is not possible with MRI or CT techniques except perhaps in some cases of melanoma. In the majority of melanomas that contain melanin, the neoplasms may be hyperintense to gray matter on unenhanced T1-weighted images, with more variable signal characteristics on a corresponding T2-weighted MRI.[114–119]

Differentiating Secretions and Inflammatory Changes from a Tumor

One of the advantages of MRI over CT is its ability to help discern complex sinonasal secretions and inflammatory disease from a tumor (**Fig. 3.2A,B**).[7,73,76,102,120–124] Secretions and mucosal disease frequently have a high water content yielding high signal intensity on T2-weighted images with peripheral enhancement (**Fig. 3.3A,B**).

A combination of T1- and T2-weighted images is extremely useful in distinguishing secretions and mucosal inflammation from neoplasm.[122] Both pulse sequences are important due to the marked variability in the signal intensity of sinonasal secretions, which is the result of variable protein concentrations, the presence and extent of mobile water protons, and viscosity. The changes in signal intensity associated with increasing protein concentrations are likely due to extensive cross-linking of the glycoproteins present within hyperproteinaceous secretions. As a result, the relative amount of mobile water protons decreases. In the presence of low protein concentrations (less than 10%) and high free water content, secretions in the paranasal sinuses are typically hypointense on T1-weighted images and hyperintense on T2-weighted images.[57] As the protein concentration increases, secretions on T1-weighted images become more hyperintense. When concentrations approach 20 to 25%, secretions typically are hyperintense on both T1-weighted and T2-weighted sequences. When protein concentrations exceed 25%, they are hyperintense on T1-weighted and hypointense on T2-weighted images (**Fig. 3.18A,B**). Finally, when protein concentrations are extremely high (exceeding 28%) such as is seen in aggressive fungal infections, they are hypointense on both T1- and T2-weighted sequences and can mimic an "aerated sinus" (**Fig. 3.19A,B**).

Bone Destruction

The hallmark of malignancies involving the sinonasal cavity is the presence of osseous destruction most commonly seen with carcinomas (**Fig. 3.20**).[111] Bone involvement is seen in ~80% of CT scans assessing sinonasal squamous cell carcinomas. Esthesioneuroblastomas occur in the upper nasal cavity/ethmoid vault, arising from the olfactory nerves. They have a marked propensity for eroding the cribriform plate and extending intracranially.[121,125] Although less common, bone destruction may also be seen with lymphomas (**Fig. 3.21A**), metastases, and sarcomas. Sclerosis secondary to a tumor is rare. The presence of such is normally related to coexistent chronic inflammatory changes. Although uncommon, osteomyelitis may occur and is usually associated with rarefaction and sclerosis of bone. Calcification of sinonasal tumors is uncommon. Although prior literature has suggested that the presence of calcification with certain tumors is typical, it is more likely that in many cases that the findings interpreted as calcifications actually corresponded to fragmented bone.[126]

A

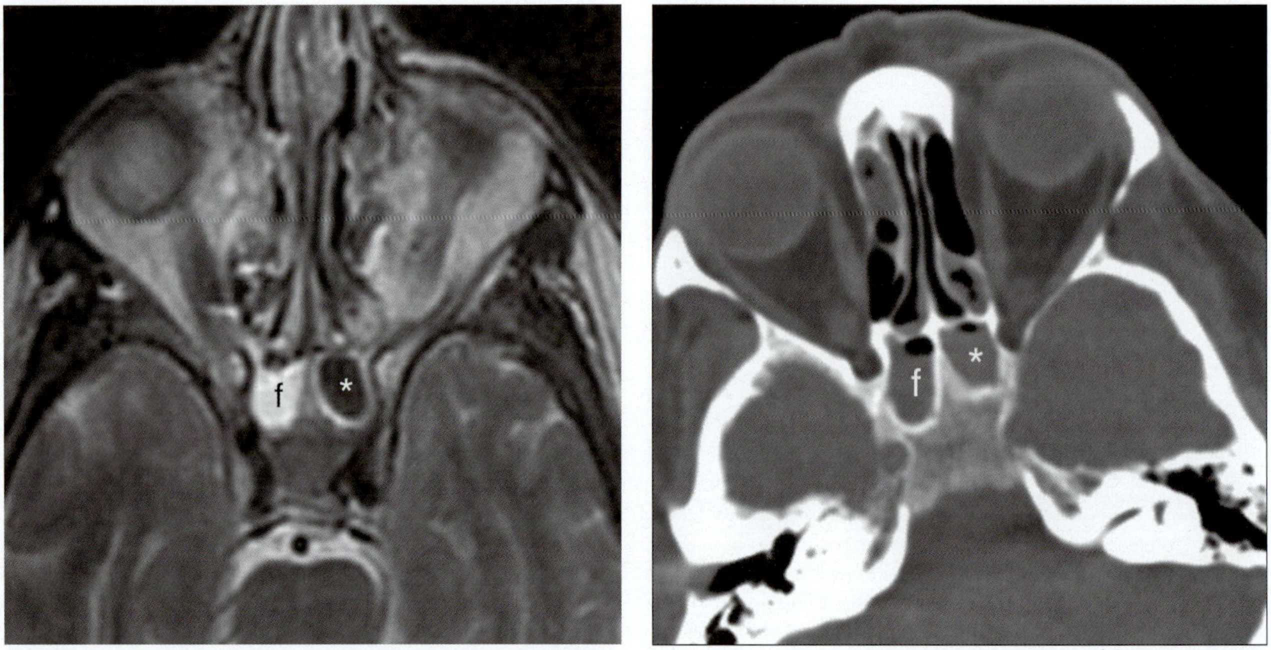

B

Fig. 3.19 Actinomycosis fungal infection in a lung transplant recipient mimicking "aerated sinus" on magnetic resonance imaging (MRI). **(A)** Axial T2-weighted MRI shows hyperintense (*bright*) fluid in the right sphenoid sinus (*f*). Low signal intensity in the left sphenoid sinus (*) appears to represent an aerated sinus. **(B)** Axial unenhanced computed tomography (CT) scan performed the same day as the MRI shows the fluid in the right sphenoid sinus (*f*), but also shows opacification of the left sphenoid sinus (*). A highly proteinaceous material such as fungus may appear markedly hypointense on T2-weighted imaging and may mimic an aerated sinus, as in this case. This case emphasizes the importance of obtaining a CT scan in all patients in whom invasive fungal infection is a diagnostic consideration.

Skull Base Invasion

Sinonasal masses that frequently erode the skull base and spread intracranially include carcinomas (squamous cell, poorly, or undifferentiated), esthesioneuroblastoma, lymphoma, and sarcomas.[74] Benign lesions that may erode the skull base include inverted papillomas, polyps, and mucoceles. The pattern of osseous destruction for benign and malignant lesions is similar at the central skull base.

Although CT may detect cortical erosion of the skull base (**Fig. 3.20**),[25,69] MRI is probably more sensitive in assessing skull base invasion.[127] It is particularly well suited to study bone marrow because it can differentiate fat from other tissues. The signal intensity is directly related to the relative amounts of fat, water, and cells in the marrow. In adults, marrow in the normal skull base and cranium is hyperintense on unenhanced T1-weighted images because it predominantly contains fat.[128–130] Skull base involvement by a tumor may be detected when the normal hyperintense appearance due to fat is replaced with hypointense tissue.[131] However, the presence of hypointense tissue does not always mean the presence of a tumor. It may also correspond to an edema or hematopoietic marrow.[128,132,133] In the presence of an abnormal hypointense T1 signal, it is important to assess the corresponding T2-weighted and enhanced images, which may help in differentiating a tumor from nonmalignant changes.

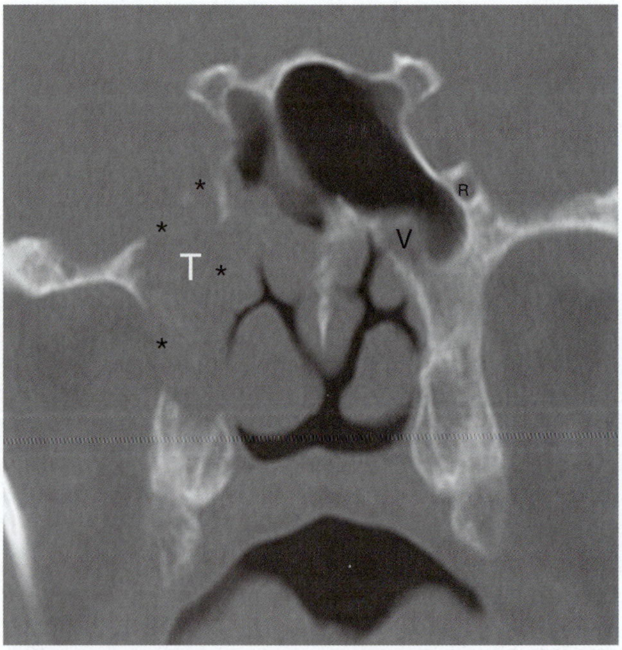

Fig. 3.20 Spindle cell carcinoma of the sphenoid sinus and skull base. There is a tumor replacing the floor and lateral recess of the right sphenoid sinus (*T*). Note the extensive bone destruction (*) consistent with an aggressive lesion. There is involvement of the right vidian canal and foramen rotundum. *R*, normal left foramen rotundum; *V*, normal left vidian canal.

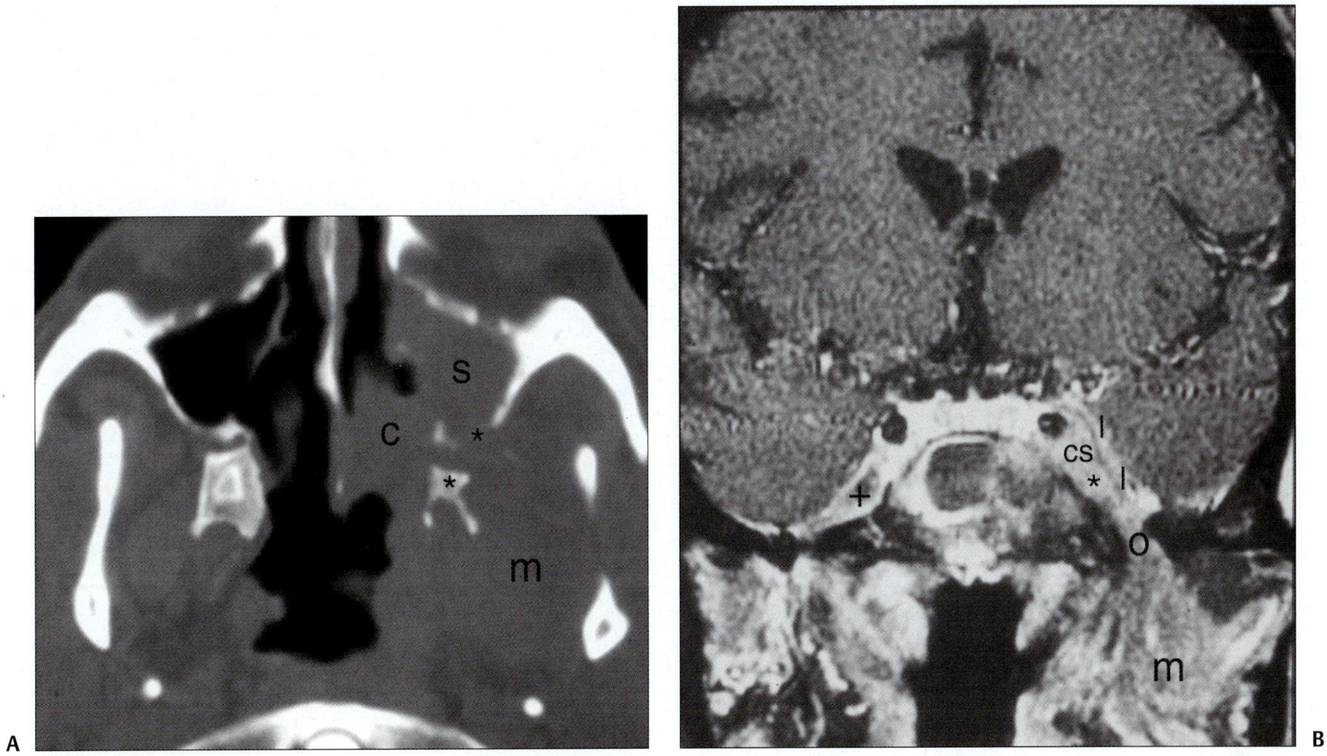

Fig. 3.21 Posttransplantation lymphoproliferative disorder in a transplant recipient with rapidly progressive facial pain and numbness. **(A)** Axial unenhanced computed tomography image in bone detail shows opacification of the left maxillary sinus (*s*) and nasal choana (*c*), with an extension of the disease outside of the sinonasal cavity into the deep left masticator space (*m*). Note the destruction of bone (*). **(B)** Coronal contrast-enhanced T1-weighted magnetic resonance image shows a tumor in the left deep masticator space (*m*), with extension through foramen ovale (*o*) into the intracranial compartment. A tumor is seen in the left Meckel's cave (*) and cavernous sinus (*cs*). +, normal right Meckel's cave; the hypointense line lateral to the left cavernous sinus (*l*), lateral dural margin. This patient had B cell lymphoma.

Perineural Spread

An especially important anatomic location for the detection of tumor spread is the pterygopalatine fossa (PPF).[64,134,135] When sinonasal tumors spread to the PPF, extension into the adjacent orbit, infratemporal fossa, skull base, and intracranial compartment may subsequently occur.[24,64,111] Specifically, a tumor may spread from the PPF to the pterygomaxillary fissure allowing for subsequent extension into the infratemporal fossa. From the PPF, a tumor may extend to the inferior orbital fissure and the orbital apex, or from the PPF to the foramen rotundum. In addition, the foramen ovale may serve as a conduit of spread from the masticator space to the intracranial compartment. In such cases, patients may present with a fifth cranial neuropathy (**Fig. 3.21B**). From the foramen rotundum, perineural spread of a tumor to the inferior orbital fissure, the orbital apex, the superior orbital fissure, and subsequently the intracranial compartment/cavernous sinus may occur (**Fig. 3.17A,B**).

Orbital Invasion

Tumor involvement of the orbit and nasolacrimal system impacts negatively upon prognosis and alters surgical planning.[98] The orbit is a cone-shaped space contained within the frontal bone, the greater and lesser wings of the sphenoid bone, the ethmoid bone, the lacrimal bone, the zygoma, and the maxilla.[136] The periorbita is comprised of the periosteum of these bones. It is continuous with the dura mater at the superior orbital fissure and the optic foramen.[136] Erosion of sinonasal malignancies through the orbital bone without an invasion of the periorbita often can be managed with orbital preservation.[137–140] There is also a lower risk of local recurrence.[96,108,141,142] When a tumor involves a limited amount of periorbita, the eye may be preserved without increasing the chance of local recurrence.[97,138–140]

When tumor penetrates through the periorbita, exenteration is usually required to obtain tumor-free margins if the patient is a surgical candidate.[137,138] CT and MRI each offer their own advantages and pitfalls. Osseous destruction with direct involvement of the orbital fat is one of the hallmarks used to suggest orbital invasion. However, some investigators have found a significant false-negative rates.[22] Therefore, the absence of abnormality in the orbital fat cannot completely exclude invasion. Other criteria evaluated include the relationship between the tumor and the periorbita (abutting, displacing, or bowing the periorbita) (**Fig. 3.22A,B**), the presence of nodularity

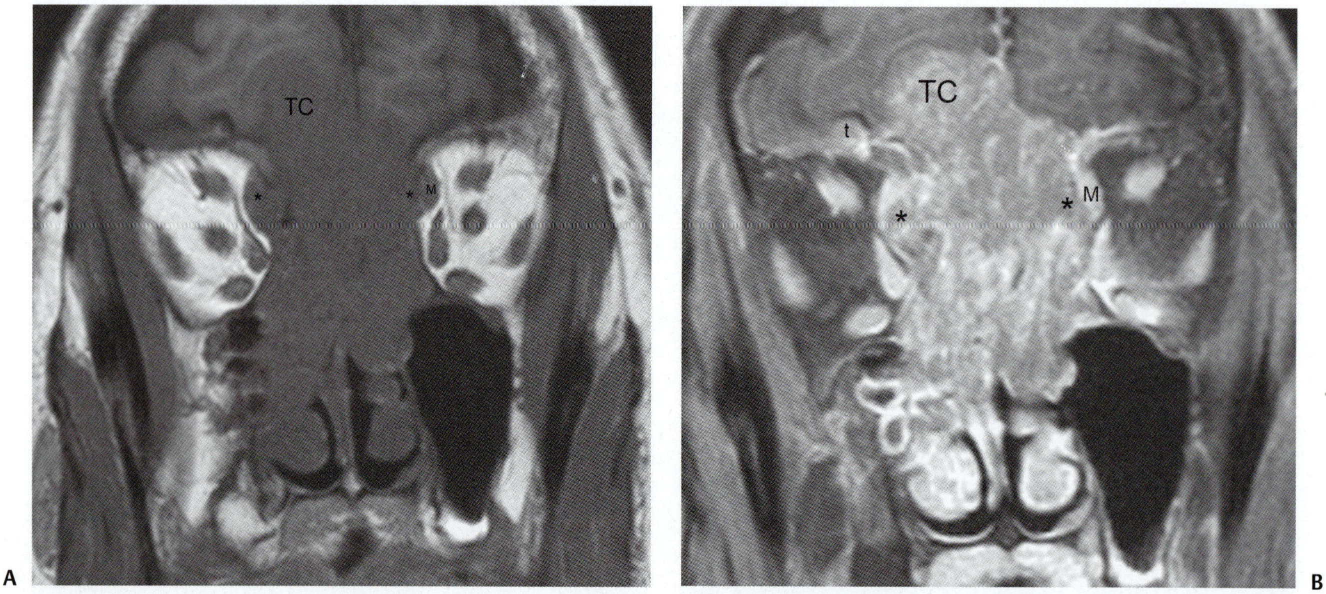

Fig. 3.22 Sinonasal undifferentiated carcinoma with extension through the periorbita and intracranial spread. Coronal unenhanced **(A)** and fat-suppressed enhanced **(B)** T1-weighted magnetic resonance images show a large mass in the bilateral sinonasal cavity. The patient presented with nasal stuffiness. There is extension of the tumor through the periorbita (*), and transcranially through the anterior cranial fossa (cribriform plate) into the intracranial compartment (*TC*). Note thick, nodular dural invasion (*t*). *M*, medial rectus muscle.

at the interface between the tumor and the periorbita, an assessment of the extraocular muscles (enlargement, displacement, and signal abnormality), and an evaluation of the integrity of the osseous structures comprising the orbital walls adjacent to the tumor.[22] None of these criteria is very accurate (each less than or equal to 65%). The strength of CT is its ability to evaluate both bone and fat; however, it is difficult to distinguish a tumor that compresses versus invades the periorbita.[103] MRI tends to underestimate orbital invasion in part because it cannot distinguish periorbita from bone, as both are hypointense on imaging. In cases where imaging is ambiguous, an intraoperative assessment with histology on frozen section remains the gold standard for determining invasion of the periorbita.

Intracranial and Dural Invasion

Contrast-enhanced MRI allows better identification of tumor extension intracranially, including the optic canal, cavernous sinus, as well as perineural spread at the skull base (**Figs. 3.17A,B and 3.21B**). MRI also provides more detailed and accurate information than CT in assessing for the presence of dural, pial, and parenchymal brain invasion (**Fig. 3.22A,B**). Smooth, continuous linear enhancement of the dura may be present in the setting of malignant infiltration; however, this appearance may also be seen in benign reactive and/or fibrovascular changes.[23] MRI findings that favor the presence of malignant involvement of the dura include the presence of discontinuous dural enhancement (multiple regions of enhancement with skip areas), thickening and/or nodularity greater than 5 mm (**Figs. 3.22A,B and 3.23A**), and the presence of T2 hyperintensity (edema) in the adjacent brain.[23] In the setting of pial invasion (subarachnoid seeding), multifocal areas of peripheral enhancement in the subarachnoid spaces are present (**Fig. 3.23B**). Such spread may occur from direct extension of the lesion or as a consequence of surgery.

Metastases

Lymphatic Drainage and Nodal Metastases

Lymph node drainage for sinonasal neoplasms is dependent on the origin of the neoplasm, the stage of the neoplasm, and the histology. Although the primary nodal drainage site for the paranasal sinuses is to the lateral retropharyngeal nodes, these lymphatics may be inconstant. Therefore, the upper internal jugular and submandibular nodes are common sites for nodal metastases. Regional lymph node metastases from sinonasal malignancies are relatively uncommon, but when present are a poor prognostic sign and usually indicative of tumor extension outside of the sinonasal cavity.[143] Cervical nodal metastases are most common with tumors originating from the maxillary antrum, seen at presentation in up to 15% of cases. Nodal metastases are uncommon with ethmoid cancers, and rare with sphenoid and frontal sinus neoplasms. Up to 40% of patients with a sinonasal melanoma have cervical nodal metastases at presentation.

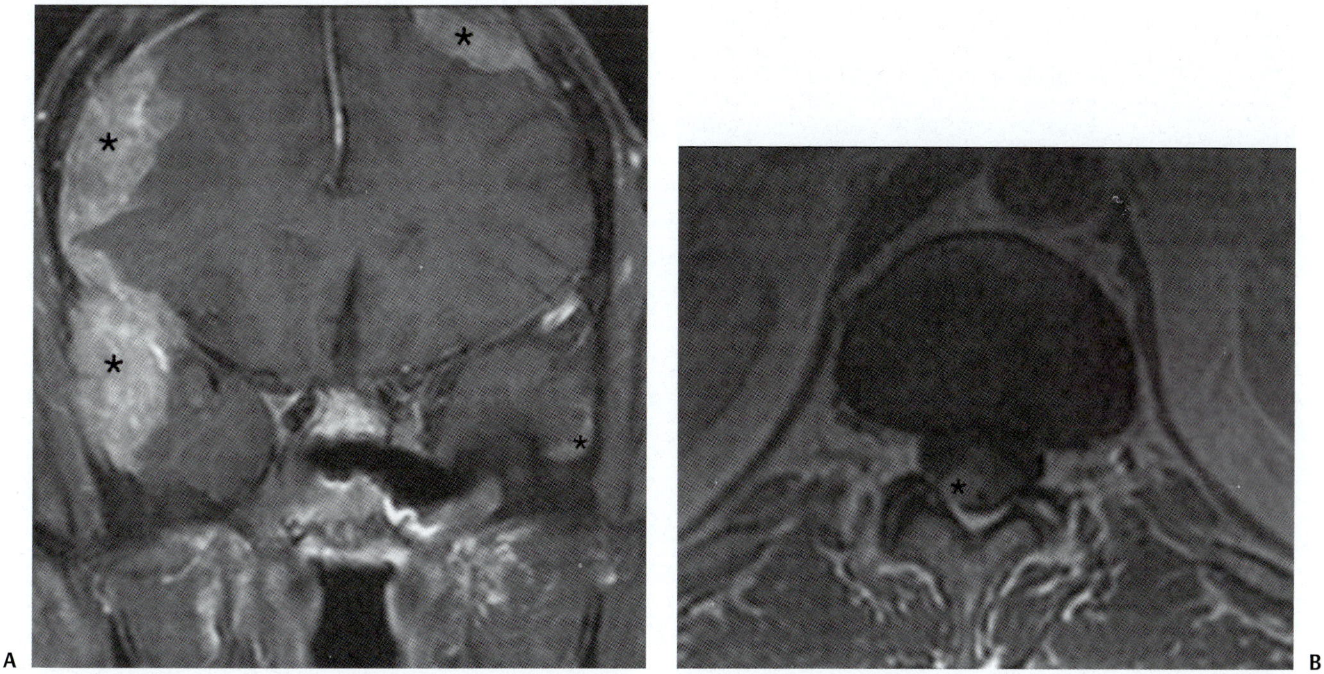

Fig. 3.23 Dural metastases with drop metastases to the spine in a sinonasal undifferentiated carcinoma. **(A)** Coronal enhanced T1-weighted magnetic resonance image (MRI) shows extensive dural metastases (*). **(B)** Axial enhanced T1-weighted MRI of the spine shows drop metastases (*) along the cauda equina in the thecal sac.

Distant Metastases

Less than 10% of all sinonasal carcinomas have systemic metastases. Hematogenous spread to the lungs is most common, with occasional bone metastases. The presence of cervical nodal disease places the patient at increased risk for distant metastases.[143] Approximately one-half of patients with adenoid cystic carcinomas have distant metastases, most commonly to the lungs, brain, and bone.[83] Hematogenous metastases are not uncommon with melanoma and affect the brain, liver, and skin. Therefore, CT imaging of the chest, abdomen, and pelvis should be included in the routine evaluation of these patients.

Imaging Following Treatment

The follow-up of patients is focused on the early detection of residual and recurrent tumors. Clinical assessment and cross-sectional imaging play complementary roles. Issues include distinguishing treatment changes from a tumor, as well as managing treatment-related complications such as cerebral radiation necrosis,[144–149] carotid artery stenosis,[149] xerostomia related to changes in the salivary glands included in the radiation field (associated with prominent enhancement followed by atrophy), and cranial nerve palsies.[150–157]

Tumor Recurrence Versus Treatment Change

Tumor recurrence implies that the patient has had a clinically and radiologically documented disease-free interval following treatment. Incomplete resolution of disease after surgery and/or radiation therapy is completed represents residual (not recurrent) neoplasm.

One of the most significant challenges facing the radiologist is distinguishing a neoplasm from a scar. CT in this regard has limited utility as treatment sequels, scars, muscles, and tumors frequently have overlapping densities, making their distinction difficult. MRI can be more sensitive. Postoperative granulation tissues, scars, and fibroses are dynamic tissues that may have a wide range of intensity and enhancement characteristics. In the paranasal sinuses, scar material may also have overlapping imaging characteristics with mucosal and inflammatory changes.[158] Early scar and granulation tissues tend to be hyperintense on T2-weighted images and enhance following contrast administration. A baseline posttreatment scan is useful, allowing the radiologist to assess on subsequent exams for increased mass effect in the surgical bed suggesting a recurrent tumor versus a contraction of tissue, which favors scars but does not entirely exclude tumors. A stable appearance or retraction of tissue on serial examinations provides reassurance that the changes are related to treatment and not recurrent disease. A mature scar can usually be distinguished from a tumor because it typically has little or no mass effect, is hypointense on T2-weighted images due to the presence of a fibrosis, and does not avidly enhance. However, in some instances, one is not able to exclude residual or recurrent neoplasm, and in these cases, biopsy or positron emission tomography (PET) is necessary (**Fig. 3.24A–C**).[159–161]

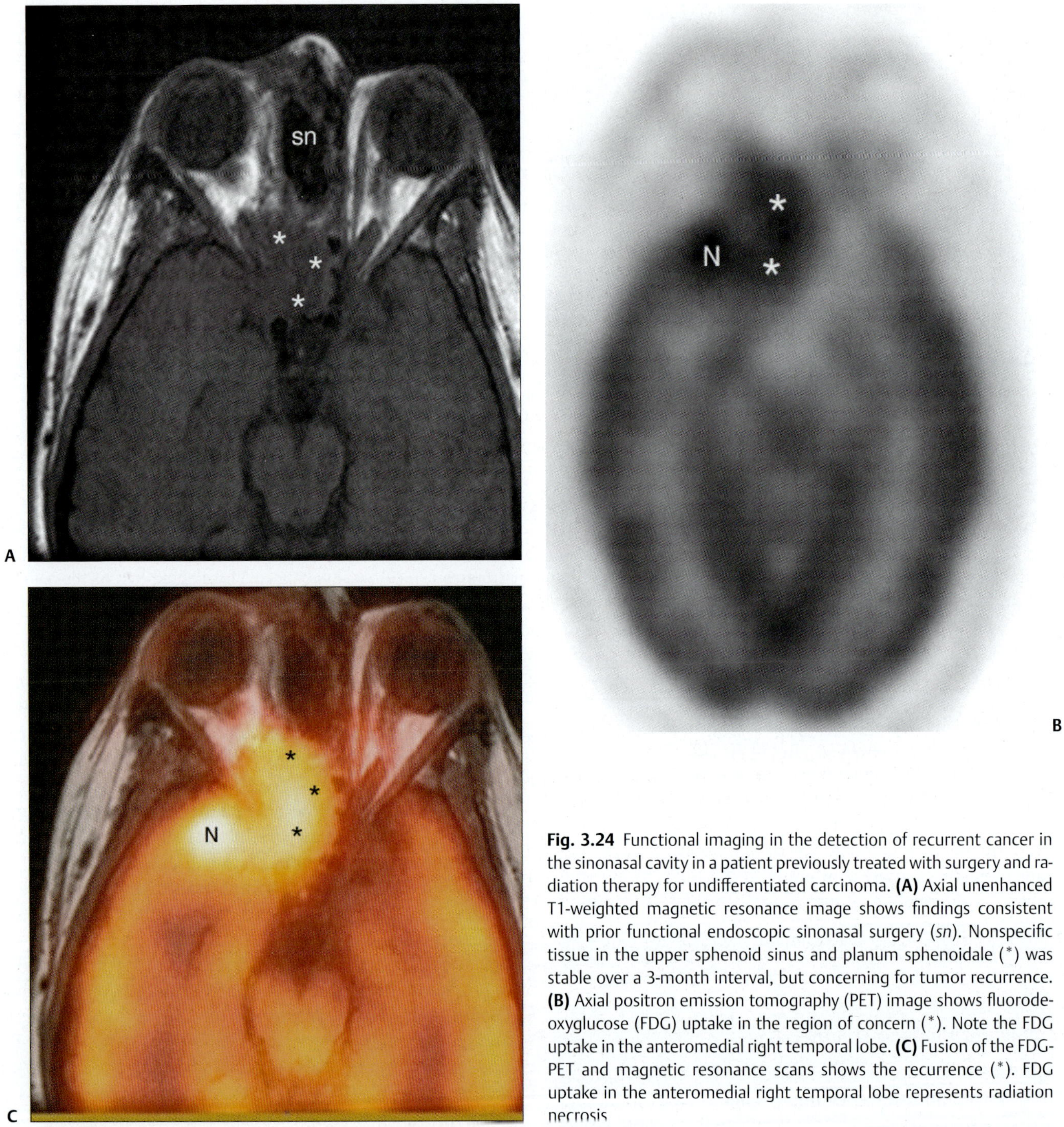

Fig. 3.24 Functional imaging in the detection of recurrent cancer in the sinonasal cavity in a patient previously treated with surgery and radiation therapy for undifferentiated carcinoma. **(A)** Axial unenhanced T1-weighted magnetic resonance image shows findings consistent with prior functional endoscopic sinonasal surgery (*sn*). Nonspecific tissue in the upper sphenoid sinus and planum sphenoidale (*) was stable over a 3-month interval, but concerning for tumor recurrence. **(B)** Axial positron emission tomography (PET) image shows fluorodeoxyglucose (FDG) uptake in the region of concern (*). Note the FDG uptake in the anteromedial right temporal lobe. **(C)** Fusion of the FDG-PET and magnetic resonance scans shows the recurrence (*). FDG uptake in the anteromedial right temporal lobe represents radiation necrosis.

Functional Imaging in the Treated Patient

New imaging techniques outside of cross-sectional imaging have focused on the physiologic properties of tumors rather than anatomic details. Positron emission tomography using 2-[^{18}F] fluoro-2-deoxy-D-glucose (FDG PET) relies on the metabolic activity of neoplasms relative to adjacent tissues (normal neck soft tissues, scar, fibrosis, inflammatory changes) in positively identifying the presence of a tumor. In sinonasal cancers, PET may be useful in guiding endoscopic biopsies, evaluating recurrent tumors,[159,160,162] and in distinguishing recurrent neoplasms from radiation changes (**Fig. 3.24A–C**). One of the potential pitfalls of CT and MRI is their inability to distinguish treatment change from recurrent tumor. In general, recurrent neoplasms have significant uptake of FDG compared with fibrotic tissue and radiation-induced changes[159–165]; however, occasionally radiation changes may demonstrate increased metabolic activity resulting in significant FDG uptake.[166] Furthermore, the timing of PET following irradiation is important in the distinction of treatment sequela from a tumor. PET performed shortly after radiotherapy is very sensitive but not specific. Both residual tumors and granulation tissues may be FDG avid. Over time, PET has increasing specificity, being quite accurate if performed at least 12 weeks following completion of therapy.[160,167–169]

Complications of Treatment

Radiation Necrosis

Radiation necrosis is not an infrequent complication of nasopharyngeal, sinonasal, and skull base neoplasms treated with irradiation.[144–149,170] Due to the field covered, the temporal lobes are most commonly affected (**Fig. 3.25A,B**), followed by the frontal lobes. The total dose, duration, and fractionation of radiation play an important role in the development of radiation necrosis.[149,171] The incidence of radiation necrosis following the treatment of head and neck cancer and skull base neoplasms ranges from 3 to 10%.[149,171,172] However, radiation necrosis is probably more common than reported, as many patients are asymptomatic and therefore are not imaged leading to underdetection. Irradiation can also result in radiation vasculitis affecting the deep perforating arteries leading to ischemic sequela in the basal ganglia, thalami, brainstem, and the deep white matter. Symptoms of radiation arteritis are dependent on the regions of the brain affected and may include changes in mental status, focal neurologic deficits, and occasionally, seizures.

Changes in the brain due to radiation necrosis may occur early (during therapy) or be delayed. Delayed radiation changes can be further divided into early (within 3 to 4 months of therapy) and late (months to years following therapy). In early as well as early delayed injury, MRI typically shows T2 hyperintensity representing edema that is frequently reversible.[172,173] Late delayed injury is usually related to vascular injury, demyelination, and inflammatory infiltrates. This is characterized on MRI by T2 hyperintensity, mass effect, and enhancement that may be solid or ringlike (peripheral enhancement around a necrotic cavity) (**Fig. 3.25A,B**).[172,173] In burnt out radiation necrosis, there frequently is temporal lobe encephalomalacia. Although the differential diagnosis of radiation necrosis includes metastatic disease, in the setting of primary head and neck or skull base malignancies, cerebral metastases are relatively uncommon. Intracranial extension of these neoplasms usually presents with extra-axial (extracerebral) masses, whereas the changes of radiation necrosis are intracerebral.

Cranial Neuropathies

The cranial nerves are relatively radioresistant. The optic and hypoglossal nerves are most commonly affected.[152,154,156,174] Cranial nerve XII palsies may present with fasciculations, weakness, tongue deviation, and problems with deglutition.[151,154] On imaging, ipsilateral edema may be present in the early stages, followed later by fatty replacement and atrophy.[154] Optic neuritis due to irradiation may present with visual loss, with enlargement and enhancement of the involved optic tracts or chiasm on MRI.[152,174] Cranial nerves IV through VII are less commonly affected. Their involvement may be related to changes in the nerves themselves or sequela of brainstem injury from radiation vasculitis.

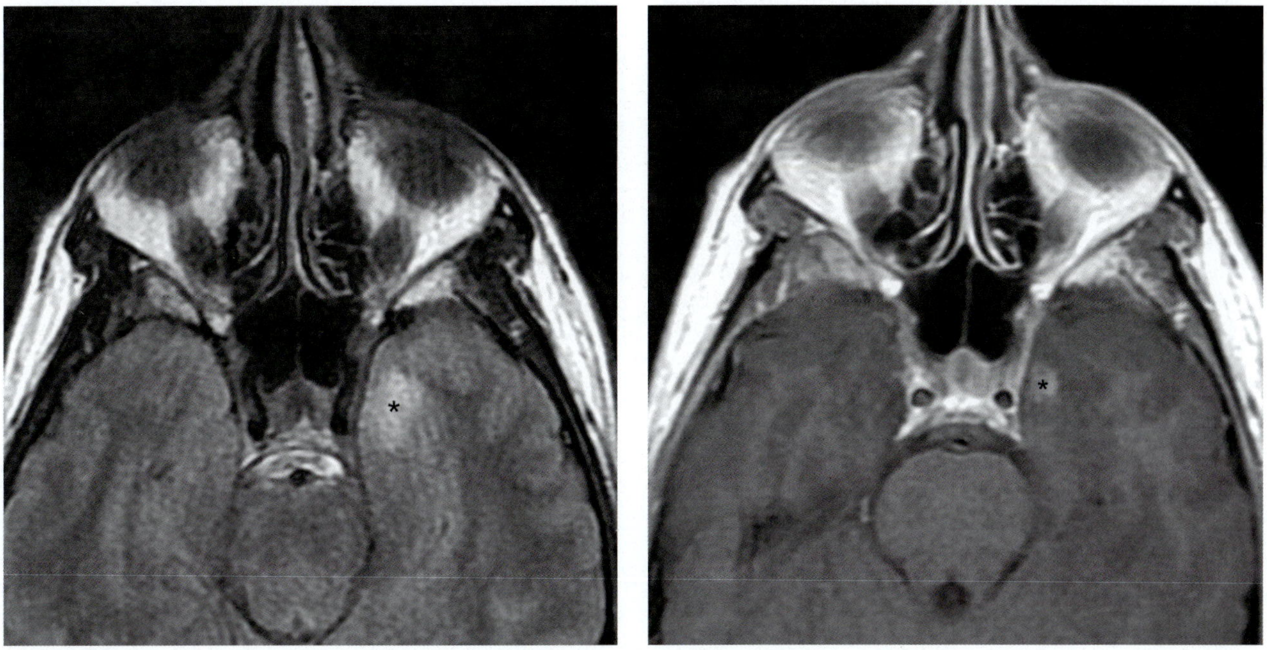

A B

Fig. 3.25 Radiation necrosis in medial left temporal lobe in a patient previously irradiated for carcinoma. **(A)** Axial flair magnetic resonance image (MRI) shows hyperintensity consistent with edema in the medial left temporal lobe (*). **(B)** Axial contrast-enhanced T1-weighted MRI shows enhancement in the radiation damage.

Radiation-Induced Neoplasms

Radiation-associated/induced neoplasms typically occur in the radiated field. Criteria in diagnosing a tumor induced by irradiation include histology different from the primary tumor treated, as well as a latency period of at least 5 years. A wide spectrum of radiation-induced neoplasms have been reported including meningiomas, sarcomas, schwannomas, minor salivary tumors, and squamous cell carcinomas.[172,174–183]

Conclusion

Sinusitis is among the most common ailments in the United States. CT is the most widely utilized imaging modality to assess this as well as other disease processes of the sinonasal cavity. The use of plain film radiographs is relatively obsolete. To understand the pathogenesis of sinusitis and other pathologic processes that may affect the paranasal sinuses, some understanding of sinonasal development and anatomy as it pertains to mucociliary clearance is essential. A focused imaging assessment of disease processes in the sinuses is invaluable when used correctly. Indications for performing MRI include CT findings like bone destruction or an extension of disease outside the sinonasal cavity that raise concern for an aggressive infection or neoplasm. For many lesions, including complicated sinusitis, encephaloceles, and neoplasms, CT and MRI play complementary roles.

Assessment of sinonasal malignancies requires a multidisciplinary team approach. Advances in pretherapeutic imaging have significantly contributed to the management of sinonasal tumors. CT and MRI play complementary roles in the assessment and staging of these malignancies by determining the presence or absence of an extension of disease into the skull base and its foramina, the orbit, and the intracranial compartment.

References

1. Zinreich SJ. Functional anatomy and computed tomography imaging of the paranasal sinuses. Am J Med Sci 1998;316(1):2–12
2. Rao VM, el-Noueam KI. Sinonasal imaging. Anatomy and pathology. Radiol Clin North Am 1998;36(5):921–939, vi
3. Kennedy DW, Zinreich SJ, Rosenbaum AE, Johns ME. Functional endoscopic sinus surgery. Theory and diagnostic evaluation. Arch Otolaryngol 1985;111(9):576–582
4. Kantarci M, Karasen RM, Alper F, Onbas O, Okur A, Karaman A. Remarkable anatomic variations in paranasal sinus region and their clinical importance. Eur J Radiol 2004;50(3):296–302
5. Hatipoğlu HG, Cetin MA, Yüksel E. Concha bullosa types: their relationship with sinusitis, ostiomeatal and frontal recess disease. Diagn Interv Radiol 2005;11(3):145–149
6. Nadas S, Duvoisin B, Landry M, Schnyder P. Concha bullosa: frequency and appearances on CT and correlations with sinus disease in 308 patients with chronic sinusitis. Neuroradiology 1995;37(3):234–237
7. Branstetter BF IV, Weissman JL. Role of MR and CT in the paranasal sinuses. Otolaryngol Clin North Am 2005;38(6):1279–1299, x
8. Hojreh A, Czerny C, Kainberger F. Dose classification scheme for computed tomography of the paranasal sinuses. Eur J Radiol 2005;56(1):31–37
9. Hagtvedt T, Aaløkken TM, Nøtthellen J, Kolbenstvedt A. A new low-dose CT examination compared with standard-dose CT in the diagnosis of acute sinusitis. Eur Radiol 2003;13(5):976–980
10. Hein E, Rogalla P, Klingebiel R, Hamm B. Low-dose CT of the paranasal sinuses with eye lens protection: effect on image quality and radiation dose. Eur Radiol 2002;12(7):1693–1696
11. Marmolya G, Wiesen EJ, Yagan R, Haria CD, Shah AC. Paranasal sinuses: low-dose CT. Radiology 1991;181(3):689–691
12. Duvoisin B, Landry M, Chapuis L, Krayenbuhl M, Schnyder P. Low-dose CT and inflammatory disease of the paranasal sinuses. Neuroradiology 1991;33(5):403–406
13. Cagici CA, Cakmak O, Hurcan C, Tercan F. Three-slice computerized tomography for the diagnosis and follow-up of rhinosinusitis. Eur Arch Otorhinolaryngol 2005;262(9):744–750
14. Yousem DM. Imaging of sinonasal inflammatory disease. Radiology 1993;188(2):303–314
15. Wippold FJ II. Head and neck imaging: the role of CT and MRI. J Magn Reson Imaging 2007;25(3):453–465
16. Ling FT, Kountakis SE. Advances in imaging of the paranasal sinuses. Curr Allergy Asthma Rep 2006;6(6):502–507
17. Aygun N, Zinreich SJ. Imaging for functional endoscopic sinus surgery. Otolaryngol Clin North Am 2006;39(3):403–416, vii
18. Maroldi R, Ravanelli M, Borghesi A, Farina D. Paranasal sinus imaging. Eur J Radiol 2008;66(3):372–386
19. Lund VJ, Savy L, Lloyd G, Howard D. Optimum imaging and diagnosis of cerebrospinal fluid rhinorrhoea. J Laryngol Otol 2000;114(12):988–992
20. Köhrmann M, Schellinger PD, Wetter A, Hähnel S. Nasal meningoencephalocele, an unusual cause for recurrent meningitis. Case report and review of the literature. J Neurol 2007;254(2): 259 –260
21. Loevner LA, Yousem DM, Lanza DC, Kennedy DW, Goldberg AN. MR evaluation of frontal sinus osteoplastic flaps with autogenous fat grafts. AJNR Am J Neuroradiol 1995;16(8):1721–1726
22. Eisen MD, Yousem DM, Loevner LA, Thaler ER, Bilker WB, Goldberg AN. Preoperative imaging to predict orbital invasion by tumor. Head Neck 2000;22(5):456–462
23. Eisen MD, Yousem DM, Montone KT, et al. Use of preoperative MR to predict dural, perineural, and venous sinus invasion of skull base tumors. AJNR Am J Neuroradiol 1996;17(10): 1937–1945
24. Hermans R, De Vuysere S, Marchal G. Squamous cell carcinoma of the sinonasal cavities. Semin Ultrasound CT MR 1999;20(3): 150–161
25. Lloyd G, Lund VJ, Howard D, Savy L. Optimum imaging for sinonasal malignancy. J Laryngol Otol 2000;114(7):557–562
26. Loevner LA, Sonners AI. Imaging of neoplasms of the paranasal sinuses. Magn Reson Imaging Clin N Am 2002;10(3):467–493
27. Pearlman AN, Conley DB. Review of current guidelines related to the diagnosis and treatment of rhinosinusitis. Curr Opin Otolaryngol Head Neck Surg 2008;16(3):226–230
28. Anzai Y, Jarvik JG, Sullivan SD, Hollingworth W. The cost-effectiveness of the management of acute sinusitis. Am J Rhinol 2007;21(4):444–451
29. Desrosiers M. Diagnosis and management of acute rhinosinusitis. Postgrad Med 2009;121(3):83–89
30. Madani G, Beale TJ. Sinonasal inflammatory disease. Semin Ultrasound CT MR 2009;30(1):17–24

31. Mafee MF, Tran BH, Chapa AR. Imaging of rhinosinusitis and its complications: plain film, CT, and MRI. Clin Rev Allergy Immunol 2006;30(3):165–186
32. Rosenfeld RM, Andes D, Bhattacharyya N, et al. Clinical practice guideline: adult sinusitis. Otolaryngol Head Neck Surg 2007; 137(3, Suppl)S1–S31
33. Zinreich SJ. Imaging for staging of rhinosinusitis. Ann Otol Rhinol Laryngol Suppl 2004;193:19–23
34. Eggesbø HB. Radiological imaging of inflammatory lesions in the nasal cavity and paranasal sinuses. Eur Radiol 2006;16(4): 872–888
35. Dalziel K, Stein K, Round A, Garside R, Royle P. Endoscopic sinus surgery for the excision of nasal polyps: A systematic review of safety and effectiveness. Am J Rhinol 2006;20(5):506–519
36. Bhatti MT, Schmalfuss IM, Mancuso AA. Orbital complications of functional endoscopic sinus surgery: MR and CT findings. Clin Radiol 2005;60(8):894–904
37. Huang CM, Meyer DR, Patrinely JR, et al. Medial rectus muscle injuries associated with functional endoscopic sinus surgery: characterization and management. Ophthal Plast Reconstr Surg 2003;19(1):25–37
38. Carton A, Hislop S. Orbital floor injury with extraocular muscle entrapment following functional endoscopic sinus surgery. Br J Oral Maxillofac Surg 2000;38(1):82–83
39. Corey JP, Bumsted R, Panje W, Namon A. Orbital complications in functional endoscopic sinus surgery. Otolaryngol Head Neck Surg 1993;109(5):814–820
40. Hudgins PA, Browning DG, Gallups J, et al. Endoscopic paranasal sinus surgery: radiographic evaluation of severe complications. AJNR Am J Neuroradiol 1992;13(4):1161–1167
41. Brook I. Sinusitis. Periodontol 2000 2009;49:126–139
42. Osborn MK, Steinberg JP. Subdural empyema and other suppurative complications of paranasal sinusitis. Lancet Infect Dis 2007;7(1):62–67
43. Reid JR. Complications of pediatric paranasal sinusitis. Pediatr Radiol 2004;34(12):933–942
44. Rosenfeld EA, Rowley AH. Infectious intracranial complications of sinusitis, other than meningitis, in children: 12-year review. Clin Infect Dis 1994;18(5):750–754
45. Younis RT, Anand VK, Davidson B. The role of computed tomography and magnetic resonance imaging in patients with sinusitis with complications. Laryngoscope 2002;112(2):224–229
46. Arrué P, Kany MT, Serrano E, et al. Mucoceles of the paranasal sinuses: uncommon location. J Laryngol Otol 1998;112(9): 840–844
47. Loo JL, Looi AL, Seah LL. Visual outcomes in patients with paranasal mucoceles. Ophthal Plast Reconstr Surg 2009;25(2): 126–129
48. Lloyd G, Lund VJ, Savy L, Howard D. Optimum imaging for mucoceles. J Laryngol Otol 2000;114(3):233–236
49. Suri A, Mahapatra AK, Gaikwad S, Sarkar C. Giant mucoceles of the frontal sinus: a series and review. J Clin Neurosci 2004;11(2):214–218
50. Ada S, Yalamanchili M, Kambhampati G. Frontal sinus mucopyocele. Arch Intern Med 2002;162(21):2487–2488
51. Yokoyama T, Inoue S, Imamura J, et al. Sphenoethmoidal mucoceles with intracranial extension—three case reports. Neurol Med Chir (Tokyo) 1996;36(11):822–828
52. Voegels RL, Balbani AP, Santos Júnior RC, Butugan O. Frontoethmoidal mucocele with intracranial extension: a case report. Ear Nose Throat J 1998;77(2):117–120
53. Kawaguchi S, Sakaki T, Okuno S, Ida Y, Nishi N. Giant frontal mucocele extending into the anterior cranial fossa. J Clin Neurosci 2002;9(1):86–89
54. Cultrera F, Giuffrida M, Mancuso P. Delayed post-traumatic frontal sinus mucopyocoele presenting with meningitis. J Craniomaxillofac Surg 2006;34(8):502–504
55. Lanzieri CF, Shah M, Krauss D, Lavertu P. Use of gadolinium-enhanced MR imaging for differentiating mucoceles from neoplasms in the paranasal sinuses. Radiology 1991;178(2):425–428
56. Dillon WP, Som PM, Fullerton GD. Hypointense MR signal in chronically inspissated sinonasal secretions. Radiology 1990; 174(1):73–78
57. Som PM, Dillon WP, Fullerton GD, Zimmerman RA, Rajagopalan B, Marom Z. Chronically obstructed sinonasal secretions: observations on T1 and T2 shortening. Radiology 1989;172(2):515–520
58. McComb JG. Spinal and cranial neural tube defects. Semin Pediatr Neurol 1997;4(3):156–166
59. Hoving EW. Nasal encephaloceles. Childs Nerv Syst 2000;16 (10-11):702–706
60. Guion-Almeida ML, Richieri-Costa A. Frontonasal dysplasia, severe neuropsychological delay, and midline central nervous system anomalies: report of 10 Brazilian male patients. Am J Med Genet A 2009;149A(5):1006–1011
61. Bhattacharjee A, Chakraborty A, Purkaystha P. Frontoethmoidal encephalomeningocoele with colpocephaly: case report and clinical review. J Laryngol Otol 2008;122(3):321–323
62. Rojas L, Melvin JJ, Faerber EN, Valencia I. Anterior encephalocele associated with subependymal nodular heterotopia, cortical dysplasia and epilepsy: case report and review of the literature. Eur J Paediatr Neurol 2006;10(5-6):227–229
63. Mahapatra AK, Suri A. Anterior encephaloceles: a study of 92 cases. Pediatr Neurosurg 2002;36(3):113–118
64. Curtin HD, Williams R, Johnson J. CT of perineural tumor extension: pterygopalatine fossa. AJR Am J Roentgenol 1985;144(1): 163–169
65. Goldenberg D, Golz A, Fradis M, Mârtu D, Netzer A, Joachims HZ. Malignant tumors of the nose and paranasal sinuses: a retrospective review of 291 cases. Ear Nose Throat J 2001;80(4):272–277
66. Hermans R, De Vuysere S, Marchal G. Squamous cell carcinoma of the sinonasal cavities. Semin Ultrasound CT MR 1999;20(3): 150–161
67. Hudgins PA. Sinonasal imaging. Neuroimaging Clin N Am 1996;6(2):319–331
68. Jeans WD, Gilani S, Bullimore J. The effects of CT scanning on staging of tumours of the paranasal sinuses. Clin Radiol 1982;33(2):173–179
69. Kraus DH, Lanzieri CF, Wanamaker JR, Little JR, Lavertu P. Complementary use of computed tomography and magnetic resonance imaging in assessing skull base lesions. Laryngoscope 1992;102(6):623–629
70. Maroldi R, Farina D, Battaglia G, Maculotti P, Nicolai P, Chiesa A. MR of malignant nasosinusal neoplasms. Frequently asked questions. Eur J Radiol 1997;24(3):181–190
71. Phillips CD. Current status and new developments in techniques for imaging the nose and sinuses. Otolaryngol Clin North Am 1997;30(3):371–387
72. Rao VM, el-Noueam KI. Sinonasal imaging. Anatomy and pathology. Radiol Clin North Am 1998;36(5):921–939, vi
73. Raghavan P, Phillips CD. Magnetic resonance imaging of sinonasal malignancies. Top Magn Reson Imaging 2007;18(4):259–267
74. Curtin HD, Hirsch WL. Base of the skull. In: Atlas SW, ed. Magnetic Resonance Imaging of the Brain and Spine. New York: Raven Press; 1991: 668–706
75. Hähnel S, Ertl-Wagner B, Tasman AJ, Forsting M, Jansen O. Relative value of MR imaging as compared with CT in the diagnosis of inflammatory paranasal sinus disease. Radiology 1999;210(1):171–176

76. Rao VM, Sharma D, Madan A. Imaging of frontal sinus disease: concepts, interpretation, and technology. Otolaryngol Clin North Am 2001;34(1):23–39
77. Krouse JH. Endoscopic treatment of inverted papilloma: safety and efficacy. Am J Otolaryngol 2001;22(2):87–99
78. Mirza S, Bradley PJ, Acharya A, Stacey M, Jones NS. Sinonasal inverted papillomas: recurrence, and synchronous and metachronous malignancy. J Laryngol Otol 2007;121(9):857–864
79. Jeon TY, Kim HJ, Chung SK, et al. Sinonasal inverted papilloma: value of convoluted cerebriform pattern on MR imaging. AJNR Am J Neuroradiol 2008;29(8):1556–1560
80. Eggers G, Mühling J, Hassfeld S. Inverted papilloma of paranasal sinuses. J Craniomaxillofac Surg 2007;35(1):21–29
81. Lund VJ. Optimum management of inverted papilloma. J Laryngol Otol 2000;114(3):194–197
82. Som PM, Lawson W, Lidov MW. Simulated aggressive skull base erosion in response to benign sinonasal disease. Radiology 1991;180(3):755–759
83. Barnes L, Verbin RS, Gnepp DR. Diseases of the nose, paranasal sinuses, and nasopharynx. In: Barnes L, ed. Surgical Pathology of the Head and Neck. New York: Marcel Dekker Inc; 1985:403–451
84. Muir C, Weiland L. Upper aerodigestive tract cancers. Cancer 1995;75(1, Suppl)147–153
85. Keane WM, Atkins JP Jr, Wetmore R, Vidas M. Epidemiology of head and neck cancer. Laryngoscope 1981;91(12):2037–2045
86. Goepfert H, Luna MA, Lindberg RD, White AK. Malignant salivary gland tumors of the paranasal sinuses and nasal cavity. Arch Otolaryngol 1983;109(10):662–668
87. Spiro RH, Koss LG, Hajdu SI, Strong EW. Tumors of minor salivary origin. A clinicopathologic study of 492 cases. Cancer 1973;31(1):117–129
88. Klintenberg C, Olofsson J, Hellquist H, Sökjer H. Adenocarcinoma of the ethmoid sinuses. A review of 28 cases with special reference to wood dust exposure. Cancer 1984;54(3):482–488
89. Bimbi G, Saraceno MS, Riccio S, Gatta G, Licitra L, Cantù G. Adenocarcinoma of ethmoid sinus: an occupational disease. Acta Otorhinolaryngol Ital 2004;24(4):199–203
90. Wax MK, Yun KJ, Wetmore SJ, Lu X, Kaufman HH. Adenocarcinoma of the ethmoid sinus. Head Neck 1995;17(4):303–311
91. Osguthorpe JD, Patel S. Craniofacial approaches to sinus malignancy. Otolaryngol Clin North Am 1995;28(6):1239–1257
92. Liu JK, Decker D, Schaefer SD, et al. Zones of approach for craniofacial resection: minimizing facial incisions for resection of anterior cranial base and paranasal sinus tumors. Neurosurgery 2003;53(5):1126–1135, discussion 1135–1137
93. Osguthorpe JD, Patel S. Craniofacial approaches to tumors of the anterior skull base. Otolaryngol Clin North Am 2001;34(6): 1123–1142, ix
94. Sakai S, Hohki A, Fuchihata H, Tanaka Y. Multidisciplinary treatment of maxillary sinus carcinoma. Cancer 1983;52(8):1360–1364
95. Shidnia H, Hornback NB, Saghafi N, Sayoc E, Lingeman R, Hamaker R. The role of radiation therapy in the treatment of malignant tumors of the paranasal sinuses. Laryngoscope 1984;94(1): 102–106
96. Som ML. Surgical management of carcinoma of the maxilla. Arch Otolaryngol 1974;99(4):270–273
97. McCary WS, Levine PA. Management of the eye in the treatment of sinonasal cancers. Otolaryngol Clin North Am 1995;28(6): 1231–1238
98. Van Tuyl R, Gussack GS. Prognostic factors in craniofacial surgery. Laryngoscope 1991;101(3):240–244
99. Alvarez I, Suárez C, Rodrigo JP, Nuñez F, Caminero MJ. Prognostic factors in paranasal sinus cancer. Am J Otolaryngol 1995;16(2):109–114
100. Jeans WD, Gilani S, Bullimore J. The effects of CT scanning on staging of tumours of the paranasal sinuses. Clin Radiol 1982;33(2):173–179
101. Allbery SM, Chaljub G, Cho NL, Rassekh CH, John SD, Guinto FC. MR imaging of nasal masses. Radiographics 1995;15(6): 1311–1327
102. Hasso AN, Lambert D. Magnetic resonance imaging of the paranasal sinuses and nasal cavities. Top Magn Reson Imaging 1994;6(4):209–223
103. Gil Z, Carlson DL, Gupta A, et al. Patterns and incidence of neural invasion in patients with cancers of the paranasal sinuses. Arch Otolaryngol Head Neck Surg 2009;135(2):173–179
104. Waldron J, Witterick I. Paranasal sinus cancer: caveats and controversies. World J Surg 2003;27(7):849–855
105. Graamans K, Slootweg PJ. Orbital exenteration in surgery of malignant neoplasms of the paranasal sinuses. The value of preoperative computed tomography. Arch Otolaryngol Head Neck Surg 1989;115(8):977–980
106. McCary WS, Levine PA. Management of the eye in the treatment of sinonasal cancers. Otolaryngol Clin North Am 1995;28(6): 1231–1238
107. Perry C, Levine PA, Williamson BR, Cantrell RW. Preservation of the eye in paranasal sinus cancer surgery. Arch Otolaryngol Head Neck Surg 1988;114(6):632–634
108. Wu X, Tang P, Qi Y. Management of the orbital contents in radical surgery for squamous cell carcinoma of the maxillary sinus. Chin Med J (Engl) 1995;108(2):123–125
109. Nassab RS, Thomas SS, Murray D. Orbital exenteration for advanced periorbital skin cancers: 20 years experience. J Plast Reconstr Aesthet Surg 2007;60(10):1103–1109
110. Iannetti G, Valentini V, Rinna C, Ventucci E, Marianetti TM. Ethmoido-orbital tumors: our experience. J Craniofac Surg 2005;16(6):1085–1091
111. Phillips CD, Futterer SF, Lipper MH, Levine PA. Sinonasal undifferentiated carcinoma: CT and MR imaging of an uncommon neoplasm of the nasal cavity. Radiology 1997;202(2):477–480
112. Madani G, Beale TJ, Lund VJ. Imaging of sinonasal tumors. Semin Ultrasound CT MR 2009;30(1):25–38
113. Rumboldt Z, Gordon L, Gordon L, Bonsall R, Ackermann S. Imaging in head and neck cancer. Curr Treat Options Oncol 2006;7(1):23–34
114. Enochs WS, Hyslop WB, Bennett HF, Brown RD III, Koenig SH, Swartz HM. Sources of the increased longitudinal relaxation rates observed in melanotic melanoma. An in vitro study of synthetic melanins. Invest Radiol 1989;24(10):794–804
115. Gomori JM, Grossman RI, Shields JA, Augsburger JJ, Joseph PM, DeSimeone D. Choroidal melanomas: correlation of NMR spectroscopy and MR imaging. Radiology 1986;158(2):443–445
116. Hammersmith SM, Terk MR, Jeffrey PB, Connolly SG, Colletti PM. Magnetic resonance imaging of nasopharyngeal and paranasal sinus melanoma. Magn Reson Imaging 1990;8(3):245–253
117. Mafee MF, Carter BL. Nasal cavity and paranasal sinuses. In: Imaging of the Head and Neck. Stuttgart: Thieme; 1995: 248–331
118. Matias C, Corde J, Soares J. Primary malignant melanoma of the nasal cavity: a clinicopathologic study of nine cases. J Surg Oncol 1988;39(1):29–32
119. Yousem DM, Li C, Montone KT, et al. Primary malignant melanoma of the sinonasal cavity: MR imaging evaluation. Radiographics 1996;16(5):1101–1110
120. Chong VF, Fan YF, Khoo JB. Computed tomographic and magnetic resonance imaging findings in paranasal sinus involvement in nasopharyngeal carcinoma. Ann Acad Med Singapore 1998;27(6):800–804

121. Schuster JJ, Phillips CD, Levine PA. MR of esthesioneuroblastoma (olfactory neuroblastoma) and appearance after craniofacial resection. AJNR Am J Neuroradiol 1994;15(6):1169–1177
122. Som PM, Shapiro MD, Biller HF, Sasaki C, Lawson W. Sinonasal tumors and inflammatory tissues: differentiation with MR imaging. Radiology 1988;167(3):803–808
123. Ling FT, Kountakis SE. Advances in imaging of the paranasal sinuses. Curr Allergy Asthma Rep 2006;6(6):502–507
124. Madani G, Beale TJ. Differential diagnosis in sinonasal disease. Semin Ultrasound CT MR 2009;30(1):39–45
125. Som PM, Lidov M, Brandwein M, Catalano P, Biller HF. Sinonasal esthesioneuroblastoma with intracranial extension: marginal tumor cysts as a diagnostic MR finding. AJNR Am J Neuroradiol 1994;15(7):1259–1262
126. Som PM, Lidov M. The significance of sinonasal radiodensities: ossification, calcification, or residual bone? AJNR Am J Neuroradiol 1994;15(5):917–922
127. Nishioka T, Shirato H, Kagei K, et al. Skull-base invasion of nasopharyngeal carcinoma: magnetic resonance imaging findings and therapeutic implications. Int J Radiat Oncol Biol Phys 2000;47(2):395–400
128. Kimura F, Kim KS, Friedman H, Russell EJ, Breit R. MR imaging of the normal and abnormal clivus. AJR Am J Roentgenol 1990;155(6):1285–1291
129. Okada Y, Aoki S, Barkovich AJ, et al. Cranial bone marrow in children: assessment of normal development with MR imaging. Radiology 1989;171(1):161–164
130. Ricci C, Cova M, Kang YS, et al. Normal age-related patterns of cellular and fatty bone marrow distribution in the axial skeleton: MR imaging study. Radiology 1990;177(1):83–88
131. Daffner RH, Lupetin AR, Dash N, Deeb ZL, Sefczek RJ, Schapiro RL. MRI in the detection of malignant infiltration of bone marrow. AJR Am J Roentgenol 1986;146(2):353–358
132. Poulton TB, Murphy WD, Duerk JL, Chapek CC, Feiglin DH. Bone marrow reconversion in adults who are smokers: MR Imaging findings. AJR Am J Roentgenol 1993;161(6):1217–1221
133. Shellock FG, Morris E, Deutsch AL, Mink JH, Kerr R, Boden SD. Hematopoietic bone marrow hyperplasia: high prevalence on MR images of the knee in asymptomatic marathon runners. AJR Am J Roentgenol 1992;158(2):335–338
134. Tomura N, Hirano H, Kato K, et al. Comparison of MR imaging with CT in depiction of tumour extension into the pterygopalatine fossa. Clin Radiol 1999;54(6):361–366
135. Pandolfo I, Gaeta M, Blandino A, Longo M, Faranda C. Perineural spread of nasopharyngeal carcinoma: radiological and CT demonstration. Eur J Radiol 1988;8(4):231–235
136. Weisman RA. Surgical anatomy of the orbit. Otolaryngol Clin North Am 1988;21(1):1–12
137. McCary WS, Levine PA. Management of the eye in the treatment of sinonasal cancers. Otolaryngol Clin North Am 1995;28(6):1231–1238
138. Suárez C, Ferlito A, Lund VJ, et al. Management of the orbit in malignant sinonasal tumors. Head Neck 2008;30(2):242–250
139. Imola MJ, Schramm VL Jr. Orbital preservation in surgical management of sinonasal malignancy. Laryngoscope 2002;112(8 Pt 1):1357–1365
140. Essig GF, Newman SA, Levine PA. Sparing the eye in craniofacial surgery for superior nasal vault malignant neoplasms: analysis of benefit. Arch Facial Plast Surg 2007;9(6):406–411
141. Perry C, Levine PA, Williamson BR, Cantrell RW. Preservation of the eye in paranasal sinus cancer surgery. Arch Otolaryngol Head Neck Surg 1988;114(6):632–634
142. Sisson GA. Symposium: 3. Treatment of malignancies of paranasal sinuses. Discussion and summary. Laryngoscope 1970;80(6):945–953
143. Nishijima W, Takooda S, Tokita N, Takayama S, Sakura M. Analyses of distant metastases in squamous cell carcinoma of the head and neck and lesions above the clavicle at autopsy. Arch Otolaryngol Head Neck Surg 1993;119(1):65–68
144. Chong VE, Fan YF. Radiation-induced temporal lobe necrosis. AJNR Am J Neuroradiol 1997;18(4):784–785
145. Chong VF, Fan YF, Chan LL. Temporal lobe necrosis in nasopharyngeal carcinoma: pictorial essay. Australas Radiol 1997;41(4):392–397
146. Chong VF, Rumpel H, Aw YS, Ho GL, Fan YF, Chua EJ. Temporal lobe necrosis following radiation therapy for nasopharyngeal carcinoma: 1H MR spectroscopic findings. Int J Radiat Oncol Biol Phys 1999;45(3):699–705
147. Chan YL, Leung SF, King AD, Choi PH, Metreweli C. Late radiation injury to the temporal lobes: morphologic evaluation at MR imaging. Radiology 1999;213(3):800–807
148. Leung GK, Chan SK, Hung KN. Triology of neurosurgical complications after radiotherapy for nasopharyngeal carcinoma. Surg Neurol 2007;68(4):466–470, discussion 470
149. Lee AW, Foo W, Chappell R, et al. Effect of time, dose, and fractionation on temporal lobe necrosis following radiotherapy for nasopharyngeal carcinoma. Int J Radiat Oncol Biol Phys 1998;40(1):35–42
150. Bacskulin A, Guthoff R. Neuromyotonia of the abducens nerve after hypophysectomy and radiation. Strabismus 1999;7(1):37–40
151. Dejaeger E, Goethals P. Deglutition disorder as a late sequel of radiotherapy for a pharyngeal tumor. Am J Gastroenterol 1995;90(3):493–495
152. Ebner R, Slamovits TL, Friedland S, Pearlman JL, Fowble B. Visual loss following treatment of sphenoid sinus carcinoma. Surv Ophthalmol 1995;40(1):62–68
153. Fu ER. Ocular neuromyotonia—an unusual ocular motility complication after radiation therapy for nasopharyngeal carcinoma. Ann Acad Med Singapore 1995;24(6):895–897
154. King AD, Ahuja A, Leung SF, Chan YL, Lam WW, Metreweli C. MR features of the denervated tongue in radiation induced neuropathy. Br J Radiol 1999;72(856):349–353
155. Kato K, Tomura N, Takahashi S, Watarai J. Motor denervation of tumors of the head and neck: changes in MR appearance. Magn Reson Med Sci 2002;1(3):157–164
156. Leber KA, Berglöff J, Langmann G, Mokry M, Schröttner O, Pendl G. Radiation sensitivity of visual and oculomotor pathways. Stereotact Funct Neurosurg 1995;64(Suppl 1):233–238
157. Leber KA, Berglöff J, Pendl G. Dose-response tolerance of the visual pathways and cranial nerves of the cavernous sinus to stereotactic radiosurgery. J Neurosurg 1998;88(1):43–50
158. Loevner LA, Yousem DM, Lanza DC, Kennedy DW, Goldberg AN. MR evaluation of frontal sinus osteoplastic flaps with autogenous fat grafts. AJNR Am J Neuroradiol 1995;16(8):1721–1726
159. Anzai Y, Carroll WR, Quint DJ, et al. Recurrence of head and neck cancer after surgery or irradiation: prospective comparison of 2-deoxy-2-[F-18]fluoro-D-glucose PET and MR imaging diagnoses. Radiology 1996;200(1):135–141
160. Greven KM, Williams DW III, Keyes JW Jr, et al. Positron emission tomography of patients with head and neck carcinoma before and after high dose irradiation. Cancer 1994;74(4):1355–1359
161. Mukherji SK, Drane WE, Mancuso AA, Parsons JT, Mendenhall WM, Stringer S. Occult primary tumors of the head and neck: detection with 2-[F-18] fluoro-2-deoxy-D-glucose SPECT. Radiology 1996;199(3):761–766
162. Shintani SA, Foote RL, Lowe VJ, Brown PD, Garces YI, Kasperbauer JL. Utility of PET/CT imaging performed early

after surgical resection in the adjuvant treatment planning for head and neck cancer. Int J Radiat Oncol Biol Phys 2008;70(2): 322–329
163. Abgral R, Querellou S, Potard G, et al. Does 18F-FDG PET/CT improve the detection of posttreatment recurrence of head and neck squamous cell carcinoma in patients negative for disease on clinical follow-up? J Nucl Med 2009;50(1):24–29
164. Wong RJ. Current status of FDG-PET for head and neck cancer. J Surg Oncol 2008;97(8):649–652
165. Rankin SC. PET in face and neck tumours. Cancer Imaging 2006;6:S89–S95
166. Fischman AJ, Thornton AF, Frosch MP, Swearinger B, Gonzalez RG, Alpert NM. FDG hypermetabolism associated with inflammatory necrotic changes following radiation of meningioma. J Nucl Med 1997;38(7):1027–1029
167. Lapela M, Grénman R, Kurki T, et al. Head and neck cancer: detection of recurrence with PET and 2-[F-18]fluoro-2-deoxy-D-glucose. Radiology 1995;197(1):205–211
168. Kao J, Vu HL, Genden EM, et al. The diagnostic and prognostic utility of positron emission tomography/computed tomography-based follow-up after radiotherapy for head and neck cancer. Cancer 2009;115(19):4586–4594 epub ahead of print
169. Isles MG, McConkey C, Mehanna HM. A systematic review and meta-analysis of the role of positron emission tomography in the follow up of head and neck squamous cell carcinoma following radiotherapy or chemoradiotherapy. Clin Otolaryngol 2008;33(3):210–222
170. Lee AW, Ng WT, Hung WM, et al. Major late toxicities after conformal radiotherapy for nasopharyngeal carcinoma—patient- and treatment-related risk factors. Int J Radiat Oncol Biol Phys 2009;73(4):1121–1128
171. Lee AW, Ng SH, Ho JH, et al. Clinical diagnosis of late temporal lobe necrosis following radiation therapy for nasopharyngeal carcinoma. Cancer 1988;61(8):1535–1542
172. Rabin BM, Meyer JR, Berlin JW, Marymount MH, Palka PS, Russell EJ. Radiation-induced changes in the central nervous system and head and neck. Radiographics 1996;16(5):1055–1072
173. Hecht-Leavitt C, Grossman RI, Curran WJ Jr, et al. MR of brain radiation injury: experimental studies in cats. AJNR Am J Neuroradiol 1987;8(3):427–430
174. Piquemal R, Cottier JP, Arsène S, et al. Radiation-induced optic neuropathy 4 years after radiation: report of a case followed up with MRI. Neuroradiology 1998;40(7):439–441
175. Makimoto Y, Yamamoto S, Takano H, et al. Imaging findings of radiation-induced sarcoma of the head and neck. Br J Radiol 2007;80(958):790–797
176. Mark RJ, Bailet JW, Poen J, et al. Postirradiation sarcoma of the head and neck. Cancer 1993;72(3):887–893
177. Abrigo JM, King AD, Leung SF, et al. MRI of radiation-induced tumors of the head and neck in post-radiation nasopharyngeal carcinoma. Eur Radiol 2009;19(5):1197–1205
178. Rubinstein AB, Reichenthal E, Borohov H. Radiation-induced schwannomas. Neurosurgery 1989;24(6):929–932
179. Sznajder L, Abrahams C, Parry DM, Gierlowski TC, Shore-Freedman E, Schneider AB. Multiple schwannomas and meningiomas associated with irradiation in childhood. Arch Intern Med 1996;156(16):1873–1878
180. Salvati M, Caroli E, Brogna C, Orlando ER, Delfini R. High-dose radiation-induced meningiomas. Report of five cases and critical review of the literature. Tumori 2003;89(4):443–447
181. Steeves RA, Bataini JP. Neoplasms induced by megavoltage radiation in the head and neck region. Cancer 1981;47(7): 1770–1774
182. van der Laan BF, Baris G, Gregor RT, Hilgers FJ, Balm AJ. Radiation-induced tumours of the head and neck. J Laryngol Otol 1995;109(4):346–349
183. Huber GF, Matthews TW, Dort JC. Radiation-induced soft tissue sarcomas of the head and neck. J Otolaryngol 2007;36(2):93–97

4 Olfaction and Taste

Erin K. O'Brien, Jose G. Gurrola II, and Donald A. Leopold

The sense of smell plays an important role in the enjoyment of life, from the flavor of food, to social interactions, to the appreciation of one's surroundings. Loss or disruption of olfaction has a significant impact on a person's life with studies showing significant reduction in quality of life scores, increased depression, weight changes, and decreased social interactions.[1–3] Patients with olfactory disorders report increased incidence of olfactory-related hazardous events, such as an inability to detect fires, spoiled food, gas leaks, or cooking-related incidents.[4] For some, loss of the sense of smell may impact their ability to work, such as firemen or plumbers, or affect their ability to care for their families, as in the case of food preparation. Patients with olfactory dysfunction may present with primary complaints of smell or taste (flavor) disruptions, but disorders of chemoreception are common in patients who are unaware of their disability, especially with increasing age.[5–8] This chapter reviews the anatomy and physiology of the olfactory system and describes causes of olfactory dysfunction. The evaluation and testing of olfactory and taste disorders are discussed, as well as treatment and counseling for patients, including the issues of safety and quality of life.

■ Anatomy of the Olfactory System

The olfactory epithelium resides in an area of a few square centimeters in the superior nasal cavity on the cribriform plate, upper septum, and medial superior and middle turbinates in the olfactory cleft. The pseudostratified columnar epithelium is thicker than the surrounding respiratory epithelium and can be visualized in the upper nasal cavity as paler in appearance than the pinker surrounding respiratory epithelium. In human fetuses, the olfactory mucosa is a continuous zone of olfactory epithelium, but in adults, clumps of respiratory epithelium are mixed with the olfactory epithelium. This intermixed respiratory mucosa increases with age, presumably due to a loss of primary olfactory neurons.

The olfactory epithelium consists of the olfactory mucosa and the underlying lamina propria, which are separated by a basal lamella. The cell types of the mucosa consist of the olfactory receptor neurons, the sustentacular and microvillar cells, and the basal cells (**Figs. 4.1 and 4.2**). The olfactory receptor neurons (ORN) are bipolar neurons with dendrites extending to the epithelial surface and axons extending intracranially and synapsing at the olfactory bulb. The dendrite has a thickened ending or knob containing nonmotile cilia which increase the functional surface area of the olfactory epithelium to 22 cm^2 and hold the olfactory receptors that bind odorants. The unmyelinated axon of each ORN joins other axons to form myelinated fascicles or fibers (filae olfactoria). The ~50 filae of cranial nerve (CN) I travel through the foramina of the cribriform plate to synapse in the olfactory bulb. The sustentacular cells insulate the bipolar receptor neurons and regulate the composition of the mucus covering the epithelium. They also feature high concentrations of cytochrome P450, responsible for metabolizing foreign molecules and protecting the olfactory epithelium. The function of the microvillar cells is currently unknown. Located within the lamina propria are Bowman's glands, which send ducts through the basal lamella to the surface of the epithelium. These glands provide the mucus layer, which covers the cilia of the ORN dendrites. Hydrophilic odorant substances dissolve in the aqueous mucus, whereas hydrophobic molecules interact with olfactory binding proteins before binding with olfactory receptors.

Olfactory epithelium is unique in its ability to replace damaged or injured neural tissue. Two types of basal cells, globose and horizontal cells, are responsible for regeneration of the olfactory epithelium. After injury, basal cells can divide and differentiate into all cell lineages, including olfactory neurons. The ability of the olfactory epithelium to regenerate appears to decrease with age or with increasing severity of injury, resulting in increased replacement with respiratory epithelium.

In 2004, the Nobel Prize for Physiology or Medicine was awarded to Richard Axel and Linda B. Buck for the discoveries of the family of genes coding for the olfactory receptors and the description of the organization of the olfactory system.[9] The identification and characterization of mammalian odorant receptors has been reviewed by Reed.[10] The olfactory receptors on the cilia of the ORNs are transmembrane G-protein coupled receptors. After the binding of an odorant to the receptor, cAMP is generated, resulting in depolarization of the cell and firing of an action potential along the axon. Each ORN contains only one type of olfactory receptor. The human genome contains 1,000 olfactory receptor genes, of which 350 functionally code for unique receptors.

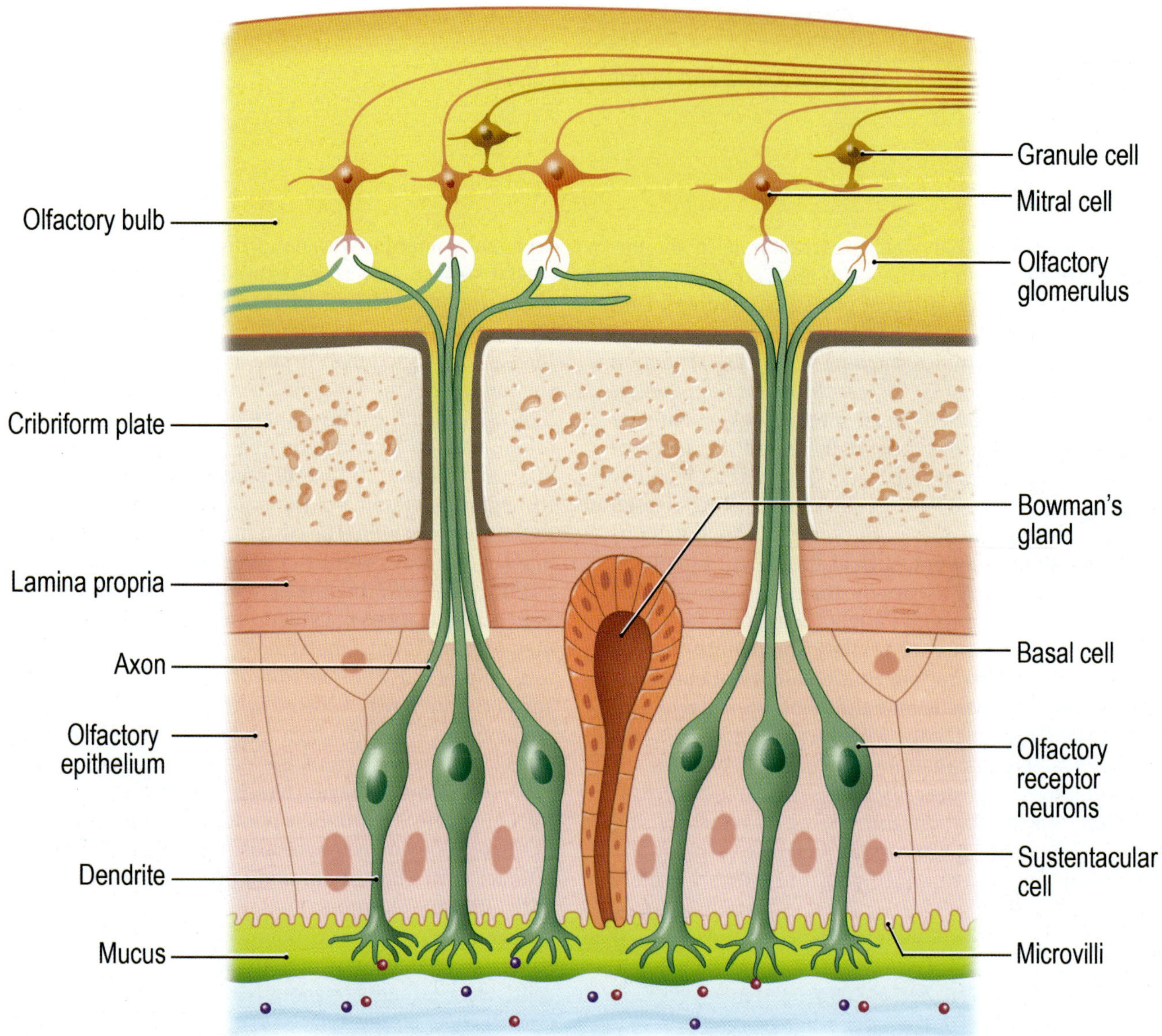

Fig. 4.1 Illustration of the olfactory epithelium and the olfactory bulb.

Most odorants can bind to and stimulate multiple olfactory receptors, whereas each receptor can likely bind multiple odorants; this combination allows for the identification of thousands of different odors by humans. The axons of ORNs expressing the same olfactory receptors converge and synapse on the same glomerulus within the olfactory bulb.

The olfactory bulb lies in the anterior cranial fossa inferior to the frontal lobe (**Fig. 4.3**). Olfactory nerve bundles synapse with the second-order neurons within thousands of glomeruli of the bulb. Within the bulb are located principal cells (mitral and tufted cells) and intrinsic neurons or interneurons. Axons from mitral and tufted cells leave the bulb as the lateral olfactory tract. These extend to the olfactory cortex, which includes the anterior olfactory cortex connecting the two olfactory bulbs, olfactory tubercle, the pyriform cortex (the main olfactory discrimination area), the cortical nucleus of the amygdala, and the entorhinal area, which projects to the hippocampus. Further connections include the medial dorsal nucleus of the thalamus, which is involved in conscious perception of odors, whereas the limbic system connections may be involved in the formation of strong olfactory memories.

Odorants reach the olfactory cleft and olfactory epithelium either anteriorly through the nares or retronasally through the oropharynx and nasopharynx into the nasal cavity. This retronasal airflow is responsible for the appreciation of the flavor of food and is why patients with olfactory disorders may present initially with complaints about taste, even with intact taste

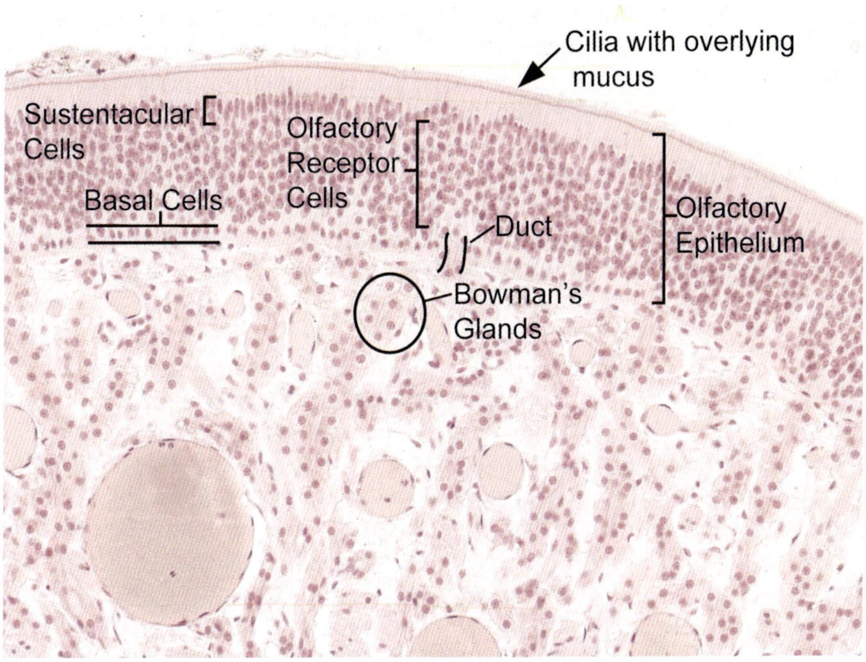

Fig. 4.2 Histology of the olfactory epithelium at 20× magnification. (Courtesy of the University of Iowa's Department of Pathology Virtual Slidebox.)

discrimination.[11] Ophthalmic and maxillary branches of the trigeminal nerve are present within the nasal cavity and respond to chemical irritants, including ammonia, and are responsible for resulting nasal mucosal edema, mucous secretion, tearing, and sneezing.

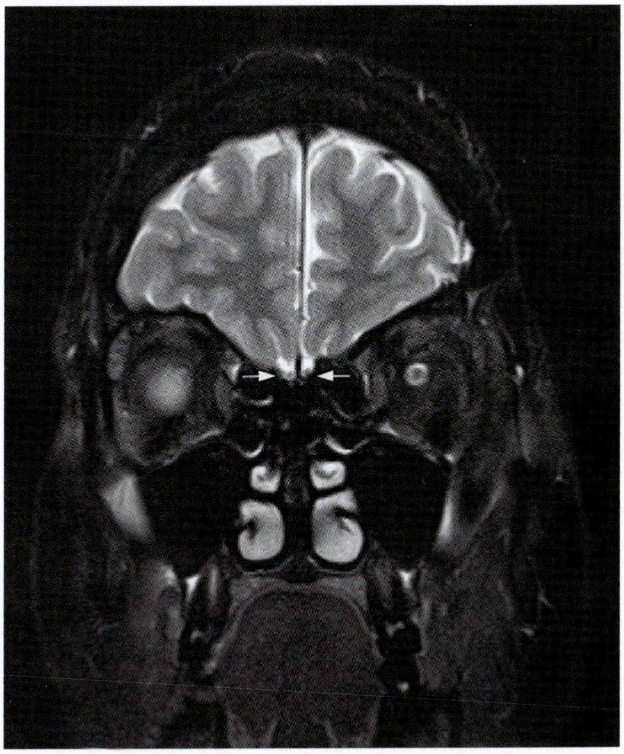

Fig. 4.3 High-resolution T2-weighted magnetic resonance image in the coronal plane demonstrates the olfactory bulb/tracts (*arrows*) in the anterior cranial fossa inferior to the frontal lobe.

Clinical Olfactory Disorders

Olfactory disorders can be classified as either the loss of ability to detect odorants or the distortion of odors and are classified as "-osmias." Anosmia refers to complete loss of the ability to detect odorants, whereas hyposmia is a decreased ability to smell. Dysosmia refers to distortion of the quality of odors, and includes parosmia, the perception of an altered sense of smell. Patients may complain that a particular odorant now has a new, often unpleasant odor, such as food smelling foul or putrid, and can be associated with loss of smell sensitivity. Phantosmia, another form of dysosmia, is the perception of an odor when no odorant is present. Dysosmias are far less common than either hyposmia or anosmia. However, parosmia and phantosmia can be significantly disruptive for patients, as the odors they perceive tend to be quite unpleasant and may smell like leaking gas, burning, or rotten fumes and may not be masked by foods, thus affecting their ability to eat or enjoy daily activities.[12,13]

Surveys of randomly selected adults have found a 1.4% prevalence of self-reported olfactory disorders in the general population.[6] The actual prevalence of olfactory disorders, as identified by odor identification objective testing, occurs at a much higher range of up to 20%, with nearly 5% with anosmia and 15% with hyposmia.[7,8] This discrepancy may be due partly to older adults not recognizing their loss of olfactory ability. Although only 1% of the population younger than 65 years has major olfactory dysfunction, the sense of smell decreases significantly with age, with a 50% incidence of olfactory loss in persons between 65 and 80 years and over 60% incidence after age 80.[3,5]

Similar to the classification of hearing loss, disorders of olfaction can also be divided into conductive or sensorineural loss, including both peripheral and central causes (**Table 4.1**). Epidemiologic studies of olfactory disorders find the most common causes to include post-upper respiratory infection (URI; 26–36%); nasal and sinus disease (both obstructive polypoid disease and inflammatory disease of the neural olfactory epithelium; 15–21%); head trauma (17–18%); and toxins/drugs, congenital, and idiopathic (18–22%). However, reviews of olfactory disorders have listed over 200 etiologies.[1]

Conductive Olfactory Disorders

The presence of sinonasal polyps can decrease nasal airflow and block the access of odorants to the olfactory epithelium; however, patients may still have some retronasal airflow, allowing the ability to detect the flavor of food. Other causes of decreased nasal airflow include nasal septal deformities, tracheostomy, previous laryngectomy, or nasal cavity tumors. Although rhinosinusitis may cause a conductive loss, and a change in the sense of smell is one of the most predictive symptoms of true rhinosinusitis, evidence also points to a sensorineural olfactory loss especially with long-standing inflammatory disease.[14,15] Sinonasal tumors, including esthesioneuroblastomas, inverted papillomas, or sinonasal malignancies, may cause a conductive olfactory loss and may be associated with epistaxis, headache, or airflow obstruction.

Sensorineural Olfactory Disorders

Post-Upper Respiratory Infections

Loss of olfaction after a URI is one of the most common causes of smell disorders, and occurs more commonly in women and the elderly.[1,16] Olfactory dysfunction during a URI can initially be conductive, but persistence of loss of smell after resolution of other symptoms indicates sensorineural injury to the olfactory epithelium. In patients with post-viral olfactory dysfunction, the presence of rhinovirus, coronavirus, parainfluenza virus, and Epstein-Barr virus have been detected in the nasal discharge.[17] Patients may present with hyposmia, anosmia, or dysosmia, with a higher incidence of hyposmia than is seen with other sensorineural causes of olfactory disorders and more parosmias than other causes.[1,16] The exact mechanism of injury is unknown, but biopsies of olfactory epithelium reveal patchy degeneration, suggesting direct injury to the olfactory epithelium, either from viral injury or the inflammatory reaction. The epithelium exhibits marked disorganization with few receptors in patients with anosmia and reduced numbers of receptors in patches in patients with hyposmia, and the olfactory bulb has decreased volume.[18,19] Patients with post-URI loss can experience some degree of recovery, but the likelihood of recovery decreases with increasing age, severity of loss, and duration of loss. Improvement varies in different studies, with 32 to 67% of patients showing significant improvement after URI olfactory loss, but less than 10% improve into the absolute normal range and less than 15% into the age-adjusted normal range.[20–22]

The viral-associated loss of olfactory neurons may actually be protective; the death of virally infected olfactory neurons may prevent the passage of viruses to the central nervous system (CNS). Certain viruses can enter the brain through an olfactory route, as the olfactory neurons provide a direct connection from the environment at the epithelial level to their first synapse within the olfactory bulb.[23,24] During the polio outbreak of the early 20th century, poliovirus was initially thought to penetrate the CNS through the olfactory epithelium, and in North America, attempts to prevent polio infection in children included treatment of the nose with zinc sulfate and Pontocaine. This did not prevent spread of the infection (later found to spread by fecal-oral transmission) and left ~10 to 15% of the patients anosmic.[25] Some strains of influenza A have been found in the brains of mice infected through an olfactory transmission, whereas other strains of the virus cause apoptosis of olfactory neurons. The viral particles are enclosed in apoptotic bodies of dying cells and cleared by the surrounding olfactory epithelium and are not transmitted to the olfactory bulb. Herpes simplex virus (HSV) causing encephalitis localizes to the frontotemporal regions of the brain, and HSV antigen has been found in the olfactory tract and cortex. These findings support the theory that virally infected olfactory epithelium undergoes apoptosis to prevent viral CNS infection, resulting in a loss of olfactory neurons and olfactory dysfunction after URI.[23,24] Although the mechanism of injury may differ from direct viral invasion of the olfactory epithelium, patients infected with HIV exhibit increased olfactory thresholds early in the disease.[26]

Table 4.1 Common Causes of Olfactory Dysfunction

Conductive	
	Rhinosinusitis
	Nasal polyposis
	Nasal cavity tumor
Sensorineural	
	Post-URI/viral
	Trauma and head injury
	Congenital
	Toxins
	Medications
	Aging
	Neurodegenerative disorders
	Alzheimer disease
	Parkinson disease

Abbreviations: URI, upper respiratory infection.

Trauma and Head Injury

Posttraumatic loss of smell is characterized by a sudden onset of olfactory dysfunction. Unlike post-URI loss, traumatic injury more commonly results in complete anosmia or dysosmia.[1–3] The mechanism includes injury anywhere along the olfactory tract, including stretching or shearing of olfactory fibers through the cribriform plate, injury to the olfactory bulb or frontal cortex, or central brain trauma to the olfactory regions. A mouse model of traumatic injury includes surgical removal of the olfactory bulb or olfactory nerve axotomy in mice, causing retrograde degeneration of the olfactory receptor neurons. Regenerating ORNs attempts to regrow them through the cribriform plate to resynapse with the olfactory bulb, but if they are unable to reconnect, the ORNs do not survive.[27] Biopsies in patients with posttraumatic olfactory dysfunction reveal disorganization of the epithelium with fewer mature neurons and an increased number of immature neurons lacking projecting cilia with receptors.[18] A disordered reconnection of olfactory neuron axons to the olfactory bulb or a loss of some of the receptors responsible for complex odor identification is hypothesized to be responsible for dysosmias following traumatic injury with perception of changes in odor, similar to synkinesis after a facial nerve injury.[27]

The severity of head injury is associated with the severity of olfactory loss. Loss of consciousness, facial or skull fractures, or occipital and lateral blows are more likely to be associated with anosmia than less severe head injuries or frontal blows.[28–30] Although some studies have found a lower rate of recovery of olfactory ability after head trauma compared with URI olfactory loss, more recent research has found a similar likelihood of recovery.[20–22] The authors concluded that the amount of olfactory loss, not the origin or causative factor, is the determinant of prognosis, and more severe loss is less likely to improve significantly.[20] Due to comorbidities associated with significant head injury, olfactory deficits may not be noted at the time of the trauma and patients may not present until after recovery from other injuries. Sinonasal fractures causing conductive loss are extremely rare. Finally, iatrogenic injury to the olfactory nerves or bulb may occur with an anterior craniotomy or neurosurgical procedures, resulting in anosmia.

Congenital Loss

Congenital anosmia accounts for ~3% of anosmia and is usually an isolated finding. These patients often present during their preteen or teenage years with an inability to smell, often discovered by family members. Patients with a congenital lack of olfactory ability may not recognize their olfactory dysfunction and have no recollection of detecting odors. They may have distinct food preferences due to their inability to appreciate the flavor of food while retaining the ability to detect the fundamental taste sensations from the taste buds. Recent studies have demonstrated that genetic mutations in the gene *SCN9A*, which encodes the voltage-gated sodium channel $Na_v1.7$, cause congenital anosmia.[31] *SCN9A* loss of function mutations were originally studied in patients with congenital analgesia, although studies in both humans and mice have demonstrated patients with these mutations also have an inability to detect odors.

Although most congenital losses are isolated, associations exist between congenital anosmia and several abnormalities including Kallmann syndrome, holoprosencephaly, anterior neuropore anomalies, and Turner syndrome. Kallmann syndrome consists of anosmia and hypogonadotropic hypogonadism and has autosomal or X-linked forms. Patients usually lack olfactory bulbs and the gonadotropin-releasing hormone, resulting in hypogonadism. The defects are due to a lack of migration of GnRH-releasing cells from the olfactory placode to the hypothalamus and a lack of migration of the olfactory neurons to the olfactory bulb and hypothalamus.[32] Depending on the cause of anosmia, magnetic resonance imaging (MRI) findings may reveal aplasia or hypoplasia of the olfactory bulb, or associated encephalocele or abnormality in the frontal lobe (**Fig. 4.4**).

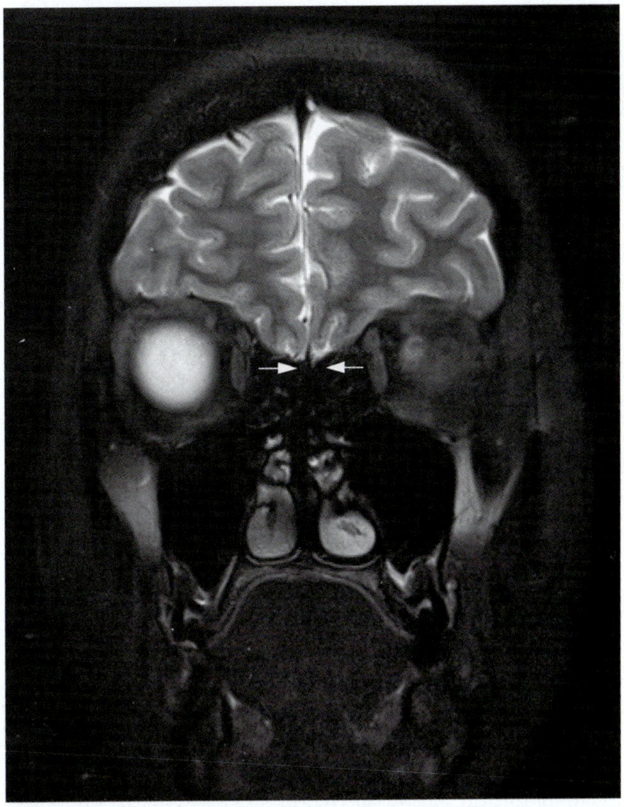

Fig. 4.4 Lack of olfactory bulbs or tracts (*arrows*) in a 21-year-old woman with congenital anosmia on a T2-weighted high-resolution coronal magnetic resonance image.

Toxins

The number of patients with olfactory dysfunction attributed to toxin exposure is relatively low (2%), but a large number of toxins are associated with olfactory loss.[3] The olfactory receptor neurons are in direct contact with the environment, leaving them vulnerable to inhaled toxins. Damage to the olfactory epithelium can occur with acute, high levels of toxin exposure or with chronic low-level exposure, which may cause more gradual olfactory decline. If the regenerating cells are spared, the olfactory neurons may regenerate after acute toxic injury, but with more severe injury to the olfactory epithelium or with chronic injury and increasing age, the regenerative potential may decrease, causing noticeable olfactory loss. In addition to direct environmental exposure, systemic toxins may cause injury to the olfactory epithelium and neurons. Within the supporting cells and Bowman's glands are high levels of xenobiotic enzymes, including cytochrome P450 monooxygenases and other biotransformation enzymes.[33] These enzymes detoxify inhaled or systemic substances, presumably to protect the olfactory neurons and CNS, or to process odorant molecules for receptor activation. Byproducts of these enzymes may include toxic metabolites, which themselves may damage the olfactory epithelium.

Specific metals, gases, and solvents have all been associated with olfactory dysfunction. Metals, in the form of dust or fumes, can be toxic to the olfactory system. The most well-known is cadmium, used in the production of batteries, semiconductors, and electroplating, and studies have documented olfactory deficits in workers exposed to cadmium, including correlating deficits in olfactory scores and cadmium levels.[34,35] Factory workers exposed to chromium, which is often used with nickel in industrial manufacturing and steel production, can have increased olfactory thresholds.[36] Additional metals linked to olfactory loss include manganese, mercury, aluminum, and lead. Gas exposure from industrial plants or pollution may damage the olfactory epithelium, either from acute high-dose or chronic low-dose exposure, and can include formaldehyde, methyl bromide, and styrene. Solvents including toluene and paint solvents have also been linked to decreased olfactory function.[37]

Tobacco smoke exposure is associated with hyposmia in active smokers.[38] Rat studies find increased olfactory receptor neuron apoptosis with tobacco smoke exposure, suggesting that the smoke causes increased cell death from toxic exposure.[39] In one study, the olfactory scores of former smokers were not significantly different than the scores in lifelong nonsmokers, suggesting that the olfactory ability can return with cessation of smoking.[5]

In addition to specific industrial toxins and tobacco smoke, exposure to elevated levels of airborne environmental pollution may lead to changes in olfaction. The specific makeup of air pollution varies by region, but is likely to include a variety of gases, large and fine particulate matter, organic compounds, and even various nanoparticles depending on the local industry and environment. Studies examining populations in busy urban centers exposed to chronically increased levels of environmental pollution show that these patients have increased olfactory and trigeminal thresholds.[40,41] Although their ability to detect and identify odorants and respond to irritants remains intact, the levels at which these patients respond to these stimuli are much higher than in control populations. In the aftermath of the collapse of the World Trade Center (WTC) on September 11, 2001, nearby residents and early responders experienced exposure to levels of pollution well beyond those typically found even in large, urban city centers. Similar to the populations exposed to lower, although still chronically elevated, levels of pollution, initial studies of people near the WTC collapse indicated changes in olfactory and trigeminal nerve irritation thresholds.[42] Participants in this initial study did not demonstrate a deficit of odorant detection when compared with control groups based on a 20-odor smell identification test. However, a more recent study used the Smell Identification Test to evaluate a similar group exposed to very high levels of pollution following the WTC collapse. A statistically significant decrease in odorant identification was seen in those patients exposed to high levels of pollution.[43] The results of these studies suggest both chronic exposure to elevated levels of air pollution and short-term exposure to dramatically increased levels of air pollution could significantly impact olfaction.

Medications

Hundreds of medications list chemosensory disturbances as possible side effects of the drugs, although there are few clinical studies as to the causality of medications and smell disorders. The effect of medication on olfaction may affect the olfactory epithelium and mucus, neurotransmission, or higher CNS processing. Several major classes of medications may cause smell disturbances or changes in taste (discussed later). The clinician should differentiate a change in flavor, which is olfactory, versus a gustatory change with taste loss—including sweet, sour, bitter, or salty—or the presence of a bad taste, with more medications causing gustatory dysfunction. If possible, changing or removing medication may reverse the effects on chemosensory perception.

The use of intranasal zinc gluconate for the treatment of URIs has been associated with a loss in the sense of smell, although this has been debated in the literature. The common scenario includes the use of the zinc gluconate followed by a burning sensation in the nose and a loss in the sense of smell.[44,45] Rodent studies have found only transient effects of zinc gluconate on the olfactory mucosa, but some children treated with intranasal zinc sulfate during the polio outbreak in the last century did develop permanent anosmia.[25,46] Because the use of intranasal zinc gluconate corresponds with the presence of a URI, a known cause of smell disorders, it may be difficult to differentiate the exact mechanism of olfactory loss.

Aging and Neurodegenerative Disorders

Decline in olfactory ability is found with increasing age and is responsible for significant impairment in the quality of life for older patients. Within the population, 20% of those 65 years of age experience olfactory dysfunction, and this increases to more than half by 80 years of age.[5] Olfactory loss is associated with less olfactory epithelium and a decreased size of the olfactory bulb with increasing age.[27,47] The regenerative ability of the olfactory epithelium appears to decline with age, possibly from a lifetime of insults from toxins, viruses, and medications. Olfactory neurons routinely die in 3- to 7-week cycles, but with diminished regeneration, the olfactory epithelium is gradually replaced with respiratory epithelium. Although olfactory dysfunction is common in the elderly population, self-reporting of olfactory deficits can be significantly underestimated, putting the elderly population at higher risk of accidents from fires, gas leaks, or spoiled food.[1,5] Loss of flavor perception also decreases the enjoyment of food and may cause decreased or poor nutritional intake.

In patients with Alzheimer and Parkinson diseases, ~90% exhibit olfactory dysfunction in the early stages of the diseases. Olfactory loss may be the first clinical sign of these neurodegenerative diseases, preceding signs of dementia in Alzheimer disease (AD) or motor symptoms in Parkinson disease (PD) by several years.[48,49] Neurofibrillary tangles and neuritic plaques appear in the olfactory bulb, anterior olfactory nucleus, and olfactory cortex in patients with AD, and olfactory neurons show signs of oxidative stress in the epithelium of patients with AD.[50] Apolipoprotein ϵ4 allele is associated with AD, and elderly patients with one allele without the signs of dementia exhibit significant decline in odor identification over a 4-year period.[51] In patients with one allele and anosmia, the risk of cognitive decline was twice that of patients with one allele with normosmia over a 2-year period and nearly five times the risk of cognitive decline seen in patients without anosmia and without the ϵ4 allele.[52] First-degree family members of patients with AD were found to have significantly reduced smell identification scores, pointing to genetic predisposition in the development of the disease.[53] In addition to poor odor identification, unawareness of smell impairment is also associated with AD; patients do not usually present with complaints of smell or flavor dysfunction. Olfactory testing may be more useful than tests of global cognition in predicting cognitive decline.[52] Although a home screening test for AD with a 12-item smell identification test is commercially available and sold to the public, the test has not been evaluated for reliability or validity and lacks appropriate counseling or professional oversight.[54]

Olfactory dysfunction is seen in both treated and untreated patients with idiopathic PD, and Lewy pathology is found in the olfactory bulb and tract early in the disease.[55,56] Smell deficits are more commonly seen in PD than in other diseases with parkinsonian symptoms and may help differentiate PD from other diseases such as essential tremor.[57–59] Smell identification is the most accurate predictor of the presence of PD compared with healthy controls in motor and nonmotor diagnostic tests for PD.[60] Because of the implication of viruses and environmental toxins in the development of AD and PD with the finding of early olfactory loss, some theorize that these diseases may be caused by agents entering the brain through an olfactory route.[61] Huntington disease is also characterized by olfactory deficits and findings of degeneration of central olfactory degeneration.[62] Odor detection and identification scores are decreased in patients with HIV and cognitive decline and may be early indicators of HIV-associated dementia.[26,63] Olfactory deficits are also present in patients with schizophrenia and in their asymptomatic first-degree relatives.[64]

Previous case reports and studies have suggested changes in olfactory function in patients with multiple sclerosis (MS), including a case report with parageusia and smell disturbances as the initial presenting clinical symptoms.[65,66] A more recent study suggested that almost 50% of patients within a known MS study group demonstrated hyposmia.[67] Almost 20% of this MS patient group demonstrated taste disorders as well. Although many patients may present with other clinical symptoms well before changes in taste and smell, patients with acute changes should be considered for the possibility of MS. Likewise, clinicians should be prepared to counsel patients with MS regarding alterations in and loss of taste and smell.

Intracranial Aneurysm/Subarachnoid Hemorrhage

Olfactory disturbances have been described in patients with intracranial aneurysms, particularly aneurysms involving the anterior communicating artery. Damage to the olfactory system may occur as a result of the treatment of an unruptured aneurysm, as the result of aneurysmal-related subarachnoid hemorrhage (SAH) itself or as a result of the treatment of a ruptured aneurysm.

Olfactory changes have been shown to occur in patient populations undergoing unruptured aneurysm treatment as well as in patients with ruptured aneurysms presenting with SAH.[68–70] In one study, surgical clipping of unruptured aneurysms led to olfactory dysfunction in several patients postoperatively, whereas patients who underwent endovascular coiling of unruptured aneurysms did not demonstrate olfactory dysfunction.[68] The location of the olfactory bulb and nerve make them susceptible to damage via the open approach required for surgical clipping. In patients with aneurysmal SAH, studies demonstrate that olfactory dysfunction may occur in patients treated with either surgical clipping or endovascular coiling.[68–70] At least one study has demonstrated that patients who underwent endovascular coiling of ruptured aneurysms recovered olfactory function more frequently than those who underwent surgical clipping, although patients from both groups experienced olfactory changes. The presence of dysfunction postrupture with endovascular coiling emphasizes the potential for SAH itself to cause changes in olfactory function.[69,70] Cerebral vasospasm and frontal lobe lesions have also been described as factors related to worse olfactory performance in patients treated with endovascular coiling.[69] Although further studies are necessary to determine the risk of specific treatment measures on unruptured aneurysms, it is clear that both preemptive aneurysmal and post-SAH surgical interventions can lead to olfactory dysfunction. In addition to the other neurologic symptoms these patients may seek treatment for after the acute phase of their treatment, it is important to recognize the counseling and social interventions that should occur as related to their olfactory dysfunction.

Workup and Therapeutic Options

Clinical History

A detailed history should include the duration and degree of olfactory loss and an inquiry in the status of chemosensory ability prior to the present complaint of olfactory dysfunction. Patients may present with taste alteration, but may be experiencing decreased flavor due to an olfactory disorder with the preservation of taste perceptions of sweet, bitter, sour, and salt. True gustatory loss is much less common than olfactory loss. Events occurring around the time of the noticed loss of olfactory ability may include URI, head injury, toxin or fume exposure, or surgery. In patients with a fluctuating smell ability or a gradual onset of dysfunction, rhinosinusitis or polyps may be the cause and nasal symptoms should be assessed. Patients should provide examples of what they can smell or should attempt to describe the odors they perceive with dysosmias. For patients with phantosmia, there may be a history of triggers or periods during the day when the smell is not present. Other pertinent history includes epistaxis or nasal airway obstruction, CNS complaints, endocrine abnormalities, occupational or tobacco exposure, or a history of neurodegenerative disorders in the patient or in the family history, as well as a review of medications.

Physical exam should consist of a complete ear, nose, and throat examination with an emphasis on nasal airway evaluation. Nasal endoscopy is warranted for the evaluation of nasal airflow obstruction blocking access to the olfactory cleft from septal deviation or polyps, the presence of tumors, mucosal edema or postoperative changes, crusting, or scarring. For patients with parosmia or phantosmia localized to one nostril, blocking that nostril to airflow may change the patient's perception of the abnormal smell. Cranial nerve function should be assessed as well as an evaluation of mental status for AD or motor function for PD.

Imaging

Computed tomography (CT) scans of the nasal cavity, paranasal sinuses, and anterior skull base may be indicated in the evaluation of olfactory disorders when the symptoms or olfactory tests do not fit a particular diagnosis. Coronal scans can evaluate the patency of the olfactory cleft and can help to rule out tumors or deformities in the anterior cranial fossa. MRI can further evaluate the extent of soft tissue masses or aid in the evaluation of the CNS, including olfactory tracts and olfactory bulbs (**Fig. 4.3**). Olfactory bulbs are absent in anosmia with Kallmann syndrome (**Fig. 4.4**), and bulbs may have decreased volume in patients with trauma-induced anosmia or olfactory disorders with schizophrenia.[29,71]

Olfactory Testing

An assessment of olfactory ability is necessary for establishing the degree of olfactory loss and allows for objective monitoring of changes in olfactory ability over time. In addition, testing may help detect malingerers or establish compensation for permanent disability. Psychophysical tests include self-administered tests that are clinically useful in the diagnosis of olfactory disorders and are widely commercially available. Smell identification tests require the patient to smell an odorant and choose the correct name from a multiple-choice test. One such test is the Smell Identification Test (SIT, also known as the University of Pennsylvania Smell Identification Test or UPSIT) that was noted previously, which includes 40 "scratch and sniff" odorants with four possible answers and is self-administered. Norms have been established by age and gender and have been classified as normosmia, microsomia, or anosmia, with scores below 5 to 6 suggesting malingering (as 10 out of 40 is considered chance performance).[72] The Cross-Cultural Smell Identification Test (CC-SIT), also known as the Brief Smell Identification Test (B-SIT), is a 12-item version of the SIT, which includes odors most consistently identified by subjects in various countries and is a useful screening tool for more rapid screening.[73] The "Sniffin' Sticks" test incorporates odor threshold or the lowest concentration of detectable odorants, odor discrimination or ability to correctly choose a target odorant, and odor identification using multiple choices for a combination score for threshold, discrimination, and identification (TDI). Normative data have also been established for normal and affected patients based on TDI scores.[74] These tests can be administered bilaterally or unilaterally by occluding one nostril to assess for laterality of olfactory deficits when appropriate.

Electrophysiological tests are available but are primarily used for research purposes. Odor event-related potentials measure brain-evoked potentials from electroencephalograms averaged after multiple exposures to an odorant.[75] Another procedure is the electro-olfactogram, which involves placing an electrode directly on the olfactory epithelium. A slow-negative shift in voltage is detected with the introduction of an odorant to stimulate the olfactory receptor neurons. The placement of these electrodes can be unpleasant for the patient and can be technically difficult in the endoscopic manipulation of the electrode and an inability to confirm placement in the olfactory rather than the respiratory epithelium.[76] Recent studies have found preliminary evidence of an intrinsic optical signal, which is visible using 600 to 700 nm wavelength light when the olfactory epithelium is stimulated by odorants. This may be useful for evaluating the function of a region of the epithelium rather than one isolated spot as is measured with an electrode in an electro-olfactogram.[77]

Therapy

Once the diagnosis of an olfactory disorder has been established, both therapy and management of the deficit should be addressed. For patients with a decreased smell ability, the physician must counsel the patient concerning necessary safety issues. Multiple functional smoke detectors are a patient's best protection against fires in the home or workplace. If a patient lives in a home with a natural gas furnace or appliances, a natural gas detector should be purchased and installed close to the appliances, as the patient will not detect the mercaptan or sulfur-based odor added to the odorless gas in the event of a leak. If practical, replacing gas appliances with electric is advisable. Patients should be aware of the expiration date of foods and ask a family member or friend to help them monitor for spoiled food in their refrigerator and potentially advise them on personal hygiene. For patients with both anosmia and dementia, these safety issues can be even more important and need to be addressed with caregivers.

For conductive causes of olfactory loss, the correction of the obstruction may result in improvement in olfactory ability, such as an ethmoidectomy or the treatment of nasal polyposis. Olfactory loss secondary to chronic rhinosinusitis may resolve with medical or surgical treatment of the underlying disease, such as allergy management, antibiotics, or functional endoscopic sinonasal surgery. Treatment with steroids may benefit conductive loss; although long-term systemic steroid therapy is not advised secondary to side effects, the application of topical steroid drops in a head-down position may be useful for reaching the olfactory cleft. Steroid nasal sprays have not been shown to be effective in the treatment of olfactory disorders because the spray fails to reach the olfactory epithelium.

For sensorineural olfactory loss, increased severity and duration of olfactory loss point to a poorer prognosis for recovery of olfactory ability. Repeating olfactory testing after an initial assessment may be helpful in counseling a patient as to the prognosis of their dysfunction. Improvement in scores after an olfactory loss from an upper respiratory infection or trauma may occur before the patient notices perceivable improvement. Except in the rare cases of olfactory disorders caused by vitamin or mineral deficits, no studies have found conclusive benefit from vitamin or mineral therapy or the use of drugs for the improvement of sensorineural olfactory loss above the level of spontaneous recovery.

The loss of food flavor can significantly affect patients' quality of life and can impact their nutritional status. Patients should experiment with new textures, colors, spiciness, and other taste cues in their foods and may find that foods they previously did not enjoy are more palatable. Oversalting may be a substitute for the lost flavor and should be avoided. For patients with hyposmia, repeated exposure to odors may help "retrain" their nose to identify odorants, such as smelling spice jars or foods.

The diagnosis and explanation of olfactory disorders can be reassuring to patients who now have a better understanding of their disorder as well as assurance that they are not alone. For patients with parosmias, their perception of foul and unpleasant odors may improve over time, but for others, this disorder can be significantly disruptive in their lives, affecting their ability to eat, concentrate, and enjoy life. The use of gabapentin or clonazepam may be beneficial in the treatment of parosmias, although this is an off-label use of these medications. Some patients have benefited from obstruction or removal of the olfactory epithelium with improvement in the parosmia, although patients should be counseled that they might lose all olfactory ability with this procedure.[78]

Taste Disorders

Patients presenting with taste complaints may in fact have olfactory dysfunction with abnormal flavor perception due to the loss of retronasal olfaction. With loss of flavor, a person may, for example, not perceive the strawberry flavor of ice cream but may still detect its sweetness. True taste loss includes a loss of perception of salty, bitter, sour, sweet, or savory (umami). Taste disorders can also include the perception of bad or metallic tastes. Taste perception occurs through the taste buds on the tongue, pharynx, larynx, and soft palate. All taste buds can perceive all taste qualities; the notion of a tongue "taste map" is a myth. Taste receptors are innervated by branches of the facial (CN VII), glossopharyngeal (CN IX), and vagus (CN X) cranial nerves to the nucleus of the solitary tract. Taste disorders include loss of taste (ageusia), partial loss of taste (hypogeusia), or altered taste (dysgeusia), including distortion with stimulus (parageusia) or without stimulus (phantogeusia). Taste disturbances can be due to local effects on the tongue, including local infection, injury to the papillae, mucositis, alterations in saliva, or poor oral hygiene. Injury to the chorda tympani, from trauma, ear surgery, or middle ear disease, can also affect taste. Strokes, particularly strokes involving the frontal lobe or those of the partial anterior circulation subtype, have been associated with taste disorders.[79] Renal disease or diabetes may affect taste perception, as may nutritional deficiencies. Medications that can commonly affect taste include antimicrobials, anticholinergics, antidepressants, and antihypertensives such as angiotensin-converting enzyme inhibitors, although a large number of medications include altered taste as a possible side effect. Chemotherapy and radiation to the head and neck are commonly associated with taste disorders due to effects on the saliva and changes to the mucosa.

Evaluation of taste disorders includes olfactory testing as well as the assessment of perception of salty, bitter, sweet, and sour stimuli on the tongue, and a thorough head and neck exam with radiographic imaging as indicated. Treatment of taste disorders involves treatment of underlying infections, improvement of oral hygiene and saliva, changes in medication, or treatment of systemic illness. Patients with a loss of taste can be counseled to the use of flavorings or flavor enhancers and varying color, texture, and temperature of food to maximize the enjoyment of food and to avoid nutritional deficiencies.

Conclusion

Olfactory disorders are common in the population and may be due to conductive or sensorineural causes. Evaluating smell disorders includes examining the nasal cavity and objective smell testing. Smell dysfunction can be the presenting sign of sinonasal disease, nasal masses, neurodegenerative disorders, or neurological insults. Loss of sense of smell can have serious implications for a patient's quality of life and safety, including an inability to detect gas leaks, fires, or spoiled food. As research into chemosensory function continues to expand, our greater understanding of taste and smell will likely provide more insight into the treatment of disorders of olfaction and gustation.

References

1. Temmel AF, Quint C, Schickinger-Fischer B, Klimek L, Stoller E, Hummel T. Characteristics of olfactory disorders in relation to major causes of olfactory loss. Arch Otolaryngol Head Neck Surg 2002;128(6):635–641
2. Brämerson A, Nordin S, Bende M. Clinical experience with patients with olfactory complaints, and their quality of life. Acta Otolaryngol 2007;127(2):167–174
3. Deems DA, Doty RL, Settle RG, et al. Smell and taste disorders, a study of 750 patients from the University of Pennsylvania Smell and Taste Center. Arch Otolaryngol Head Neck Surg 1991;117(5):519–528
4. Santos DV, Reiter ER, DiNardo LJ, Costanzo RM. Hazardous events associated with impaired olfactory function. Arch Otolaryngol Head Neck Surg 2004;130(3):317–319
5. Murphy C, Schubert CR, Cruickshanks KJ, Klein BE, Klein R, Nondahl DM. Prevalence of olfactory impairment in older adults. JAMA 2002;288(18):2307–2312
6. Hoffman HJ, Ishii EK, MacTurk RH. Age-related changes in the prevalence of smell/taste problems among the United States adult population. Results of the 1994 disability supplement to the National Health Interview Survey (NHIS). Ann N Y Acad Sci 1998;855:716–722
7. Brämerson A, Johansson L, Ek L, Nordin S, Bende M. Prevalence of olfactory dysfunction: the skövde population-based study. Laryngoscope 2004;114(4):733–737
8. Landis BN, Konnerth CG, Hummel T. A study on the frequency of olfactory dysfunction. Laryngoscope 2004;114(10):1764–1769
9. Buck L, Axel R. A novel multigene family may encode odorant receptors: a molecular basis for odor recognition. Cell 1991;65(1):175–187
10. Reed RR. After the holy grail: establishing a molecular basis for Mammalian olfaction. Cell 2004;116(2):329–336
11. Small DM, Gerber JC, Mak YE, Hummel T. Differential neural responses evoked by orthonasal versus retronasal odorant perception in humans. Neuron 2005;47(4):593–605
12. Bonfils P, Avan P, Faulcon P, Malinvaud D. Distorted odorant perception: analysis of a series of 56 patients with parosmia. Arch Otolaryngol Head Neck Surg 2005;131(2):107–112
13. Leopold D. Distortion of olfactory perception: diagnosis and treatment. Chem Senses 2002;27(7):611–615
14. Bhattacharyya N. Clinical and symptom criteria for the accurate diagnosis of chronic rhinosinusitis. Laryngoscope 2006; 116(7 Pt 2, Suppl 110)1–22
15. Kern RC. Chronic sinusitis and anosmia: pathologic changes in the olfactory mucosa. Laryngoscope 2000;110(7):1071–1077
16. Harris R, Davidson TM, Murphy C, Gilbert PE, Chen M. Clinical evaluation and symptoms of chemosensory impairment: one thousand consecutive cases from the Nasal Dysfunction Clinic in San Diego. Am J Rhinol 2006;20(1):101–108
17. Suzuki M, Saito K, Min WP, et al. Identification of viruses in patients with postviral olfactory dysfunction. Laryngoscope 2007;117(2):272–277
18. Jafek BW, Murrow B, Michaels R, Restrepo D, Linschoten M. Biopsies of human olfactory epithelium. Chem Senses 2002;27(7):623–628
19. Rombaux P, Mouraux A, Bertrand B, Nicolas G, Duprez T, Hummel T. Olfactory function and olfactory bulb volume in patients with postinfectious olfactory loss. Laryngoscope 2006;116(3):436–439
20. London B, Nabet B, Fisher AR, White B, Sammel MD, Doty RL. Predictors of prognosis in patients with olfactory disturbance. Ann Neurol 2008;63(2):159–166
21. Reden J, Mueller A, Mueller C, et al. Recovery of olfactory function following closed head injury or infections of the upper respiratory tract. Arch Otolaryngol Head Neck Surg 2006;132(3):265–269
22. Duncan HJ, Seiden AM. Long-term follow-up of olfactory loss secondary to head trauma and upper respiratory tract infection. Arch Otolaryngol Head Neck Surg 1995;121(10):1183–1187
23. Mori I, Nishiyama Y, Yokochi T, Kimura Y. Olfactory transmission of neurotropic viruses. J Neurovirol 2005;11(2):129–137
24. Mori I, Nishiyama Y, Yokochi T, Kimura Y. Virus-induced neuronal apoptosis as pathological and protective responses of the host. Rev Med Virol 2004;14(4):209–216
25. Rutty CJ. The middle-class plague: epidemic polio and the Canadian state, 1936-37. Can Bull Med Hist 1996;13(2):277–314
26. Mueller C, Temmel AF, Quint C, Rieger A, Hummel T. Olfactory function in HIV-positive subjects. Acta Otolaryngol 2002;122(1):67–71
27. Kern RC, Conley DB, Haines GK III, Robinson AM. Pathology of the olfactory mucosa: implications for the treatment of olfactory dysfunction. Laryngoscope 2004;114(2):279–285

28. Renzi G, Carboni A, Gasparini G, Perugini M, Becelli R. Taste and olfactory disturbances after upper and middle third facial fractures: a preliminary study. Ann Plast Surg 2002;48(4): 355–358
29. Doty RL, Yousem DM, Pham LT, Kreshak AA, Geckle R, Lee WW. Olfactory dysfunction in patients with head trauma. Arch Neurol 1997;54(9):1131–1140
30. Sandford AA, Davidson TM, Herrera N, et al. Olfactory dysfunction: a sequela of pediatric blunt head trauma. Int J Pediatr Otorhinolaryngol 2006;70(6):1015–1025
31. Weiss J, Pyrski M, Jacobi E, et al. Loss-of-function mutations in sodium channel Nav1.7 cause anosmia. Nature 2011;472(7342): 186–190
32. Kim HG, Bhagavath B, Layman LC. Clinical manifestations of impaired GnRH neuron development and function. Neurosignals 2008;16(2-3):165–182
33. Ling G, Gu J, Genter MB, Zhuo X, Ding X. Regulation of cytochrome P450 gene expression in the olfactory mucosa. Chem Biol Interact 2004;147(3):247–258
34. Sulkowski WJ, Rydzewski B, Miarzynska M. Smell impairment in workers occupationally exposed to cadmium. Acta Otolaryngol 2000;120(2):316–318
35. Mascagni P, Consonni D, Bregante G, Chiappino G, Toffoletto F. Olfactory function in workers exposed to moderate airborne cadmium levels. Neurotoxicology 2003;24(4-5):717–724
36. Kitamura F, Yokoyama K, Araki S, et al. Increase of olfactory threshold in plating factory workers exposed to chromium in Korea. Ind Health 2003;41(3):279–285
37. Gobba F. Olfactory toxicity: long-term effects of occupational exposures. Int Arch Occup Environ Health 2006;79(4):322–331
38. Sugiyama K, Hasegawa Y, Sugiyama N, Suzuki M, Watanabe N, Murakami S. Smoking-induced olfactory dysfunction in chronic sinusitis and assessment of brief University of Pennsylvania Smell Identification Test and T&T methods. Am J Rhinol 2006;20(5):439–444
39. Vent J, Robinson AM, Gentry-Nielsen MJ, et al. Pathology of the olfactory epithelium: smoking and ethanol exposure. Laryngoscope 2004;114(8):1383–1388
40. Hudson R, Arriola A, Martínez-Gómez M, Distel H. Effect of air pollution on olfactory function in residents of Mexico City. Chem Senses 2006;31(1):79–85
41. Guarneros M, Hummel T, Martínez-Gómez M, Hudson R. Mexico City air pollution adversely affects olfactory function and intranasal trigeminal sensitivity. Chem Senses 2009;34(9): 819–826
42. Dalton PH, Opiekun RE, Gould M, et al. Chemosensory loss: functional consequences of the world trade center disaster. Environ Health Perspect 2010;118(9):1251–1256
43. Altman KW, Desai SC, Moline J, et al. Odor identification ability and self-reported upper respiratory symptoms in workers at the post-9/11 World Trade Center site. Int Arch Occup Environ Health 2011;84(2):131–137
44. Alexander TH, Davidson TM. Intranasal zinc and anosmia: the zinc-induced anosmia syndrome. Laryngoscope 2006;116(2):217–220
45. Jafek BW, Linschoten MR, Murrow BW. Anosmia after intranasal zinc gluconate use. Am J Rhinol 2004;18(3):137–141
46. Slotnick B, Sanguino A, Husband S, Marquino G, Silberberg A. Olfaction and olfactory epithelium in mice treated with zinc gluconate. Laryngoscope 2007;117(4):743–749
47. Wang J, Eslinger PJ, Smith MB, Yang QX. Functional magnetic resonance imaging study of human olfaction and normal aging. J Gerontol A Biol Sci Med Sci 2005;60(4):510–514
48. Doty RL, Perl DP, Steele JC, et al. Olfactory dysfunction in three neurodegenerative diseases. Geriatrics 1991;46(Suppl 1):47–51
49. Mesholam RI, Moberg PJ, Mahr RN, Doty RL. Olfaction in neurodegenerative disease: a meta-analysis of olfactory functioning in Alzheimer's and Parkinson's diseases. Arch Neurol 1998;55(1):84–90
50. Perry G, Castellani RJ, Smith MA, et al. Oxidative damage in the olfactory system in Alzheimer's disease. Acta Neuropathol 2003;106(6):552–556
51. Calhoun-Haney R, Murphy C. Apolipoprotein epsilon4 is associated with more rapid decline in odor identification than in odor threshold or Dementia Rating Scale scores. Brain Cogn 2005;58(2):178–182
52. Graves AB, Bowen JD, Rajaram L, et al. Impaired olfaction as a marker for cognitive decline: interaction with apolipoprotein E epsilon4 status. Neurology 1999;53(7):1480–1487
53. Serby M, Mohan C, Aryan M, Williams L, Mohs RC, Davis KL. Olfactory identification deficits in relatives of Alzheimer's disease patients. Biol Psychiatry 1996;39(5):375–377
54. Kier FJ, Molinari V. "Do-it-yourself" dementia testing: issues regarding an Alzheimer's home screening test. Gerontologist 2003;43(3):295–301
55. Doty RL, Stern MB, Pfeiffer C, Gollomp SM, Hurtig HI. Bilateral olfactory dysfunction in early stage treated and untreated idiopathic Parkinson's disease. J Neurol Neurosurg Psychiatry 1992;55(2):138–142
56. Braak H, Del Tredici K, Rüb U, de Vos RA, Jansen Steur EN, Braak E. Staging of brain pathology related to sporadic Parkinson's disease. Neurobiol Aging 2003;24(2):197–211
57. Stern MB, Doty RL, Dotti M, et al. Olfactory function in Parkinson's disease subtypes. Neurology 1994;44(2):266–268
58. Shah M, Muhammed N, Findley LJ, Hawkes CH. Olfactory tests in the diagnosis of essential tremor. Parkinsonism Relat Disord 2008;14(7):563–568
59. McKinnon JH, Demaerschalk BM, Caviness JN, Wellik KE, Adler CH, Wingerchuk DM. Sniffing out Parkinson disease: can olfactory testing differentiate parkinsonian disorders? Neurologist 2007;13(6):382–385
60. Bohnen NI, Studenski SA, Constantine GM, Moore RY. Diagnostic performance of clinical motor and non-motor tests of Parkinson disease: a matched case-control study. Eur J Neurol 2008;15(7):685–691
61. Doty RL. The olfactory vector hypothesis of neurodegenerative disease: is it viable? Ann Neurol 2008;63(1):7–15
62. Barrios FA, Gonzalez L, Favila R, et al. Olfaction and neurodegeneration in HD. Neuroreport 2007;18(1):73–76
63. Zucco GM, Ingegneri G. Olfactory deficits in HIV-infected patients with and without AIDS dementia complex. Physiol Behav 2004;80(5):669–674
64. Turetsky BI, Kohler CG, Gur RE, Moberg PJ. Olfactory physiological impairment in first-degree relatives of schizophrenia patients. Schizophr Res 2008;102(1-3):220–229
65. Nocentini U, Giordano A, Castriota-Scanderbeg A, Caltagirone C. Parageusia: an unusual presentation of multiple sclerosis. Eur Neurol 2004;51(2):123–124
66. Constantinescu CS, Raps EC, Cohen JA, West SE, Doty RL. Olfactory disturbances as the initial or most prominent symptom of multiple sclerosis. J Neurol Neurosurg Psychiatry 1994;57(8):1011–1012
67. Fleiner F, Dahlslett SB, Schmidt F, Harms L, Goektas O. Olfactory and gustatory function in patients with multiple sclerosis. Am J Rhinol Allergy 2010;24(5):e93–e97
68. Moman MR, Verweij BH, Buwalda J, Rinkel GJ. Anosmia after endovascular and open surgical treatment of intracranial aneurysms. J Neurosurg 2009;110(3):482–486
69. Martin GE, Junqué C, Juncadella M, Gabarrós A, de Miquel MA, Rubio F. Olfactory dysfunction after subarachnoid hemorrhage

caused by ruptured aneurysms of the anterior communicating artery. Clinical article. J Neurosurg 2009;111(5):958–962

70. Wermer MJ, Donswijk M, Greebe P, Verweij BH, Rinkel GJ. Anosmia after aneurysmal subarachnoid hemorrhage. Neurosurgery 2007;61(5):918–922, discussion 922–923
71. Turetsky BI, Moberg PJ, Yousem DM, Doty RL, Arnold SE, Gur RE. Reduced olfactory bulb volume in patients with schizophrenia. Am J Psychiatry 2000;157(5):828–830
72. Doty RL, Shaman P, Dann M. Development of the University of Pennsylvania Smell Identification Test: a standardized microencapsulated test of olfactory function. Physiol Behav 1984;32(3):489–502
73. Doty RL, Marcus A, Lee WW. Development of the 12-item Cross-Cultural Smell Identification Test (CC-SIT). Laryngoscope 1996;106(3 Pt 1):353–356
74. Hummel T, Sekinger B, Wolf SR, Pauli E, Kobal G. 'Sniffin' sticks': olfactory performance assessed by the combined testing of odor identification, odor discrimination and olfactory threshold. Chem Senses 1997;22(1):39–52
75. Thesen T, Murphy C. Reliability analysis of event-related brain potentials to olfactory stimuli. Psychophysiology 2002;39(6):733–738
76. Knecht M, Hummel T. Recording of the human electro-olfactogram. Physiol Behav 2004;83(1):13–19
77. Ishimaru T, Reden J, Krone F, Scheibe M. Optical recordings from the human nasal mucosa in response to olfactory stimulation. Neurosci Lett 2007;423(3):231–235
78. Leopold DA, Schwob JE, Youngentob SL, Hornung DE, Wright HN, Mozell MM. Successful treatment of phantosmia with preservation of olfaction. Arch Otolaryngol Head Neck Surg 1991;117(12):1402–1406
79. Heckmann JG, Stössel C, Lang CJ, Neundörfer B, Tomandl B, Hummel T. Taste disorders in acute stroke: a prospective observational study on taste disorders in 102 stroke patients. Stroke 2005;36(8):1690–1694

5 Objective Measures of Nasal Function

John F. Pallanch

It has been said, "You wouldn't think of operating on a patient's ear without an audiogram, so why would you operate on a patient's nose without objective testing?" Despite a rapid advancement in technology that is increasing the sophistication and capability of nasal testing equipment, objective assessment of the nasal airway has largely been relegated to research in nasal physiology and clinical outcomes studies. This chapter deals with the objective assessment of nasal breathing function. For information regarding the objective assessment of other nasal functions, see Chapter 2 regarding mucociliary clearance, and Chapter 4 regarding olfaction.

Patient Selection and Indications for Testing

Candidates for nasal airway testing include patients who have nasal obstruction, or those in whom nasal airway pathology is suspected of contributing to other conditions such as sleep disordered breathing, voice problems, or allergy. Objective airway testing is also used for research.

Like any test, nasal airway testing should be used in those cases in which it can reveal information that may change the course of action taken for a given patient. Objective assessment can be particularly helpful when the clinician is faced with conflicting information (e.g., severe symptoms but an unremarkable exam). Objective testing can also yield an accurate objective measure of changes from medical or surgical therapy and thus can be a useful tool to monitor the progress of therapy.

Diagnostic Workup of the Symptoms of Nasal Obstruction

History

The patient is asked specifically about the side of obstruction, severity, frequency, duration, exacerbating factors, and maneuvers that can improve nasal breathing. Symptom and quality of life questionnaires may be used.[1]

Examination

Anterior rhinoscopy is done with a speculum and a headlight or a head mirror and by looking for any areas of restriction, assessing the cross-sectional area of the airway, and the condition of the nasal mucosa. In addition, endoscopy is done either with a small flexible or rigid scope. Endoscopy has the advantage of seeing into parts of the nasal airway that may not be visualized with a headlight and a speculum and may reveal polyps or other pathology. The scope may also be used to visualize the area of the internal valve without any distortion from retraction by the nasal speculum.

There are some maneuvers that can be performed as part of the physical examination that can help to elucidate the nature of the nasal obstruction. One simple test is to occlude each side of the patient's nose and ask the patient to compare the nasal breathing through each side. It is important that the examiner then looks to see if the visual assessment of the airway matches the patient's subjective impression. To assess the contribution of the nasal valve, the patient's cheek can be drawn back (similar to the maneuver done by a patient with positive Cottle sign) to see whether a significant improvement in breathing occurs. Alternatively, the internal and external nasal valve area can be gently widened with a wax curette. These tests require subjective appraisal by the patient and clinician and thus their effects are not easy to quantify objectively.

Types of Objective Testing of Nasal Function

Over a century ago, methods used for the objective assessment of the nasal airway included breathing on a mirror or glass plate (rhinohygrometry), assessing the sound of a forced expiration through the nose, and evaluating the pitch of the sound made by a patient humming while first one and then the other side of the nose was occluded. By the mid-20th century, rhinomanometry was used to measure transnasal pressure and flow. Starting in the late 1970s, the computerization of airway testing allowed for simultaneous storage, calculation, analysis, and printing of test results.[2,3] In the early 1980s, the first reports of acoustic rhinometry emerged. Because of its relative ease of use, it became the more widespread method for objective nasal airway assessment in some countries.

Today, the most commonly used tests are rhinomanometry, peak flow, and acoustic rhinometry. Rhinomanometry measures the actual continuum of airflow that results from the increasing and decreasing transnasal pressures that occur in the course of respiration. Rhinomanometry, when performed using the pressure drop across the entire nose, primarily reflects the narrowest effective cross-sectional area of the nasal airway because the greatest part of the resistance drop occurs at the narrowest site.[4] Nasal peak flow is typically measured upon maximal inspiration with a peak flow meter, which is available in many offices that treat allergy and asthma patients. It does not yield the corresponding pressure needed to generate the measured flow. Acoustic rhinometry uses sound waves to measure the cross-sectional area of the nasal airway rather than the actual movement of air through the nasal passage. It has the advantage of being somewhat easier for some technicians to perform than rhinomanometry and of giving a distance to areas of maximal narrowing. Acoustic rhinometric measurements yield an area distance display that allows the measurement of the smallest cross-sectional area for the anatomic presentation of the sound wave from the instrument and yields the distance to that narrowest area.

Computed tomography (CT) scanning done for assessing the sinuses can also give excellent information about the dimensions of the nasal airway. Most recently, computational fluid dynamics (CFD) has been applied to CT images of the nasal airway.[5] This entails using computer software to define the airspace of the nose from high resolution CT images, then using CFD computer software to predict the fluid dynamics of the airspace.

The reproducibility of the results obtained from any method of objective assessment of the nasal airway can be affected by the nasal cycle, secretions in the nose, exertion close to the time of testing (can increase airway dimension),

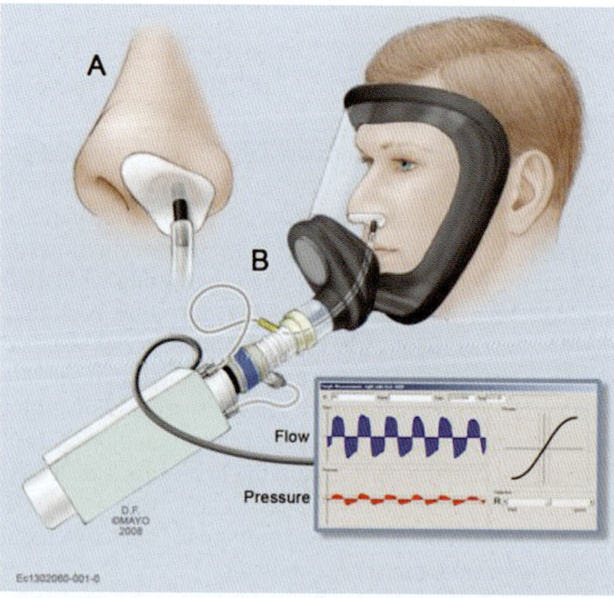

Fig. 5.1 (A,B) Nasal airflow is measured by a device attached to the front of the mask. Transnasal pressure is measured between the pressure in the mask and the pressure in the nasopharynx detected through a tube attached to the opposite nostril. (By permission of Mayo Foundation for Medical Education and Research. All rights reserved.)

temperature (cold air can reduce the airway), hyperventilation (can increase the airway), time of day (the airway can be less open at night and in the early morning), and the use of certain medications. Some have found an increase in the airway with increase in height, with increasing age in children, and in the elderly.

In light of these variables, patients should avoid exercise and exposure to climatic extremes for 30 minutes before testing. Patients should not be taking any interfering medications. Distortion of the alae should be avoided. The measurement should be performed in a comfortable, stable, nonirritating environment with constant temperature and humidity. The patient should have no tobacco or coffee before the test. The test procedure and equipment should be explained to the patient first to help alleviate patient anxiety.

Rhinomanometry

Technique

Nasal airflow is best measured using a face mask that is large enough that it does not distort the external nasal structures. The nasal airflow is measured by a device attached to the front of the mask (**Fig. 5.1B**) that sends the flow readings to the computer. For pressure detection, silastic tubing is secured by tape to the side of the nose not being measured (**Fig. 5.1A,B**). The following steps are followed:

1. The patient is in a sitting position.
2. The patient's name, clinic number, and other information are entered into the computer database on the rhinomanometer.
3. The patient is given the mask to hold, and then is instructed to put it on his or her face with the chin in the appropriate location and to take several breaths with the mouth closed. This relieves any apprehension about wearing the mask and also verifies an appropriate fit.
4. If the machine requires a baseline collection (similar to adjusting a digital bathroom scale to zero) this is done before any connection to the device.
5. The right nasal airway is tested first. The appropriately shaped tape to cover the left nostril is fastened to the pressure tube that comes into the inside of the mask. This in turn is attached to the left nostril for pressure detection to the nasopharynx while leaving the right nostril open for testing.
6. The mask is then put in place on the patient's face and the pressure tubing is adjusted as the tester views it through the mask and verifies that it is correctly positioned and not kinked.
7. The patient is instructed to close his or her mouth and to breathe in and out. The pressure-flow curve is visualized on the computer display and any needed adjustments are made. Deviation from the normal shape of the curve could alert one to the

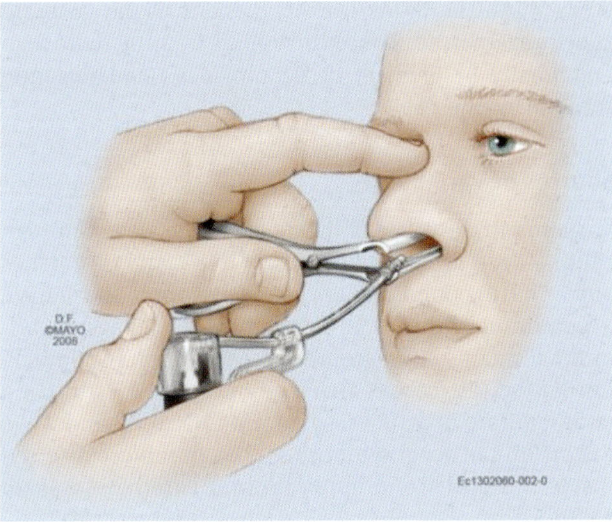

Fig. 5.2 Application of a decongestant spray. This is repeated after 5 minutes. Measurements are then made 10 minutes later. (By permission of Mayo Foundation for Medical Education and Research. All rights reserved.)

presence of a tape or mask leak. The collection is completed and the computer saves the pressure-flow data.

8. The mask is removed, and the tape is removed from the left nostril. The left nasal airway is then tested in a similar fashion.

If testing is not going to be done with dilators but is going to be done after decongestion, application of a decongestant spray (**Fig. 5.2**) to the patient's nasal tissues is usually done twice, 15 and 10 minutes prior, with either phenylephrine or oxymetazoline. If testing will be done with dilating plastic strips or other dilating devices, these are placed and the previously listed procedures are repeated for both sides of the nose. If testing will be done following both dilation and nasal decongestion, testing with dilation alone precedes the testing with dilation and decongestion so that the dilating strips will remain in a consistent position. In this case, testing with decongestion alone is done last.

For children, a smaller face mask can be used, but the test is performed in the same way as for adults. For patients whose chief complaint is nasal obstruction when recumbent, additional studies can be performed in the supine, right-side lying, and left-side lying positions, preferably with appropriate delay after positioning before testing. For patients with suspected allergic rhinitis, nasal provocation testing can be performed.

Reporting Results

One way to evaluate the results of the test is to examine the pressure-flow curve. The plot is usually an S-shaped curve (**Fig. 5.1B**). The amount of curvature can vary. A flattening of the curve may represent flow limitation from an airway restriction (e.g., valve area collapse). Looping of the curve may be evident, particularly with the high resolution rhinomanometry (HRR) of Vogt.[6] Curves representing a more obstructed airway will lie closer to the pressure (*x*- or horizontal) axis. The curvature is due to smaller increases in flow (*y*-axis) for each increase in pressure at points farther from the origin. Resistance (pressure divided by flow) values therefore increase at more distal points on the pressure-flow curve because of this nonlinear relationship.

Various parameters can be calculated from the pressure and flow data that were stored by the computer. The most common result reported is nasal resistance, which is the ratio of pressure divided by flow and sometimes abbreviated as NAR or Rn. The International Committee on Standardization of Rhinomanometry[6,7] recommends that rhinomanometric values should be expressed in SI metric units, with pressure expressed in pascals (100 Pa = 1.0 cm H_2O) and flow expressed in cm^3/sec (1,000 cm^3/sec = 1 L/sec). Nasal resistance is reported as Pa/cm^3/sec (0.1 Pa/cm^3/sec = 1 cm H_2O/L/sec).

A commonly reported parameter is the flow corresponding to a pressure of 150 Pa. Using this parameter from both the right and left sides of the airway, the total nasal airflow at 150 Pa may be calculated by adding the two flows that were obtained at the same pressure. Another important parameter is the resistance at the peak pressure and flow point called the maximum resistance[1,8,9] or the vertex resistance by Vogt.[6] An advantage of obtaining resistance from this point on the curve is that a result can be obtained in all patients because it is not necessary to reach a designated point. This parameter was also found to correlate best with the symptom of nasal obstruction when compared with a wide array of other proposed parameters.[9]

Sources of Variability

It is important to understand potential causes of variability in rhinomanometry. The equipment can be out of calibration. If the patient laughs, speaks, or opens his or her mouth during the test, then it will cause an error in the recording. Some variability can result from movement of the nasal alae. In many patients, this would be minimal because the alar muscles tend to work toward stabilization of the vestibular wall.[4] In the patient with a valve abnormality or disruption of the alar muscles (e.g., after rhinoplasty), alar movement may cause variability. Some variability has been attributed to mask use, but in general, masks distort the alae much less than do nozzles, and different mask shapes and volumes do not significantly affect rhinomanometric measurements.

To minimize the variability while performing a rhinomanometry, the apparatus should first be at room temperature and then should be properly calibrated. The mask, which is preferred to nozzles, should fit without an air leak throughout the test. It is best to view the display of the pressure-flow curve in real time so that mask leaks or other artifacts may be detected and addressed during the exam. The patient should be instructed to keep his or her mouth closed and to not speak during the test.

Acoustic Rhinometry

Technique

The equipment used in acoustic rhinometry has been described by Hilberg et al.[10] An acoustic pulse from a spark or a click from a trigger module travels through a wave tube and through a nosepiece in contact with the nasal inlet. Variations in the cross-sectional area of the nose affect the reflectance of the sound. A microphone detects the reflected sound, and the signal from the microphone is processed and then converted to digital data. A computer then calculates and plots an area-distance function from the data, yielding a profile of the cross-sectional areas through each side of the nose.

The patient is seated, and a nosepiece on the tube is applied to the patient's nose so that there is no noise leak and no distortion of the anterior nasal structures. Surgical lubricant is used on the nosepiece that touches the nostril rim to help ensure a seal. The acoustic pulse is then generated while the nosepiece is held still for 10 seconds. The test is repeated after decongestant spray.

Reporting Results

The acoustic rhinometer calculates and displays an area-distance curve. The curve usually shows two notches after the straight line that corresponds to the nosepiece. The first dip in the curve has been called the I-notch.[11] The I stands for isthmus nasi, and it occurs at the first part of the valve region. The second depression in the curve has been called the C-notch. The C stands for concha, and this depression corresponds with the anterior tip (head) of the inferior turbinate. Lenders and Pirsig[11] found that the part measured by the I-notch was always the narrowest segment in normal patients, with the second narrowest segment occurring at the C-notch. The display for this result has the pattern of the first notch lower than the second ("the climbing W"). They also found that the second constriction improved with decongestion, but the first did not. In patients with allergic rhinitis and in patients with habitual snoring, the second constriction was the smallest ("the descending W").

The parameters most commonly reported are the size of the airway at these two notches and a third that is the next posterior dip in the curve (CSA1, the valve area; CSA2, the head of the inferior turbinate; and CSA3, sometimes the head of the middle turbinate). Other parameters that might be reported include the volume of the nose on each side, the distance to each of the notches, and the cross-sectional area at various distances from the nosepiece (e.g., 2, 4, and 6 cm). For the total nasal minimal cross-sectional area (MCA), the MCAs from both sides of the nose are added together.[12] A consensus report from the European Community by Clement et al.[6] provides standardization recommendations.

Sources of Variability

Variation in the angle of incidence of the wave tube can cause a decrease in the depths of the I- and C- notches and a shifting of both anteriorly. Operator bias can have a significant effect on all parameters if tracings of suboptimal quality are accepted. Breathing or swallowing during the test causes a change in the MCA estimation or a high rate of artifactual traces.[13] Nasal tip and valve distortion can occur with the use of a nosepiece inserted inside the nostril. An application of external nasal tip adaptors can also cause distortion of the nasal tip structures. The size of the nosepiece can affect the results if an acoustic seal with the nostril is not achieved. Other causes of results variability include: head position, probe position, probe movement, measurement beyond a restriction or beyond 6 cm, measurements of regions with a great rate of change in the cross-sectional area, and motion of the soft palate. Hilberg et al.[10] found that, in general, if the anterior area is less than 0.7 cm^2, then there will be significant error for more distal (from the nosepiece) measurements. Because this is the normal dimension for the adult nose, one might expect inaccuracies posterior to the MCA from pathologic restrictions or in children's noses.

To reduce variability in acoustic rhinometry, some investigators have found it desirable to use a special stand for the patient to rest his or her head, maintaining a constant angle of incidence with the device to improve the reliability of serial measurements. Operator bias can be reduced by using the average of at least three consecutive traces. It is important that the patient hold his or her breath and not swallow during the measurement. Nosepieces that go inside the nose are avoided now by most investigators by using a nasal adaptor that fits on the rim of the nostril. Even with the external nasal adaptor, care must be taken to avoid distortion of the compliant vestibular region as contact is maintained during the test. A layer of water-soluble jelly is recommended to provide an acoustic seal.

Comparison of Acoustic Rhinometry and Rhinomanometry

Hilberg et al.[10] believed that acoustic rhinometry provided less variability of results than those obtained with rhinomanometry. Further, they noted that the method requires little cooperation by the patient, is noninvasive, and is easy to perform. It was noted that acoustic rhinometry is rapid and would be particularly useful for the evaluation of children because it required minimal cooperation from the subject. However, Fisher[13] noted that the many sources of variability in performing acoustic rhinometry dampened the original enthusiasm about the possibility of acoustic rhinometry providing superior reproducibility as compared with other objective tests. In addition, he noted that the repeat tests needed to minimize variability "detract from the perceived speed of acoustic rhinometry."

Peak Nasal Airflow

The readily available peak expiratory flow meter has been used to assess the nasal airway. Results have been shown to correlate with results from rhinomanometry but Connell found that the method was unreliable.[14] A nasal peak *inspiratory* flow meter continues to be used in some clinics. This was found to have a drawback in children in that it depended on the degree of cooperation of the child and on the subjective impression of the observer as to when a maximal effort had been made. Measurement of peak inspiratory flow was found to be less sensitive than rhinomanometry for detecting changes in nasal patency after a histamine challenge or following increasing doses of xylometazoline.

Computed Tomography Scanning for Airway Analysis and Computational Fluid Dynamics

CT scanning yields a very accurate assessment of the nasal airway. Current three-dimensional (3D) tools allow for the study of the airway from any angle. **Figure 5.3A** shows the 3D shape of the airway obtained from high resolution CT data. **Figure 5.4** shows the graph of the cross-sectional areas of a patient's nose at regular intervals perpendicular to the line following the center of the air passage for each side of the nose in **Fig. 5.3B**. The corresponding measurements from rhinomanometry performed coincident with the time of the CT are shown in **Fig. 5.5**. Note that the greatest nasal resistance values and symptoms correspond to the side with the smallest cross-sectional area overall. Although in the anterior nose the right side is smaller than the left, in the posterior nose, the left side has the smallest cross-sectional area of either side, which corresponds with the patient's symptoms of the left side being the most restricted. Acoustic rhinometry yields a cross-sectional area curve that is an approximation of this type of analysis, though it is less accurate beyond any area of constriction.

CFD allows for a more detailed study of the theoretical nasal airstream than ever before (**Fig. 5.6**).[5] This entails creating an airway volume from CT data and then using fluid dynamic software to create the airflow vectors for the various parts of that airway. It is too early in the application of CFD to know the manner in which useful parameters that correlate with symptoms will be obtained from these many flow vectors.

Other Methods of Objective Assessment of the Nasal Airway

Other objective tests of the nasal airway include rhinostereometry, Doppler velocimetry, manometric rhinometry, forced oscillation rhinomanometry, and nasometry.[15]

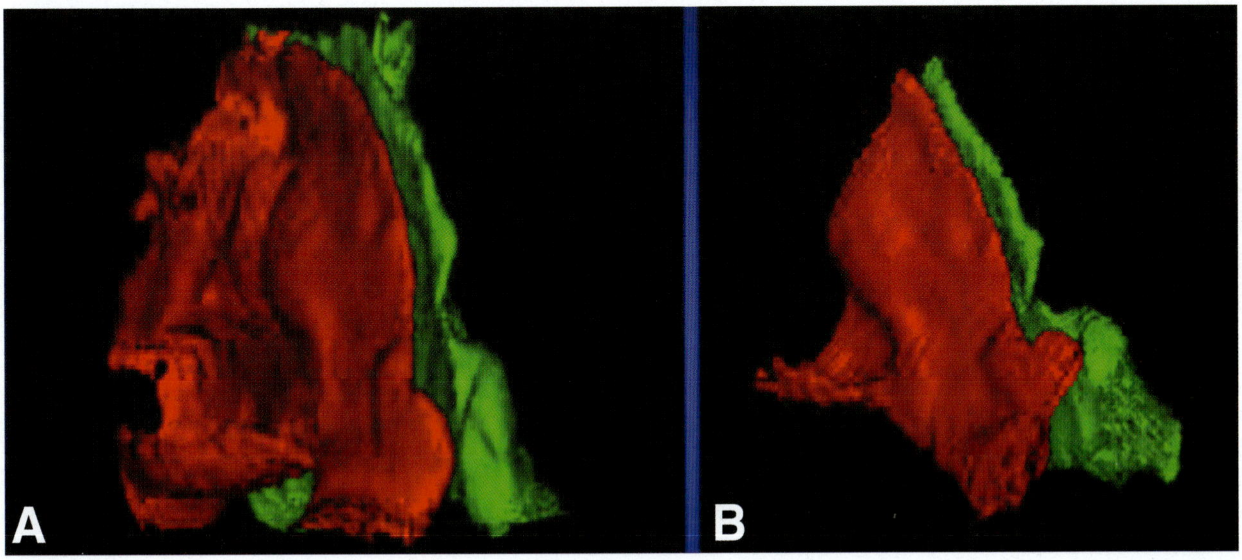

Fig. 5.3 Three-dimensional airway depiction. **(A)** The shape of the right (*red*) and left (*green*) nasal airways. Reconstruction was done from high resolution computed tomography images using Analyze 6.0 (Mayo Biomedical Imaging Resource). **(B)** The stacked cross-sections that would be obtained at 1 mm intervals if each section was perpendicular to the overall axis of the direction of airflow.

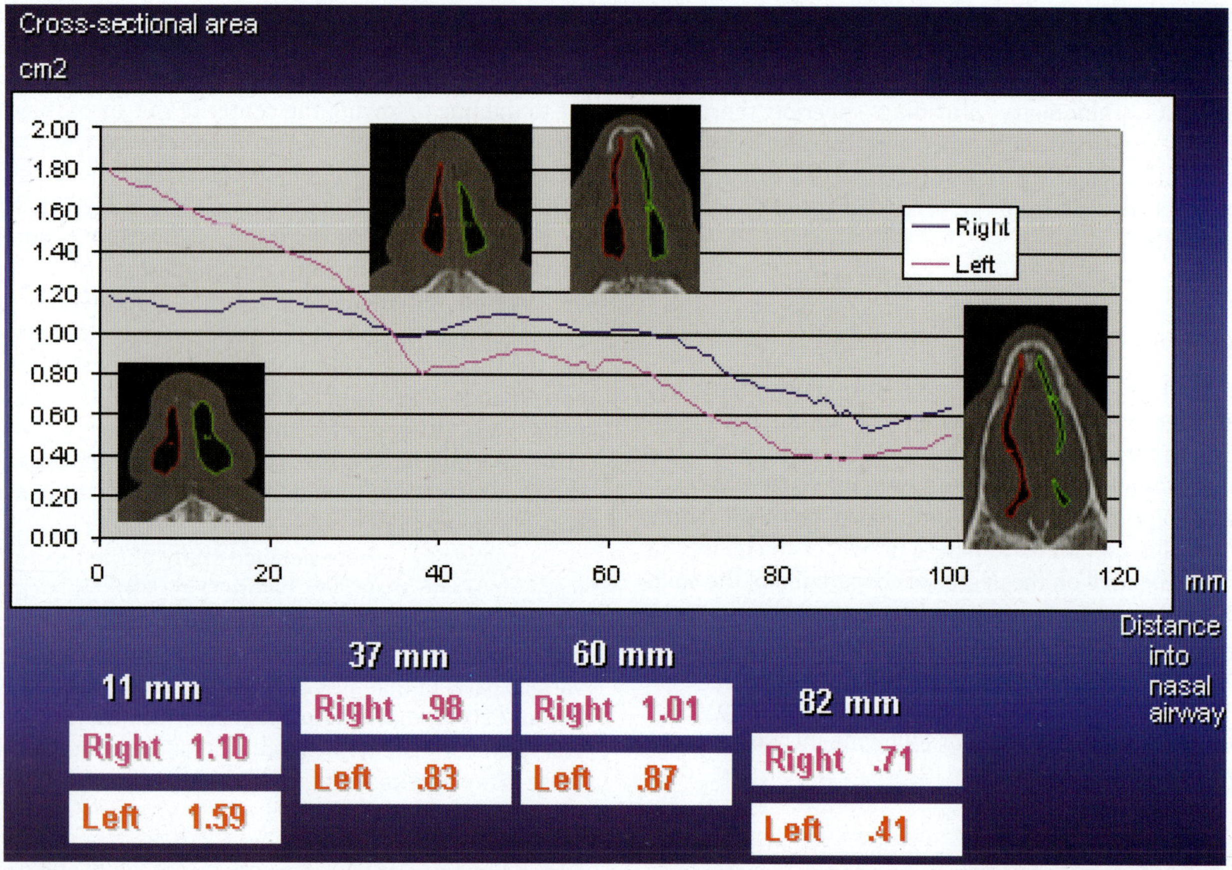

Fig. 5.4 Plot of the right (*blue*) and left (*red*) cross-sectional areas at increasing distances from the nasal opening. Examples of the cross-sectional views for slices that are perpendicular to the central axis of the airstream for given distances (in mm) along the airstream axis. At 11 mm the view is upward into the nostrils, and the cross-sectional airway on the left is greater than the right. On the graph, note that the right airway is less open than the left until 37 mm into the nose. At 37 mm, the two sides are almost the same cross-sectional airway. Beyond that the left becomes the narrower side as seen in the views at 60 mm and 82 mm.

Applications of Objective Nasal Airway Testing

Sleep Disordered Breathing

Objective testing of the nasal airway can be used for the evaluation of patients with snoring and sleep apnea. Rhinomanometry has been used to study the change in resistance that occurs when the patient is supine and has been found to be more severe in patients with sleep apnea. Patients with allergic rhinitis, those with snoring, and mild sleep apnea had significantly greater congestion at the anterior portion of the inferior turbinate as measured by acoustic rhinometry and less subjective improvement with nasal decongestion. Patients with habitual snoring (some with sleep apnea) had an MCA located at the C-notch (turbinate), whereas in normal subjects the MCA was located at the I-notch. Even with decongestion, the C-notch of the patients who snored did not reach normal size. Increasing the objective measurement of the nasal airway with a dilator can reduce the apnea index in some patients. Furthermore, in a group of habitual snorers, 65% were found to have elevated nasal resistance but only 19% complained of the symptom of nasal obstruction. The role of objective nasal airway testing in helping to assess the contribution of the nasal airway in patients with snoring and sleep apnea will continue to evolve as investigators look at questions such as the role of airway testing in predicting compliance with continuous positive airway pressure (CPAP) and the impact of varying degrees of nasal obstruction on sleep disordered breathing in certain patients.

Nasal Challenge Testing in Allergic Rhinitis

Nasal challenge testing is performed by introducing a specific allergen into the nose to directly assess nasal mucosal responses rather than indirect reactions manifested by skin tests.[16] Both acoustic rhinometry and rhinomanometry have yielded comparable results in nasal challenge testing.[17] Intranasal allergen challenges with ragweed

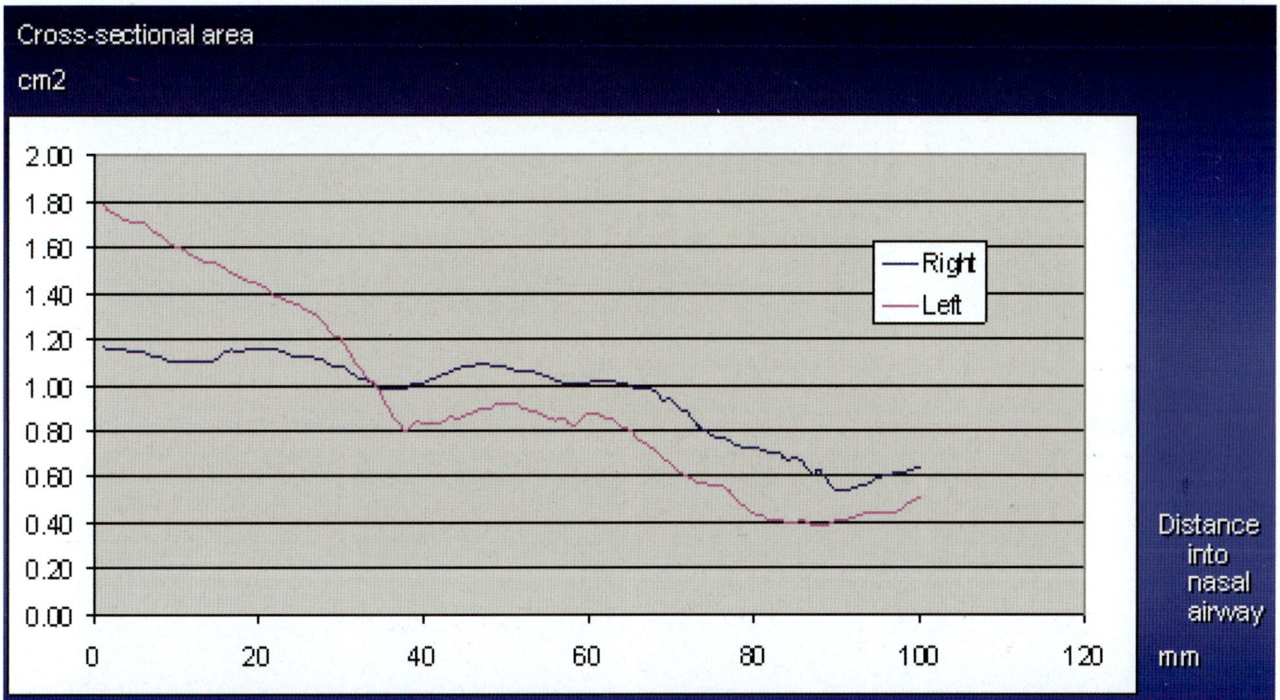

	Flow150	Res150	Reff Ins	VR Rvert Ins	Sx side	Sxs subj
right	526	0.29	0.33	0.37		50
left	404	0.37	0.45	0.50	left worst	36

Fig. 5.5 Plot of the right (*blue*) and left (*red*) cross-sectional areas at increasing distances from the nasal opening in the same patient as shown in **Fig. 5.4**. The table at the bottom of this figure shows results from rhinomanometries done corresponding to the time of the patient's computed tomography scan. The values measured by rhinomanometry show the left side to have the higher resistance (and lower flow), which likely reflects the narrowest dimension of the airway at 80 mm where the left airway is smaller than the right. The patient's symptoms at the time of the tests were left worse than right nasal obstruction, corresponding with the side with the narrower dimension. The significant turbinate swelling in this patient caused the less typical situation of the narrowest airway dimension being more posterior.

pollen in patients with ragweed allergy reproducibly caused an increase in nasal resistance with an increased dose of ragweed. The advantage of objective testing in challenge testing is that it enables the calculation of percent change from a baseline value, which would be difficult to assess with symptom scores alone. Lenders and Pirsig[11] thought that acoustic rhinometry could be more sensitive than rhinomanometry in detecting allergic rhinitis because it might reveal mucosal changes even when no change in resistance had occurred.

Assessing the Effect of Medical and Surgical Therapy

Objective testing of the nasal airway has been a useful way to assess the effect of intranasal medications because it does not rely on subjective assessment by the patient or the clinician. Objective testing has been used to demonstrate improvement in the nasal airway after septoplasty,[18–22] after turbinate surgery,[11] and after rhinoplasty.

Objective testing has been proposed as a way to select patients who would have the best chance of success with surgery.[23] Patients with high preoperative resistance or low preoperative MCA were more satisfied with surgery than those with preoperatively lower resistance or higher preoperative MCA. Grymer et al.,[12] using acoustic rhinometry, found that the patient's satisfaction was correlated with the improvement in the size of the MCA after the septoplasty. Bachmann[24] outlined rhinomanometric indications for and against surgery and noted that "when constant stenosis exists and 'total flow (at 150 Pa)' is below 700 cm^3/sec, then there exists a clear indication for surgery."

Some clinicians have wanted a means of obtaining an objective assessment that would demonstrate the need for surgery to managed care reviewers. Although objective testing might support the decision for surgery or help verify the area to be addressed, the results of objective testing should never be required or used by third-party payers for decisions regarding coverage for surgery because it is the experience and recommendation of the surgeon that is most important in deciding when surgery can be pursued.

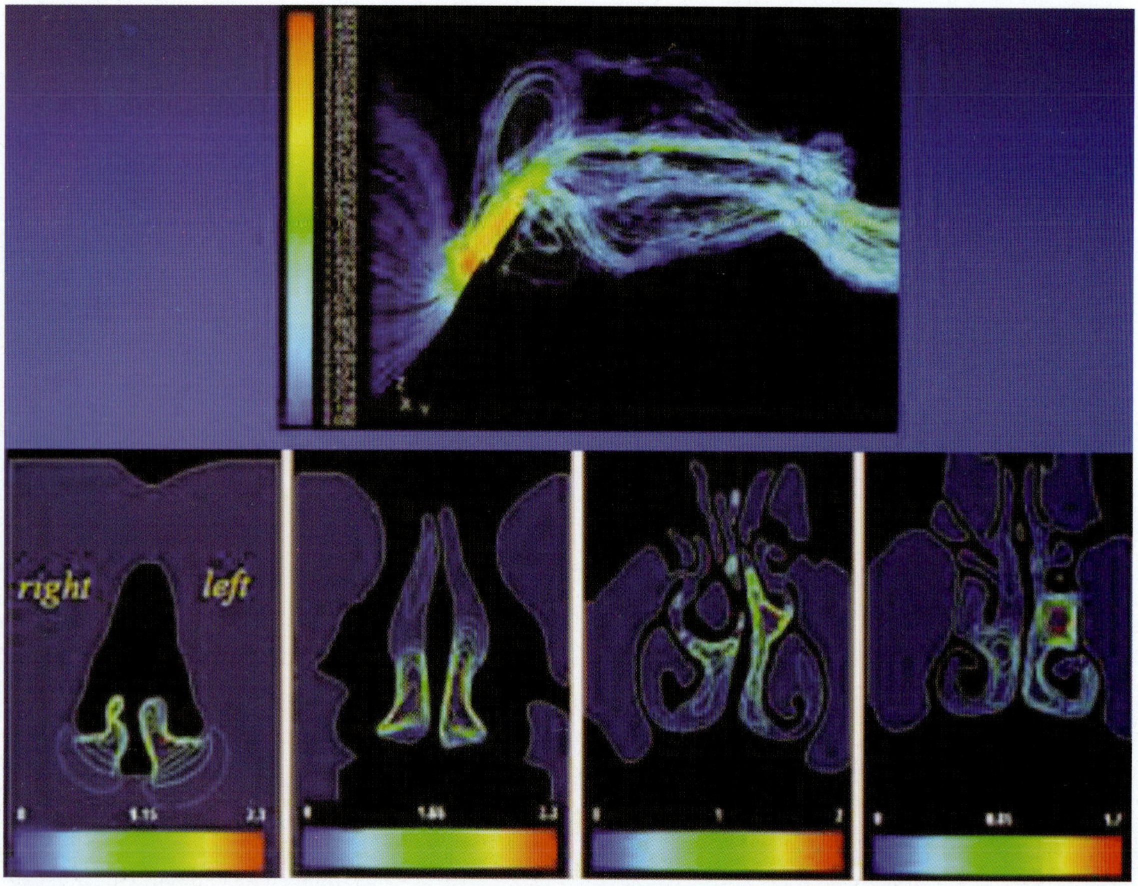

Fig. 5.6 Computational fluid dynamics. An example of one of the many ways to display the airflow through the nasal airway. The *red airstream lines* have the greatest velocity. Colors can also represent temperature, surface shear, and pressure. The anatomic dimensions are constructed from the computed tomography scan of the patient's nasal airway. (Courtesy of ANSYS Inc., Canonsburg, PA.)

Nasal Obstruction: Diagnosis

Airway testing results may agree or disagree with a patient's symptoms and the nasal pathology noted by the physician. Bachmann[24] has emphasized that rhinoscopy and objective testing should be performed together because the synthesis of the simultaneous information they provide can help uncover more about the nature of the pathology that is causing a patient's complaint of nasal airway obstruction.

Because the patient's description of symptoms and the clinician's assessment of the airway are both subjective, an objective assessment of the airway can provide additional information that might change the diagnosis or choice of treatment. The airway testing results prove particularly useful when there are conflicting findings in the evaluation of symptoms, rhinoscopy, and the effect of decongestion and of valve area dilators. Bachmann[24] noted that, rather than dismiss the use of objective testing because of the times that the results do not match symptoms, "one should rather examine the causes of discrepancy," because "these causes are of considerable clinical interest." Similarly, cases in which the airway testing results do not match the physician's rhinoscopic assessment of the nasal airway are the ones in which objective testing may be most useful.

If no airway restriction is objectively identified in a symptomatic patient, then other causes need to be looked for. Obstructive symptoms can be present in a person with an open airway—that is, due to atrophic rhinitis, inflammation, sinusitis, psychogenic causes, or pulmonary disease. These patients will have the least chance of being helped by treatment that is directed at enlarging the dimension of the nasal airway. If other causes are not found, a menthol-type nasal inhaler might be tried to stimulate the airflow receptors. If testing reveals that some airway restriction is present but is of notably less severity than the patient's symptoms, the patient may have a low threshold for the symptom of nasal obstruction. Consequently, the patient can be counselled that the odds of success at alleviating his or her symptoms might be less than maximal.

If the physician can see only minor pathology on exam to explain the patient's symptoms but the airway testing shows a significant restriction, then the physician may wish to reconsider the clinical significance of the findings seen. A second look may be considered, and the physician may have greater confidence that surgically addressing the pathology would relieve the patient's symptoms.

A less frequent scenario can occur in which airway restriction is found in a patient who presented for problems other than nasal obstruction. Typically, significant appearing pathology is seen by the examiner. Some patients are sent for an evaluation because they have voice problems attributed to their chronic mouth breathing, and some have CPAP intolerance with a suspected contribution from nasal obstruction. If airway testing reveals significant airway restriction, this additional information can be helpful in identifying additional therapeutic targets.

Nasal Obstruction: Selection of Surgical Approach

Airway testing can help in selecting treatment by demonstrating the effect of modifications in the airway using decongestion and nasal dilators. When decongestion or dilation is performed with testing, a profile is obtained of the relative effect of each type of intervention at the different sites as well as the combined effect of the two on the amount of airflow through the nose (**Fig. 5.7**).

The external and internal valves can be static or dynamic components of obstruction. When dilators are used during testing, one can see the effect of opening a valve area narrowed by a septal deflection or other pathology, or the effect of stabilizing a flaccid valve area.

Historically, if the airway did not improve with decongestion, any obstruction was attributed to a problem with the intranasal "structure." Complete relief of symptoms with decongestion indicated a "mucosal" cause. In actuality, most nasal obstruction occurs with a combination of structural and mucosal components. It should also be noted that not all patients respond to the decongestant with a decrease in mucosal thickness. Naito[25] found that 10% of 86 patients had a slight increase in nasal resistance after decongestion.

The septum, turbinate bone, and bony side walls are structural components that are static, but the mucosal portions are dynamic and change with the amount of congestion

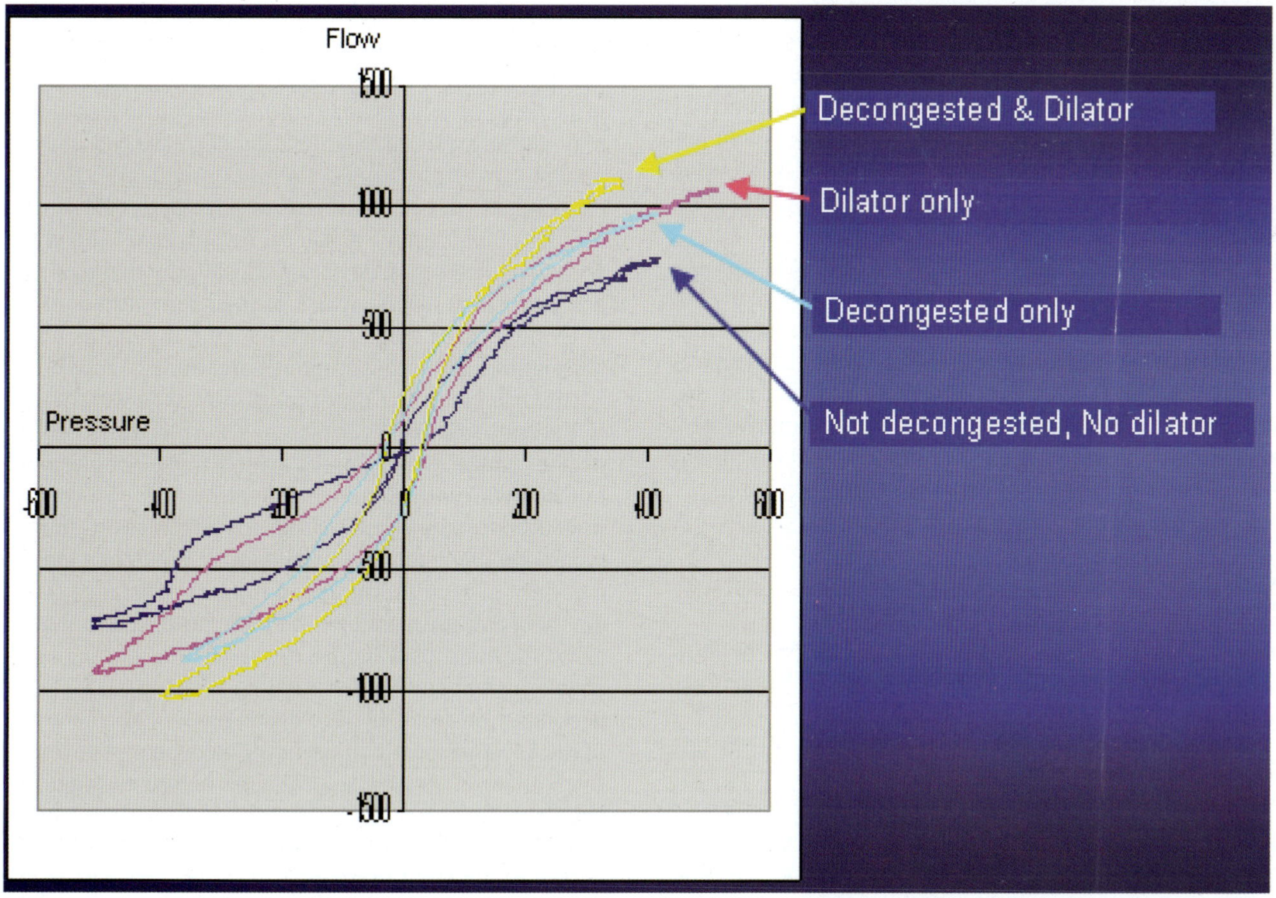

Fig. 5.7 Pressure-flow curves (color-coded by intervention) for rhinomanometric measurements of a patient's left nasal airway. The closer the curve is to the pressure (x) axis, the greater the resistance and obstruction. The curves for different interventions are shown in different colors. In this particular unilateral nasal airway, the effect of a dilator alone is comparable to the effect of a decongestant alone, but the combination of both decongestion and a dilator results in the most open airway.

or decongestion of the nasal tissues. A person whose nasal airway is at the edge of the threshold of comfortable breathing will more likely be aware of worsening with recumbency or improvement with exercise. This can occur because of increased mucosal reactivity or because of structural narrowing that lowers the patient's tolerance for mucosal swelling.

Objective improvements in nasal function with decongestion and dilation, when correlated with subjective improvements, can guide the selection of optimal treatment for any given patient. If the nasal dilator has a significantly larger effect on the airway testing results than decongestion, this would reinforce the importance of intervention in the valve area. If decongestion has a much greater effect on the airway than the dilator, this would suggest that any surgery (if medical therapy was inadequate) should be particularly directed at sites of mucosal congestion (e.g., inferior turbinate tissues). This information is useful both in treatment planning and in counseling the patient about therapeutic options and expectations regarding the success of treatment.[26]

Postoperative Persistence of Nasal Obstruction

In a patient who shows no symptom improvement after surgical treatment, objective testing may be helpful to confirm that the intervention did in fact change the airway dynamics. If the objective test shows no improvement and the patient remains symptomatic, the examiner knows to take a second look to see if the site of the significant restriction can be identified.

If the objective result is improved but not the symptoms, the physician is alerted to the possibility that there may be additional causes for the patient's symptoms other than the targeted site of airway restriction. Without the airway testing, the physician might have assumed that the reason the intervention had not resulted in an improvement in symptoms was because it had not changed the airway enough to overcome the effect of the pathology noted.

■ Pitfalls in Objective Nasal Airway Testing

Potential pitfalls in objective airway testing can be illustrated by comparisons to a more widely used functional test: audiometry.

Problem 1: The Airway Being Tested is Variable

Because of the nasal cycle, unilateral nasal airway testing has inherent variability (although total nasal resistance remains relatively constant).[1] This would be like doing an audiogram on a patient who has hearing that fluctuates. Despite this variability, it is still meaningful to measure each side of the nose. Total airway values are derived from the results from each side. Total resistance has been noted to correlate best with overall symptoms of nasal obstruction[1] and may be the most important determinant of the patient's sense of well-being.[24] Furthermore, unilateral data are still desirable to assess the effect of specific pathologies observed and to compare with symptoms.

The problem of variability can be addressed by obtaining data about the patient's current symptoms and exam at the time of the test so that comparisons can be made between simultaneous symptoms, exam, and test results. Comparisons of pre- and postdecongestion testing can also be helpful in revealing the effect of the nasal cycle.

Problem 2: Population Data for Normal and Abnormal Results Are Not Well Defined

It is apparent that there is a difference between a group of obstructed individuals and a group with no symptoms of nasal obstruction; however, there is a sizeable overlap between the airway values for these two groups.[1] This overlap appears to be greater than the one encountered in audiometry, although most of us have experienced telling a patient with presbycusis that they have a significant 35-dB hearing loss only to have them tell us that they feel that their hearing is fine.

A person who has not experienced a sudden change in hearing, or who never could hear well to begin with, may not be aware of their hearing decrease, yet it can be apparent to those around them. Consequently, they are encouraged to seek treatment to have better hearing for reasons of education and safety. Yet someone who is born with a marked septal deviation causing restriction of their breathing may not be aware of their diminished airway, nor would those around them notice it unless the person had significant snoring or mouth breathing.

This brings up the question of how a "normal range" is determined. For hearing, the "normal range" is the decibel range of hearing at which most people would not be aware of a significant hearing loss. We can also find a "normal range" for nasal resistance in subjects who deny having nasal obstruction.[27] When one looks at a variety of studies, the mean normal resistance (in Pa/cm^3/sec) at a pressure of 150 Pa ranges for the unilateral airway around 0.54 before decongestion and 0.33 after decongestion, and for the total nasal airway 0.27 before decongestion and 0.15 after decongestion. Normal values of MCA from acoustic rhinometry have been reported for the unilateral airway at 0.72 cm^2 before decongestion and 0.94 cm^2 after decongestion, and for the total airway at 1.46 cm^2 before decongestion and 1.88 cm^2 after decongestion.[28,29] The subjects in these studies were usually "normal" on the basis of lack of symptoms. Palma and Sulsenti[30] recommend that subjects described as normal also be "rhinoscopically normal." Should the group of "abnormals" include those who have pathology causing airway restriction although they do not complain of nasal obstruction because they have felt this way since birth, yet who would notice improvement if the restriction was opened? Including them in the "abnormal" group would decrease the proportion of the population in the area of overlap.

Although the range of thresholds at which a patient first experiences nasal obstruction may be broader than the range of thresholds at which one appreciates a hearing loss, the information can still be useful. We start by knowing the reference range for the population who do not feel obstruction. Examples of reference ranges of "normals" are the plots of the 5th to 95th percentiles of the pressure-flow curve, which can be shown in shadow behind the pressure-flow curves. If an individual is in the range at which there is overlap between "normal" and "abnormal," then there will not be as certain a prediction of the significance of the airway values. Yet if a patient's results are well into the "normal" or "abnormal" range, then there is increased utility of the results.

Problem 3: Controversy Exists about the Correlation between Airway Test Results and Patients' Symptoms

To believe that an audiogram is meaningful, we trust that if an audiogram is abnormal then that person is experiencing decreased hearing. With airway testing, however, there are some who believe that the results do not correlate with symptoms.[31–37] However, studies have successfully shown that there is a correlation between airway testing results and symptoms in patients who have nasal obstruction.[1,9,39] As would be expected, a correlation between nasal resistance and the symptom of obstruction has been found more easily in symptomatic patients than in subjects who do not have nasal obstruction.

There will be patients whose results do not seem to show a correlation (e.g., symptoms staying the same though airflow improves after decongestion) and those are the very patients for whom the test is most useful. If a patient complains of nasal obstruction but the airway testing shows that the airway is widely patent, then the physician knows to look for other causes for the symptoms than airway obstruction.

Problem 4: Objective Nasal Airway Testing Does Not Reflect Subjective Aspects of Patients' Comfort

It is typical for an audiogram to measure whether someone can hear at a certain level, but not if he or she is comfortable with his or her hearing at that level (although that can be quantified by *most comfortable loudness*—a parameter that can be important for hearing aid fitting). Yet, in nasal airway testing, physicians often will expect the test to not only show the level of breathing that is present, but also tell whether that level of nasal breathing is comfortable for the patient. If the patient is not comfortable with his or her breathing at a "normal" level of resistance, then the test is said to be less useful because there is not a perfect correlation between resistance and comfort.

The art of having satisfied patients after treatment goes beyond the numbers obtained with the test, yet can be enhanced by the information provided by the test. It is helpful to know that ranges of airway resistance have been correlated to different levels of breathing comfort in the general population. An example of the reference ranges for airway values for various degrees of nasal obstruction symptoms are the ranges of flow values (at a pressure of 150 Pa) in **Table 5.1**.[38,39] Ranges of resistance values corresponding to VAS levels of obstructive symptoms have been recently described by Vogt.[39]

If a patient has a resistance value that is significantly different from others with a similar level of symptoms, then attaining a satisfied patient with airway treatment may have higher or lower odds of success. Patients who feel that their airway restriction is far more severe than others with the same measured level may be harder to please with treatment, whereas patients who have a large degree of airway restriction yet think that their symptoms are mild can have a greater chance of being happy after treatment.

Problem 5: Nasal Resistance is Measured Based on a Continuum Rather than Thresholds

We can measure the dB level at which someone can hear a sound, but when we measure their airway, we are usually measuring a point on a gradation of airway values. A 20-dB hearing loss is readily grasped, but it is less clear what it means to breathe with a resistance level of "0.3 Pa/cm^3/sec."

Table 5.1 The Range of Flow Values (at 150 Pa) for Unilateral and Total Nasal Airways That Corresponds on Average to Each Degree of Symptoms of Nasal Obstruction

Degree of Nasal Obstruction	Unilateral Flow at 150 Pa	Total Flow at 150 Pa
No obstruction	>500	>800
Slight obstruction	300–500	500–800
Moderate obstruction	180–300	300–500
Severe obstruction	60–180	100–300
Airway closed	<60	<100

If a person cannot hear, they may be deleteriously affected in school or traffic, and others around them may notice that they do not respond. If a person's nasal breathing is diminished, it does not always affect performance in a way that is as easy to recognize, yet it could affect such things as tolerance of CPAP, craniofacial development, or drying of laryngeal structures that adversely affect voice. The clinician must therefore recognize that nasal resistance will not have a single cutoff point for performance, but rather needs to be considered in relationship to how it fits into a continuum of values.

Problem 6: Other Obstacles to Utilization

There are some additional reasons that nasal airway testing has not been widely adopted in some locations. In some states, insurance companies do not to reimburse for the test, making it difficult for clinicians to cover the costs to perform it. There is wider use of rhinomanometry in countries such as Japan, where there is reimbursement for a designated number of tests. Also, there is some training required to administer the test, as well as equipment costs and personnel costs. In addition, the desirability of documenting the exam contemporaneously with the testing and symptoms puts further demands on the clinician's time, which is already stretched thin. Furthermore, patient scheduling becomes more complex to accommodate the testing time and revisit or call back time. Lastly, physicians are not aware of how the test may benefit their evaluation of patients.

Conclusion

Objective testing can further explain the relationship between symptoms and physical findings.[40] Simultaneous rhinoscopic evaluation, symptom assessment, and objective testing are key elements.

Diagnosis, patient counseling, and treatment can be enhanced by the additional information provided by objective testing. In addition, objective testing can provide further information regarding the changes brought about by surgery, the effects of nasal challenge in patients with allergic rhinitis, and the role of the nasal airway in the disturbance of breathing during sleep.

Future work will further define and refine the clinical applications of objective testing. Those who wish to obtain all available information about the nasal airway when assessing patients who complain of nasal obstruction will continue to use objective methods of assessing nasal patency for the wider understanding of nasal functions.[8]

References

1. McCaffrey TV, Kern EB. Clinical evaluation of nasal obstruction. A study of 1,000 patients. Arch Otolaryngol 1979;105(9):542–545
2. Cole P, Fastag O, Niinimaa V. Computer-aided rhinometry. A research rhinometer for clinical trial. Acta Otolaryngol 1980;90(1-2):139–142
3. Pallanch JF. Nasal resistance: a comparison of the methods used for obtaining normal values and a comparison of proposed models of the transnasal pressure-flow curves. Thesis. Rochester, NY; 1984
4. Haight JS, Cole P. The site and function of the nasal valve. Laryngoscope 1983;93(1):49–55
5. Bailie N, Hanna B, Watterson J, Gallagher G. An overview of numerical modelling of nasal airflow. Rhinology 2006;44(1):53–57
6. Clement PA, Gordts F; Standardisation Committee on Objective Assessment of the Nasal Airway, IRS, and ERS. Consensus report on acoustic rhinometry and rhinomanometry. Rhinology 2005;43(3):169–179
7. Kern EB. Committee report on standardization of rhinomanometry. Rhinology 1981;19(4):231–236
8. Cottle M. Rhino-sphygmomanometry: an aid in physical diagnosis. Int Rhinol 1968;6:7–26
9. Pallanch JF. Comparison of the Relative Strength of Correlation of Various Rhinomanometric Parameters with the Symptom of Nasal Obstruction. Omaha, NE: Triologic Society; 1995
10. Hilberg O, Jackson AC, Swift DL, Pedersen OF. Acoustic rhinometry: evaluation of nasal cavity geometry by acoustic reflection. J Appl Physiol 1989;66(1):295–303
11. Lenders H, Pirsig W. Diagnostic value of acoustic rhinometry: patients with allergic and vasomotor rhinitis compared with normal controls. Rhinology 1990;28(1):5–16
12. Grymer LF, Hilberg O, Elbrønd O, Pedersen OF. Acoustic rhinometry: evaluation of the nasal cavity with septal deviations, before and after septoplasty. Laryngoscope 1989;99(11):1180–1187
13. Fisher EW, Morris DP, Biemans JM, Palmer CR, Lund VJ. Practical aspects of acoustic rhinometry: problems and solutions. Rhinology 1995;33(4):219–223
14. Connell JT. Rhinometry: measurement of nasal patency. Ann Allergy 1982;49(4):179–185
15. Lund VJ. Objective assessment of nasal obstruction. Otolaryngol Clin North Am 1989;22(2):279–290
16. Schumacher MJ, Pain MC. Nasal challenge testing in grass pollen hay fever. J Allergy Clin Immunol 1979;64(3):202–208
17. Scadding GK, Darby YC, Austin CE. Acoustic rhinometry compared with anterior rhinomanometry in the assessment of the response to nasal allergen challenge. Clin Otolaryngol Allied Sci 1994;19(5):451–454
18. Gordon AS, McCaffrey TV, Kern EB, Pallanch JF. Rhinomanometry for preoperative and postoperative assessment of nasal obstruction. Otolaryngol Head Neck Surg 1989;101(1):20–26
19. Broms P, Jonson B, Malm L. Rhinomanometry. IV. A pre- and postoperative evaluation in functional septoplasty. Acta Otolaryngol 1982;94(5-6):523–529
20. Jalowayski AA, Yuh YS, Koziol JA, Davidson TM. Surgery for nasal obstruction—evaluation by rhinomanometry. Laryngoscope 1983;93(3):341–345
21. Sulsenti G, Palma P. Nasal valve surgery through hemitransfixion incision: functional results assessed by rhinomanometry. Facial Plast Surg 1990;7(4):315–326
22. Moore M, Eccles R. Objective evidence for the efficacy of surgical management of the deviated septum as a treatment for chronic nasal obstruction: a systemic review. Clin Otolaryngol 2011; 36(2):106–113
23. Malm L. Rhinomanometric assessment for rhinologic surgery. Ear Nose Throat J 1992;71(1):11–16, 19

24. Bachmann W. Differential diagnosis in patients with nasal obstruction: rhinomanometric indications for surgery. Facial Plast Surg 1990;7:274
25. Naito K. Comparison of subjective and objective nasal patency before and after decongestion of the nasal mucosa. Am J Otolaryngol 1991;5(3):113–115
26. Holstrom M. The use of objective measures in selecting patients for septal surgery. Rhinology 2010; 48:387–393
27. Pallanch JF, McCaffrey TV, Kern EB. Normal nasal resistance. Otolaryngol Head Neck Surg 1985;93(6):778–785
28. Grymer LF, Hilberg O, Pedersen OF, Rasmussen TR. Acoustic rhinometry: values from adults with subjective normal nasal patency. Rhinology 1991;29(1):35–47
29. Corey JP, Gungor A, Nelson R, Liu X, Fredberg J. Normative standards for nasal cross-sectional areas by race as measured by acoustic rhinometry. Otolaryngol Head Neck Surg 1998;119(4):389–393
30. Palma P, Papalexiou AH, Sulsenti G. Nasal resistance in healthy subjects. Presentation at Plenary Session on Rhinomanometry. 13th Congress European Rhinologic Society; June 24–29, 1990; London, England.
31. André RF, Vuyk HD, Ahmed A, et al. Correlation between subjective and objective evaluation of the nasal airway. A systematic review of the highest level of evidence. Clin Otolaryngol 2009;34(6):518–525
32. Hopkins C. Re: Correlation between subjective and objective evaluation of the nasal airway. Clin Otolaryngol 2010; 35(2):147–148
33. Eccles R, Doddi NM, Leong S. Re: Correlation between subjective and objective evaluation of the nasal airway. Clin Otolaryngol 2010;35(2):149
34. Williams J, Kulendra K, Hanif J. Re: Correlation between subjective and objective evaluation of the nasal airway. Clin Otolaryngol 2010;35(2):150–151
35. Barnes ML, White PS, Gardiner Q. Re: Correlation between subjective and objective evaluation of the nasal airway. Clin Otolaryngol 2010;35(2):152–153
36. Hopkins C, Earnshaw J, Roberts D. Re: Correlation between subjective and objective evaluation of the nasal airway. Clin Otolaryngol 2010;35(4):337–338
37. Nivatvongs W, Earnshaw J, Roberts D, Hopkins. Re: Correlation between subjective and objective evaluation of the nasal airway. Clin Otolaryngol. 2011;36(2):181–182
38. Vogt K, et al. Computergestutztes System zur rhinologischen Funktionsdiagnostik. HNO 1990;38(3):110–115
39. Vogt K, Jalowayski AA, Althaus W, et al. 4-Phase-Rhinomanometry (4PR)—basics and practice 2010. Rhinol Suppl 2010;(21):25–31
40. Williams H. The history of rhinometry in North America. Int Rhinol 1968;6:34–49

6 Allergic and Nonallergic Rhinitis

Marie-Noëlle Corriveau and Claus Bachert

Rhinitis is a common disease with widespread morbidities that can seriously affect patients' quality of life and work performance; its socioeconomic burden is heavily underestimated. The term rhinitis comprises heterogeneous diseases, of which allergic rhinitis is the best understood. Rhinitis is usually defined as an inflammation of the nose with one or more of the following symptoms: anterior or posterior rhinorrhea, sneezing, nasal congestion, and nasal itching. These symptoms must last for at least two consecutive days and for more than one hour most days.[1,2] Allergic rhinitis (AR) results from immunoglobin E (IgE) -dependent events; its diagnosis requires a systematic approach and an evaluation of comorbidities. Treatment of rhinitis depends not only on the type of disease, but also on symptoms described by the patient. Therapy therefore must be individualized and can become challenging for those patients with more severe disease.

Epidemiology and Risk Factors

Rhinitis is a common problem that causes disabilities worldwide. In industrialized countries, AR affects around 10 to 30% of the population with various prevalence rates according to recent studies.[1] In Belgium, the adjusted prevalence of AR is around 28% of the population, with another 10% suffering from noninfectious, nonallergic rhinitis.[3] The European Community Respiratory Health Survey collected data on adults aged 20 to 40 years in 15 countries. The prevalence of nasal allergy was estimated to be around 25% of the whole population (varying from 12 to 46% per country).[4] In the United States, it is estimated that AR affects 30 to 60 million people annually.[2,5] For children, the International Study of Asthma and Allergies in Childhood (ISAAC) study group estimated that the prevalence of nasal symptoms was around 32%.[6] The same study group showed a worldwide trend toward increasing prevalence of AR in both children and adolescents.[7] Seasonal rhinitis is more prevalent among children, but adults are more affected by perennial rhinitis. AR usually develops before the age of 20, and boys are more affected before adulthood.[2] Less is known about nonallergic rhinitis. One recent Danish study found that around 25% of rhinitis was classified as nonallergic. They also found an increased prevalence of this disease in women.[8] In the United States, nonallergic rhinitis is estimated to affect around 19 million people.[5]

Epidemiologic studies have identified several factors that increase the risk of developing AR. These include: family history of atopy, a serum total IgE higher than 100 IU/mL before the age of 6 years, higher socioeconomic class, and positive allergy skin prick tests.[2] Other factors mentioned are firstborn children and early exposure to food formulas, allergens, and cigarette smoke.[9]

Pathophysiology

Allergic mechanisms leading to rhinitis are far more understood than nonallergic pathways. AR is mediated by IgE antibodies and associated with nasal inflammation (type I reaction in Gell and Coombs classification). The production of allergen-specific IgE needs an initial exposure to an allergen under defined circumstances. The allergen is processed by dendritic cells in the nasal mucosa and presented via major histocompatibility complex (MHC) class II molecules to T helper (TH2) lymphocytes.[2] TH2 cells produce inflammatory mediators such as interleukin (IL)-4, IL-5, IL-13, and others that promote the differentiation of B cells to plasma cells, producing specific IgE antibodies.[1] TH2 cells control the synthesis of IgE and, furthermore, the regulation of eosinophils, basophils, and mast cells. Specific antibodies bind to mast cell surface structures, high affinity IgE receptors, and, upon bridging two adjacent IgE molecules, induce degranulation of the mast cell. Those cells release histamine, leukotrienes, prostaglandins, and other mediators, which cause the early phase reaction, consisting of watery discharge, sneezing and itching, and nasal congestion. There is evidence now that specific allergens such as *Dermatophagoides pteronyssinus* directly activate epithelial cells and lead to a TH2 immune response via their enzymatic activities.[1] The late phase reaction involves mast cells and other inflammatory cells such as T cells and eosinophils, which are recruited into the mucosal site, releasing mediators including IL-4, IL-13, cysteinyl leukotrienes, and neurotrophins, which orchestrate neural hyperresponsiveness and persistent nasal blockage.[1,2]

The hygiene hypothesis suggests that the lack of early exposure to infectious agents may bias the development of an immune response to TH2 cells and thus favor allergic diseases. Vice versa, the exposure to specific bacteria (such as found in farming environments) might induce the release of IL-12 and interferon (INF) production and, thus, increase the activity of T-regulatory cells. This hypothesis is not universally accepted, however, and therapeutic approaches derived from it are still in their infancy.[1,2]

Unlike AR, the physiopathology of nonallergic rhinitis remains elusive. Idiopathic rhinitis, previously called vasomotor rhinitis, is thought to be linked to an imbalance of the autonomic system. Hyporesponsiveness of the sympathetic system results in a decrease of norepinephrine and neuropeptide Y. Hyperactivity of the parasympathetic system implies an increase of acetylcholine and vasoactive intestinal peptide (VIP). This imbalance may lead to glandular hyperactivity and nasal congestion. Other hypotheses imply C-fiber hyperactivity, or the release of increased amounts of neuropeptides (substance P and neurokinins) that promote nasal congestion and nasal secretion production.[10–12] Occupational rhinitis can result from allergic or irritant responses, which elicit eosinophilic or neutrophilic inflammation.[2]

Clinical Presentation

Rhinitis Classification

In 2008, the Allergic Rhinitis and its Impact on Asthma (ARIA) position statement, originally introducing a new AR classification, was updated.[1] The terms *seasonal* and *perennial* were replaced by *intermittent* and *persistent* AR. Also, the assessment of the severity of disease has changed from symptoms only to quality-of-life issues, and forms an important aspect of the new classification (**Table 6.1**). Nonallergic rhinitis encompasses several heterogeneous diseases. **Table 6.2** summarizes the classification of those pathologies according to the ARIA update[1] and the Joint Task Force practice parameters.[2] Occupational rhinitis can be caused by allergic or nonallergic mechanisms.

History

The history of patients with rhinitis should include main nasal complaints such as rhinorrhea, congestion, decreased smell, sneezing, and itching. Duration and frequency of the symptoms, triggers, and associated symptoms like headaches, facial pain, snoring, throat pain, chronic cough, and ear or ocular symptoms must be noted. Past medical and familial history involving eczema, food allergy, and aspirin-exacerbated respiratory disease is relevant. Children may also experience general malaise, disturbed sleep, and episodes of otitis media with effusion. Especially in moderate-to-severe AR, the asthmatic status should be obtained because rhinitis is a powerful predictor of asthma comorbidity with an adjusted relative risk of 2.71 for nonallergic rhinitis and 3.53 for allergic rhinitis[13]—10 to 40% of patients with rhinitis also have asthma.[1] Any past use of medications and their efficacy should be noted. Details about environmental exposures, including tobacco and work-related exposures, should be obtained. Symptoms usually not associated with rhinitis, requiring referral to a specialist, include unilateral symptoms, nasal obstruction as single symptom, mucopurulent rhinorrhea, pain, recurrent epistaxis, and anosmia.[1] Specific presentations associated with each type of rhinitis are described in **Table 6.1** and **Table 6.2**. Severity of the symptoms should be assessed using the Rhinoconjunctivitis Quality of Life Questionnaire (RQLQ) according to ARIA or with a simple visual analogue scale (0 to 10) from "not bothersome" to "very bothersome."[1] Quality of life impairment is of great concern to the patient, as rhinitis often causes sleep disorders, impairment at work and school, and limitations of activities or social dysfunction. Also, ocular symptoms should not be underestimated, as they affect the quality of life of patients with AR. Understanding the sequelae of the disease helps to select and evaluate further therapy.

Differential Diagnosis

Several pathologies of the nose and sinuses should be evaluated before establishing the diagnosis of rhinitis. Chronic rhinosinusitis with or without polyps, anatomic abnormalities including septal deviations, foreign bodies, choanal atresia, adenoidal hypertrophy, or tumors (benign or malignant) usually can be excluded by a meticulous nasal examination, and may require specific imaging studies. If nasal polyps are visualized in children, cystic fibrosis must be excluded. Granulomatous diseases can mimic rhinitis and suspicion is raised with systemic complaints. Those include tuberculosis, Wegener disease, sarcoidosis, Churg-Strauss syndrome, relapsing polychondritis,

Table 6.1 Classification of Allergic Rhinitis

Classification	Definition	Specific Presentations
Intermittent	Symptoms <4 days/week or for <4 consecutive weeks	Primary symptoms are sneezing (paroxysmal ≥4 consecutive), itching, congestion, and clear rhinorrhea, bilateral symptoms; often associated with eye symptoms (bilateral, itching, red eyes, no photophobia); exposition to allergens triggers symptoms; onset usually before the age of 20 years; positive family history of atopic diseases
Persistent	Symptoms >4 days/week or for >4 consecutive weeks	
Mild severity	No sleep disturbance; no impairment of daily activities, leisure, or sport; no impairment of school or work; symptoms present but are not troublesome	
Moderate/severe	Sleep disturbance; impairment of daily activities, leisure, or sport; impairment of school or work; troublesome symptoms	

Source: Data from Bousquet J, Khaltaev N, Cruz AA, et al. Allergic Rhinitis and its Impact on Asthma (ARIA) 2008 update (in collaboration with the World Health Organization, GA[2]LEN and AllerGen). Allergy 2008;63(Suppl 86):8–160.

Table 6.2 Classification of Nonallergic Rhinitis

Type	Classification	Definition	Specific Presentations
Infectious	Viral	Adenovirus, influenza, RSV, parainfluenza, coronavirus	Associated with facial pain and pressure, nasal obstruction; <7–10 days
	Bacterial	*Streptococcus, Haemophilus*	Purulent rhinorrhea, persistent, and fever
Occupational	Caused by work	Inflammatory disease of the nose causing intermittent or persistent symptoms arising out of causes and conditions attributable to a particular work environment; can be elicited by single or multiple exposures; corrosive rhinitis is the most severe form, which causes a permanent inflammation of the nasal mucosa (high concentration of soluble chemicals)	Frequently associated with concurrent asthma; nonallergic form is without latency; nasal challenge tests confirm the diagnosis Agents include: *High molecular weight*: grain dust, flour, latex, biological enzymes, fish and seafood proteins, animals *Low molecular weight*: diisocyanate, anhydrides, wood dust, metals, drugs, chemicals
	Exacerbated by work	Preexisting or concurrent rhinitis exacerbated by workplace exposures	
Drug induced	NSAIDs and ASA	Intense eosinophilic inflammation with an overproduction of cysteinyl leukotrienes and other prostanoids	Profuse rhinorrhea, red eyes, periorbital edema, asthma attacks after ingestion; associated with NP and asthma
	Others	Beta-blockers, ACE inhibitors, methyldopa, reserpine, guanethidine, phentolamine, alpha-adrenoreceptor antagonists, chlorpromazine, oral contraceptives	
	Medicamentosa	Persistent nasal obstruction after using nasal sympathomimetics >5–10 days (oxymetazoline, phenylephrine, xylometazoline, etc.)	Rebound nasal congestion if the medication is stopped
		Cocaine abuse	Septal perforation often associated
Hormonal	Pregnancy, menstruation, puberty	Nasal congestion present during pregnancy without other cause, disappearing within 2 weeks after delivery	Rhinorrhea and nasal obstruction
	Hypothyroidism, acromegaly	Edema of turbinate secondary to thyrotropic hormone release	Nasal congestion
Idiopathic	Vasomotor rhinitis	Diagnosis of exclusion, not IgE-mediated, not infectious, and not associated with nasal eosinophilia	Chronic nasal symptoms triggered by cold air, change in humidity, exposure to tobacco smoke, strong odor, stress, or exercise
Other	NARES	Presence of rhinitis with eosinophils (5–25/HPF) in nasal smears in the absence of demonstrable allergy; precursor of aspirin triad?	Persistent symptoms of nasal congestion, sneezing, rhinorrhea, nasal pruritus, and hyposmia; no history of atopy
	Gustatory rhinitis	Profuse watery rhinorrhea within few hours of oral ingestion	Copious rhinorrhea associated with eating, usually spicy food
	Atrophic	Primary: *Klebsiella ozaenae*	Atrophy of the nasal mucosa with copious smelling crusts
		Secondary: post-excessive nasal surgery, granulomatosis, post radiotherapy or trauma	Atrophy of the nasal mucosa

Source: Data from[1,2,16]
Abbreviations: ACE, angiotensin-converting enzyme; ASA, acetylsalicylic acid; NARES, nonallergic rhinitis with eosinophilia syndrome; NP, nasal polyposis; NSAIDs, nonsteroidal anti-inflammatory drugs; RSV, respiratory syncytial virus.

and amyloidosis. A primary ciliary defect is suspected in cases of persistent infections in childhood and should be differentiated from secondary defects (i.e., post-viral or post-surgery). Refractory clear rhinorrhea could be an indication of a cerebrospinal fluid leak, especially if unilateral with a history of trauma or prior surgery.

Diagnostic Workup

Examination

The general appearance of a patient should be observed; an obstructed nose can induce mouth breathing, and tumors may cause swelling of the face or proptosis. Children may present with obstructed breathing features including malocclusion, long face, a high arch palate, and upper lip elevation. Conjunctival infection with increased lacrimation, Dennie-Morgan lines (creases in the lower eyelid), allergic shiners (blue-gray discoloration below the eyelids), and transverse nasal crease are characteristics of allergic rhinitis patients. Anterior rhinoscopy often reveals hypertrophic turbinates and a pale or bluish mucosa. Hyperemic mucosa points more in the direction of infection or overuse of topical decongestants. However, the appearance of the mucosa cannot be relied upon to differentiate allergic from nonallergic rhinitis. The type and quantity of nasal secretion should be noted. Crusts and inflamed mucosa may suggest atrophic rhinitis or systemic disease. A full head and neck examination should be performed, including a rigid endoscopy to exclude pathologies listed in the differential diagnosis section.

Investigation

To differentiate allergic from nonallergic rhinitis, allergy testing based on the history must be performed. Skin tests are usually preferred to in vitro immunoassays, as they are fast and cheap; however, their results may be influenced by the experience of the investigator and any medication used prior to testing. In brief, antihistamine drugs must be withdrawn 48 hours before the test, and topical steroids must be stopped 3 to 6 days before. The test should not be performed if specific immunotherapy is ongoing. If skin prick tests and serum allergen-specific IgE antibodies to the most common inhalant allergens are negative, rhinitis is unlikely to be allergic. Positive tests need to be linked to the history of the patient, as the sensitization might be clinically irrelevant.

Nasal provocation tests (NPTs) are mainly required for the diagnosis of occupational rhinitis to confirm the causality between symptoms and exposure. Nasal provocation tests are also indicated in the following situations: to support the diagnosis of AR before starting immunotherapy, when symptoms do not correlate with allergic test results, or when there is a nonspecific hyperreactivity. NPTs can also be used as a substitute for oral aspirin provocation tests (however, a negative test does not exclude the diagnosis of aspirin-exacerbated respiratory disease).[14] A positive test usually includes an increase in symptom score and a variation of objective nasal measurements (nasal patency, airflow resistance, volume or weight of secretions).[14] Isotonic and buffered solutions must be at room temperature to avoid unspecific reactions, and a control solution is tested first to exclude hyperresponsiveness of the mucosa. Meter-dose pump sprays should be used to apply the allergens, with deep inspiration performed before the spray to avoid deposition of the substance in the lower airways. One or both nostrils can be tested.

Functional tests can be used to objectively assess the severity of rhinitis by the measurement of nasal obstruction (peak nasal inspiratory flow [PNIF], rhinomanometry, or acoustic rhinometry). PNIF is interesting in the clinical setting and can be used at patients' homes because it is easy to perform, reasonably reproducible, and correlates to the symptoms.[1] Nasal cytology may be performed, using a swab or lavage techniques followed by a hematoxylin and eosin secretion staining. The eosinophil count is often increased in AR, parasitic infections, and nonallergic rhinitis with eosinophilia syndrome (NARES). Mucociliary function tests (e.g., the saccharin test) can help in the diagnosis of mucociliary dysfunction. Suspicious lesions of the nasal mucosa must be biopsied to exclude neoplastic or granulomatous diseases. Other nasal tests are currently evaluated and are, for the moment, useful in research settings (e.g., exhaled nasal nitric oxide).

A computerized tomography (CT) scan is indicated to exclude conditions such as chronic rhinosinusitis and tumors, in the case of unilateral rhinitis, when there is no response to the treatment or when a complication is suspected.[1] Plain radiographs are nowadays not considered useful any more.

Treatment

Treatment of rhinitis should be individualized and should target symptoms as well as improve the quality of life of patients. Age, severity of the disease, presence of comorbidities, and patient preferences are important factors to include in treatment decisions. Educating and counseling patients is crucial; they must understand the chronicity of the disease and how to adapt their treatment to their symptoms. Monitoring treatment should be accomplished after 2 to 4 weeks; control of symptoms is achieved if there is no interference with daily activities and nasal complaints are negligible. In this situation, treatment may be maintained or stepped-down for the following month. However, if patients present with remaining symptoms interfering with their daily activities, a step-up approach using the combination of medications should be initiated. Eventually, the diagnosis needs to be revised and a reevaluation of the patient is mandatory.[2] Some of the medications used for AR can also be employed for nonallergic rhinitis (**Table 6.3**).

Nonallergic Rhinitis

The first-line treatment of nonallergic rhinitis is individualized and usually targets the most bothersome symptoms. Avoidance of irritants such as cigarette smoke can be applied for every type of rhinitis. Intranasal corticosteroids may be effective at relieving nasal obstruction in idiopathic rhinitis and in NARES. Topical decongestants can also be used; however, their usage should be limited to 7 days to avoid abuse.

Table 6.3 Treatment of Rhinitis According to the Type of Rhinitis

Class of Agents	Allergic	Occupational	Drug Induced	Hormonal	Idiopathic	NARES	Atrophic	Symptoms Improved
Topical steroid	✓	+/−	✓		✓	✓		Congestion, rhinorrhea, sneezing, itching eye symptoms
Antihistamine	✓	+/−			Topical			Rhinorrhea, sneezing, itching (eye symptoms if oral)
Anticholinergic	+/−				✓			Rhinorrhea
Oral decongestant	+/−	+/−				+/−		Obstruction
Cromolyn	✓			✓				Prevention if allergen exposure, short action, modest effects
Saline	+/−				✓		✓	Crusts, dryness
Montelukast	✓							Weak effect if alone
Omalizumab	+/−							If asthma comorbidity, nasal and eye symptoms
Treatment comments	See text	Avoid exposure to offending agents	Stop offending drug, +/− oral steroid if rhinitis medicamentosa		Capsaicin may help by desensitization; avoid irritants	Symptomatic, high dose of topical steroid	Symptomatic, debridement, +/− topical antibiotic	

Source: Data from[1,2,10,12,16,22,23,27]

Patients with rhinitis medicamentosa need to progressively withdraw decongestant agents, and topical corticosteroids are usually required. In severe cases, even a short course of oral prednisone may be necessary,[2] and sometimes surgery cannot be avoided. Intranasal anticholinergics are potent at reducing rhinorrhea and are useful in gustatory rhinitis. Those anticholinergics constitute the first-line of treatment for rhinorrhea in elderly patients.[15] Treatment trials should last for 6 weeks before an evaluation of its efficiency can be performed.[10] Intranasal antihistamines (especially azelastine) have been shown to decrease nasal obstruction and rhinorrhea in patients with idiopathic rhinitis and combined "allergic and nonallergic" forms[15]; mere oral antihistamine formulas are usually not indicated in this situation. If treatments mentioned fail, a nasal application of capsaicin can reduce nasal hyperreactivity through desensitization of C-fibers.[10] However, more studies are needed to evaluate precise dosages and the long-term efficacy.

Occupational rhinitis is of special interest with regard to its close relationship with occupational asthma. Complete avoidance of the offending agent is the most effective option. When complete avoidance is not possible and patients have a low risk of developing asthma, a reduction in exposure and pharmacologic agents used in AR can be tried. A close follow-up of those patients is essential to detect the first signs of occupational asthma. In allergic occupational rhinitis, there are some reported improvements with immunotherapy with purified rodent proteins, wheat flour extracts, and natural rubber latex in specific exposure professions.[16]

Allergic Rhinitis

Treatment of AR includes education and environment control, pharmacotherapy, and immunotherapy. Principles of immunotherapy are covered in Chapter 7. There is controversy about the efficacy of environmental measures to control symptoms in AR. Even if there is some evidence of decreased allergen levels, the majority of preventive measures studied have failed to show meaningful clinical benefit.[1] However, general recommendations are usually made: limit exposure to outdoor allergens and pets (air filters for cars and houses), improve ventilation and cleaning the house, avoid carpets, and control moisture and sources of pollution.[1,2] Single interventions for dust mite control usually are ineffective. The combination of measures such as bedding covers, high efficiency particulate air vacuuming of carpets, and using acaricides may be of some benefit and should be considered for severely ill patients.[17] Increased interest in the primary prevention of allergic diseases has led scientists to study the role of probiotics[18]; however, firm recommendations are not yet possible.

The most effective pharmacologic treatment of AR remains the use of newest generation topical glucocorticosteroids (GCS), followed by oral nonsedating second-generation antihistamines or topical drugs. These two agents are recommended as first-line treatments for all forms of AR,[1] with GCS being more efficacious for any nasal symptoms. First-generation antihistamines are not recommended anymore because of their sedative effects. If nasal congestion is important, oral decongestants may be used in combination with oral antihistamines. Antileukotrienes are mostly indicated if patients have asthma associated with seasonal AR. In severe cases of AR, a short course of oral corticosteroids may be needed. If allergic conjunctivitis is present, oral or intraocular antihistamines or chromone (cromolyn) eye drops may be added. In patients with moderate-to-severe rhinitis, the combination of topical GCS with topical antihistamines had been proven effective in one study.[19] A summary of the treatment algorithm published by the updated ARIA workshop is shown in **Fig. 6.1**.

Pharmacotherapy

Nasal corticosteroids are useful to reduce nasal congestion, pruritus, rhinorrhea, eye symptoms, and sneezing for adults and children.[20,21] They potentially reduce nasal inflammation and are known as the most effective treatment of AR. However, they have a slow onset of action compared with antihistamines, and a trial of 1 week should be attempted.[2] Also, their effect on lower airway disease in comorbid asthma

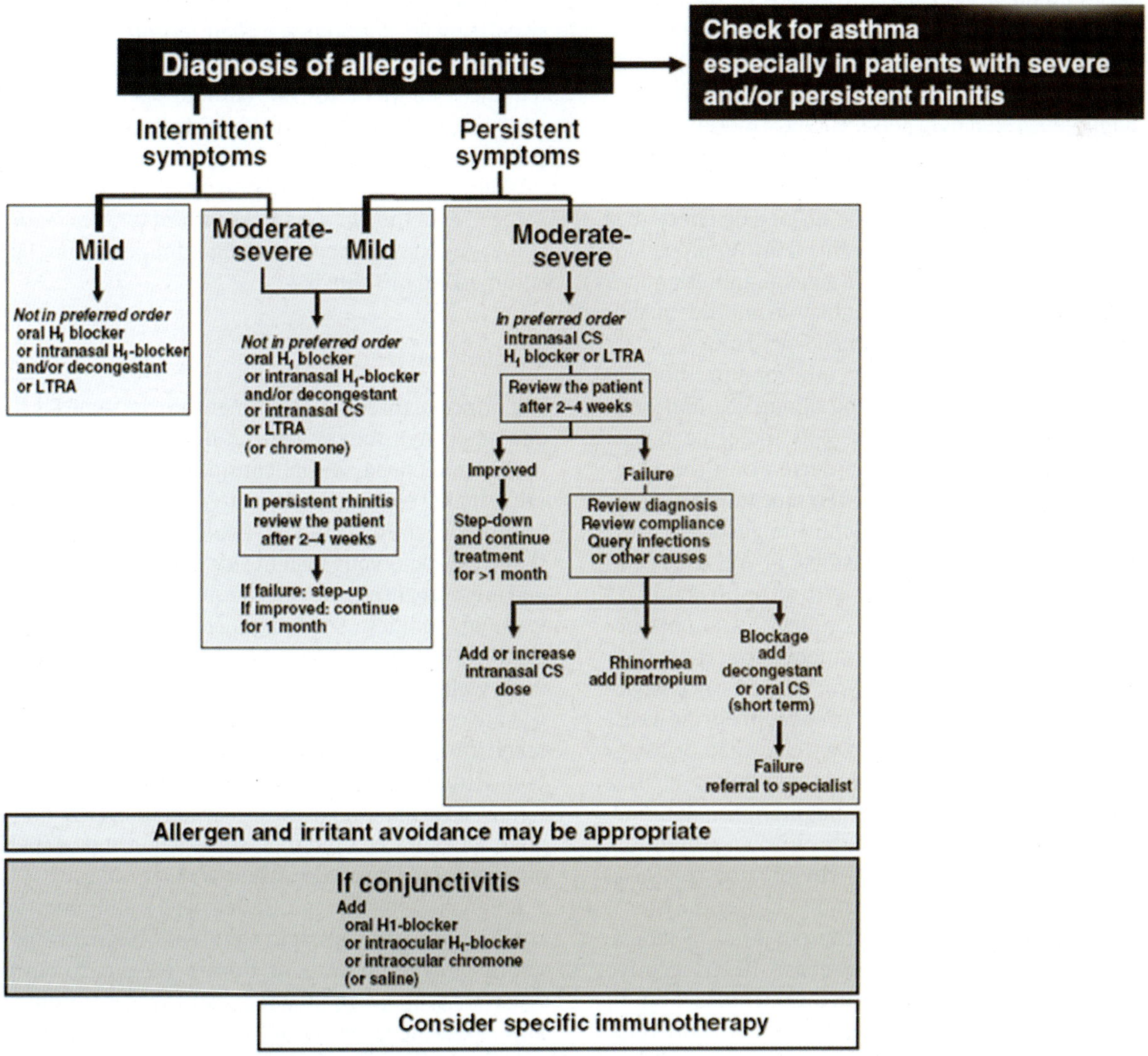

Fig. 6.1 Algorithm for allergic rhinitis. *CS*, corticosteroid; *LTRA*, leukotriene receptor antagonist. (Reprinted with permission from Bousquet J, Khaltaev N, Cruz AA, et al. Allergic Rhinitis and its Impact on Asthma [ARIA] 2008 update [in collaboration with the World Health Organization, GA(2)LEN, and AllerGen]. Allergy 2008;63[Suppl 86]:70.)

still is debated. Minor local side effects such as nasal irritation and bleeding are rare, and septal perforations are an exception. These side effects can be avoided by counseling the patient, and a proper technique of administration is taught. No growth retardation was noted in children after 1 year of applications of either fluticasone propionate or mometasone furoate at appropriate dosages,[1] but caution must be taken with older GCS, such as beclomethasone dipropionate, in the long-term treatment of children.[22,23]

Antihistamines act by blocking H1 receptors on smooth muscle cells, nerve endings, and glandular cells. Second-generation antihistamines are preferred over first-generation drugs because they poorly penetrate the central nervous system, inducing much less sedation, and the higher specificity for the H1 receptor decreases anticholinergic and antiserotonergic side effects.[12] Antihistamines with possible cardiotoxic effects (terfenadine, astemizole) should be avoided and are nowadays restricted in use by health authorities.[24] Antihistamines may have antiallergic and anti-inflammatory properties,[24] although the clinical relevance of such activities is not clear. Last-generation oral formulas act rapidly; are effective against pruritus, sneezing, rhinorrhea, and ocular symptoms; and also affect nasal obstruction, as demonstrated in recent long-term studies in persistent AR.[25] Intranasal antihistamines are also effective for nasal symptoms and may be more effective against nasal congestion than oral formulas, have a safe profile (bitter taste is the major side effect), but need a twice-a-day regimen.[1] Azelastine is also approved for the treatment of idiopathic rhinitis. In general, antihistamines are not as effective as topical GCS, but they do improve quality of life and school performance in patients with AR.

Nasal anticholinergics such as ipratropium bromide 0.03% are effective against anterior rhinorrhea, but does not affect other nasal symptoms. This molecule blocks muscarinic receptors, leading to a decrease in the parasympathetic function. Minor side effects include headache, epistaxis, and nasal dryness. It is helpful for gustatory rhinitis, idiopathic rhinitis with rhinorrhea, or AR, usually in combination with a topical GCS or with an antihistamine.[2]

Local or systemic decongestants relieve nasal obstruction according to their sympathomimetic properties. They act on alpha-adrenergic vessels, producing vasoconstriction. Oral decongestants such as pseudoephedrine must be used with caution for patients with cardiac diseases, glaucoma, urinary retention problems, and thyrotoxicosis. Side effects include hypertension, palpitations, agitation, tremor, insomnia, headache, dry mucosa, urinary retention, and exacerbation of glaucoma or thyrotoxicosis.[1] Nasal administration of topical decongestants causes only local side effects; however, they have the potential to induce rebound congestion if used for more than 10 consecutive days, which may lead to rhinitis medicamentosa. Topical decongestants are therefore only indicated for short-term courses and usually in the case of acute infectious rhinitis; and oral treatment can be used in combination with oral antihistamines to relieve nasal congestion in AR.

Intranasal sodium cromoglycate is an inhibitor of mast cell degranulation, but shows varying responsiveness in different organs. Although chromones are well tolerated and shown to be effective in the prevention and treatment of AR,[2] they are clearly less effective than topical GCS or topical and oral antihistamines, and need to be applied four times a day. Therefore, nasal use is limited, but ocular formulas are helpful in treating allergic conjunctivitis in AR patients.

Leukotriene receptor antagonists are indicated for the treatment of AR in adults and children. Montelukast is the only agent approved for the treatment of AR and is a selective and competitive receptor antagonist for the activity of leukotriene D4 and E4. A recent meta-analysis showed that montelukast provides a benefit over placebo to treat nasal and ocular symptoms, but is less effective than antihistamines or topical steroids. Even with the combination of montelukast and oral antihistamine, control of symptoms was less than that with topical GCS.[26,27]

Omalizumab is a humanized antibody that binds to circulating IgE antibodies at their receptor-binding region. For the moment, this molecule has not been approved for the treatment of AR without concomitant severe and uncontrolled asthma. Its high cost would probably preclude regular use.[12]

Child and adult dosages as well as pregnancy risk categories of the main drugs approved for the treatment of rhinitis by the US Food and Drug Administration (FDA) are summarized in **Table 6.4**.

Special Considerations

The principles of rhinitis treatment are the same for children and adults, but the dosage and possible side effects of the medications need special consideration. Oral medications are usually easier to administer than nasal ones. First-generation antihistamines should be avoided because of their central nervous system side effects including sedation and impairment of performance, leading to further impaired learning abilities. Second-generation antihistamines do produce less side effects and their safety in children has been well studied.[1] Nasal steroids in the appropriate dosage are considered to be safe for children. Caution must be taken if inhaled steroids are added when there is concomitant asthma. No growth delay was identified in a 1-year follow-up of children using last-generation GCS.[1] Intranasal chromones are safe, but their short action and relative weak activity should discourage their widespread use.

Pregnant women can suffer from different types of rhinitis; however, allergic rhinitis is frequent and often affords further treatment during pregnancy. **Table 6.4** illustrates the pregnancy risk categories according to the FDA. Treatment of those patients with drugs requires evaluating the effect of the untreated diseases compared with the potential risk to the fetus. Drugs should be avoided during the first trimester because of the fetus's

Table 6.4 FDA-Approved Drugs for Rhinitis Management

Category	Generic Name	Indications in Rhinitis	Adult Dosage per Nostril (≥12 years)	Pediatric Dosage per Nostril (6–11 years)	Pregnancy Risk
Intranasal steroids	Beclomethasone dipropionate 42 µg/spray	AR and NAR ≥6 years	1–2 sprays BID	1 spray BID	**C**
	Budesonide 32 µg/spray	AR ≥6 years	1–4 sprays DIE	1–2 spray DIE	**B**
	Ciclesonide 50 µg/spray	Seasonal AR ≥6 years Perennial AR ≥12 years	2 sprays DIE	2 sprays DIE	**C**
	Flunisolide 25 µg/spray	AR ≥6 years	(≥15 years) 2 sprays BID ad TID	(6–14 years) 2 sprays BID	**C**
	Fluticasone furoate 27.5 µg/spray	AR ≥2 years	2 sprays DIE	(2–11 years) 1 spray DIE	**C**
	Fluticasone propionate 50 µg/spray	AR and NAR ≥4 years	1 spray BID or 2 sprays DIE	(4–11 years) 1 spray DIE	**C**
	Mometasone furoate 50 µg/spray	AR ≥2 years, prophylaxis of seasonal AR ≥12 years	2 sprays DIE	(2–11 years) 1 spray DIE	**C**
	Triamcinolone acetonide 55 µg/spray	AR ≥2 years	2 sprays DIE	(2–5 years) 1 spray DIE (6–12 years) 1–2 sprays DIE	**C**
Intranasal antihistamines	Azelastine 137 µg/spray	Seasonal AR ≥5 years NAR ≥12 years	2 sprays BID	(5–11 years) 1 spray BID	**C**
	Olopatadine hydrochloride 0.6%	Seasonal AR ≥6 years	2 sprays BID	1 spray BID	**C**
Intranasal anticholinergics	Ipratropium bromide 0.03%	AR and NAR ≥6 years	2 sprays BID to TID	2 sprays BID to TID	**B**
Intranasal chromones	Cromolyn sodium 5.2 mg/spray	AR and prophylaxis before exposure ≥2 years	1 spray TID to QID	(2–11 years) 1 spray TID to QID	**B**
Oral antihistamines, second generation	Acrivastine	Seasonal AR ≥12 years	8 mg QID	–	**B**
	Cetirizine	Seasonal AR ≥ 2 years Perennial AR ≥ 6 months	5–10 mg DIE	(6 months –2 years) 2.5 mg DIE (2–5 years) 2.5–5 mg DIE (6–11 years) 5–10 mg DIE	**B**
	Desloratadine	Seasonal AR ≥ 2 years Perennial AR ≥ 6 months	5 mg DIE	(6–11 months) 1 mg DIE (1–5 years) 1.25 mg DIE (6–11 years) 2.5 mg DIE	**C**
	Fexofenadine	Seasonal AR ≥2 years	60 mg BID	(2–11 years) 30 mg BID	**C**
	Levocetirizine	Seasonal AR ≥2 years Perennial AR ≥6 months	5 mg DIE	(6 months–5 years) 1.25 mg DIE (6–11 years) 2.5 mg DIE	**B**
	Loratadine	Seasonal AR ≥2 years	10 mg DIE	(2–5 years) 5 mg DIE (6–11 years) 10 mg DIE	**B**
Oral decongestants	Pseudoephedrine	AR and NAR ≥2 years	30–60 mg each 4–6 hours	See specific products	**C Not last trimester**
	Phenylephrine	AR and NAR ≥2 years	10–20 mg each 4–6 hours	See specific products	**C Not last trimester**
Leukotriene antagonists	Montelukast	Seasonal AR ≥2 years Perennial AR ≥6 months	(≥15 years) 10 mg DIE	(6 months–5 years) 4 mg DIE (6–14 years) 5 mg DIE	**B**

Source: US Food and Drug Administration Web site: www.fda.gov/cder/info/healthcare.htm 2011.
Abbreviations: AR, allergic rhinitis; NAR, nonallergic rhinitis; BID, twice per day; DIE, once a day; TID, three times per day; QID, four times per day.

organogenesis, and the lowest effective dose should be used if unavoidable. Decongestants and oral GCS certainly need to be avoided. New-generation oral antihistamines and low bioavailability topical GCS are usually considered safe even if most of them were given a category C by the FDA, meaning that animal studies have shown adverse effects (this risk has not been confirmed for humans).[2] However, intranasal steroids are not useful in rhinitis induced by pregnancy, which best is treated by saline douches.

Moreover, athletes are of special concern because some drugs usually used to treat rhinitis are not allowed in competitions. No medication should be used that can modify the athlete's performance. In general, all oral decongestants are banned. Oral antihistamines and intranasal steroids are usually tolerated, but sometimes on a case-to-case basis.[2]

Surgery

Surgery is indicated as an adjuvant therapy if there is a structural problem. A septoplasty is indicated in the case of a function-impairing nasoseptal deviation associated with bothersome nasal obstruction. A partial inferior conchotomy may be performed in the case of therapy-resistant rhinitis medicamentosa or other forms of drug-resistant turbinate hypertrophy. Endoscopic sinus surgery is reserved for comorbidities of rhinitis such as chronic rhinosinusitis or nasal polyposis. Vidian neurectomies have been replaced by medical treatments, which are as effective to treat idiopathic rhinitis, but without surgical complications.

Outcomes

The impact of rhinitis on a patient's health-related quality of life is now better investigated. Several studies using validated questionnaires revealed a diminished quality of life, sleeping disorders, trouble with concentration, lower performance at work, and difficult social relationships among patients with AR.[28] Pharmacologic treatment of AR not only improves symptoms, but also improves quality of life of the patients with moderate/severe rhinitis. For oral last-generation nonsedating antihistamines, a sustained effect on the quality of life has been demonstrated; a larger effect seems to be given by topical GCS, but more studies are needed here.[28] It is to be noted that the quality of life of patients with prominent allergic ocular symptoms can be increased when olopatadine hydrochloride ophthalmic solution is added to the treatment.[29] Oral GCS needs to be reserved for severe cases of seasonal AR and needs to be restricted to a short period followed by topical use—intramuscular GCS should not be used. A control visit of patients is needed to ensure that the treatment is effective to modify AR symptoms and its sequelae sufficiently. It is not clear if the treatment of rhinitis with pharmacotherapy can prevent or modulate asthma. As AR is a risk factor for the development of asthma, the clinical examination should include screening for asthma comorbidity in moderate-to-severe disease.

As for other chronic diseases, compliance with medications is of concern. According to an American survey, more than half of patients with AR use over-the-counter medications to relieve their symptoms[19]; emphasis must therefore be put on individualized treatment algorithms to help patients choose the best drug. Up to one-quarter of patients stop their treatment because of side effects.[19] Nasal sprays have different forms and components and may be confused, wrongly applied, or just disliked. All of these factors may contribute to a low compliance and may undermine treatment success. Counseling measures are therefore of great importance.

Despite adequate treatments and compliance, there are some patients whose symptoms are inadequately controlled. Those patients can be classified as having severe chronic upper airway diseases (SCUADs), which include AR, nonallergic rhinitis, occupational rhinitis, and chronic rhinosinusitis. In severe persistent AR, 20% of patients are expected to have uncontrolled symptoms with pharmacologic treatments based on guidelines.[30] The proportion of patients having SCUADs in nonallergic rhinitis and occupational rhinitis is unknown. Comorbidities in SCUADs are common and these patients have impaired quality of life and working performance.

Conclusion

Rhinitis is a highly prevalent condition worldwide. It can be generally classified into allergic, infectious, and nonallergic, but an accurate diagnosis is essential, in particular between the subtypes of nonallergic rhinitis. Pharmacologic treatments should target symptoms to improve quality of life for patients. Although this condition is frequent, more studies are needed to have a more accurate view of the prevalence, phenotype, and treatments of rhinitis. In particular, understanding the pathophysiology of nonallergic rhinitis and AR would lead to an improved medical management of those diseases. Moreover, SCUADs need to be better defined, and novel treatments are required.

References

1. Bousquet J, Khaltaev N, Cruz AA, et al; World Health Organization; GA(2)LEN; AllerGen. Allergic Rhinitis and its Impact on Asthma (ARIA) 2008 update (in collaboration with the World Health Organization, GA(2)LEN and AllerGen). Allergy 2008;63(Suppl 86):8–160
2. Wallace DV, Dykewicz MS, Bernstein DI, et al; Joint Task Force on Practice; American Academy of Allergy; Asthma & Immunology; American College of Allergy; Asthma and Immunology; Joint Council of Allergy, Asthma and Immunology. The diagnosis and management of rhinitis: an updated practice parameter. J Allergy Clin Immunol 2008;122(2, Suppl)S1–S84
3. Bachert C, van Cauwenberge P, Olbrecht J, van Schoor J. Prevalence, classification and perception of allergic and nonallergic rhinitis in Belgium. Allergy 2006;61(6):693–698

4. Bousquet PJ, Leynaert B, Neukirch F, et al. Geographical distribution of atopic rhinitis in the European Community Respiratory Health Survey I. Allergy 2008;63(10):1301–1309
5. Settipane RA, Charnock DR. Epidemiology of rhinitis: allergic and nonallergic. Clin Allergy Immunol 2007;19:23–34
6. Aït-Khaled N, Pearce N, Anderson HR, Ellwood P, Montefort S, Shah J; ISAAC Phase Three Study Group. Global map of the prevalence of symptoms of rhinoconjunctivitis in children: The International Study of Asthma and Allergies in Childhood (ISAAC) Phase Three. Allergy 2009;64(1):123–148
7. Asher MI, Montefort S, Björkstén B, et al; ISAAC Phase Three Study Group. Worldwide time trends in the prevalence of symptoms of asthma, allergic rhinoconjunctivitis, and eczema in childhood: ISAAC Phases One and Three repeat multicountry cross-sectional surveys. Lancet 2006;368(9537):733–743
8. Mølgaard E, Thomsen SF, Lund T, Pedersen L, Nolte H, Backer V. Differences between allergic and nonallergic rhinitis in a large sample of adolescents and adults. Allergy 2007;62(9):1033–1037
9. Skoner DP. Allergic rhinitis: definition, epidemiology, pathophysiology, detection, and diagnosis. J Allergy Clin Immunol 2001;108(1, Suppl)S2–S8
10. van Rijswijk JB, Blom HM, Fokkens WJ. Idiopathic rhinitis, the ongoing quest. Allergy 2005;60(12):1471–1481
11. Salib RJ, Harries PG, Nair SB, Howarth PH. Mechanisms and mediators of nasal symptoms in non-allergic rhinitis. Clin Exp Allergy 2008;38(3):393–404
12. Greiner AN, Meltzer EO. Pharmacologic rationale for treating allergic and nonallergic rhinitis. J Allergy Clin Immunol 2006;118(5):985–998
13. Shaaban R, Zureik M, Soussan D, et al. Rhinitis and onset of asthma: a longitudinal population-based study. Lancet 2008;372(9643):1049–1057
14. Malm L, Gerth van Wijk R, Bachert C. Guidelines for nasal provocations with aspects on nasal patency, airflow, and airflow resistance. International Committee on Objective Assessment of the Nasal Airways, International Rhinologic Society. Rhinology 2000;38(1):1–6
15. Gehanno P, Deschamps E, Garay E, Baehre M, Garay RP. Vasomotor rhinitis: clinical efficacy of azelastine nasal spray in comparison with placebo. ORL J Otorhinolaryngol Relat Spec 2001;63(2):76–81
16. Moscato G, Vandenplas O, Gerth Van Wijk R, et al; EAACI Task Force on Occupational Rhinitis. Occupational rhinitis. Allergy 2008;63(8):969–980
17. Sheikh A, Hurwitz B, Shehata Y. House dust mite avoidance measures for perennial allergic rhinitis. Cochrane Database Syst Rev 2007; (1):CD001563
18. Kuitunen M, Kukkonen K, Juntunen-Backman K, et al. Probiotics prevent IgE-associated allergy until age 5 years in cesarean-delivered children but not in the total cohort. J Allergy Clin Immunol 2009;123(2):335–341
19. Carr WW, Nelson MR, Hadley JA. Managing rhinitis: Strategies for improved patient outcomes. Allergy Asthma Proc 2008;29(4):349–357
20. Origlieri C, Bielory L. Intranasal corticosteroids and allergic rhinoconjunctivitis. Curr Opin Allergy Clin Immunol 2008;8(5):450–456
21. Penagos M, Compalati E, Tarantini F, Baena-Cagnani CE, Passalacqua G, Canonica GW. Efficacy of mometasone furoate nasal spray in the treatment of allergic rhinitis. Meta-analysis of randomized, double-blind, placebo-controlled, clinical trials. Allergy 2008;63(10):1280–1291
22. Plaut M, Valentine MD. Clinical practice. Allergic rhinitis. N Engl J Med 2005;353(18):1934–1944
23. Bousquet J, Reid J, van Weel C, et al. Allergic rhinitis management pocket reference 2008. Allergy 2008;63(8):990–996
24. Simons FE. Advances in H1-antihistamines. N Engl J Med 2004;351(21):2203–2217
25. Canonica GW, Tarantini F, Compalati E, Penagos M. Efficacy of desloratadine in the treatment of allergic rhinitis: a meta-analysis of randomized, double-blind, controlled trials. Allergy 2007;62(4):359–366
26. Grainger J, Drake-Lee A. Montelukast in allergic rhinitis: a systematic review and meta-analysis. Clin Otolaryngol 2006;31(5):360–367
27. Wilson AM, O'Byrne PM, Parameswaran K. Leukotriene receptor antagonists for allergic rhinitis: a systematic review and meta-analysis. Am J Med 2004;116(5):338–344
28. Baiardini I, Braido F, Tarantini F, et al; GA2LEN. ARIA-suggested drugs for allergic rhinitis: what impact on quality of life? A GA2LEN review. Allergy 2008;63(6):660–669
29. Berger W, Abelson MB, Gomes PJ, et al. Effects of adjuvant therapy with 0.1% olopatadine hydrochloride ophthalmic solution on quality of life in patients with allergic rhinitis using systemic or nasal therapy. Ann Allergy Asthma Immunol 2005;95(4):361–371
30. Bousquet J, Bachert C, Canonica GW, et al; Extended Gobal Allergy and Asthma European Network, World Allergy Organization and Allergic Rhinitis and its Impact on Asthma Study Group. Unmet needs in severe chronic upper airway disease (SCUAD). J Allergy Clin Immunol 2009;124(3):428–433

7 Principles of Allergy Skin Testing and Immunotherapy

Daniel L. Hamilos

Allergy skin and in vitro testing are designed to detect classic type I immunoglobulin E (IgE)-mediated immediate hypersensitivity reactions. This chapter focuses on the use of skin testing and in vitro testing for the diagnosis of inhalant allergies relevant to otorhinolaryngology—head and neck surgery. Similar principles apply to the diagnosis of other types of IgE-mediated allergies. It is implied that allergy testing should only be performed when the patient elicits an appropriate or suggestive history or physical findings suggesting of an allergic disease. Allergy testing should not substitute for an appropriate clinical history and environmental survey of potential allergen exposures, because patients may have positive tests in the absence of clinical symptoms either because of target organ insensitivity—that is, false-positive tests or lack of allergen exposure.

■ The Immunologic Basis for Allergic Responses

Allergic responses require the presence of allergen-specific IgE antibodies. The development of allergen-specific IgE antibodies requires allergen exposure, antigen processing by subepithelial and intraepithelial antigen-presenting dendritic cells, and activation of T helper cells down a "Th2 pathway." The precise determinants leading T helper cells to differentiate toward the Th2 pathway are incompletely understood. Components include: genetic susceptibility factors, route and dose of allergen exposure, signaling through the innate immune system, and intrinsic allergen properties. With regard to signaling through the innate immune system, the protein thymic stromal lymphopoietin (TSLP)—produced by epithelial cells, fibroblasts, and mast cells—has been found to be a "master switch" toward Th2 cell development.[1–3] TSLP modulates dendritic cell antigen-presenting cell (APC) capacity resulting in a "polarized" Th2 activation. With regard to intrinsic allergenic properties, certain allergens, such as the dust mite protease Der p2, have the capacity to cleave tight junctions in airway epithelium increasing their penetration and uptake by antigen presenting dendritic cells, activate protease-activated receptors, such as PAR-2,[4] and interact with other components of the innate immune system, such as MD-2, thereby signaling via the toll-like receptor 4 (TLR-4) on epithelial cells and dendritic cells.[5] Each of these properties of dust mite proteases has been shown in experimental animals to be important in inducing a Th2 polarized immune response.

Once activated down the Th2 pathway, the Th2 cells produce characteristic Th2 cytokines, including interleukin (IL)-4, IL-5, IL-9, and IL-13. IL-4 is a potent B lymphocyte activation and differentiation factor that promotes antibody isotype switching toward the production of allergen-specific IgE.

Allergen-specific IgE antibodies elicit allergic responses via binding to cells expressing the high-affinity FcεRI IgE receptor. In the skin, FcεRI are expressed primarily on mast cells. Immediate allergic responses, which occur within 15 minutes of placement of an allergy skin test, are a mast cell event elicited by cross-linking of two FcεRI receptors on the mast cell surface. FcεRI cross-linking leads to degranulation with the release of preformed mediators, most notably histamine, proteases (tryptase, chymotrypsin, carboxypeptidase A, and chymase), and certain cytokines (e.g., tumor necrosis factor [TNF]-α).[6] FcεRI cross-linking also leads to mast cell activation and production of newly formed mediators, cytokines, and chemokines. The newly formed mediators include: prostaglandin D2 (PgD2), leukotrienes (LTC4, LTD4), thromboxanes (TXA2), and platelet activating factor (PAF). Activated mast cells have the capacity to produce multiple cytokines, including TNF-α, IL-4, IL-5, IL-13, and chemokines, including MCP-1 (CCL2) and the CXC chemokine IL-8 (CXCL8).[6] The immediate allergic skin test response is classically described as a "wheal and flare" response.

Release of mediators and production of cytokines and chemokines help the mast cell contribute to an inflammatory response known as the late-phase response (LPR).[7] The LPR typically occurs 3 to 24 hours following allergen exposure and is characterized by a local edema formation and inflammatory cell infiltration. It can be demonstrated experimentally in the skin, conjunctiva, nose, and lungs. Key inflammatory features of the allergic LPR include an infiltration of Th2 T lymphocytes, monocytes, eosinophils, basophils, and eosinophil/basophil progenitor cells.[8] Mature basophils contribute to histamine release during the LPR due to their expression of FcεRI. The allergic LPR is reminiscent of the histopathologic appearance of chronic allergic inflammation in response to natural allergen exposure. The immediate and late-phase allergic responses are distinct events, but allergen-specific IgE contributes to both responses.[7]

Figure 7.1 summarizes the salient features of the allergic response, including the process of allergen sensitization and the effector pathways of immediate and late-phase allergic responses.

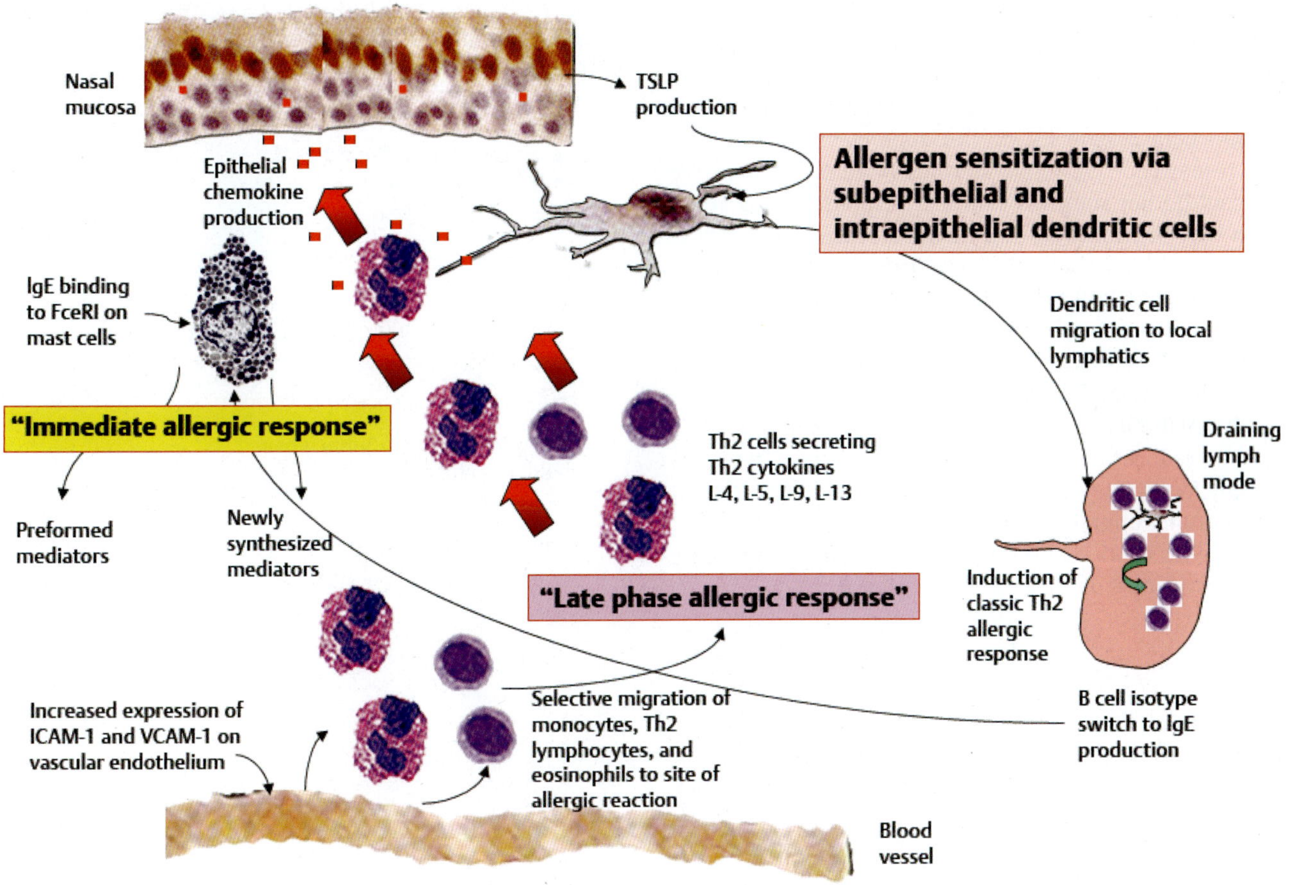

Fig. 7.1 Schematic of the allergic response. Salient features of the allergic response are illustrated, including the process of allergen sensitization with the induction of allergen-specific Th2 lymphocytes and the effector pathways of immediate and late-phase allergic responses. The immediate and late-phase allergic responses are distinct events, but allergen-specific IgE contributes to both responses.

Allergic Skin Testing Procedures and Devices

Skin testing has traditionally been the most popular allergy testing method and remains so despite considerable improvements in in vitro testing over the past two decades. Compared with in vitro testing by the IgE ImmunoCAP Radioallergosorbent Test (CAP-RAST) method, allergy skin testing is faster, less expensive, and slightly more sensitive.[9] By comparison, in vitro IgE CAP-RAST testing offers certain advantages, including (1) the fact that it can be performed in patients who are receiving antihistamines or who are dermographic; (2) the fact that it provides more quantitative results (that may have clinical significance, for instance, in predicting the likelihood of anaphylaxis from food allergens); and (3) that it is absolutely safe (although skin testing is nearly always safe).

Factors That Increase or Decrease Allergy Skin Testing Responses

Certain conditions may cause a nonspecific increase[10] in skin testing responsiveness. These include: dermographism (also referred to as dermatographism), application of skin tests too close together (at least 2.5 cm apart is recommended), use of systemic beta-blocker drugs, and perhaps ingestion of foods that cross-react with inhalant allergens. In contrast, an increase in allergen-specific skin test responsiveness is seen immediately following pollen allergy season that is associated with an increase in allergen-specific IgE in the serum.[11,12]

Other conditions may cause a nonspecific decrease in skin testing responsiveness. The most common condition is use of an antihistamine. As a rule, patients in our clinic are instructed to withhold antihistamines for 1 week prior to skin testing, although the required period of withholding varies somewhat from one antihistamine to another. Topical application of azelastine (Astelin) nasal spray suppresses skin test responses if administered within 48 hours of testing.[13] Certain nontraditional antihistamines also possess potent antihistaminic effects. Most notable are tricyclic antidepressants (e.g., amitriptyline, nortriptyline, doxepin) and possibly newer antidepressants, such as venlafaxine (Effexor). Depending on the patient's need for these medications, it may or may not be advisable to withhold them for 1 week before skin testing. Systemic beta-agonists (e.g., terbutaline) and theophylline are also reported to suppress skin test responses, although the degree of suppression is weak. H2 antihistamines cause mild skin test suppression and are recommended to be withheld for 24 hours.[14] Other drugs, such as proton pump inhibitors, leukotriene blockers, cromolyn, and inhaled beta-2 agonists, do not appreciably inhibit skin test responses.[15] Systemic steroids (e.g., prednisone, 30 mg/day) do not suppress skin test responses if given for up to 1 week prior to testing. However, chronic use of systemic steroids or the topical application of high potency topical steroids for greater than 3 weeks may cause some degree of suppression of responses.[16] Immunotherapy may decrease allergen-specific IgE responses, but this is not a consistent finding.[17,18] The anti-IgE monoclonal antibody, omalizumab (Xolair), administered for a minimum of 3 months reduces both circulating and mucosal allergen-specific free IgE levels.[19] For these reasons, skin testing in patients on immunotherapy or omalizumab must be interpreted with caution and is not recommended to evaluate the effectiveness of these treatments.

Prick Testing

Prick skin testing is typically performed using a commercially supplied needle or lancet. Several different devices are available, including hypodermic needles, solid bore needles, lancets with or without a bifurcated tip, and multiple-head devices. None of these devices is clearly superior to the others.[14] The needle is either dipped in the allergenic extract first or pricked through a drop of extract on the skin. The needle is introduced at a 45- to 60-degree angle to the skin and then gently lifted to allow the allergen to enter the epidermis. Alternatively, using a puncture technique, the skin is punctured at a 90-degree angle using a device that typically has a shoulder to prevent penetration into the dermis (e.g., Morrow-Brown type needle). Individual skin tests are spaced a minimum of 2 to 2.5 cm apart to prevent interference. Tests are also placed a minimum of 5 cm from the wrist and 3 cm from the antecubital fossa.[14] Positive (histamine dihydrochloride 10 mg/mL) and negative (saline or 50% glycerinated HSA-saline) controls are also performed. Because some prick testing allergens contain 50% glycerine, a 50% glycerine control test is also performed. Most clinicians use disposable devices rather than traditional solid bore needles that can be wiped and reused. The wheal responses in prick skin testing are read at 15 to 20 minutes.

An alternative epicutaneous technique is scratch testing, in which a drop of allergen is first placed on the skin followed by scratching the skin through it with a needle without drawing blood. Scratch testing is more uncomfortable and less reproducible than prick testing and is no longer commonly used.[9]

Although studies comparing the various devices used for prick or puncture testing have failed to reveal any clear-cut advantage for any particular device, the wheal size elicited in response to saline and histamine varies with the device.

Table 7.1 Size of Wheals That Are Larger Than 99% of Wheals with Saline Using the Same Device on the Patient's Back Performed by the Same Operator

Device	Wheal Size, mm
Devices for which a 3-mm wheal would be significant	
Quintest (HS) puncture	0
Smallpox needle (HS) prick	0
DuoTip (Lincoln) prick	1.5
Lancet (HS) puncture	2.0
Lancet (ALK) puncture	3.0
Derma PICK II (BioMedx)	0
Devices for which a >3-mm wheal would be significant	
DuoTip (Lincoln) twist	3.5
Bifurcated needle (ALO) prick	4.0
MultiTest (Lincoln) puncture	4.0
Bifurcated needle (ALK) puncture	4.5
Quick Test (Pantrex)	4.0
Greer Track (Greer)	3.5

Abbreviations: BioMedx, Seattle, WA: HS, Hollister Stier, Spokane, WA; Greer, Greer Laboratories, Lenoir, NC; Lincoln, Lincoln Diagnostics, Decatur, IL; ALK, ALK America, Round Rock, TX; ALO, Allergy Laboratories of Ohio, Columbus, OH. (Used with permission from Oppenheimer J, Nelson HS. Skin testing. Ann Allergy Asthma Immunol 2006;96(2 Suppl 1):S6–12.)

Therefore, the user should become familiar with the size of the wheal elicited by saline and histamine with whatever device is used. A summary of wheal sizes elicited by different commercially available devices is summarized in **Table 7.1**. A procedure for assessing a technician's proficiency with a particular skin testing device has been published.[14] The results of prick testing are highly reproducible over 1 to 2 years of observation.[20,21]

Multiheaded Skin Testing Device Testing

Multiheaded testing devices allow up to eight prick or percutaneous tests to be performed simultaneously. These devices may have single tips or multipronged tips. The testing devices vary in the amount of trauma they produce and the wheal size greater than the saline control to be regarded as a positive test (**Table 7.1**).

A comparative study of multiheaded test devices found that the Multitest II (Lincoln Diagnostics, Decatur, IL), DermaPik II (BioMedx, Spokane, WA), Quick Test (Panatex, Placentia, CA), and Greer Track (Greer Laboratories, Lenoir, NC) had a high rate of consistency in producing negative reactions to saline. However, the Quick Test and Greer Track had higher numbers of false-negative reactions to histamine.[22] Generally, using multiheaded devices, wheal sizes >3 mm larger than the saline reaction are required to confidently represent positive reactions.[23]

Intradermal (Intracutaneous) Single Dilution Skin Testing

Intradermal (ID) single dilution skin testing is done with a 26-gauge hypodermic needle. Approximately 0.01 to 0.02 mL of allergen solution is injected intradermally resulting in a wheal of 4 to 5 mm. The wheal response in intradermal testing is read at 10 to 15 minutes.[24] Positive (histamine 0.004 mg/mL) and negative (saline) control tests are performed simultaneously. The histamine control should elicit ≥7 mm wheal. The diagnostic accuracy of intradermal testing is reported to be greater than prick/puncture tests when testing with insect venom or certain drugs.[14] The concentration of allergens used in ID testing by board-certified allergists is typically 1/100th of that used for skin prick testing. This is different from what is typically used in intradermal dilutional testing (see the following).

Intradermal Dilutional Testing

Intradermal dilutional testing (IDT), formerly known as skin endpoint titration (SET) testing, has been the traditional method of allergy skin testing in otorhinolaryngology for the past half-century.[25] IDT is performed using serial 1:5 dilutions of the prick testing reagents. Phenolated saline or human serum albumin (HSA) are used to prepare dilutions. **Table 7.2** summarizes the allergen concentrations used in IDT testing. All allergens are first tested at dilution # 6, representing a dilution of 1:3.125 from the concentrated extract. Wheal size is measured at 10 minutes. If the tests are negative, progressively stronger dilutions are tested until a positive wheal is elicited. All test dilutions are injected with the needle bevel down with an injection of sufficient volume to raise a 4 to 5 mm wheal (~0.01 to 0.02 mL). Testing is stopped at dilution #2 (1:5 dilution of concentrated extract). The endpoint is the allergen concentration at which a progressively positive wheal reaction commences. A positive response is usually accompanied by erythema. The endpoint is confirmed by testing one concentration above the endpoint and confirming a larger wheal size. The major advantages of endpoint titration are (1) determining the patient's degree of allergic sensitivity, and (2) determining the concentration of extract at which allergen immunotherapy can be started.[26] The saline control and negative allergen responses may increase in size from 4 to 5 mm due to physical spreading but should not increase in size beyond that and should not elicit erythema. Because dilution #2 may contain 2% glycerine, a 2% glycerine control test is also recommended.

Some allergens, particularly intradermally injected mold extracts, may elicit either a combined immediate and delayed positive response or an isolated delayed positive response within 24 hours. It has been presumed, but never proven, that the delayed responses represent the equivalent of an IgE-dependent late-phase allergic response.[27]

Table 7.2 Comparison of Allergen Concentrations Typically Used for Intradermal Dilutional Testing Versus Single Concentration Intradermal Testing

Dilution	Allergen Dilution (weight/volume)	Concentration Typically Used for Single ID Testing
Concentrate	1/20 w/v	1/100th of the concentration used for prick testing*
1	1/100 w/v	
2	1/500 w/v	
3	1/2,500 w/v	
4	1/12,500 w/v	
5	1/62,500 w/v	
6	1/312,500 w/v	

*Some manufacturers supply allergens for ID testing at 500 PNU/mL.
Abbreviations: ID, intradermal.

Differences in Results From Intradermal and Intradermal Dilutional Skin Testing Procedures

In a conventional allergy practice, allergens for intradermal testing are prepared from concentrated extracts or purchased commercially. Commercial extracts are typically prepared at 1/100th dilution of the fully concentrated prick testing reagents. A recent survey of board-certified allergists in the United States revealed great variability in the concentration of ID test reagents used in practice.[23] The equivalencies of prick and ID testing reagents are only estimates because prick testing reagents are often supplied in w/v units, whereas ID reagents are supplied in PNU/mL. Nonetheless, considering that ID testing is roughly 500- to 1000-fold more sensitive than prick testing, the use of ID extracts at 1/100th the prick testing concentration explains why these ID tests are more sensitive than prick tests.

Because fivefold dilutions are used for IDT, dilution #3 (1:125th of the concentrated extract) is roughly equivalent to the allergen concentration used by allergists for ID testing. Dilution #2 represents a considerably higher allergen concentration than that used by allergists. This explains the lack of agreement between ID and IDT testing results. Considering that several studies have shown a lack of correlation of positive ID tests with allergen challenge procedures, it is to be expected that positive IDT tests with dilution #2 would often be clinically irrelevant.

The clinical relevance of positive skin test responses can only be assessed by determining how well the test predicts target organ sensitivity (nose or lungs). This type of verification, done by nasal or bronchial allergen challenge testing, has established a high degree of positive predictive value (PPV) for a positive prick test but a low PPV for a positive intradermal test (see the following).

In Vitro CAP-RAST Testing (IgE CAP-RAST Test)

The state of the art in vitro specific IgE assay is the ImmunoCAP (Pharmacia Diagnostics, Uppsala, Sweden) or the Immulite (Diagnostics Product Corporation, Los Angeles, CA).[24] These tests are based on a solid-phase immunoassay in which the allergen is bound to a hydrophilic carrier polymer encased in a capsule. Pharmacia developed the ImmunoCAP in 1989, and this method received US Food and Drug Administration (FDA) approval to quantify allergen-specific IgE down to a detection limit of 0.1 kU/L. The ImmunoCAP polymer consists of a CNBr-activated cellulose derivative that has a much higher protein binding capacity than traditional paper disks used in earlier versions of the RAST test. The Immulite 2000 uses a chemiluminescent enzyme-labeled sequential immunoassay for detection of allergen-specific IgE. The sensitivity and specificity of these state of the art assays are roughly equivalent to those of skin prick testing.

Sensitivity and Specificity of Prick and Intradermal Testing Procedures

The sensitivity of skin prick tests, as judged by the frequency of positive skin test responses to allergens known to be allergenic by history and positive bronchial challenge, is ~80%.[28] The corresponding specificity of a negative skin prick test is estimated at 95%.[29] The sensitivity of prick testing can be increased by avoidance of glycerinated extracts or by adding a small concentration of Tween 80 (0.0005%); however, these are not typically used in clinical practice. False-positive prick skin tests are immunologically specific but clinically silent, and may represent "latent" allergies or portend future sensitivities.[30] By comparison, traditional intradermal skin testing using allergens diluted to 1/100th (1/1000 w/v) of the concentration used for prick skin testing has a sensitivity greater than 90% but a lower specificity. Therefore, a positive intradermal test has a lower likelihood of predicting a positive nasal or bronchial challenge test. In a study by Spector and Farr,[31] positive ID skin tests at 1/1000 w/v (compared with prick testing at 1/10 w/v) were associated with a positive bronchial challenge test in only 27% of cases, whereas positive prick tests eliciting a wheal size >9 mm were associated with a positive bronchial challenge test in 50% of cases. This is an argument for cautious interpretation of positive ID skin test results, including positive IDT elicited only at the highest dilution (bottle 2) (see later). In the study by Spector and Farr, only 4% of subjects with a negative intradermal skin test at 1/1000 w/v had a positive bronchial challenge.

It is interesting to note that in the study by Spector and Farr, the highest percentage of positive bronchial challenge tests occurred in subjects with a positive intradermal test at 1/100,000 w/v, but was only 61% in this subgroup. Thus, not all highly allergic subjects respond to an allergen challenge.

Similar studies have been conducted of nasal allergen challenges in patients with perennial allergic rhinitis (PAR) and dust mite allergy. One study revealed that positive nasal allergen challenges occurred in 62% of those with positive prick skin tests.[32] Although nonallergic controls were not included in this study, the confirmation rate of 62% was consistent with the earlier study of bronchial allergen challenge.[31] In another study, only subjects with 4+ skin prick test responses to dust mite allergen consistently responded to nasal allergen challenge.[33] The latter study further showed that high doses of dust mite nasal allergen challenges could elicit nonspecific responses in some nonallergic subjects. Another study showed that conjunctival provocation testing elicited similar responses to nasal allergen challenges and suggested that this type of challenge may be easier for a confirmation of target organ allergic responses.[34]

Intradermal testing is more sensitive by a factor of 500- to 1000-fold.[9,35] It is considered especially useful for the evaluation of anaphylaxis due to a drug (such as penicillin) or Hymenoptera venom. In a typical allergists office, intradermal tests are applied at 1/100th of the concentration used for prick testing. This explains why intradermal tests have greater sensitivity than prick tests. Prick testing can be performed with extracts containing 50% glycerine (e.g., dust mite allergens), whereas intradermal testing cannot use 50% glycerine due to irritant effects and false-positive results.[9]

A study by Nelson et al.[36] assessed the utility of intradermal testing in the diagnosis of grass pollen allergy. Three groups of patients with a history suggestive of seasonal allergic rhinitis during grass pollen season in Denver, Colorado, were studied: one with positive prick tests to timothy grass, one with negative prick but positive intradermal tests to timothy, and one with negative prick and ID tests to timothy grass. A healthy nonallergic control group was also studied. All subjects underwent nasal allergen challenges with timothy grass pollen. The percentage of patients with a positive nasal allergen challenge in the four groups is summarized in **Table 7.3**. The authors

Table 7.3 Nasal Allergen Challenge Results in Patients with Suspected Allergic Rhinitis During Grass Pollen Season in Denver, Colorado

Study Group Based on Results of Prick and Intradermal Skin Tests to Timothy Grass	Positive Nasal Allergen Challenge
SAR with positive prick test	68%
SAR with negative prick but positive intradermal test	11%
SAR with negative prick and intradermal test	11%
Healthy nonallergic control	0%

Abbreviations: SAR, seasonal allergic rhinitis.
Source: Data from Nelson HS, Oppenheimer J, Buchmeier A, Kordash TR, Freshwater LL. An assessment of the role of intradermal skin testing in the diagnosis of clinically relevant allergy to timothy grass. J Allergy Clin Immunol 1996;97(6):1193–1201.

concluded that in the absence of a positive prick test, the presence of a positive ID test to timothy grass did not predict clinically relevant allergy.

A similar study was performed with cat allergen.[37] Patients were exposed in a room with a domestic cat for 1 hour. Patients with a positive prick skin test had a 92.7% rate of positive nasal or bronchial allergic reactions. All patients with a positive IgE CAP-RAST test (n = 27) also had a positive skin prick test, and in this group, 100% had a positive nasal or bronchial allergic reaction (**Table 7.4**). In contrast, a positive allergen challenge was seen in only 6/26 patients with a positive ID test (23%) and in only 4/13 patients with a negative ID skin test (31%).

A study by Schwindt et al.[38] compared the utility of prick tests, multitests (percutaneous testing), and ID tests in the diagnosis of "clinically relevant respiratory allergy." In this study, clinical history was used as the "gold standard" for diagnosis. The sensitivity of positive prick and multitest reactions for the diagnosis of allergy was 62% and 77%, respectively. Patients with negative prick and multitest responses but positive ID tests underwent nasal allergen challenges. None of the latter nasal allergen challenges were positive. It was concluded that the multitest device was more sensitive than prick testing at detecting clinically relevant allergy without losing specificity. However, because none of the patients with positive multitest responses underwent nasal allergen challenges, this conclusion could be challenged. A study by Simons et al.[39] directly compared the prevalence of positive reactions using a Multi-Test II device with IDT in 34 patients. Of the 408 antigens tested, IDTs were positive in 56.3%, whereas the Multi-Test II tests were positive in only 16.9%. The vast majority of positive IDTs had an endpoint of 2 or 3. These and other studies show that multitest devices have a sensitivity intermediate between prick and IDTs.

The extent to which bronchial or nasal allergen challenges truly predict clinical allergic sensitivity is unknown and difficult to assess. The results summarized here could be interpreted to mean that clinical sensitivity is lower (roughly 60%) than that predicted by positive allergy skin tests. However, bronchial or nasal allergen challenges may not be the ideal way to confirm sensitivity to allergens, especially perennial allergens to which patients are exposed in low concentrations for prolonged periods of time. Studies that have analyzed the sensitivity and specificity of prick skin testing relative to either (1) clinical history with or without physical findings or (2) results of nasal or bronchial allergen challenges have failed to demonstrate a strong predictive value of a positive prick test for the presence of allergic rhinitis or asthma.[14] This is partly due to the fact that positive prick tests often occur in the absence of clinical allergic rhinitis or asthma (false-positive test).

Table 7.4 A Summary of Positive Upper or Lower Airway Cat Allergen Challenge Tests Based on Results of Allergy Skin Testing or RAST Tests to Cat Allergens

Study Group Based on Results of Prick and ID Skin Tests or RAST Test to Cat	No. Subjects (Total: 120)	Positive Upper or Lower Airway Cat Allergen Challenge*
Positive skin prick test	81	38/41
Negative prick but positive ID test	26	6/26
Negative prick test and negative ID test	13	4/13
Positive skin prick and positive RAST test	27	27/27
Negative prick and negative RAST test	44	12/44

*Cat allergen challenge was performed in a 13.7 m^3 room with two domestic cats, a bed, and a small carpet for 1 hour. Subjects recorded upper and lower respiratory symptoms every 5 minutes, and spirometry was recorded every 15 minutes during the exposure.

Abbreviations: ID, intradermal; RAST, radioallergosorbent.

Source: Data from Wood RA, Phipatanakul W, Hamilton RG, Eggleston PA. A comparison of skin prick tests, intradermal skin tests, and RASTs in the diagnosis of cat allergy. J Allergy Clin Immunol 1999;103(5 Pt 1):773–779. [IgE CAP RAST tests were positive in 45 of 51 patients with a positive skin prick test and negative in all subjects with a negative skin prick test.]

Local Allergy

The studies discussed suggest that the rate of "false-negative" allergy skin tests is low. However, occasionally, there are patients who present with classic allergic symptoms following allergen exposure but who fail to demonstrate a positive allergy skin or RAST tests. Huggins and Brostoff[40] reported on a series of 14 patients with a clinical history suggestive of allergy to house dust mites despite negative prick skin tests and negative RAST tests. They were found to have mite-specific IgE detectable in their nasal secretions and a positive nasal allergen challenge with *Dermatophagoides pteronyssinus* extract. Because ID testing was not done, it is unknown whether these patients would have had a positive ID skin test. Nevertheless, this and other studies[41] have raised the possibility of a "local" IgE-mediated allergy as a disease mechanism. The frequency of this phenomenon is believed to be low.[14]

Allergy Testing in the Otorhinolaryngologist's and Allergist's Office

The optimal method of allergy skin testing has been an area of controversy between allergists and otorhinolaryngologists for decades, although more recent consensus conferences have indicated an evolution toward closer agreement on the methods employed.

Approach 1: Skin Endpoint Titration/Intradermal Dilutional Testing

The historic approach of otolaryngic allergists was skin endpoint titration (SET) testing. The term SET was recently replaced by intradermal dilutional testing (IDT). The main advantage of IDT is determining the patient's level of sensitivity, which can be used to determine allergen starting dose for immunotherapy, thus perhaps reducing the potential for an allergic reaction. IDT is more quantitative but also more time-consuming and labor intensive than prick and single intradermal skin testing.

Approach 2

The traditional approach employed by allergists is prick skin testing followed by single ID testing for allergens that are negative by prick testing but potentially clinically relevant. The single ID tests are done at a concentration of 1/100th of the prick testing concentrations. No IDT testing is done to assess the patient's level of sensitivity prior to starting immunotherapy. Instead, immunotherapy is started at a fixed dose except in cases where the clinical history suggests severe allergic sensitivity, in which case the dose may be reduced 10-fold.

An example of routine prick and intradermal skin testing in an allergist's office is shown in **Fig. 7.2**.

Approach 3: Revised Otolaryngic Allergist Approach

Prick skin testing is now the preferred initial means of testing for otolaryngic allergies.[42] A typical prick test screening battery in the midwestern United States is summarized in **Table 7.5**. Other allergens may be added to this list depending on local pollen counts.[42] The prick test screening battery used in the author's clinic in Boston, Massachusetts, is summarized in **Table 7.6**. The screening battery may be followed by IDTs for selected antigens that are negative on prick testing but for which significant clinical suspicion exists. IDTs are only performed for allergens that are negative by prick testing.[42] However, if immunotherapy is to be given, IDTs are still performed in many otorhinolaryngologist's offices to assess the level of sensitivity prior to starting immunotherapy. This abbreviated hybrid form of IDT is called modified quantitative testing (MQT). MQT uses an algorithm to estimate the safe starting dose of immunotherapy based on the wheal size from screening skin prick testing. Endpoint determination using MQT has been shown to have strong agreement with endpoints using IDT for common allergens.[43]

In some cases, it may be necessary to substitute in vitro IgE CAP-RAST testing (e.g., Pharmacia ImmunoCAP, Phadia, Uppsala, Sweden) for skin testing. If in vitro testing is used as the basis for immunotherapy, a similar panel of allergens is ordered as in **Table 7.6**.

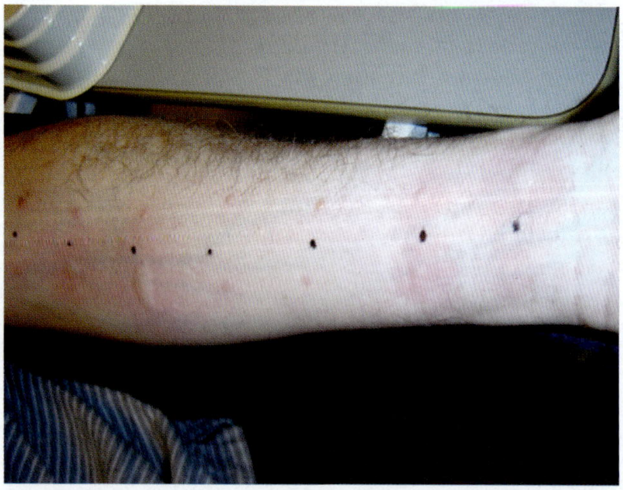

Fig. 7.2 A typical appearance of allergy prick skin testing results in a highly allergic patient. Strong wheal and flare responses are seen to several allergens, especially on the upper portion of the forearm. The histamine positive control is nearest to the wrist (ulnar aspect).

Table 7.5 Typical Screening Prick Skin Test Battery in the Midwestern United States

Timothy grass	*Helminthosporium*
Bermuda grass	*Penicillium*
Short ragweed	*Dermatophagoides pteronyssinus*
White oak	*Dermatophagoides farinae*
Eastern cottonwood	American cockroach
Alternaria	Cat

Source: Data from Krouse JH, Mabry RL. Skin testing for inhalant allergy 2003: current strategies. Otolaryngol Head Neck Surg 2003;129(4 Suppl):S33–49.

Implications of Different Skin Testing Methods

The two major implications of using different skin testing methods are (1) *diagnostic*, namely determining what constitutes a clinically relevant allergy, and (2) *therapeutic*,

Table 7.6 Allergy Skin Test Battery Used in the Author's Clinic in Boston, Massachusetts

White ash	Raqweed mixture
Birch mixture	Sorrel/yellow dock
Common cottonwood	*Dermatophagoides farinae*
Red cedar	*Dermatophagoides farinae*
American elm	American cockroach
Hickory shagbark	Cat hair
Maple, hard/sugar	Dog hair and dander
Black willow	*Aspergillus fumigatus/niger* mixture
Red oak	*Alternaria*
Northern grass mixture	*Fusarium vasinfectum*
Bermuda grass	*Helminthosporium*
Lambs quarters	*Hormodendrum*
Mugwort/sage	*Penicillium*
Pigweed/careless weed	

namely determining the starting allergen dose for immunotherapy.

In terms of diagnostic interpretation, the skin testing methods differ only in terms of the allergen concentrations used for intradermal skin testing. IDT tests are continued up to a 1:5 dilution (dilution 1) from the prick testing concentrations, whereas ID testing is done only at 1/100th of the prick testing concentrations.

Excessive reliance on IDT tests positive at the highest dilution (dilution 2) may lead to overinterpretation of an allergy and overuse of immunotherapy. This is suggested in the study by Lane et al.[44] in which the results of skin testing from ~3,300 patients were reviewed. In this clinic, 85% of patients had positive tests; however, 56% of positives occurred at the lowest dilution of the allergen. Overall, 75.7% of the patients were placed on IT. Considering that positive ID tests have not been shown to reliably correlate with positive allergen challenge tests, it could be argued that immunotherapy was overused in this clinic. Analogously, if excessive reliance is given to positive ID tests in an allergist's office, the result will be a similar overuse of immunotherapy. It has been my observation that patients treated with immunotherapy based solely on positive ID or IDT tests at the highest dilution often fail to receive benefit. This could be predicted by their low level of allergen sensitivity prior to the immunotherapy.

In the author's opinion, ID testing is most useful for detecting allergies to dust mites, animal dander, or molds, especially if the criterion used for a positive test is a wheal size of ≥10 mm.[35]

Allergen Immunotherapy

What is Allergen Immunotherapy?

Allergen immunotherapy is defined as the administration of aqueous extracts of allergens to an allergic patient in an incremental, dose escalation pattern to reduce the symptoms and objective evidence of allergic response to allergen exposure. The effects are allergen specific, and the procedure is also referred to as specific immunotherapy (SIT).[45]

The goal of immunotherapy is to induce a state of immunologic tolerance to the allergens administered such that, under conditions of natural allergen exposure, the allergic response will be attenuated or eliminated. Tolerance has been demonstrated when the doses of allergen are sufficiently high and is not achieved at lower dose levels (see following text).

The mechanism of action of immunotherapy has been the subject of numerous investigations, reflecting the evolution of our understanding of mechanisms of immune tolerance induction. Immune tolerance has been demonstrated in several ways, including: (1) down modulation of target organ sensitivity to the allergen; (2) a decrease in late-phase allergic response to the allergen; (3) a modest reduction in allergen-specific IgE levels; (4) a shift in Th1/Th2 cytokine balance in favor of Th1 (IFN-gamma); (5) induction of Th2 cell anergy; and (6) induction of regulatory T cells (commonly known as "Tregs") that mediate allergen-specific tolerance through the production of IL-10.[46-48] The latter has received the most attention recently.

Usual Method of Administration of Allergen Immunotherapy

Conventional immunotherapy (IT) has been in existence since the time of Noon et al.[49] Conventional IT is administered weekly in gradually increasing incremental doses until the maintenance dose is reached. This typically requires several months. The final maintenance dose is usually 1000 to 10,000 times the starting dose and is often close to the highest tolerated dose.

The incremental doses of conventional IT can be administered several times per week to accelerate the process. This is known as "modified rush" immunotherapy. Rarely, immunotherapy is administered several times per day in incremental doses to reach the maintenance dose after several days. This "rush" technique is used mostly in research settings. In general, with all immunotherapy protocols, tolerance induction occurs once the maintenance dose of allergen is reached.

Indications for Immunotherapy

Immunotherapy is indicated for the treatment of allergic rhinitis or asthma in patients with a documented allergy to clinically relevant allergens and in whom environmental control measures and pharmacotherapy fail to provide adequate control of symptoms. In special circumstances, immunotherapy may be given to overcome occupational allergen sensitivities (e.g., laboratory worker sensitive to mouse antigen).

Evidence supporting the benefit of immunotherapy has been the subject of several comprehensive reviews. For instance, a review of multiple randomized controlled trials of immunotherapy for asthma conducted between 1954 and 2001 concluded that overall, immunotherapy reduced allergic symptoms, medication use, and airway responses to allergen challenge but had no consistent effect on pulmonary function tests.[10] In a systematic review of immunotherapy studies in children, it was concluded that immunotherapy produced no added benefit in children already receiving optimal medical therapy for asthma.[50] However, not all experts agree with this assessment,[51,52] and early intervention with immunotherapy may offer more promise of benefit. Immunotherapy may have other benefits, such as preventing the development of new allergen sensitivities in children. Also, immunotherapy may attenuate preexisting asthma or may delay or prevent the onset of asthma.[53,54] As with other asthma therapies, it is important to pay attention to other factors that impact asthma control, such as environmental control measures. Compared with immunotherapy, allergen avoidance is cheaper, has more immediate impact, and has been shown to be an effective means of improving asthma.[55,56]

Allergens for Immunotherapy

Most commercially available allergen extracts are not standardized. Their contents are expressed with a confusing array of units, such as protein nitrogen units (PNU) per milliliter, weight per volume (w/v), or milligram per milliliter. These remain in common use for skin testing and immunotherapy. Given their lack of standardization, extracts with nominally equivalent PNU/mL or w/v concentrations can vary widely in terms of biologic activities.[57-59]

There is a strong impetus to standardize allergen extracts. In the United States, a procedure has been adopted that uses reference standards and assesses the potency of a new extract by performing quantitative intradermal dilutional testing in 15 to 20 highly sensitive allergic subjects. Serial threefold dilutions of 0.05 mL of extract are applied, and the dose that elicits a sum of the longest plus midpoint diameter of erythema of 50 mm is assigned a potency of 1 BAU/mL. Certain extracts, such as dust mites, were originally standardized by inhibition radioimmunoassay (RIA) and assigned units of allergy units per milliliter. It was later determined by ID50EAL testing that allergy units per milliliter were bioequivalent to bioequivalent allergy units per milliliter.[60] The following standardized extracts are currently available: cat hair, cat pelt, *Dermatophagoides farinae, Dermatophagoides pteronyssinus*, short ragweed, Bermuda grass, Kentucky bluegrass, perennial rye grass, orchard grass, timothy grass, meadow fescue grass, red top grass, sweet vernal grass, and Hymenoptera venoms.[60]

The predominant allergenic proteins within extracts have been determined for most allergens. A procedure for naming allergens has also been established.[61] For instance, for birch pollen, the major allergen Bet v 1 is so named from the genus name (*Betula*), the first letter of the species name (*verrucosa*), and the first allergen identified. Similarly, the cat allergen Fel d 1 is so named from the genus name (*Felis*), the first letter of the species name (*domesticus*), and the first allergen identified.

Clinically Relevant Cross-Reacting Allergens

Significant cross-reactions exist among pollens that impact the choice of allergens used for skin testing and immunotherapy. There is generally a high degree of cross-allergenicity between species of the same genus and some degree of cross-allergenicity between plants of the same tribe. However, there is rarely significant cross-allergenicity between plants of the same family. Most notably, northern grasses, such as timothy, perennial rye, and meadow fescue, are highly cross-reactive and can be regarded as interchangeable for skin testing and immunotherapy. Certain tree families cross-react, such as the cypress family Cupressaceae (juniper, cedar, and cypress), the birch family Betulaceae (birch, alder, hazel), and oak Fagaceae (oak, beech, chestnut). Among the weeds, the most cross-reactive are the Amaranthaceae family, including pigweed, red root pigweed, and amaranth. The ragweeds (genus *Ambrosia*) are highly cross-reactive, including short, giant, false, and western. However, southern and slender ragweed are not cross-reactive with these and should be considered distinct.

Most important is the high degree of cross-reactivity between the different northern grasses, such as timothy, perennial rye, Kentucky blue, johnsongrass, and meadow fescue. These are allergenically distinct from the southern grasses, such as Bermuda grass. The two most common species of dust mites (*D. farinae* and *D. pteronyssinus*) are also highly cross-reactive but are often mixed 50:50 in allergen immunotherapy.

Preparation and Administration of Immunotherapy

Allergen mixtures for immunotherapy should be prepared while mindful of the fact that certain extracts, including cockroach, mite, and molds, contain proteases that degrade pollens and animal danders. Pollen extracts can be mixed, and danders can be mixed with pollens. Mold extracts can be mixed with other molds but should not be mixed with pollens or danders. Dust mites can be mixed with molds. Dust mites can be mixed with pollens or danders provided the glycerine content is ≥25%; however, such a high content of glycerine is usually not employed because it induces a local burning sensation. For a patient with multiple allergen sensitivities, it may be necessary to prepare one pollen mixture, one dust mite/cockroach/mold mixture, and one animal dander mixture.

In an allergist's practice, immunotherapy is administered in the outpatient clinic by an experienced health-care professional. Patients are first asked if they are having problems with asthma. If there is uncertainty about the patient's asthma status, a peak flow or spirometry is obtained, and immunotherapy is not given unless the asthma is considered stable. After immunotherapy is administered, the patient is observed for a minimum of 30 minutes for signs of an adverse reaction, such as hives, angioedema, bronchospasm, light-headedness, or anaphylactic shock. The staff is familiar with recognition of acute allergic reactions and the use of epinephrine.

It has been shown that 3 years of immunotherapy provides lasting benefit that can be measured as long as 6 years after stopping immunotherapy.[62,63] Therefore, the current recommendation is that immunotherapy should be administered for a minimum of 3 years at a maintenance dose after which time the treatment should be reevaluated.

Outcomes of Immunotherapy

Immunotherapy Based on the Rinkel Method

A method of IT administration was popularized by Rinkel[64] who is also credited with developing the SET method.[65] This method, traditionally known as the "Rinkel method," used SET testing to determine the starting dose of IT and also to redefine the patient's allergen sensitivity during IT. In a double-blind, multicenter, placebo-controlled trial sponsored by the American Academy of Allergy in 1981, the efficacy of Rinkel IT versus histamine-placebo IT was compared.[66] No statistically significant improvement in allergic rhinitis symptoms was found in patients receiving Rinkel IT versus placebo. This study found that the mean cumulative dose of ragweed allergen administered by Rinkel IT was only 18.55 PNU, which is far lower than the average cumulative preseasonal dose of ragweed allergen typically administered (9,483 PNU) by conventional IT.[67] Considering that studies of conventional IT have shown that higher maintenance doses of allergens are more effective (see Conventional Immunotherapy, which follows), it is not surprising that the Rinkel IT would have been ineffective in this study.

IDT-Based Immunotherapy

The efficacy of IDT-based immunotherapy has been the subject of three studies.[68-70] In the study by Lee and Kniker,[68] subjects in San Antonio were randomly assigned to receive coseasonal immunotherapy with mountain cedar pollen based on SDET, traditional immunotherapy, or placebo. The groups were comparable at baseline in terms of age, gender distribution, and SDET endpoint. Subjects receiving IT by SDET had a higher starting dose (SDET mean of 6.99 PNU versus traditional IT mean of 0.16 PNU) and a higher final dose achieved at the end of the pollen season (245 versus 82 PNU). The cumulative allergen dose was also higher in the SDET group versus the traditional IT group (2745 versus 251 PNU). The incidence of local and systemic allergic reactions from IT was comparable in both active treatment groups. At the end of the study, none of the groups showed reduced sensitivity to mountain cedar by SDET; however, the SDET group showed the smallest increase in sensitivity. Improvement in symptom and medication scores slightly favored the SDET treatment group, but the difference was not statistically significant. This study suggests that IT based on SDET does not slow down the buildup toward a maintenance dose of IT, although it could be argued that this study did not aim to achieve a fixed IT maintenance dose.

In the study by Trevino,[69] three methods of determining the starting dose of IT were compared, namely based on results of scratch testing, prick testing, or SET testing. IT based on positive scratch tests was begun at 0.05 mL of 1:50,000 w/v. IT based on positive prick tests was begun at 0.05 mL of 1:500,000 w/v. IT based on positive SET tests was begun at the endpoint titration dose. All IT was given in progressive weekly increments of 0.05 mL up to the maximum tolerated dose—that is, the dose that caused pain or a local reaction at the site of injection. Treatment was continued for 6 months, after which symptom relief was compared between groups. None of the patients treated based on scratch tests or prick tests experienced benefit, whereas 9 of 10 subjects treated based on SET testing experienced complete relief of symptoms. This study has been quoted as a validation of IT based on SET testing. However, the study is problematic for many reasons. First, local pain and local reactions to IT have not been shown to correlate with a risk for a systemic reaction to IT,[70] and most allergists continue to advance the dose of IT despite moderately large immediate local reactions. Second, the author did not provide information on the doses of IT administered in each treatment arm. Without this, it is unclear why patients treated with conventional IT failed to improve.

In the study by Krouse and Krouse,[71] a group of five patients received IT based on SET testing to a panel of allergens including three experimental allergens, short ragweed, and either oak or *Dermatophagoides pteronyssinus*. The control group received IT to all other allergens that were positive with the exception of these test allergens. Each group of five patients received twice weekly IT injections with a similar pattern of dose escalation. At the end of 6 months, all patients had an endoscopic assessment and a nasal allergen challenge with short ragweed. Both groups showed an improvement in endoscopic score and a reduction in response to the nasal ragweed challenge. This study is quoted as a validation of IT based on SET testing. However, the authors did not provide information about the starting dose or the total dose of experimental allergens administered.

Conventional Immunotherapy

Immunotherapy administered using a fixed schedule of dose escalation and a "target" maintenance dose of allergen is typically referred to in allergy as "conventional" immunotherapy. The efficacy of conventional immunotherapy has been established in several studies.[67,72-76] The most important determinant of the efficacy of immunotherapy is the dose of allergen administered. For instance, in a study of ragweed immunotherapy, a maintenance dose of 1 of 12 μg of Amb was more effective than a dose of 1.94 μg.[77,78] Effective maintenance doses of IT using unstandardized extracts are in the range of 10 to 20 μg of specific allergen for ragweed, dust mite, cat, and timothy grass.

Conclusion

Inhalant allergies impact several otorhinolaryngologic disorders including, but not limited to, allergic rhinitis and rhinoconjunctivitis, chronic rhinosinusitis, and otitis media. Accurate diagnosis of IgE-mediated allergy is important for the comprehensive management of these conditions. Allergy skin testing remains the most commonly used method of diagnosing an allergy. Although specialists in allergy and otorhinolaryngology–head and neck surgery have traditionally taken different approaches to skin testing, their approaches have become more uniform in recent years. Prick skin testing is the preferred initial method. In patients with a suggestive history of allergy, a positive prick skin test is the best means of detecting clinically relevant allergies. Intradermal skin testing, using either single intradermal testing or IDT, is also useful, especially for detecting clinically relevant perennial allergies. IDT testing offers the advantage of determining the degree of allergen sensitivity. However, studies of allergen immunotherapy strongly suggest that the most important determinant of the efficacy of allergen immunotherapy is reaching a sufficiently high maintenance dose for each allergen administered.

References

1. Zhou B, Comeau MR, De Smedt T, et al. Thymic stromal lymphopoietin as a key initiator of allergic airway inflammation in mice. Nat Immunol 2005;6(10):1047–1053
2. Al-Shami A, Spolski R, Kelly J, Keane-Myers A, Leonard WJ. A role for TSLP in the development of inflammation in an asthma model. J Exp Med 2005;202(6):829–839
3. Liu YJ. Thymic stromal lymphopoietin: master switch for allergic inflammation. J Exp Med 2006;203(2):269–273
4. Hammad H, Lambrecht BN. Dendritic cells and epithelial cells: linking innate and adaptive immunity in asthma. Nat Rev Immunol 2008;8(3):193–204
5. Trompette A, Divanovic S, Visintin A, et al. Allergenicity resulting from functional mimicry of a Toll-like receptor complex protein. Nature 2009;457(7229):585–588
6. Gurish M, Castells MC. Mast cell derived mediators. http://www.uptodate.com/contents/mast-cell-derived-mediators. Accessed August 29, 2011
7. Togawa M, Kiniwa M, Nagai H. The roles of IL-4, IL-5 and mast cells in the accumulation of eosinophils during allergic cutaneous late phase reaction in mice. Life Sci 2001;69(6): 699–705
8. Allakhverdi Z, Comeau MR, Smith DE, et al. CD34+ hemopoietic progenitor cells are potent effectors of allergic inflammation. J Allergy Clin Immunol 2009;123(2):472–478
9. Oppenheimer J, Nelson HS. Skin testing. Ann Allergy Asthma Immunol 2006; 96(2, Suppl 1)S6–S12
10. Abramson MJ, Puy RM, Weiner JM. Allergen immunotherapy for asthma. Cochrane Database Syst Rev 2003;4(4):CD001186
11. Oppenheimer JJ, Nelson HS. Seasonal variation in immediate skin test reactions. Ann Allergy 1993;71(3):227–229
12. Henderson LL, Larson JB, Gleich GJ. Maximal rise in IgE antibody following ragweed pollination season. J Allergy Clin Immunol 1975;55(1):10–15
13. Pearlman DS, Grossman J, Meltzer EO. Histamine skin test reactivity following single and multiple doses of azelastine nasal spray in patients with seasonal allergic rhinitis. Ann Allergy Asthma Immunol 2003;91(3):258–262
14. Bernstein IL, Li JT, Bernstein DI, et al; American Academy of Allergy, Asthma and Immunology; American College of Allergy, Asthma and Immunology. Allergy diagnostic testing: an updated practice parameter. Ann Allergy Asthma Immunol 2008;100(3, Suppl 3)S1–S148
15. Simons FE, Johnston L, Gu X, Simons KJ. Suppression of the early and late cutaneous allergic responses using fexofenadine and montelukast. Ann Allergy Asthma Immunol 2001;86(1):44–50
16. Slott RI, Zweiman B. A controlled study of the effect of corticosteroids on immediate skin test reactivity. J Allergy Clin Immunol 1974;54(4):229–234
17. Nelson HS, Brown G, O'Barr TP, Branch LB, Spaulding H, Black JW. Clinical and immunological studies of timothy antigen D immunotherapy. J Allergy Clin Immunol 1976;57(5):463–472
18. Tipton WR, Nelson HS. Experience with daily immunotherapy in 59 adult allergic patients. J Allergy Clin Immunol 1982;69(2): 194–199
19. Casale TB. Experience with monoclonal antibodies in allergic mediated disease: seasonal allergic rhinitis. J Allergy Clin Immunol 2001;108(2, Suppl)S84–S88
20. Illi S, Garcia-Marcos L, Hernando V, Guillen JJ, Liese A, von Mutius E. Reproducibility of skin prick test results in epidemiologic studies: a comparison of two devices. Allergy 1998;53(4):353–358
21. Johnston SL, Clough JB, Pattemore PK, Smith S, Holgate ST. Longitudinal changes in skin-prick test reactivity over 2 years in a population of schoolchildren with respiratory symptoms. Clin Exp Allergy 1992;22(10):948–957
22. Nelson HS, Kolehmainen C, Lahr J, Murphy J, Buchmeier A. A comparison of multiheaded devices for allergy skin testing. J Allergy Clin Immunol 2004;113(6):1218–1219
23. Oppenheimer J, Nelson HS. Skin testing: a survey of allergists. Ann Allergy Asthma Immunol 2006;96(1):19–23
24. Wallace DV, Bahna SL, Goldstein S, Hamilton RG, Cohn JR. American Academy of Allergy, Asthma & Immunology Work Group Report: allergy diagnosis in clinical practice. J Allergy Clin Immunol 2007;120(4):967–969
25. Anon JB. Otolaryngic allergy. The last half-century. Otolaryngol Clin North Am 1992;25(1):1–12
26. Mabry RL. Blending skin endpoint titration and in vitro methods in clinical practice. Otolaryngol Clin North Am 1992;25(1):61–70
27. Frew AJ, Kay AB. The relationship between infiltrating CD4+ lymphocytes, activated eosinophils, and the magnitude of the allergen-induced late phase cutaneous reaction in man. J Immunol 1988;141(12):4158–4164
28. Eriksson NE. Diagnosis of reaginic allergy with house dust, animal dander and pollen allergens in adult patients. III. Case histories and combinations of case histories, skin tests and the radioallergosorbent test, RAST, compared with provocation tests. Int Arch Allergy Appl Immunol 1977;53(5):441–449
29. Curran WS, Goldman G. The incidence of immediately reacting allergy skin tests in a "normal" adult population. Ann Intern Med 1961;55:777–783
30. Bodtger U, Poulsen LK, Malling HJ. Asymptomatic skin sensitization to birch predicts later development of birch pollen allergy in adults: a 3-year follow-up study. J Allergy Clin Immunol 2003;111(1):149–154
31. Spector S, Farr R. Bronchial inhalation challenge with antigens. J Allergy Clin Immunol 1979;64(6 pt 2):580–586
32. Damps I, Mincewicz G, Poławska K, Kurowski W, Stankiewicz C, Słomiński JM. Nasal provocation tests with house dust mite in patients with perennial rhinitis. Otolaryngol Pol 2003;57(1):69–74
33. Kanthawatana S, Maturim W, Fooanan S, Trakultivakorn M. Skin prick reaction and nasal provocation response in diagnosis of nasal allergy to the house dust mite. Ann Allergy Asthma Immunol 1997;79(5):427–430
34. Riechelmann H, Epple B, Gropper G. Comparison of conjunctival and nasal provocation test in allergic rhinitis to house dust mite. Int Arch Allergy Immunol 2003;130(1):51–59
35. Voorhorst R, Van Krieken H. Atopic skin test reevaluated. I. Perfection of skin testing technique. Ann Allergy 1973;31(3): 137–142

36. Nelson HS, Oppenheimer J, Buchmeier A, Kordash TR, Freshwater LL. An assessment of the role of intradermal skin testing in the diagnosis of clinically relevant allergy to timothy grass. J Allergy Clin Immunol 1996;97(6):1193–1201
37. Wood RA, Phipatanakul W, Hamilton RG, Eggleston PA. A comparison of skin prick tests, intradermal skin tests, and RASTs in the diagnosis of cat allergy. J Allergy Clin Immunol 1999;103(5 Pt 1): 773–779
38. Schwindt CD, Hutcheson PS, Leu SY, Dykewicz MS. Role of intradermal skin tests in the evaluation of clinically relevant respiratory allergy assessed using patient history and nasal challenges. Ann Allergy Asthma Immunol 2005;94(6):627–633
39. Simons JP, Rubinstein EN, Kogut VJ, Melfi PJ, Ferguson BJ. Comparison of Multi-Test II skin prick testing to intradermal dilutional testing. Otolaryngol Head Neck Surg 2004;130(5):536–544
40. Huggins KG, Brostoff J. Local production of specific IgE antibodies in allergic-rhinitis patients with negative skin tests. Lancet 1975;2(7926):148–150
41. Marcucci F, Passalacqua G, Canonica GW, et al. Measurement of nasal IgE in an epidemiological study: assessment of its diagnostic value in respiratory allergy. Eur Ann Allergy Clin Immunol 2004;36(6):225–231
42. Krouse JH, Mabry RL. Skin testing for inhalant allergy 2003: current strategies. Otolaryngol Head Neck Surg 2003;129(4, Suppl)S33–S49
43. Peltier J, Ryan MW. Comparison of intradermal dilutional testing, skin prick testing, and modified quantitative testing for common allergens. Otolaryngol Head Neck Surg 2007;137(2):246–249
44. Lane AP, Pine HS, Pillsbury HC III. Allergy testing and immunotherapy in an academic otolaryngology practice: a 20-year review. Otolaryngol Head Neck Surg 2001;124(1):9–15
45. Bousquet J, Lockey R, Malling HJ, et al. Allergen immunotherapy: therapeutic vaccines for allergic diseases. World Health Organization. American Academy of Allergy, Asthma and Immunology. Ann Allergy Asthma Immunol 1998;81(5 Pt 1):401–405
46. Akdis M, Blaser K, Akdis CA. T regulatory cells in allergy: novel concepts in the pathogenesis, prevention, and treatment of allergic diseases. J Allergy Clin Immunol 2005;116(5):961–968, quiz 969
47. Akdis M, Akdis CA. Mechanisms of allergen-specific immunotherapy. J Allergy Clin Immunol 2007;119(4):780–791
48. Bacchetta R, Gambineri E, Roncarolo MG. Role of regulatory T cells and FOXP3 in human diseases. J Allergy Clin Immunol 2007;120(2):227–235, quiz 236–237
49. Noon L. Prophylactic inoculation against hay fever (historical document). Ann Allergy 1955;13(6):713–716
50. Adkinson NF Jr, Eggleston PA, Eney D, et al. A controlled trial of immunotherapy for asthma in allergic children. N Engl J Med 1997;336(5):324–331
51. Creticos PS. The consideration of immunotherapy in the treatment of allergic asthma. J Allergy Clin Immunol 2000;105 (2 Pt 2):S559–S574
52. Nelson HS. Efficacy and safety of allergen immunotherapy in children. Ann Allergy Asthma Immunol 2006;96(2, Suppl 1)S2–S5
53. Des Roches A, Paradis L, Menardo JL, Bouges S, Daurés JP, Bousquet J. Immunotherapy with a standardized Dermatophagoides pteronyssinus extract. VI. Specific immunotherapy prevents the onset of new sensitizations in children. J Allergy Clin Immunol 1997;99(4):450–453
54. Boquete M, Carballada F, Expósito F, González A. Preventive immunotherapy. Allergol Immunopathol (Madr) 2000;28(3): 89–93
55. Platts-Mills TA, Tovey ER, Mitchell EB, Moszoro H, Nock P, Wilkins SR. Reduction of bronchial hyperreactivity during prolonged allergen avoidance. Lancet 1982;2(8300):675–678
56. Platts-Mills TA. Allergen avoidance in the treatment of asthma and rhinitis. N Engl J Med 2003;349(3):207–208
57. Baer H, Godfrey H, Maloney CJ, Norman PS, Lichtenstein LM. The potency and antigen E content of commercially prepared ragweed extracts. J Allergy 1970;45(6):347–354
58. Baer H, Maloney CJ, Norman PS, Marsh DG. The potency and Group I antigen content of six commercially prepared grass pollen extracts. J Allergy Clin Immunol 1974;54(3):157–164
59. Greenert S, Bernstein IL, Michael JG. Immune responses of nonatopic individuals to prolonged immunisation with ragweed extract. Lancet 1971;2(7734):1121–1123
60. Joint Task Force on Practice Parameters; American Academy of Allergy, Asthma and Immunology; American College of Allergy, Asthma and Immunology; Joint Council of Allergy, Asthma and Immunology. Allergen immunotherapy: a practice parameter second update. J Allergy Clin Immunol 2007;120(3, Suppl)S25–S85
61. Hoffman D, Lowenstin H, Marsh DG, Platts-Mills TAE, Thomas W. Allergen nomenclature by the WHO/IUIS Allergen Nomenclature Sub-Committee. http://www.allergen.org/Allergen.aspx. Accessed August 30, 2011.
62. Naclerio RM, Proud D, Moylan B, et al. A double-blind study of the discontinuation of ragweed immunotherapy. J Allergy Clin Immunol 1997;100(3):293–300
63. Durham SR, Walker SM, Varga EM, et al. Long-term clinical efficacy of grass-pollen immunotherapy. N Engl J Med 1999;341(7):468–475
64. Rinkel HJ. Inhalant allergy; the coseasonal application of serial dilution testing (titration). Ann Allergy 1949;7(5):639–645
65. Rinkel HJ. Inhalant allergy; the whealing response of the skin to serial dilution testing. Ann Allergy 1949;7(5):625–630
66. Hirsch SR, Kalbfleisch JH, Golbert TM, et al. Rinkel injection therapy: a multicenter controlled study. J Allergy Clin Immunol 1981;68(2):133–155
67. Norman PS, Winkenwerder WL, Lichtenstein LM. Immunotherapy of hay fever with ragweed antigen E: comparisons with whole pollen extract and placebos. J Allergy 1968;42(2):93–108
68. Lee LK, Kniker WT, Campos T. Aggressive coseasonal immunotherapy in mountain cedar pollen allergy. Arch Otolaryngol 1982;108(12):787–794
69. Trevino RJ. Comparison of results of immunotherapy based on skin end-point titration, prick testing, and scratch testing. Otolaryngol Head Neck Surg 1994;111(5):550–552
70. Lockey RF, Benedict LM, Turkeltaub PC, Bukantz SC. Fatalities from immunotherapy (IT) and skin testing (ST). J Allergy Clin Immunol 1987;79(4):660–677
71. Krouse JH, Krouse HJ. Efficacy of immunotherapy based on skin endpoint titration. Otolaryngol Head Neck Surg 2000;123(3):183–187
72. Franklin W, Lowell FC. Comparison of two dosages of ragweed extract in the treatment of pollenosis. JAMA 1967;201(12):915–917
73. Lowell FC, Franklin W. A double-blind study of the effectiveness and specificity of injecton therapy in ragweed hay fever. N Engl J Med 1965;273(13):675–679
74. Lichtenstein LM, Norman PS, Winkenwerder WL. A single year of immunotherapy for ragweed hay fever. Immunologic and clinical studies. Ann Intern Med 1971;75(5):663–671
75. Norman PS, Winkenwerder WL, Lichtenstein LM. Maintenance immunotherapy in ragweed hay fever. Booster injections at six week intervals. J Allergy 1971;47(5):273–282
76. Norman PS, Winkenwerder WL, Lichtenstein LM. Maintenance immunotherapy in ragweed hay fever. Booster injections at six week intervals. J Allergy 1971;47(5):273–282
77. Iliopoulos O, Proud D, Adkinson NF Jr, et al. Effects of immunotherapy on the early, late, and rechallenge nasal reaction to provocation with allergen: changes in inflammatory mediators and cells. J Allergy Clin Immunol 1991;87(4):855–866
78. Naclerio RM, Proud D, Moylan B, et al. A double-blind study of the discontinuation of ragweed immunotherapy. J Allergy Clin Immunol 1997;100(3):293–300

8 Unified Airway Disease

Elina Toskala

Allergic rhinitis (AR) is a global health problem that causes major illness and disability worldwide. Patients from all countries, all ethnic groups, and all ages may suffer from AR. AR affects social life, sleep, school, and work. The economic impact of AR is often underestimated because the disease does not induce elevated direct costs. However, the indirect costs are substantial. Both AR and asthma are systemic inflammatory conditions and often are comorbidities.[1,2]

The results and conclusions of the World Health Organization's (WHO) workshop ARIA (Allergic Rhinitis and Its Impact on Asthma) are as follows:

- AR is a major respiratory disease due to its prevalence, impact on quality of life, impact on work/school performance and productivity, economic burden, and links to asthma.
- In addition, AR is associated with sinusitis and other comorbidities such as conjunctivitis.
- AR should be considered as a risk for asthma along with other known risk factors.
- A new subcategory of AR has been proposed: "intermittent and persistent."
- The severity of AR has been classified as mild or moderate/severe.
- Depending from subcategorization and severity of AR, a stepwise therapeutic approach has been proposed.
- The treatment of AR combines allergy avoidance, pharmacotherapy, immunotherapy, and education.
- Patients with persistent AR should be evaluated for asthma by history, chest examination, and, if possible and when necessary, the assessment of airflow obstruction before and after use of a bronchodilator.
- Patients with asthma should be appropriately evaluated (history and physical examination) for rhinitis.
- A combined strategy should ideally be used to treat the upper and lower airway diseases in terms of efficacy and safety.

Epidemiology

AR is the most common chronic recurrent disease of the developed world and is increasingly important in developing countries. An estimated 600 million people worldwide suffer from AR, with 200 million of them suffering concomitantly from asthma (PG1) and further large numbers suffering from nasal hyperreactivity.[3,4]

Interactions between the lower and the upper airways are well-known and have been extensively studied for over a decade. It is clear that rhinitis is a risk factor for asthma independent of allergy. Epidemiological studies have also shown that asthma and rhinitis often coexist in the same patient.[5] It is known that over 80% of asthmatic patients also have rhinitis and that up to 40% of patients with rhinitis also have asthma.[1] The fact that most patients with asthma also have rhinitis supports the concept of "one airway disease." However, not all patients with rhinitis present with asthma, and there are differences between asthma and rhinitis.[6,7]

Asthma is more frequently associated with perennial allergic rhinitis and more severe asthma and is more likely to be associated with perennial compared with seasonal AR. In children, AR is often diagnosed later than asthma,[8] which might be due to the tendency to ignore rhinitis symptoms in childhood. However, most studies support the view that rhinitis frequently precedes the development of asthma.[9,10]

Risk factors for AR have been identified. Indoor and outdoor allergens as well as occupational agents cause rhinitis and other allergic diseases. In occupational respiratory diseases, many patients begin with rhinitis symptoms and only later develop asthma. It is known that occupational rhinitis increases the risk for occupational asthma later three- to sevenfold if the exposure continues. The highest risk is among farmers and wood workers. The early recognition of occupational rhinitis may prevent the development of occupational asthma and is essential in preventing the onset of severe persistent asthma, which may progress even after the occupational agent has been removed.[11] Many studies have shown that viral upper respiratory tract infections are very common triggers of asthma exacerbations.[12]

According to ARIA, the epidemiological links between rhinitis and asthma include the following:

- The vast majority of asthmatics have rhinitis.
- Many patients with rhinitis have asthma.
- Asthma prevalence is increased in rhinitis and particularly so in persistent and/or moderate/severe rhinitis.
- Allergy is associated with rhinitis and asthma.
- Occupational agents can cause rhinitis and asthma.
- Nonallergic rhinitis is associated with asthma.
- Allergic and nonallergic rhinitis are risk factors for asthma.

- Rhinitis may be associated with nonspecific bronchial hyperreactivity.
- The coexistence of rhinitis and asthma appears to impair asthma control.
- Most asthmatic exacerbations are associated with nasal viral infection.

Pathophysiology

Rhinitis and bronchial asthma are both manifestations of an inflammatory process within a continuous airway system. The upper and lower airways may be considered as a unique entity influenced by a common and often evolving inflammation process. This inflammation process can be sustained and amplified by different mechanisms of several risk factors (**Fig. 8.1**).[13]

Nasal and bronchial epithelium share many histological features. Both are characterized by a pseudostratified epithelium with columnar, ciliated cells resting on a basement membrane. In the submucosa, vessels and mucous glands are present with structural cells (fibroblasts), inflammatory cells (essentially, monocytic cells, lymphocytes, and mast cells), and nerves. However, there are also differences. In the nose, there is a large subepithelial capillary and arterial system and venous cavernous sinusoids, and the nasal epithelium has high degree of vascularization leading to severe nasal obstruction in the inflammation. The nose does not have airway smooth muscle, which in the trachea accounts for bronchoconstriction (**Fig. 8.1**).

Breathing through the nose rather than through the mouth is the more natural way of breathing and protects the lower airways against contaminants in inhaled air. The nose also warms and humidifies the inhaled air before it

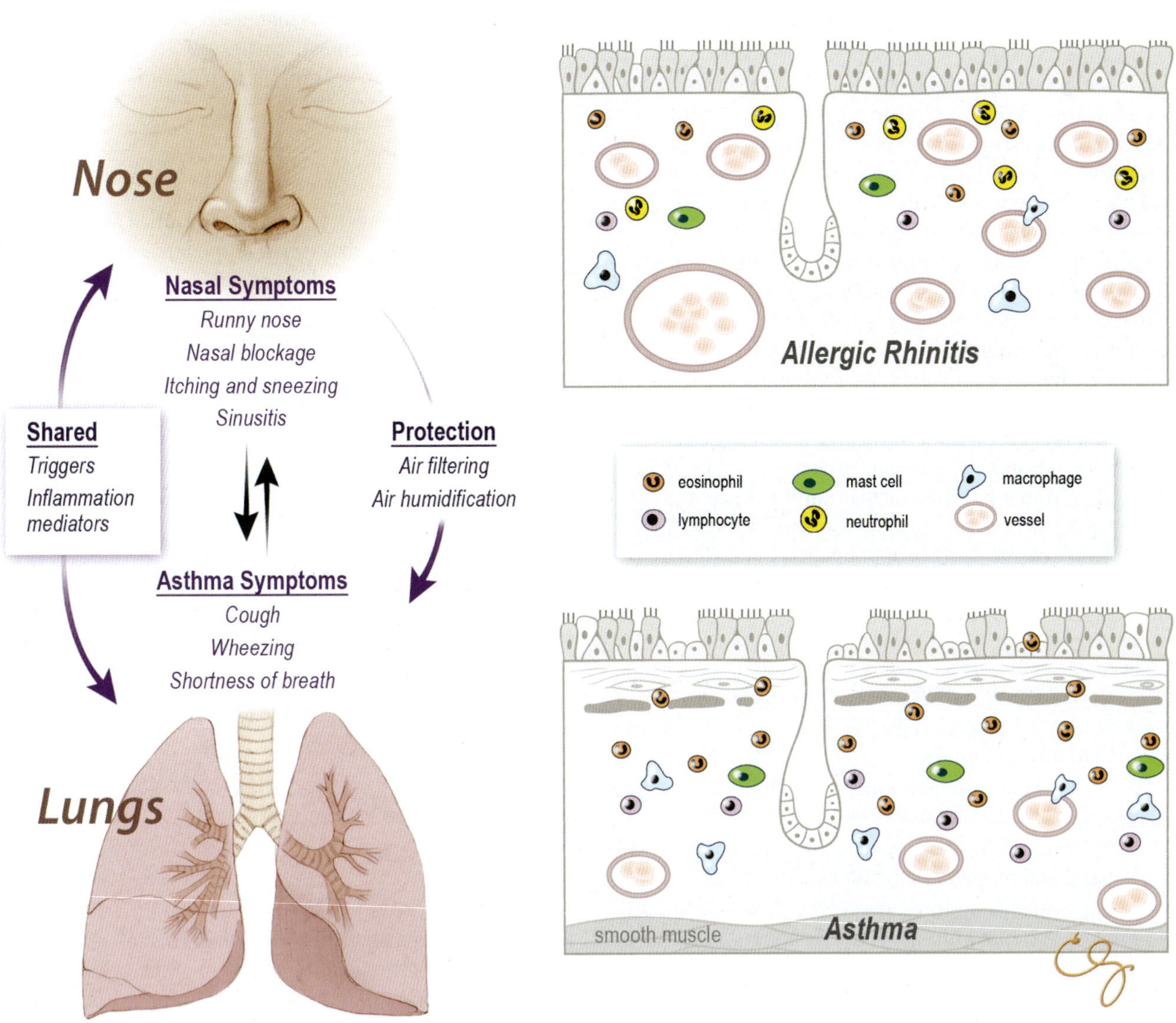

Fig. 8.1 Allergic rhinitis and asthma demonstrate clinical and histologic relatedness.

enters the lungs. When rhinitis causes obstruction of the nose (e.g., during the pollen season), the inhaled particles then reach the bronchial epithelium more easily and cause asthma symptoms. There is evidence of inflammation in the bronchial mucosa in seasonal rhinitis, and exposure to allergens through the nose causes an inflammatory response both in the nose and in the lungs. However, remodelling of the bronchi is usually absent in seasonal asthma compared with perennial asthma.

Inflammatory processes are similar in AR and asthma. Mast cells, basophils, and eosinophils have important roles, and imbalance between the T-helper (Th)1 and Th2 cells is characteristically in favor of Th2 cells. Th2 cells play a crucial role in regulating immunoglobin E (IgE) synthesis and cell recruitment to the allergic inflammation site. In allergic rhinitis and asthma, the submucosa and the epithelium are infiltrated with T lymphocytes (CD4+ T cells and CD25+ T cells).[14]

Inflammation of the nasal mucosa may worsen the bronchial asthma through several mechanisms. In the biopsies of nasal and bronchial epithelium, the same inflammatory cells and Th2-like cytokines have been found in both, and the number of eosinophils in nasal smears correlate well with abnormal pulmonary function test results as well as nonspecific bronchial hyperresponsiveness in methacholine inhalation challenge. When patients with AR but without asthma had segmental bronchial allergen provocation, it resulted in nasal inflammation with tissue eosinophilia and up regulated eosinophil-specific adhesion molecule VCAM-1 (vascular cell adhesion molecule-1).[15]

There are several proposals for explaining the link between the nose and the lungs in AR and asthma. One explanation is the existence of a neural nasobronchial reflex, whereas other options are the possible postnasal drip of inflammatory cells and mediators from the nose to the lower airways, or the absorption of inflammatory cells from the nasal epithelium to the systemic circulation and from there to bronchial mucosa.[16] The nasal challenge with house dust mites has shown that similar early and late-phase responses are produced in the nose and the lungs.[17]

According to ARIA, the commonalities and differences in mechanisms between rhinitis and asthma include the following:

- Most asthmatics have rhinosinusitis as demonstrated by computed tomography (CT) scans.
- Severe asthmatics have more severe rhinosinusitis than mild asthmatics.
- Eosinophilic inflammation is present in the nasal and bronchial mucosa of asthmatics.
- Epithelium and basement membrane differ in the nasal and bronchial mucosa of asthmatics.
- The bronchial and nasal mucosa of chronic obstructive pulmonary disease (COPD) patients appear to be similar.
- Endobronchial challenge in rhinitis patients induces a bronchial reaction.
- A bronchial challenge induces nasal inflammation.
- A nasal challenge induces bronchial inflammation.
- Allergic inflammation has a systemic component.

Clinical Presentation

Rhinitis

Rhinitis symptoms include rhinorrhea, nasal obstruction, nasal itching, and sneezing. Postnasal drip can occur either with profuse anterior rhinorrhea or alone. AR symptoms are classified as intermittent when symptoms are present less than 4 days a week or less than 4 consecutive weeks and are persistent when symptoms are present more than 4 days a week for longer than 4 consecutive weeks. AR is moderate/severe when one or more of the following symptoms are present: sleep disturbance; impaired daily activities, leisure/sport, school, or work; or if patients feel the symptoms are troublesome. AR is mild when none of these symptoms are present. Rhinitis can be infectious, allergic, occupational, drug-induced, or hormonal; can be caused by irritants, food, or emotion; and can be atrophic or idiopathic.

Asthma

Asthma symptoms can include episodic breathlessness, wheezing, and chest tightness. Seasonal variability of symptoms, atopic disease, and positive family history are often related. According to GINA (Global Initiative of Asthma), important questions to consider for the diagnosis of asthma include the following:

- Has the patient had an attack or recurrent attacks of wheezing?
- Does the patient have a troublesome cough at night?
- Does the patient have a wheeze or cough after exercise?
- Does the patient have a wheeze, chest tightness, or cough after exposure to airborne allergens or pollutants?
- Do the patient's colds "go to the chest" or take more than 10 days to clear up?
- Are symptoms improved by appropriate anti-asthma treatment?

Diagnostic Evaluation

History

History-taking is key for the diagnosis of rhinitis and asthma. The nature and the duration of the symptoms distinguish rhinitis and asthma from symptoms of acute upper respiratory tract infections. Symptom triggers, symptom severity, and the impact of symptoms should be recorded and an appropriate differential diagnosis should be kept in mind. Family history, contact with animals and other triggers, the work environment, night time incidences, and exercise-induced symptoms should also be recorded.

Nasal symptoms for rhinitis can vary and may include sneezing; a runny, itchy, blocked nose; crusting; and hyposmia depending on the status of the disease. Asthma symptoms can include dyspnea, airflow limitation (wheeze), and hyperinflation during the symptomatic period. Troublesome cough at night, wheezing, coughing after exercise, and prolonged infections where a cough continues are typical for asthma and should also be inquired about.

Physical Examination

Otorhinolaryngological status, rhinoscopy, and exclusion of sinusitis are standard for the diagnosis of rhinitis. For diagnosis of asthma, an auscultation of the lungs should be included. Specific IgE antibody determination is a necessary step for the diagnosis of allergic rhinitis and asthma. It can be done with a skin prick test (SPT) or the determination of allergen-specific IgE radioallergosorbent test (RAST). Lung function tests with a measurement of hyperresponsiveness are most helpful in the diagnosis of asthma.

According to GINA, key points for the diagnosis and classification of asthma include the following:

- Asthma is underdiagnosed throughout the world.
- Asthma can often be diagnosed on the basis of symptoms. However, measurements of lung function and, particularly, the reversibility of lung function abnormalities greatly enhance diagnostic confidence.
- Lung function measurements that are most helpful for the diagnosis of asthma (in patients over 5 years of age) include forced expiratory volume in 1 second (FEV_1), forced vital capacity (FVC), peak expiratory flow (PEF), and airway hyperresponsiveness.
- Asthma severity is classified by the presence of clinical features before treatment is started and/or by the amount of daily medication required for optimal treatment.
- Measurements of allergic status add little to the diagnosis of asthma but can help in the identification of risk factors so that the appropriate environmental control measures can be recommended.
- Special care should be given to diagnosing asthma in children, in individuals with recurrent cough, in the elderly, and in individuals exposed to occupational agents known to cause asthma.

Treatment

An adequate treatment of AR in asthmatics has been shown to improve asthma symptoms and pulmonary function test results, and to reduce costs. The risk of emergency room treatment or hospitalizations, exercise-induced asthma, and bronchial hyperresponsiveness has been shown to be reduced also. Inadequately controlled AR in asthmatic patients can cause exacerbations of asthma and poorer symptom control.[18]

Oral antihistamines are the first-line treatment for AR but have only modest effect on asthma symptoms. They may reduce peak seasonal wheezing but are not sufficient alone to treat asthma, whereas inhaled corticosteroids and bronchodilatators are the first-line treatment for asthma.[19] Intranasal glucocorticoids (GCS) have been shown to moderately improve asthma, but they do not treat asthma symptoms sufficiently and therefore intranasal GCS with a combination of inhaled corticosteroids are needed for the treatment of AR and asthma.[20] Oral GCS are very effective in treating both AR and asthma, but they should be used only for a short time and for the exacerbation phases of asthma due to their side effects. Antileukotrienes are effective in the treatment of mild and moderate asthma and of the symptoms of rhinitis. Use of antileukotrienes also reduces the need for other asthma and rhinitis medications in some, but not all, patients. Accordingly, patient response to antileukotrienes should be tested with individual patients to identify who benefits from the treatment.[21] Anti-IgE medication (omalizumab) has been shown to be effective in the treatment of concomitant asthma and persistent AR, but because of its cost, it cannot be considered as a first-line treatment option.[22]

Specific immunotherapy is effective for patients with perennial AR with asthma, and it significantly improves their lung function.[23] The treatment of AR may reduce the risk of development of asthma. Immunotherapy for 3 years with standardized allergen extracts of grass and/or birch showed long-term clinical effects and had a preventive effect on the development of asthma in children with seasonal rhinoconjunctivitis.[24] Similar results with lower asthma risk have been shown in adult patients with AR treated with allergen immunotherapy.[25] Also, sublingual immunotherapy has been shown to be beneficial for the treatment of asthma and AR.[26] The mechanisms are not quite clear yet and new data are needed to identify susceptible patients. Also, the differences between the sublingual and subcutaneous routes still need more studies with more patients and longer follow-up times.

There are several studies of combination therapies for rhinitis and asthma, but fewer studies of costs compared with benefits. In general, the combination of intranasal and inhaled GCS is needed to control seasonal nasal and asthma symptoms.[27] Some data show that combination therapy with antihistamines and antileukotrienes may be as effective as GCS in patients with seasonal AR and asthma.[28] Other combination therapies are commonly used, and more studies are needed.

There are no guidelines for treatment of concomitant rhinitis and asthma, and both conditions are usually treated independently. Patients with rhinitis develop asthma more often than those patients without the disease and, therefore, regular follow-up should be included and asthma symptoms should be inquired about from patients during every follow-up visit. If an otorhinolaryngologist–head and neck surgeon does not have the necessary equipment to measure lung function or is not accustomed to treating asthma, patients should be referred to a pulmonologist when diagnosed.

The treatment of rhinitis and asthma using a single approach according to ARIA is as follows:

- Oral H1-antihistamines are not recommended, but not contraindicated in the treatment of asthma.
- Intranasal glucocorticosteroids are, at best, moderately effective in asthma.
- Intranasal glucocorticosteroids may be effective in reducing asthma exacerbations and hospitalization.
- The role of intrabronchial glucocorticosteroids in rhinitis is unknown.
- Montelukast is effective in the treatment of AR and asthma in patients over 6 years of age.
- Subcutaneous immunotherapy is recommended for both rhinitis and asthma in adults, but it is burdened by side effects, in particular in asthmatics.
- Anti-IgE monoclonal antibody is effective for both rhinitis and asthma.

Conclusion

It is important to recognize and treat rhinitis patients with bronchial asthma because it improves the patient's symptoms and quality of life. While recognizing that there is at this time only limited data existing for the possible preventive role of early treatment of rhinitis in preventing asthma development, there are some encouraging indications from long-term studies of allergen immunotherapy. Otorhinolaryngologists see many patients with upper airway symptoms, rhinitis, and sinusitis and therefore have a key role in diagnosing and referring patients who also have lower airway symptoms and are suspicious for asthma. However, these symptoms may not come up in routine discussion and in the evaluation of a patient unless patients are specifically asked about lower airway symptoms.

References

1. Bousquet J, Khaltaev N, Cruz AA, et al; World Health Organization; GA(2)LEN; AllerGen. Allergic Rhinitis and its Impact on Asthma (ARIA) 2008 update (in collaboration with the World Health Organization, GA(2)LEN and AllerGen). Allergy 2008;63 (Suppl 86):8–160
2. Van Cauwenberge P, Watelet JB, Van Zele T, et al; GA2LEN workpackages 3.2 and 3.3. Does rhinitis lead to asthma? Rhinology 2007;45(2):112–121
3. Bousquet J, Clark TJ, Hurd S, et al. GINA guidelines on asthma and beyond. Allergy 2007;62(2):102–112
4. Settipane RA, Lieberman P. Update on nonallergic rhinitis. Ann Allergy Asthma Immunol 2001;86(5):494–507, quiz 507–508
5. Valovirta E, Jacobsen L, Ljørring C, Koivikko A, Savolainen J. Clinical efficacy and safety of sublingual immunotherapy with tree pollen extract in children. Allergy 2006;61(10):1177–1183
6. Bousquet J, Jacot W, Vignola AM, Bachert C, Van Cauwenberge P. Allergic rhinitis: a disease remodeling the upper airways? J Allergy Clin Immunol 2004;113(1):43–49
7. Bachert C, Vignola AM, Gevaert P, Leynaert B, Van Cauwenberge P, Bousquet J. Allergic rhinitis, rhinosinusitis, and asthma: one airway disease. Immunol Allergy Clin North Am 2004;24(1):19–43
8. Sherman CB, Tosteson TD, Tager IB, Speizer FE, Weiss ST. Early childhood predictors of asthma. Am J Epidemiol 1990; 132(1):83–95
9. Leynaert B, Bousquet J, Neukirch C, Liard R, Neukirch F. Perennial rhinitis: An independent risk factor for asthma in nonatopic subjects: results from the European Community Respiratory Health Survey. J Allergy Clin Immunol 1999;104(2 Pt 1):301–304
10. Huovinen E, Kaprio J, Laitinen LA, Koskenvuo M. Incidence and prevalence of asthma among adult Finnish men and women of the Finnish Twin Cohort from 1975 to 1990, and their relation to hay fever and chronic bronchitis. Chest 1999;115(4):928–936
11. Karjalainen A, Martikainen R, Klaukka T, Saarinen K, Uitti J. Risk of asthma among Finnish patients with occupational rhinitis. Chest 2003;123(1):283–288
12. Lemanske RF Jr, Busse WW. 6. Asthma: factors underlying inception, exacerbation, and disease progression. J Allergy Clin Immunol 2006;117(2, Suppl Mini-Primer)S456–S461
13. Chakir J, Laviolette M, Turcotte H, Boutet M, Boulet LP. Cytokine expression in the lower airways of nonasthmatic subjects with allergic rhinitis: influence of natural allergen exposure. J Allergy Clin Immunol 2000;106(5):904–910
14. Varney VA, Jacobson MR, Sudderick RM, et al. Immunohistology of the nasal mucosa following allergen-induced rhinitis. Identification of activated T lymphocytes, eosinophils, and neutrophils. Am Rev Respir Dis 1992;146(1):170–176
15. Braunstahl GJ, Overbeek SE, Kleinjan A, Prins JB, Hoogsteden HC, Fokkens WJ. Nasal allergen provocation induces adhesion molecule expression and tissue eosinophilia in upper and lower airways. J Allergy Clin Immunol 2001;107(3):469–476
16. Bousquet J, Vignola AM, Demoly P. Links between rhinitis and asthma. Allergy 2003;58(8):691–706
17. Wang DY, Goh DY, Ho AK, Chew FT, Yeoh KH, Lee BW. The upper and lower airway responses to nasal challenge with house-dust mite Blomia tropicalis. Allergy 2003;58(1):78–82
18. Meltzer EO. The relationships of rhinitis and asthma. Allergy Asthma Proc 2005;26(5):336–340
19. Van Ganse E, Kaufman L, Derde MP, Yernault JC, Delaunois L, Vincken W. Effects of antihistamines in adult asthma: a meta-analysis of clinical trials. Eur Respir J 1997;10(10):2216–2224
20. Taramarcaz P, Gibson PG. Intranasal corticosteroids for asthma control in people with coexisting asthma and rhinitis. Cochrane Database Syst Rev 2003;(4):CD003570
21. Virchow JC, Bachert C. Efficacy and safety of montelukast in adults with asthma and allergic rhinitis. Respir Med 2006; 100(11):1952–1959
22. Vignola AM, Humbert M, Bousquet J, et al. Efficacy and tolerability of anti-immunoglobulin E therapy with omalizumab in patients with concomitant allergic asthma and persistent allergic rhinitis: SOLAR. Allergy 2004;59(7):709–717

23. Alvarez-Cuesta E, Bousquet J, Canonica GW, Durham SR, Malling HJ, Valovirta E; EAACI, Immunotherapy Task Force. Standards for practical allergen-specific immunotherapy. Allergy 2006;61(Suppl 82):1–20
24. Niggemann B, Jacobsen L, Dreborg S, et al; PAT Investigator Group. Five-year follow-up on the PAT study: specific immunotherapy and long-term prevention of asthma in children. Allergy 2006;61(7):855–859
25. Abramson MJ, Puy RM, Weiner JM. Allergen immunotherapy for asthma. Cochrane Database Syst Rev 2003;(4):CD001186
26. Calamita Z, Saconato H, Pelá AB, Atallah AN. Efficacy of sublingual immunotherapy in asthma: systematic review of randomized-clinical trials using the Cochrane Collaboration method. Allergy 2006;61(10):1162–1172
27. Dahl R, Nielsen LP, Kips J, et al; SPIRA Study Group. Intranasal and inhaled fluticasone propionate for pollen-induced rhinitis and asthma. Allergy 2005;60(7):875–881
28. Walsh GM. Second-generation antihistamines in asthma therapy: is there a protective effect? Am J Respir Med 2002; 1(1):27–34

9 The Diagnosis of Rhinosinusitis

Victoria A. Epstein and Donald C. Lanza

Rhinosinusitis is an inflammatory condition affecting the lining of the sinuses and nasal passages that can be variable in its clinical presentation. Proper diagnosis and classification of this disorder is important for at least two distinct reasons. First, the prognosis and recommended treatment strategies can be different for each form of rhinosinusitis. Second, because of its high prevalence and inconsistent presentation, rhinosinusitis can be mistaken for other common disorders such as headache syndromes or allergies. Alternately, it can be misdiagnosed in place of rare conditions such as sinus malignancy. Adding to the diagnostic challenge, rhinosinusitis in a given individual can have multiple etiologies (**Table 9.1**) and/or comorbidities. For example, a patient with chronic rhinosinusitis may also have the diagnosis of inhalant allergy, cystic fibrosis, and/or immunodeficiency. Classifying rhinosinusitis is also important to enable healthcare professionals to accurately communicate complexity, duration, etiology, and to advance general understanding of the disorder.

The most widely accepted classification systems of rhinosinusitis are consensus statements from panels of experts in the field.[1–5] Categorizations are based predominantly on the clinical presentation. In these classification systems, diagnostic criteria for rhinosinusitis have been set forth to aid the clinician with a diagnosis. For all forms of rhinosinusitis, diagnosis hinges on obtaining a careful medical history and performing a physical examination. However, certain types of rhinosinusitis can also require either nasal endoscopy or computerized tomography (CT) imaging to assert the presence of this disorder. Other tests can be used to further characterize rhinosinusitis and to identify comorbidities. The goals of this chapter are to classify varied forms of rhinosinusitis based on existing guidelines[1–5] and to describe methods that are used to appropriately diagnose and evaluate rhinosinusitis (**Table 9.2**).

Table 9.1 Etiology of Rhinosinusitis

Host Factors	Environmental
Genetic/congenital • Cystic fibrosis • Ciliary dyskinesia	Infectious • Viral • Bacterial • Fungal
Allergic/ immune	Trauma
Anatomic	Noxious chemicals
Systemic disease • Endocrine • Autoimmune	Iatrogenic • Medications • Surgery
Neoplasm	

In this chapter, adult rhinosinusitis is the primary focus of discussion. Pediatric rhinosinusitis has unique features related to both the relative immaturity of the immune system and to its microbiology. Fungal rhinosinusitis is another category of rhinosinusitis also not thoroughly reviewed here. Variations associated within this form of rhinosinusitis are delineated in **Table 9.3**.[6]

Classification of Rhinosinusitis

Presenting symptoms are an important part of properly classifying varied forms of rhinosinusitis. Specifically, certain types of rhinosinusitis are more likely to present with a specific symptom complex and therefore certain diagnostic criteria apply (as discussed later). General symptoms of rhinosinusitis include: nasal obstruction/ congestion, nasal discharge, nasal purulence, postnasal drip, facial pressure/pain, headache, dental pain, altered sense of smell, cough, fever, halitosis, fatigue, pharyngitis, and otologic symptoms such as ear fullness or popping. Nighttime cough can be an important sign of this disorder in children.

Acute Rhinosinusitis

Acute rhinosinusitis is a condition whereby nasal and sinus inflammation occurs and lasts for up to 4 weeks. Patients can describe a variety of symptoms, but its cardinal diagnostic features are (1) mucopurulent/purulent nasal or postnasal drainage, and either (2) nasal obstruction or (3) facial pressure/pain. Objective evidence for the diagnosis of acute rhinosinusitis includes: (1) visualized nasal/sinus passage purulent or mucopurulent discharge, (2) posterior pharyngeal purulence, or (3) radiographic evidence of sinus soft tissue swelling/inflammation (plain film or CT imaging).[2]

The majority of clinically significant episodes of acute rhinosinusitis are secondary to a predominant microbe. These can be viral, bacterial, and/or fungal. Inhalation of irritating substances such as chemicals, smoke, and allergens can also be associated with acute sinus inflammation. By far the most common form of acute rhinosinusitis is associated with a viral infection that results in self-limited upper respiratory symptoms (nasal discharge, congestion, and cough).[2] One explanation for the high incidence of viral etiologies of acute rhinosinusitis is that the common cold has been shown to affect the paranasal sinuses in addition

Table 9.2 Classification of Rhinosinusitis

Type of Rhinosinusitis		Criteria for Diagnosis		
		Duration	**Symptoms for Diagnosis**	**Objective Documentation**
Acute	AVRS	Present for <10 days and symptoms are not worsening[2,5]	Requires: (1) and [(2) or (3)][2,5] (1) Anterior and/or posterior mucopurulent drainage (2) Nasal obstruction (3) Facial pain/ pressure/ fullness	Requires either[2]: (1) Nasal airway examination for mucopurulent drainage (2) Radiographic evidence of acute rhinosinusitis
	ABRS	Present for 10 days to 4 weeks OR worsening disease within 10 days after an initial improvement[2,5]		
	AIFRS	Present for <4 weeks[6,66]	Typically immunosuppressed patients with symptoms of fever, facial or orbital swelling, pain, numbness, unilateral nerve damage, acute visual changes with altered motility or declining vision[6]	Requires both: (1) Radiological imaging showing mucosal thickening of sinonasal passages (2) Histopathological evidence of hyphal forms within sinus mucosa, submucosa, blood vessels, or bone[67]
Recurrent Acute		≥4 episodes/year + each episode lasts from 10 days up to 4 weeks[1,2]	Same as ABRS absence of signs or symptoms of rhinosinusitis between episodes[1,2]	Each episode must meet criteria for ABRS[2,5]
Subacute		Present for 4–12 weeks[1]	Same as ABRS	Same as ABRS
Chronic	CRSsNP	Present for ≥12 weeks[1,2]	Requires ≥2 of the following[2]: (1) Anterior and/or posterior mucopurulent drainage (2) Nasal obstruction (3) Facial pain/ pressure/ fullness	Requires nasal endoscopy to exclude presence of polyps and to document the presence of inflammation.[2] Sinus CT imaging is not required but should be strongly considered.[2]
	CRSwNP	Present for ≥12 weeks[1,2]	Requires ≥ 2 of the following[2]: (1) Anterior and/or posterior mucopurulent drainage (2) Nasal obstruction (3) Decreased sense of smell	Requires nasal endoscopy to exclude presence of polyps and to document the presence of inflammation.[2] Sinus CT imaging is not required but should be strongly considered.[2]
	AFRS	Present for ≥12 weeks[1,2]	Requires ≥1 of the following[2]: (1) Anterior and/or posterior mucopurulent drainage (2) Nasal obstruction (3) Decreased sense of smell (4) Facial pain/ pressure/ fullness	Requires[2]: (1) Endoscopy to document presence of allergic mucin (fungal hyphae with degranulating eosinophils) and inflammation (2) Fungal specific IgE (3) No histologic evidence of fungal invasion Other possible but not required documentation measures[2]: (4) Fungal culture (5) Total serum IgE (6) Imaging by more than one technique (CT or MRI) highly suggestive of AFRS Sinus CT imaging is not required but is highly recommended (bony erosion and extension of disease into adjacent anatomic areas).[2]
Acute Exacerbation of Chronic		Sudden worsening of CRS, with return to baseline after treatment[1]	Has features of ABRS superimposed on CRS	Nasal endoscopy to document presence of inflammation. Sinus CT imaging is not required but should be strongly considered.

Abbreviations: ABRS, acute bacterial rhinosinusitis; AFRS, allergic fungal rhinosinusitis; AIFRS, acute invasive fungal rhinosinusitis; AVRS, acute viral rhinosinusitis; CRSsNP, chronic rhinosinusitis without nasal polyps; CRSwNP, chronic rhinosinusitis with nasal polyps; CT, computed tomography; IgE, immunoglobulin E; MRI, magnetic resonance imaging.

to the nasal cavity. In one study of 31 adults with the common cold, nearly 90% had CT evidence of sinus mucosal thickening.[7] Additionally, secondary bacterial infection of the sinuses in the face of viral infection has been shown to be possible by forceful nose blowing.[8]

Acute bacterial rhinosinusitis without preceding viral infection is believed far less common, and when it is related to dental disease, it arises first within the maxillary sinus (**Fig. 9.1**). Regardless if it is virally or bacterially mediated, acute rhinosinusitis symptoms completely resolve within 4 weeks. Depending on its etiology, resolution may occur with or without treatment.

Interestingly, patients and clinicians can find it difficult to distinguish acute bacterial rhinosinusitis (ABRS) from

Table 9.3 Classification of Fungal Rhinosinusitis

Extramucosal (Noninvasive) Fungal Rhinosinusitis	Invasive Fungal Rhinosinusitis
• Superficial sinonasal mycosis	• Acute (fulminant) invasive fungal rhinosinusitis
• Fungal ball	• Chronic invasive fungal rhinosinusitis
• Allergic fungal rhinosinusitis	• Granulomatous invasive fungal rhinosinusitis

acute viral rhinosinusitis (AVRS) because these clinical entities can overlap in presentation, especially in the first 10 days of illness. AVRS is diagnosed when symptoms or signs of acute rhinosinusitis are present less than 10 days and the symptoms are not worsening.[5] It does not require the prescription of an antibiotic. Medical evaluation by a healthcare professional for acute rhinosinusitis is recommended when any of the following occur:

1. Symptoms or signs are present for 10 or more days
2. Symptoms or signs worsen within 10 days after an initial improvement
3. Inadequate hydration
4. Fever >38.9°C (102°F)
5. Eye pain or swelling and/or vision changes
6. Severe head or facial pain
7. Other comorbidities that place the patient at risk for complications (e.g., immune compromise)

Acute (Fulminant) Invasive Fungal Rhinosinusitis

Acute invasive fungal rhinosinusitis (AIFRS) is a result of aggressive and rapid tissue invasion by fungal organisms (**Table 9.3**). It is almost exclusively observed in immunocompromised patients (e.g., diabetic, transplant, HIV). The symptom complex of AIFRS can be very different than that of acute bacterial or viral rhinosinusitis. Its presentation can be missed until it is advanced. AIFRS can present with nasal blockage, facial pain/headache, diplopia, proptosis, loss of vision, and or anesthesia/paresthesias of face and palate. Whitish necrotic debris (typically nonmucor) or black eschar (typically mucor) that resembles a scab is typically seen within the nasal or sinus passages on physical examination. Diagnosis of AIFRS is objectively confirmed by tissue biopsy demonstrating invasion by fungus. Vascular invasion and necrosis are common hallmark findings.[6]

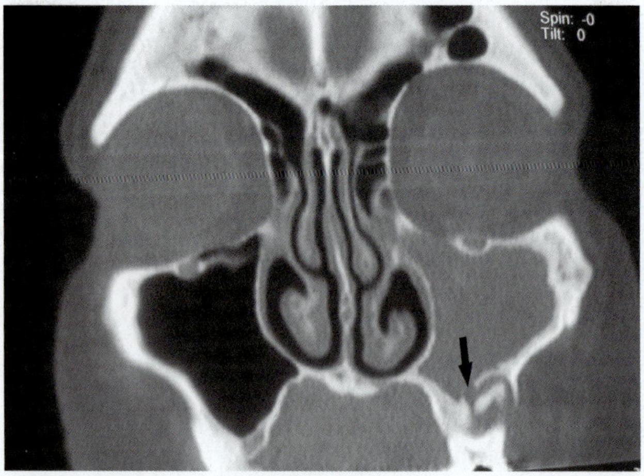

Fig. 9.1 Coronal reformatted computed tomography scan of left maxillary sinusitis secondary to periapical abscess; the black arrow demonstrates erosion into the sinus.

Recurrent Acute Rhinosinusitis

Recurrent acute rhinosinusitis is diagnosed when a patient experiences four or more episodes of acute rhinosinusitis per year. Symptoms and physical findings are consistent with acute rhinosinusitis, with each episode lasting 10 days to 4 weeks. Between episodes, symptoms are absent. Diagnostic criteria are otherwise identical to those for acute rhinosinusitis.[1,2,5] This diagnosis can be associated with:

- Frequent contact with viruses from:
  - Exposure to young children in daycare or early school years up to age 10
  - Frequent air travel or hand shaking without hand washing
  - Exposure to infected individuals—for example, healthcare workers
- Naturally occurring or surgically created recirculation of sinus mucus
- Recurring exposure to a respiratory irritant(s)
- Immune deficiency (e.g., common variable immune deficiency)

Clinical experience suggests that certain conditions can mimic recurrent, acute rhinosinusitis. These include undiagnosed or undertreated inhalant allergy, undiagnosed or undertreated chronic rhinosinusitis, and extraesophageal reflux triggering recurrent sinonasal swelling. Occasionally, headache or facial pain syndromes masquerade as rhinosinusitis.

Subacute Rhinosinusitis

Subacute rhinosinusitis represents the natural progression of acute rhinosinusitis that has not yet resolved. It is diagnosed after 4 weeks' duration of acute rhinosinusitis and lasts for up to 12 weeks. Subacute rhinosinusitis is not known to represent a discrete histopathological entity. Although patients may or may not have been treated for the acute phase of disease their symptoms tend to be less severe than in acute rhinosinusitis. Typically, it is thought that subacute rhinosinusitis resolves completely after an effective medical regimen.[1]

Chronic Rhinosinusitis

Chronic rhinosinusitis (CRS) is diagnosed by signs and symptoms of rhinosinusitis lasting more than 12 weeks. CRS has at least three distinct categories based on clinical presentation and diagnostic criteria[2]:

1. CRS without nasal polyps (CRSsNP)
2. CRS with nasal polyps (CRSwNP)
3. Allergic fungal rhinosinusitis (AFRS)

It is unclear whether these three clinical entities represent different phases of the same disease or instead discrete entities with different pathophysiologies. In light of the multiple etiologies that can occur in a given individual with CRS, this condition has been described as a syndrome instead of a distinct disease entity.[1]

Patients with CRSsNP will have two or more of the following symptoms present: (1) mucopurulent discharge (anterior or posterior); (2) nasal obstruction; and/or (3) facial pressure/pain. Patients with CRSwNP will instead have two or more of the following symptoms present: (1) mucopurulent discharge (anterior or posterior); (2) nasal obstruction; and/or (3) decreased sense of smell. Facial pain/pressure is not considered a defining symptom for CRSwNP in the absence of other nasal factors. This is related to the fact that nasal polyps are depleted of substance P, a neurotransmitter associated with sensory C fibers, which mediate pain through the trigeminal system.[9]

All patients with possible CRS require documentation of objective findings of sinonasal inflammation, either by physical exam or radiologic exam, to confirm the diagnosis. Physical examination should be performed to determine the presence or absence of polyps, edema, or sinus discharge, whether it be mucopus or eosinophilic mucin. Endoscopically directed cultures (see later) may be of particular value in all forms of CRS to identify associated resistant microbial flora. In many cases, nasal endoscopy is needed to perform an adequate evaluation because anterior rhinoscopy can be limited (as described later). Alternately, imaging with CT can be used to establish the diagnosis of CRS by demonstrating mucosal thickening in the paranasal sinuses.

Allergic Fungal Rhinosinusitis

Acute fungal rhinosinusitis (AFRS) appears to be a subset of CRS in which patients will have evidence of a fungal allergy to their colonizing fungus. Those patients with AFRS typically demonstrate five characteristics: gross production of eosinophilic mucin containing noninvasive fungal hyphae seen on endoscopy; nasal polyposis; characteristic radiographic findings; immunocompetence; and an allergy to cultured fungi.[2]

Acute Exacerbation of Chronic Rhinosinusitis

This represents a sudden deterioration of the baseline chronic rhinosinusitis with either worsening or new symptoms. There is typically complete resolution of the acute symptoms between occurrences.[1] Due to the underlying chronic nature of this condition, unusual or resistant bacterial and fungal species may be implicated; thus, endoscopically guided cultures may be particularly helpful in guiding antimicrobial therapy.

History and Physical Exam

Medical history should document all relevant symptoms, their time course, and their severity. Screening for host and environmental predisposing factors[1] is critical as part of history taking. Past medical/surgical history, review of systems, allergies, social/work history, and family history are also essential elements of the evaluation. A history of recurring pneumonia, otitis media, and rhinosinusitis in an adult suggests the possibility of a common variable immune deficiency, other immunocompromised states, or ciliary dyskinesia. A family history of cystic fibrosis or allergy also has implications for additional diagnostic testing. Diagnoses such as extraesophageal reflux or aspirin hypersensitivity may be missed without careful, directed questioning. Careful history can also influence the selection of treatments. For example, a patient with CRS and allergies who has a past medical history of shingles and prostatic hypertrophy may be a poor candidate for either systemic steroids (reactivation of shingles) or antihistamines (acute urinary retention).

Physical examination should encompass the head and neck and should include an otoscopy, an anterior rhinoscopy, and an oropharyngeal and laryngeal examination.

Anterior Rhinoscopy

Anterior rhinoscopy is typically performed with illumination via nasal speculum. It is advisable to perform anterior rhinoscopy before decongestion with an agent such as oxymetazoline to determine the baseline extent of soft tissue edema and erythema. Structural causes of nasal obstruction such as septal deviation, nasal valve collapse, and turbinate hypertrophy may have a markedly different appearance pre- and post-decongestion. Decongestion will permit most clinicians with illumination (head lighting) to see much further into the nasal airway. The extent of what can be visualized is variable and partly dependent on the severity of septal deviation, narrowness of the nasal airway, and extent of disease. It should be noted that one study reports the incidence of septal deviation/spur in humans to be as high as 79%.[10] Occasionally, the middle meatus and even the nasopharynx can be partly evaluated with an anterior rhinoscopy. Nasal purulence is the most significant physical finding for the diagnosis of rhinosinusitis. Additional evidence of rhinosinusitis includes polyps (**Fig. 9.2**), erythema, edema, crusting, and golden sticky mucus referred to as eosinophilic mucin.

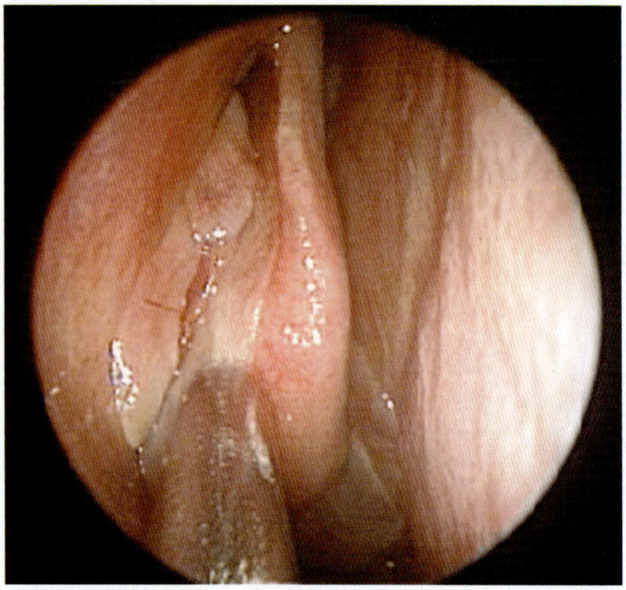

Fig. 9.2 A right-sided rigid nasal endoscopy demonstrating middle meatal polyps.

Nasal Endoscopy

In contrast to anterior rhinoscopy, endoscopy introduces brilliant illumination and permits greatly improved, magnified direct visualization of the nasal cavity, turbinates, septum, drainage pathways of the paranasal sinuses, and, in postsurgical patients, the sinus cavities themselves. There are two types of endoscopes that are widely available for evaluating the sinonasal passages—flexible fiberoptic endoscopes and rigid endoscopes/telescopes (**Fig. 9.3**). Flexible endoscopes allow for more comfortable visualization of the nasopharynx, eustachian tube orifices, as well as the larynx to detect signs of extraesophageal reflux. In patients with prior sinus surgery, flexible endoscopes provide greater visualization into the maxillary, sphenoid, and frontal sinuses. This is especially true for lateral recesses of the sphenoid and frontal sinuses as well as the floor of the maxillary sinus.

Although the imaging quality of flexible endoscopes has been significantly enhanced by digital video chip technology, rigid endoscopes still offer superior image clarity. Furthermore, rigid endoscopy greatly facilitates surgical instrumentation of the nose and sinuses, such as obtaining cultures or biopsies, controlling epistaxis, or performing surgery. The zero-degree endoscope is the easiest to maneuver in the nasal cavity, whereas angled rigid endoscopes (e.g., 30-degree nasal endoscope) can be used to visualize structures that are not in the direct line of sight and offer superior visualization of the lateral nasal wall, skull base, and frontal recess. The 45-, 70-, and 90-degree endoscopes are used for the visualization of challenging frontal recess and maxillary sinus pathology.

Unless contraindicated, topical vasoconstrictive and anesthetic agents are typically used to facilitate nasal endoscopy. Some clinicians and patients, however, prefer not to use topical anesthesia. This does help demonstrate active mucociliary clearance in vivo because the ciliary function is deactivated by topical anesthesia; however, intolerance of endoscopy without anesthesia may limit the completeness of the evaluation. Although endoscopy is generally a very safe and well-tolerated procedure, the most common adverse effects of endoscopy are patient discomfort/

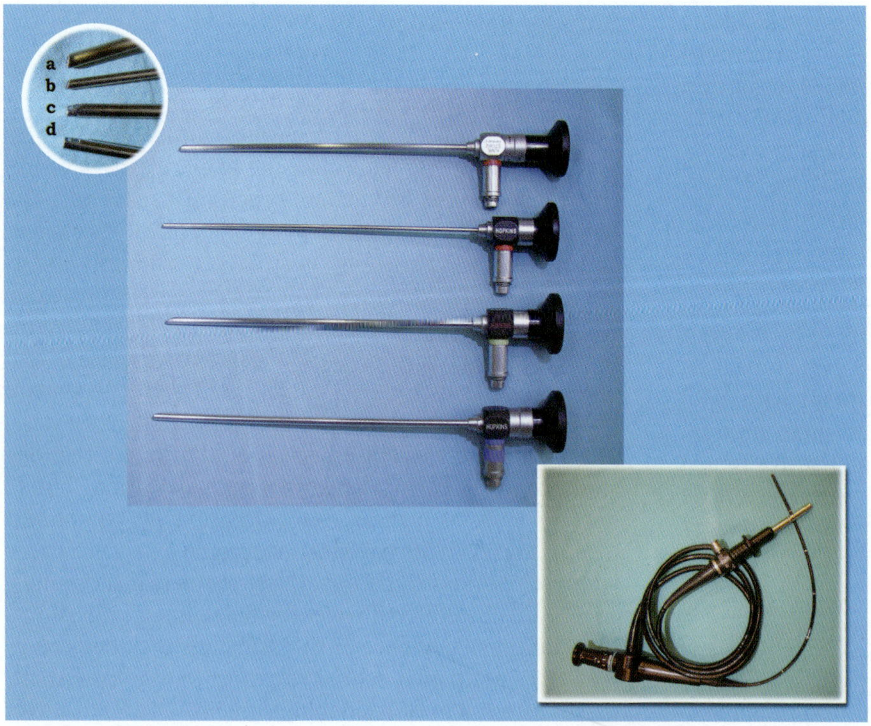

Fig. 9.3 Rigid Karl Storz endoscopes and an Olympus flexible endoscope. *Insert*, the left upper corner shows a magnified view of the tips of the rigid endoscopes: *a*, 30 degrees 4 mm; *b*, 30 degrees 2.7 mm; *c*, 70 degrees 4 mm; and *d*, 90 degrees 4 mm).

pain, nasal bleeding, and feeling faint or lightheaded from anxiety. Smaller diameter telescopes and flexible scopes are recommended for pediatric use or for use in patients with difficult nasal anatomy.

Indications for Nasal Endoscopy

Indications for nasal endoscopy include (but are not limited to) the following[11]:

1. Sinonasal symptoms refractory to appropriate empiric therapy or in suspected chronic rhinosinusitis
2. Unilateral disease without septal deviation
3. Severe and disabling symptoms attributed to the nose or sinuses
4. Actual or impending complications of sinonasal disease
5. Immunocompromised patients who have sinonasal complaints (transplant, diabetes, leukemia, etc.)
6. Evaluation of surgical treatments after sinus surgery and/or trauma

Among rhinologists, there are six tenets of nasal endoscopy that apply[11]:

1. Patient symptoms can be an unreliable gauge of disease (especially in CRSwNP).
2. Discolored drainage (yellow to green) represents a pathological process draining through the nasal passageways.
3. Endoscopy is well tolerated and generally safe but is not without risk.
4. Endoscopy facilitates proper diagnosis and can detect disease missed on a routine history and physical examination or even missed on imaging studies.
5. Properly obtained, endoscopic cultures are useful in identifying organisms that may be responsible for certain forms of rhinosinusitis.
6. The most important role of endoscopy is in the assessment and treatment of patients with refractory or chronic symptoms, and in patients who are threatened by impending or existing complications of rhinosinusitis.

A systematic approach to the nasal endoscopy is traditionally divided into three phases[12]:

1. The inferior examination consists of passing the nasal endoscope along the floor of the nose to visualize the floor of the nasal cavity, the inferior turbinate/meatus, nasal septum, and the eustachian tube orifice as well as the nasopharynx. Occasionally, the lacrimal drainage at Hasner's valve can be observed within the inferior meatus.
2. The second passage of the telescope evaluates the nasal valve anteriorly and superiorly, the nasal septum, the anterior middle turbinate, the olfactory cleft, the sphenoethmoid recess, the superior turbinate, and occasionally, the sphenoid sinus ostium.
3. The third passage occurs by rolling the endoscope into the middle meatus posteriorly and examining the basal lamella attachment of the middle turbinate to the lateral wall as well as the ostiomeatal complex, the uncinate process, and possibly, the anterior ethmoid bulla.[12]

A general description of the nasal airway size, shape, and configuration is pursued. Septal deviation/spurs/perforation, concha bullosa, as well as nonspecific mucosal findings are described that may include a bluish discoloration, edema, erythema, and cobblestoning. The nature of the mucus and moisture/dryness of the nasal airway is considered while looking for mucus stasis or stranding of mucus across the nasal cavity. Quality of sinus drainage/purulence, color, and site of origin are noted in addition to the presence of polyps, eosinophilic or inspissated sinus debris, fungal hyphae growing directly on tissue or retained secretions, and even tissue necrosis from invasive bacterial and fungal pathogens. Purulent or mucopurulent drainage above or below the eustachian tube orifice has significance as to its points of origin. Typically, drainage that passes below the eustachian orifice originated from the middle meatus (drainage of the anterior ethmoid, maxillary, and/or frontal sinuses) and that above the eustachian tube originated from the superior meatus and/or sphenoethmoidal recess. Sinus mucus recirculation can be an important cause of recurrent acute rhinosinusitis. This occurs when mucus leaving a given sinus returns back into that sinus of origin via a patent accessory ostium (most commonly seen in the maxillary sinus). This recirculation of mucus permits relative stagnation and secondary colonization leading to local infection. Additional findings suggesting other diseases include granulomas, telangiectasias, foreign body (young children or mentally impaired), or nonpolyp masses suspicious for tumors. Although imaging studies can characterize the degree of obstruction of unoperated sinuses (whereas endoscopy is typically ineffective), qualitative assessment of the surface nasal and sinus mucosa is best achieved with endoscopy. Therefore, it is important to remember that endoscopy and imaging are complementary methods of patient evaluation.

Endoscopically Obtained Sinus Culture and Sensitivities

Endoscopic culture techniques allow direct sampling of abnormal-appearing discharge emanating from the paranasal sinuses. This is strongly preferred to undirected swabbing of the nasal vestibule, nasal cavity, or nasopharynx, which is subject to contamination with commensal organisms. Endoscopic cultures are obtained transnasally and may be performed with either a sterile swab or a sterile suction trap (**Fig. 9.4**).[13] Care must be taken to minimize contamination of the swab, usually achieved by retraction of the nasal ala by the endoscope and by careful passage of the swab under endoscopic visualization.

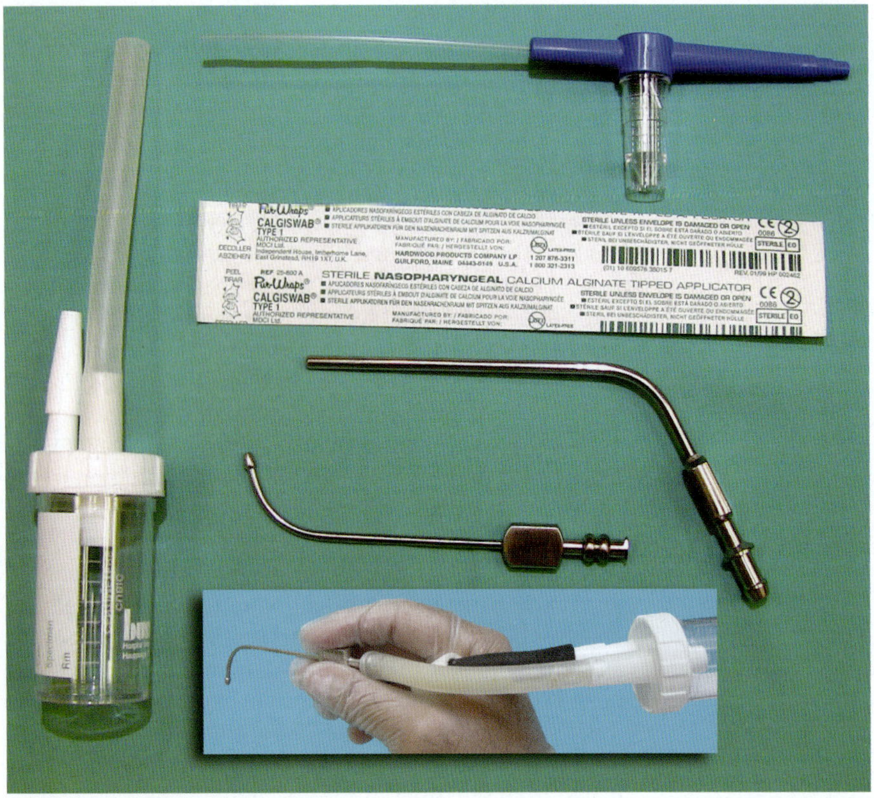

Fig. 9.4 Endoscopic culture equipment, including a sterile ARGYLE Lukens specimen trap (Covidien, Mansfield, MA), a Medtronic Tami Sinus Secretion Collector (Minneapolis, MN), a calcium alginate swab, a Frazier, and olive-tipped Eiken suction cannulas.

The emergence of antibiotic resistance has increased concern over the use of empiric antimicrobial therapy for rhinosinusitis.[14] Thus, more specialists use endoscopically guided bacterial/fungal cultures and antibacterial sensitivities to guide care (**Fig. 9.5**). Less frequently, cultures for anaerobic bacteria and acid fast bacilli (AFB) may be sought.[15] Using standard techniques, it can take up to 4 weeks to obtain identification for fungus and AFB. Specialized mycology methods can grow fungus more rapidly in 100% of normal subjects, and therefore, a positive result is difficult to interpret without other supporting information. Cincik and Ferguson[16] reported that endoscopically guided culture results directed a change in therapy in 51.4% of patients with CRS. Benninger et al.[17] performed meta-analysis with pooled data consisting of 126 patients with 131 "culture pairs" obtained from maxillary sinus taps and endoscopically obtained sinus cultures. For known pathogenic bacteria in ABRS, endoscopically directed middle meatal cultures had a sensitivity of 80.9%, a specificity of 90.5%, a positive predictive value of 82.6%, a negative predictive value of 89.4%, and an overall accuracy of 87.0% as compared with maxillary sinus tap.

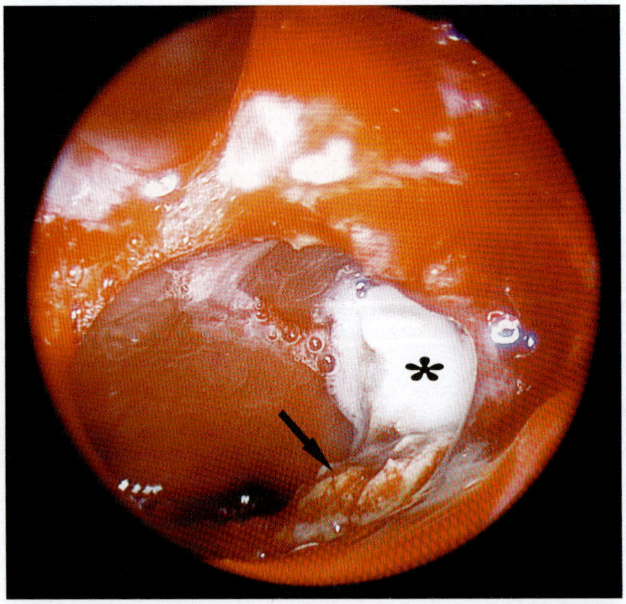

Fig. 9.5 A left-sided rigid nasal endoscopy showing a surgically enlarged sphenoid ostium with evidence of a fungal ball (*black arrow*), erythema, and purulence (*asterisk*). Purulence was sent for Gram stain, aerobic, and anaerobic cultures. Surgical pathology was requested to confirm the diagnosis of a fungal ball.

Imaging

Computerized Tomography Scans

Currently, CT scans are considered the standard of care for imaging the paranasal sinuses and have replaced conventional radiographs for the assessment of rhinosinusitis. Conventional plain X-ray films have a poor sensitivity for mucosal disease in the maxillary sinuses.[18] They do not allow for a robust analysis of anatomic variants, such as secondary ostia (recirculation) and concha bullosa. Despite this, but due to its wide availability, plain X-rays are still used by some clinicians as a screening tool for acute rhinosinusitis. Indications for obtaining sinus CT scans resemble those for nasal endoscopy (see previous text), but CT imaging and endoscopy should be viewed as complementary methods of patient evaluation. Repeat CT imaging to assess the interval change or response to treatment may be advisable when there is a paucity of findings on nasal endoscopy but persistent sinus mucosal disease is suspected.

CT scans provide excellent bone detail, and when using the proper windowing, they are sensitive in detecting small amounts of mucosal swelling. CT scans provide useful anatomic information for operative planning and can be integrated into surgery as part of image guidance (aka computer-aided surgery).

There are now many modalities for obtaining CT images, including screening sinus CT, spiral CT, and point-of-service cone beam CT. These vary in radiation dose, cost, image detail, and clarity. CT images obtained in the axial or coronal plane, using bone window algorithm, are generally sufficient to establish the diagnosis of rhinosinusitis. Triplanar reconstruction and soft tissue windows provide additional important anatomic detail but are not required for the diagnosis of rhinosinusitis. Intravenous contrast usually is not required unless there is a concern about tumors or an infectious orbital or intracranial complication.

The risk of radiation from sinus CT imaging is generally perceived to be small. However, the growing use of this technology has raised concern over radiation exposure related to repeat imaging, especially in children. The organs most likely to be affected by a cumulative radiation dose are the lens of the eye and the thyroid gland. According to the US Food and Drug Administration (FDA),[19] standard head CT leads to 2 mSv (effective dose in milli-sieverts) of radiation . This is equivalent to approximately the effective radiation dose from 100 chest X-rays or the natural background radiation an individual would be exposed to in 243 days. CT of the sinuses with cone beam technology in the office setting is estimated to substantially decrease effective dose (MiniCAT [Xoran Technologies, Ann Arbor, MI] sinus 40 second algorithm leads to 0.13 mSv)[20] but image quality and resolution may be diminished.

Appearance of CT images is affected by "window width" and "window center" that are arranged according to Hounsfield units (HU: unit of X-ray attenuation based on water where air has a value of −1,000; water, 0; and compact bone/metallic density, +1,000). Bone windowing for sinus disease is generally evaluated with a window width of ~2,300 and a center level of 300 HU (**Fig. 9.6**). The windowing can be adjusted in many CT image software systems to enhance the contrast between high-density areas and surrounding inflammatory tissue. If the windowing is improperly applied, misinterpretations of findings on CT scans are possible. For example, with soft tissue windowing, which was developed for evaluating the orbit or brain, fine bone detail is lost and soft tissue swelling of the sinus mucosa could be more difficult to evaluate.

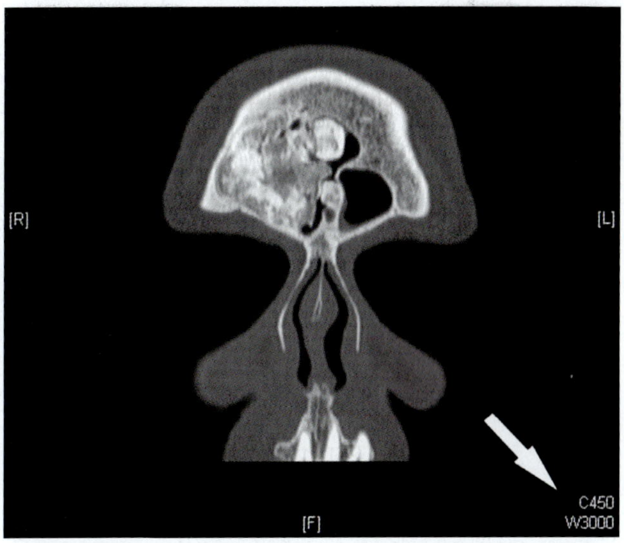

Fig. 9.6 A coronal reformatted computed tomography scan with fibro-osseous lesion nearly completely filling the right frontal sinus. The *white arrow* points to the right bottom corner where window center (*c*) and window width (*w*) numbers are displayed, corresponding to "bone windows."

CT scan can provide important diagnostic information. Soft tissue swelling or thickening within the lumen of a sinus is consistent with rhinosinusitis. When an air-fluid level is present, it is suggestive of acute rhinosinusitis associated with purulence. Irregularities within the lumen can have a rounded appearance as with a polyp or cyst or irregular surface as may be consistent with extramucosal fungus. High-density material detected within the sinus lumen can also represent inspissated pus or fungal material (**Fig. 9.7A,B**). Osteitic bone (**Fig. 9.8**) and anatomic variations are also sought to explain persistence of disease. Inverted papilloma is suspected on CT scans when a middle meatal mass is continuous through an expanded maxillary ostium into the adjacent maxillary antrum (**Fig. 9.9**). The mass may contain areas of high density or calcification, and there may be sclerosis of the wall of the affected sinus.[21] Additional interesting CT findings are depicted in **Fig. 9.10A,B.**

There has been substantial interest in the usefulness of the CT scan in staging patients with CRS for research purposes. Currently, the most widely used system is the Lund-Mackay CT staging system due to its simplicity as well as its excellent inter- and intraobserver agreement.[22]

Magnetic Resonance Imaging

Magnetic resonance imaging (MRI) can be a useful adjunct to CT scans, but it is more expensive and time consuming. Soft tissue tumors and impending or actual orbital/intracranial complications of rhinosinusitis are indications for MRI. MRI excels at delineating soft tissues but does not depict fine bone architecture. MRI permits the assessment of various fluid compositions and often allows scar tissue to be more readily distinguished from

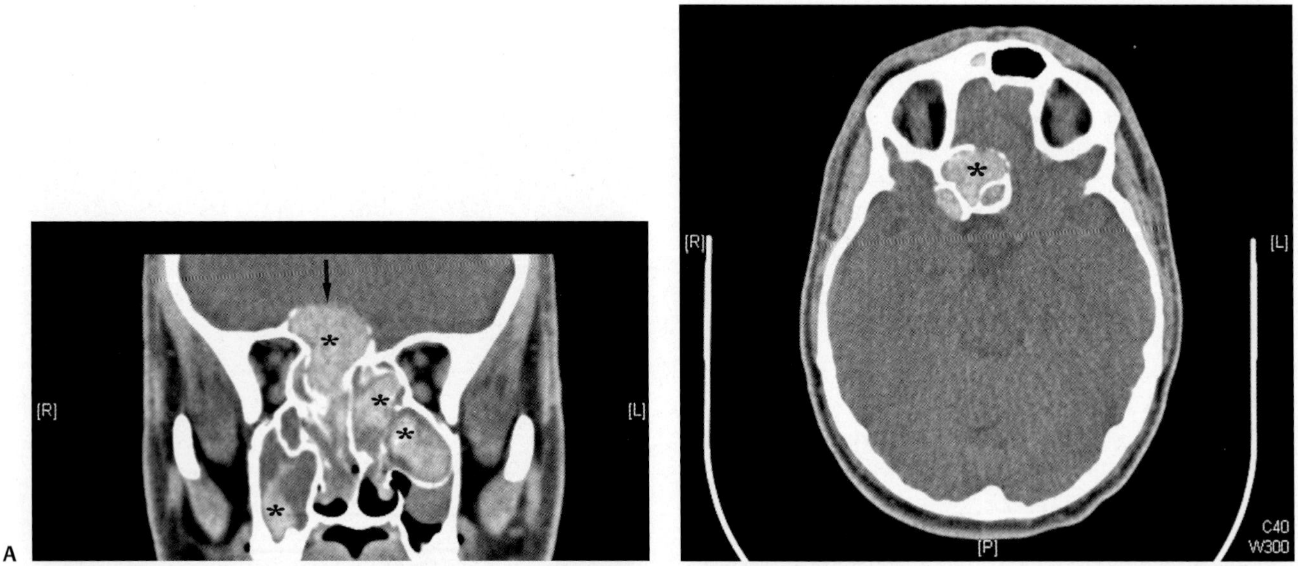

Fig. 9.7 Coronal reformatted **(A)** and axial **(B)** computed tomography scan images of allergic fungal rhinosinusitis. There is diffuse and extensive sinus disease with increased soft tissue density (*asterisks*) within bilateral maxillary, ethmoid, and sphenoid sinuses. A right posterior ethmoid cell is dehiscent of bone (**A**, *black arrow*) and is expanded with high density material extending epidurally into the floor of the anterior cranial fossa, best seen on axial **(B)** view.

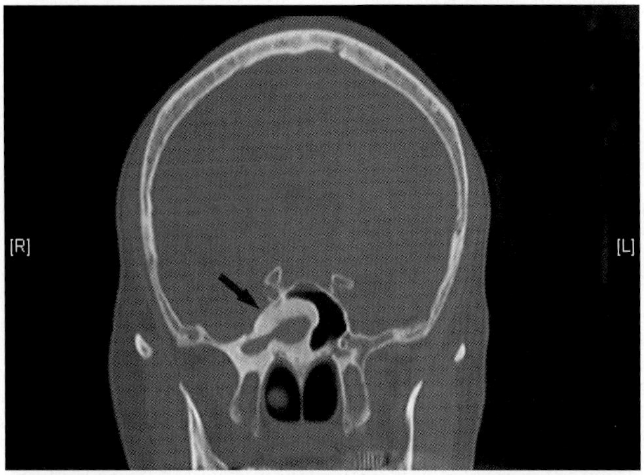

Fig. 9.8 Coronal reformatted computed tomography scan of complete opacification of the right sphenoid sinus. Note the marked bony wall thickening at the right sphenoid sinus (*black arrow*).

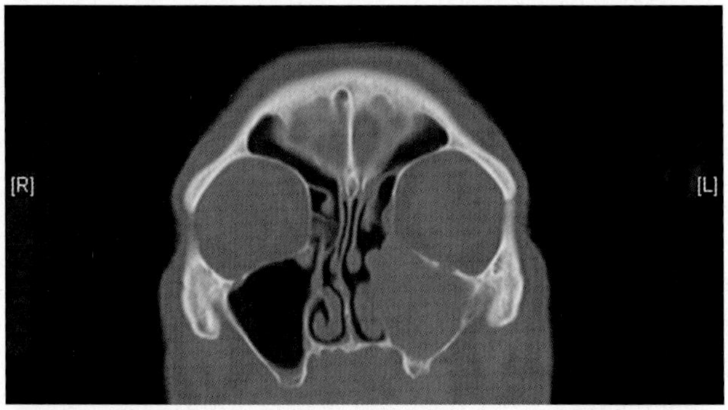

Fig. 9.9 Coronal reformatted computed tomography scan of a patient with inverted papilloma filling the left maxillary sinus. Note the bone resorption of the left medial wall of the maxillary sinus. There is extension of soft tissue from the maxillary sinus into the left nasal cavity.

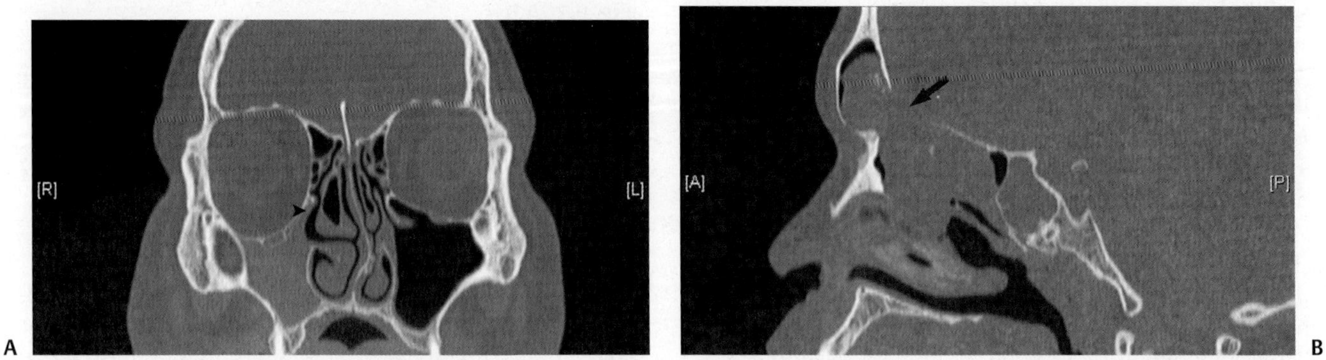

Fig. 9.10 **(A)** Coronal reformatted computed tomography (CT) scan of silent sinus syndrome. Note the contracted right maxillary sinus with downward displacement of the orbital floor. The uncinate process (*arrowhead*) is laterally displaced and is directly apposing the inferomedial orbital wall. **(B)** Sagittal reformatted CT scan of a patient with a large encephalocele presenting 10 years after sustaining a closed head injury. A bony dehiscence (*black arrow*) extends from the posterior table of the frontal sinus to the cribriform plate and measures 1.7 cm in the anteroposterior dimension. Encephaloceles may be mistaken for polyps; radiographic imaging studies can greatly facilitate the diagnosis.

other forms of soft tissue disease and recurrent tumors. T1-weighted (T1W) images tend to brighten tissues with fat density and T2-weighted (T2W) brighten those with characteristics of water. Depending on the degree of desiccation of sinus debris, the T1W and T2W signals may be hyperintense or hypointense. AFRS is classically identified by low signal intensity on T1W imaging and marked hypointensity (dark) with T2W weighting (**Fig. 9.11A–D**). Fungi accumulate heavy metals, such as zinc, magnesium, manganese, and iron. Decreased signal intensity on a T2W MRI may be associated with these metals.[23] However, the presence of inspissated mucosal

Fig. 9.11 Computed tomography (CT) and magnetic resonance images (MRI) of an intracranial complication of a right sphenoid fungal and bacterial infection. Coronal reformatted CT scan **(A)** showing increased density (*black arrow*) corresponding to fungal concretion. T2-weighted fat suppressed coronal MRI **(B)** with decreased signal intensity/signal void (*black arrow*) corresponding to fungal concretion on CT scan. Gadolinium-enhanced T1-weighted fat suppressed coronal and sagittal MRI **(C,D)** demonstrating a sinogenic abscess (*white arrows*) within the left inferior frontal lobe.

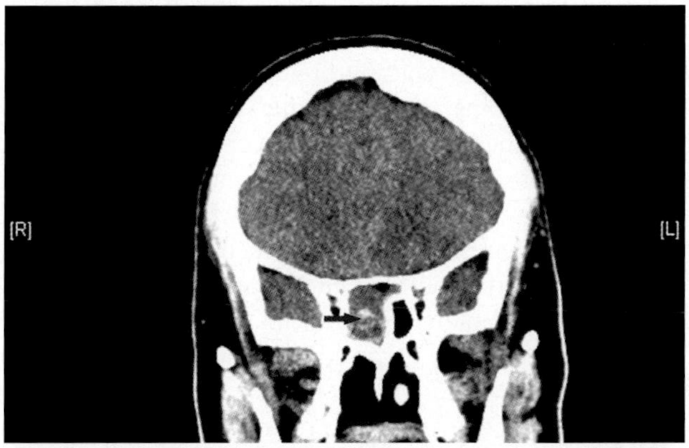

A

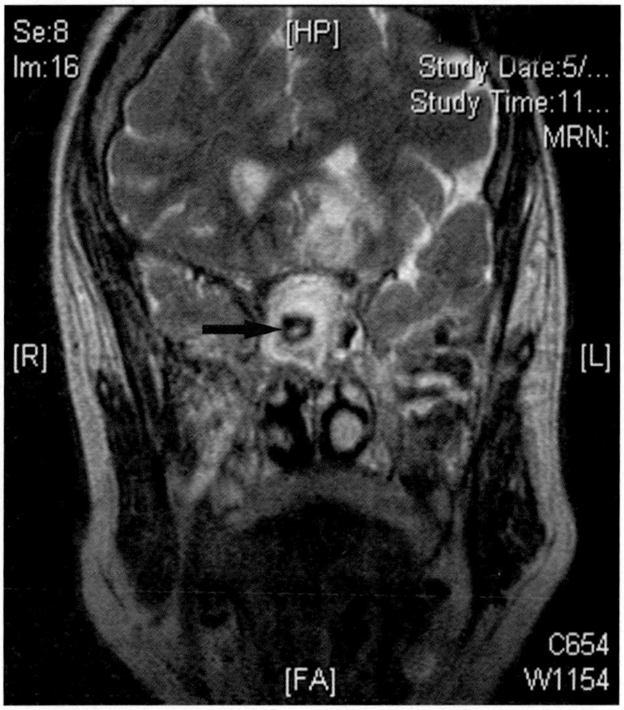

B

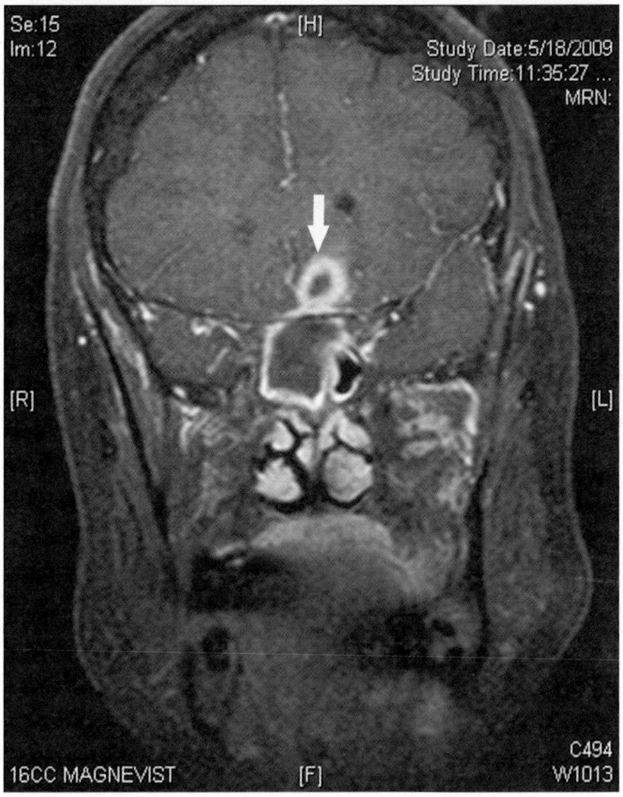

C

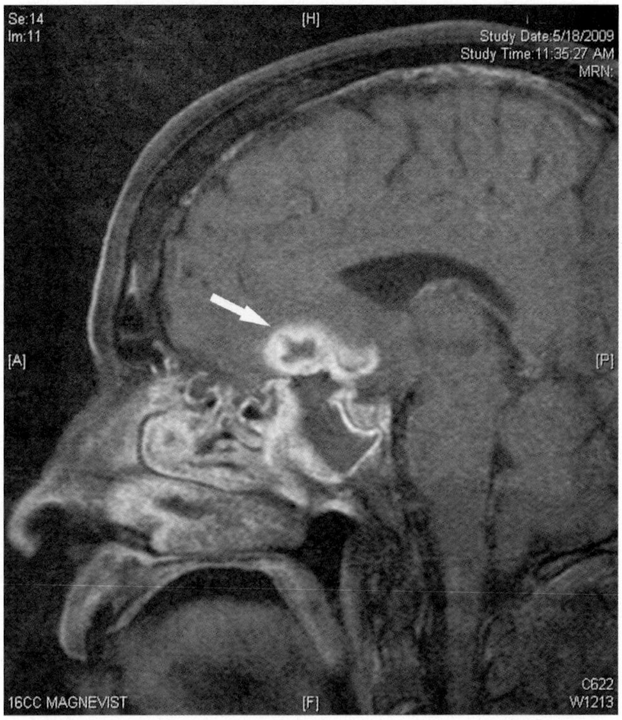

D

secretions within the sinus cavity can also result in a markedly hypointense T2W signal.[24] Contrast-enhanced MRI may be useful to distinguish a mucopyocele from a tumor.[18]

Ultrasound

Ultrasound (US) has been used in the diagnosis of rhinosinusitis primarily in Europe.[25–28] The main advantages of US are the lack of radiation exposure, low cost, and wide availability. The sensitivity of US for maxillary sinus disease was found to be 66.7% and the specificity was 94.9% compared with CT. As a result, the role of US in the diagnosis of rhinosinusitis, like plain films, is fading.

Laboratory Studies

Routine Blood Work

Complete Blood Count With Differential

A complete blood count (CBC) with differential can point to important alterations in white blood cell counts and can identify anemia. Specific elevations in various kinds of blood cells will be helpful in understanding the pathogenesis of ARS and CRS.

Eosinophils

Eosinophils are especially known to be involved in allergic inflammation but also are known to be the predominant inflammatory cell type in studies of sinus tissue from some patients with CRS. Inflammatory mediators released by eosinophils, such as major basic protein and eosinophilic cationic protein, have toxic effects on respiratory epithelium.[29] Substantial elevations in serum eosinophils should raise the suspicion of Churg-Strauss syndrome in the proper clinical setting. Serum eosinophilia may also have prognostic significance because serum eosinophilia (total eosinophil count greater than 200/μL)[30] correlates with extensive sinus disease and a worse prognosis.[31–34]

Comprehensive Metabolic Panel

A comprehensive metabolic panel will help identify multiple aberrations in chemistries, blood glucose, and renal and liver function—all of which can be associated with chronic illness.

In Vitro mRAST and Cutaneous Allergy Testing

Allergic inflammation has been identified consistently as one factor contributing to both acute and chronic rhinosinusitis.[35] If the history and a physical exam indicate the presence of inhalant allergy, diagnostic allergy testing is often recommended. Evaluation of the allergic patient is covered in greater detail in Chapter 7 of this book.

Briefly, screening tests for the detection of inhalant allergy can be performed with commercially available modified radioallergosorbent tests (mRAST) via ImmunoCAP (Pharmacia Diagnostics, Clayton, NC) or Phadezym-RAST (Pharmacia Diagnostics). They can also be performed using in vivo tests through epicutaneous tests (prick/puncture techniques and scratch testing) or percutaneous tests (single-dilutional and multidilutional intradermal techniques).[30] The number of antigens used in screening evaluations varies but could be as low as 8 to 12 antigens. Selection of antigens should reflect local geography and should contain one or two grasses, weeds, trees, two or three molds, cat allergen, and one dust mite allergen.

The sensitivity of in vitro testing can be less than prick/intradermal combinations, but in vitro testing produces few false-positive results.[36] Per allergen evaluated, in vitro testing is more expensive than cutaneous testing. In vitro testing is typically preferred for patients with a preference against needle testing, a history of anaphylaxis, an angioedema or laryngeal edema, an active use of beta-blockers, who are pregnant, who have skin abnormalities (e.g., dermatographia), or when skin reactivity might be suppressed by existing medications, and in any situation where an allergic challenge might be potentially dangerous.[37] In many instances, in vitro testing combined with cutaneous testing can add significantly to the allergic diagnostic evaluation.[36]

Total serum IgE levels are not reliable in measuring the presence of allergy but can be helpful markers to follow in severe refractory allergy (e.g., AFRS). Elevated total IgE levels have a high correlation with the presence of inhaled allergy but low levels do not rule out clinically important allergic disease.[30]

Immunoglobulin Evaluation

Immunodeficiency should be considered in patients with chronic and recurrent rhinosinusitis refractory to treatment when other causes have been excluded, especially when rhinosinusitis is associated with otitis media, bronchitis, bronchiectasis, or pneumonia.[5] Common diseases such as variable immune deficiency or selective immunoglobulin subclass deficiencies should be considered, and consultation with an immunologist and/or infectious disease specialist may be advised. Common immunodeficiencies that are identified include decreases in serum IgA, IgG, and its subclasses, and abnormalities in markers of T-lymphocyte function.[38,39] An evaluation includes measurements of quantitative IgA, total IgG, and IgG subclass levels, complete blood cell count with differential, and responses to immunization with protein (e.g., diphtheria and tetanus toxoid), and polysaccharide (e.g., Pneumovax) antigens. HIV testing is also considered in the appropriate clinical setting. Identification of immune defects will often affect treatment considerations. Prophylactic antibiotic therapy can reduce or resolve symptoms in patients with mild immune deficits, and intravenous immunoglobulin can be added in more refractory diseases with beneficial results.

Genetic and Sweat Chloride Testing for Cystic Fibrosis

Patients with cystic fibrosis (CF) are typically identified early in life with sweat chloride testing. However, it is now recognized that some patients can escape early detection either due to a less severe form of the disease or a false-negative sweat test.[40] The association between CF and CRS is well established, with a 43% prevalence of nasal polyps in CF patients.[41,42] CF testing should be considered in adult patients with a history of lifelong respiratory disturbances including CRS and digestive or fertility disorders. Although sweat chloride testing is the most commonly used screening test for CF diagnosis, genetic testing currently offers specific serologic testing for known CF mutations and plays an important adjunctive role in CF diagnosis.[40]

Histopathology

Histopathology can be used to evaluate mucosal tissue as well as mucus and debris. Eosinophilic mucin (**Fig. 9.12**) and fungal balls can be readily identified through this method. In addition, fungal stains can complement culture techniques for fungi. Special stains such as the Gomori methenamine silver stain, potassium hydroxide prep, or calcofluor white stain may be employed. Chitin, an abundant polysaccharide found in fungal cell walls, can also be identified with special staining.[43] Tissue can also be analyzed for eosinophilia, granulomas (**Fig. 9.13**), and tissue invasion by bacteria or fungi. A tissue biopsy of unilateral nasal polyps or a nasal mass can be important to rule out an inverted papilloma or sinus malignancy (after ruling out a meningoencephalocele, for which a biopsy is contraindicated). An electron microscopy of respiratory epithelium can reveal ultrastructural ciliary defects, leading to a diagnosis of primary ciliary dyskinesia.

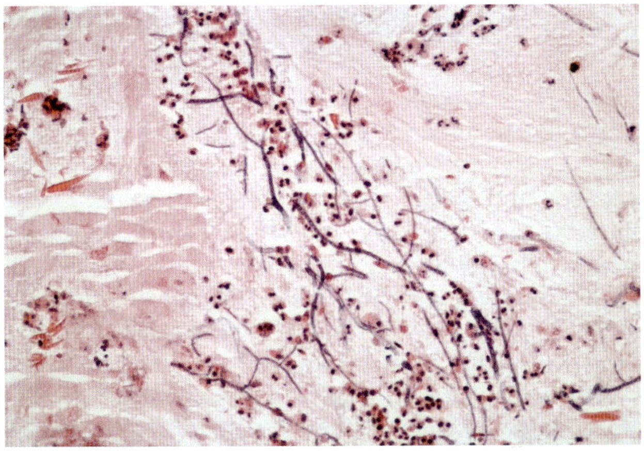

Fig. 9.12 A histopathology demonstrating fungal hyphae in mucin, with eosinophils clustering adjacent to hyphae.

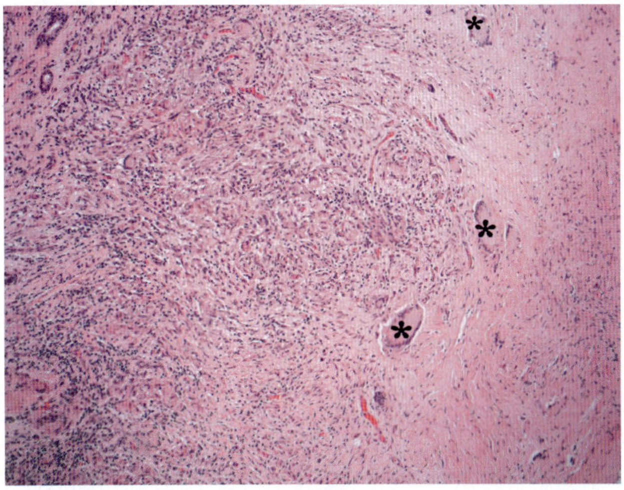

Fig. 9.13 Hematoxylin-eosin staining (10× magnification) of lateral nasal wall mucosa from a patient with chronic rhinosinusitis without nasal polyps demonstrating granulomatous inflammation with multinucleated giant cells (*asterisks*). (Courtesy of Dr. Kern M. Davis, St. Petersburg, FL.)

Nasal Function Studies

Nasal function tests can be used to further characterize or measure the severity of rhinosinusitis as well as to advance research. Pulmonary function studies (not reviewed here) are also valuable to comprehensively evaluate the patient with lower airway symptoms.

Olfactory Testing

Chronic rhinosinusitis is a common cause of olfactory dysfunction, believed to account for at least 25% of smell loss cases and affecting more than 10 million people.[44] CRS can cause a diminished sense of smell through two known mechanisms: by decreased conduction of odorants to the olfactory neuroepithelium and by associated neuroepithelial inflammation.[45,46] Again, loss of the sense of smell is a clinically important criterion for the diagnosis of CRSwNP. Although most clinical assessments of smell function tend to be subjective, well validated objective tests of olfaction do exist. The instrument most widely used by specialists for olfactory testing is the smell identification test (SIT), a "scratch and sniff" test formerly known as the University of Pennsylvania Smell Identification Test (UPSIT). In Europe, a commonly used test uses odorant-impregnated, reusable, felt-tipped pens (Sniffin' Sticks).[47] For additional information regarding olfactory testing, please refer to Chapter 4 of this book.

Saccharin Test

The saccharin test is used to evaluate mucociliary clearance from the nasal airway—in particular, to help determine the need for a biopsy to rule out ciliary dyskinesia syndrome. It is performed by placing a small amount of saccharin at the leading edge of the inferior turbinate and determining how long it takes for sweetness to be detected by the study subject. The normal time ranges between 6 and 30 minutes.[48] There is a fairly high correlation between the saccharin test results, the measurement of nitric oxide levels, and electron microscopy in patients with primary ciliary dyskinesia.[49]

Nitric Oxide

Nitric oxide (NO) is a biologically produced gas that is an important signaling molecule in humans for a variety of physiologic activities, including phagocytosis, smooth muscle relaxation, and ciliary motility. Therefore, for a variety of reasons, it can be found elevated or depressed in the respiratory tree. Nonetheless, NO is growing in popularity as a clinical marker of airway inflammation. There was once thought to be a direct relationship between exhaled NO and sputum eosinophils but it is now known to be imperfect. An elevation in exhaled NO can be due to a simple viral cold or atopy, or it can even be constitutional. Levels of nasal NO are found to be significantly lower in patients with CRSwNP as compared with patients who have CRSsNP ($p < 0.001$).[50] NO levels are also significantly reduced in primary ciliary dyskinesia, sinobronchial syndrome, and Young syndrome.[49]

Measurement of Nasal Patency

Nasal obstruction is an important symptom of rhinosinusitis. The subjective sensation of nasal obstruction can be difficult to quantify. Patient perceptions of nasal obstruction vary considerably and can have no bearing to the actual resistance to airflow in the nose. As a result, objective methods were developed to assess nasal patency.[51] Acoustic rhinometry[52] has replaced rhinomanometry as the leading method used to assess nasal airway obstruction. A major advantage of acoustic rhinometry, which measures the nasal cross-sectional area as a result of reflected sound waves, is that it is a very simple technique and requires minimal patient cooperation.[53] Rhinomanometry involves the simultaneous measurement of nasal airflow and the pressure required to achieve that flow, from which nasal airway resistance is calculated.[53]

Quality of Life Measurement Tools

It is generally recommended that physical, functional, and emotional problems associated with rhinosinusitis be measured. Validated instruments for this evaluation are used to measure quality of life (QOL). This is essential for good outcome studies of rhinosinusitis. Relevant QOL measurement tools that are disease-specific for rhinosinusitis include the Rhinosinusitis Outcomes Measure-31, the Sino-Nasal Outcome Test-22 (SNOT-22), the Chronic Sinusitis Survey, and the Rhinosinusitis Disability Index (RSDI).

Evolving Diagnostic Studies

Major Basic Protein

Major basic protein (MBP) is a cytotoxic protein released by the eosinophil granules. In vitro, MBP has been shown to directly damage respiratory and sinus epithelium.[54] A commercially available MBP assay of nasal mucus is in development to help determine the severity of disease and how the levels are influenced by therapy.

Superantigens

Superantigens are secreted proteins that can be produced by bacteria, fungi, or viruses that can stimulate hyperresponsiveness of the immune system. Superantigenic toxins have been detected in the tissues of patients with CRSwNP.[55,56] Testing for superantigens in the nasal cavities of patients with CRS has not yet been incorporated into clinical practice.

Detection of Biofilm

Biofilms are structured communities of microbes (bacteria and/or fungi) encased in a self-produced glycocalyx and are firmly attached to an inert or living surface. They are now known to exist in some patients with chronic rhinosinusitis.[57,58] Biofilms are very difficult to culture using standard techniques and are extremely resistant to host defenses and conventional antibiotic therapy.[59] There are no commercially available techniques for use in the outpatient clinic to assert the presence of biofilms in rhinosinusitis.

Contact Endoscopy

Contact rhinoscopes (Karl Storz Inc., Tuttlingen, Germany) are used in conjunction with methylene blue (1%) as a vital colorant to identify squamous epithelium, ciliated epithelium, glandular orifices, mucus layers, microvascular networks, inflammatory cell infiltrates, impregnated inclusions, and fungal hyphae. It has been used to diagnose nasopharyngeal carcinoma[60]; to delineate the angioarchitecture of the nasal mucosa in hereditary hemorrhagic telangiectasia (aka Osler-Weber-Rendu syndrome)[61]; and to differentiate between inverted schneiderian papilloma and inflammatory polyps.[62] The potential of contact endoscopy is promising for the study of rhinosinusitis.

The Electronic Nose

The electronic nose (E-nose) is an experimental tool that replicates chemical senses by the detection of volatile compounds to detect the presence of pathology. An E-nose can differentiate among various common bacterial pathogens of the upper respiratory tract, including *Staphylococcusaureus*, *Streptococcus pneumoniae*, *Haemophilus influenzae*, and *Pseudomonas aeruginosa*.[63] An E-nose is able to distinguish between patients with and without bacterial rhinosinusitis and those with cerebrospinal fluid leaks.[64] An E-nose has also been applied to the detection of biofilms.[65]

Conclusion

Rhinosinusitis is a complex disorder that can have a variable presentation and should be properly categorized into its various types. Proper diagnosis is critical because prognosis and recommended treatment strategies can differ for each form of rhinosinusitis. Moreover, given the overlapping clinical presentation of CRS with other conditions, such as allergy or headache syndromes, failure to use the aforementioned criteria for rhinosinusitis can lead to a misdiagnosis. A classification system based on presenting symptoms and objective criteria is presented in this chapter. A wide variety of technologies are available to characterize the type of rhinosinusitis that may be present. Careful medical history and physical examination are essential to diagnose all forms of rhinosinusitis. Due to limitations associated with anterior rhinoscopy, nasal endoscopy and/or CT imaging are often required to assert the presence of CRS.

Despite the importance of a meaningful classification, the International Statistical Classification of Diseases version 9 and 10 (ICD-9 &10) and the FDA have lagged behind physician organizations in establishing useful classifications of rhinosinusitis. One explanation for this is related to the limited amount of controlled bench and clinical research available to make certain delineations. A consequence of this deficiency in ICD coding and FDA guidelines is that the pharmaceutical industry has not invested in new treatment strategies for this pervasive health care problem. In fact, as of 2009, there is only one medication that is FDA approved for the treatment of chronic rhinosinusitis: a topical nasal steroid (mometasone furoate).

Consensus guidelines are published jointly by five national societies: the American Academy of Otolaryngology–Head Neck Surgery Foundation (AAO-HNS); the American Rhinologic Society (ARS); the American Academy of Otolaryngic Allergy (AAOA); the American Academy of Asthma, Allergy, & Immunology (AAAAI); and the American College of Asthma Allergy and Immunology (ACAAI).[2,3] These guidelines, including the 2007 AAO-HNS clinical practice guidelines[5] and the 2007 European Position Paper on Rhinosinusitis and Nasal Polyps,[4] are advised readings for those interested in more detail.

References

1. Lanza DC, Kennedy DW. Adult rhinosinusitis defined. Otolaryngol Head Neck Surg 1997;117(3 Pt 2):S1–S7
2. Meltzer EO, Hamilos DL, Hadley JA, et al; American Academy of Allergy, Asthma and Immunology; American Academy of Otolaryngic Allergy; American Academy of Otolaryngology-Head and Neck Surgery; American College of Allergy, Asthma and Immunology; American Rhinologic Society. Rhinosinusitis: establishing definitions for clinical research and patient care. Otolaryngol Head Neck Surg 2004;131(6, Suppl)S1–S62
3. Meltzer EO, Hamilos DL, Hadley JA, et al; Rhinosinusitis Initiative. Rhinosinusitis: developing guidance for clinical trials. Otolaryngol Head Neck Surg 2006;135(5, Suppl)S31–S80
4. Fokkens W, Lund V, Mullol J; European Position Paper on Rhinosinusitis and Nasal Polyps Group. EP3OS 2007: European position paper on rhinosinusitis and nasal polyps 2007. A summary for otorhinolaryngologists. Rhinology 2007;45(2):97–101
5. Rosenfeld RM, Andes D, Bhattacharyya N, et al. Clinical practice guideline: adult sinusitis. Otolaryngol Head Neck Surg 2007; 137(3, Suppl)S1–S31
6. Dhong HJ, Lanza DC. Fungal rhinosinusitis. In: Kennedy DW, Bolger WE, Zinreich SJ, ed. Diseases of the Sinuses: Diagnosis and Management. Hamilton, Ontario: BC Decker Inc.; 2001:179–194
7. Gwaltney JM Jr, Phillips CD, Miller RD, Riker DK. Computed tomographic study of the common cold. N Engl J Med 1994; 330(1):25–30
8. Gwaltney JM Jr, Hendley JO, Phillips CD, Bass CR, Mygind N, Winther B. Nose blowing propels nasal fluid into the paranasal sinuses. Clin Infect Dis 2000;30(2):387–391
9. Gungor A, Baroody FM, Naclerio RM, White SR, Corey JP. Decreased neuropeptide release may play a role in the pathogenesis of nasal polyps. Otolaryngol Head Neck Surg 1999;121(5):585–590
10. Gray LP. Deviated nasal septum. Incidence and etiology. Ann Otol Rhinol Laryngol Suppl 1978;87(3 Pt 3, Suppl 50)3–20
11. Lanza DC. Diagnosis of chronic rhinosinusitis. Ann Otol Rhinol Laryngol Suppl 2004;193:10–14
12. Lanza DC, Kennedy DW. Endoscopic sinus surgery. In: Bailey BJ, ed. Head & Neck Surgery- Otolaryngology. Vol 1. 3 ed. Philadelphia: Lippincott Williams & Wilkins; 2001:371–382
13. Tantilipikorn P, Fritz M, Tanabodee J, Lanza DC, Kennedy DW. A comparison of endoscopic culture techniques for chronic rhinosinusitis. Am J Rhinol 2002;16(5):255–260
14. Hsu J, Lanza DC, Kennedy DW. Antimicrobial resistance in bacterial chronic sinusitis. Am J Rhinol 1998;12(4):243–248
15. Nadel DM, Lanza DC, Kennedy DW. Endoscopically guided cultures in chronic sinusitis. Am J Rhinol 1998;12(4):233–241
16. Cincik H, Ferguson BJ. The impact of endoscopic cultures on care in rhinosinusitis. Laryngoscope 2006;116(9):1562–1568
17. Benninger MS, Payne SC, Ferguson BJ, Hadley JA, Ahmad N. Endoscopically directed middle meatal cultures versus maxillary sinus taps in acute bacterial maxillary rhinosinusitis: a meta-analysis. Otolaryngol Head Neck Surg 2006;134(1):3–9
18. Branstetter BF IV, Weissman JL. Role of MR and CT in the paranasal sinuses. Otolaryngol Clin North Am 2005;38(6):1279–1299
19. U.S. Food and Drug Administration, Center for Devices and Radiological Health. What are the Radiation Risks from CT? http://www.fda.gov/Radiation-EmittingProducts/Radiation

EmittingProductsandProcedures/MedicalImaging/Medical X-Rays/ucm115329.htm. Accessed July 17, 2009
20. Xoran Technologies. MiniCAT™ Effective Patient Radiation Dose. https://www.xorantech.com/Products/minicat_radiationdose.aspx. Accessed July 18, 2009
21. Savy L, Lloyd G, Lund VJ, Howard D. Optimum imaging for inverted papilloma. J Laryngol Otol 2000;114(11):891–893
22. Hopkins C, Browne JP, Slack R, Lund V, Brown P. The Lund-Mackay staging system for chronic rhinosinusitis: how is it used and what does it predict? Otolaryngol Head Neck Surg 2007;137(4): 555–561
23. Zinreich SJ, Kennedy DW, Malat J, et al. Fungal sinusitis: diagnosis with CT and MR imaging. Radiology 1988;169(2):439–444
24. Som PM, Curtin HD. Chronic inflammatory sinonasal diseases including fungal infections. The role of imaging. Radiol Clin North Am 1993;31(1):33–44
25. Karantanas AH, Sandris V. Maxillary sinus inflammatory disease: ultrasound compared to computed tomography. Comput Med Imaging Graph 1997;21(4):233–241
26. Vento SI, Ertama LO, Hytönen ML, Malmberg CH. A-mode ultrasound in the diagnosis of chronic polypous sinusitis. Acta Otolaryngol 1999;119(8):916–920
27. Savolainen S, Pietola M, Kiukaanniemi H, Lappalainen E, Salminen M, Mikkonen P. An ultrasound device in the diagnosis of acute maxillary sinusitis. Acta Otolaryngol Suppl 1997;529: 148–152
28. Haapaniemi J, Laurikainen E. Ultrasound and antral lavage in the examination of maxillary sinuses. Rhinology 2001;39(1):39–42
29. Ponikau JU, Sherris DA, Kephart GM, et al. Striking deposition of toxic eosinophil major basic protein in mucus: implications for chronic rhinosinusitis. J Allergy Clin Immunol 2005;116(2): 362–369
30. Krouse JH, Stachler RJ, Shah A. Current in vivo and in vitro screens for inhalant allergy. Otolaryngol Clin North Am 2003;36(5): 855–868
31. Newman LJ, Platts-Mills TA, Phillips CD, Hazen KC, Gross CW. Chronic sinusitis. Relationship of computed tomographic findings to allergy, asthma, and eosinophilia. JAMA 1994;271(5): 363–367
32. Kountakis SE, Arango P, Bradley D, Wade ZK, Borish L. Molecular and cellular staging for the severity of chronic rhinosinusitis. Laryngoscope 2004;114(11):1895–1905
33. Poznanovic SA, Kingdom TT. Total IgE levels and peripheral eosinophilia: correlation with mucosal disease based on computed tomographic imaging of the paranasal sinus. Arch Otolaryngol Head Neck Surg 2007;133(7):701–704
34. Zadeh MH, Banthia V, Anand VK, Huang C. Significance of eosinophilia in chronic rhinosinusitis. Am J Rhinol 2002;16(6): 313–317
35. Spector SL. The role of allergy in sinusitis in adults. J Allergy Clin Immunol 1992;90(3 Pt 2):518–520
36. Kelso JM, Sodhi N, Gosselin VA, Yunginger JW. Diagnostic performance characteristics of the standard Phadebas RAST, modified RAST, and pharmacia CAP system versus skin testing. Ann Allergy 1991;67(5):511–514
37. Emanuel IA. In vitro testing for allergy diagnosis. Otolaryngol Clin North Am 2003;36(5):879–893
38. Chee L, Graham SM, Carothers DG, Ballas ZK. Immune dysfunction in refractory sinusitis in a tertiary care setting. Laryngoscope 2001;111(2):233–235
39. Sethi DS, Winkelstein JA, Lederman H, Loury MC. Immunologic defects in patients with chronic recurrent sinusitis: diagnosis and management. Otolaryngol Head Neck Surg 1995;112(2): 242–247
40. Farrell PM, Rosenstein BJ, White TB, et al; Cystic Fibrosis Foundation. Guidelines for diagnosis of cystic fibrosis in newborns through older adults: Cystic Fibrosis Foundation consensus report. J Pediatr 2008;153(2):S4–S14
41. Coste A, Gilain L, Roger G, et al. Endoscopic and CT-scan evaluation of rhinosinusitis in cystic fibrosis. Rhinology 1995;33(3): 152–156
42. Slavin RG. Resistant rhinosinusitis: what to do when usual measures fail. Allergy Asthma Proc 2003;24(5):303–306
43. Taylor MJ, Ponikau JU, Sherris DA, et al. Detection of fungal organisms in eosinophilic mucin using a fluorescein-labeled chitin-specific binding protein. Otolaryngol Head Neck Surg 2002; 127(5):377–383
44. Cullen MM, Leopold DA. Disorders of smell and taste. Med Clin North Am 1999;83(1):57–74
45. Kern RC. Chronic sinusitis and anosmia: pathologic changes in the olfactory mucosa. Laryngoscope 2000;110(7):1071–1077
46. Kern RC, Conley DB, Haines GK III, Robinson AM. Pathology of the olfactory mucosa: implications for the treatment of olfactory dysfunction. Laryngoscope 2004;114(2):279–285
47. Kobal G, Hummel T, Sekinger B, Barz S, Roscher S, Wolf S. "Sniffin' sticks": screening of olfactory performance. Rhinology 1996; 34(4):222–226
48. Stanley P, MacWilliam L, Greenstone M, Mackay I, Cole P. Efficacy of a saccharin test for screening to detect abnormal mucociliary clearance. Br J Dis Chest 1984;78(1):62–65
49. Tamaoki J, Taira M, Nishimura K, Nakata J, Nagai A. Impairment of airway mucociliary transport in patients with sinobronchial syndrome: role of nitric oxide. J Aerosol Med 2000;13(3):239–244
50. Bommarito L, Guida G, Heffler E, et al. Nasal nitric oxide concentration in suspected chronic rhinosinusitis. Ann Allergy Asthma Immunol 2008;101(4):358–362
51. Panagou P, Loukides S, Tsipra S, Syrigou K, Anastasakis C, Kalogeropoulos N. Evaluation of nasal patency: comparison of patient and clinician assessments with rhinomanometry. Acta Otolaryngol 1998;118(6):847–851
52. Lane AP, Zweiman B, Lanza DC, et al. Acoustic rhinometry in the study of the acute nasal allergic response. Ann Otol Rhinol Laryngol 1996;105(10):811–818
53. Nathan RA, Eccles R, Howarth PH, Steinsvåg SK, Togias A. Objective monitoring of nasal patency and nasal physiology in rhinitis. J Allergy Clin Immunol 2005;115(3, Suppl 1) S442–S459
54. Frigas E, Loegering DA, Gleich GJ. Cytotoxic effects of the guinea pig eosinophil major basic protein on tracheal epithelium. Lab Invest 1980;42(1):35–43
55. Bachert C, Gevaert P, van Cauwenberge P. Staphylococcus aureus superantigens and airway disease. Curr Allergy Asthma Rep 2002;2(3):252–258
56. Seiberling KA, Conley DB, Tripathi A, et al. Superantigens and chronic rhinosinusitis: detection of staphylococcal exotoxins in nasal polyps. Laryngoscope 2005;115(9):1580–1585
57. Ferguson BJ, Stolz DB. Demonstration of biofilm in human bacterial chronic rhinosinusitis. Am J Rhinol 2005;19(5):452–457
58. Ramadan HH, Sanclement JA, Thomas JG. Chronic rhinosinusitis and biofilms. Otolaryngol Head Neck Surg 2005;132(3):414–417
59. Psaltis AJ, Ha KR, Beule AG, Tan LW, Wormald PJ. Confocal scanning laser microscopy evidence of biofilms in patients with chronic rhinosinusitis. Laryngoscope 2007;117(7):1302–1306
60. Pak MW, To KF, Leung SF, van Hasselt CA. In vivo diagnosis of nasopharyngeal carcinoma using contact rhinoscopy. Laryngoscope 2001;111(8):1453–1458
61. Folz BJ, Werner JA. Contact endoscopy of the nose in patients with Rendu-Osler-Weber syndrome. Auris Nasus Larynx 2007; 34(1):45–48

62. Romano FR, Voegels RL, Goto EY, Prado FA, Butugan O. Nasal contact endoscopy for the in vivo diagnosis of inverted schneiderian papilloma and unilateral inflammatory nasal polyps. Am J Rhinol 2007;21(2):137–144
63. Lai SY, Deffenderfer OF, Hanson W, Phillips MP, Thaler ER. Identification of upper respiratory bacterial pathogens with the electronic nose. Laryngoscope 2002;112(6):975–979
64. Thaler ER, Hanson CW. Use of an electronic nose to diagnose bacterial sinusitis. Am J Rhinol 2006;20(2):170–172
65. Thaler ER, Huang D, Giebeig L, et al. Use of an electronic nose for detection of biofilms. Am J Rhinol 2008;22(1):29–33
66. Chakrabarti A, Denning DW, Ferguson BJ, et al. Fungal rhinosinusitis: a categorization and definitional schema addressing current controversies. Laryngoscope 2009;119(9):1809–1818
67. deShazo RD, O'Brien M, Chapin K, Soto-Aguilar M, Gardner L, Swain R. A new classification and diagnostic criteria for invasive fungal sinusitis. Arch Otolaryngol Head Neck Surg 1997; 123(11):1181–1188

10 Sinonasal Manifestations of Systemic Disease

Shaun J. Kilty, Reza Alizadehfar, and Martin Desrosiers

The identification of a particular systemic illness affecting the sinonasal cavity can be difficult at times to demonstrate. Even when there is overt evidence of a systemic illness affecting this region, diagnostic serologic testing may not be supportive of our clinical impression (**Fig. 10.1**). Occasionally, even with clinical findings serology only becomes positive after following an individual over time. Given that these illnesses are systemic, complementary specialty medical services should be actively involved in the diagnosis and management of these illnesses because the therapies prescribed for treatment are often not customary to rhinologic practice.

Ciliopathy and Cystic Fibrosis

Primary Ciliary Dyskinesia

Primary ciliary dyskinesia (PCD) is a genetic disorder causing a systemic disease in which ciliary dysmotility results in chronic otosinonasal and pulmonary disease, infertility, and in some cases, laterality defects. PCD was previously referred to as immotile cilia syndrome. It is now recognized that "immotile cilia" is a misnomer, because the disease encompasses a wide variety of ciliary movement disorders; true immotility of cilia is much less common than motile but dyskinetic cilia. Kartagener syndrome (KS), a subset of PCD, consists of a triad of clinical findings due to cilia dysfunction—specifically, chronic sinusitis, bronchiectasis, and situs inversus totalis.

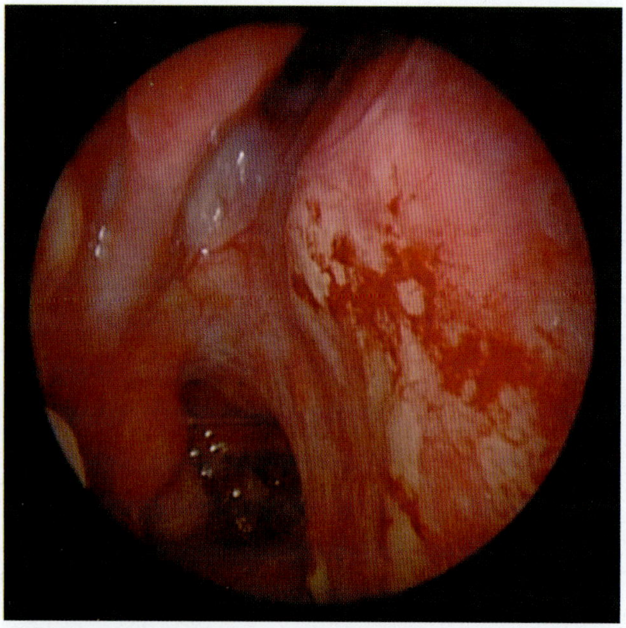

Fig. 10.1 Vasculitis-like lesions of the mucosa in a patient with a normal serologic profile.

Epidemiology

The incidence of PCD is 1 in 15,000 to 30,000 live births, which may be an underestimate of the incidence of the disease in the general population. There is no predilection for sex, nor is there a racial predisposition. PCD demonstrates an autosomal recessive mode of inheritance, although rare cases of autosomal dominant and X-linked inheritances have been reported.

Pathophysiology

For a complete review of cilia ultrastructure, function, and physiology, the reader is referred to Chapter 2. Given that ciliary motion occurs in the form of a wave, any disturbance of this wave can result in disease. In theory, a mutation of the gene encoding for any of the constituent proteins of a cilium could result in a wave disturbance, making identification of the causative mutation problematic. A genetic mutation identified in 10% of PCD patients is an insertion defect in the *DNAI1* gene. This mutation results in outer dynein arm defects and functional ciliary abnormalities.

Clinical Presentation

The initial presentation of individuals with PCD is usually due to conditions affecting the respiratory tract. The severity of the ciliary defect will usually dictate the age of presentation; most patients present after a period of prolonged, recurrent illness. Patients often have a history of recurrent pneumonia, otitis media, and chronic rhinosinusitis (CRS). Other diagnoses that must be excluded in the workup of patients with this condition include cystic fibrosis (CF), immunodeficiency, and secondary (acquired) ciliary dysfunction.

Diagnostic Workup

Given the pulmonary manifestations of this disease, it is important that these patients be evaluated in concert with a pulmonologist. Notably, a belated diagnosis of PCD is affiliated with a greater impairment of lung function, thus making an earlier diagnosis crucial. After a diagnosis has been made, consultation with a geneticist should be discussed with every patient given the inheritance pattern. Assessment of sinonasal disease in PCD is not that dissimilar from that done for any other patient. A thorough history, endoscopic evaluation, and computed tomography (CT) examination of the sinonasal airway should be performed. A chest X-ray may demonstrate dextrocardia in up to 50% of patients with PCD.

The saccharin test serves as a screening test for PCD. A small particle of saccharin is placed 1 cm from the anterior end of the inferior turbinate. The patient is instructed to not sniff, blow the nose, eat, or drink. If the patient tastes the sweetness of the saccharin after greater than 60 minutes, the saccharin test is considered abnormal and may reflect ciliary dysfunction.[1] Another potential screening test requiring more specialized equipment is the measurement of nitric oxide (NO), which typically yields low levels of exhaled NO in patients with PCD. Confirmatory testing for PCD requires cilia examination by light and electron microscopy to identify structural defects of the cilia. A sample can be obtained by tracheal biopsy or, alternatively, nasal brushing. Other analyses of this sample can include an assessment of the ciliary beat frequency and pattern using high-speed video photography and, lastly, measurement of the ciliary orientation. For cases that are difficult to diagnose due to damage from infection or inflammation, cell culture and regrowth of the ciliated respiratory epithelium is an option. Approximately 10% of initial tests are indefinite, but repeat brushing will provide a diagnosis in 50% of these patients. For adolescents and adult males, microscopic examination of the sperm to demonstrate anomalies of motility can be helpful.

Treatment

Due to the rarity of this disease, there are no evidence-based recommendations for the long-term management of these patients. However, current recommendations, largely based on clinical experience with CF, suggest that infections of the upper and lower respiratory tract should be treated aggressively. Patients should undergo routine monitoring of respiratory function, and should also participate in airway clearance activities either with a physiotherapist or via regular physical activity.

Management of chronic rhinorrhea is generally with saline irrigation, and topical steroids may be tried in an effort to control mucosal inflammation. If recurrent acute or chronic sinusitis occurs, endoscopic sinus surgery (ESS) may be an option to reestablish ventilation and to allow for the irrigation of the operated paranasal sinuses. The placement of ventilation tubes for otitis media with effusion (OME) may result in chronic otorrhea without a significant hearing benefit.

Outcome

When PCD is identified early and appropriate treatments are implemented, life expectancy is not felt to be altered. Once a thorough pulmonary treatment is implemented, lung function should stabilize, as treatments are generally more successful than with CF. In the upper respiratory tract, the longitudinal study of children with PCD has demonstrated that OME usually spontaneously resolves by 13 years of age.

Cystic Fibrosis

CF is a genetically inherited autosomal recessive disease of the cystic fibrosis transmembrane regulator (*CFTR*) gene located at the q31.2 locus of chromosome 7, first discovered at the Hospital for Sick Children in Toronto, Canada. This gene is responsible for a protein involved in chloride transport, which has widespread clinical implications, most importantly in the respiratory and gastrointestinal systems.

Epidemiology

CF occurs in 1:3300 live births among the Caucasian population. This disease occurs predominantly in Caucasians of European descent and in Ashkenazi Jews. Given that the inheritance is autosomal recessive, there is no sex predilection. Of the over 1400 identified mutations, 70% of cases worldwide and 90% of cases in the United States occur due to the ΔF508 mutation, which results in the loss of the amino acid phenylalanine at the 508 position of this protein.

Pathophysiology

The *CFTR* gene codes for a transmembrane chloride channel that is anchored to the outer membrane of cells of all affected organs. This protein normally regulates the passage of chloride out of the cell; however, in the mutant form, chloride cannot pass out of the cell and, as a result, positively charged ions such as sodium are not able to enter the cell. The net result is thickened secretions, which block the lumen of exocrine glands, resulting in end-organ damage. In the lung, this leads to remodeling and chronic infection; in the pancreas, duct obstruction and autodigestion occur; and there is impaired intestinal function of the bowel.

Clinical Presentation

Because this disease primarily affects the respiratory and digestive systems, signs of CF may be present as early as birth. Initial signs include meconium ileus, failure to thrive, and recurrent pneumonia. In childhood, recurrent ear and sinus infections, poor growth, and diarrhea predominate. Male infertility is due to the congenital absence of the vas deferens. Recurrent sinusitis or nasal polyposis may be the initial presenting sign in childhood. CT often demonstrates hypoplasia of the paranasal sinuses and mucosal thickening

(**Figs. 10.2 and 10.3**); however, CT may also demonstrate bilateral maxillary sinus involvement with bulging of the medial wall sufficient to narrow the nasal passages. A presentation of recurrent sinusitis and/or nasal polyposis in childhood should prompt an investigation for CF, PCD, or possible immune deficiency. Early diagnosis of CF will allow for the institution of aggressive treatment, which has been demonstrated to improve outcomes.

Diagnostic Workup

Postnatal diagnosis of CF may be made using the sweat chloride test, with two positive chloride levels on two separate tests being diagnostic for CF. However, given that milder variants of CF do exist, borderline test results may warrant further testing to diagnose CF. Chloride values greater than 60 mEq/L are positive, whereas values between 40 to 60 mEq/L are borderline. Genetic testing can be used to verify these results and to identify the common genetic mutations.

Treatment

The treatment of patients with CF requires a multidisciplinary team given the multisystem nature of this disease. Although there is variability in the severity of this illness, many patients require intensive medical therapy for both the preventative and therapeutic measures that are employed in the treatment of the various manifestations of this disease.

Given that many individuals have CRS, often with polyps, ESS may be indicated. However, some CF patients have very few symptoms, and function rather well from a sinonasal perspective. Thus, the mere presence of nasal polyposis is not an indication for surgical management. For those patients with significant symptoms, ESS is typically well tolerated and can often be performed on an outpatient basis. Postoperatively, these patients can expect clinical improvements but may be particularly prone to the formation of mucoceles, which can occur in all paranasal sinus locations in this population.

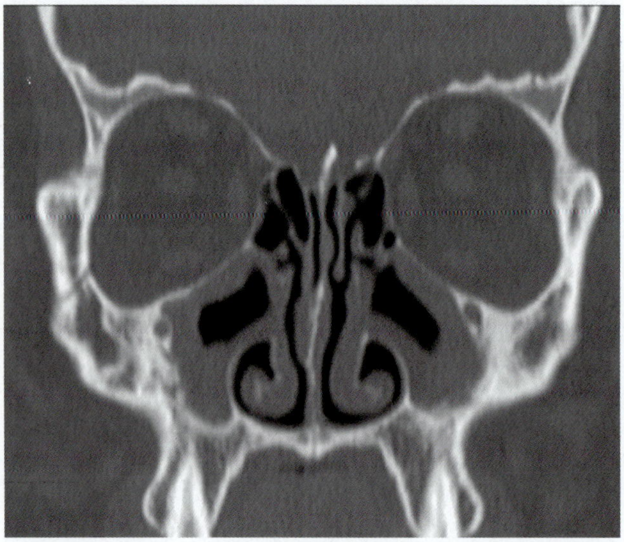

Fig. 10.2 Maxillary sinus hypoplasia and mucosal thickening typical of cystic fibrosis.

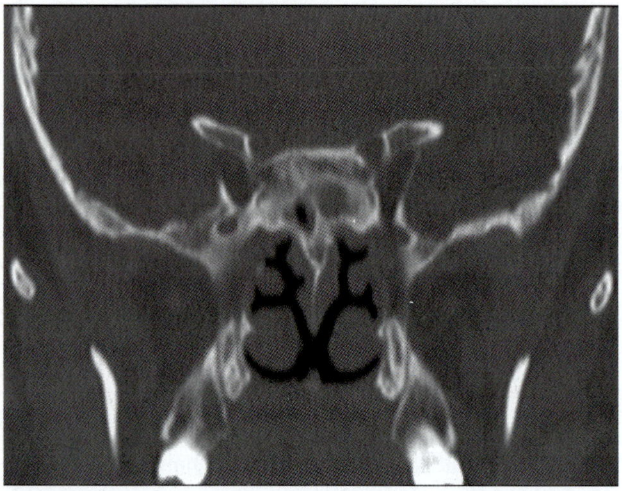

Fig. 10.3 Sphenoid sinus hypoplasia typical of cystic fibrosis.

In choosing an antimicrobial for the treatment of a sinus infection, one would surmise that whatever organism that was most recently cultured from the lung during bronchoalveolar lavage (BAL) is likely that which is causing the bacterial sinusitis. However, this may not be true. In children, the BAL has been shown to have a positive predictive value (PPV) of only 65 to 75% depending on the organism. Similarly, although *Pseudomonas aeruginosa* is commonly recovered in CF, *Staphylococcus aureus* and *Haemophilus influenzae* are also important causes of bacterial sinusitis in children with CF.[2]

Finally, patients with CF who are being considered as candidates for lung transplantation are often referred for preoperative assessment of the need for ESS preceding transplantation. The reasoning is that pretreatment of the sinuses will prevent colonization of the lung transplant and will therefore prolong the recipient's use of the lung. However, no prospective study has evaluated this theory and the available evidence does not suggest that ESS prior to a lung transplantation has a proven benefit.[3] However, the presence of complications such as a mucocele should be considered for surgical correction pretransplantation, given that the leading cause of morbidity posttransplant is pulmonary bacterial and opportunistic infections.[4]

Noninfectious Granulomatous Disease

Wegener Granulomatosis

Wegener granulomatosis (WG) is a systemic illness that usually affects the upper and lower respiratory tract as well as the renal system. It is named for the German pathologist Friedreich Wegener who, in 1936, was the first to describe the disease using specific clinical and histopathological criteria.

Epidemiology

WG occurs infrequently, with an incidence of ~10 cases per million population per year. Diagnosis typically occurs during the fourth and fifth decades of life, but WG does occur in the pediatric age group. Up to 90% of patients are Caucasian and predominantly male, at a ratio of 2:1. The 1-year mortality of untreated WG is 18 to 20%, and is mostly related to renal disease.

Pathophysiology

WG is an idiopathic, possibly autoimmune, systemic illness that initially begins as a granulomatous disease of the respiratory tract prior to becoming a systemic small-to-medium vessel vasculitis. This transition is accompanied by the development of proteinase 3-specific antineutrophil cytoplasmic autoantibodies (PR3-ANCA), which are responsible for the autoimmune vasculitis.[5] The inciting event for this intolerance of PR3 remains to be determined. The PR3-ANCA systemic vasculitis produces inflammatory lesions of the affected organs, which promotes the self-perpetuating pathology of inflammation and PR3 autoimmunity.

Clinical Presentation

The majority of patients (up to 90%) with WG will present with otorhinolaryngologic symptoms. However, patients often have chronic, nonspecific constitutional symptoms such as fatigue, fever, malaise, arthralgias, and weight loss. Specific to rhinology practice, 85% of patients will present with symptoms of CRS and a lesser percentage will present with rhinitis. Characteristically, these are resistant to standard medical treatment. Sinonasal manifestations include septal perforation, which, if neglected, can result in the classic saddle-nose deformity. More commonly, patients will report nasal obstruction, mucosal crusting, a purulent nasal discharge, or recurrent epistaxis (**Figs. 10.4 and 10.5**). Other sites of head and neck involvement include the middle ear (serous effusion) and the larynx (subglottic stenosis). In limited form WG, the patient may have only head and neck manifestations with normal pulmonary and renal examinations. In classic multisystem WG, pulmonary manifestations include dyspnea, cough, and hemoptysis. Renal manifestations include hematuria and oliguria. Peripheral and central nervous symptoms may occur secondary to vasculitis; cranial nerve palsy is a rare presenting finding. Ophthalmologic manifestations include episcleritis and lacrimal obstruction. Less commonly, various cutaneous eruptions or ulcerations may be seen.

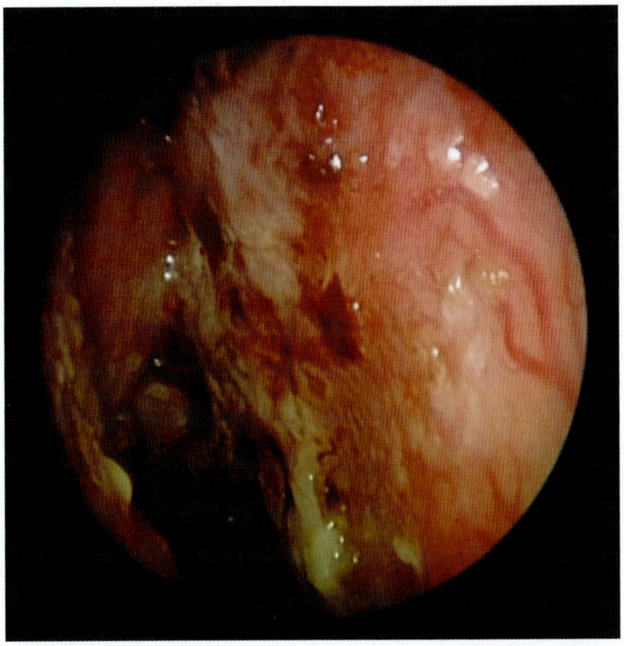

Fig. 10.4 The fragile and crusted mucosa of the nasal septum in Wegener granulomatosis.

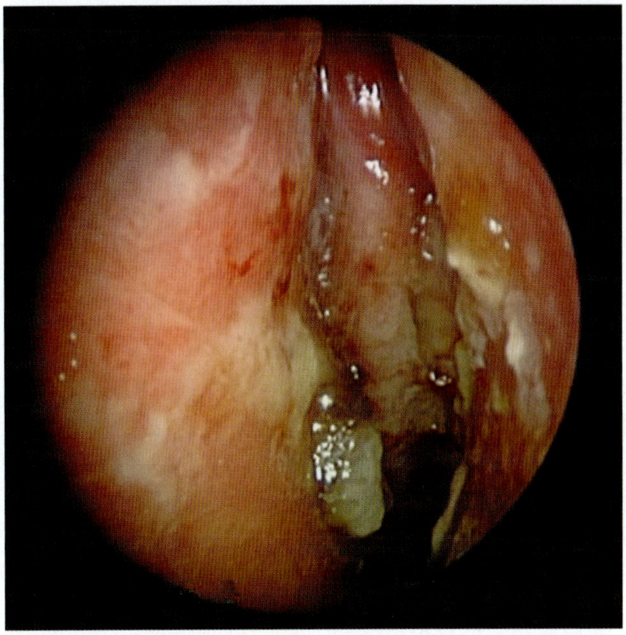

Fig. 10.5 Crusting of the middle turbinate and lateral nasal wall in Wegener granulomatosis.

Diagnostic Workup

It is essential that the evaluation of these patients be performed in concert with a rheumatologist given the systemic nature of this disease and the therapies used in its treatment. In 1990, the American College of Rheumatology published criteria for WG, with two or more positive criteria having a sensitivity of 88.2% and a specificity of 92.0% (**Table 10.1**).[6]

Table 10.1 Diagnostic Criteria for Wegener Granulomatosis

Criterion	Finding
Oral or nasal inflammation	Oral ulcers or purulent rhinorrhea or epistaxis
Abnormal chest X-ray	Nodules, cavities, or fixed infiltrates
Urinary sediment	>5 RBC/hpf or red cell casts
Biopsy with granulomatous inflammation	Perivascular granulomatous inflammation

Abbreviations: RBC, red blood cell; hpf, high power field.

Laboratory evaluation should include a PR3(c)-ANCA, as this is specific for WG and positive in up to 95% of active cases. A p-ANCA may be positive in up to 25% of active cases. A complete blood count (CBC) may demonstrate anemia and leukocytosis. An erythrocyte sedimentation rate (ESR) may be elevated, as may the rheumatoid factor (RF). Elevated blood urea nitrogen (BUN) and creatinine or creatinine clearance (CrCl) levels indicate possible renal involvement. In such a case, urinalysis will reveal hematuria, casts, and albumin. Sinus mucosal biopsy can be used for a pathologic confirmation of WG disease. However, negative results may be misleading because the diagnostic yield is generally low for the nasal mucosa (20%) and only somewhat better for the paranasal sinuses (55%).

Imaging with a CT scan often reveals nonspecific findings such as sinonasal mucosal thickening with or without sinus opacification, bone erosion (especially septal), sclerosing osteitis, and neo-osteogenesis.[7] Advanced WG often demonstrates nasal septal destruction with concurrent destruction of the inferior and middle turbinate, lamina papyracea, medial maxillary wall, and cribriform plate. Magnetic resonance imaging (MRI) reveals nonspecific mucosal thickening and T2 hyperintensity of the mucosa early in the disease. Advanced disease will demonstrate hypointensity on both T1 and T2 sequences, with variable enhancement. This represents the submucosal accumulation of collagen, which occurs with granuloma formation.[8]

Treatment

Treatment is chosen according to the severity and systemic effects of the disease. The goals of treatment are to induce a rapid remission using high drug doses followed by tapering the dose or switching to alternate, less toxic maintenance drug therapy in an effort to prevent a relapse.[9] For localized disease affecting only the upper or lower respiratory tract without constitutional symptoms, treatment with oral prednisone or with trimethoprim/sulfamethoxazole (TMP/SMX) may be adequate. The treatment of systemic or localized disease with constitutional symptoms necessitates the addition of chemotherapies such as cyclophosphamide (CYC) for severe disease or methotrexate (MTX) for nonsevere disease in combination with steroids. Patients with a severe renal disease or an imminently life-threatening disease may respond to the addition of plasmapheresis. Recent evidence has demonstrated improved relapse prevention when using leflunomide (LEF) or azathioprine.[10]

Because up to 50% of patients will have a relapse of vasculitis, reinvestigation of the patient at that time is essential because the relapse may be secondary to the adverse effects of the treatment agent, or it may suggest an alternate diagnosis. Colonization of the upper respiratory tract by *S. aureus* has been shown to increase the risk of relapse. Long-term treatment with TMP/SMX, when added to conventional immunosuppressive therapy, has been shown to decrease the risk of relapse in the respiratory tract. Similarly, concomitant treatment with TMP/SMX for patients undergoing immunosuppressive therapy is useful for prophylaxis against *Pneumocystis jiroveci* pneumonia.[9]

In the treatment of sinonasal manifestations of WG, medical therapy predominates as a treatment modality. Management of crusting with saline irrigation and nasal lubricants is most important. Antibiotic treatment of infectious sinusitis should be prescribed using culture-guided therapy. Endoscopic sinus surgery is not suggested to be a useful therapeutic modality in the setting of active vasculitic disease unless it is being used for the treatment of an infectious complication of sinusitis. However, ESS may be useful for the management of WG-related sinusitis where there has been remission of active vasculitis. Reconstructive surgery for severe nasal deformities may only be considered after remission of active vasculitis.

Complications

Given the high incidence of subglottic stenosis associated with WG, CT evaluation of the larynx should be obtained prior to general anesthesia to avoid a difficult airway situation during intubation or following extubation.

Sarcoidosis

Sarcoidosis is an idiopathic systemic granulomatous disease that most frequently involves the lower respiratory tract (90%), with involvement of the upper respiratory tract occurring in 1 to 6% of patients.[11] Sinus involvement by sarcoidosis is less common than nasal cavity involvement, although there may be secondary obstruction of sinus drainage pathways from nasal sarcoidosis.

Epidemiology

Sarcoidosis occurs with a prevalence range of 1 to 40 per 100,000 persons. Worldwide, it is most prevalent and more severe in the Scandinavian countries, but in North America, it is more commonly found in individuals of African descent than in Caucasians, with notably higher morbidity and mortality rates. The greatest incidence of sarcoidosis is in individuals less than 50 years of age, with the peak occurrence in the 20 to 40 years of age range, with a slight female preponderance.

Pathophysiology

Sarcoidosis is best characterized by the formation of noncaseating granulomas. The inciting event for their formation remains elusive but it is believed that there is an interaction involving a host's genetic susceptibility with environmental exposure. Immune abnormalities in affected patients have been noted, and it is theorized that immune dysregulation due to a persistent antigen of low virulence (environmental or autoimmune) results in a chronic T-helper cell, Th1 subtype, response. These cells then secrete interleukin (IL)-2 and interferon (IFN)-gamma, stimulating macrophage tumor necrosis factor (TNF-alpha) production and augmenting the local cellular immune response, which predisposes to granuloma formation.[12] After prolonged inflammation, fibrosis occurs due to a Th2 T-cell response, thereby stimulating fibroblast proliferation and collagen production, causing end-organ dysfunction or failure. In those patients with sinonasal sarcoidosis (SNS), symptoms are believed to represent a loss or impairment of ciliated respiratory mucosal function as a result of the granulomatous infiltration.

Clinical Presentation

This is extremely variable given the systemic nature of this illness. Patients tend to present in winter or spring, suggesting a possible environmental trigger. Up to one third of patients will have constitutional symptoms of fever, fatigue, and weight loss, and a similar number of patients present with palpable nontender lymphadenopathy. Half of patients will have lower respiratory tract symptoms, including dyspnea, chest pain, or a chronic nonproductive cough. Anterior uveitis can occur; when present with parotid hypertrophy and fever, uveoparotid fever is diagnosed. Myocardial involvement occurs in ~5% of patients and central nervous system involvement (neurosarcoidosis) in up to 10%, where facial nerve palsy is the most common finding. Cutaneous involvement can be present in 25% of patients but is rarely noted as an isolated finding. Lupus pernio is the most notable head and neck sarcoidal skin lesion and is associated with granulomatous involvement of the lower and upper respiratory tract in 75 and 50% of cases, respectively.

The most common sinonasal complaints usually consist of nasal obstruction, anosmia, rhinorrhea, and crusting. Typical nasal findings include mucosal hypertrophy with an irregular surface characterized by a purple-red coloration of the mucosa with pale yellow nodules typically located on the nasal septum and inferior turbinates (**Fig. 10.6**).[11] The appearance of these mucosal changes can help to differentiate SNS from the other granulomatous diseases, including WG, tuberculosis, syphilis, and berylliosis.

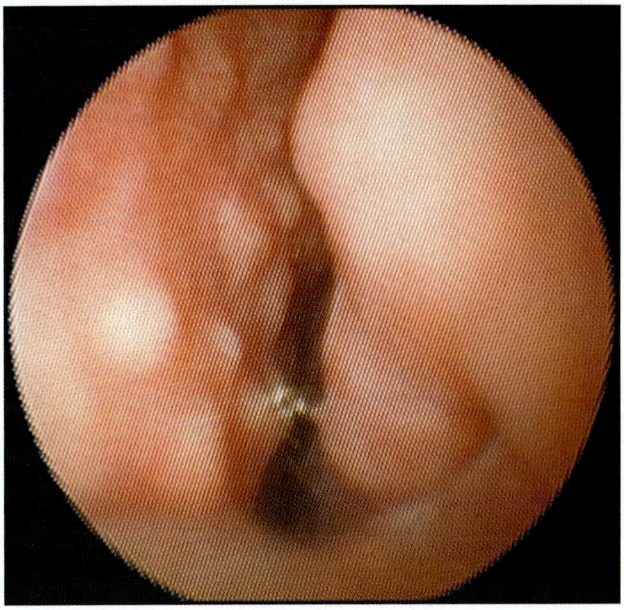

Fig. 10.6 Nodular left nasal septal mucosa typical of sarcoidosis.

However, appearance may vary and may only be evident on biopsy. Further differentiation between these diagnoses is only possible with mucosal biopsy results and radiographic findings, as well as laboratory evaluations. Sinonasal involvement may be an indicator of severe systemic disease.

Diagnostic Workup

It is less of a challenge to identify patients already diagnosed with sarcoidosis who present with sinonasal manifestations of the disease than those presenting with unusual rhinitis of unknown origin where symptoms may mimic those of severe CRS. The diagnosis of sarcoidosis is founded on clinical and radiologic evidence that is supported by histologic findings. Specific radiologic findings in sarcoidosis include hilar adenopathy, pulmonary infiltrates, or fibrosis on chest X-ray.[13] Sinus CT characteristically can show lytic lesions of the septum and inferior turbinates, although mucosal hypertrophy and sinus opacification of the anterior ethmoid and maxillary sinuses are typically present. ^{18}F-fluorodeoxyglucose positron emission tomography (^{18}FDG-PET) may be helpful in assessing the extent of organ involvement and in identifying regions that could be biopsied.

Laboratory evaluation is of limited usefulness in diagnosis as there is no specific test for sarcoidosis, but it may help to identify involved organ systems. Tests of liver and renal function, CBC looking for anemia and thrombocytopenia, and electrolytes must be measured. Patients typically are hypercalcemic. A serum angiotensin converting enzyme (ACE) level is elevated in at least 50% of patients, but it lacks adequate sensitivity and specificity to be a diagnostic test. In SNS with systemic involvement, nearly 75% of patients can be expected to have an elevated ACE, whereas in patients with isolated SNS, only 25% may have an elevation of this enzyme.[11] A biopsy of nasal mucosa or another affected tissue can detect noncaseating granulomas, which differentiate sarcoidosis from other granulomatous diseases. Langhans cells with asteroid bodies or lamellar (Schaumann bodies) inclusions may be present, but are not unique to sarcoidosis. A gallium-67 scan is a nonspecific test that can demonstrate an increased uptake in the salivary glands, the nasopharynx, and the lacrimal glands, thus producing a "panda" sign. The Kveim-Siltzbach test, now not commonly used, involves injecting homogenates of sarcoid spleen or lymph node tissue intradermally and then biopsying this area in 4 to 6 weeks looking pathologically for characteristic granuloma formation. Given the multisystem involvement characteristic of this disease, patients need an assessment and treatment by multiple medical specialists with pulmonologists and rheumatologists assuming a central role given the usual pulmonary implications and systemic therapies that can be required.

Treatment

Attempts at management of SNS symptoms with nasal saline irrigation and topical steroids are generally unsatisfactory. Irrigation or nebulization with topical steroid solutions may improve responses. Patients may nevertheless require oral therapy—typically a prolonged course of oral corticosteroids—to manage their sinonasal and systemic disease manifestations.[11]

Therapy for systemic involvement is initiated when there is evidence or the possibility of impending organ dysfunction. Again, therapy typically consists of systemic corticosteroids, although the use of combined therapy is common. The addition of methotrexate allows for lower doses of corticosteroids, to be used. Hydroxychloroquine can be used as a combined therapy in the setting of hypercalcemia and dermatologic and/or neurologic involvement, whereas nonsteroidal anti-inflammatory drugs (NSAIDs) and thalidomide have also been employed for dermatologic manifestations. The need for ESS is limited in these patients. In one series, only 7% of patients required ESS to remove granulomatous disease-causing sinus ostial obstruction, thereby improving the ventilation of the affected sinuses.[14] If ESS has been performed for diagnostic purposes, this may improve access of irrigation solutions to the affected areas and improve response.

Outcomes

The evolution for each patient with sarcoidosis is tremendously variable as there are limited acute forms and chronic debilitating forms of the disease. Up to 50% of patients with sarcoidosis enter a remission within 3 years of diagnosis, and two thirds of patients by 10 years. Less than 5% of patients suffer from a recurrence after a 1-year remission. However, a third of patients will have an unrelenting and progressive form of disease that will result in end-organ impairment. The mortality rate from sarcoidosis, ~6%, is mainly due to pulmonary fibrosis or cardiac or neurologic involvement.

Churg-Strauss Syndrome

Churg-Strauss syndrome (CSS) is a systemic necrotizing vasculitic disorder of small blood vessels presumed to be of an autoimmune origin. It is characterized by asthma, nasal polyposis, hypereosinophilia, and vascular or extravascular necrotizing granulomas.[15]

Epidemiology

This disease is rare, and it occurs with an incidence of 1 to 3 cases per 100,000 adults per year. The age at diagnosis is 50 years, with a sex ratio of 1:1.[16]

Pathophysiology

The pathogenesis of CSS is, in effect, due to the prolonged survival of eosinophils and the release of their cytotoxic enzymes, which cause direct tissue injury. Their survival may be related to alterations in the tumor necrosis factor-related apoptosis (TRAIL) receptor 3 expression of eosinophils.[17]

Clinical Presentation

The syndrome can be divided into three phases of disease, although the progression through each stage for a given patient is variable. The first, or prodromal, phase is characterized by asthma and sinonasal (allergic) manifestations; phase two is characterized by the eosinophilic infiltration of various tissues; and patients in the third, or systemic, phase demonstrate necrotizing vasculitis of the integumentary, peripheral neurologic, and renal systems usually within 4 years of the development of asthma.[16]

Patients with CSS often present with the systemic symptoms of fever and weight loss, but the pulmonary manifestations, particularly asthma, are the most common presentation for this disease. The respiratory symptoms usually precede the onset of other symptoms, and their severity is variable. However, up to 60% of patients will have sinonasal complaints at the time of their asthma diagnosis.[18] Up to 70% of patients will be diagnosed with nasal polyposis or allergic rhinitis, and relatively few present with chronic rhinosinusitis without polyps.[16,18] Other common presenting manifestations include peripheral neuropathy and skin lesions—particularly, palpable purpura of the lower extremities.

Diagnostic Workup

The diagnosis of CSS is made by identifying at least four out of six criteria published by the American College of Rheumatology.[19] These criteria include asthma, serum eosinophilia >10%, mono- or polyneuropathy, pulmonary infiltrates (nonfixed), a paranasal sinus abnormality, and extravascular eosinophils. Identifying at least four criteria provides a diagnostic sensitivity of 85% and a specificity of 99.7%. However, even with these criteria, CSS can be difficult to diagnose because there is usually a temporal development of symptomatology; hence, at the initial presentation, a patient may not present with an adequate disease spectrum for the diagnosis of this debilitating disease. Other factors that may impede a clinical diagnosis include the intermittent treatment of a patient's asthma with immunosuppressant medications such as prednisone. These treatments may mask the other symptoms of the disease and may impede their clinical declaration. This makes repeated examinations and the further investigation of these patients, for which there is a clinical suspicion of this disorder, extremely important. Notable findings on serologic investigations include marked peripheral eosinophilia and, usually, an elevated immunoglobulin E (IgE). An elevated IgG is usually also found as is a positive cytoplasmic antineutrophil cytoplasmic antibodies (c-ANCA) in up to 50% of patients.[16] Tests for ESR, rheumatoid factor, and C-reactive protein (CRP) are usually positive. The importance of renal function tests and a thorough systemic investigation coordinated by a rheumatologist cannot be overemphasized. The majority of patients will have chest X-rays that demonstrate patchy lung infiltrates.

Treatment

The treatment of CSS is based on the use of high-dose corticosteroids, but other immunosuppressant therapy may be used when poor prognostic indicators are present.[20] Initially, prednisone may be administered for up to 6 months prior to being tapered to a lower dose. Even once CSS is in remission, it is common for asthma to persist and necessitate inhaled or oral corticosteroid therapy.[21] Relapses of disease are common and often necessitate the addition of another immunosuppressant, such as cyclophosphamide.

The treatment of sinonasal disease cannot occur in isolation of the other systemic manifestations. Once the diagnosis of CSS is made, a response to systemic therapy is anticipated. To avoid a rapid recurrence, embarking on surgical treatments for sinonasal complaints when the overall disease is uncontrolled is not recommended, unless there are acute complications of sinusitis. Once CSS is in remission, nasal polyposis can be treated with endoscopic surgical techniques if required, although no studies have specifically addressed the role of surgical treatment or topical medical treatments for the sinonasal manifestations of this disease.

Outcomes

Importantly, CSS is a multisystem disease often causing gastrointestinal tract symptoms, renal disease (focal segmental glomerulonephritis), and cardiac disease. The main cause of death for these patients is uncontrolled vasculitis, the majority of which is due to cardiac involvement, making an early referral of suspected cases to a rheumatologist imperative.[16]

Immune Deficiency

Primary Immune Deficiency

Primary immune deficiencies (PID) are a group of inherited disorders characterized by either a dysfunctional or a nonfunctional segment of the immune system. In contrast, secondary immune deficiencies are due to external influences on the immune system, which lead to its compromise—for example, the effects of chemotherapy agents or viral illnesses such as HIV.

Epidemiology

The incidence of PID is highly variable as there are over 150 different primary immune deficiencies that have been recognized by the World Health Organization (WHO). PID has an estimated prevalence of 1:10,000, which may be an underestimate given the occurrence of asymptomatic individuals with deficiencies such as selective immunoglobulin A deficiency (SID) and its prevalence of ~1:500 persons.

Pathophysiology

This is directly related to the underlying disorder of the immune system. Some of the most commonly encountered PIDs are discussed as they relate to disease (**Table 10.2**). Many of the organisms that are involved in infections of patients with a given immunodeficiency reflect the underlying immune deficiency.[22] These defects may involve the humoral (B lymphocytes), cellular (T lymphocytes), phagocytic, or the complement arm of the immune system.

Clinical Presentation

Commonly, untreated PID presents as recurrent, potentially life-threatening infections and debilitating illnesses. Patients with common variable immune deficiency (CVID) typically present with recurrent infections of both the upper and lower respiratory tract. By comparison, the clinical course for patients with SID is quite variable with most being asymptomatic or having only mild illnesses, whereas others may suffer from severe recurrent or chronic

Table 10.2 Characteristics of Select Primary Immune Deficiencies

Immune Deficiency (Impairment)	Clinical Manifestations	Infective Agents	Screening Tests
CVID (IgG, IgA, ± IgM)	Recurrent infections	Encapsulated organisms	Ig levels; B-cell phenotype by flow cytometry; vaccine Ig response (tetanus, polio, pneumococcus)
Selective IgA (IgA±IgG2 and/ or IgG4)	Recurrent RTI; chronic diarrhea; 25% AID	Encapsulated organisms	A/A; AID, CBC, renal and thyroid function tests; allergy
Combined (T- and B-cell defect)	Recurrent viral, fungal, bacterial, OI	Fungi, viruses, OI agents, bacteria, mycobacteria	B-cell workup; T-cell number by flow cytometry; anergy screen (PPD, etc.); T-cell proliferation to mitogens
HIES (humoral or phagocytic defect)	Skin abscesses; RTI; scoliosis and fractures; pneumatoceles	*S. aureus*; *Candida* species	Mainly a clinical diagnosis; IgE >2,000 IU/mL; CBC with differential (hypereosinophilia)
Phagocytic cell (neutrophils)	Neutropenia; chronic granulomatous disease	*S. aureus*, GNB, *Aspergillus*, *Nocardia*	CBC with differential; 1,2,3-dihydrorhodamine; adhesion molecule expression by flow cytometry
Complement *Early* (C2, C4, C3) *Late* (C5-C9)	CVD or similar to B-cell deficiency; neisserial infections	Encapsulated organisms NM or *N. gonorrheae*	Total hemolytic complement (CH_{50}); AH50; mannose binding lectin, C3,C4; other selected levels

Abbreviations: A/A, as above; AID, autoimmune disease; CBC, complete blood count; CVD, collagen vascular disease; encapsulated organisms, *S. pneumoniae*, *H. influenzae*, *M, catarrhalis*, *Giardia*, *Campylobacter*; GNB, Gram-negative bacteria; HIES, hyper-IgE syndrome; Ig, immunoglobulin; NM, *Neisseria meningitides*; OI, opportunistic infections; RTI, respiratory tract infections.

infections (**Fig. 10.7**). Allergy is also common in these individuals, occurring in 10 to 15% of these patients, as is asthma, often of a severe form. Patients with a specific antibody deficiency also present with recurrent infections of the upper and lower respiratory tract, typically starting as early as 2 years of age.

Diagnostic Workup

The diagnostic assessment of individuals with primary immune B cell deficiency is nearly identical regardless of the underlying deficiency. Patients with refractory sinusitis should be assessed for PID as the literature has shown that a significant percentage of these individuals may have an undiagnosed immune deficiency.[23] Assessment in conjunction with an immunologist is helpful not only in making the initial diagnosis, but also for implementing long-term therapy for individuals with recurrent or severe infections.

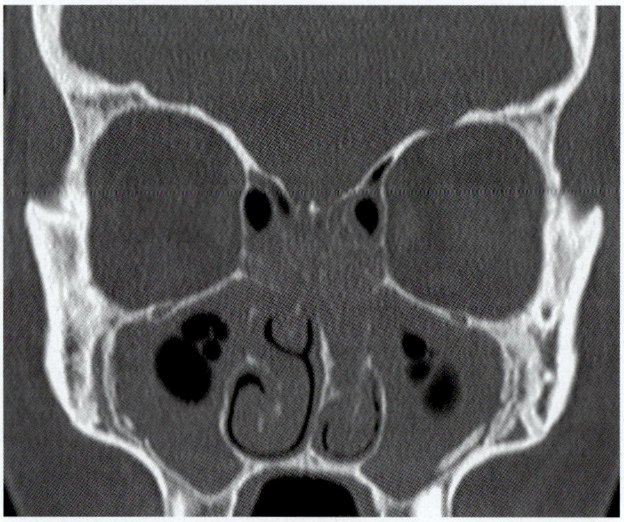

Fig. 10.7 Coronal computed tomography scan demonstrating pansinusitis in a patient with IgA and IgG2 deficiency.

Treatment

The treatment of B-cell PID typically consists of intravenous immunoglobulin (IVIG), which brings about significant improvement unless there is an associated T-lymphocyte defect or an end-organ injury. Serial administration of IVIG is typically required for best clinical effect. Chronic sinus disease is often managed with antibiotic therapy and ESS as required. ESS can improve sinus ventilation and access to the sinus cavities for regular irrigation and topical steroid application as part of maintenance therapy. Culture directed antibiotic therapy for rhinosinusitis should be used for these individuals, as they often receive prophylactic antibiotics and/or numerous antibiotic treatment courses.

Outcome

In general, clinical outcomes vary with the type of deficiency, the delay in patient diagnosis, and the degree of end-organ injury prior to the initiation of therapy. A health status can be sustained once appropriate therapy (IVIG, antibiotics, etc.) is begun. However, given the wide variability of the clinical severity of disease involved in these different immune defects, it is difficult to predict an outcome for any particular patient. The outcome for these patients may be more related to the associated autoimmune and neoplastic complications that accompany the deficiency.

Secondary Immune Deficiency: HIV

The early North American epidemic for HIV/AIDS of the 1980s occurred not only in individuals who engaged in male-to-male sexual contact (MMS), but also in those who were injection drug users (IDU). Although the epidemic continues to affect IDU and MMS groups, there is now a greater representation of women and racial minority groups.

Epidemiology

By the end of 2003, just over 1 million people in the United States were living with HIV/AIDS and an estimated 25% of these cases were unaware of their infection. Currently, the three most common methods for HIV transmission are MMS (44%), heterosexual contact (34%), and IDU (17%).

Pathophysiology

The HIV retrovirus has two viral envelope glycoproteins, gp41 and gp120, which are responsible for binding to the CD4 molecule on the surface of T-helper lymphocytes and other cells of a monocyte/macrophage lineage. After binding, there is membrane fusion and resultant infection with the HIV nucleoprotein complex that enters the host cell cytoplasm. The RNA genome then replicates via reverse transcription and undergoes nuclear localization and uncoating. Within the nucleus, the double-stranded DNA is integrated with the host's DNA, transcribed, spliced, and the RNA is exported to the cytoplasm. Here it undergoes translation, modification, and assembly budding prior to its maturation to infect other cells.

Clinical Presentation

There is a strong correlation between the occurrence of infection and the CD4 lymphocyte count. As such, there are three categories of CD4 count. A CD4 count greater than 500 cells/mm^3, category one, is usually not associated with opportunistic infections (OI). In category two, a CD4 count between 200 and 500 cells/mm^3 can be associated with oral candidiasis, bacterial pneumonia, tuberculosis, and non-Hodgkin lymphoma (NHL). *Pneumocystis* pneumonia, fungal esophagitis, and cryptococcal meningitis typically occur in category three, when the CD4 count is less than 200 cells/mm^3, and disseminated fungal, mycobacterial, and cytomegalovirus (CMV) infections typically occur with CD4 counts below 50 cells/mm^3.[24]

Patients with HIV often suffer from rhinitis with or without episodes of recurrent acute or chronic rhinosinusitis. In fact, up to 20 to 60% of individuals will have chronic sinus disease during the course of their illness. Clinically, there is often an elevated serum IgE level, which is sometimes accompanied with eosinophilia and is most commonly seen in individuals with a category two or three CD4 count. The predisposition to sinusitis is likely multifactorial and is related both to HIV infection, its cellular and resultant humoral immune dysfunction, mucociliary clearance abnormalities, as well as possible substance abuse such as cocaine in some individuals. However, HIV patients with category one and two CD4 counts can be expected to have typical infectious organisms for their illness given the relatively normal function of their immune system. These include *Staphylococcus* and *Streptococcus* species, as well as *H. influenzae*. Patients with category three CD4 counts more commonly have OI, and sampling of the infectious agent from the involved sinus(es) is suggested to provide targeted therapy. Possible infectious agents to consider include viruses (CMV, herpes simplex, varicella zoster), fungi (*Candida*, *Pneumocystis*, *Cryptococcus*, and *Rhizopus* species), atypical aerobic and anaerobic bacteria, and mycobacteria. In addition to their predisposition for infectious agents, these patients are also at an increased risk for autoimmune and neoplastic complications.

Diagnostic Workup

Following HIV transmission, seroconversion can typically be detected by 6 to 12 weeks (95% of individuals seroconvert by 6 months). HIV positivity is determined by the detection of antibodies using enzyme-linked immunosorbent assay (ELISA) testing and confirmed by Western blot. There is also a rapid RNA of p24 antigen test available for recently exposed individuals. The HIV viral load is measured using the polymerase chain reaction (PCR) because this information is used to monitor the status of the disease, to guide therapy, and for prognostication.

The investigation of patients presenting with sinusitis and HIV should include imaging studies such as CT to document the extent of sinusitis and to rule out the possibility of either invasive infectious disease or neoplasia. If there is evidence of extrasinus extension of disease, MRI should be employed to guide further clinical management. Treatment of bacterial sinusitis in the presence of a category three CD4 count or in the event of an OI occurring in the paranasal sinuses should be culture-directed, given the possibility of atypical organisms in at least a third of these patients. Consultation with an infectious disease specialist should also be considered. A biopsy of tissue from an affected sinus should also be considered to rule out neoplasms such as NHL or Kaposi sarcoma, or to rule out invasive fungal disease. These entities may initially masquerade as bacterial sinusitis, ultimately being nonresponsive to conventional antibiotic therapy.

Treatment

Antibiotic treatment for category three CD4 count HIV (AIDS) patients should be prolonged up to 3 weeks for acute infection and 6 weeks for CRS. Antimicrobial therapy should be culture-directed whenever possible. Saline irrigation and topical steroids should be used for both acute and CRS except if there is a concurrent OI or the CD4 count is below 50 cells/mm^3. Category one and two patients can be treated with typical antimicrobial therapy with the caveat that these individuals may be more likely to have a staphylococcal or pseudomonal organism that is perhaps related to impaired cellular immunity. A further consideration for antibiotic therapy is in the form of prophylaxis. Specifically, when used in HIV patients with category three CD4 counts, TMP-SMX has been demonstrated to significantly decrease the risk of sinusitis over a 39-month observation period.[25] Rhinitis secondary to HIV infection may be responsive to a trial of topical nasal steroids.

HIV or AIDS patients with chronic sinus disease who are nonresponsive to sufficient medical therapy may receive benefit from ESS. This will provide better ventilation of the sinus cavities as well as access for topical medical therapies. There is some anecdotal and retrospective evidence for symptomatic improvement of HIV patients post-ESS, with fewer infections and a decrease in the symptom severity.

Outcome

Untreated, the average individual with AIDS will die within 1 to 3 years. However, the advent of highly active antiretroviral therapy (HAART) in 1996 has allowed for a significant delayed onset of AIDS, decreased morbidity, and prolonged survival.

Infectious Illnesses

Numerous systemic infectious illnesses can affect the sinonasal tract. These infections may start in the nose or they may first be demonstrable in another location. Given the numerous infectious possibilities and the finite limits of this chapter, pertinent summaries of these illnesses will be provided.

Bacteria

Rhinoscleroma

Rhinoscleroma is a chronic infectious, granulomatous disease that occurs in the nose and sinus cavities in at least 95% of cases and is caused by *Klebsiella rhinoscleromatis*. This disease can affect the entire respiratory tract, with delayed diagnosis potentially resulting in obstructive laryngotracheobronchial disease. Rhinoscleroma occurs most commonly in Central and South America, central and eastern Europe, and southeast Asia and Africa, but the migration and mobility of individuals worldwide makes knowledge of this entity essential.[26] Transmission of disease occurs through direct contact with the transfer of respiratory droplets or by direct inhalation of the pathogen. There are three clinicopathologic stages to this illness (**Table 10.3**), with the initial symptom of rhinorrhea progressing to nasal and facial deformity with progressive nasal obstruction. Diagnostic evaluation consists of nasal culture and a biopsy specimen because pathology can help to differentiate this lesion from other granulomatous infections and diseases, as well as neoplasms such as natural killer (NK) T-cell lymphoma (**Figs. 10.8 and 10.9**) that can present with rhinorrhea as a primary symptom in the clinical setting of rhinitis.[27] Treatment is with long-term ciprofloxacin therapy, although surgical therapy may be needed for airway reconstruction given the stenotic effects of this disease on the respiratory tract.

Table 10.3 Clinicopathologic Stages of Rhinoscleroma

Stage	Clinical Findings	Pathologic Events
1. Catarrhal	Rhinitis, nasal crusting, purulent rhinorrhea	Mucosal inflammation; neutrophils, granulation tissue; squamous metaplasia of the epithelium
2. Granulomatous or proliferative	Granulomatous nodules, nasal (Hebra) deformity, uvular hypertrophy, anosmia, dysphonia	Submucosal chronic granulomatous; inflammation of mixed cellularity; Russell bodies and Mikulicz cells
3. Fibrotic	Scarring, deformity, and stenosis	Fibrosis and scleroma

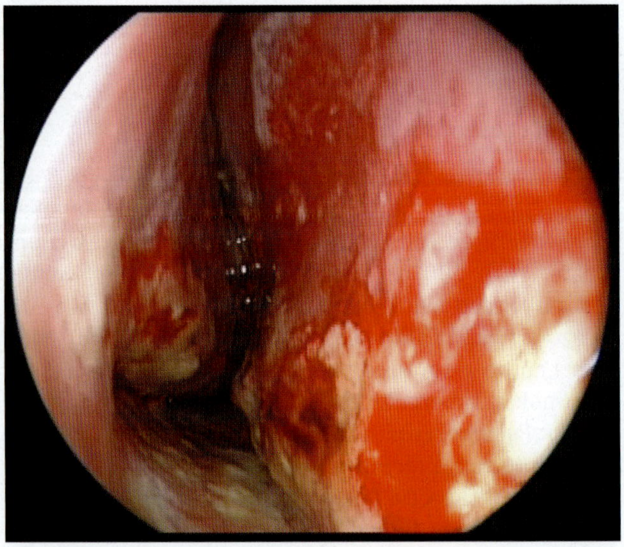

Fig. 10.8 NK-cell lymphoma evident on the nasal septum, nasal floor, and inferior turbinate. (Courtesy of Dr. F. Lavigne.)

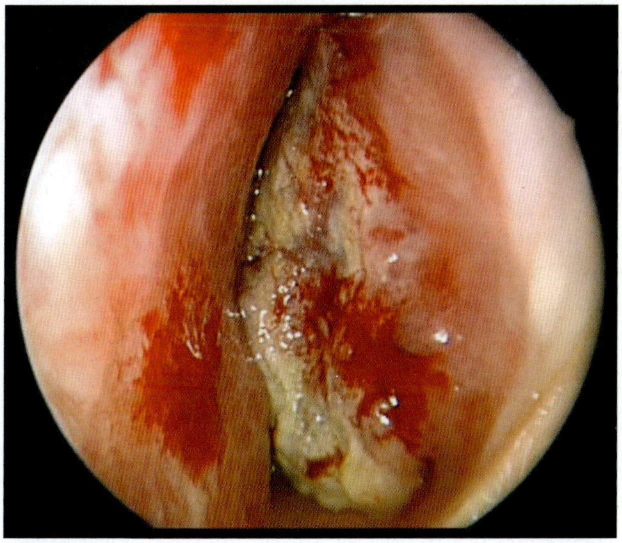

Fig. 10.9 NK-cell lymphoma of the left inferior turbinate. (Courtesy of Dr. F. Lavigne.)

Syphilis

Syphilis is caused by the spirochete *Treponema pallidum*, and it has four forms: congenital, primary, secondary, and tertiary. The nasal findings in congenital syphilis are diffuse mucosal inflammation. In primary syphilis, there may be a chancre of the septum or vestibule as well as diffuse mucosal edema. Vestibular fissures are the nasal hallmark of secondary syphilis, whereas in tertiary syphilis, there may be diffuse swelling, causing facial bone and soft tissue necrosis, septal perforation, or a solitary gumma that causes septal perforation. Diagnosis can be made using a combination of a nasal culture, a biopsy, and serum testing using the venereal disease research laboratory (VDRL) and fluorescent treponemal antibody absorbed (FTA-ABS) tests. Therapy for syphilis requires treatment with penicillin, and there may be a role for reconstructive surgery.

Leprosy

Mycobacterium leprae is the cause of this chronic disease also known as Hansen disease. Nasal findings in these patients include mucosal nodular thickening, ulcers, and crusting. Other notable findings include septal perforation, atrophic rhinitis, oronasal fistulae, and Bergen syndrome (or "facies leprosa," the atrophy of both the anterior nasal spine and premaxillary alveolar process with endonasal inflammatory changes). The nose and sinuses may act as a potential reservoir for this disease. Diagnosis is based on clinical exam, culture, lesional biopsy, and the Lepromin skin test may also be of value. Treatment consists of multidrug antibiotic therapy, but irrigations and lubricants can also be useful in the management of sinonasal disease.

Tuberculosis

Due primarily to *Mycobacterium tuberculosis*, tuberculosis (TB) is transmitted by aerosol droplets. In either primary or secondary TB, there may be septal or inferior turbinate mucosal hypertrophy or ulcers, crusting, or septal perforation. Purulent rhinorrhea, nasal fissure, and occasionally, lupus vulgaris (a painful nodular tuberculoid lesion commonly around the nose or ears) may occur. Diagnostic assessment for TB includes microbiological smears and cultures of acid-fast bacilli, tissue biopsy, PCR, chest X-ray, and a Mantoux test. An HIV test should also be considered. Treatment consists of prolonged multidrug therapy.

Actinomycosis

This is an uncommon infection of the nose and paranasal sinuses caused by *Actinomyces israelii*. Nasal findings include inflammatory polyps, purulence, or a keratin-like mass. Infection is usually related to poor oral hygiene. Diagnosis is made with an anaerobic culture and/or a lesional biopsy. A CT scan will demonstrate the extent of disease. Treatment is based on surgical drainage and debridement of the infected areas, as well as systemic penicillin therapy.

Protozoan

Leishmaniasis

This is due to a protozoan parasite of the *Leishmania* species, which is transmitted by sand flies. It is endemic in the regions of southern Europe, the Middle East, southwest Asia, and Africa. It can also be found in the southern United States right through to South America. Findings of mucocutaneous leishmaniasis include erythema and edema of the mucosa, sometimes with ulcers and secondary infections (**Figs. 10.10 and 10.11**). This often results in scarring. Diagnosis is based on a history of travel to an affected region, tissue smears, a serum or urine agglutination test, and the Montenegro skin test (a test of cell mediated immunity). The use of bed netting and insecticides may prevent transmission, whereas an intralesional injection of pentavalent antimony is an option for the treatment for active disease.

Rhinosporidiosis

This is a chronic granulomatous disease that commonly affects the nasal mucosa and ocular conjunctiva. Intranasal polyps occur with infection of the sinonasal region. Cutaneous and disseminated forms of the disease also occur. Inoculation occurs through contact with water containing the aquatic protozoan *Rhinosporidium seeberi*. Formerly thought to be a fungus, *Rhinosporidium* is now attributed to a novel class of waterborne protozoan parasites called *Mesomycetozoea*. Diagnosis is clinical or with a pathological analysis of the excised lesion because no culture methods exist. There is no medical treatment, and lesions must be excised as the sole form of treatment.

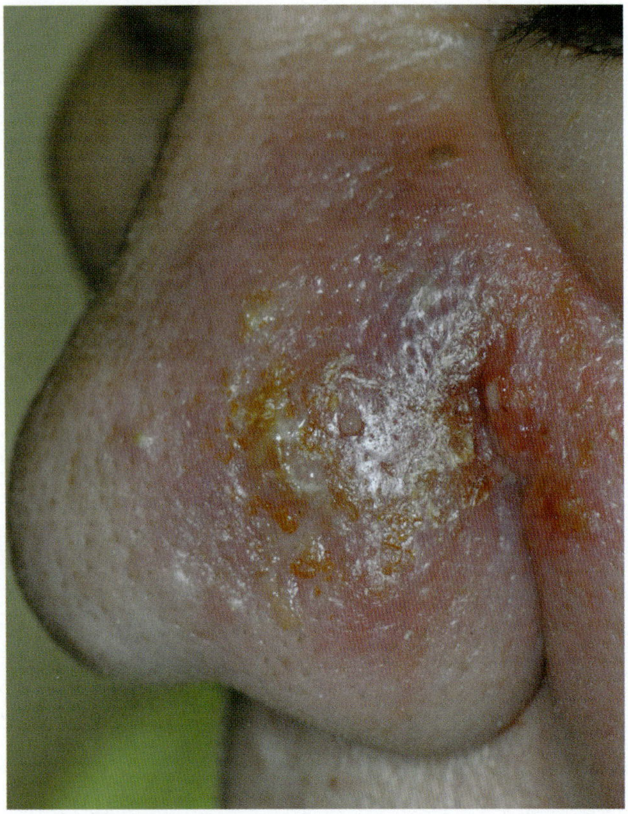

Fig. 10.10 External nasal appearance of a patient with leishmaniasis.

Fungal

Histoplasmosis

The infectious organism is *Histoplasma capsulatum*, which is a dimorphic ubiquitous soil-dwelling fungus found most commonly in central and eastern Canada and the United States, Central and South America, and Africa.

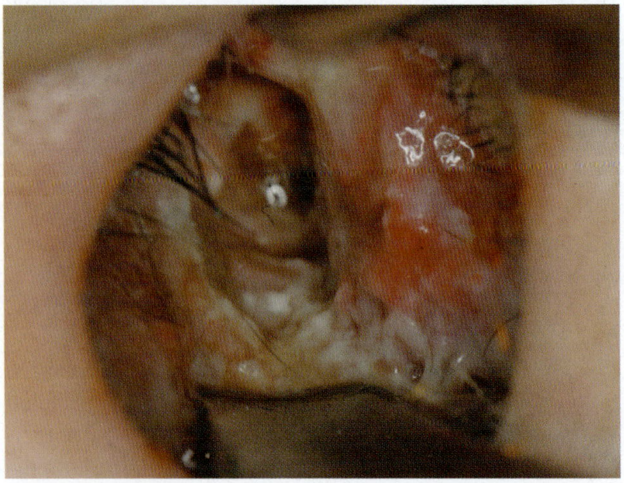

Fig. 10.11 Anterior rhinoscopy appearance of left nasal mucosa of a patient with leishmaniasis.

It most commonly occurs as an asymptomatic pulmonary infection, but in the setting of immune compromise, it can become disseminated. Mucocutaneous forms of disease are usually associated with AIDS. Isolated sinonasal infection is not common but it can manifest as mucosal ulceration of the nasal floor, inferior turbinate, or septum, which can be associated with crusting. The organism can be identified by culture, fine needle aspiration biopsy (FNAB) or incisional biopsy of a lesion, or by lymph node excision. A chest X-ray is required given its affinity for the lungs. Treatment of an isolated nonsevere infection in an immune competent host is usually with an oral triazole such as itraconazole.

Blastomycosis

This is another dimorphic fungal infection due to *Blastomyces dermatitidis*. It too is ubiquitous to soil and its primary form of infection occurs in the lungs. Its location throughout North America is not dissimilar to histoplasmosis. It less commonly presents in the head and neck region, but it may occur as a friable mucocutaneous lesion or even a papillomatous intranasal mass. Patient evaluation, diagnosis, and treatment are the same as for histoplasmosis.

Mucormycosis

Rhinocerebral mucormycosis is caused by *Rhizopus oryzae*. Diagnosis of this infection usually requires clinical suspicion in a patient with immune or metabolic deficiency. Definitive diagnosis is made with a biopsy while identifying nonseptate hyphae with a 90-degree branching pattern, angioinvasion, and a polymorphonuclear infiltrate. Initially, sites of infection of the nasal mucosa may demonstrate pallor before the onset of black necrotic eschar and pus. A CT or MRI may help to delimit the extent of the infection. Urgent treatment is required to manage this infection and consists of surgical debridement, intravenous liposomal amphotericin B, and hyperbaric oxygen therapy, if available. Early aggressive therapy and serial monitoring by endoscopy and radiography are essential to attain a positive outcome.

Vascular Disorder: Hereditary Hemorrhagic Telangiectasia

Hereditary hemorrhagic telangiectasia (HHT), or Osler-Weber-Rendu disease, is an autosomal-dominant inherited multisystem vascular dysplasia disorder. This illness was first described over a century ago and numerous advances have since been made in our understanding of the origin of the disorder as well as in the treatment of its clinical manifestations.

Epidemiology

The incidence of HHT is approximately 1/5000 individuals in North America and worldwide. This disorder affects both sexes and it occurs in all racial and ethnic groups. Recurrent acute epistaxis occurs in up to 95% of individuals and its onset is by the third decade.

Pathophysiology

HHT is due to the occurrence of mutations in the *endoglin* (chromosome 9, HHT type 1) and *ALK1* (chromosome 12, HHT type 2) genes, the proteins of which are endothelial receptors of the transforming growth factor (TGF)-beta family. They are essential for vascular integrity as TGF-beta serves a pivotal role in angiogenesis. These genetic mutations result in impaired control of endothelial cell migration and proliferation with an end result of disrupted or abnormal angiogenesis seen clinically as small vessel fragility and resultant bleeding.[28]

Diagnostic Workup

Definitive diagnosis of an individual with HHT requires the identification of three out of the four possible criteria (**Table 10.4**).[29] Other conditions that demonstrate telangiectasia and that should be considered include scleroderma and CREST (calcinosis, Raynaud phenomenon, esophageal dysmotility, sclerodactlyl, telangiectasia) syndrome, hereditary benign telangiectasia, and chronic liver disease. Once diagnosed, if not already performed, individuals should undergo imaging studies in an effort to identify important arteriovenous malformations (more common in HHT type 1) that can cause life-threatening complications (brain, lung, liver). Given the multisystem manifestations of HHT, medical care needs to be coordinated with the appropriate medical specialists. In recognition of this need and in an effort to improve care for those affected individuals, the HHT Foundation International (see www.hht.org) has identified worldwide centers of excellence for comprehensive and coordinated medical care for HHT.

Treatment

Due to its common occurrence, the preventative treatment of recurrent epistaxis in HHT has been covered extensively in the literature. To determine the clinical severity of epistaxis, an online tool has been developed that assesses epistaxis characteristics of an HHT patient over 3 months (www2.drexelmed.edu/hht-ess/). However, it does not dictate treatment alternatives based on this score. To date, the gold standard for treatment of severe epistaxis is septal dermoplasty, where the septal mucosa containing telangiectasia is stripped and then replaced with a split-thickness skin graft. This treatment can be expected to significantly decrease the occurrence of epistaxis and the resultant need for blood transfusions while improving an individual's perceived quality of life.[30]

Table 10.4 Criteria for the Diagnosis of HHT

1. Occurrence of spontaneous recurrent epistaxis
2. Multiple telangiectasia located on the lips, oral and nasal mucosa, and fingers
3. Visceral AVM of the hepatic, pulmonary, and CNS vascular systems
4. First-degree familial occurrence

Abbreviations: AVM, arteriovenous malformation; CNS, central nervous system.

Numerous other therapies have also been described. Lasers have been used extensively and the neodymium-yttrium, aluminum, and garnet (Nd-YAG) laser, in particular, is well suited for the treatment of telangiectasias and vascular malformations.[31] Other options include the argon laser, the argon plasma coagulation, and possibly, bipolar cautery. Endovascular treatment is only recommended for acute severe hemorrhage because its effect is not long lasting. For women, the systemic use of estrogen therapy in the form of the birth control pill offers a means of possibly decreasing the occurrence of epistaxis, whereas topical-use estrogen or estriol products, which induce squamous metaplasia of the nasal mucosa may take advantage of mucosal beta-estrogen receptors. This therapy can be used in combination with a variety of the aforementioned treatments. Lastly, nasal closure (otherwise known as Young's procedure) may be an option for patients with epistaxis when treatment fails with the other alternatives.

Outcome

Long-term follow-up of individuals with HHT is required due to the multisystem nature of their illness. Although there are risks such as cardiac failure and life-threatening hemorrhage, this disorder is compatible with a long and full life. Genetic counseling is a consideration for prospective parents with a family history of HHT. Screening of first degree relatives should also be considered in patients who have been newly diagnosed with HHT.

Autoimmune Diseases

The vast majority of these diseases have overt findings that are present in other organ systems prior to the occurrence of sinonasal manifestations. Similarly, the presentation of these diseases solely or initially in the sinonasal tract is very uncommon. Systemic lupus erythematosus (SLE), a connective tissue disease, may cause ulceration of the septal mucosa with possible perforation and a resultant saddle nose deformity. However, other signs of SLE will have been diagnosed long before the occurrence of these findings, and SLE will more commonly demonstrate involvement of the skin of the nasal dorsum and nasal vestibule. Behçet disease may similarly cause septal mucosal ulceration, but it may be accompanied by typical orogenital findings among others. Relapsing polychondritis can demonstrate chondritis of the auricular, nasal, and laryngeal cartilages, but the occurrence of disease at all three locations simultaneously is the exception. A presentation of recurrent auricular swelling and pain would be more common than a nasal presentation for this exceedingly uncommon disease. Lastly, pemphigoid, pemphigus, and cicatricial pemphigoid may all cause ulceration of septal mucosa, but their accompanying findings and biopsy results are more revealing than are the nasal findings.

Conclusion

The manifestation of systemic diseases in the nose and paranasal sinuses is an infrequent occurrence. However, the early identification of these illnesses by recognizing their sinonasal manifestations can lead to their early diagnosis and subsequent treatment. Establishing a network of complementary specialists for the diagnosis and management of these patients could better meet the needs of these patients with these multisystem and complex diseases.

References

1. Stanley P, MacWilliam L, Greenstone M, Mackay I, Cole P. Efficacy of a saccharin test for screening to detect abnormal mucociliary clearance. Br J Dis Chest 1984;78(1):62–65
2. Muhlebach MS, Miller MB, Moore C, Wedd JP, Drake AF, Leigh MW. Are lower airway or throat cultures predictive of sinus bacteriology in cystic fibrosis? Pediatr Pulmonol 2006;41(5):445–451
3. Leung MK, Rachakonda L, Weill D, Hwang PH. Effects of sinus surgery on lung transplantation outcomes in cystic fibrosis. Am J Rhinol 2008;22(2):192–196
4. Quattrucci S, Rolla M, Cimino G, et al. Lung transplantation for cystic fibrosis: 6-year follow-up. J Cyst Fibros 2005;4(2):107–114
5. Haubitz M. ANCA-associated vasculitis: diagnosis, clinical characteristics and treatment. Vasa 2007;36(2):81–89
6. Leavitt RY, Fauci AS, Bloch DA, et al. The American College of Rheumatology 1990 criteria for the classification of Wegener's granulomatosis. Arthritis Rheum 1990;33(8):1101–1107
7. Yang C, Talbot JM, Hwang PH. Bony abnormalities of the paranasal sinuses in patients with Wegener's granulomatosis. Am J Rhinol 2001;15(2):121–125
8. Silvera S, Vignaux O, Legmann P. Sinonasal and cerebral imaging findings in Wegener's granulomatosis. Presse Med 2007;36 (5 Pt 2):913–921
9. Langford CA. Small-vessel vasculitis: therapeutic management. Curr Rheumatol Rep 2007;9(4):328–335
10. Metzler C, Miehle N, Manger K, et al; German Network of Rheumatic Diseases. Elevated relapse rate under oral methotrexate versus leflunomide for maintenance of remission in Wegener's granulomatosis. Rheumatology (Oxford) 2007;46(7):1087–1091
11. Aubart FC, Ouayoun M, Brauner M, et al. Sinonasal involvement in sarcoidosis: a case-control study of 20 patients. Medicine (Baltimore) 2006;85(6):365–371
12. Zissel G, Prasse A, Müller-Quernheim J. Sarcoidosis—immunopathogenetic concepts. Semin Respir Crit Care Med 2007;28(1):3–14
13. Hunninghake GW, Costabel U, Ando M, et al; American Thoracic Society/European Respiratory Society/World Association of Sarcoidosis and Other Granulomatous Disorders. ATS/ERS/WASOG statement on sarcoidosis. Sarcoidosis Vasc Diffuse Lung Dis 1999;16(2):149–173
14. Kay DJ, Har-El G. The role of endoscopic sinus surgery in chronic sinonasal sarcoidosis. Am J Rhinol 2001;15(4):249–254
15. Churg J, Strauss L. Allergic granulomatosis, allergic angiitis, and periarteritis nodosa. Am J Pathol 1951;27(2):277–301
16. Pagnoux C, Guilpain P, Guillevin L. Churg-Strauss syndrome. Curr Opin Rheumatol 2007;19(1):25–32
17. Mitsuyama H, Matsuyama W, Watanabe M, et al. Increased expression of TRAIL receptor 3 on eosinophils in Churg-Strauss syndrome. Arthritis Rheum 2007;56(2):662–673
18. Masi AT, Hunder GG, Lie JT, et al. The American College of Rheumatology 1990 criteria for the classification of Churg-Strauss syndrome (allergic granulomatosis and angiitis). Arthritis Rheum 1990;33(8):1094–1100
19. Bacciu A, Bacciu S, Mercante G, et al. Ear, nose and throat manifestations of Churg-Strauss syndrome. Acta Otolaryngol 2006;126(5):503–509
20. Guillevin L, Lhote F, Gayraud M, et al. Prognostic factors in polyarteritis nodosa and Churg-Strauss syndrome. A prospective study in 342 patients. Medicine (Baltimore) 1996;75(1):17–28
21. Guillevin L, Cohen P, Gayraud M, Lhote F, Jarrousse B, Casassus P. Churg-Strauss syndrome. Clinical study and long-term follow-up of 96 patients. Medicine (Baltimore) 1999;78(1):26–37
22. Azar AE, Ballas ZK. Evaluation of the adult with suspected immunodeficiency. Am J Med 2007;120(9):764–768
23. Chee L, Graham SM, Carothers DG, Ballas ZK. Immune dysfunction in refractory sinusitis in a tertiary care setting. Laryngoscope 2001;111(2):233–235
24. Centers for Disease Control. 1993 revised classification system for HIV infection and expanded surveillance case definition for AIDS among adolescents and adults. MMWR Recomm Rep 1992;41(RR-17):1–19
25. DiRienzo AG, van Der Horst C, Finkelstein DM, Frame P, Bozzette SA, Tashima KT. Efficacy of trimethoprim-sulfamethoxazole for the prevention of bacterial infections in a randomized prophylaxis trial of patients with advanced HIV infection. AIDS Res Hum Retroviruses 2002;18(2):89–94
26. Chan TV, Spiegel JH. Klebsiella rhinoscleromatis of the membranous nasal septum. J Laryngol Otol 2007;121(10):998–1002
27. Sands NB, Tewfik MA, Hwang SY, Desrosiers M. Extranodal T-cell lymphoma of the sinonasal tract presenting as severe rhinitis: a case series. J Otolaryngol 2008; In press
28. Lebrin F, Deckers M, Bertolino P, Ten Dijke P. TGF-beta receptor function in the endothelium. Cardiovasc Res 2005;65(3):599–608
29. Shovlin CL, Guttmacher AE, Buscarini E, et al. Diagnostic criteria for hereditary hemorrhagic telangiectasia (Rendu-Osler-Weber syndrome). Am J Med Genet 2000;91(1):66–67
30. Fiorella ML, Ross D, Henderson KJ, White RI Jr. Outcome of septal dermoplasty in patients with hereditary hemorrhagic telangiectasia. Laryngoscope 2005;115(2):301–305
31. Mahoney EJ, Shapshay SM. New classification of nasal vasculature patterns in hereditary hemorrhagic telangiectasia. Am J Rhinol 2006;20(1):87–90

11 Infectious Rhinitis

Jayant M. Pinto, Fuad M. Baroody, and Robert M. Naclerio

Upper respiratory tract infections (URIs) are perhaps the most common short-term maladies that plague humankind. URIs are characterized by inflammation through some or all parts of the respiratory tract, such as the nose, sinuses, pharynx, larynx, trachea, and bronchi. Many of these infections occur in the nasal passages, a fact that has important implications from both epidemiologic and public health perspectives. Indeed, the burden of these illnesses is heavy both on the individual level (symptoms, quality of life), and on society. They lead to an increased use of medications (over-the-counter and prescription), a large number of physician visits, workplace absenteeism, and lost productivity.[1,2] Therefore, the topic of infectious rhinitis remains very important.

The diagnosis and treatment of infectious rhinitis must focus on distinguishing the cause,[3,4] because many etiologies of rhinitis (allergic, rhinosinusitis, and nonallergic with its subtypes) may present with similar symptom complexes.[2] Because of the proximity of the nose and paranasal sinuses, it is not surprising that inflammatory conditions span these anatomic locations. Indeed, it has been shown on imaging that the common cold typically causes changes in the sinus mucosa.[5] This has led to the adoption of the term "rhinosinusitis" to reflect the fact that sinusitis rarely occurs without rhinitis. For brevity, we will use the term rhinitis in this chapter.

A host of organisms, including bacteria, fungi, and parasites, can cause infectious rhinitis. In the United States, a viral etiology predominates. In developing nations, other etiologies become important as their prevalence increases. In this chapter, we review the pathogenesis of infectious rhinitis with an emphasis on viral causes, and we discuss the management of viral infection in the nose, therapies available, and future directions of research in this field.

Viruses

Viral rhinitis refers to inflammation of the sinonasal mucosa caused by viral infection. Commonly referred to as "the common cold," this disease is estimated to occur ~2 to 4 times per year in adults and 4 to 10 times per year in children, with higher frequency in families with multiple children.[6,7] Although the frequency of this disease varies widely, the burden of illness is enormous, with estimates of 1 billion colds and 22 million lost school days annually in the United States, and $40 billion in direct and indirect annual costs.[8–10] Sex-based differences in incidence have been reported,[11] and the frequency of illness diminishes with age.[12] Another important factor is the season, with increased frequency of infection starting in autumn, continuing throughout winter, and declining in spring. In the tropics, the peak occurs during the rainy season. There is some variation within the specific season with different viruses, although the pattern of increase in the winter is common.[13] For example, both respiratory syncytial virus (RSV) and influenza infections have their peak prevalence in January to March, whereas parainfluenza viruses peak in the spring or autumn/early winter, depending on the type.[13] Rhinovirus and adenovirus cause viral rhinitis throughout the year.

In children, their presence in daycare is a major risk factor for increased frequency of infections.[14,15] Interestingly, early life exposures such as episodes of viral rhinitis may alter the developing immune system.[16] These viral illnesses can affect the development of immunologic diseases such as asthma and allergies later in life, as shown in birth-cohort studies.[17,18] Current data show a paradox in that severe respiratory viral infections are involved in wheezing illness in young children and serve as a marker of asthma development later in life on the one hand, whereas early life viral infections are also clearly associated with protection from allergic diseases in some circumstances.[19,20] In general, the body of data linking infection and allergic disease supports the hygiene hypothesis regarding the development of atopic disease. Indeed, T-helper (Th) 1 and Th2 balance may be affected by viral infection and may also be the cause of susceptibility in children.[21] Additionally, responses to viruses may perturb the immune system, causing dysregulated immunity.[22,23] Other factors that increase the susceptibility to viral rhinitis, but lack strong supporting evidence, include psychological stress, humidity, allergies, and physical activity.[8,24,25] Viral rhinitis is often the trigger for exacerbation of lower airway disease such as asthma. This topic is complex and is a subject of ongoing investigation worldwide.

More than 200 different viruses are known to cause the symptoms of the common cold,[8] the most common of which are rhinovirus and coronaviruses, which together account for ~50% of all colds.[13] Other causative viruses include parainfluenza, RSV, adenoviruses, coxsackieviruses, echoviruses, influenza viruses (A and B), and enteroviruses. Historically, no organism can be isolated in many instances, although this is changing with the advent of sophisticated polymerase chain reaction (PCR)-based assays[26,27] (see later, Novel Diagnostics) and other technologies (e.g., next generation sequencing) for the detection of viruses in human samples. It is thought that the agents that cause adult and pediatric disease are similar, although studies are limited in children because of the difficulty in obtaining specimens. In some cases, these viruses cause more severe lower airway than upper airway disease, depending on age (e.g., RSV in children).

The transmission of viral rhinitis can occur through either contact via hands (direct or via inanimate objects) or through aerosolization of infected secretions. Although in daily life and clinical practice these are likely to be common to all viruses and difficult to distinguish, there is some evidence that routes of transmission vary by agent. For example, rhinovirus is thought to be transmitted mostly through hand contact and self-inoculation,[28] whereas influenza is spread by aerosol.[29,30] School-age children introduce rhinovirus infections into their families three times more frequently than do working adults.[31] These differences have important relevance for prevention, education, and public health strategies that minimize the spread of disease.

The pathogenesis of viral rhinitis is incompletely understood. Some pathogens cause minimal epithelial damage (e.g., rhinovirus[32]), whereas others cause more significant injury (e.g., influenza and RSV, mainly to the lower airway[29,30]). Perhaps most is known about rhinovirus, the most common pathogen involved in viral rhinitis; this virus may serve as a model for understanding the pathobiology of viral rhinitis. After deposition on the nasal epithelium or conjunctiva, rhinovirus attaches to the surface intercellular adhesion molecule-1 (ICAM-1) receptor, with a resultant increase in nasal secretions.[33] The virus then invades the host cells, co-opts the cellular machinery, and replicates. Viral replication kinetics is rapid, occurring between 3 and 10 hours, and leading to inflammatory responses and symptoms. The site of initial infection seems to be the adenoid, where the ciliated epithelium expresses ICAM-1 highly, with subsequent anterograde spread of the infection from the nasopharynx forward.[34]

Host immune defense responses to this infection play a critical role in symptoms of viral rhinitis. Cytokines are involved in all aspects of inflammatory responses and in all forms of viral rhinitis in an interrelated and complex fashion. Responses may begin with the release of nonspecific mediators such as tumor necrosis factor (TNF)-α and interleukin (IL)-1, resulting in local and systemic responses and symptoms.[35] Recruitment of other inflammatory cells then occurs with resultant secretion of new mediators that amplify the inflammatory effects. These include neurogenic inflammation, vascular permeability, and other responses with resultant symptoms. Some of these mediators activate nociceptive nerves leading to local mucosal axon responses and the subsequent release of inflammatory peptides and resultant neurogenic inflammation. Neural reflexes may be involved in nasal irritation, sneezing, engorgement of venous sinusoids, increased vascular permeability, glandular exocytosis, cellular inflammation, and reflexive problems in nearby anatomic sites.[35]

These interactions result in the stimulation of immune responses and the release of mediators such as kinins, leukotrienes, histamines, interleukins such as IL-1, -6, and -8, and chemokines such as RANTES[36] and others.[37] These mediators are thought to cause local and systemic symptoms.[38–41] Other viruses invade the respiratory epithelium by using other receptors but are thought to have a similar disease biology in terms of binding, replication, and inflammatory consequences. For example, the coronaviruses that infect humans gain access via human aminopeptidase N, hemagglutinin-esterase, and spike glycoproteins. In a similar fashion, these and other viruses cause symptoms.

In vitro and in vivo studies have demonstrated the production of mainly Th1-derived proinflammatory cytokines such as IL-1β, IL-6, tumor necrosis factor (TNF)-α, and interferon (IFN)-γ in viral rhinitis.[42,43] Klemens and colleagues studied nasal secretions in patients with various forms of rhinitis and in controls.[44] They found that, in viral rhinitis, a predominantly proinflammatory profile included IL-8, granulocytic colony simulating factor (G-CSF), and elastase, suggesting that neutrophil granulocytes may be important in mounting a response to infection. Additionally, IL-5, eosinophilic catonic protein (ECP), and granulocyte macrophage colony stimulating factor (GM-CSF), and IL-4 and IL-13 were also elevated; hence, no clear Th1/Th2 dichotomy could be determined. Interestingly, data suggested that IL-10 may play a role in limiting the inflammatory response in the nasal mucosa during the infection. These preliminary studies attest to the complexity of the cytokine pattern in viral rhinitis.

Symptoms of viral rhinitis are associated with elevated levels of several cytokines (IL-1β, IL-6, IL-8, or IFN-γ[42,45]) in contrast to asymptomatic colds,[46] suggesting that cytokine responses are responsible for the symptoms. Indeed, nasal secretion levels of bradykinin, leukotrienes (LTs), IFN-α, IFN-β, IFN-γ, IL-1, IL-6, IL-8, IL-11, TNF, and nitric oxide are all elevated in viral rhinitis.[35] Nasal symptoms are directly correlated with the expression of IL-1, IL-6, and bradykinin. Thus, therapies directed toward production of anti-inflammatory cytokines represent a theoretically attractive strategy for alleviating or preventing inflammation-related symptoms. However, efficacy trials using synthesis inhibitors or pathway blockade toward relevant cytokines have failed, in part due to power, study design, interactions among mediators, inadequate knowledge of systems biology, redundancy of cytokine profiles, or issues of drug potency or delivery.[35]

Interestingly, in experimental human models of rhinovirus infection, asthmatic patients show increased levels of IL-8 in nasal lavage, which correlates with the level of airway responsiveness.[47] These and other data suggest that rhinovirus infection of airway epithelial cells may potentiate preexisting proinflammatory pathways, enhancing chemokine production and airway inflammation. Rhinovirus and cytokines seem to combine to induce augmented airway epithelial-cell chemokine expression, thus promoting further inflammation. Herschenson used a cellular system to study the combined effects of rhinovirus and TNF-α on airway epithelial cell proinflammatory gene expression.[48] This group found that costimulation of epithelial cell lines and primary tracheal epithelial cells with rhinovirus and TNF-α induced synergistic increases in cytokine production and transcription, suggesting that cooperative increases in epithelial cell chemokine expression may provide a cellular mechanism for rhinovirus-induced exacerbations of lower airway disease (see Rhinovirus and Asthma).[48] This probably has relevance for the upper airway as well.

TNF-α and IL-1 are thought to have central roles in viral rhinitis.[35] TNF-α is the first cytokine to be up regulated, with peak levels within several hours; IL-1 follows, with levels peaking after 24 to 48 hours. These events then cause up regulation of other cytokines (e.g., IL-6, IL-8, and IL-10). Of interest, the severity of URI symptoms and the development of complications such as bacterial sinusitis are linked to the cascade of production of these various proinflammatory cytokines.[49,50] The pleiotropic effects of TNF-α, which include fever, relaxation of smooth muscle, the induction of endothelial cytokine expression, an enhanced vascular permeability, and cell adhesion, are all consistent with a primary role of TNF-α in the pathogenesis of virally induced rhinitis.[51–54] IL-1 has many of the same activities as TNF-α.[51] As with TNF-α, the timing of release in nasal lavage correlates with peak periods of symptom expression and resolution, supporting the hypotheses that IL-1 contributes to the pathogenesis of viral rhinitis and that IL-1 receptor antagonist (ra) plays an important role in disease resolution.[35]

More recent data shed more light on the timing and sequence of these mediators in response to viral infection. Hayden et al. measured IL-1β, IL-2, IL-6, IL-8, IFN-α, TGF-β, and TNF-α in nasal lavage fluid, plasma, and serum in a human experimental model of influenza A, and they correlated these levels with various measures of infection and illness severity.[50] With this pathogen and in this setting, IL-6 and IFN-α levels in nasal lavage fluids peaked early (day 2) and correlated directly with viral titers, temperature, mucus production, and symptom scores. In contrast, TNF-α responses peaked later (days 3 to 4), when viral shedding and symptoms were subsiding. Similarly, IL-8 peaked late (days 4 to 6) and correlated only with lower respiratory symptoms. In these studies, IL-1β, IL-2, or transforming growth factor (TGF)-β levels did not increase significantly. These data implicate IL-6 and IFN-α as key factors in both symptom formation and host defense in influenza.[50] How this relates to other pathogens is not clear, but it serves as a model for further studies. Simplistically, these and other data suggest that IFN-α levels correlate with virus detection and mucosal defense alert, IL-1 and IL-6 correlate with the up regulation of the resultant inflammatory response, TNF-α is an antiviral response, and IL-8 and IL-10 reflect regulatory responses to decrease inflammation.[2] Indeed, suppression of inflammatory responses is critical to a host of diseases, especially those like viral rhinitis in which the response is part of the problem. IL-10 is considered to be an intrinsic anti-inflammatory and immunosuppressive cytokine that is important in T-regulatory cell function. Increases in local IL-10 production were reported during experimental viral rhinitis, and maximal IL-10 levels typically coincide with the onset of resolution of viral URI–induced symptoms.[55]

In support of the concept of cytokine production being relevant for disease symptoms, increases in local IL-6 production have also been reported during URIs caused by rhinovirus, influenza, and RSV, and they coincide with peaks in symptomatology and pathophysiology.[35] IL-6 results in increased nasal secretions after topical application.[56] IL-8 is a neutrophil-chemotactic cytokine whose production by monocytes, fibroblasts, endothelial cells, epithelial cells, and neutrophils is induced by IL-1 and TNF-α. It has been detected in nasal secretions of volunteers infected with rhinovirus, influenza, and RSV.[35] This cytokine has been associated with disease severity during experimental rhinovirus infection.[57] Rhinovirus infections in asthmatics are associated with a selective recruitment of neutrophils and, to a lesser extent, of lymphocytes to the lower airways. The degree of neutrophil degranulation correlates with symptom severity in virus-induced exacerbations of asthma. Airway neutrophilia is a prominent feature of chronic obstructive pulmonary disease (COPD) and asthma exacerbations, consistent with a viral etiology. One mediator that has been implicated is IL-8, which is involved in neutrophil chemoattraction in the lower airway in these settings. Experimental models of RV-induced COPD exacerbations are being investigated.[58]

Insights into innate immunity are offering fresh perspectives on the pathogenesis of viral infection by shedding light on the responses of this physiologic arm of the immune system that triggers inflammation and subsequent specific immune responses.[59] As the first line of defense against viral pathogens, innate immune responses play a critical role in viral rhinitis.[60] Critical parts of this system include toll-like receptors (TLR), RNA helicases, and cytosolic DNA sensors. Airway epithelial cells express several functional TLRs. Double stranded (ds) RNA and RNA viruses are recognized by TLR3 and also by the RNA helicases retinoic-acid-inducible gene (RIG-I) and melanoma differentiation-associated gene-5 (MDA5), and the serine-threonine kinase PKR, all in the cytoplasm.[61,62] The role played by epithelial cells in the initiation, maintenance, and regulation of both innate and adaptive immune responses is now being understood.[63] Not only do these cells serve a barrier function, but they also clear pathogens through mucociliary clearance, produce substances that destroy or inhibit microorganisms directly, and produce immunostimulatory mediators to trigger further immune responses through the use of a variety of pathogen-recognition receptors. These molecules, such as TLRs, and others, such as helicases (RIG-I, MDA5) and kinases (PKR), recognize pathogens including viruses.[64] Epithelial cells can regulate the activation and differentiation of dendritic cells (DCs), B cells, and T cells.

Intense interest in TLRs has provided data showing their role in the initiation of the immune responses to viral infection. Kurt Jones noted the role of TLR4 in triggering the inflammatory response to RSV infection.[65] With this pathogen, the response appears to be directed toward the fusion protein of the virus. TLR3 has been shown to interact with dsRNA, providing a mechanism for responding to viruses that have this type of genome.[66] Similarly, TLR7 has been demonstrated to stimulate cytokine production via interactions with single stranded (ss) RNA viral genomes such as influenza A.[67] Knockout studies in mice showed that picornaviruses are sensed by MDA5,[68] a helicase that triggers antiviral cellular responses. Another gene in this pathway, RIG-I, recognizes viral RNA, including influenza A[69–71] and promotes caspase function and inflammation. Other components of innate immunity are being actively investigated: DCs play an important role in IFN-α production in the lower airway in RSV-infected mice,[72] and TLR3 stimulates chemokine and cytokine production in RSV infection of human epithelial cells in vitro.[73] Because of this new information supporting the important role of the innate immune system in viral diseases, pharmaceutical companies are developing therapies for infectious and immune diseases that target innate immunity. For example, TLR4 antagonists can block responses to viral vaccines in animal models.[74] The development of pharmaceutical agonists for innate immunity molecules may allow for more rapid responses to viral pathogens and may abort clinical infection and/or result in abbreviated symptoms.

Extracellular (most TLRs) and intracellular (helicases, etc.) components of innate immunity may work in separate compartments. For example, TLR4 recognizes the F protein on the RSV surface outside the host cell, whereas inside the cell, other molecules, such as RIG-I and TLR3, recognize viral replication intermediates.[75] In this way, innate immunity can protect from both viral entry and subsequent developments inside the cell. Recently, Medzhitov described a new component of the innate immune system—the cytosolic DNA sensor[76] which may be involved in recognition of intracellular viral DNA. After binding host cells, RSV triggers the host cellular response by using viral proteins that bind TLR4, leading to up regulation of the transcriptional programs of genes involved in the antiviral response,[77,78] such as mediators.[79,80] Similarly, surveillance is enhanced through prominent up regulation of cell-adhesion molecules such as ICAM-1 that are involved in cellular recruitment[81] and antigen-presenting molecules like major histocompatability complex (MHC)-I[82] on the cell surface of lung epithelial cells.

As another example, a rhinovirus infection of airway epithelial cells induces the production of a host of cytokines and several adhesion molecules resulting in inflammatory cell infiltrates and inflammation in situ.[83–86] Recently, Schliemer and Kim reported testing the ability of the human rhinovirus to alter the expression of the costimulatory molecules on human airway epithelial cells by using flow cytometry and real-time PCR, using both in vivo and in vitro methods.[87] This group showed that rhinovirus infection or exposure to dsRNA induces epithelial expression of costimulatory molecules, thus providing support for the concept that innate immune responses are linked to adaptive immunity in viral infection in the nose. Other molecules such as thymic stromal lymphopoietin (TSLP), which is elevated in asthma and triggers dendritic cell-mediated activation of Th2 inflammatory responses, are also induced in in vitro infection with rhinovirus in human bronchial epithelial cells.[88] Knockdown approaches implicated nuclear factor kappaB (NF-κB) and IFN regulatory factor 3 (IRF-3) signaling via TLR3 in this process, effects that were suppressed by glucocorticoids. This work supports the idea that respiratory viral infection and the recruitment of Th2 cytokine-producing cells may amplify Th2 inflammation via the induction of TSLP in the asthmatic airway. Because in humans TSLP activates dendritic cells,[89,90] which are involved in antigen presentation and the regulation of immune responses, its involvement in responses to viral infection or exposure to dsRNA indicates a mechanism by which the airway epithelium can stimulate dendritic cells to generate responses to viral pathogens and cause inflammation that results in symptoms.

Some avian influenza A strains induce intense cytokine and inflammatory responses in humans with a high fatality rate. Both TLR3 and TLR7 interact with influenza A virus with resultant cytokine production.[67,91] In the human lung and in epithelial and alveolar cell lines, TLR3 has been implicated in cytokine responses to influenza A.[92] Other studies have shed light on the role of TLR3 in responses to influenza through classic inflammatory pathways such as NF-κB and others,[69,93,94] such as RIG-I and its adapter.[95]

Because respiratory viruses target nasal and airway epithelial cells, they can cause damage to the barrier function of these cells, with resultant increased epithelial permeability. Perhaps more importantly, epithelial cells serve as guardians in defending against infection, where they are now thought to regulate immune responses by producing mediators and stimulating immune cells. This involves innate immune responses and the generation of cytokines, which work to generate adapative responses as well. Further investigation of this important area will provide fresh insights into targets for therapeutic development.

With the advent of the genome era, examination of the association of genetic variation with disease has come to the forefront of biomedicine. Recent studies demonstrated associations between variation in cytokine and receptor genes. For example, genetic variation associated with a high production of TNF-α or IL-1β is associated with increased susceptibility to several inflammatory conditions.[96] In RSV infection, polymorphisms in IL-8, IL-4, IL-9, IL-10, CD14, protein surfactant D, and TLR4 are associated with the type and severity of clinical disease.[97–103] These results suggest that specific polymorphisms in cytokine and other relevant genes or receptors may be associated with increased susceptibility to viral rhinitis and its complications.

Clinical Manifestations of Viral Rhinitis

Viruses that cause rhinitis include rhinovirus, adenovirus, influenza virus, parainfluenza virus, coxsackievirus, enterovirus, and RSV. All of these viruses cause local symptoms with similar presentations, but they vary in the extent of systemic involvement. This variation may reflect tissue tropism, pathogenicity, or inflammatory host response. For example, influenza can infect leukocytes and therefore may be associated with systemic dissemination and manifestations. Commonality of symptoms caused by different pathogens represents the consequences of a generalized host response to viral infection of the nasal mucosa. How to differentiate among types of rhinitis remains an understudied art. In general, obtaining a thorough history usually suggests the correct diagnosis. An acute onset (1 week or less) has a limited differential and usually suggests a viral etiology, although viral symptoms can persist for up to 14 days. Viral rhinitis will cause generalized symptoms and occasional fevers.

Clinically, viral rhinitis includes symptoms of watery rhinorrhea, sneezing, nasal congestion, as well as related symptoms of the common cold such as pharyngitis, sneezing, hoarseness, and cough. Other typical symptoms include temporary olfactory loss, headache, sore throat, malaise, and sweats. Fever is present in some patients but does not predict bacterial infection as an isolated diagnostic criterion. Secretion color should not be used for assessing the need for antibiotic therapy, because color is related to the presence of neutrophils, not of bacteria, which often appear in the nasal discharge of patients with viral rhinitis.[104]

Symptoms of viral rhinitis occur 2 to 3 days after the infection and usually last for 2 to 10 days or sometimes longer.[105] The duration of symptoms after rhinovirus infections takes the following course: fever is the earliest and shortest lasting symptom, peaking at day 2 of illness and all but resolving by day 6; sore throat also starts early, with a peak at day 2 of illness and almost complete resolution by 10 days; nasal drainage and cough start a little later in the course of the disease, peaking at around the 3rd to 4th day, and can last up to 14 days.[106] In healthy subjects, the illness is generally self-limited. However, viral rhinitis is associated with complications in patients with comorbidities, especially in those with immunosuppression,[107] and can cause severe consequences in the very old or young.[108] Viral infection in the nose is also associated with infection in related structures, in particular the sinuses[5] and middle ear[109] and also the lower airways.[110] Although it has been difficult to culture viruses from these other sites (sinus, lung, or middle ear), the development of concomitant infection has been associated with the extension of the inflammatory response to these adjacent sites. The use of modern techniques has enhanced the ability to identify the evidence of viral infection in these sites.

A focused physical examination will provide data for distinguishing other causes and confirming a viral pathology. A careful examination of the nose is important for identifying any structural abnormalities, obvious polyps, mucosal swelling, and discharge, and excluding other causes (see later). Nasal endoscopy provides the best evaluation but is not necessary unless unusual or persistent symptoms or the medical history warrant it. Enlarged tonsils, pharyngeal inflammation, or postnasal drip can also be confirmatory signs, but they are nonspecific. Similarly, conjunctivitis can be a component of viral rhinitis. Lymphadenopathy may be present in either viral or bacterial rhinitis.

Recent, multidisciplinary consensus panels have attempted to provide guidelines on issues regarding the management of acute rhinitis, including viral rhinitis.[111] This group states that a clinician should diagnose viral rhinitis when symptoms or signs of acute rhinosinusitis are present for less than 10 days and the symptoms are not worsening. The diagnosis of bacterial processes is discussed elsewhere in this text, but it should be noted that transition from viral to bacterial infection is thought to occur in only ~0.5 to 2.0% of episodes of viral rhinitis.[112] There is a gray zone between slow resolution of viral rhinitis and the development of bacterial disease, which is why the symptom trajectory (worsening or improving) is helpful during this period.[113] One must not forget that a majority of acute bacterial sinus infections resolve spontaneously.

Abnormalities in nasal airflow and mucociliary clearance have been shown during natural episodes of viral rhinitis and were associated with sinus disease, a finding that was especially prevalent in allergic subjects.[114–116] Allergic rhinitis is a condition that has been suggested to increase susceptibility to recurrent sinusitis.[117] In fact, impairment of sinus ventilation and mucociliary clearance have been considered key factors in the development of bacterial sinusitis for more than 20 years.[118] Similar results have been found in experimentally induced viral colds.[109,119–121] The relationship between rhinovirus infection and allergic rhinitis and asthma is complex,[122] but some data suggest that allergic responses are potentiated by experimental rhinovirus infections in subjects with allergic rhinitis despite a lack of increase in nasal symptoms. Fireman suggests that the host immune response plays a major role in the genesis of symptoms via intracellular signaling pathways that lead to enhanced inflammation. Overall, however, symptoms may not differ between viral rhinitis with and without allergic rhinitis.[120]

Typically, viral rhinitis is treated without laboratory testing, but serologic, tissue culture, and PCR-based assays for a host of agents are available. In children and in certain clinical situations (e.g., immunosuppression), viral identification may be useful and is obtained using nasal swabs or nasopharyngeal aspirates. Recently, RT-PCR has been shown to increase the sensitivity of the detection of rhinovirus in nasal aspirates compared with conventional techniques.[123] In the vast majority of cases of viral rhinitis, laboratory testing is not performed clinically and remains a research tool.

Causative Viruses in Rhinitis

Rhinoviruses

Rhinoviruses are small, positive-sense, ssRNA molecules surrounded by a protein capsid.[124] Variability in the proteins in the capsid reflects the antigenic diversity found in these pathogens and explains the challenge for the development of vaccines. More than 100 serotypes of rhinoviruses have been identified to date. The vast majority of these attach to cells through ICAM-1,[125] and the minority bind the low density lipoprotein (LDL) receptor.[126] The A species predominate over the B by ~3:1. A new class of rhinovirus (C) was recently discovered and characterized.[127]

Rhinoviruses cause ~50% of common colds, but the precise fraction remains unknown. These pathogens cause disease worldwide, year-round, and are not age specific. Perhaps because of the lack of useful therapies, these viruses are responsible for the widespread overuse of antibiotics.[128]

Rhinoviruses cause sinonasal mucosal inflammation, which is detectable by imaging and which resolves without antibiotics. Perhaps more than 1.2 billion episodes of the common cold occur in the United States annually, but only a small percentage are thought to be complicated by secondary bacterial infection.[112] On the other hand, most cases of bacterial rhinosinusitis are thought to follow a preceding viral infection. Nose blowing has been shown to cause nasal/nasopharyngeal secretions to enter into the sinuses,[129] representing another mechanism that might make acute bacterial sinus disease a complication of viral rhinitis.

Rhinoviruses are stable at a variety of temperatures and are able to withstand drying on the skin and household objects.[28,130] The introduction of rhinovirus into a household causes disease in about two thirds of other family members.[31,131] Transmission via objects from the hands of an infected person to another by autoinoculation into the nose or eye is thought to account for most disease spread.[130]

Coronaviruses

Coronaviruses are positive ssRNA viruses that are divided into three groups. Perhaps the most famous coronavirus is the one responsible for the severe acute respiratory syndrome (SARS), SARS-CoV,[132] which caused the 2002 to 2003 SARS epidemic.[133,134] This health crisis affected more than 8,000 individuals and caused 774 fatalities.[135,136] Clinically, SARS included a progressive atypical pneumonia that was refractory to conventional antibiotics. Isolation and quarantine eventually helped control the epidemic.[137]

Most, but not all, group I coronaviruses use CD13 (human aminopeptidase N) as their cellular receptor, and others use angiotensin-converting enzyme 2 (ACE2).[138,139] Both of these receptors can be found on ciliated nasal epithelial cells. After surface spike proteins bind these receptors, the viral particles are internalized, and the replication cycle begins.

Coronaviruses are estimated to cause ~10 to 15% of adult common colds with epidemics occurring every 2 to 3 years.[12,140] Like the rhinovirus, they have been linked to asthma and COPD exacerbations. Lower respiratory tract coronavirus infections (bronchitis, bronchiolitis, pneumonia) were far more common than those in the upper respiratory tract (rhinitis, pharyngitis, laryngitis) in one prospective study.[124] Additionally, some data suggest that coinfection with a second virus can result in severe lower airways disease.

Typically, coronaviruses are not tested for in clinical practice. As with other viral agents, such testing requires special cell lines or organ culture, efforts that are impractical, insensitive, and not cost-effective. Other available options include RT-PCR, antibody assays, complement-fixing assays, and enzyme-linked immunosorbent assays (ELISAs); most of these currently serve as research tools. Serologic testing is available for suspected cases of SARS-CoV.[141]

Parainfluenza Viruses

Human parainfluenza viruses are an important cause of serious respiratory tract disease in infants and young children.[142–144] Approximately 25% of children under the age of 5 years experience a significant parainfluenza infection annually, and some of these infections require hospitalization. Four types are associated with respiratory illness in young infants and children, especially type 3, which causes pneumonia and bronchiolitis, with parainfluenza ranking second only to RSV as a cause of bronchiolitis and pneumonia in infants <6 months of age.[145] The type 3 virus can cause severe disease in the very young, and almost all children have been infected by age 4. Overall, this type is thought to be responsible for ~11% of hospitalizations for pediatric respiratory illness in the United States.[146]

Adenoviruses

Adenovirus is a nonenveloped dsDNA virus that causes both rhinitis and lower respiratory tract disease. The early region 1A (E1A) gene of this virus has been associated with enhancing host inflammatory mediators through NF-κB activation. Adenovirus infection causes induction of inflammatory cytokines, and their levels correlate with the severity of disease.[147] In immunocompromised patients, the disease can progress systemically and be fatal.

Adenovirus has a remarkable capacity to spread because of the large number of viral particles present in secretions and the low number of particles required to transmit the illness. In most cases, infected persons remain asymptomatic despite proof of infection by viral culture or serology. Ten percent of exposed persons may become ill, and some of these patients may have lower airway disease such as pneumonia.[148] Outbreaks can occur in close environments such as schools or in the military. Fever and conjunctivitis are common features.

Adenoviruses are antigenically stable, which lowers the opportunity for epidemic spread. Generally, infection stimulates long lasting protective immunity to the relevant serotype. Hence, genetic stability, the frequency of subclinical infection, and long-term immunity may explain why the adenovirus does not cause epidemic disease.[148] These viruses account for ~2 to 5% of episodes of viral rhinitis.

Respiratory Syncytial Viruses

RSV is a negative-sense, enveloped RNA virus, which is unstable in the environment and is readily inactivated with soap and water. Two subgroups, A and B, have been identified. RSV causes acute respiratory disease in all age groups, but the burden of disease is highest in children.[149] Natural resistance does not occur in RSV infection because of antigenic variation among strains and also because of unclear humoral and cellular immune factors.

RSV is the leading cause of bronchiolitis in infants and young children. The World Health Organization (WHO) estimates that there are 64 million infections annually worldwide, with 160,000 deaths.[59] Every year, ~100,000 infants are hospitalized with RSV in the United States.[150] This infection can spread easily, especially in school or daycare settings,[151] by transmission of large-particle aerosols to the nasal mucosa or conjunctivae, or by self-inoculation of secretions from the hands.[152] The diagnosis of an RSV infection is generally made by the use of antigen detection assays from swabs or nasopharyngeal aspirates, although techniques of virus isolation, detection of viral RNA, and serologic tests are also available. Newer diagnostic techniques using nucleic acids are emerging.[153]

There is evidence that certain viruses, such as rhinovirus and RSV, may play a causal role in the development of acute bacterial rhinosinusitis, which has been suggested to be caused by RSV-induced priming of a hyperimmune response.[154]

Influenza

Influenza A and B viruses are members of the orthomyxovirus group. Influenza A virus, a negative-sense ssRNA virus, causes morbidity every winter. They are designated by two major antigenic determinants (hemagglutinin and neuraminidase), which are transmembrane glycoproteins. In recent years, there has been widespread concern about the potential for pandemic spread because of the possibility of animal-to-human and subsequent human-to-human transmission.[97]

Transmission of the influenza virus is by aerosol or direct contact inhalation. As few as three infective particles can transmit the infection, and the majority of infected persons have the symptoms of disease, which, in turn, enhance the likelihood of contagion.[97] This virus is spread in the home and also in poorly ventilated spaces such as ships or airplanes. Antigenic shift—a major change in pathogenic antigens—may lead to epidemic or pandemic infections. The H5N1 variant is an influenza A virus subtype that occurs mainly in birds. Although it usually does not infect people, infections with these viruses have occurred in humans, mostly in those with direct or close contact with H5N1-infected poultry or contaminated surfaces.[155] The strain that infected large numbers of birds in Hong Kong in 1997 failed to cause epidemics because it was minimally infective for humans. Despite widespread exposure, disease in humans remains very rare with only 340 cases confirmed to date.[156]

More than 500,000 people in the United States are hospitalized annually with influenza-associated disease and up to 40,000 patients, primarily high-risk groups such as children and the elderly, die from this infection and its sequelae.[157] Two types of influenza vaccines are currently available: an intramuscular one consisting of three inactivated viruses and an intranasally delivered one that contains live, attenuated influenza virus. Of course, the efficacy of the vaccine can vary with the "match" of virus strains in the vaccine and those in circulation in the population, something which varies from year to year.[158] The recommended age for vaccination has been decreasing in recent years and is as low as 6 months for the inactivated vaccine.

Therapy for Viral Rhinitis

Other than for specific, limited applications (e.g., influenza, herpes), there are currently no approved antiviral medications for the typical, isolated case of viral rhinitis, and thus supportive, symptomatic therapy remains the only option available for patients and their treating physicians. Analgesics and antipyretics are useful for fevers and aches. Topical or systemic decongestants may offer additional symptomatic relief, but they do not prevent progression to bacterial disease. Topical decongestants can provide more symptom relief than do oral decongestants because of greater potency, but their use should be limited to prevent rhinitis medicamentosa. Systemic steroid therapy has not been shown to be effective for viral rhinitis. Many remedial measures such as decongestants, vitamin C, interferon, and traditional remedies play a role in the treatment of viral rhinitis (see later). Others include anticholinergic medications (intranasal ipratroprium), which reduce rhinorrhea, and first-generation antihistamines, which relieve sneezing and reduce secretions, either through anticholinergic effects or via inhibition of histamine pathways.[159–161]

Antihistamines

First-generation antihistamines (e.g., diphenhydramine, triprolidine, chlorpheniramine, brompheniramine, hydroxyzine) are effective[159,161] and in widespread use for rhinorrhea and sneezing associated with viral rhinitis, especially because they are sold over the counter. Because they are lipophilic, they cross the blood-brain barrier and induce central nervous system effects such as sedation, which limits their benefits. Second-generation antihistamines (loratadine, cetirizine, and fexofenadine) are available over the counter, but none are approved by the U.S. Food and Drug Adminstration (FDA) for use in viral rhinitis. In general, these agents are much less sedating than are the first-generation antihistamines, but they are less effective for rhinorrhea, probably because they lack anticholinergic and antimuscarinic effects.[162] Interestingly, these antihistamines down regulate the expression of ICAM-1 in vitro[163]; however, clinical benefits related to this effect remain unclear. Perhaps, in this regard, topical antihistamines may be effective, but there are few data on this possibility.

Anticholinergics

Intranasal ipratropium bromide is another FDA-approved, topical therapeutic agent that is effective for the treatment of rhinorrhea associated with viral rhinitis via its effects on reducing glandular secretions. Nasal irritation and epistaxis may occur with its use. Ipratropium leads to an ~30% reduction in secretions[164,165] and has been examined in combination with oxymetzaoline.[166] Intranasal ipratropium is marketed in two concentrations: 0.03% (approved for treatment of rhinorrhea associated with allergic rhinitis) and 0.06% (approved for treatment of rhinorrhea associated with the common cold).

Decongestants

Other supportive medications in widespread use but of unclear efficacy, include topical and systemic decongestants. Both topical (e.g., phenylephrine, oxymetazoline, naphazoline, tetrahydrozoline, zylometazoline) and oral (pseudoephedrine and phenylephrine) adrenergic agents are widely used for the treatment of nasal congestion. Recent data have suggested that the use of oral decongestants for the common cold is not efficacious.[167] Prolonged use of topical agents may cause rhinitis medicamentosa. One report suggested that oxymetazoline has inhibitory effects on the rhinovirus, but this remains to be confirmed.[168]

Steroids

The evidence in support of the use of intranasal steroids for viral rhinitis is weak.[169] In the lower airway, pretreatment with inhaled budesonide did not significantly affect experimentally induced rhinovirus-16-associated changes in the numbers of any of the inflammatory cell types in mild asthmatics,[170] suggesting that pretreatment with steroids was not sufficient to inhibit this type of low level inflammation, at least in the lower airway. Data suggest that in the nose, steroid prophylaxis suppresses inflammation and cold symptoms during the first 2 days, but not subsequently.[171] The data on steroid use in viral rhinitis present an interesting challenge, especially because steroids down regulate cytokine expression.[172] Barnes and colleagues suggested that some cytokines counteract the glucocorticoid-induced inhibition of the effects of IL-1β,[173,174] a pivotal cytokine in the rhinovirus-induced immune response.[175] Other investigators concluded that rhinovirus infection by itself induces only subtle worsening of airway inflammation in patients with asthma, which is not improved or is worsened by inhaled corticosteroids.[169] The latter finding is in keeping with the limited protection of inhaled corticosteroids against acute exacerbations of asthma.

In a randomized, placebo-controlled, double-blind clinical trial examining kinin levels and symptoms in experimental rhinovirus colds, a 5-day course of oral steroids reduced kinin levels but provided no significant reduction of symptoms. Viral growth was enhanced in the steroid group.[176] The interaction of glucocorticoids, viral rhinitis, and allergic inflammation is likely to be complex and remains understudied.

Other Pharmacotherapies (Over-the-Counter)

Because cough is a common symptom, nonprescription cough remedies may be helpful, as may nonsteroidal anti-inflammatory drugs (NSAIDs), which control related systemic symptoms such as pain, myalgias, and fever.

Complementary and Alternative Medicine

Other, nonpharmacologic therapies suggested but which are not proven to be successful include heated, humidified steam[177,178]; nasal saline; and herbal remedies.

Steam

Heated, humidified steam is a common home remedy for viral rhinitis that is widely considered to provide relief.[179] Its use stems from the simple premise that steam may help secretion drainage and that heat may inhibit or inactivate viral pathogens. Some data suggest that raising the mucosal temperature will inhibit rhinovirus replication.[180] Rhinotherm is a commercially available device that was developed for delivering such therapy, but studies on its use have shown conflicting results. In a Cochrane review, Singh assessed the effects of inhaling steam in the treatment of the common cold by comparing symptoms, viral shedding, and nasal resistance.[178] Of the six trials meeting the inclusion criteria of this rigorous review, three showed benefits of steam for symptom relief. Results on symptom indices were equivocal. The treatments were universally safe, with minor side effects and no worsening of symptom scores. Results on nasal resistance were varied, with one study showing improvement and one showing no improvement. One study examined viral shedding and antibody titers but no differences between the placebo and the active treatment were found. Singh concluded that steam inhalations are not recommended in the routine treatment of the common cold, pending double-blind, randomized clinical trials. Duration, temperature, delivery method, timing, humidity, and ambient climate remain variables that may affect the results of such investigations. Hot, humid air can be delivered by hot water, tea, or soup, in addition to steam showers and inhalation devices.

Echinacea

Alternative medications, such as *Echinacea* preparations or zinc lozenges, have been tested in several trials, but have not been found to be effective. Native American tribes discovered the potential of *Echinacea* in the treatment of cough, sore throat, snake bites, and pain.[181] A wide body of literature is devoted to the role of *Echinacea* in the prevention and treatment of the common cold, including viral rhinitis. *Echinacea* is one of the best-selling herbal medications in the United States, with annual sales of more than $300 million.[182] Preparations made from these plants are widely used worldwide for the prevention and treatment of colds. Hundreds of studies have detailed *Echinacea*'s properties and examined its clinical effects[183] with inconclusive results.

Preparations mainly include various parts of the plant from three species: *Echinacea purpurea, E. angustifolia,* and *E. pallida*. These may include refined or unrefined preparations; flowers, leaves, stems, and roots, or other parts of the plant; and/or mixtures with other products. The extracts are manufactured by a variety of methods and are delivered in a variety of ways.[184]

Overall, the literature is equivocal regarding the efficacy of *Echinacea*, perhaps because of the study designs and quality, patient heterogeneity, variability in preparation, lack of objective improvement by validated outcome measures, lack of clear definitions in randomization and blinding, limited sample size and power, and limited generalizability.[182–188] A recent Cochrane review concluded from five randomized trials that there was still insufficient evidence to recommend *Echinacea* preparations for the prevention of the common cold. In addition, observed effect sizes (~15%) may be clinically irrelevant.[189] Schoop et al. performed a meta-analysis that suggested that standardized extracts of *Echinacea* were more effective in the prevention of symptoms of the common cold after clinical inoculation as compared with a placebo.[190] Definitive large, prospective clinical trials are required for confirmation of this finding. The best data are consistent with a 10 to 15% reduction in relative risk in the prevention of colds.[191] *Echinacea* may have a beneficial effect on virus-inducing inflammation, perhaps by reducing the relevant cytokine levels in the nose.[192,193] The effects of *Echinacea* on such proinflammatory cytokines in nasal secretions during colds has not been shown in vivo to date.

Zinc

Zinc lozenges have long been marketed for reducing the symptoms and duration of the common cold. Numerous studies have examined the efficacy of zinc for the treatment of viral rhinitis. Zinc preparations have been shown to inhibit viral replication in vitro, but not in vivo, and clinical studies have yielded variable results.[194–197] Further, significantly more adverse events have been reported among school-age children who were taking zinc in a placebo-controlled RCT.[198] Topical preparations of zinc have been associated with loss of olfaction, although these reports are confounded by the fact that viral rhinitis itself can cause olfactory loss. A more common side effect is a bad taste in the mouth.

Nasal Saline

Nasal irrigation with sodium chloride solutions is thought to reduce nasal dryness, facilitate the clearing of secretions, and provide symptomatic relief. A variety of modalities are available for delivery[199,200] and a recent Cochrane analysis suggested a benefit in patients with chronic rhinosinusitis.[201,202] One study showed some benefit in patients with URIs[203]; further study is required for clear indications. This therapy is a good adjunctive with minimal risks.[199]

Acidic Buffers

Gern and colleagues reported that a low pH inhibited replication of several rhinovirus serotypes as well as the influenza virus in vitro.[204] Additionally, preliminary experiments demonstrated the ability to lower the pH of the human nasopharynx by topical administration of citrate/phosphate buffers. These sprays were well tolerated and were able to reduce viral shedding, although respiratory symptoms were not reduced significantly. Animal models provide supportive data for this form of therapy.[205] This represents another therapeutic venue that may reduce rates of viral transmission in the future.

Antibiotics

Antibiotics are not recommended because they are ineffective for viral illness and do not relieve symptoms. The unnecessary use of antibiotics for viral rhinitis has an adverse impact on cost and has the potential for side effects, drug–drug interactions, and bacterial resistance.

Immunomodulators

In the research setting, several immunomodulators have been studied as therapy for viral rhinitis.[124] These include immunostimulants such as intranasal IFN-α2,[206–211] agents that block virus uncoating such as pleconaril,[212] molecules that target the viral genome coding region such as enviroxime,[213] and protease inhibitors.[214,215] Some of these agents have shown promise, but they are limited by toxicity, their side effect profile, or a lack of efficacy in the natural setting.[216]

Vaccines, Monoclonals, and Antiviral Therapies

A limited arsenal of vaccines and antiviral agents exists in the treatment of viral illness, but these weapons are directed primarily at major illnesses in the lower airway rather than nasal disease. Patients at risk for severe influenza-induced lower respiratory illness can be actively immunized with influenza vaccines.[217] However, the development of vaccines for the prevention of viral rhinitis has been limited by the biological challenges of the large number of viruses that have great antigenic variability, by concerns about resistance, and by the complexity of host-pathogen interaction. Currently, clinical trials of live-attenuated parainfluenza type 3 and type 1 vaccines are being conducted.[218]

Palivizumab is a monoclonal antibody that exhibits neutralizing and fusion-inhibitory activity against RSV. This biologic agent reduces pulmonary RSV replication 100-fold in animal models and has been shown in human in vivo studies to have neutralizing activity in the lungs in randomized trials.[219] In the United States, indications for use include lower airway disease in children under 2 years of age who have chronic lung disease, a history of prematurity, or significant congenital heart disease.[220] Prophylactic intravenous infusion is performed monthly during the RSV season (typically November to April or early May). Interestingly, rhinitis is reported to be one side effect of this medication. Additionally, anti-RSV immunoglobulin is available in some countries (but no longer in the United States) for passive immunization (see later).[221,222]

Ribavirin has long been known as a broad-spectrum antiviral agent. Even though it was used in SARS patients, its efficacy in this setting remains questionable, and in vitro studies did not show significant antiviral activity in this disease.[223] Current data do not support the use of ribavirin for treating SARS in humans. It is currently indicated for lower airway RSV infection.

Two classes of antiviral chemotherapeutic agents are currently available for treatment of influenza: the M2 ion-channel inhibitors (amantadine and rimantadine) and the neuraminidase inhibitors (oseltamivir and zanamivir). The neuraminidase inhibitors are effective for the treatment and prophylaxis of influenza A and B, whereas the M2 ion channel inhibitors are active only against influenza A viruses. Only the neuraminidase inhibitors are currently recommended for use in influenza as a result of surveillance data on drug resistance. Indications for these agents include both therapy and prophylaxis. Guidelines are available and are updated annually based on current data.[224] These medications may be given systemically or in aerolized forms; they can reduce the severity of illness and shorten the duration of illness and may prevent serious complications, but they must be started within 48 hours of the onset of symptoms. A detailed study of efficacy is not yet available for some of these agents,[225] and they are not indicated for isolated viral rhinitis.

Prevention

Prevention is perhaps the best approach to viral rhinitis.[226] Because the spread of rhinovirus and coronavirus occurs through hand-to-hand transmission, frequent hand washing and avoiding contact with mucous membranes are critical in the prevention of transmission. Topical preparations that eliminate the virus on human skin are in development,[227] generally taking advantage of the use of the inhibitory effects of organic acids on viral proteins.

Reducing aerosol spread and improving hand hygiene are key public health measures for the prevention of spread. Infrequent hand washing has been associated with higher frequencies of URIs. Hence, simple, frequent hand washing is a critical step that should be recommended by physicians because intervention studies show up to a 44% risk reduction in transmission in institutional settings.[228,229] In contrast, in the home, a randomized, double-blind clinical trial showed no benefit to antimicrobial cleaning/hygiene products in the transmission of URIs.[230] Another randomized trial[231] showed a trend toward lower household transmission of URIs with increased use of an alcohol-based cleanser. Nevertheless, several studies have shown that the use of alcohol and other products (e.g., benzalkonium rinses) can reduce absenteeism caused by illness as well as reduce URI symptoms and the number of URIs.[231–235]

Current recommendations include the use of alcohol-based hand sanitizers and environmental interventions such as washing fomites. Additionally, the reduction of aerosol spread can be promoted through education on aseptic nose wiping and cough etiquette protocols.

■ Other Pathogens

A host of other pathogens may cause rhinitis. Most of these include unusual symptoms or physical findings in the nose and occur in the context of disease in other body locations. The range of these pathogens is broad and includes bacteria, fungi, protozoa, and parasites.[236] These agents are prevalent in many developing countries and are rare in the United States, although they may be more prevalent in areas with a large number of recent immigrants from endemic areas.

Bacterial infection is discussed elsewhere in this text. Outside the context of the typical acute rhinosinusitis pathogens, other infectious agents include *Actinomyces, Corynebacterium, Mycobacterium tuberculosis, Klebsiella* (the cause of rhinoscleroma), and *Treponema* species. Protozoa such as the *Leshmania* species can produce nasal symptoms, as can parasites such as *Chryosomyia* and *Rhinosporidium*. A host of fungal organisms can cause rhinitis, including *Aspergillus, Mucor, Cryptococcus, Histoplasma, Sporothrix*, and *Candida* species.

New Horizons

Human Models

Human experimental models of infection have been used for studies of a variety of factors in viral upper respiratory tract infections for more than 40 years.[237–241] Human volunteer studies of rhinovirus infections have clarified important aspects related to virus transmission, infectivity, culture, serologic responses, and immunity in normal subjects.[242,243] Modern applications of these techniques have been invaluable.[109,120,244–246] Experimental disease studies in volunteers have elucidated important aspects of the pathogenesis of viral diseases and associated lung complications in humans, including mediators involved, symptomatology, serologic and immune responses, duration of illness, transmission of disease, and efficacy of medications and of other interventions. The genesis of modern studies dates from those that employed virus inocula from tissue cultures and also from nasal washings from volunteers or from groups living in isolation (e.g., the Common Cold Unit, Salisbury, UK).[247] A fascinating account of this work was recently published.[248]

One curious finding in these studies has been that not all inoculated subjects become infected, and not all subjects who are infected become symptomatic.[243] These methods have shown that the severity of viral rhinitis may be related to the local production of proinflammatory cytokines. As an example, Skoner compared the pattern of nasal proinflammatory cytokine elaboration in asymptomatic and symptomatic subjects who were experimentally infected with rhinovirus.[49] He showed elevations in certain locally produced cytokines during symptomatic but not asymptomatic respiratory rhinovirus infection. Clear delineation of the precise cytokines involved in disease and symptom genesis could lead to the development of novel, targeted therapies, even though redundancies in the system may prove difficult to surmount.

Another method of studying viral respiratory tract infections in human subjects is the use of ex vivo studies. For example, recent work has demonstrated a deficient induction of interferons in lung cells obtained from asthmatic donors in response to rhinovirus infection.[249,250]

Despite some limitations, human models of viral rhinitis will continue to provide opportunities for translational research on viral rhinitis and related problems such as COPD and asthma exacerbations in the relevant species. One exciting example of this is a recent report of a biomarker, IFN-γ induced protein 10 (IP-10), the release of which has been suggested to be specific to acute virus-induced asthma. This study suggests the possibility of a serum assay for markers that may predict a viral trigger for acute asthma.[251]

Animal Models

Rhinovirus

Attempts to develop animal models of rhinovirus infections in many animal species have failed,[252] an obstacle that has severely hampered research into molecular pathophysiology and therapeutic design. Because 10% of rhinovirus serotypes can use both the human and mouse forms of the receptor to enter cells of either species, these serotypes can be manipulated directly in the mouse. Bartlett et al. have developed an in vivo mouse model rhinovirus-induced asthma exacerbation by using the species-common rhinovirus infection as well as transgenic models of human-specific serotypes.[252] These models have several relevant disease-related features such as lower airway neutrophilic and lymphocytic inflammation, mucin secretion, and chemokine and proinflammatory cytokine responses.

Respiratory Syncytial Virus

Initial work on a model development for RSV was limited.[253] However, Coates and Chanock demonstrated susceptibility of the ferret to RSV in a search for animal models involving several other species[254]; work that was replicated by Prince and Porter.[255] This model was left derelict due to a lack of bronchiolar involvement, which limited its usefulness; nevertheless, it should be noted that the virus was identified in the nasal turbinates and that age had an influence on susceptibility to infection.

Newer studies of RSV infection in mice have been used for investigation of innate immunity, including dendritic cell development. Beyer demonstrated a continuous increase in the number of mature dendritic cells after the establishment of infection,[256] suggesting that immune responses are important in viral infection. From these data and studies on human RSV infection, it seems that RSV may induce DC maturation, but disables their ability to secrete IL-12. In this way, RSV infection biases the immune system toward a Th2-type response by inhibiting DC function and altering the cytokine microenvironment.[257] These models allow for molecular immunologic dissection of immune responses to this important pathogen.

In mouse models, intranasal infection with RSV results in viral replication in the lower airway, with resultant inflammation[258,259] and airway hyperresponsiveness.[260–262] Such models have shown that RSV infection facilitates the development of allergic airway inflammation and lower airway hyperresponsiveness.

The common cotton rat has also been employed as an experimental host for RSV infection.[263] Unlike the ferret, in the rats lower airway, disease could be generated. This model was confirmed by a second group.[264] Newer work has demonstrated the utility of the cotton rat as a tool for studying influenza pathogenesis, including innate and adaptive responses.[265] These models are not only devoted to dissecting pathophysiology, but also used in preclinical trials of therapies.

Parainfluenza

Experimental parainfluenza type 3 virus infections in hamsters were developed by Buthala.[266] Guinea pigs are known to be susceptible to parainfluenza infection, but they can develop immunity and may require colonies devoid of exposure.[267] More recently, transgenic approaches have been used for the development of modern models of infection with this pathogen.[268]

Influenza

Several groups have published studies on mouse models of influenza infection[269] that included the study of innate immunity.[270] The development of the current concepts of immunity to influenza, and the role of the secretory immune system in mucosal defense against it, relied extensively on these models. As an example, in mice deficient for IL-6 or in those treated with IL-1ra, symptoms of influenza were partially reduced.[271] Moreover, mortality was reduced in animals treated with IL-1ra. In perhaps a more pressing example, recent data demonstrated that ribavirin enhanced the infectivity of SARS-CoV in mice.[272] The effects of ribvarins have been questionable in human studies that were compromised by the nature of clinical work in humans.

Osterhaus developed primate models of other viral respiratory diseases in response to worldwide efforts to prepare for epidemics. For example, this group investigated the use of influenza A virus vaccines in macaques. Some protection was observed in this model.[273] Similar prevention studies of vaccines have been reported in mouse models.[274] Other studies have provided insights into innate immune responses to influenza. Murine studies with the use of reconstructed 1918 influenza virus showed elevated innate immune responses, including high cytokine levels and severe pulmonary pathology,[275,276] providing hints as to one reason why the epidemic affected primarily young, healthy adults and killed millions of people worldwide. A detailed analysis of the nasal passages has not been performed in these models.

Sendai Virus

Naclerio's group developed a mouse model of rhinosinusitis and used it to study viral rhinitis.[277] Mice were inoculated intranasally with the Sendai virus (a murine parainfluenza virus) or the ultraviolet-inactivated Sendai virus. Nasal lavage was employed for viral cultures, and inflammation in tissue was monitored by flow cytometry. Culture data demonstrated early virus growth and subsequent clearance by 10 days. This process corresponded to inflammatory cell infiltrates and symptoms such as sneezing and nasal irritation as measured by nose rubs. Not only did this model show acute symptoms, but abnormalities on histamine challenges persisted for up to 36 days. This mouse model has some parallels to chronic rhinosinusitis after a viral infection in humans. Further development of this model may allow molecular manipulation of factors involved in the pathophysiology.[277]

SARS-CoV

In response to the SARS epidemic, several groups infected macaques with SARS-CoV to develop models of this important viral illness.[278,279] These models showed effects that were similar pathologically to human SARS. This health crisis led to the development of animal models for the testing of vaccines and antiviral therapies. More recent studies demonstrated that ribavirin even enhanced the infectivity of SARS-CoV in mice.[272] Newer methods under study in these models for use in SARS include target virus entry, fusion with host cells, replication machinery, viral proteases using small molecules, RNA interference, interferons, and other drugs.

In summary, animal models represent an opportunity to understand disease biology and to manipulate therapeutic strategies. As in most diseases, they entail some limitations regarding the applicability of the results to humans because of inherent species differences.

Genome Studies

Recent molecular genetic analyses of the rhinovirus have begun to unravel the relationships between serotypes, the functionality of the variation in the pathogen genome, and the pathobiology of disease.[280–287] A sophisticated evolutionary analysis of the rhinovirus genome has begun to provide a better understanding of the genetic diversity and evolutionary pressures affecting this pathogen and its relationship to other viruses.[288,289] This knowledge may begin the process of genome-directed, targeted therapy. Rhinoviruses share extensive genomic sequence similarity with enteroviruses, and both are part of the picornavirus family. Nevertheless, they differ significantly at the phenotypic level. Surprisingly, little is known about their genetic variability. Some critical regions have been sequenced for a large number of rhinovirus serotypes (capsid proteins, etc.), but a number remain to be analyzed. Some genome data are available online,[290] and newer data are emerging with the number of full-length sequences that are available increasing,[289] thus allowing for new insights into the molecular genetics of this important pathogen.

Zdobnov et al. recently reported the complete genome sequences of 12 rhinovirus serotypes, more than doubling the current number of available rhinovirus sequences.[291] Phylogenetic analysis suggests that HRV-B and human enteroviruses diverged from the last common ancestor after their separation from HRV-A. This group also identified the presence of a replication element present in one serotype (B), but not in another (A). These data allow for the future study of how genomic differences in these and related pathogens account for both biological similarities and differences (e.g., tissue tropism, temperature adaptation, acid lability) of these viruses. The isolation of rhinovirus C along with sequencing-based classification methods are allowing for a new discussion of how to distinguish these pathogens.[292] Genomic approaches may elucidate the evolutionary biology of this important pathogen and allow the development of targeted agents for this virus and related ones.[291]

The full genome sequence analysis of the rhinovirus supports the current classification of rhinovirus into two distinct species reflective of the capsid type, but this classification does not reflect variation in all parts of the rhinovirus genome.[291] The rhinovirus genome consists of ~7200 base pairs. Rhinoviruses belong to the *Picornaviridae* family and are closely related to the enterovirus, but the pathogens remain distinct clinically and phenotypically, both in vivo and in vitro. The genome organization of *Picornaviridae* is conserved among family members with a long 5′-untranslated region, a single open reading frame encoding a polyprotein, a short 3′ untranslated segment, and a polyA tail.[293–296] Exact methods employed by the rhinovirus for invasion and replication are not well understood.

Relationship to Lower Airway Disease

Asthma

Recent epidemiologic studies have suggested that the rhinovirus may be associated with the majority of exacerbations of asthma.[297] Peaks in asthma hospitalization in school-age children have been linked with a return to school after summer vacation.[298] Analysis of these data revealed that the magnitude of the peak increased up to age 7 years, declined from age 7 to 18, and remained stable until age 50. Interestingly, there was a geographic variation with an earlier peak in northern latitudes, perhaps suggesting the close contact that would predispose one to the transmission of a viral infection. Viral infections have been shown to be associated with as high as 80% of asthma exacerbations in this age group. The strong correlation with a return to school in older children suggested that returning to school may accelerate the transmission of rhinovirus infections. Similar results have been obtained from countries with different return-to-school times, with peaks in asthma hospitalizations occurring 2 to 3 weeks after school return. In Scotland and Sweden, the peaks are of lesser amplitude than are those in Canada and England.[299]

Using a case control approach in patients with emergency room exacerbations versus patients with similarly severe asthma who did not get an exacerbation, Sears et al. used questionnaires, skin-prick allergen testing, and microbiological testing of nasal mucus for human rhinoviruses, adenoviruses, influenza A and B viruses, parainfluenza viruses, coronaviruses, respiratory syncytial viruses A and B, *Chlamydia pneumoniae*, and *Mycoplasma pneumoniae* to evaluate these patients. Of asthma cases, 62% had an identifiable respiratory virus infection compared with 42% of controls.[300]

Up to 80% of asthma exacerbations are associated with viral upper respiratory tract infections.[301,302] This is true both in young children, most obviously with RSV,[303] and in adults.[304] In the majority of cases, rhinoviruses are implicated, but similar problems can occur secondary to coronaviruses, influenza viruses, parainfluenza viruses, RSV, and metapneumovirus—a recently discovered pathogen (see Novel Pathogens).[305] Growing interest will require new human volunteer studies for examining this observation in greater depth. Significant increases in T cells and eosinophils are seen in biopsy studies of the lower airway during rhinovirus infections. Experimental studies of rhinovirus infections in allergic individuals have demonstrated new late asthmatic reactions to allergen provocation in association with infections[47,302,306] and, in allergics, potentiated airway inflammation after bronchoprovocation,[307] highlighting the value of examining this issue in vivo. These and other studies have shown that airway obstruction, airway inflammation, and airway responsiveness are induced following rhinovirus infections in asthmatic subjects.

By the use of immunohistochemistry and quantitative PCR, a rhinovirus can be detected in the lower airway (sputum and biopsy) in a large number of subjects during a cold,[308] suggesting another link between upper and lower airway disease. Papadopoulos detected rhinovirus in the lower airways after intranasal inoculation,[309] and in situ hybridization showed the replicative strand of rhinovirus present in the lower airways in experimental studies.[310]

Clinical studies, which have been replicated in vitro, suggest that the rhinovirus stimulates exacerbations of asthma by inducing bronchial epithelial cell production of IL-8, a neutrophil chemoattractant, leading to a neutrophilic inflammatory response.[48,85,311–314] Other cytokines are likely to be involved in lower airway responses to viral rhinitis as well. For example, Proud's recent data suggest that IL-17A can modify epithelial responses to the rhinovirus that would favor the recruitment of neutrophils, immature dendritic cells, and memory T cells to the airways.[315] IL-17A is a proinflammatory cytokine whose receptor is present on a wide range of cell types, including epithelial cells.[316] The numbers of IL-17A-expressing T cells are increased in the airways of patients with asthma,[317] and levels of IL-17A detected in the sputum of patients with asthma and chronic bronchitis correlate with airway hyperresponsiveness.[318] IL-17A plays a role in host defense and neutrophil recruitment and strongly induces the production of a defensin from human epithelial cells,[319] providing a link between the innate and specific immune responses to a rhinovirus.[320] Innate immune responses may be defective in bronchial epithelial cells from asthmatic subjects. Additionally, these epithelial cells show impaired production of interferon and apoptosis, which may predispose one to increased rhinovirus replication.[250,321] This body of literature provides a link between innate and adaptive immune systems and also links clinical viral infection in the upper and lower airway.[322]

Thus, the previously listed data suggest that the effects of viral URIs on the lower airway could have several mechanisms at play. Among the more direct mechanisms would be aspiration of secretions from the upper airway to the lower airway, with a resultant transmission of infection or direct deposition of viruses in the lower airway at the time of an upper respiratory illness. Indirectly, the negative effect of URIs on the lower airway could be related to systemic inflammatory responses, or to neurogenic mechanisms linking the upper to the lower airway.

Chronic Obstructive Pulmonary Disease

As with asthma, epidemiologic studies have documented the involvement of viral rhinitis in exacerbations of chronic bronchitis,[262,323] including rhinovirus and CoV. The mechanisms may reflect upregulation of ICAM-1 in the bronchial mucosa of patients with COPD, production of inflammatory mediators,[324] or the interaction of respiratory virus with bacterial pathogens.[124]

Novel Diagnostics

Recently, a DNA microarray bearing the most conserved sequences of all known viruses of humans, animals, plants, and microbes has been developed.[325,326] This technology and others like it have the advantage of being comprehensive and able to detect new pathogens by cross-hybridization.[327,328] Boushey's group applied this microarray to study the diversity of viral pathogens in viral rhinitis in adults with and without asthma.[288] This test detected viruses in a higher proportion of samples than did culture isolation, with comparable sensitivity and specificity to pathogen-specific PCR. The breadth of this technology—to determine in a single test, the entire spectrum of known respiratory viral pathogens—presents the possibility for an advanced understanding of the viral pathophysiology in upper respiratory tract infections and related diseases.

Other novel diagnostic technologies have been reported. The Respiratory MultiCode-PLx Assay (EraGen Biosciences, Madison, WI) is a new multitarget, high-throughput detection platform technology that can be adapted to multiple uses, including the detection of viral genomes.[329–331] This technology uses multiplex PCR chemistry coupled with high-throughput microsphere flow cytometry and has been employed for detecting the presence of the conserved sequences of all available respiratory virus sequences for eight distinct groups: rhinovirus, RSV, parainfluenza virus, influenza virus, metapneumovirus, adenovirus, coronavirus, and enterovirus.[332] Preliminary work with this technology has shown it to be an accurate, sensitive, and practical test.[333] These and other technologies hold promise for practical use in large clinical studies of respiratory viruses and, with further development, for routine clinical use in diagnostic virology laboratories. They may also be useful for the surveillance of emerging or reemerging respiratory viruses, such as SARS-CoV or the avian influenza virus.[334]

As another example, using a multiplex MassTag PCR platform, Lamson recently detected numerous pathogens in samples that had been submitted for laboratory diagnosis but that had tested negative during a routine diagnostic assessment.[335] Several rhinoviruses were identified, and genetic analysis indicated that a large fraction of these viruses represent a previously uncharacterized type of rhinovirus that is divergent from the two common lineages/serotype categories. In a subsequent report, they found that infections with the novel rhinovirus were associated with rhinitis and also with bronchitis, bronchiolitis, and pneumonia.[336] It is likely that similar tools will allow novel community- and hospital-based laboratory tests for use in research and in clinical practice.

Lastly, advances in second- and third-generation sequencing techologies bring the possibility of DNA- and RNA-based diagnostic tools for clinical use.

Novel Viruses

Several new respiratory viruses have recently been discovered, including most infamously the SARS CoV, which emerged in 2002, as well as the bocavirus.[258] MPV and CoV NL63 were also discovered recently.[337,338] Discovered in 2001, human metapneumovirus (hMPV) is a member of the paramyxovirus family. This pathogen has been associated with upper and lower respiratory tract infections, most commonly in young children, elderly subjects, and immunocompromised patients, and can account for up to 10% of hospitalizations of children suffering from acute respiratory tract infections.[339] Clinically, these infections mimic RSV,[340] but they cause greater pathology in the lower airway and less in the upper airway, including the nasopharynx, which shows less marked changes in inflammatory markers.[341] Manifestations range from common colds and mild URIs to more severe lower airway diseases (bronchiolitis and pneumonia). Other symptoms include those typical for a URI (cough, wheezing, coryza, fever) and may include disorders in related anatomic sites, such as acute otitis media.[341] This area is under intense study.[342]

The precise role of these new pathogens in disease has yet to be elucidated, but advances in molecular genetics and genomics are likely to lead to broader coverage of viral species and deeper insights into their role in viral rhinitis and other forms of atypical nasal complaints.

Conclusion

In this chapter, we focused on infectious rhinitis of viral etiology, which is the most common cause of infections of the upper respiratory tract. We discussed and described the different offending viruses as well as the pathophysiology of their effects. The clinical presentation of this disease and treatment measures were described. For the most part, these consist of supportive symptomatic treatment. Finally, new frontiers in research related to these viruses and their effects on the nose and the lower airway were discussed, which allows a peek into the future of this exciting area of rhinology.

Acknowledgments

Jamie Phillips assisted with the preparation of this work. Elisabeth Lanzl provided editorial assistance. Jayant M. Pinto is supported by an American Geriatrics Society Dennis W. Jahnigen Career Development Scholars Award, a New Investigator Award from the American Rhinologic Society, and the McHugh Otolaryngology Research Fund.

References

1. National Center for Health Statistics. Current Estimates from National Health Interview Survey. Vital Health Stat 10 1985;10:854–1578
2. Doyle WJ, Gentile DA, Skoner DP. Viral and bacterial rhinitis. Clin Allergy Immunol 2007;19:177–195
3. Quillen DM, Feller DB. Diagnosing rhinitis: allergic vs. nonallergic. Am Fam Physician 2006;73(9):1583–1590
4. Dykewicz MS, Fineman S, Skoner DP, et al. Diagnosis and management of rhinitis: complete guidelines of the Joint Task Force on Practice Parameters in Allergy, Asthma and Immunology. American Academy of Allergy, Asthma, and Immunology. Ann Allergy Asthma Immunol 1998;81(5 Pt 2):478–518
5. Gwaltney JM Jr, Phillips CD, Miller RD, Riker DK. Computed tomographic study of the common cold. N Engl J Med 1994;330(1):25–30
6. Monto AS, Ullman BM. Acute respiratory illness in an American community. The Tecumseh study. JAMA 1974;227(2):164–169
7. Gwaltney JM Jr. Epidemiology of the common cold. Ann N Y Acad Sci 1980;353:54–60
8. National Institute of Allergy and Infectious Disease. Common cold. http://www.niaid.nih.gov/topics/commonCold/Pages/default.aspx. Accessed September 7, 2011
9. Fendrick AM, Monto AS, Nightengale B, Sarnes M. The economic burden of non-influenza-related viral respiratory tract infection in the United States. Arch Intern Med 2003;163(4):487–494
10. Centers for Disease Control and Prevention. Stopping germs at home, work, and school. http://www.cdc.gov/germstopper/home_work_school.htm. Accessed September 7, 2011
11. Monto AS, Sullivan KM. Acute respiratory illness in the community. Frequency of illness and the agents involved. Epidemiol Infect 1993;110(1):145–160
12. Monto AS. Medical reviews. Coronaviruses. Yale J Biol Med 1974;47(4):234–251
13. Wat D. The common cold: a review of the literature. Eur J Intern Med 2004;15(2):79–88
14. Wald ER, Dashefsky B, Byers C, Guerra N, Taylor F. Frequency and severity of infections in day care. J Pediatr 1988;112(4):540–546
15. Alho OP, Koivu M, Sorri M, Rantakallio P. Risk factors for recurrent acute otitis media and respiratory infection in infancy. Int J Pediatr Otorhinolaryngol 1990;19(2):151–161
16. Stein RT, Sherrill D, Morgan WJ, et al. Respiratory syncytial virus in early life and risk of wheeze and allergy by age 13 years. Lancet 1999;354(9178):541–545
17. Hoffjan S, Nicolae D, Ostrovnaya I, et al. Gene-environment interaction effects on the development of immune responses in the 1st year of life. Am J Hum Genet 2005;76(4):696–704
18. Taussig LM, Wright AL, Holberg CJ, Halonen M, Morgan WJ, Martinez FD. Tucson Children's Respiratory Study: 1980 to present. J Allergy Clin Immunol 2003;111(4):661–675, quiz 676
19. Copenhaver CC, Gern JE, Li Z, et al. Cytokine response patterns, exposure to viruses, and respiratory infections in the first year of life. Am J Respir Crit Care Med 2004;170(2):175–180
20. Walton RP, Johnston SL. Role of respiratory viral infections in the development of atopic conditions. Curr Opin Allergy Clin Immunol 2008;8(2):150–153
21. van Benten IJ, van Drunen CM, Koevoet JL, et al. Reduced nasal IL-10 and enhanced TNFalpha responses during rhinovirus and RSV-induced upper respiratory tract infection in atopic and non-atopic infants. J Med Virol 2005;75(2):348–357
22. Kirchberger S, Majdic O, Stockl J. Modulation of the immune system by human rhinoviruses. Int Arch Allergy Immunol 2007;142(1):1–10
23. Gern JE, Brooks GD, Meyer P, et al. Bidirectional interactions between viral respiratory illnesses and cytokine responses in the first year of life. J Allergy Clin Immunol 2006;117(1):72–78
24. Cohen S, Doyle WJ, Skoner DP. Psychological stress, cytokine production, and severity of upper respiratory illness. Psychosom Med 1999;61(2):175–180
25. Cohen S, Alper CM, Doyle WJ, Treanor JJ, Turner RB. Positive emotional style predicts resistance to illness after experimental exposure to rhinovirus or influenza a virus. Psychosom Med 2006;68(6):809–815
26. Mäkelä MJ, Puhakka T, Ruuskanen O, et al. Viruses and bacteria in the etiology of the common cold. J Clin Microbiol 1998;36(2):539–542
27. Arruda E, Pitkäranta A, Witek TJ Jr, Doyle CA, Hayden FG. Frequency and natural history of rhinovirus infections in adults during autumn. J Clin Microbiol 1997;35(11):2864–2868
28. Gwaltney JM Jr, Hendley JO. Rhinovirus transmission: one if by air, two if by hand. Am J Epidemiol 1978;107(5):357–361
29. Tristram DA, Hicks W Jr, Hard R. Respiratory syncytial virus and human bronchial epithelium. Arch Otolaryngol Head Neck Surg 1998;124(7):777–783
30. Nicholson K. Human Influenza. Oxford: Blackwell; 1998: 219–264
31. Hendley JO, Gwaltney JM Jr, Jordan WS Jr. Rhinovirus infections in an industrial population. IV. Infections within families of employees during two fall peaks of respiratory illness. Am J Epidemiol 1969;89(2):184–196
32. Winther B, Gwaltney JM Jr, Mygind N, Turner RB, Hendley JO. Sites of rhinovirus recovery after point inoculation of the upper airway. JAMA 1986;256(13):1763–1767

33. Winther B. Effects on the nasal mucosa of upper respiratory viruses (common cold). Dan Med Bull 1994;41(2):193–204
34. Gwaltney JM Jr. Rhinovirus infection of the normal human airway. Am J Respir Crit Care Med 1995;152(4 Pt 2):S36–S39
35. Gentile DA, Skoner DP. Viral rhinitis. Curr Allergy Asthma Rep 2001;1(3):227–234
36. Fritz RS, Hayden FG, Calfee DP, et al. Nasal cytokine and chemokine responses in experimental influenza A virus infection: results of a placebo-controlled trial of intravenous zanamivir treatment. J Infect Dis 1999;180(3):586–593
37. Doyle WJ, Skoner DP, Gentile D. Nasal cytokines as mediators of illness during the common cold. Curr Allergy Asthma Rep 2005;5(3):173–181
38. Proud D, Naclerio RM, Gwaltney JM, Hendley JO. Kinins are generated in nasal secretions during natural rhinovirus colds. J Infect Dis 1990;161(1):120–123
39. Naclerio RM, Proud D, Lichtenstein LM, et al. Kinins are generated during experimental rhinovirus colds. J Infect Dis 1988;157(1):133–142
40. Naclerio RM, Proud D, Kagey-Sobotka A, Lichtenstein LM, Hendley JO, Gwaltney JM Jr. Is histamine responsible for the symptoms of rhinovirus colds? A look at the inflammatory mediators following infection. Pediatr Infect Dis J 1988;7(3):218–222
41. Hsia J, Goldstein AL, Simon GL, Sztein M, Hayden FG. Peripheral blood mononuclear cell interleukin-2 and interferon-gamma production, cytotoxicity, and antigen-stimulated blastogenesis during experimental rhinovirus infection. J Infect Dis 1990;162(3): 591–597
42. Röseler S, Holtappels G, Wagenmann M, Bachert C. Elevated levels of interleukins IL-1 beta, IL-6 and IL-8 in naturally acquired viral rhinitis. Eur Arch Otorhinolaryngol 1995;252(Suppl 1):S61–S63
43. Bachert C, van Kempen MJ, Höpken K, Holtappels G, Wagenmann M. Elevated levels of myeloperoxidase, pro-inflammatory cytokines and chemokines in naturally acquired upper respiratory tract infections. Eur Arch Otorhinolaryngol 2001;258(8):406–412
44. Klemens C, Rasp G, Jund F, et al. Mediators and cytokines in allergic and viral-triggered rhinitis. Allergy Asthma Proc 2007;28(4):434–441
45. van Kempen M, Bachert C, Van Cauwenberge P. An update on the pathophysiology of rhinovirus upper respiratory tract infections. Rhinology 1999;37(3):97–103
46. Gentile DA, Villalobos E, Angelini B, Skoner D. Cytokine levels during symptomatic viral upper respiratory tract infection. Ann Allergy Asthma Immunol 2003;91(4):362–367
47. Grünberg K, Timmers MC, Smits HH, et al. Effect of experimental rhinovirus 16 colds on airway hyperresponsiveness to histamine and interleukin-8 in nasal lavage in asthmatic subjects in vivo. Clin Exp Allergy 1997;27(1):36–45
48. Newcomb DC, Sajjan US, Nagarkar DR, Goldsmith AM, Bentley JK, Hershenson MB. Cooperative effects of rhinovirus and TNF-alpha on airway epithelial cell chemokine expression. Am J Physiol Lung Cell Mol Physiol 2007;293(4):L1021–L1028
49. Skoner DP, Gentile DA, Patel A, Doyle WJ. Evidence for cytokine mediation of disease expression in adults experimentally infected with influenza A virus. J Infect Dis 1999;180(1):10–14
50. Hayden FG, Fritz R, Lobo MC, Alvord W, Strober W, Straus SE. Local and systemic cytokine responses during experimental human influenza A virus infection. Relation to symptom formation and host defense. J Clin Invest 1998;101(3):643–649
51. Yoon HJ, Zhu Z, Gwaltney JM Jr, Elias JA. Rhinovirus regulation of IL-1 receptor antagonist in vivo and in vitro: a potential mechanism of symptom resolution. J Immunol 1999;162(12):7461–7469
52. Raza MW, Essery SD, Weir DM, Ogilvie MM, Elton RA, Blackwell CC. Infection with respiratory syncytial virus and water-soluble components of cigarette smoke alter production of tumour necrosis factor alpha and nitric oxide by human blood monocytes. FEMS Immunol Med Microbiol 1999;24(4):387–394
53. Matsuda K, Tsutsumi H, Okamoto Y, Chiba C. Development of interleukin 6 and tumor necrosis factor alpha activity in nasopharyngeal secretions of infants and children during infection with respiratory syncytial virus. Clin Diagn Lab Immunol 1995;2(3):322–324
54. Hornsleth A, Klug B, Nir M, et al. Severity of respiratory syncytial virus disease related to type and genotype of virus and to cytokine values in nasopharyngeal secretions. Pediatr Infect Dis J 1998;17(12):1114–1121
55. Gentile DA, Patel A, Ollila C, et al. Diminished IL-10 production in subjects with allergy after infection with influenza A virus. J Allergy Clin Immunol 1999;103(6):1045–1048
56. Gentile DA, Yokitis J, Angelini BL, Doyle WJ, Skoner DP. Effect of intranasal challenge with interleukin-6 on upper airway symptomatology and physiology in allergic and nonallergic patients. Ann Allergy Asthma Immunol 2001;86(5):531–536
57. Turner RB, Weingand KW, Yeh CH, Leedy DW. Association between interleukin-8 concentration in nasal secretions and severity of symptoms of experimental rhinovirus colds. Clin Infect Dis 1998;26(4):840–846
58. Mallia P, Message SD, Gielen V, et al. Experimental rhinovirus infection as a human model of chronic obstructive pulmonary disease exacerbation. Am J Respir Crit Care Med 2011;183(6):734–742
59. van Drunen Littel-van den Hurk S, Mapletoft JW, Arsic N, Kovacs-Nolan J. Immunopathology of RSV infection: prospects for developing vaccines without this complication. Rev Med Virol 2007;17(1):5–34
60. Wang JP, Kurt-Jones EA, Finberg RW. Innate immunity to respiratory viruses. Cell Microbiol 2007;9(7):1641–1646
61. Schliemer RP. Glucocorticoids: Part A: Mechanism of action in allergic diseases. In: Yundinger JW, Adkinson NF, Busse WW, Bochner BS, eds. Middleton's Allergy: Principles and Practice. Saint Louis: Mosby; 2003
62. Meylan E, Tschopp J. Toll-like receptors and RNA helicases: two parallel ways to trigger antiviral responses. Mol Cell 2006;22(5):561–569
63. Schleimer RP, Kato A, Kern R, Kuperman D, Avila PC. Epithelium: at the interface of innate and adaptive immune responses. J Allergy Clin Immunol 2007;120(6):1279–1284
64. Yu M, Levine SJ. Toll-like receptor, RIG-I-like receptors and the NLRP3 inflammasome: key modulators of innate immune responses to double-stranded RNA viruses. Cytokine Growth Factor Rev 2011;22(2, Issue 2)63–72
65. Kurt-Jones EA, Popova L, Kwinn L, et al. Pattern recognition receptors TLR4 and CD14 mediate response to respiratory syncytial virus. Nat Immunol 2000;1(5):398–401
66. Alexopoulou L, Holt AC, Medzhitov R, Flavell RA. Recognition of double-stranded RNA and activation of NF-kappaB by Toll-like receptor 3. Nature 2001;413(6857):732–738
67. Diebold SS, Kaisho T, Hemmi H, Akira S, Reis e Sousa C. Innate antiviral responses by means of TLR7-mediated recognition of single-stranded RNA. Science 2004;303(5663):1529–1531
68. Kang DC, Gopalkrishnan RV, Lin L, et al. Expression analysis and genomic characterization of human melanoma differentiation associated gene-5, mda-5: a novel type I interferon-responsive apoptosis-inducing gene. Oncogene 2004;23(9):1789–1800
69. Pichlmair A, Schulz O, Tan CP, et al. RIG-I-mediated antiviral responses to single-stranded RNA bearing 5′-phosphates. Science 2006;314(5801):997–1001
70. Kato H, Takeuchi O, Akira S. Cell type specific involvement of RIG-I in antiviral responses. Nippon Rinsho 2006;64(7):1244–1247

71. Hornung V, Ellegast J, Kim S, et al. 5′-Triphosphate RNA is the ligand for RIG-I. Science 2006;314(5801):994–997
72. Smit JJ, Rudd BD, Lukacs NW. Plasmacytoid dendritic cells inhibit pulmonary immunopathology and promote clearance of respiratory syncytial virus. J Exp Med 2006;203(5):1153–1159
73. Rudd BD, Burstein E, Duckett CS, Li X, Lukacs NW. Differential role for TLR3 in respiratory syncytial virus-induced chemokine expression. J Virol 2005;79(6):3350–3357
74. Boukhvalova MS, Prince GA, Soroush L, Harrigan DC, Vogel SN, Blanco JC. The TLR4 agonist, monophosphoryl lipid A, attenuates the cytokine storm associated with respiratory syncytial virus vaccine-enhanced disease. Vaccine 2006;24(23):5027–5035
75. Liu P, Jamaluddin M, Li K, Garofalo RP, Casola A, Brasier AR. Retinoic acid-inducible gene I mediates early antiviral response and Toll-like receptor 3 expression in respiratory syncytial virus-infected airway epithelial cells. J Virol 2007;81(3):1401–1411
76. Stetson DB, Medzhitov R. Recognition of cytosolic DNA activates an IRF3-dependent innate immune response. Immunity 2006;24(1):93–103
77. Haeberle HA, Casola A, Gatalica Z, et al. IkappaB kinase is a critical regulator of chemokine expression and lung inflammation in respiratory syncytial virus infection. J Virol 2004;78(5):2232–2241
78. Bitko V, Velazquez A, Yang L, Yang YC, Barik S. Transcriptional induction of multiple cytokines by human respiratory syncytial virus requires activation of NF-kappa B and is inhibited by sodium salicylate and aspirin. Virology 1997;232(2):369–378
79. Noah TL, Becker S. Respiratory syncytial virus-induced cytokine production by a human bronchial epithelial cell line. Am J Physiol 1993;265(5 Pt 1):L472–L478
80. Monick MM, Yarovinsky TO, Powers LS, et al. Respiratory syncytial virus up-regulates TLR4 and sensitizes airway epithelial cells to endotoxin. J Biol Chem 2003;278(52):53035–53044
81. Arnold R, Konig W. ICAM-1 expression and low-molecular-weight G-protein activation of human bronchial epithelial cells (A549) infected with RSV. J Leukoc Biol 1996;60(6):766–771
82. Garofalo R, Mei F, Espejo R, et al. Respiratory syncytial virus infection of human respiratory epithelial cells up-regulates class I MHC expression through the induction of IFN-beta and IL-1 alpha. J Immunol 1996;157(6):2506–2513
83. Wang X, Lau C, Wiehler S, et al. Syk is downstream of intercellular adhesion molecule-1 and mediates human rhinovirus activation of p38 MAPK in airway epithelial cells. J Immunol 2006;177(10):6859–6870
84. Papadopoulos NG, Papi A, Meyer J, et al. Rhinovirus infection up-regulates eotaxin and eotaxin-2 expression in bronchial epithelial cells. Clin Exp Allergy 2001;31(7):1060–1066
85. Gern JE, Vrtis R, Grindle KA, Swenson C, Busse WW. Relationship of upper and lower airway cytokines to outcome of experimental rhinovirus infection. Am J Respir Crit Care Med 2000;162(6):2226–2231
86. Einarsson O, Geba GP, Zhu Z, Landry M, Elias JA. Interleukin-11: stimulation in vivo and in vitro by respiratory viruses and induction of airways hyperresponsiveness. J Clin Invest 1996;97(4):915–924
87. Heinecke L, Proud D, Sanders S, Schleimer RP, Kim J. Induction of B7-H1 and B7-DC expression on airway epithelial cells by the Toll-like receptor 3 agonist double-stranded RNA and human rhinovirus infection: In vivo and in vitro studies. J Allergy Clin Immunol 2008;121(5):1155–1160
88. Kato A, Favoreto S Jr, Avila PC, Schleimer RP. TLR3- and Th2 cytokine-dependent production of thymic stromal lymphopoietin in human airway epithelial cells. J Immunol 2007;179(2):1080–1087
89. Reche PA, Soumelis V, Gorman DM, et al. Human thymic stromal lymphopoietin preferentially stimulates myeloid cells. J Immunol 2001;167(1):336–343
90. Liu YJ, Soumelis V, Watanabe N, et al. TSLP: an epithelial cell cytokine that regulates T cell differentiation by conditioning dendritic cell maturation. Annu Rev Immunol 2007;25:193–219
91. Lund JM, Alexopoulou L, Sato A, et al. Recognition of single-stranded RNA viruses by Toll-like receptor 7. Proc Natl Acad Sci U S A 2004;101(15):5598–5603
92. Guillot L, Le Goffic R, Bloch S, et al. Involvement of toll-like receptor 3 in the immune response of lung epithelial cells to double-stranded RNA and influenza A virus. J Biol Chem 2005;280(7):5571–5580
93. Diebold SS, Montoya M, Unger H, et al. Viral infection switches non-plasmacytoid dendritic cells into high interferon producers. Nature 2003;424(6946):324–328
94. Opitz B, Rejaibi A, Dauber B, et al. IFNbeta induction by influenza A virus is mediated by RIG-I which is regulated by the viral NS1 protein. Cell Microbiol 2007;9(4):930–938
95. Le Goffic R, Pothlichet J, Vitour D, et al. Cutting edge: Influenza A virus activates TLR3-dependent inflammatory and RIG-I-dependent antiviral responses in human lung epithelial cells. J Immunol 2007;178(6):3368–3372
96. Mira JP, Cariou A, Grall F, et al. Association of TNF2, a TNF-alpha promoter polymorphism, with septic shock susceptibility and mortality: a multicenter study. JAMA 1999;282(6):561–568
97. Tal G, Mandelberg A, Dalal I, et al. Association between common Toll-like receptor 4 mutations and severe respiratory syncytial virus disease. J Infect Dis 2004;189(11):2057–2063
98. Soferman R, Bar-Zohar D, Jurgenson U, Fireman E. Soluble CD14 as a predictor of subsequent development of recurrent wheezing in hospitalized young children with respiratory syncytial virus-induced bronchiolitis. Ann Allergy Asthma Immunol 2004;92(5):545–548
99. Lahti M, Lofgren J, Marttila R, et al. Surfactant protein D gene polymorphism associated with severe respiratory syncytial virus infection. Pediatr Res 2002;51(6):696–699
100. Hoebee B, Bont L, Rietveld E, et al. Influence of promoter variants of interleukin-10, interleukin-9, and tumor necrosis factor-alpha genes on respiratory syncytial virus bronchiolitis. J Infect Dis 2004;189(2):239–247
101. Hacking D, Knight JC, Rockett K, et al. Increased in vivo transcription of an IL-8 haplotype associated with respiratory syncytial virus disease-susceptibility. Genes Immun 2004;5(4):274–282
102. Goetghebuer T, Isles K, Moore C, Thomson A, Kwiatkowski D, Hull J. Genetic predisposition to wheeze following respiratory syncytial virus bronchiolitis. Clin Exp Allergy 2004;34(5):801–803
103. Choi EH, Lee HJ, Yoo T, Chanock SJ. A common haplotype of interleukin-4 gene IL4 is associated with severe respiratory syncytial virus disease in Korean children. J Infect Dis 2002;186(9):1207–1211
104. Lacroix JS, Ricchetti A, Lew D, et al. Symptoms and clinical and radiological signs predicting the presence of pathogenic bacteria in acute rhinosinusitis. Acta Otolaryngol 2002;122(2):192–196
105. Gwaltney JM Jr, Hendley JO, Simon G, Jordan WS Jr. Rhinovirus infections in an industrial population. II. Characteristics of illness and antibody response. JAMA 1967;202(6):494–500
106. Sinus and Allergy Health Partnership. Antimicrobial treatment guidelines for acute bacterial rhinosinusitis. Otolaryngol Head Neck Surg 2000;123(1 Pt 2):5–31
107. Kaiser L, Fritz RS, Straus SE, Gubareva L, Hayden FG. Symptom pathogenesis during acute influenza: interleukin-6 and other cytokine responses. J Med Virol 2001;64(3):262–268
108. Lemanske RF Jr, Jackson DJ, Gangnon RE, et al. Rhinovirus illnesses during infancy predict subsequent childhood wheezing. J Allergy Clin Immunol 2005;116(3):571–577
109. Doyle WJ, Skoner DP, Hayden FG, Buchman CA, Seroky JT, Fireman P. Nasal and otologic effects of experimental influenza A virus infection. Ann Otol Rhinol Laryngol 1994;103(1):59–69

110. Wos M, Sanak M, Soja J, Olechnowicz H, Busse WW, Szczeklik A. The presence of rhinovirus in lower airways of patients with bronchial asthma. Am J Respir Crit Care Med 2008;177(10):1082–1089
111. Rosenfeld RM, Andes D, Bhattacharyya N, et al. Clinical practice guideline: adult sinusitis. Otolaryngol Head Neck Surg 2007;137(3, Suppl)S1–S31
112. Gwaltney JM Jr. Acute community-acquired sinusitis. Clin Infect Dis 1996;23(6):1209–1223, quiz 1224–1225
113. Williams JW Jr, Simel DL, Roberts L, Samsa GP. Clinical evaluation for sinusitis. Making the diagnosis by history and physical examination. Ann Intern Med 1992;117(9):705–710
114. Alho OP, Karttunen TJ, Karttunen R, et al. Subjects with allergic rhinitis show signs of more severely impaired paranasal sinus functioning during viral colds than nonallergic subjects. Allergy 2003;58(8):767–771
115. Alho OP, Karttunen R, Karttunen TJ. Nasal mucosa in natural colds: effects of allergic rhinitis and susceptibility to recurrent sinusitis. Clin Exp Immunol 2004;137(2):366–372
116. Alho OP. Nasal airflow, mucociliary clearance, and sinus functioning during viral colds: effects of allergic rhinitis and susceptibility to recurrent sinusitis. Am J Rhinol 2004;18(6):349–355
117. Alho OP, Ylitalo K, Jokinen K, et al. The common cold in patients with a history of recurrent sinusitis: increased symptoms and radiologic sinusitislike findings. J Fam Pract 2001;50(1):26–31
118. Stammberger H. Endoscopic endonasal surgery—concepts in treatment of recurring rhinosinusitis. Part II. Surgical technique. Otolaryngol Head Neck Surg 1986;94(2):147–156
119. Eccles R, Reilly M, Eccles KS. Changes in the amplitude of the nasal cycle associated with symptoms of acute upper respiratory tract infection. Acta Otolaryngol 1996;116(1):77–81
120. Doyle WJ, Skoner DP, Fireman P, et al. Rhinovirus 39 infection in allergic and nonallergic subjects. J Allergy Clin Immunol 1992;89(5):968–978
121. Bende M, Barrow I, Heptonstall J, et al. Changes in human nasal mucosa during experimental coronavirus common colds. Acta Otolaryngol 1989;107(3-4):262–269
122. Fireman P. Virus-provoked rhinitis in patients who have allergies. Allergy Asthma Proc 2002;23(2):99–102
123. Jang YJ, Kwon HJ, Park HW, Lee BJ. Detection of rhinovirus in turbinate epithelial cells of chronic sinusitis. Am J Rhinol 2006;20(6):634–636
124. Greenberg SB. Rhinovirus and coronavirus infections. Semin Respir Crit Care Med 2007;28(2):182–192
125. Greve JM, Davis G, Meyer AM, et al. The major human rhinovirus receptor is ICAM-1. Cell 1989;56(5):839–847
126. Hofer F, Gruenberger M, Kowalski H, et al. Members of the low density lipoprotein receptor family mediate cell entry of a minor-group common cold virus. Proc Natl Acad Sci U S A 1994;91(5):1839–1842
127. Bochkov YA, Palmenberg AC, Lee WM, et al. Molecular modeling, organ culture and reverse genetics for a newly identified human rhinovirus C. Nat Med 2011;17(5):627–632
128. Sharp HJ, Denman D, Puumala S, Leopold DA. Treatment of acute and chronic rhinosinusitis in the United States, 1999-2002. Arch Otolaryngol Head Neck Surg 2007;133(3):260–265
129. Gwaltney JM Jr, Hendley JO, Phillips CD, Bass CR, Mygind N, Winther B. Nose blowing propels nasal fluid into the paranasal sinuses. Clin Infect Dis 2000;30(2):387–391
130. Hendley JO, Wenzel RP, Gwaltney JM Jr. Transmission of rhinovirus colds by self-inoculation. N Engl J Med 1973;288(26):1361–1364
131. Gwaltney JM. Clinical significance and pathogenesis of viral respiratory infections. Am J Med 2002;112(Suppl 6A):13S–18S
132. Rota PA, Oberste MS, Monroe SS, et al. Characterization of a novel coronavirus associated with severe acute respiratory syndrome. Science 2003;300(5624):1394–1399
133. Peiris JS, Lai ST, Poon LL, et al; SARS study group. Coronavirus as a possible cause of severe acute respiratory syndrome. Lancet 2003;361(9366):1319–1325
134. Muller MP, McGeer A. Severe acute respiratory syndrome (SARS) coronavirus. Semin Respir Crit Care Med 2007;28(2):201–212
135. Poon LL, Guan Y, Nicholls JM, Yuen KY, Peiris JS. The aetiology, origins, and diagnosis of severe acute respiratory syndrome. Lancet Infect Dis 2004;4(11):663–671
136. Peiris JS, Yuen KY, Osterhaus AD, Stöhr K. The severe acute respiratory syndrome. N Engl J Med 2003;349(25):2431–2441
137. Haagmans BL, Osterhaus AD. Coronaviruses and their therapy. Antiviral Res 2006;71(2-3):397–403
138. Yeager CL, Ashmun RA, Williams RK, et al. Human aminopeptidase N is a receptor for human coronavirus 229E. Nature 1992;357(6377):420–422
139. Hofmann H, Pyrc K, van der Hoek L, Geier M, Berkhout B, Pöhlmann S. Human coronavirus NL63 employs the severe acute respiratory syndrome coronavirus receptor for cellular entry. Proc Natl Acad Sci U S A 2005;102(22):7988–7993
140. McIntosh K, Kapikian AZ, Turner HC, Hartley JW, Parrott RH, Chanock RM. Seroepidemiologic studies of coronavirus infection in adults and children. Am J Epidemiol 1970;91(6):585–592
141. Tang P, Louie M, Richardson SE, et al; Ontario Laboratory Working Group for the Rapid Diagnosis of Emerging Infections. Interpretation of diagnostic laboratory tests for severe acute respiratory syndrome: the Toronto experience. CMAJ 2004;170(1):47–54
142. Reed G, Jewett PH, Thompson J, Tollefson S, Wright PF. Epidemiology and clinical impact of parainfluenza virus infections in otherwise healthy infants and young children $<$ 5 years old. J Infect Dis 1997;175(4):807–813
143. Glezen P, Denny FW. Epidemiology of acute lower respiratory disease in children. N Engl J Med 1973;288(10):498–505
144. Chanock RMMB, Collins PL. Parainfluenza Viruses. Philadelphia: Lippincott Williams and Wilkins, 2001:11341–11380.
145. Henrickson KJ, Hoover S, Kehl KS, Hua W. National disease burden of respiratory viruses detected in children by polymerase chain reaction. Pediatr Infect Dis J 2004;23(1, Suppl)S11–S18
146. Medicine Io. Establishing priorities: diseases of importance in the United States New Vaccine Development. Washington, DC: National Academies Press; 1988
147. Mistchenko AS, Diez RA, Mariani AL, et al. Cytokines in adenoviral disease in children: association of interleukin-6, interleukin-8, and tumor necrosis factor alpha levels with clinical outcome. J Pediatr 1994;124(5 Pt 1):714–720
148. Musher DM. How contagious are common respiratory tract infections? N Engl J Med 2003;348(13):1256–1266
149. Everard ML, Milner AD. The respiratory syncitial virus and its role in acute bronchiolitis. Eur J Pediatr 1992;151(9):638–651
150. Garofalo RP, Haeberle H. Epithelial regulation of innate immunity to respiratory syncytial virus. Am J Respir Cell Mol Biol 2000;23(5):581–585
151. Henderson FW, Collier AM, Clyde WA Jr, Denny FW. Respiratory-syncytial-virus infections, reinfections and immunity. A prospective, longitudinal study in young children. N Engl J Med 1979;300(10):530–534
152. Hall CB, Douglas RG Jr, Schnabel KC, Geiman JM. Infectivity of respiratory syncytial virus by various routes of inoculation. Infect Immun 1981;33(3):779–783
153. Henrickson KJ, Hall CB. Diagnostic assays for respiratory syncytial virus disease. Pediatr Infect Dis J 2007;26(11, Suppl)S36–S40
154. Das S, Palmer OP, Leight WD, et al. Cytokine amplification by respiratory syncytial virus infection in human nasal epithelial cells. Laryngoscope 2005;115(5):764–768

155. Centers for Disease Control and Prevention. Key facts about avian influenza (bird flu) and highly pathogenic avian influenza (H5N1) virus. http://www.cdc.gov/flu/avian/gen-info/facts.htm. September 7, 2011
156. Abdel-Ghafar AN, Chotpitayasunondh T, Gao Z, et al; Writing Committee of the Second World Health Organization Consultation on Clinical Aspects of Human Infection with Avian Influenza A (H5N1) Virus. Update on avian influenza A (H5N1) virus infection in humans. N Engl J Med 2008;358(3):261–273
157. Thompson WW, Shay DK, Weintraub E, et al. Mortality associated with influenza and respiratory syncytial virus in the United States. JAMA 2003;289(2):179–186
158. Centers for Disease Control and Prevention (CDC). Interim within-season estimate of the effectiveness of trivalent inactivated influenza vaccine—Marshfield, Wisconsin, 2007-08 influenza season. MMWR Morb Mortal Wkly Rep 2008;57(15):393–398
159. Doyle WJ, McBride TP, Skoner DP, Maddern BR, Gwaltney JM Jr, Uhrin M. A double-blind, placebo-controlled clinical trial of the effect of chlorpheniramine on the response of the nasal airway, middle ear and eustachian tube to provocative rhinovirus challenge. Pediatr Infect Dis J 1988;7(3):229–238
160. Gwaltney JM Jr, Druce HM. Efficacy of brompheniramine maleate for the treatment of rhinovirus colds. Clin Infect Dis 1997;25(5):1188–1194
161. Gwaltney JM Jr, Park J, Paul RA, Edelman DA, O'Connor RR, Turner RB. Randomized controlled trial of clemastine fumarate for treatment of experimental rhinovirus colds. Clin Infect Dis 1996;22(4):656–662
162. Berkowitz RB, Tinkelman DG. Evaluation of oral terfenadine for treatment of the common cold. Ann Allergy 1991;67(6):593–597
163. Paolieri F, Battifora M, Riccio AM, et al. Terfenadine and fexofenadine reduce in vitro ICAM-1 expression on human continuous cell lines. Ann Allergy Asthma Immunol 1998;81(6):601–607
164. Dockhorn R, Grossman J, Posner M, Zinny M, Tinkleman D. A double-blind, placebo-controlled study of the safety and efficacy of ipratropium bromide nasal spray versus placebo in patients with the common cold. J Allergy Clin Immunol 1992;90(6 Pt 2): 1076–1082
165. Gaffey MJ, Hayden FG, Boyd JC, Gwaltney JM Jr. Ipratropium bromide treatment of experimental rhinovirus infection. Antimicrob Agents Chemother 1988;32(11):1644–1647
166. Pitkäranta A, Wecker MT, Korts DC, Hayden FG. Combined intranasal ipratropium bromide and oxymetazoline in experimental rhinovirus infection. Am J Rhinol 1998;12(2):125–129
167. Latte J, Taverner D. Clinical trial of 3 days of treatment with oral pseudoephedrine for the common cold in the southern hemisphere. Am J Rhinol 2007;21(4):452–455
168. Koelsch S, Tschaikin M, Sacher F. Anti-rhinovirus-specific activity of the alpha-sympathomimetic oxymetazoline. Arzneimittelforschung 2007;57(7):475–482
169. Malm L. Pharmacological background to decongesting and anti-inflammatory treatment of rhinitis and sinusitis. Acta Otolaryngol Suppl 1994;515:53–55, discussion 55–56
170. Grünberg K, Sharon RF, Sont JK, et al. Rhinovirus-induced airway inflammation in asthma: effect of treatment with inhaled corticosteroids before and during experimental infection. Am J Respir Crit Care Med 2001;164(10 Pt 1):1816–1822
171. Farr BM, Gwaltney JM Jr, Hendley JO, et al. A randomized controlled trial of glucocorticoid prophylaxis against experimental rhinovirus infection. J Infect Dis 1990;162(5):1173–1177
172. Barnes PJ. Anti-inflammatory actions of glucocorticoids: molecular mechanisms. Clin Sci (Lond) 1998;94(6):557–572
173. Chizzolini C, Chicheportiche R, Burger D, Dayer JM. Human Th1 cells preferentially induce interleukin (IL)-1beta while Th2 cells induce IL-1 receptor antagonist production upon cell/cell contact with monocytes. Eur J Immunol 1997;27(1):171–177
174. Kovalovsky D, Páez Pereda M, Sauer J, et al. The Th1 and Th2 cytokines IFN-gamma and IL-4 antagonize the inhibition of monocyte IL-1 receptor antagonist by glucocorticoids: involvement of IL-1. Eur J Immunol 1998;28(7):2075–2085
175. Gern JE, Dick EC, Lee WM, et al. Rhinovirus enters but does not replicate inside monocytes and airway macrophages. J Immunol 1996;156(2):621–627
176. Gustafson LM, Proud D, Hendley JO, Hayden FG, Gwaltney JM Jr. Oral prednisone therapy in experimental rhinovirus infections. J Allergy Clin Immunol 1996;97(4):1009–1014
177. Singh M. Heated, humidified air for the common cold. Cochrane Database Syst Rev 2004;(2):CD001728
178. Singh M. Heated, humidified air for the common cold. Cochrane Database Syst Rev 2006;3:CD001728
179. Saketkhoo K, Januszkiewicz A, Sackner MA. Effects of drinking hot water, cold water, and chicken soup on nasal mucus velocity and nasal airflow resistance. Chest 1978;74(4):408–410
180. Forstall GJ, Macknin ML, Yen-Lieberman BR, Medendrop SV. Effect of inhaling heated vapor on symptoms of the common cold. JAMA 1994;271(14):1109–1111
181. Smith HH. Ethnobotany of the Meswaki Indians. Bull Pub Museum Milwaukee 1928;4:175–326
182. Breevort P. The booming U.S. botanicals market. HerbalGram 1998;44:33–46
183. Barrett B. Medicinal properties of Echinacea: a critical review. Phytomedicine 2003;10(1):66–86
184. Barnes J, Anderson LA, Gibbons S, Phillipson JD. Echinacea species (Echinacea angustifolia (DC.) Hell., Echinacea pallida (Nutt.) Nutt., Echinacea purpurea (L.) Moench): a review of their chemistry, pharmacology and clinical properties. J Pharm Pharmacol 2005;57(8):929–954
185. Barrett BP, Brown RL, Locken K, Maberry R, Bobula JA, D'Alessio D. Treatment of the common cold with unrefined echinacea. A randomized, double-blind, placebo-controlled trial. Ann Intern Med 2002;137(12):939–946
186. Caruso TJ, Gwaltney JM Jr. Treatment of the common cold with echinacea: a structured review. Clin Infect Dis 2005;40(6): 807–810
187. Taylor JA, Weber W, Standish L, et al. Efficacy and safety of echinacea in treating upper respiratory tract infections in children: a randomized controlled trial. JAMA 2003;290(21):2824–2830
188. Wichtl M. Herbal drugs and phytopharmaceuticals. In: Wichtl M, ed. A Handbook for Practice on a Scientific Basis. Stuttgart, Germany: Medpharm Scientific; 2004
189. Linde K, Barrett B, Wölkart K, Bauer R, Melchart D. Echinacea for preventing and treating the common cold. Cochrane Database Syst Rev 2006; (1):CD000530
190. Schoop R, Klein P, Suter A, Johnston SL. Echinacea in the prevention of induced rhinovirus colds: a meta-analysis. Clin Ther 2006;28(2):174–183
191. Melchart D, Walther E, Linde K, Brandmaier R, Lersch C. Echinacea root extracts for the prevention of upper respiratory tract infections: a double-blind, placebo-controlled randomized trial. Arch Fam Med 1998;7(6):541–545
192. Barak V, Birkenfeld S, Halperin T, Kalickman I. The effect of herbal remedies on the production of human inflammatory and anti-inflammatory cytokines. Isr Med Assoc J 2002;4(11, Suppl) 919–922
193. Gertsch J, Schoop R, Kuenzle U, Suter A. Echinacea alkylamides modulate TNF-alpha gene expression via cannabinoid receptor CB2 and multiple signal transduction pathways. FEBS Lett 2004;577(3):563–569

194. Eby GA. Zinc ion availability—the determinant of efficacy in zinc lozenge treatment of common colds. J Antimicrob Chemother 1997;40(4):483–493
195. Hulisz D. Efficacy of zinc against common cold viruses: an overview. J Am Pharm Assoc (2003) 2004;44(5):594–603
196. Prasad AS, Fitzgerald JT, Bao B, Beck FW, Chandrasekar PH. Duration of symptoms and plasma cytokine levels in patients with the common cold treated with zinc acetate. A randomized, double-blind, placebo-controlled trial. Ann Intern Med 2000;133(4): 245–252
197. Marshall I. Zinc for the common cold. Cochrane Database Syst Rev 2000; (2):CD001364
198. Macknin ML, Piedmonte M, Calendine C, Janosky J, Wald E. Zinc gluconate lozenges for treating the common cold in children: a randomized controlled trial. JAMA 1998;279(24):1962–1967
199. Papsin B, McTavish A. Saline nasal irrigation: Its role as an adjunct treatment. Can Fam Physician 2003;49:168–173
200. Passàli D, Damiani V, Passàli FM, Passàli GC, Bellussi L. Atomized nasal douche vs nasal lavage in acute viral rhinitis. Arch Otolaryngol Head Neck Surg 2005;131(9):788–790
201. Harvey R, Hannan SA, Badia L, Scadding G. Nasal saline irrigations for the symptoms of chronic rhinosinusitis. Cochrane Database Syst Rev 2007;(3):CD006394
202. Slapak I, Skoupá J, Strnad P, Horník P. Efficacy of isotonic nasal wash (seawater) in the treatment and prevention of rhinitis in children. Arch Otolaryngol Head Neck Surg 2008;134(1):67–74
203. Adam P, Stiffman M, Blake RL Jr. A clinical trial of hypertonic saline nasal spray in subjects with the common cold or rhinosinusitis. Arch Fam Med 1998;7(1):39–43
204. Gern JE, Mosser AG, Swenson CA, et al. Inhibition of rhinovirus replication in vitro and in vivo by acid-buffered saline. J Infect Dis 2007;195(8):1137–1143
205. Rennie P, Bowtell P, Hull D, Charbonneau D, Lambkin-Williams R, Oxford J. Low pH gel intranasal sprays inactivate influenza viruses in vitro and protect ferrets against influenza infection. Respir Res 2007;8:38
206. Douglas RM, Albrecht JK, Miles HB, et al. Intranasal interferon-alpha 2 prophylaxis of natural respiratory virus infection. J Infect Dis 1985;151(4):731–736
207. Hayden FG, Gwaltney JM Jr. Intranasal interferon alpha 2 for prevention of rhinovirus infection and illness. J Infect Dis 1983;148(3):543–550
208. Hayden FG, Gwaltney JM Jr. Intranasal interferon-alpha 2 treatment of experimental rhinoviral colds. J Infect Dis 1984;150(2):174–180
209. Higgins PG, Phillpotts RJ, Scott GM, Wallace J, Bernhardt LL, Tyrrell DA. Intranasal interferon as protection against experimental respiratory coronavirus infection in volunteers. Antimicrob Agents Chemother 1983;24(5):713–715
210. Monto AS, Shope TC, Schwartz SA, Albrecht JK. Intranasal interferon-alpha 2b for seasonal prophylaxis of respiratory infection. J Infect Dis 1986;154(1):128–133
211. Samo TC, Greenberg SB, Palmer JM, Couch RB, Harmon MW, Johnson PE. Intranasally applied recombinant leukocyte A interferon in normal volunteers. II. Determination of minimal effective and tolerable dose. J Infect Dis 1984;150(2):181–188
212. Hayden FG, Herrington DT, Coats TL, et al; Pleconaril Respiratory Infection Study Group. Efficacy and safety of oral pleconaril for treatment of colds due to picornaviruses in adults: results of 2 double-blind, randomized, placebo-controlled trials. Clin Infect Dis 2003;36(12):1523–1532
213. Kahn JS, McIntosh K. History and recent advances in coronavirus discovery. Pediatr Infect Dis J 2005;24(11, Suppl)S223–S227, discussion S226
214. Hayden FG, Turner RB, Gwaltney JM, et al. Phase II, randomized, double-blind, placebo-controlled studies of ruprintrivir nasal spray 2-percent suspension for prevention and treatment of experimentally induced rhinovirus colds in healthy volunteers. Antimicrob Agents Chemother 2003;47(12):3907–3916
215. Patick AK, Brothers MA, Maldonado F, et al. In vitro antiviral activity and single-dose pharmacokinetics in humans of a novel, orally bioavailable inhibitor of human rhinovirus 3C protease. Antimicrob Agents Chemother 2005;49(6):2267–2275
216. Gwaltney JM Jr. Combined antiviral and antimediator treatment of rhinovirus colds. J Infect Dis 1992;166(4):776–782
217. Deguchi Y, Takasugi Y. Efficacy of influenza vaccine in the elderly: reduction in risks of mortality and morbidity during an influenza A (H3N2) epidemic for the elderly in nursing homes. Int J Clin Lab Res 2000;30(1):1–4
218. Belshe RB, Newman FK, Tsai TF, et al. Phase 2 evaluation of parainfluenza type 3 cold passage mutant 45 live attenuated vaccine in healthy children 6-18 months old. J Infect Dis 2004;189(3):462–470
219. Micromedex. Palivizumab, 2008. http:// www.thompsonhc.com/ micromedexz, librarian
220. Meissner HC, Long SS; American Academy of Pediatrics Committee on Infectious Diseases and Committee on Fetus and Newborn. Revised indications for the use of palivizumab and respiratory syncytial virus immune globulin intravenous for the prevention of respiratory syncytial virus infections. Pediatrics 2003;112 (6 Pt 1):1447–1452
221. Sawyer LA. Antibodies for the prevention and treatment of viral diseases. Antiviral Res 2000;47(2):57–77
222. DeVincenzo J. Passive antibody prophylaxis for RSV. Pediatr Infect Dis J 2008;27(1):69–70
223. Cinatl J, Morgenstern B, Bauer G, Chandra P, Rabenau H, Doerr HW. Treatment of SARS with human interferons. Lancet 2003; 362(9380):293–294
224. Centers for Disease Control and Prevention. Antiviral drugs. http://www.cdc.gov/flu/professionals/antivirals/index.htm. Accessed September 7, 2011
225. Alves Galvão MG, Rocha Crispino Santos MA, Alves da Cunha AJ. Amantadine and rimantadine for influenza A in children and the elderly. Cochrane Database Syst Rev 2008;(1):CD002745
226. Larson EL. Warned, but not well armed: preventing viral upper respiratory infections in households. Public Health Nurs 2007;24(1):48–59
227. Turner RB, Hendley JO. Virucidal hand treatments for prevention of rhinovirus infection. J Antimicrob Chemother 2005;56(5):805–807
228. McCutcheon H, Fitzgerald M. The public health problem of acute respiratory illness in childcare. J Clin Nurs 2001;10(3):305–310
229. Rabie T, Curtis V. Handwashing and risk of respiratory infections: a quantitative systematic review. Trop Med Int Health 2006;11(3):258–267
230. Larson EL, Lin SX, Gomez-Pichardo C, Della-Latta P. Effect of antibacterial home cleaning and handwashing products on infectious disease symptoms: a randomized, double-blind trial. Ann Intern Med 2004;140(5):321–329
231. Sandora TJ, Taveras EM, Shih MC, et al. A randomized, controlled trial of a multifaceted intervention including alcohol-based hand sanitizer and hand-hygiene education to reduce illness transmission in the home. Pediatrics 2005;116(3):587–594
232. Pönkä A, Poussa T, Laosmaa M. The effect of enhanced hygiene practices on absences due to infectious diseases among children in day care centers in Helsinki. Infection 2004;32(1):2–7
233. White C, Kolble R, Carlson R, Lipson N. The impact of a health campaign on hand hygiene and upper respiratory illness among college students living in residence halls. J Am Coll Health 2005;53(4):175–181

234. White C, Kolble R, Carlson R, et al. The effect of hand hygiene on illness rate among students in university residence halls. Am J Infect Control 2003;31(6):364–370
235. White CG, Shinder FS, Shinder AL, Dyer DL. Reduction of illness absenteeism in elementary schools using an alcohol-free instant hand sanitizer. J Sch Nurs 2001;17(5):258–265
236. Lund VJ. Acute and chronic nasal disorders. In: Snow JB, Ballenger JJ, eds. Otorhinolaryngology–Head and Neck Surgery. Hamilton, Ontario: BC Decker; 2003: 745
237. Couch RB, Cate TR, Douglas RG Jr, Gerone PJ, Knight V. Effect of route of inoculation on experimental respiratory viral disease in volunteers and evidence for airborne transmission. Bacteriol Rev 1966;30(3):517–529
238. Halperin SA, Eggleston PA, Hendley JO, Suratt PM, Gröschel DH, Gwaltney JM Jr. Pathogenesis of lower respiratory tract symptoms in experimental rhinovirus infection. Am Rev Respir Dis 1983;128(5):806–810
239. Meschievitz CK, Schultz SB, Dick EC. A model for obtaining predictable natural transmission of rhinoviruses in human volunteers. J Infect Dis 1984;150(2):195–201
240. Mufson MA, Ludwig WM, James HD Jr, et al. Effect of neutralizing antibody on experimental rhinovirus infection. JAMA 1963;186: 578–584
241. Summers QA, Higgins PG, Barrow IG, Tyrrell DA, Holgate ST. Bronchial reactivity to histamine and bradykinin is unchanged after rhinovirus infection in normal subjects. Eur Respir J 1992;5(3):313–317
242. Bardin PG, Fraenkel DJ, Sanderson G, et al. Amplified rhinovirus colds in atopic subjects. Clin Exp Allergy 1994;24(5):457–464
243. Bardin PG, Sanderson G, Robinson BS, Holgate ST, Tyrrell DA. Experimental rhinovirus infection in volunteers. Eur Respir J 1996;9(11):2250–2255
244. Buchman CA, Doyle WJ, Pilcher O, Gentile DA, Skoner DP. Nasal and otologic effects of experimental respiratory syncytial virus infection in adults. Am J Otolaryngol 2002;23(2):70–75
245. Hayden FG, Gwaltney JM Jr. Prophylactic activity of intranasal enviroxime against experimentally induced rhinovirus type 39 infection. Antimicrob Agents Chemother 1982;21(6):892–897
246. Turner RB, Hendley JO, Gwaltney JM Jr. Shedding of infected ciliated epithelial cells in rhinovirus colds. J Infect Dis 1982;145(6): 849–853
247. Jackson GG, Dowling HF, Spiesman IG, Boand AV. Transmission of the common cold to volunteers under controlled conditions. I. The common cold as a clinical entity. AMA Arch Intern Med 1958;101(2):267–278
248. Tyrrell D, Fielder M. Cold Wars: The Fight against the Common Cold. New York: Oxford University Press; 2002
249. Contoli M, Message SD, Laza-Stanca V, et al. Role of deficient type III interferon-lambda production in asthma exacerbations. Nat Med 2006;12(9):1023–1026
250. Wark PA, Johnston SL, Bucchieri F, et al. Asthmatic bronchial epithelial cells have a deficient innate immune response to infection with rhinovirus. J Exp Med 2005;201(6):937–947
251. Wark PA, Bucchieri F, Johnston SL, et al. IFN-gamma-induced protein 10 is a novel biomarker of rhinovirus-induced asthma exacerbations. J Allergy Clin Immunol 2007;120(3):586–593
252. Bartlett NW, Walton RP, Edwards MR, et al. Mouse models of rhinovirus-induced disease and exacerbation of allergic airway inflammation. Nat Med 2008;14(2):199–204
253. Clyde WA Jr. Experimental models for study of common respiratory viruses. Environ Health Perspect 1980;35:107–112
254. Coates HV, Chanock RM. Experimental infection with respiratory syncytial virus in several species of animals. Am J Hyg 1962;76: 302–312
255. Prince GA, Porter DD. The pathogenesis of respiratory syncytial virus infection in infant ferrets. Am J Pathol 1976;82(2):339–352
256. Beyer M, Bartz H, Hörner K, Doths S, Koerner-Rettberg C, Schwarze J. Sustained increases in numbers of pulmonary dendritic cells after respiratory syncytial virus infection. J Allergy Clin Immunol 2004;113(1):127–133
257. Bartz H, Türkel O, Hoffjan S, Rothoeft T, Gonschorek A, Schauer U. Respiratory syncytial virus decreases the capacity of myeloid dendritic cells to induce interferon-gamma in naïve T cells. Immunology 2003;109(1):49–57
258. Allander T, Tammi MT, Eriksson M, Bjerkner A, Tiveljung-Lindell A, Andersson B. Cloning of a human parvovirus by molecular screening of respiratory tract samples. Proc Natl Acad Sci U S A 2005;102(36):12891–12896
259. Graham BS, Tang YW, Gruber WC. Topical immunoprophylaxis of respiratory syncytial virus (RSV)-challenged mice with RSV-specific immune globulin. J Infect Dis 1995;171(6):1468–1474
260. Schwarze J, Cieslewicz G, Joetham A, Ikemura T, Hamelmann E, Gelfand EW. CD8 T cells are essential in the development of respiratory syncytial virus-induced lung eosinophilia and airway hyperresponsiveness. J Immunol 1999;162(7):4207–4211
261. Schwarze J, Hamelmann E, Bradley KL, Takeda K, Gelfand EW. Respiratory syncytial virus infection results in airway hyperresponsiveness and enhanced airway sensitization to allergen. J Clin Invest 1997;100(1):226–233
262. Schwarze J, Mäkelä M, Cieslewicz G, et al. Transfer of the enhancing effect of respiratory syncytial virus infection on subsequent allergic airway sensitization by T lymphocytes. J Immunol 1999;163(10):5729–5734
263. Dreĭzin RS, Vyshnevetskaia LO, Bagdamian EE, Iankevich OD, Tarasova LB. Experimental RS virus infection of cotton rats. A viral and immunofluorescent study. Vopr Virusol 1971;16(6): 670–676
264. Prince GA, Jenson AB, Horswood RL, Camargo E, Chanock RM. The pathogenesis of respiratory syncytial virus infection in cotton rats. Am J Pathol 1978;93(3):771–791
265. Eichelberger MC. The cotton rat as a model to study influenza pathogenesis and immunity. Viral Immunol 2007;20(2):243–249
266. Buthala DA, Soret MG. Parainfluenza type 3 virus infection in hamsters: Virologic, serologic, and pathologic studies. J Infect Dis 1964;114:226–234
267. Welch BG, Snow EJ Jr, Hegner JR, Adams SR Jr, Quist KD. Development of a guinea pig colony free of complement-fixing antibodies to parainfluenza virus. Lab Anim Sci 1977;27(6):976–979
268. Kraus TA, Garza L, Horvath CM. Enabled interferon signaling evasion in an immune-competent transgenic mouse model of parainfluenza virus 5 infection. Virology 2008;371(1):196–205
269. Renegar KB. Influenza virus infections and immunity: a review of human and animal models. Lab Anim Sci 1992;42(3):222–232
270. Yamamoto N, Suzuki S, Shirai A, et al. Dendritic cells are associated with augmentation of antigen sensitization by influenza A virus infection in mice. Eur J Immunol 2000;30(1):316–326
271. Swiergiel AH, Smagin GN, Johnson LJ, Dunn AJ. The role of cytokines in the behavioral responses to endotoxin and influenza virus infection in mice: effects of acute and chronic administration of the interleukin-1-receptor antagonist (IL-1ra). Brain Res 1997;776(1-2):96–104
272. Barnard DL, Day CW, Bailey K, et al. Enhancement of the infectivity of SARS-CoV in BALB/c mice by IMP dehydrogenase inhibitors, including ribavirin. Antiviral Res 2006;71(1):53–63
273. Ruat C, Caillet C, Bidaut A, Simon J, Osterhaus AD. Vaccination of macaques with adjuvanted formalin-inactivated influenza A virus (H5N1) vaccines: protection against H5N1 challenge without disease enhancement. J Virol 2008;82(5):2565–2569

274. Ichinohe T, Tamura S, Kawaguchi A, et al. Cross-protection against H5N1 influenza virus infection is afforded by intranasal inoculation with seasonal trivalent inactivated influenza vaccine. J Infect Dis 2007;196(9):1313–1320
275. Kash JC, Tumpey TM, Proll SC, et al. Genomic analysis of increased host immune and cell death responses induced by 1918 influenza virus. Nature 2006;443(7111):578–581
276. Kobasa D, Jones SM, Shinya K, et al. Aberrant innate immune response in lethal infection of macaques with the 1918 influenza virus. Nature 2007;445(7125):319–323
277. Klemens JJ, Thompson K, Langerman A, Naclerio RM. Persistent inflammation and hyperresponsiveness following viral rhinosinusitis. Laryngoscope 2006;116(7):1236–1240
278. Fouchier RA, Kuiken T, Schutten M, et al. Aetiology: Koch's postulates fulfilled for SARS virus. Nature 2003;423(6937):240
279. Kuiken T, Fouchier RA, Schutten M, et al. Newly discovered coronavirus as the primary cause of severe acute respiratory syndrome. Lancet 2003;362(9380):263–270
280. Abraham G, Colonno RJ. Many rhinovirus serotypes share the same cellular receptor. J Virol 1984;51(2):340–345
281. Binford SL, Maldonado F, Brothers MA, et al. Conservation of amino acids in human rhinovirus 3C protease correlates with broad-spectrum antiviral activity of rupintrivir, a novel human rhinovirus 3C protease inhibitor. Antimicrob Agents Chemother 2005;49(2):619–626
282. Deffernez C, Wunderli W, Thomas Y, Yerly S, Perrin L, Kaiser L. Amplicon sequencing and improved detection of human rhinovirus in respiratory samples. J Clin Microbiol 2004;42(7):3212–3218
283. Horsnell C, Gama RE, Hughes PJ, Stanway G. Molecular relationships between 21 human rhinovirus serotypes. J Gen Virol 1995;76(Pt 10):2549–2555
284. Ledford RM, Patel NR, Demenczuk TM, et al. VP1 sequencing of all human rhinovirus serotypes: insights into genus phylogeny and susceptibility to antiviral capsid-binding compounds. J Virol 2004;78(7):3663–3674
285. Loens K, Ieven M, Ursi D, et al. Improved detection of rhinoviruses by nucleic acid sequence-based amplification after nucleotide sequence determination of the 5′ noncoding regions of additional rhinovirus strains. J Clin Microbiol 2003;41(5):1971–1976
286. Savolainen C, Blomqvist S, Mulders MN, Hovi T. Genetic clustering of all 102 human rhinovirus prototype strains: serotype 87 is close to human enterovirus 70. J Gen Virol 2002;83(Pt 2):333–340
287. Savolainen C, Laine P, Mulders MN, Hovi T. Sequence analysis of human rhinoviruses in the RNA-dependent RNA polymerase coding region reveals large within-species variation. J Gen Virol 2004;85(Pt 8):2271–2277
288. Kistler A, Avila PC, Rouskin S, et al. Pan-viral screening of respiratory tract infections in adults with and without asthma reveals unexpected human coronavirus and human rhinovirus diversity. J Infect Dis 2007;196(6):817–825
289. Kistler AL, Webster DR, Rouskin S, et al. Genome-wide diversity and selective pressure in the human rhinovirus. Virol J 2007;4:40
290. The Picornaviridae Database, 2008. http://www.viprbrc.org/brc/home.do?decorator=picorna
291. Tapparel C, Junier T, Gerlach D, et al. New complete genome sequences of human rhinoviruses shed light on their phylogeny and genomic features. BMC Genomics 2007;8:224
292. Simmonds P, McIntyre C, Savolainen-Kopra C, Tapparel C, Mackay IM, Hovi T. Proposals for the classification of human rhinovirus species C into genotypically assigned types. J Gen Virol 2010;91(Pt 10):2409–2419
293. Kitamura N, Semler BL, Rothberg PG, et al. Primary structure, gene organization and polypeptide expression of poliovirus RNA. Nature 1981;291(5816):547–553
294. Paul AV, van Boom JH, Filippov D, Wimmer E. Protein-primed RNA synthesis by purified poliovirus RNA polymerase. Nature 1998;393(6682):280–284
295. Rohll JB, Percy N, Ley R, Evans DJ, Almond JW, Barclay WS. The 5′-untranslated regions of picornavirus RNAs contain independent functional domains essential for RNA replication and translation. J Virol 1994;68(7):4384–4391
296. Semler BL, Wimmer E. Molecular Biology of Picornaviruses. Washington, DC: ASM Press; 2002: 227–246
297. Van Cauwenberge PB, Vermeiren JS, van Kempen MJ. Viral rhinitis and asthma. Curr Opin Allergy Clin Immunol 2001;1(1):21–25
298. Sears MR, Johnston NW. Understanding the September asthma epidemic. J Allergy Clin Immunol 2007;120(3):526–529
299. Johnston NW, Sears MR. Asthma exacerbations. 1: epidemiology. Thorax 2006;61(8):722–728
300. Johnston NW, Johnston SL, Duncan JM, et al. The September epidemic of asthma exacerbations in children: a search for etiology. J Allergy Clin Immunol 2005;115(1):132–138
301. Johnston SL, Pattemore PK, Sanderson G, et al. The relationship between upper respiratory infections and hospital admissions for asthma: a time-trend analysis. Am J Respir Crit Care Med 1996;154(3 Pt 1):654–660
302. Johnston SL, Pattemore PK, Sanderson G, et al. Community study of role of viral infections in exacerbations of asthma in 9-11 year old children. BMJ 1995;310(6989):1225–1229
303. Message SD, Johnston SL. Viruses in asthma. Br Med Bull 2002;61:29–43
304. Nicholson KG. Respiratory Viruses and Exacerbations of Asthma in Adults. Textbook of Influenza. Oxford: Blackwell; 1998: 219–264
305. Tan WC. Viruses in asthma exacerbations. Curr Opin Pulm Med 2005;11(1):21–26
306. Lemanske RF Jr, Dick EC, Swenson CA, Vrtis RF, Busse WW. Rhinovirus upper respiratory infection increases airway hyperreactivity and late asthmatic reactions. J Clin Invest 1989;83(1):1–10
307. Calhoun WJ, Dick EC, Schwartz LB, Busse WW. A common cold virus, rhinovirus 16, potentiates airway inflammation after segmental antigen bronchoprovocation in allergic subjects. J Clin Invest 1994;94(6):2200–2208
308. Mosser AG, Vrtis R, Burchell L, et al. Quantitative and qualitative analysis of rhinovirus infection in bronchial tissues. Am J Respir Crit Care Med 2005;171(6):645–651
309. Papadopoulos NG, Bates PJ, Bardin PG, et al. Rhinoviruses infect the lower airways. J Infect Dis 2000;181(6):1875–1884
310. Gern JE, Galagan DM, Jarjour NN, Dick EC, Busse WW. Detection of rhinovirus RNA in lower airway cells during experimentally induced infection. Am J Respir Crit Care Med 1997;155(3):1159–1161
311. Fleming HE, Little FF, Schnurr D, et al. Rhinovirus-16 colds in healthy and in asthmatic subjects: similar changes in upper and lower airways. Am J Respir Crit Care Med 1999;160(1):100–108
312. Garofalo R, Sabry M, Jamaluddin M, et al. Transcriptional activation of the interleukin-8 gene by respiratory syncytial virus infection in alveolar epithelial cells: nuclear translocation of the RelA transcription factor as a mechanism producing airway mucosal inflammation. J Virol 1996;70(12):8773–8781
313. Schroth MK, Grimm E, Frindt P, et al. Rhinovirus replication causes RANTES production in primary bronchial epithelial cells. Am J Respir Cell Mol Biol 1999;20(6):1220–1228
314. Subauste MC, Jacoby DB, Richards SM, Proud D. Infection of a human respiratory epithelial cell line with rhinovirus. Induction of cytokine release and modulation of susceptibility to infection by cytokine exposure. J Clin Invest 1995;96(1):549–557
315. Wiehler S, Proud D. Interleukin-17A modulates human airway epithelial responses to human rhinovirus infection. Am J Physiol Lung Cell Mol Physiol 2007;293(2):L505–L515

316. Yao Z, Fanslow WC, Seldin MF, et al. Herpesvirus Saimiri encodes a new cytokine, IL-17, which binds to a novel cytokine receptor. Immunity 1995;3(6):811–821
317. Molet S, Hamid Q, Davoine F, et al. IL-17 is increased in asthmatic airways and induces human bronchial fibroblasts to produce cytokines. J Allergy Clin Immunol 2001;108(3):430–438
318. Barczyk A, Pierzchala W, Sozañska E. Interleukin-17 in sputum correlates with airway hyperresponsiveness to methacholine. Respir Med 2003;97(6):726–733
319. Kao CY, Chen Y, Thai P, et al. IL-17 markedly up-regulates beta-defensin-2 expression in human airway epithelium via JAK and NF-kappaB signaling pathways. J Immunol 2004;173(5):3482–3491
320. Proud D, Sanders SP, Wiehler S. Human rhinovirus infection induces airway epithelial cell production of human beta-defensin 2 both in vitro and in vivo. J Immunol 2004;172(7):4637–4645
321. Cheung D, Dick EC, Timmers MC, de Klerk EP, Spaan WJ, Sterk PJ. Rhinovirus inhalation causes long-lasting excessive airway narrowing in response to methacholine in asthmatic subjects in vivo. Am J Respir Crit Care Med 1995;152(5 Pt 1):1490–1496
322. Wark PA, Gibson PG. Asthma exacerbations. 3: Pathogenesis. Thorax 2006;61(10):909–915
323. Smith CB, Golden CA, Kanner RE, Renzetti AD Jr. Association of viral and Mycoplasma pneumoniae infections with acute respiratory illness in patients with chronic obstructive pulmonary diseases. Am Rev Respir Dis 1980;121(2):225–232
324. Keatings VM, Collins PD, Scott DM, Barnes PJ. Differences in interleukin-8 and tumor necrosis factor-alpha in induced sputum from patients with chronic obstructive pulmonary disease or asthma. Am J Respir Crit Care Med 1996;153(2):530–534
325. Wang D, Coscoy L, Zylberberg M, et al. Microarray-based detection and genotyping of viral pathogens. Proc Natl Acad Sci U S A 2002;99(24):15687–15692
326. Wang D, Urisman A, Liu YT, et al. Viral discovery and sequence recovery using DNA microarrays. PLoS Biol 2003;1(2):E2
327. Chiu CY, Rouskin S, Koshy A, et al. Microarray detection of human parainfluenzavirus 4 infection associated with respiratory failure in an immunocompetent adult. Clin Infect Dis 2006;43(8):e71–e76
328. Urisman A, Molinaro RJ, Fischer N, et al. Identification of a novel Gammaretrovirus in prostate tumors of patients homozygous for R462Q RNASEL variant. PLoS Pathog 2006;2(3):e25
329. Johnson SC, Marshall DJ, Harms G, et al. Multiplexed genetic analysis using an expanded genetic alphabet. Clin Chem 2004;50(11): 2019–2027
330. Novinska MS, Pietz BC, Ellis TM, Newman DK, Newman PJ. The alleles of PECAM-1. Gene 2006;376(1):95–101
331. Pietz BC, Warden MB, DuChateau BK, Ellis TM. Multiplex genotyping of human minor histocompatibility antigens. Hum Immunol 2005;66(11):1174–1182
332. Lee WM, Grindle K, Pappas T, et al. High-throughput, sensitive, and accurate multiplex PCR-microsphere flow cytometry system for large-scale comprehensive detection of respiratory viruses. J Clin Microbiol 2007;45(8):2626–2634
333. Lee WM, Kiesner C, Pappas T, et al. A diverse group of previously unrecognized human rhinoviruses are common causes of respiratory illnesses in infants. PLoS ONE 2007;2(10):e966
334. Mahony J, Chong S, Merante F, et al. Development of a respiratory virus panel test for detection of twenty human respiratory viruses by use of multiplex PCR and a fluid microbead-based assay. J Clin Microbiol 2007;45(9):2965–2970
335. Lamson D, Renwick N, Kapoor V, et al. MassTag polymerase-chain-reaction detection of respiratory pathogens, including a new rhinovirus genotype, that caused influenza-like illness in New York State during 2004-2005. J Infect Dis 2006;194(10): 1398–1402
336. Renwick N, Schweiger B, Kapoor V, et al. A recently identified rhinovirus genotype is associated with severe respiratory-tract infection in children in Germany. J Infect Dis 2007;196(12): 1754–1760
337. van den Hoogen BG, de Jong JC, Groen J, et al. A newly discovered human pneumovirus isolated from young children with respiratory tract disease. Nat Med 2001;7(6):719–724
338. van der Hoek L, Pyrc K, Jebbink MF, et al. Identification of a new human coronavirus. Nat Med 2004;10(4):368–373
339. Deffrasnes C, Hamelin ME, Boivin G. Human metapneumovirus. Semin Respir Crit Care Med 2007;28(2):213–221
340. Maggi F, Pifferi M, Vatteroni M, et al. Human metapneumovirus associated with respiratory tract infections in a 3-year study of nasal swabs from infants in Italy. J Clin Microbiol 2003;41(7):2987–2991
341. Boivin G, De Serres G, Côté S, et al. Human metapneumovirus infections in hospitalized children. Emerg Infect Dis 2003;9(6): 634–640
342. Williams JV, Harris PA, Tollefson SJ, et al. Human metapneumovirus and lower respiratory tract disease in otherwise healthy infants and children. N Engl J Med 2004;350(5): 443–450

12 Acute Rhinosinusitis

Joseph K. Han and Stephen M. Wold

Rhinosinusitis is very common in the general population of the United States, accounting for an estimated 25 million ambulatory visits in 1996.[1] Rhinosinusitis is the fifth most common reason for the prescribing of antibiotics.[2] The direct and indirect costs associated with rhinosinusitis are tremendous, stemming from the use of diagnostic and therapeutic resources, procedures, prescriptions, and lost productivity.[3]

In the majority of sinusitis, there is inflammation of the nasal cavity in addition to the mucosal lining of the paranasal sinuses; therefore, the term "rhinosinusitis" is preferred over "sinusitis." Rhinosinusitis is divided into acute, subacute, and chronic based on the duration of symptoms. Acute bacterial rhinosinusitis (ABRS) is defined as inflammation of the sinonasal cavity due to bacterial infection with clinical symptoms that last 4 weeks or less.[4] Acute rhinosinusitis differs from chronic rhinosinusitis on multiple levels such as clinical presentation, microbiology, histopathology, pathophysiology, and progression of disease.

Epidemiology

About 25 million people in the United States are diagnosed with rhinosinusitis each year, making it one of the top reasons for presentation to a primary care physician or otolaryngologist.[2,3] The prevalence of rhinosinusitis is slightly higher among females than males.[5] Lower socioeconomic status and cigarette smoking are also associated with a higher prevalence of rhinosinusitis.

In general, although some geographic and population-based variability exists among the spectrum of etiologies for acute rhinosinusitis, the most frequently implicated offenders are viruses such as rhinovirus, influenza, and parainfluenza. Approximately 0.5 to 2% of adult and up to 10% of pediatric cases of viral rhinosinusitis develop into bacterial infection of the sinuses.[6] The majority of pediatric ABRS is secondary to upper respiratory viral infection.[7] The second highest factor contributing to pediatric ABRS is allergy exacerbation.

The most common bacterial pathogens in ABRS are *Streptococcus pneumoniae*, *Haemophilus influenzae*, and *Moraxella catarrhalis*, the last being more commonly seen in pediatric patients. Aspiration studies from the maxillary sinus of patients with suspected acute bacterial rhinosinusitis have identified *S. pneumoniae* in 20 to 43%, *H. influenzae* in 22 to 35%, and *M. catarrhalis* in 2 to 10% of cultures.[8,9] Although an earlier study[9] showed that beta hemolytic streptococci and *S. pneumoniae* were the most frequent isolates, more recent studies have shown that *S. pneumoniae* and *H. influenzae* are the most frequent bacterial pathogens in ABRS.

Due in part to the often indiscriminate prescribing of antibiotics for acute and chronic respiratory infections, drug-resistant organisms have increased in prevalence in the past few decades, especially *S. pneumoniae*.[10] Between 1994 and 2004, the prevalence of penicillin-resistant *S. pneumoniae* increased from 24 to 35%. Macrolide resistance in *S. pneumoniae* also increased from 9 to 39% during that time. Antibiotic resistance has leveled off in recent years, but the antibiotic resistance rate remains high. Antibiotic resistance rates can vary widely depending on geographic location, so local antibiograms should be reviewed to be cognizant of locoregional trends in antimicrobial resistance.

Pathophysiology

Appreciation of the pathophysiology of acute bacterial rhinosinusitis first demands familiarity with the regional anatomy. Frequently implicated in ABRS is obstruction of

Table 12.1 Causative Agents for Acute Bacterial Rhinosinusitis

Mucosal injury
Inhalant allergen exposure
Laryngopharyngeal reflux
Hormonal change
Pregnancy
Infectious
Bacteria
Fungus
Virus
Obstructive anatomic structure
Infraorbital ethmoid cell
Frontal cell
Narrow ostiomeatal complex
Neoplasm
Sinonasal trauma
Tumors
Systemic disease
Aspirin triad
Ciliary dysfunction
Cystic fibrosis
Immunodeficiency
Sarcoidosis
Wegener's granulomatosis

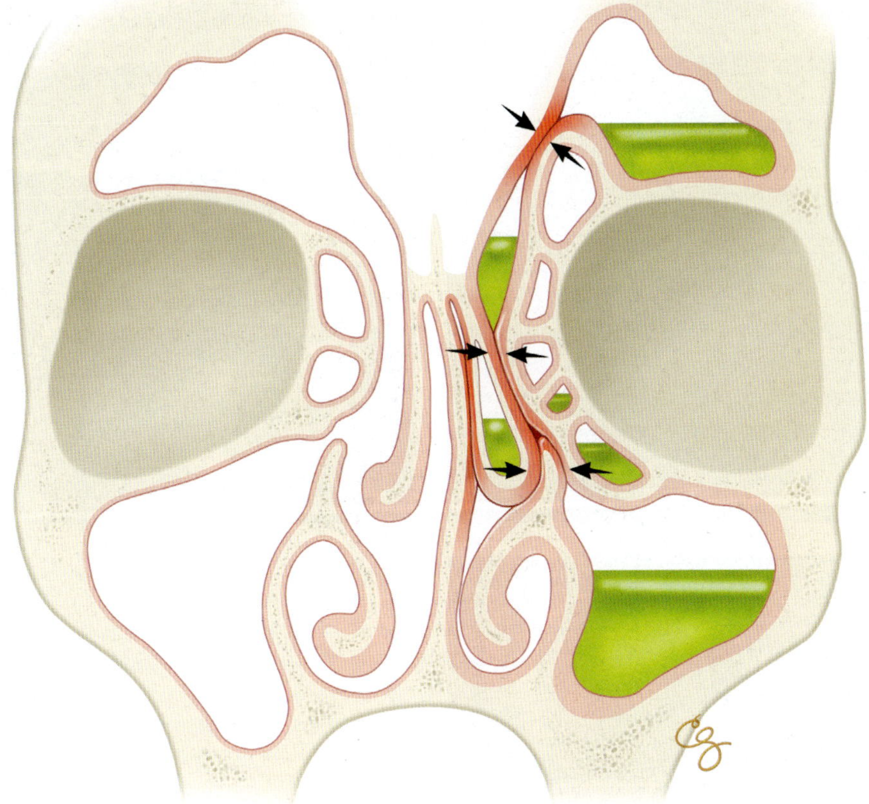

Fig. 12.1 Illustration demonstrating obstruction of the left ostiomeatal complex due to the deviated septum to the left side as well as a left concha bullosa. The left maxillary, anterior ethmoid, and frontal sinuses are involved. Also, a type III frontal cell is contributing to the obstruction of the left frontal sinus.

the ostiomeatal complex (OMC), a regional confluence of drainage pathways of the frontal sinus, anterior ethmoid sinus, and maxillary sinus (**Fig. 12.1**). Certain anatomic abnormalities can contribute to physical obstruction of the OMC and may predispose individuals to a more frequent or protracted disease course. Presence of anatomic variations such as septal deviation, concha bullosa, infraorbital ethmoid cell, interfrontal sinus septal air cell, and frontal cell are more likely to encourage the development of obstructive rhinosinusitis.[11] When these anatomic variants are larger in size, the probability of developing rhinosinusitis is higher. Other obstructive etiologies include nasal polyps, neoplasm, indwelling nasotracheal or nasogastric tubes, and nasal foreign bodies.

Although there is a significant list of inciting factors (**Table 12.1**) that may lead to acute bacterial rhinosinusitis, the common pathway is obstruction of the sinus ostium. When an instigating event such as a viral infection occurs, the mucosa is damaged and expands (**Fig. 12.2**). An ostium, which is already narrow due to anatomic variants such as an infraorbital ethmoid cell, is further narrowed by the swollen mucosa. The obstructed ostium allows for mucus to gather within the sinus. Hypoxia and subatmospheric pressure develop within the sinus due to Dalton's law of partial pressure of gas. This leads to vasodilation and the release of vascular endothelial growth factor, which causes transudation of fluid and thickening of the mucosal lining in the paranasal sinus (**Fig. 12.3**).[12]

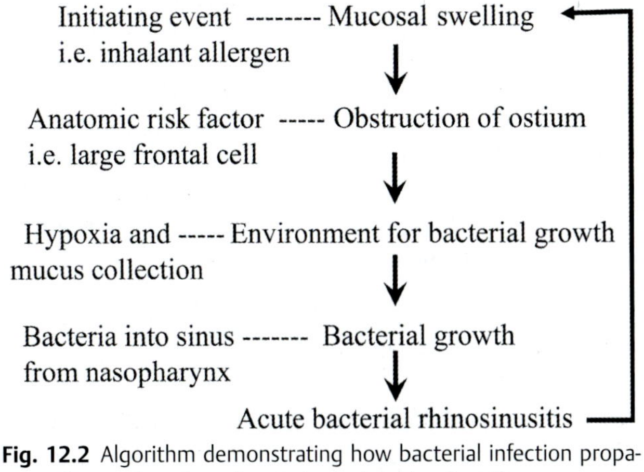

Fig. 12.2 Algorithm demonstrating how bacterial infection propagates the continuation of acute bacterial rhinosinusitis.

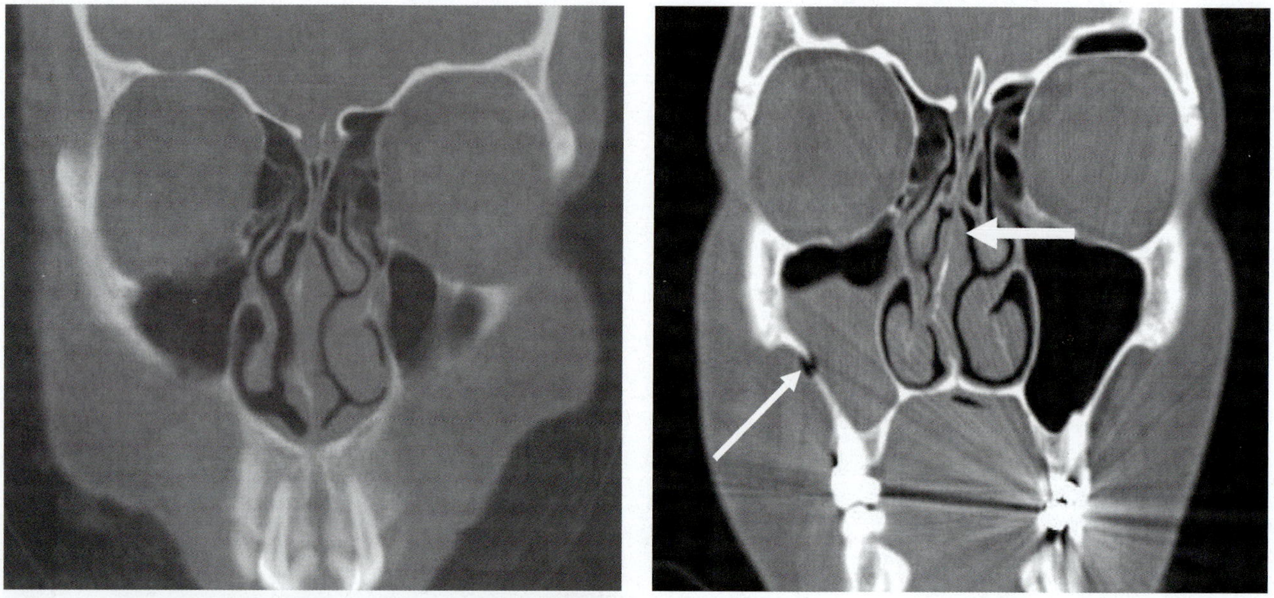

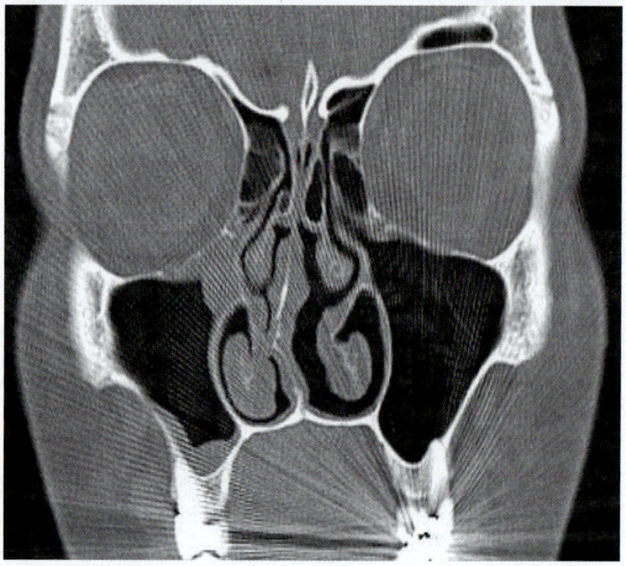

Fig. 12.3 (A) Coronal computed tomography (CT) of a sinus from a patient with a complaint of nasal obstruction. The right side of the nasal cavity is normal. **(B)** CT of the sinus after trauma to the right maxilla. Notice the fracture of the maxillary sinus (*arrow*) and shifted ostiomeatal complex (*large arrow*). **(C)** CT of the sinus 3 months after the facial trauma. There is inspissated mucus and swollen mucosa of the right maxillary sinus.

The collection of mucus is normally sterile.[8] The bacterial pathogens that cause ABRS normally inhabit the nasopharynx or nasal cavity and are absent from the OMC. Bacterial transfer into the OMC occurs when the nose is blown, seeding the sinuses that have inspissated mucus. The bacteria flourish within the sinus cavity and develop into a sinus infection. The inflammation associated with the infection damages the mucosal lining of the sinus, which then propagates mucociliary compromise.

Clinical Presentation

When considering the diagnosis of suspected ABRS, one must also consider a differential diagnosis that includes rhinitis medicamentosa, allergic rhinitis, migraines, vasomotor rhinitis, and viral rhinosinusitis. Rhinitis medicamentosa can be excluded if there is no history of topical vasoconstrictor use. Allergic rhinitis is usually accompanied with pruritic eyes and nose, symptoms that are not associated with ABRS. Should the diagnosis of allergic rhinitis still be in question, a simple challenge with an antihistamine should clear the symptoms. Another quick measure would be to check a serum level of total IgE during the presentation of the disease process. Although elevated IgE is seen in allergic disease, there may be other causes for elevated total serum IgE.

Migraine headaches can be confused with ABRS. Migraine headaches can present with facial pain or headache, nasal congestion, rhinorrhea, and even postnasal drainage. Therefore, it is imperative that a close investigation of exacerbating and alleviating causes is taken during the office visit. Acute bacterial rhinosinusitis features do not worsen with bright light or loud noise. Taking a nap or lying in a dark closed room does not alleviate ABRS symptoms. These characteristics are likely indicators of a migraine. Atypical migraines can be more challenging to diagnose; selected patients may benefit from consultation with a neurologist.

Vasomotor rhinitis is less common than allergic rhinitis and is not associated with inhalant allergens. Instead, vasomotor rhinitis is an umbrella term for a heterogeneous group of nasal cavity diseases characterized by engorgement of the nasal mucosa. The mucosal swelling is typically induced by changes in ambient air temperature, but can also be due to a change in hormone levels, such as in hypothyroidism or pregnancy. Vasomotor rhinitis can also be due to an imbalance of the autonomic innervation of the nasal cavity, such as in gustatory rhinitis in which rhinorrhea and nasal congestion are associated with eating. Differentiation of vasomotor rhinitides from ABRS can be made by clinical history.

To distinguish between rhinosinusitis resulting from acute bacterial infection versus viral illness alone, this task may prove quite difficult because the clinical presentations are typically quite similar, particularly within the first 3 to 5 days. For this reason, much of the diagnostic focus is placed on characterizing the clinical course and duration rather than the presence or absence of specific factors. Symptoms or signs present for a total of less than 10 days are more likely to represent acute viral rhinosinusitis (AVRS), which tends to peak early then slowly wane.[13] Whenever findings persist for greater than 10 days that are atypically severe or display worsening within 10 days after an initial improvement, a heightened suspicion for bacterial infection or superimposed bacterial infection after a viral infection should be entertained.

Although numerous classification systems have been proposed and used in the past for establishing a diagnosis of rhinosinusitis, the most used method has been described by Lanza and Kennedy.[8] Based on this organization (**Table 12.2**), a diagnosis of ABRS can be made assuming that the factors have either worsened after 5 days or persisted for more than 10 days but did not extend past 4 weeks in duration. Although this categorization is based on combinations of major and minor rhinosinusitis symptoms or findings, three cardinal criteria are pointed out as highly suspicious for bacterial sinusitis: purulent nasal discharge, nasal obstruction, and facial pain, pressure, or fullness.

Table 12.2 Diagnosis of Rhinosinusitis Is Defined as Either Two More Major Factors, One Major with Two Minor Factors, or Purulence on Nasal Examination

Major Factors	Minor Factors
Facial pain or pressure	Headache
Nasal obstruction	Halitosis
Facial congestion/fullness	Fatigue
Purulent nasal discharge	Dental pain
Discolored postnasal discharge	Cough
Hyposmia or anosmia	Ear pain or pressure
Nasal purulence on exam	Fever (chronic)
Fever (acute bacterial rhinosinusitis)	

Patients with either VRS or ABRS may complain of sore throat, sneezing, rhinorrhea, cough, malaise, anosmia/hyposmia, otalgia/aural fullness, maxillary dental pain, halitosis, or fatigue. The presence of fever is a poor predictive factor and yields only ~50% specificity and sensitivity. Many patients with either VRS or ABRS will present for medical attention only after failing to obtain relief from over-the-counter medications. Some patients, particularly those with other medical comorbidities such as immunodeficiency syndromes, ciliary dyskinesias, and diabetes mellitus, may present with increasingly severe or progressive symptomatology and may appear quite acutely ill. It is within this last group that a prompt diagnosis is particularly critical, so that early treatment decisions may be made and initiated without delay.

Diagnostic Workup

In most cases of uncomplicated acute rhinosinusitis, which account for the vast majority of patients, a clinical diagnosis can be elicited from a clinical history and a physical exam without the need for additional blood tests, imaging, or invasive sampling. This is not to say that there is not any role for ancillary studies, but simply that one should be selective and ask what exactly is hoped to be gained from the test. The workup of all patients should start with a careful history and physical examination. In addition to subjective findings and time course as previously discussed, close attention should also be given to any chronic medical illnesses, history of asthma, migraine history, past craniofacial or sinonasal surgery, allergies, tobacco use, or status of immunocompetency. Physical examination should include a thorough head and neck examination, which may demonstrate a variety of findings including hyponasal voice quality, periorbital or malar edema, orbital cellulitis, proptosis, facial tenderness, pharyngeal secretions or exudates, tender maxillary dentition, middle ear effusion, reduced nasal airflow, and purulent nasal drainage. In addition to a comprehensive head and neck examination for an initial patient, a flexible or rigid nasal endoscopy should be performed to evaluate for anatomic abnormalities, nasal patency, mucosal edema, and thick or colored mucus drainage. If desired, cultures may be obtained at this time as well; however, cultures from general nasal secretions typically correlate poorly with those from the sinuses, so attempts at directly swabbing or aspirating the middle meatus near the involved sinus is preferred. The gold standard for diagnosis has long been the demonstration of bacteria (>100,000) via maxillary sinus puncture and aspiration, but this is frequently uncomfortable for the patient and does not necessarily alter management in the presence of other clinical findings. Furthermore, the timing of maxillary sinus puncture may grossly affect the likelihood of obtaining positive cultures, as samples taken within the first 10 days of acute symptoms are more frequently sterile or low in bacterial count. If cultures are desired for a diagnosis or for focusing antibiotic coverage, middle meatal swabs are much less uncomfortable than maxillary sinus puncture and demonstrate a high degree of diagnostic accuracy when purulence is present in the middle meatus.[14]

Several imaging modalities exist for evaluation of the nose and sinuses, and efforts should be made to balance cost and availability with the value of the information obtained. Although plain films are no longer recommended as a diagnostic tool for rhinosinusitis, their use may persist among primary care providers. The "sinus series" typically include anteroposterior (Caldwell), occipitomental (Waters), and lateral views, all taken with the patient in the upright position to better demonstrate air-fluid levels. Opacification, air-fluid levels, and mucosal thickening support, but do not necessarily prove, a diagnosis of ABRS. A meta-analysis of these demonstrates sensitivities and specificities ranging from 73 to 90% and 41 to 80%, respectively, for these findings.[15] Ultrasound has also been investigated as a diagnostic tool, but has failed to establish a role in routine workup given the extremely variable test accuracy, due in part to operator experience and interpretation.

Noncontrast computed tomography (CT) is the radiographic method employed most frequently in the evaluation of sinusitis, though it is generally considered unnecessary in the routine diagnosis of ABRS. Similar to plain films, CT can demonstrate mucosal thickening or air fluid levels, but CT additionally yield anatomic information of the sinuses along with better visualization of the sinuses, orbits, and brain. Although access and ease of CT scans have increased exponentially over the past 10 years, they remain significantly more costly than plain films and involve a higher dose of radiation to the patient. It should also be kept in mind that abnormalities on CT typically accompany viral rhinosinusitis, so clinical correlation is required in interpreting CT scans.[16] Contrast CT and magnetic resonance imaging (MRI) may be used to delineate extension of the disease beyond the confines of the bony sinuses themselves, such as into the orbit or intracranial cavity.[17]

In general, laboratory studies and imaging, although helpful, are typically reserved for instances when the clinical picture of suspected sinusitis is somewhat atypical, particularly severe, refractory to initial management, or to rule out other potential etiologies. In this sense, imaging may help to evaluate for intranasal masses, mucoceles, vascular compromise, fungal balls, orbital cellulitis or abscess, bony erosion, meningitis, or intracranial extension. Skin testing or immunoglobulin assays may similarly help to elucidate an allergic component to the rhinosinusitis. Autoimmune panels, although helpful in the workup of more chronic forms of disease, are typically of limited use in ABRS. One additional consideration is the testing for cystic fibrosis in the child or young adult with recurrent, severe bouts of acute bacterial sinusitis.

Treatment and Outcome

The aims of treatment may be generally simplified into two main goals: symptomatic relief and resolution of the disease process. Depending on the individual patient as well as the disease process itself, the balance between these aims may be drastically different. For example, in cases of viral rhinosinusitis, the disease process is self-limiting and by nature demands only symptomatic therapy except in the case of secondary superimposed bacterial infection. Antibiotics have not been shown to alter the clinical course of VRS and are not recommended in its treatment as these simply expose the patient to additional costs, adverse reactions, drug–drug interactions, and bacterial resistance.

In terms of symptomatic therapy, analgesics and antipyretics are a mainstay for relief, and over-the-counter acetaminophen or nonsteroidal anti-inflammatory drugs (NSAIDs) are routinely sufficient for most cases. A stronger, opioid-containing drug may be required in some patients with more severe, symptomatic disease. Systemic steroid therapy, topical nasal steroids, mucolytics, antihistamines, decongestants, and other "cold medications" are among the most extensively used agents for relief of rhinosinusitis in general, but data are sufficiently lacking regarding whether any of these truly alter disease outcomes, particularly in VRS. Meltzer et al. did demonstrate a reduction of symptom scores in patients with ABRS receiving topical mometasone versus placebo.[18] Nasal saline and sinus irrigations have been advocated as being able to reduce symptomatology, to improve mucociliary clearance, and to decrease the requirement for adjunctive treatment; however, compelling randomized control data have yet to be demonstrated.

Perhaps a disputed clinical decision is with regard to which patients should receive antibiotics and when during the clinical course they should receive them. As previously stated, antibiotics are not recommended for the treatment of VRS; thus, until a diagnosis or strong suspicion of ABRS is made, decisions regarding antibiotics should be deferred. It is thus advocated that patients presenting with less than 7 to 10 days of symptoms are more appropriately managed conservatively without antibiotics in an otherwise healthy, immunocompetent patient. It is also suggested that patients with an uncomplicated acute sinusitis may likewise be observed for up to a week following the diagnosis of suspected ABRS because many of these episodes may resolve spontaneously as well.[19] A meta-analysis of randomized placebo-controlled antibiotic trials demonstrated that antibiotics provided no significant added benefit to disease improvement or resolution at days 3 to 5 or 14 to 15 compared with placebo.[18] Patients may experience improvement or resolution of symptoms several days earlier when receiving antibiotics, but this must be balanced against the cost, the risk of increased bacterial resistance, and the adverse drug effects, which are more frequent within this group.[18] Additional considerations in deciding which patients may be suitable for watchful waiting include medical comorbidities, general health, age, symptom severity, and reliability for follow-up and reevaluation should the condition fail to improve or become worse.

The empiric use of antibiotics for ABRS has been widely studied, frequently via placebo or drug comparison randomized control trials (RCTs). A systematic Cochrane review failed to identify significant differences in clinical outcomes between different antibiotic agents in patients with ABRS.[20] Although geographic population, bacterial resistance patterns, frequency of dosing, and individual patient tolerance may certainly play a role in antibiotic selection, amoxicillin has repeatedly been supported as a first-line agent in the outpatient management of ABRS due to its safety, efficacy, low cost, and narrow spectrum.[2,5,20–22] Trimethoprim-sulfamethoxazole and macrolides are useful agents in patients with penicillin allergy. Second- or third-generation cephalosporins, chosen primarily for their strong antipneumococcal activity, serve as alternative first-line therapy options. Amoxicillin with clavulanate is useful as a second-line agent for those failing initial measures or in patients with other systemic comorbidities, yet it has demonstrated no therapeutic advantage over amoxicillin alone in uncomplicated ABRS.[8] Additional second-line options include fluoroquinolones in adults. Intravenous antibiotics are rarely required and their use is typically more a function of the patient's overall health and medical comorbidities than of the disease process itself. The use of intravenous (IV) antibiotics may be considered in patients who are unable to take oral preparations, have developed suppurative complications of acute sinusitis, are immunocompromised, or have poor bowel absorption. Oral antibiotics are typically prescribed for a course between 5 to 10 days, although considerable variability is present in clinical practice. A systematic review of randomized control trials suggests that a shorter course of antibiotics is equally effective in resolving infection and yields fewer adverse events, though it is unclear what effect this might have on contributing to microbial drug resistance.[23]

Although the most common causative bacteria in ABRS have remained largely unchanged over time, drug resistance is a continually evolving challenge to practitioners. Perhaps as many as 35% of pneumococcal strains now demonstrate penicillin resistance, and this rate is likely higher in certain local distributions.[2] Penicillin resistance is even higher, sometimes nearing 100%, in strains of *Moraxella catarrhalis* and *H. influenzae*. Without specific knowledge of local resistance patterns, amoxicillin still serves as an appropriate initial therapy, and given sufficient doses will overcome some intermediate-level resistance. If cultures are obtained, susceptibility data should be reviewed to reassess and focus antibiotic selection. If a patient's condition becomes worse or fails to demonstrate improvement after 5 to 7 days of therapy, resistance should be considered and a shift to an alternative first-line or second-line agent may be reasonable. Drug cycling, in which certain classes of antibiotics with high resistance patterns are temporarily removed from clinical use and then later reintroduced, may also help to stem this increasing problem as well.[24]

Complications

Because complications of rhinosinusitis are covered in Chapter 21 in detail, only a short description of ABRS complications will be discussed here. Complications from ABRS are rare among adults and more commonly involve the pediatric population. Complications arise when there is an extension of the bacterial infection to the surrounding structures such as the orbit or cranium. Extension from the paranasal sinuses to the orbit can cause periorbital or orbital cellulitis or abscess. Extension to the cranium can cause meningitis or cranial abscess. The location of the orbital abscess helps direct the source of the bacterial sinus infection. Medially based orbital abscesses usually start from the ethmoid sinus, whereas the superior-based abscess is likely from the frontal sinus. Prognosis for the orbital abscess is dependent on the size of the abscess as well as the age of the patient. A common pathogen in pediatric bacterial sinus infection that is responsible for invasion into structures surrounding the paranasal sinuses is *S. milleri*, which is often difficult to identify and culture. Fortunately, *S. milleri* is usually penicillin susceptible, but again increasing drug resistance has been observed in this organism.[25]

Conclusion

Acute rhinosinusitis is a very common problem in the United States. The majority of acute rhinosinusitis is viral in nature. It is difficult to differentiate acute viral rhinosinusitis from acute bacterial rhinosinusitis, but prolonged course of symptoms is very suspicious of acute bacterial sinusitis. Fortunately, acute bacterial rhinosinusitis is a self-limiting infection but antibiotics can shorten the disease process. Radiographic examination is rarely indicated in acute sinusitis, unless there is a complication for the sinus infection.

References

1. Schappert SM. Ambulatory care visits to physician offices, hospital outpatient departments, and emergency departments: United States, 1996. Vital Health Stat 13 1998;134(134):1–37
2. Anon JB, Jacobs MR, Poole MD, et al; Sinus And Allergy Health Partnership. Antimicrobial treatment guidelines for acute bacterial rhinosinusitis. Otolaryngol Head Neck Surg 2004;130 (1, Suppl)1–45
3. Anand VK. Epidemiology and economic impact of rhinosinusitis. Ann Otol Rhinol Laryngol Suppl 2004;193(Suppl):3–5
4. Lanza DC, Kennedy DW. Adult rhinosinusitis defined. Otolaryngol Head Neck Surg 1997;117(3 Pt 2)S1–S7
5. Chen Y, Dales R, Lin M. The epidemiology of chronic rhinosinusitis in Canadians. Laryngoscope 2003;113(7):1199–1205
6. Gwaltney JM Jr. Acute community-acquired sinusitis. Clin Infect Dis 1996;23(6):1209–1223, quiz 1224–1225
7. Fireman P. Diagnosis of sinusitis in children: emphasis on the history and physical examination. J Allergy Clin Immunol 1992;90(3 Pt 2):433–436
8. Gwaltney JM Jr, Scheld WM, Sande MA, Sydnor A. The microbial etiology and antimicrobial therapy of adults with acute community-acquired sinusitis: a fifteen-year experience at the University of Virginia and review of other selected studies. J Allergy Clin Immunol 1992;90(3 Pt 2)457–461, discussion 462
9. Low DE, Desrosiers M, McSherry J, et al. A practical guide for the diagnosis and treatment of acute sinusitis. CMAJ 1997;156(Suppl 6):S1–S14
10. Jenkins SG, Farrell DJ, Patel M, Lavin BS. Trends in anti-bacterial resistance among Streptococcus pneumoniae isolated in the USA, 2000–2003. PROTEKT US years 1-3. J Infect 2005;51(5):355–363
11. Caughey RJ, Jameson MJ, Gross CW, Han JK. Anatomic risk factors for sinus disease: fact or fiction? Am J Rhinol 2005;19(4): 334–339
12. Early SB, Hise K, Han JK, Borish L, Steinke JW. Hypoxia stimulates inflammatory and fibrotic responses from nasal-polyp derived fibroblasts. Laryngoscope 2007;117(3):511–515
13. Rosenfeld RM, Andes D, Bhattacharyya N, et al. Clinical practice guideline: adult sinusitis. Otolaryngol Head Neck Surg 2007;137 (3, Suppl)S1–S31
14. Dubin MG, Ebert CS, Coffey CS, Melroy CT, Sonnenburg RE, Senior BA. Concordance of middle meatal swab and maxillary sinus aspirate in acute and chronic sinusitis: a meta-analysis. Am J Rhinol 2005;19(5):462–470
15. Scheid DC, Hamm RM. Acute bacterial rhinosinusitis in adults: part I. Evaluation. Am Fam Physician 2004;70(9):1685–1692
16. Gwaltney JM Jr, Phillips CD, Miller RD, Riker DK. Computed tomographic study of the common cold. N Engl J Med 1994; 330(1):25–30
17. Younis RT, Anand VK, Davidson B. The role of computed tomography and magnetic resonance imaging in patients with sinusitis with complications. Laryngoscope 2002;112(2):224–229
18. Meltzer EO, Charous BL, Busse WW, Zinreich SJ, Lorber RR, Danzig MR; The Nasonex Sinusitis Group. Added relief in the treatment of acute recurrent sinusitis with adjunctive mometasone furoate nasal spray. J Allergy Clin Immunol 2000;106(4):630–637
19. Gwaltney JM Jr, Wiesinger BA, Patrie JT. Acute community-acquired bacterial sinusitis: the value of antimicrobial treatment and the natural history. Clin Infect Dis 2004;38(2):227–233
20. Williams JW Jr, Aguilar C, Cornell J, et al. Antibiotics for acute maxillary sinusitis. Cochrane Database Syst Rev 2003;(2, Issue 2) CD000243 10.1002/14651858.
21. Snow V, Mottur-Pilson C, Hickner JM; American Academy of Family Physicians; American College of Physicians-American Society of Internal Medicine; Centers for Disease Control; Infectious Diseases Society of America. Principles of appropriate antibiotic use for acute sinusitis in adults. Ann Intern Med 2001;134(6): 495–497
22. Luterman M, Tellier G, Lasko B, Leroy B. Efficacy and tolerability of telithromycin for 5 or 10 days vs amoxicillin/clavulanic acid for 10 days in acute maxillary sinusitis. Ear Nose Throat J 2003;82(8):576–580, 82–84, 586 passim
23. Ip S, Fu L, Balk E, et al. Update on acute bacterial rhinosinusitis. Evidence report/technology assessment No. 124 (prepared by Tufts-New England Medical Center Evidence-based Practice Center under contract No. 290-02-0022). AHRQ Publications No. 05-E020-2. Rockville, MD: Agency for Healthcare Research and Quality; 2005
24. Marple BF, Brunton S, Ferguson BJ. Acute bacterial rhinosinusitis: a review of U.S. treatment guidelines. Otolaryngol Head Neck Surg 2006;135(3):341–348
25. Han JK, Kerschner JE. Streptococcus milleri: an organism for head and neck infections and abscess. Arch Otolaryngol Head Neck Surg 2001;127(6):650–654

13 Etiologic Factors in Chronic Rhinosinusitis

Andrew P. Lane and Justin H. Turner

Chronic rhinosinusitis (CRS) is an inflammatory disorder involving the mucosa of the nose and paranasal sinuses. Although not necessary for clinical diagnosis, CRS is often accompanied by the presence of infectious processes of viral, fungal, or bacterial origin. These and other environmental influences combine with host factors to produce persistent sinonasal inflammation. The precise etiologic contributors to CRS are difficult to clearly separate and identify. Certain factors can be easily associated with ongoing CRS, but often cannot be proven as direct etiologies of the disease process itself. It has become increasingly suggested in the clinical and research communities that CRS is driven by an abnormal host immune response against environmental agents. In many ways, this is not surprising. The nasal cavity is often the first point of contact between the airway mucosa and the external world. Multiple immune mechanisms exist at this critical interface to defend against a myriad of microbial and nonmicrobial elements. Thus, although diverse initiating events may ultimately contribute to the development and persistence of CRS, it is likely that a derangement of host immunity ultimately underlies the recalcitrant mucosal inflammation that characterizes the most severe forms of the disease.

Systemic Host Factors

Innate Immunity

Many innate immune mechanisms exist at the mucosal surface to defend the host against environmental pathogens. The most obvious of these is the continuously flowing mucus blanket that is regularly propelled along the sinonasal tract by ciliated epithelial cells. This continuous flow of mucus serves as a primitive defense mechanism to usher pathogens and particulates out of the nasal cavity. Additionally, sinonasal mucus contains a variety of antimicrobial products, including enzymes, permeabilizing proteins, neutralizing proteins, protease inhibitors, opsonins, defensins, surfactants, acute-phase proteins, and immunoglobulins. Innate immune effectors are produced constitutively or may be stimulated by the activation of pathogen-recognition receptors, such as Toll-like receptors (TLR), which are expressed on multiple cell types, including macrophages, dendritic cells, and epithelial cells. The role of innate immune effectors in CRS is under continued investigation. Studies have demonstrated altered expression of innate effectors such as serum amyloid A, antimicrobial cathelicidin, beta-defensins, and surfactants in the sinonasal epithelial cells of patients with CRS with or without polyps. Evidence also exists for a role of TLRs in chronic rhinosinusitis, as well as in other inflammatory disorders such as asthma and atherosclerosis. Genetic polymorphisms in TLR genes have been implicated in asthma and atopy, particularly TLR4, which appears to regulate allergic airway inflammation via mast cell activation.[1] In CRS, there is conflicting data suggesting either an up or down regulation in the expression of distinct TLRs. Other innate effectors, such as the enzyme acidic mammalian chitinase, have also been found to have altered expression in chronic sinonasal disease.[2] Disruption and/or dysregulation of these innate immune effectors likely represents a major contributor to the persistent inflammation in chronic rhinosinusitis.

Acquired/Adaptive Immunity

Adaptive immunity is a protective response to specific antigens derived from environmental pathogens. These pathways typically involve local antigen-presenting cells such as dendritic cells, as well as locally recruited T cells and B cells. Dendritic cells exist throughout the nasal and respiratory airway. These cells are situated adjacent to epithelial cells of the mucosal surface, where they contact antigenic material as it traverses the sinonasal tract. The dendritic cells then present antigen to and activate T cells, which, in turn, recruit neutrophils, basophils, and eosinophils to the mucosal surface via expression of inflammatory cytokines and chemokines. In general, T-cell responses in CRS can be divided into T-helper (Th) cells 1 or a Th2 phenotype, depending largely on the pattern of cytokine expression induced. Th1 cells secrete large amounts of interferon-γ (IFN-γ) and tumor necrosis factor α (TNF-α), which in turn activate macrophages and cytotoxic T cells. Th2 cells secrete multiple cytokines, including interleukin (IL)-4, IL-5, IL-9, and IL-13, most of which enhance the development and maturation of eosinophils and mast cells. Each pathway is distinct and capable of inhibiting the other. Previous studies have established that CRS with or without polyps is mediated via a mixed Th1/Th2 response,[3] and some evidence suggests that the precise balance between these immunogenic pathways may govern the type and severity of sinonasal disease. Abnormal immune responses appear to be a feature of chronic rhinosinusitis, and several cytokines, chiefly granulocyte macrophage colony-stimulating factor (GM-CSF), TNF-α, IL-1β, IL-4, IL-5, IL-6, and IL-13 are now thought to be associated with CRS. Furthermore, chemokines such as eotaxin 1 and 2, monocyte chemoattractant protein (MCP) 3 and 4, RANTES, and IL-8 are also associated with CRS, and are capable of inducing migration of eosinophils and/or lymphocytes. For example, sinonasal lavage from patients with treatment-resistant chronic rhinosinusitis contains elevated levels of inflammatory and regulatory cytokines, including IFN-γ, IL-5, IL-8, IL-10, and IL-18.[4] Likewise, sinonasal lavage from patients with "allergic" or "nonallergic" CRS both contain elevated levels of the inflammatory cytokine IL-13.[5] This molecule is secreted in massive amounts by Th2 lymphocytes, and is capable of recruiting and activating large numbers of eosinophils.[6]

Additional subsets of Th cells, most notably Th17 cells and regulatory T cells (T_{reg}), have more recently been identified and characterized. Th17 cells are named in reference to their ability to produce IL-17. These cells have provided new insights into basic mucosal immune responses, as well as complex autoimmune and inflammatory diseases. Many disorders that were previously defined as Th1- or Th2-mediated diseases, including encephalomyelitis, arthritis, and allergy, are now believed to also involve Th17-mediated pathways. In mouse models of atopic dermatitis, allergic rhinitis, and allergy, IL-17 and Th17 cells appear to play an important role. The involvement of Th17 cells in these disease entities suggests a similar role in CRS because these disorders share many similar histologic and pathologic features. Investigations into the role of Th17-mediated pathways in CRS have thus far been very limited. Molet et al. reported an increase in IL-17 expression in hyperplastic nasal polyps as compared with normal nasal turbinate tissue.[7] As reported by Ramanathan et al., IL-22 (a Th17-pathway cytokine) and its receptor are expressed in cultured nasal epithelial cells.[8] Furthermore, expression of this receptor was found to be reduced in individuals with recalcitrant CRS with polyps, as compared with nonrecalcitrant individuals and healthy controls. The role of T_{reg} cells in sinusitis is only beginning to be explored, although preliminary evidence seems to suggest decreased T_{reg} activity in CRS with nasal polyps.

For the purpose of this chapter, immune mechanisms contributing to CRS have been divided into those of the innate immune system and those of the adaptive immune system. In many ways this is an oversimplification, and there is really no dividing line between these two classifications. Antigen-specific stimulation of adaptive immune mechanisms can nonspecifically enhance innate immune responses. Likewise, costimulatory molecules on epithelial cells and other secreted products of the innate immune system can augment antigen-specific immune pathways under most circumstances. Thus, the integration of innate and adaptive immune pathways can ultimately be defined under the broader label of "mucosal immunity" (**Fig. 13.1**). Further investigation into the interaction of the innate and adaptive immune system will further clarify what is a complicated yet very important clinical and research subject.

Airway Hyperreactivity

It is now widely accepted that chronic rhinosinusitis and asthma are closely related disease processes. This idea is well supported by epidemiological studies showing extensive clinical, endoscopic, or radiological findings of sinusitis among asthmatics. For example, Bresciani et al. reported that 100% of severe steroid-dependent asthmatics had abnormal sinus computed tomography (CT) scans.[9] Likewise, the same cells and inflammatory mediators are found in tissue from the upper airway of patients with CRS and the lower airway of patients with chronic asthma. This relationship appears to be consistent in both adults and children and strengthens what appears to be a strong relationship between rhinosinusitis and asthma. However, controversy exists as to whether (1) chronic rhinosinusitis triggers asthma or vice versa, or (2) chronic rhinosinusitis and asthma represent upper and lower airway manifestations of the same underlying disease process. Clearly, asthma and CRS share multiple pathophysiological similarities, and the mucosal remodeling observed in CRS, particularly involving nasal polyps, is remarkably similar to that which occurs in the bronchioles of persistent asthma sufferers.[10] The nasobronchial reflex is a proposed mechanism by which irritants in the nasal cavity or upper airway can stimulate bronchoconstriction. This pathway is mediated by afferent branches of the trigeminal nerve and efferent bronchoconstriction-inducing networks derived from the vagus nerve. Though the existence of this pathway has been confirmed in multiple studies, few investigators believe that this hypothesis can explain the chronicity of symptoms associated with asthma and CRS. It has also been proposed that inflammation of the lower airways can activate the bone marrow to produce inflammatory cells that can then affect the upper airways, or vice versa. In support of this hypothesis, a study by Braunstahl et al. showed that allergic patients with rhinitis, when subjected to a bronchial allergen challenge, had increased basophils, eosinophils, and inflammatory cytokines in their nasal tissue.[11] Likewise, Denburg et al. found that the activated airway can produce hematopoietic growth factors that can drive the maturation of mast cells, basophils, and eosinophils.[12] Without a doubt, the histopathological findings and inflammatory mediators and cells found in chronic rhinosinusitis and asthma are remarkably similar. However, research outlining a clear cause-and-effect relationship between these two diagnoses has yet to be published.

Allergy

A link between allergy and CRS has been proposed for over 50 years, based largely on several epidemiologic studies. For example, in 1999, Suzuki and colleagues noted an increased prevalence of allergy among CRS patients and also found higher levels of eosinophils and inflammatory cytokines in the sinus fluids of allergic patients who

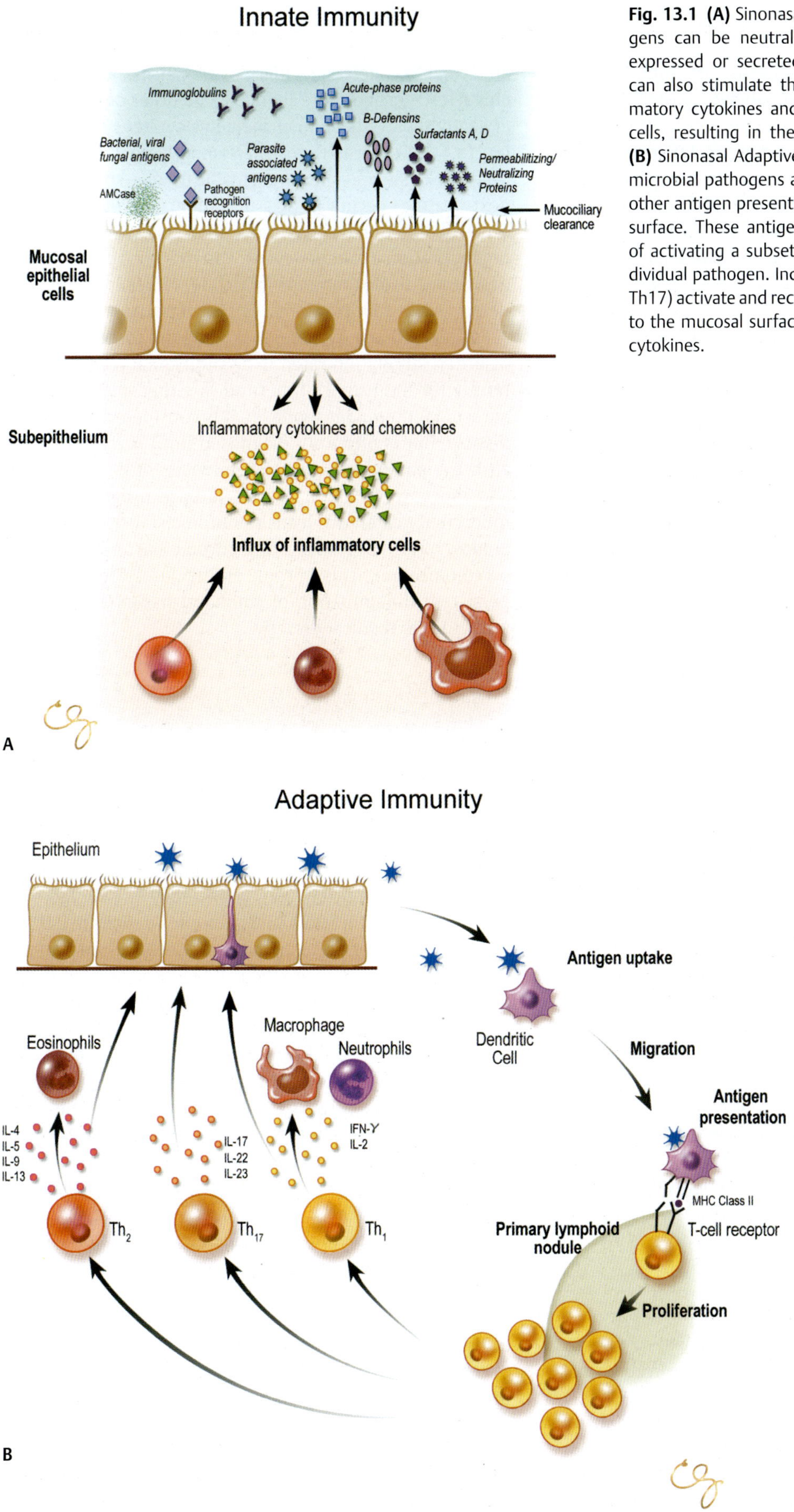

Fig. 13.1 (A) Sinonasal Innate Immunity. Microbial pathogens can be neutralized by innate immune mediators expressed or secreted from the cell surface. Pathogens can also stimulate the nonspecific expression of inflammatory cytokines and chemokines by mucosal epithelial cells, resulting in the rapid influx of inflammatory cells. **(B)** Sinonasal Adaptive Immunity. Antigens from different microbial pathogens are recognized by dendritic cells and other antigen presenting cell-types at or near the mucosal surface. These antigen-presenting cells are then capable of activating a subset of T-helper cells specific to that individual pathogen. Individual T-helper subtypes (Th1, Th2, Th17) activate and recruit other inflammatory cell subtypes to the mucosal surface through the expression of specific cytokines.

concurrently had CRS.[13] Allergic rhinitis is an immunoglobulin E (IgE)-mediated disease that affects 10 to 30% of the adult population. Patients with allergic sensitivities demonstrated by elevated total and/or specific IgE levels often have more extensive sinus disease than nonallergic patients. Likewise, patients with documented inhalant allergies are more likely to have chronic sinusitis and are more likely to undergo functional endoscopic sinus surgery.

It appears likely that allergy represents a predisposing factor for chronic rhinosinusitis. Research documenting the pathophysiological relationship between these two disease phenomena has been increasing over the last decade. In one study, allergic patients with CRS were exposed to an inhaled antigen to which they had previously tested positive by skin testing.[14] The majority of these patients developed worsening of their sinus symptoms after antigen exposure as well as radiographic changes to their sinuses. The authors subsequently proposed that exposure of allergic patients with CRS to an allergen results in increased edema, ciliary dysfunction, and increased mucus production. In a similar study, Baroody et al. found that instillation of antigen into the nasal cavity of individuals with CRS resulted in elevated lavaged eosinophils from their maxillary sinus.[15]

Aspirin Intolerance

The combination of nasal polyposis, aspirin sensitivity, and asthma is known as Samter's triad, or aspirin-exacerbated respiratory disease. This terminology emerged from studies in the late 1960s evaluating the phenomenon of aspirin-induced bronchospasm that had first been noted as early as 100 years ago. The pathophysiology behind this disease remains unclear, but may involve a disorder in arachidonic acid metabolism that renders overproduction of bronchoconstriction-inducing leukotrienes. Ingestion of non-steroidal anti-inflammatory drugs blocks prostaglandin synthesis and effectively shunts arachidonic acid metabolism towards even greater levels of leukotriene synthesis. The result is an anaphylactoid reaction that can cause serious airway compromise. Patients with aspirin-induced asthma often present with particularly severe sinonasal disease that is commonly recalcitrant to routine medical and surgical therapy. The pathophysiology of asthma with aspirin intolerance appears to be very similar to asthma without aspirin intolerance.

Mucociliary Dysfunction

Primary ciliary dyskinesia (PCD) refers to a heterogeneous group of ciliary ultrastructural defects resulting in abnormal ciliary motility. The term "immotile cilia syndrome," is no longer used to describe PCD, in acknowledgment that many forms of PCD have some retention of ciliary motility, albeit dysfunctional. Kartagener syndrome, the classic description of PCD, has been characterized in case reports since the early 20th century. Since that time, the ultrastructural abnormality, a defect in ciliary dynein arms, has been well characterized, and more than a dozen other defects in ciliary activity have been identified. Kartagener syndrome refers to a clinical triad that signals underlying PCD: sinusitis, bronchiectasis, and situs inversus. Situs inversus (including dextrocardia) occurs in 50% of patients, owing to an absence of directional ciliary movement that renders visceral organ rotation a random event. Patients with ciliary dyskinesia may also experience infertility, either from motility defects of the fallopian canal or spermatozoa.

Primary ciliary dyskinesia is thought to be a genetic disorder, largely inherited in an autosomal recessive pattern, with the balance inherited in either an X-linked or autosomal dominant mode. PCD is considered a pediatric disease, but is often not diagnosed until early adulthood after the patient has experienced years of heavy sputum and mucus production. As the disease progresses, poor mucociliary clearance leads to chronic sinusitis and nasal polyps, often with underlying chronic bacterial infection or colonization. This chronic infectious state results in persistent inflammation of sinonasal tissue that is often refractory to medical therapy.

Immunodeficiency

CRS is occasionally caused by a defect in either cell-mediated or humoral immunity. A retrospective analysis by Vanlerberghe et al. assessed the prevalence of humoral immune deficiency in 307 adult and pediatric subjects with treatment-refractory chronic rhinosinusitis. A total of 21.8% of these patients had laboratory evidence for humoral immune deficiency (IgA deficiency in 2.2%, IgG subclass deficiencies in 19.8%, and combined deficits in 2.9%).[16] Although many of these deficits were subtle, humoral immune deficiency was nonetheless proposed as an etiologic factor, particularly in chronic refractory rhinosinusitis. Patients undergoing bone marrow transplantation are also known to be more predisposed to the development of CRS. A 2006 study by Ortiz et al. found that CRS was prevalent in 49% of patients following bone marrow transplantation, none of whom had symptoms prior to transplantation.[17]

The recently described transporter associated with presentation (TAP)-deficiency syndrome is heralded by chronic rhinosinusitis and conductive hearing loss, and clinically may resemble Wegener granulomatosis in its presentation. This syndrome results from a defect in the TAP, a molecule essential for the stabilization and surface expression of human leukocyte antigen (HLA) class I molecules. Although rare, this syndrome is the most common of several defects in HLA class I pathways, all of which can present with CRS. CRS is particularly prevalent in patients infected with HIV, with studies noting an occurrence in between 20 and 68% of this patient population.[18] These patients display a gradual depletion of CD4+ T lymphocytes with a resulting blunting of the humoral immune response, as well as macrophage dysfunction. CRS in these patients is associated with significantly increased rates of staphylococcal and pseudomonal infections. The increased rates of reported CRS in HIV-positive patients may also be associated with immune dysregulation and aggressive allergic responses to previously innocuous environmental agents.

Granulomatous Diseases

CRS that continues despite extensive and adequate treatment can be secondary to multiple serious granulomatous conditions. Diseases such as Wegener granulomatosis, Churg-Strauss syndrome, and sarcoidosis are now well accepted causes of chronic nasal inflammation. Typically, these are multisystem disorders that affect pulmonary, renal, and other tissues, in addition to their effects on the sinonasal mucosa. The cause of these diseases is unknown, but research suggests that they are abnormal immune responses to some unknown environmental or host antigen. Wegener granulomatosis is a typical granulomatous vasculitis that involves the nose and paranasal sinuses, kidneys, and lungs. Significant inflammation of the turbinates and nasal mucosa results in profound edema and crusting. This disorder is often further complicated by a secondary bacterial infection, usually by *Staphylococcus aureus*, which further contributes to the inflammatory response. The precise cause of Wegener granulomatosis is unknown, but is presumed to be some form of immunological dysregulation. Like Wegener's, sarcoidosis often affects the lungs and kidneys, but can affect virtually any organ in the body. Sinonasal involvement is much less common than in Wegener granulomatosis, but when it occurs, it results in mucosal inflammation, nasal crusting, and occasionally, bacterial superinfection. Churg-Strauss is an atypical vasculitis syndrome that is defined by asthma, peripheral eosinophilia, paranasal sinusitis, pulmonary involvement, and neuropathy. Like sarcoidosis, it can ultimately affect any and all organ systems. The cause of this disorder is unknown but it is assumed to be secondary to aberrant recruitment of eosinophils to different tissues, possibly stimulated by malfunctioning neutrophils. These patients often have nasal obstruction secondary to polyps and heavy nasal crusting.

Multiple chronic indolent infections can also be direct or indirect causes of CRS. These may be bacterial, fungal, or mycobacterial in origin. For example, the bacterium *Klebsiella rhinoscleromatis* can cause a chronic sinonasal disease called rhinoscleroma that almost universally involves the nasal tissues, and infrequently, the paranasal sinuses. This Gram-negative organism endemic to Central and South America, as well as East Africa and India produces nasal granulomas that can occasionally obstruct sinus outflow. *Klebsiella ozaenae* can cause atrophic rhinitis, an erosive inflammatory condition resulting in chronic crusting and progressive tissue loss intranasally. Chronic granuloma-forming mycobacterial infections, most notably *Mycobacterium tuberculosis*, can also cause considerable intranasal inflammation that persists even after antimicrobial therapy.

Cystic Fibrosis

The highly viscous mucus secretions found in patients with cystic fibrosis (CF) lead to impaired mucociliary clearance, mucosal edema, and local tissue inflammation. Not surprisingly, the prevalence of CRS is greatly increased in CF patients. Although individual studies vary, the prevalence of chronic rhinosinusitis in patients with CF varies from 74 to 100%. However, the type of CF mutation appears to be an important factor in determining the type and characteristics of CRS present in individual patients. "Strong" mutations are much more likely, for example, to produce nasal polyps. Of even greater interest, a study by Wang et al. found that up to 7% of CRS patients are carriers of a single CF gene mutation, compared with less than 1% of normal controls.[19] These heterozygotes also appear to be predisposed to other manifestations of CF, including pancreatitis, allergic bronchopulmonary aspergillosis, and diffuse bronchiectasis. Similar results have been found in children, with a study by Raman et al. finding an increased occurrence of CFTR (cystic fibrosis transmembrane conductance regulator) mutations in children with CRS than in the general public (12% vs. 3 to 4%).[20] These individuals generally have a normal sweat chloride test but are likely to have decreased functional CFTR expression that may alter chloride transport at the cell surface. In the study by Raman et al., it was proposed that the increased prevalence of CRS in CF heterozygotes may be secondary to the role of the CFTR in innate immunity at the epithelial surface. The CFTR is known to play a role in the uptake and removal of certain bacterial and foreign pathogens from the mucosal surface. Furthermore, the altered viscosity and electrolyte content of sinus secretions in these patients may drastically alter the mucoid barrier that is essential for a functional innate immune system. This group may very well represent a segment of the general population that is predisposed to developing CRS, particularly because they are rarely aware of their carrier status.

Local Host Factors

Odontogenic Inflammation

The maxillary sinus is conveniently situated immediately adjacent to the oral cavity, making it particularly sensitive to invasion by pathogenic organisms from this area. CRS of odontogenic origin often originates from periodontal disease, dental abscesses, dental implants, or dental extractions that violate the maxillary sinus. The maxillary teeth are exceptionally close to the antrum, with the sinus cavity often separated from the tooth roots by only a thin layer of mucoperiosteum (Schneiderian membrane). Disruption of the Schneiderian membrane can result in a chronic infection and/or colonization of the maxillary sinus by a polymicrobial group of aerobic and especially anaerobic organisms.

The most common source of infection is untreated dental caries that leads to a dental abscess. Alternatively, severe periodontal disease can lead to the formation of a secondary endodontic lesion. The most common iatrogenic cause of odontogenic sinus disease is root canal therapy, which can occasionally perforate the sinus membrane. Maxillary sinusitis can also be a complication of the sinus lift procedure, which refers to surgical augmentation of the maxilla with bone grafts to facilitate dental implants. Maxillary sinusitis, both acute and chronic, is secondary to an odontogenic source in about one-tenth of cases. However, sinus inflammation of dental origin is generally considered one of the most treatable causes of CRS, and often resolves quickly after appropriate medical and surgical therapy that includes elimination of the source of infection.

Anatomic Abnormalities

Anatomic and structural anomalies of the sinonasal cavity have long been recognized as major contributors to CRS. All paranasal sinus structures require patent outflow tracts that allow for adequate mucociliary function and subsequent mucus clearance of inhaled pathogens and particulates. However, not until the widespread use of computed tomographic (CT) imaging was the true role of anatomic structural variations in CRS fully understood. There are now multiple anatomic variants known to contribute to sinus obstruction, including nasal septal deviation, infraorbital (Haller) cells, concha bullosa, craniofacial abnormalities, traumatic or iatrogenic obstacles, or narrow sinus outflow tracts. A study by Krzeski et al. examined the incidence of different anatomic variations of the lateral nasal wall in a group of 157 patients with chronic rhinosinusitis.[21] Different anatomic variations were observed in every patient in the study group. For example, Haller cells were identified in ~9% of this population, although rates in other studies have varied from 20 to 45%, whereas a pneumatized middle turbinate was found in greater than 30%. However, the incidence of these anatomic variations was not assessed or compared in asymptomatic individuals.

Particular attention has been paid to the ostiomeatal complex, the functional outflow tract that drains the frontal, maxillary, and anterior ethmoid sinuses. Obstruction of this unit can impede mucus outflow and create an environment hospitable to bacterial overgrowth and chronic inflammation. However, many studies have found a similar incidence of ostiomeatal complex obstruction in patients with CRS and the aymptomatic population. Nasal septal deviation has also long been proposed as an etiologic factor in chronic rhinosinusitis. However, the literature evaluating this hypothesis has been decidedly mixed. Yasan et al. found that nasal septal deviation is not a direct risk factor for development of CRS.[22] A comprehensive review by Collet et al. examined the role of septal deviation in the pathogenesis of CRS by exploring all associated literature between 1980 and 2001.[23] Individual authors proposed multiple pathophysiological roles for nasal septal deviation in the development of CRS, including (1) an increased angle of deviation in the ostiomeatal complex area, (2) mechanical obstruction of the ostiomeatal complex, (3) altered ciliary activity secondary to modified air flow, and (4) changes in antral ventilation. However, this comprehensive review could not establish a role for nasal septal deviation as either an associated or contributing factor in CRS. In fact, most of these studies found a similar incidence of septal deviation, as based on radiographic imaging, in patients with CRS and in healthy controls. Most recently, Orlandi conducted a systematic review of the literature and found a positive correlation between septal deviation with rhinosinusitis. He found an odds ratio of 1.47 for the association between rhinosinusitis and a having a septal deviation angle of 10 degrees or greater. Many studies in the systematic review were excluded for being inadequately powered, or for including patients with minimal deviations.[24]

It has previously been proposed that anatomic variations can also lead to altered nasal airflow that may predispose an individual to chronic sinonasal disease. Normal nasal airflow is essential for the maintenance of a healthy nasal epithelium. Although some animal models have shown that unilateral nasal obstruction can lead to rhinitis and chronic sinusitis, there exists little convincing evidence in humans that would lead to the same conclusion. In fact, the paranasal sinuses are largely protected from inspired air by their narrow ostia. It is still hypothesized by some that increased airflow causes drying of the nasal epithelium that can result in irritation and/or infection. Nevertheless, experimental support for these or other hypotheses are limited. The role of anatomic abnormalities in CRS therefore appears to be largely limited to those conditions that impinge on sinus outflow and orderly mucociliary function.

Bone Inflammation

Recent evidence suggests that the recalcitrant nature of CRS may partly result from persistent mucosal inflammation secondary to osteitis of underlying bone. Much of the support for this hypothesis comes from a few animal studies showing bony changes in models of induced sinusitis. Human clinical studies into this area are sparse. Using histomorphometric studies, Giacchi et al. examined the ethmoid bones of patients who had recently undergone endoscopic sinus surgery for CRS and found that 18 out of 19 patients had some evidence of bony resorption or remodeling.[25] Control patients showed either no evidence of bony pathology or greatly reduced changes compared with those with sinusitis. Likewise, Jang et al. were able to correlate radionucleotide studies showing increased uptake in bone of the paranasal sinuses with poor outcomes following endoscopic sinus surgery.[26] Furthermore, patients with CRS had significantly higher isotope uptake than healthy controls. The bone inflammation of CRS is thought to be secondary to bacteria that inhabit the sinus mucosa.

However, the presence of bacterial organisms within the bone itself has yet to be reported. It has been proposed that bacteria may increase local levels of inflammatory mediators, prostaglandins, and leukotrienes, which then stimulate bone remodeling by osteoblasts. The intricate system of Haversian canals provides a network for the spread of inflammation throughout the bony sinuses. Underlying bone inflammation may in turn contribute to the persistent mucosal edema of the sinus cavities that is universally seen in CRS.

Acquired Mucociliary Dysfunction

Inspired air contains large quantities of environmental pollutants, microorganisms, and particulates. Among the primary components of the innate immune system is the superficial mucosa and overlying mucus layer of the nose, paranasal sinuses, and bronchial airways. These protective layers participate in mucociliary clearance, which prevents deposition of such foreign bodies within the aerodigestive tract. Most epithelial cells are ciliated and create a continuous propulsive force that ushers mucus toward the natural ostia and prevents local irritation or inflammation. This is not a random process; rather, these cilia beat in a coordinated fashion and at a specific frequency. During times of stress, such as exercise and infection, the ciliary beat frequency increases to accelerate the clearance of mucus from the sinonasal cavity. Multiple studies have shown that patients with CRS have reduced mucociliary clearance when compared with healthy controls. Adequate mucociliary clearance requires (1) appropriate mucus production and viscoelastic properties, and (2) appropriate basal and stimulated ciliary beat frequency. CF represents one extreme example of thickened mucus and decreased clearance. Likewise, many studies have found increased mucus viscosity in patients with CRS. For example, Majima et al. found that the viscoelasticity of mucus from patients with CRS is largely dependent on elevated levels of IgG and various mucus glycoproteins.[27]

The primary contributor to acquired mucociliary dysfunction, however, appears to be changes in ciliary beat frequency. Several studies have documented decreased ciliary beat frequency in patients with CRS. Furthermore, Chen et al. found that the cholinergic- and adrenergic-stimulated ciliary beat frequency of mucosal explants from patients with CRS was also significantly diminished.[28] The mechanism by which ciliary beat frequency is altered in CRS is unclear. However, in the study by Chen et al., sinonasal epithelial cells from more than 70% of patients reverted back to their baseline stimulatory phenotype when maintained in culture for more than 72 hours, suggesting that the altered ciliary function was secondary to CRS-associated inflammation rather than genetic defects. Likewise, inflammatory cytokines such as IL-8 and IL-13 have been shown to decrease basal and/or stimulatory ciliary beat frequency in bronchial epithelial cells.

Gastroesophageal Reflux Disease

A role for gastroesophageal reflux disease (GERD) in chronic sinonasal inflammation has been proposed for several years. Patients with CRS have higher rates of GERD than the general public and many of their sinonasal symptoms often resolve after adequate medical treatment of their reflux. A small, prospective, open label study by DiBaise et al. found a modest improvement in individual sinus symptoms in 25 to 89% of patients with CRS who received a proton pump inhibitor for 3 months.[29] A placebo controlled double-blind study by Vaezi et al. found that twice daily lansoprazole improved symptoms of chronic postnasal discharge in patients without evidence of sinusitis.[30] However, convincing evidence that refluxed stomach contents actually reach the nasopharynx is limited. A 2005 study by DelGaudio found elevated reflux in the nasopharynx and upper esophageal sphincter in patients with recalcitrant CRS when compared with healthy control subjects.[31] Conversely, a 2006 study by Jecker et al. using 24-hour pH monitoring found an increase in reflux events and decreased pH in the esophagus of patients with recurrent CRS, but observed no difference in the hypopharynx.[32] However, one of the major etiologic factors in chronic reflux disease, the bacterium *Helicobacter pylori,* is detected at equal levels in diseased and nondiseased sinonasal tissue.[33] Some groups have proposed that GERD may reflect an underlying vagal dystonia and may contribute to CRS via vagus nerve-induced neuroinflammatory changes to the sinonasal mucosa; by such a theory, refluxed stomach contents would not necessarily need to reach the nasopharynx. Yet, this remains only a hypothesis, and little if any supporting data exist for this model. Although the mechanism by which GERD contributes to persistent sinonasal inflammation remains unclear, it appears likely that GERD at least represents an associated or predisposing factor for the development of CRS.

Environmental Factors

Viruses

Most cases of acute rhinosinusitis follow viral upper respiratory infections, most commonly by rhinoviruses. A very small percentage of patients with acute rhinosinusitis will go on to develop chronic disease that features bacterial colonization and persistent inflammation. Although a role for viruses in the development of ARS is well established, the role of viruses in the pathogenesis of CRS remains unclear. Using real-time polymerase chain reaction (RT-PCR), Jang et al. were able to detect rhinovirus in only 21% of turbinate epithelial cells from CRS patients.[34] Although the virus was detected in none of the control samples, there remained some question whether this represented subclinical persistence of rhinovirus from an earlier infection or true infection or colonization. Rhinovirus and other viral organisms are capable of inducing neutrophil recruitment and the inflammatory response. Further study is required to determine the precise role of viruses in CRS.

Bacteria

The mucosal and epithelial surfaces of the human sinonasal tract are colonized by aerobic and anaerobic microorganisms. Bacterial species in the nasal cavity that are considered "normal flora" include *Staphylococcus epidermidis*, *S. aureus*, alpha- and gamma-streptococci, and *Propionibacterium acnes*. Potential sinus pathogens are rarely isolated from the nasal cavities of healthy individuals. The development of upper respiratory infections into acute, and subsequently chronic, rhinosinusitis appears to involve a defined sequence of events. The first stage is a viral infection lasting from 7 to 10 days. The vast majority of these individuals will recover completely, but a limited few (usually less than 1%) will develop a secondary acute bacterial infection. Common organisms during the acute stage include aerobic and facultative bacteria such as *Streptococcus pneumoniae*, *Haemophilus influenzae*, and *Moraxella catarrhalis*. Over subsequent weeks to months, a subset of these patients will then go on to develop CRS, with anaerobic organisms of oropharyngeal origin becoming the predominant inhabitants of the nasal passages and sinuses. Support for this sequence of events comes largely from a study by Brook et al. that documented serial endoscopic cultures from the maxillary sinus of patients as they progressed from acute to chronic rhinosinusitis.[35] However, despite the documented presence of bacterial pathogens in the human sinonasal tract, it remains unclear how bacterial colonization contributes to the inflammation that is ubiquitous in patients with CRS. In fact, some investigators have proposed that the prevalence of anaerobic organisms in CRS may be simply the result of persistent edema, an acidic environment, and the decreased oxygen tension that accompanies an acute sinus infection with aerobic organisms. Much of the support for anaerobes as etiologic factors in CRS comes from animal studies in which chronic sinusitis and a profound production of immunoglobulin (Ig)G antibodies was induced in rabbits after intranasal inoculation with *Bacteroides fragilis*.[36] The ability of bacterial organisms to contribute to CRS may be largely due to complex immunologic pathways that may become dysregulated in a chronic inflammatory state.

Superantigens

A superantigen is any substance that can nonspecifically activate large numbers of T lymphocytes. Prototypical superantigens function by interacting with the beta-chain of the human T-cell receptor, thereby cross-linking the receptor to the major histocompatibility complex and circumventing the normal mechanism of T-cell activation. Using this pathway, up to 30% of circulating T cells can be activated as opposed to the 0.01%, or less that is typical of conventional antigen-specific responses. These superantigens are now associated with multiple chronic eosinophilic-lymphocytic inflammatory disorders, including atopic dermatitis, asthma, and allergic rhinitis. Superantigen stimulation can initiate the release of inflammatory cytokines (IL-4, IL-5, and IL-13) that contribute to the eosinophilia that heralds these disorders, as well as CRS with nasal polyps. *S. aureus*, a common inhabitant of the nasal mucosa, produces no less than 19 different superantigens, notably enterotoxins A and B, and toxic shock syndrome toxin 1. This organism is cultured from the nasal cavity of most patients with CRS with nasal polyps, but is found in only 25% of the general population. The first experimental evidence for superantigens as etiologic agents in CRS came from a study by Bachert et al. in 2001, which demonstrated specific IgE antibodies to *S. aureus* enterotoxins A and B in the polypoid tissue of half of all patients with CRS with nasal polyps.[37] Subsequent studies have shown that the toxins themselves are also present, at a rate approaching 50%, in the nasal mucosa of patients with CRS with nasal polyps, whereas it is only rarely present in nonpolyp CRS patients or patients with no history of CRS.

The role of bacterial superantigens in CRS remains largely unclear. At a minimum, superantigens may at least play the role of immunologic modifiers, which contribute to the lymphocytic and eosinophilic mucosal infiltrate associated with CRS with polyposis. Given that toxin-secreting *S. aureus* is a ubiquitous inhabitant of the human sinonasal tract, it appears unlikely to be the primary contributor to the development of inflammation and chronic sinus disease. Disease states associated with superantigens may depend on a genetic predisposition toward immune susceptibility. It is likely that complex genetic and environmental factors play a role in establishing an environment in which superantigens can become a significant contributor to CRS.

Biofilms

According to the Centers for Disease Control and Prevention, at least 65% of all human bacterial infectious processes involve biofilms. A biofilm is a complex aggregation of microorganisms marked by the excretion of a protective and adhesive matrix. The requirement for oxygen and nutrients is greatly reduced in this state and these assemblages are marked by increased resistance to antibiotics. Biofilms are increasingly associated with recalcitrant infections such as chronic prostatitis, chronic otitis media, infective endocarditis, and chronic adenoiditis. Likewise, the recalcitrant nature of CRS has led many to believe that biofilms may play an important role in this disease entity as well. Cryer et al. were able to identify the presence of biofilms in the sinus mucosa of CRS patients who had received appropriate surgical and medical therapy, but who had continued symptoms.[38] The dominant organism in these cases was *Pseudomonas aeruginosa*. A subsequent larger study by Sanclement et al. evaluated 30 patients with CRS and found that biofilms were present in the sinus mucosa of 80% of these patients.[39] Biofilms were not identified in any control patients. Of the dozen or so published reports associating biofilms with CRS, all identified *P. aeruginosa* as the primary cultured microbe. The importance of biofilms in chronic sinonasal infections remains largely unexplored. Particularly, it remains unclear how biofilms might contribute to the chronic inflammation that is an identifying component of CRS. Biofilms may instead represent an additional factor that contributes to the recalcitrance of CRS by creating a protective environment that is largely immune to medical treatments. Further investigation in this field is certainly forthcoming and will likely clarify what role, if any, biofilms play in CRS.

Fungi

Fungal disease was once considered to be a rare contributor to CRS, but evidence presented over the past decade has suggested that fungal pathogens may play a much more prominent role in this and other disease entities. The sentinel study involving fungal rhinosinusitis was performed at the Mayo Clinic in 1999 by Ponikau et al.[40] Using exquisitely sensitive culture techniques and immunohistological staining, fungal organisms were found in 96% of 210 patients with CRS. Confounding these results, evidence of fungal elements was also identified in healthy control subjects with no history of sinonasal disease at a rate approaching 100%. Consequently, great attention has focused on whether the detection of fungal organisms in the paranasal sinuses and nasal mucosa represents a true etiologic factor or simply a contaminant. Many fungal organisms are ubiquitous, and it is likely that the human sinonasal tract is colonized to some extent by these organisms very early on in life. In support of this hypothesis, Lackner et al. showed that fungi could be cultured from the nasal mucus of 94% of neonates at only 4 months of life.[41]

Furthermore, the composition of these organisms can be very diverse, with a study by Braun et al. identifying 88 different genera in the nasal mucin of 250 different patients, with an average of 2.4 to 3.1 different species per patient.[42] At this point in time, the role of fungi in CRS remains controversial. Given that the majority of well-designed published studies have shown no benefit to antifungal therapy in CRS, the widespread impression is that fungi are not the central etiologic agent in the disease overall, and that the presence of ubiquitous fungal organisms in the nasal mucin should not be viewed as pathologic. That being said, in some individuals, it seems that fungal antigens are capable of triggering an immune reaction, either allergic or nonallergic in nature, which may stimulate CRS or act as a disease modifier.

Allergic Fungal Eosinophilic Rhinosinusitis

Allergic fungal rhinosinusitis shares many features with allergic bronchopulmonary aspergillosis; most importantly, tissue infiltration by eosinophils that signal a late-phase allergic inflammatory response. It is now accepted dogma that fungi can elicit IgE-mediated mucosal inflammation in the absence of frank tissue invasion. Allergic fungal rhinosinusitis is diagnosed using three clinical criteria: (1) chronic sinusitis; (2) allergic mucin containing fungal hyphae; and (3) a positive skin test and/or specific IgE (RAST) to the respective fungus. There is considerable evidence to support a role for allergy in the pathogenesis of allergic fungal sinusitis. In a case-control study by Manning et al., every one of 16 patients with documented allergic fungal sinusitis was found to have a positive radioallergosorbent test to at least one fungal antigen that corresponded to the organisms cultured from their sinuses.[43] Many studies now support that allergic fungal rhinosinusitis is a fungal antigen-triggered, IgE and IgG-mediated hypersensitivity response that features a late-phase eosinophilic inflammatory reaction.

Nonallergic Fungal Eosinophilic Chronic Rhinosinusitis

Eosinophils play a major role in the immunological response to fungal antigens. However, a conventional IgE-mediated response is not consistently observed in chronic fungal rhinosinusitis, and recent evidence suggests that eosinophilic inflammation elicited by fungal organisms may be largely independent from a prototypical "allergic" IgE-mediated pathway. In support of this hypothesis, Shin et al. reported that <30% of CRS patients had elevated specific IgE antibodies to two different ubiquitous airborne fungi.[44] In contrast, IgG specific for these antigens was found to be greatly elevated when compared with normal controls. In the same study, peripheral blood lymphocytes from CRS patients, when incubated with fungal extracts, were found to produce elevated levels of the inflammatory mediators IL-5, IL-13, and IFN-γ. This response may derive from the ability of some fungal organisms, including *Aspergillus fumigatus* and *Alternaria*, to function as superantigens that can stimulate the production of inflammatory cytokines by subepithelial lymphocytes. Therefore, it may be that many CRS patients have an exaggerated response to common airborne environmental fungi that inhabit the sinonasal tract, thus resulting in sinonasal inflammation independent of allergic pathways.

Air Pollution

It has long been hypothesized that air quality is related to the development of CRS. The inherent difficulty in conducting controlled studies in this area has made proof of this hypothesis quite difficult. Previous research has been largely conflicting. A 1994 study by Luttmann et al. concluded that bronchitis and sinusitis was more prevalent in children living in urban rather than rural locations.[45] In contrast, a Korean study found no difference in the prevalence of chronic sinusitis in inhabitants of urban versus rural areas.[46] Perhaps the most comprehensive study linking urban air pollution with CRS was a retrospective analysis performed by Wolf in 2002 that found a weak but statistically significant effect of pollution on the prevalence of chronic rhinosinusitis.[47] In this study, CRS patients treated over a 10-year period were identified by the city district of their residency and linked to chemical indicators of pollution in the airborne environment of their district. Studies such as these are clearly troubled by confounding socioeconomic and demographic factors that make data analysis difficult and, at times, misleading. However, as environmental pollution becomes increasingly more of a geopolitical concern, further investigation into this area will hopefully be forthcoming.

Smoking

Tobacco smoke was convincingly associated with the development of rhinosinusitis by Lieu and Feinstein in 2000.[48] By analyzing survey data from more than 20,000 adults, they were able to conclude that primary cigarette or other tobacco product use was associated with increased self-reported rates of both acute and chronic rhinosinusitis. The same association was not found in individuals exposed to passive tobacco smoke. Multiple studies have concluded that the nasal mucosae of smoking individuals have greatly reduced mucociliary transport times, and this point was highlighted by the surgeon general as early as 1964. Alteration in mucociliary transport would be expected to result in mucostasis and, ultimately, persistent inflammation and CRS. Beyond its effect on mucociliary transport, tobacco smoke has also been found to up regulate proinflammatory cytokines such as IL-5 and IL-8, which may further contribute to the inflammation seen in CRS. Finally, Briggs et al. reported that smoking is a predictor of poor long-term outcome among CRS patients following endoscopic sinus surgery, suggesting that smoking may also adversely affect resolution of rhinosinusitis-attributed symptoms following definitive surgical treatment.[49] In sum, it appears likely that smoking is a contributor to the development and persistence of CRS, if not a true etiologic agent. Further study will no doubt be forthcoming.

Conclusion

Several factors have been proposed to contribute to the pathogenesis of CRS, with varying degrees of supporting evidence. Although a role likely exists for many of these putative etiologies in either the development or persistence of sinonasal inflammation in subsets of CRS patients, a single unifying "cause" of CRS remains elusive. Recent research implicates dysregulation of the sinonasal innate and adaptive mucosal immune system, rather than any specific inciting exogenous agent, as the most directly underlying chronic inflammation in CRS. As a greater understanding is achieved of sinonasal immune dysfunction in the diseased state, new therapies will focus on inflammatory resolution and restoration of normal mucosal homeostasis, rather than eradication of particular pathogens. In forthcoming decades, ongoing basic research promises to clarify the complex balance of environmental and host factors that drive CRS, resulting in more effective treatment options.

References

1. Yang IA, Barton SJ, Rorke S, et al. Toll-like receptor 4 polymorphism and severity of atopy in asthmatics. Genes Immun 2004; 5(1):41–45
2. Ramanathan M Jr, Lee WK, Lane AP. Increased expression of acidic mammalian chitinase in chronic rhinosinusitis with nasal polyps. Am J Rhinol 2006;20(3):330–335
3. Hamilos DL, Leung DY, Wood R, et al. Evidence for distinct cytokine expression in allergic versus nonallergic chronic sinusitis. J Allergy Clin Immunol 1995;96(4):537–544
4. Jyonouchi H, Sun S, Le H, Rimell FL. Evidence of dysregulated cytokine production by sinus lavage and peripheral blood mononuclear cells in patients with treatment-resistant chronic rhinosinusitis. Arch Otolaryngol Head Neck Surg 2001;127(12):1488–1494
5. al Ghamdi K, Ghaffar O, Small P, Frenkiel S, Hamid Q. IL-4 and IL-13 expression in chronic sinusitis: relationship with cellular infiltrate and effect of topical corticosteroid treatment. J Otolaryngol 1997;26(3):160–166
6. de Vries JE. The role of IL-13 and its receptor in allergy and inflammatory responses. J Allergy Clin Immunol 1998;102(2):165–169
7. Molet SM, Hamid QA, Hamilos DL. IL-11 and IL-17 expression in nasal polyps: relationship to collagen deposition and suppression by intranasal fluticasone propionate. Laryngoscope 2003;113(10):1803–1812
8. Ramanathan M Jr, Spannhake EW, Lane AP. Chronic rhinosinusitis with nasal polyps is associated with decreased expression of mucosal interleukin 22 receptor. Laryngoscope 2007;117(10):1839–1843
9. Bresciani M, Paradis L, Des Roches A, et al. Rhinosinusitis in severe asthma. J Allergy Clin Immunol 2001;107(1):73–80
10. Rehl RM, Balla AA, Cabay RJ, Hearp ML, Pytynia KB, Joe SA. Mucosal remodeling in chronic rhinosinusitis. Am J Rhinol 2007;21(6): 651–657
11. Braunstahl GJ, Kleinjan A, Overbeek SE, Prins JB, Hoogsteden HC, Fokkens WJ. Segmental bronchial provocation induces nasal inflammation in allergic rhinitis patients. Am J Respir Crit Care Med 2000;161(6):2051–2057
12. Denburg JA, Inman MD, Wood L, et al. Bone marrow progenitors in allergic airways diseases: studies in canine and human models. Int Arch Allergy Immunol 1997;113(1-3):181–183
13. Suzuki M, Watanabe T, Suko T, Mogi G. Comparison of sinusitis with and without allergic rhinitis: characteristics of paranasal sinus effusion and mucosa. Am J Otolaryngol 1999;20(3):143–150

14. Pelikan Z, Pelikan-Filipek M. Role of nasal allergy in chronic maxillary sinusitis—diagnostic value of nasal challenge with allergen. J Allergy Clin Immunol 1990;86(4 Pt 1):484–491
15. Baroody FM, Mucha SM, Detineo M, Naclerio RM. Nasal challenge with allergen leads to maxillary sinus inflammation. J Allergy Clin Immunol 2008;121(5):1126–1132
16. Vanlerberghe L, Joniau S, Jorissen M. The prevalence of humoral immunodeficiency in refractory rhinosinusitis: a retrospective analysis. B-ENT 2006;2(4):161–166
17. Ortiz E, Sakano E, De Souza CA, Vigorito A, Eid KA. Chronic GVHD: predictive factor for rhinosinusitis in bone marrow transplantation. Braz J Otorhinolaryngol 2006;72(3):328–332
18. Tami TA. The management of sinusitis in patients infected with the human immunodeficiency virus (HIV). Ear Nose Throat J 1995; 74(5):360–363
19. Wang X, Moylan B, Leopold DA, et al. Mutation in the gene responsible for cystic fibrosis and predisposition to chronic rhinosinusitis in the general population. JAMA 2000;284(14):1814–1819
20. Raman V, Clary R, Siegrist KL, Zehnbauer B, Chatila TA. Increased prevalence of mutations in the cystic fibrosis transmembrane conductance regulator in children with chronic rhinosinusitis. Pediatrics 2002;109(1):E13
21. Krzeski A, Tomaszewska E, Jakubczyk I, Galewicz-Zielińska A. Anatomic variations of the lateral nasal wall in the computed tomography scans of patients with chronic rhinosinusitis. Am J Rhinol 2001;15(6):371–375
22. Yasan H, Doğru H, Baykal B, Döner F, Tüz M. What is the relationship between chronic sinus disease and isolated nasal septal deviation? Otolaryngol Head Neck Surg 2005;133(2):190–193
23. Collet S, Bertrand B, Cornu S, Eloy P, Rombaux P. Is septal deviation a risk factor for chronic sinusitis? Review of literature. Acta Otorhinolaryngol Belg 2001;55(4):299–304
24. Orlandi RR, A systematic analysis of septal deviation associated with rhinosinusitis. Laryngoscope 2010 Aug; 120(8):1687–95
25. Giacchi RJ, Lebowitz RA, Yee HT, Light JP, Jacobs JB. Histopathologic evaluation of the ethmoid bone in chronic sinusitis. Am J Rhinol 2001;15(3):193–197
26. Jang YJ, Koo TW, Chung SY, Park SG. Bone involvement in chronic rhinosinusitis assessed by 99mTc-MDP bone SPECT. Clin Otolaryngol Allied Sci 2002;27(3):156–161
27. Majima Y, Hirata K, Matsubara T, Sakakura Y, Miyoshi Y. Viscoelastic properties of nasal mucus from patients with chronic sinusitis. Nippon Jibiinkoka Gakkai Kaiho 1983;86(6):644–651
28. Chen B, Antunes MB, Claire SE, et al. Reversal of chronic rhinosinusitis-associated sinonasal ciliary dysfunction. Am J Rhinol 2007;21(3):346–353
29. DiBaise JK, Olusola BF, Huerter JV, Quigley EM. Role of GERD in chronic resistant sinusitis: a prospective, open label, pilot trial. Am J Gastroenterol 2002;97(4):843–850
30. Vaezi MF, Hagaman DD, Slaughter JC, Tanner SB et al. Gastroenterology 2010 Dec; 139(6):1887–1893
31. DelGaudio JM. Direct nasopharyngeal reflux of gastric acid is a contributing factor in refractory chronic rhinosinusitis. Laryngoscope 2005;115(6):946–957
32. Jecker P, Orloff LA, Wohlfeil M, Mann WJ. Gastroesophageal reflux disease (GERD), extraesophageal reflux (EER) and recurrent chronic rhinosinusitis. Eur Arch Otorhinolaryngol 2006;263(7):664–667
33. Dinis PB, Subtil J. Helicobacter pylori and laryngopharyngeal reflux in chronic rhinosinusitis. Otolaryngol Head Neck Surg 2006;134(1):67–72
34. Jang YJ, Kwon HJ, Park HW, Lee BJ. Detection of rhinovirus in turbinate epithelial cells of chronic sinusitis. Am J Rhinol 2006;20(6): 634–636
35. Brook I, Frazier EH, Foote PA. Microbiology of chronic maxillary sinusitis: comparison between specimens obtained by sinus endoscopy and by surgical drainage. J Med Microbiol 1997;46(5): 430–432
36. Jyonouchi H, Sun S, Kennedy CA, et al. Localized sinus inflammation in a rabbit sinusitis model induced by Bacteroides fragilis is accompanied by rigorous immune responses. Otolaryngol Head Neck Surg 1999;120(6):869–875
37. Bachert C, Gevaert P, van Cauwenberge P. Staphylococcus aureus superantigens and airway disease. Curr Allergy Asthma Rep 2002;2(3):252–258
38. Cryer J, Schipor I, Perloff JR, Palmer JN. Evidence of bacterial biofilms in human chronic sinusitis. ORL J Otorhinolaryngol Relat Spec 2004;66(3):155–158
39. Sanclement JA, Webster P, Thomas J, Ramadan HH. Bacterial biofilms in surgical specimens of patients with chronic rhinosinusitis. Laryngoscope 2005;115(4):578–582
40. Ponikau JU, Sherris DA, Kern EB, et al. The diagnosis and incidence of allergic fungal sinusitis. Mayo Clin Proc 1999;74(9):877–884
41. Lackner A, Freudenschuss K, Buzina W, et al. From when on can fungi be identified in nasal mucus of humans? Laryngorhinootologie 2004;83(2):117–121
42. Braun H, Stammberger H, Buzina W, Freudenschuss K, Lackner A, Beham A. Incidence and detection of fungi and eosinophilic granulocytes in chronic rhinosinusitis. Laryngorhinootologie 2003; 82(5):330–340
43. Manning SC, Mabry RL, Schaefer SD, Close LG. Evidence of IgE-mediated hypersensitivity in allergic fungal sinusitis. Laryngoscope 1993;103(7):717–721
44. Shin SH, Ponikau JU, Sherris DA, et al. Chronic rhinosinusitis: an enhanced immune response to ubiquitous airborne fungi. J Allergy Clin Immunol 2004;114(6):1369–1375
45. Luttmann H, Grömping U, Kreienbrock L, Treiber-Klötzer C, Wichmann HE. Cohort study of respiratory diseases and lung function in school children in Southwest Germany. 4. Inner city environment influences on respiratory diseases in Mannheim. Zentralbl Hyg Umweltmed 1995;198(2): 172–189
46. Min YG, Jung HW, Kim HS, Park SK, Yoo KY. Prevalence and risk factors of chronic sinusitis in Korea: results of a nationwide survey. Eur Arch Otorhinolaryngol 1996;253(7):435–439
47. Wolf C. Urban air pollution and health: an ecological study of chronic rhinosinusitis in Cologne, Germany. Health Place 2002;8(2):129–139
48. Lieu JE, Feinstein AR. Confirmations and surprises in the association of tobacco use with sinusitis. Arch Otolaryngol Head Neck Surg 2000;126(8):940–946
49. Briggs RD, Wright ST, Cordes S, Calhoun KH. Smoking in chronic rhinosinusitis: a predictor of poor long-term outcome after endoscopic sinus surgery. Laryngoscope 2004;114(1): 126–128

14 Nasal Polyposis

Rakesh K. Chandra, David B. Conley, and Robert C. Kern

Chronic rhinosinusitis (CRS) represents a heterogeneous group of disorders that can be further classified by phenotypical presentation as either CRS without nasal polyps (CRSsNP) or CRS with nasal polyps (CRSwNP). In turn, the latter group also reflects a multitude of potential underlying pathophysiologic processes, which may even coexist in any individual patient. The development of nasal polyposis thus requires susceptibility of the host, in addition to environmental factors such as microorganisms and immunologic stimuli. The exact etiology of nasal polyposis unfortunately remains idiopathic in the preponderance of cases; however, consideration of the potential underlying pathophysiology is important in tailoring an optimal therapeutic regimen. Some of these associated conditions reflect known genetic defects, such as cystic fibrosis (CF) or aspirin-exacerbated respiratory disease (AERD, also known as ASA triad or Samter's triad); others are associated with clinical syndromes such as classic allergic fungal sinusitis (AFS). The antrochoanal polyp, which typically exists as a solitary entity, reflects a distinct pathologic entity that contrasts with CRSwNP, in which diffuse polyposis is typically encountered. The goal of the present chapter is to discuss the diagnosis and management of CRSwNP in the setting of the current state of knowledge of proposed etiologies for the condition.

Epidemiology

Current estimates suggest that CRS affects 30 to 35 million people in the United States and accounts for ~20 million physician office visits annually.[1] It is currently accepted that CRSsNP and CRSwNP are distinct disease states, and it is thus difficult to quantify the prevalence of each entity based on historical data. Furthermore, the incidence of CRS and CRSwNP are likely to vary geographically. A recent Denmark study[2] suggested that the mean incidence of *symptomatic* nasal polyps was ~1 case per 1000 population. The prevalence was greater in males and peaked in the 50 to 59 year age group, although the subset of patients with antrochoanal polyps, which accounted for 5%, tended to present at a younger age.

The prevalence of nasal polyposis must also be considered in the context of other chronic airway inflammatory diseases such as rhinitis and asthma. Allergic rhinitis is thought to be the most commonly diagnosed chronic condition, affecting 5 to 22% of the population,[3] and the prevalence of nonallergic rhinitis may be even higher. Contrary to commonly held perceptions, atopic patients are not at increased risk for developing nasal polyps. Although ~50% of patients with nasal polyps have positive skin tests, the prevalence of polyps in patients with rhinitis and/or asthma is thought to be <5% and may be lower in atopic compared with nonatopic patients.

This hypothesis was supported by a recent Greek study of over 3800 patients, which demonstrated that polyps were more prevalent in patients with nonallergic rhinitis than in patients with allergic rhinitis (8.9% vs. 1.7%). The same study revealed an even greater disparity in the incidence of nasal polyposis between nonallergic and allergic asthmatic patients (13% vs. 2.4%, respectively).[4] The preponderance of current data dispels the common misperception that atopy is the dominant mechanism linking these disorders.

Etiology of Nasal Polyposis: Current Concepts

A single final common pathway in the etiology of nasal polyposis is yet to be elucidated. Histologic examination is a first step in understanding potential mechanisms. Polyp tissue from western populations has revealed eosinophilia in the majority of CRSwNP cases. These patients appear to mount T-helper 2 (Th2) mediated inflammation, where interleukin (IL)-4, IL-5, and interferon (INF)-gamma are key cytokines, and reverse transcriptase polymerase chain reaction (RT-PCR) studies have demonstrated elevated mRNA for each of these mediators in nasal polyp tissue.[5,6] Leukotrienes are also thought to be important in the progression of Th2 pathways, eosinophilia, and polyposis. Multiple underlying etiologies have been investigated as the driving force behind this vigorous Th2-mediated inflammation including atopic disease, genetic defects in leukotriene metabolism, immune responses to fungi, and stimulation by bacterial superantigens. Others have examined the role of defects of mucosal barrier function, which may confer susceptibility to these inflammatory stimuli. When discussing the pathophysiology, it should be recalled that "typical" eosinophilic polyps must be contrasted from antrochoanal polyps and polyps from the subset of CRSwNP patients with CF. In these latter disorders, neutrophilic inflammation usually predominates and Th1 pathways have been implicated. Additionally, it should be noted that although Th1-mediated inflammation is thought to be the driving force in patients with CRSsNP,[6] small subsets of patients with CRSwNP (e.g., some Asian populations) may also manifest neutrophilic rather than eosinophilic inflammation via stimuli that are presently unclear.

Role of Systemic Atopy

The observation of eosinophilic inflammation is consistent with known clinical associations between CRS, asthma, and allergic rhinitis, which manifest similar inflammatory patterns, particularly when present comorbidly. Intuitively, it would seem that allergic rhinitis would be the prime driving force behind the development of nasal polyposis. However, it is estimated that only ~38 to 67% of patients with CRS who require functional endoscopic sinus surgery (FESS) have comorbid systemic immunoglobulin (Ig)E-mediated allergy.[7] Additionally, the enzyme-linked immunosorbent assay has revealed elevated eosinophils, eosinophil cationic protein, eotaxin, IgE, and IL-5 in nasal polyp tissue when compared with controls and CRSsNP,[6] further supporting the hypothesis that nasal polyposis is typically mediated by Th2 inflammatory pathways and eosinophils. Data from the Northwestern Sinus and Allergy Center revealed that the mean Lund-Mackay score was higher in polyp patients compared with nonpolyp patients ($p < 0.0001$), but this finding was independent of atopic status. Additionally, asthmatics were more likely than nonasthmatics to have polyps (57.6% vs. 25%; $p = 0.0015$), but this was also irrespective of atopic status. Although these observations underscore links between polyps and radiologic severity of CRS, as well as between polyps and other forms of chronic airway inflammatory disease, the data suggest that systemic IgE-mediated disease is not the sole pathophysiologic mechanism.

Defects of Leukotriene Metabolism

Examination of patients with AERD (ASA triad) has inspired exploration of the role of cysteinyl leukotrienes in CRS. Cysteinyl leukotrienes are formed by the action of 5-lipoxygenase upon arachidonic acid, which is liberated from the cell membrane by phospholipase A2. The cysteinyl leukotrienes LTC4, LTD4, and LTE4 are three end products of the lipoxygenase pathway. These leukotrienes cause mucosal inflammation, bronchoconstriction, microvascular leakage, and mucus secretion via their effects on epithelial cells, mucus secreting cells, and leukocytes. The other pathway through which arachidonic acid is metabolized involves the action of cyclooxygenase, the end products of which are prostaglandins and thromboxanes. Because aspirin is an irreversible inhibitor of the cyclooxygenase pathway, exposure to aspirin increases the substrate available for lipoxygenase activity and thus results in accelerated leukotriene synthesis. It has been hypothesized that AERD patients may have increased susceptibility to mucosal inflammation, microvascular leakage, and mucus secretion secondary to increased activity of the enzymes involved in leukotriene generation and/or increased expression of leukotriene receptors.

Although cysteinyl leukotrienes are elevated in CRS of many etiologies and clinical presentations, as well as asthma and allergic rhinitis, patients with AERD exhibit even higher levels of these mediators, and levels are even further enhanced by aspirin administration.[8] Additionally, when compared with normal controls, the cysteinyl leukotrienes type 1 receptor appears to be elevated in leukocytes of CRS patients with AERD.[9] Additional investigations demonstrated increased expression of this receptor in both polyp epithelium and stroma when compared with mucosa from controls, and this observation was apparent in patients with and without aspirin sensitivity.[10] Furthermore, in vitro studies have revealed that IL-4, IL-5, and IL-13 up regulate expression of the cysteinyl leukotriene type 1 receptor in eosinophils.[11] In summary, current data suggest that leukotriene stimulation may be a key step in the Th2-mediated cascade that has been implicated in the genesis of nasal polyposis, and that this response is even further heightened in aspirin-intolerant patients.

Immune Response to Fungi

The development of polyposis in the clinical picture of classic AFS is well-known. In this condition, chronic hypersensitivity to dematiaceous fungi is associated with nasal polyposis, ostial obstruction, and multiple sinus involvement. Initially, the immunologic processes at work in AFS were thought to involve type I, type III, and/or type IVa_2 hypersensitivity, which are also observed in allergic bronchopulmonary aspergillosis. Recent studies, however, have suggested that AFS is predominantly mediated by eosinophils, and that non-IgE mediated mechanisms of Th2 stimulation (especially IL-5 production) are most important. Furthermore, it has been hypothesized by some that the eosinophilic response to fungi, particularly *Alternaria*, may be responsible for CRS in general, whereas classic AFS merely reflects the end stage of the disease process.[12] Although it is possible that an immune response to a fungus is responsible for polyp development in a subset of patients with CRS, a direct link between fungi and polyposis is yet to be demonstrated.

Role of Superantigens

An area of active investigation involves the role of immunologic responses to *Staphylococcus aureus* enterotoxins, particularly staphylococcal enterotoxin B (SEB) in the pathophysiology of CRS. These proteins, in susceptible patients, appear to have the ability to function as "superantigens," in that they are able to cross-link the class II major histocompatibility complex of antigen presenting cells and the beta-chain variable region of the T-cell receptor. This is thought to result in vigorous production of Th2 cytokines, including IL-4, IL-5, IL-13, and eotaxin, thereby predisposing patients to nasal polyp formation.[13] In one recent investigation, polyp-derived lymphocytes from patients with CRSwNP were analyzed by flow cytometry. In a significant proportion of these patients, specificity of the T-cell receptor V beta-region was skewed toward those specific for *S. aureus* superantigens. These data support studies by other authors implicating *S. aureus* superantigens in the induction of inflammatory pathways leading to polyposis.[14]

Abnormalities of Innate Mucosal Immunity

Toll-like Receptors

Toll-like receptors (TLRs) are a family of membrane-bound pattern recognition receptors thought to be involved in innate mucosal immunity. Thirteen TLRs are recognized in humans and, in the sinonasal tract, these receptors are thought to be a mechanism of innate antimicrobial defense for the mucosal epithelial cells. Each TLR responds to a class of ligands. For example, TLR3 binds double-stranded RNA (such as that of viral origin), and TLR4 binds lipopolysaccharide. RT-PCR revealed that mRNA for TLRs and key cytokines was detected in the ethmoid mucosa of both control and CRS subjects. As compared with controls, CRS was associated with a significantly higher expression of TLR2 and the inflammatory genes macrophage-inflammatory protein alpha, RANTES, and granulocyte-macrophage colony-stimulating factor. Patients with a recurrence of polyps postsurgery had significantly decreased expression of TLR2 (which binds Gram-positive peptidoglycan) and TLR9 (which binds CpG DNA), which are markers of innate immunity, and higher macrophage-inflammatory protein alpha.[15] These observations suggest that defects in the mucosal barrier function may be associated with polyp development.

Matrix Metalloproteinases

Matrix metalloproteinases (MMPs) have been recently examined for their role in the pathogenesis of CRSwNP. MMPs constitute a group of zinc-dependent endopeptidases that are able to degrade the extracellular matrix and are possibly responsible for the development of tissue edema in CRS. A recent study using RT-PCR was conducted to determine the expression of MMP-2, MMP-9, and tissue inhibitor of matrix metalloproteinase-1 (TIMP-1) mRNA and to correlate these findings with expression of IL-5 and IL-8. The data revealed expression of both MMP-9 and IL-5 mRNA in polyp tissue. A correlation between IL-5 and TIMP-1 was also observed, indicating a role for TIMP-1 in maintaining the homeostasis in nasal polyps.[16]

Other Epithelial Genes Under Investigation

SPINK5 is an epithelial serine protease inhibitor that has been associated with allergic disease and is believed to have an important role in the balance of inflammatory effects of mast cells on the epithelial barrier. Specifically, allergens often possess serine protease activity, and diminished expression of antiproteases such as SPINK5 may influence susceptibility for atopy. RT-PCR data from our laboratory[17] have revealed reduced SPINK5 expression in tissues of patients with CRSwNP and CRSsNP. Immunohistochemistry also demonstrated decreased expression of SPINK5 in polyp tissue compared with controls. The S100 family proteins are part of the epidermal differentiation complex (EDC) on chromosome 1q21. This collection of epithelial genes is important in both antimicrobial and immunoregulatory functions. Our data have also demonstrated a down regulation of mRNA for S100A7, S100A8, and S100A9 in CRS, which could theoretically result in a decreased proliferative or aberrant regenerative capacity of the respiratory epithelium. This could hypothetically decrease the mechanical barrier effect and accentuate both sensitization and the inflammatory response to a variety of exogenous agents.

Our series of investigations has also explored the role of B cell-activating factor of the tumor necrosis factor (TNF) family (BAFF).[18] This is a cytokine that is an important regulator of class switch recombination and immunoglobulin production. Preliminary data also demonstrate that it is expressed in nasal polyp tissue by immunohistochemistry. BAFF mRNA was significantly increased in nasal polyps from patients with CRSwNP ($p < 0.001$) compared with inferior turbinate tissue from patients with CRS or healthy subjects. Expression of mRNA for BAFF in polyp tissue was significantly correlated with B lymphocyte markers CD20 and TACI, as well as IgA. These data suggest that overproduction of BAFF in nasal polyps may contribute to the pathogenesis of CRSwNP via the local induction of IgA and the activation of eosinophils.[19]

The previous findings implicate a role for dysregulation of innate mucosal defenses in conferring susceptibility to antigen exposure, sensitization, and/or aberrant host inflammatory response. Furthermore, the spectrum of investigations published to date has suggested roles for multiple (possibly coexisting) immunologic defects that may be implicated in the development of nasal polyposis. This further underscores the philosophy that nasal polyposis is an inflammatory rather than an infectious disease.

Clinical Presentation

Patients with CRS present with symptoms such as nasal airflow obstruction, rhinorrhea, postnasal discharge, smell loss, taste disturbance, and facial pain/pressure. These symptoms are consistent with the major symptom criteria

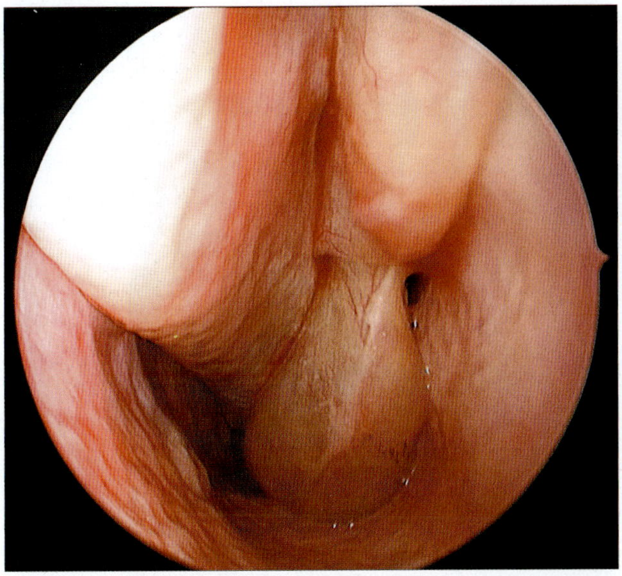

Fig. 14.1 Nasal polyposis with an obstruction of the posterior nasal airway.

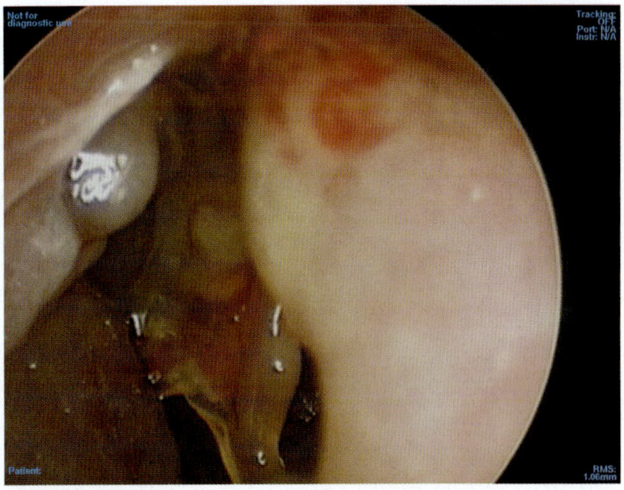

Fig. 14.2 Allergic mucin admixed with polypoid changes, as seen in a patient with allergic fungal sinusitis.

defined by the Task Force on Rhinosinusitis,[1] and minor symptom criteria such as ear fullness are possible as well. Compared with CRSsNP, CRSwNP patients are more likely to exhibit obstructive symptoms and hyposmia rather than symptoms of pain and pressure.[20] Subtle findings in many of these patients also include hyponasality of voice, sleep disturbance, mouth breathing, and occasionally, epistaxis. CRS patients with asthma are also more likely than those without asthma to exhibit polyps.[21] Occasionally, the patient will notice nasal polyps by self-examination. Advanced sinonasal polyposis may also be associated with proptosis and/or pseudotelecanthus, particularly in the setting of classic AFS.

Diagnostic Workup

A diligent history, a physical examination, computed tomography (CT), and sinonasal endoscopy are complementary tools, and findings on any of these modalities must be considered in the context of the others.

Sinonasal Endoscopy

Sinonasal endoscopy is critical in the workup of nasal polyposis (**Fig. 14.1**). In addition to providing visualization of polyps themselves, endoscopy may point to important clues regarding comorbid disease (e.g., AFS) (**Fig. 14.2**). Additionally, subtle endoscopic features may suggest other diagnoses that may grossly present as polypoid nasal masses. Conversely, masses that appear consistent with inflammatory polyposis are occasionally found to be other entities, including benign neoplasms such as inverting papillomas (**Fig. 14.3**), malignant neoplasms (**Fig. 14.4**), and encephaloceles (**Fig. 14.5**). Hemorrhagic, friable, or ulcerative features may reflect a neoplastic rather than an inflammatory origin. Additionally, masses that appear pedicled medial to the vertical lamella of the middle turbinate must be considered suspicious of noninflammatory pathology (e.g., an encephalocele) (**Fig. 14.5**).

Computed Tomography Scan

CT scans continue to be the mainstay of imaging modalities in the evaluation of CRSwNP. CT can evaluate the extent of paranasal sinus opacification and the degree of thinning,

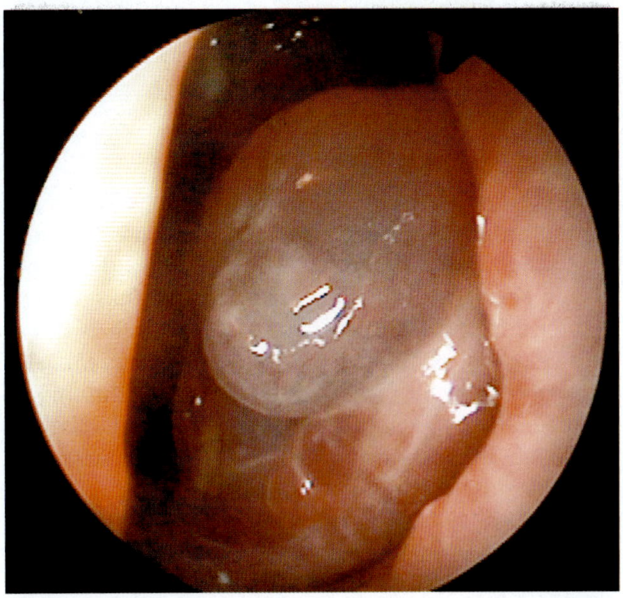

Fig. 14.3 This polyplike mass was found to be an inverting papilloma, highlighting the need for histopathologic evaluation of resected tissue.

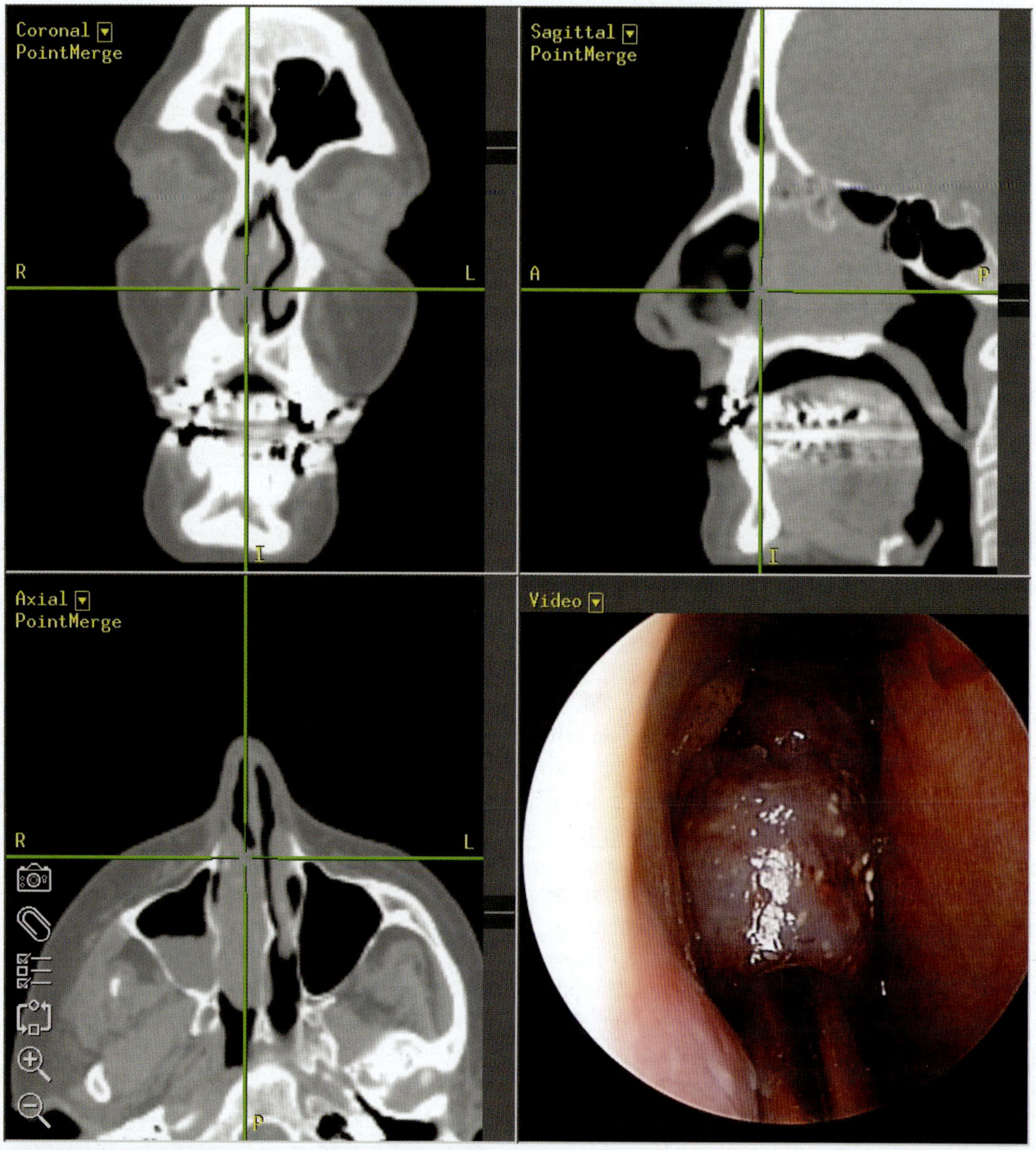

Fig. 14.4 This hemorrhagic mass was found to be an olfactory neuroblastoma. In the endoscopic view (*right lower panel*), note that the mass arises medial to the right middle turbinate, compressing this structure against the lateral nasal wall.

if any, of the adjacent bone. The sites of polyp origin can sometimes be elucidated. In typical noncontrast-enhanced bone windows on CT, polyps will be of similar radiodensity as fluid or other soft tissues (except fat). CT must also be examined for clues to comorbid pathology such as classic AFS, which will exhibit radiodense foci secondary to chelation of metals by fungal organisms (**Fig. 14.6**). This finding will be more apparent in soft tissue windows. Conditions associated with extensive polyposis, such as advanced AFS, may cause bowing or an expansion of sinus walls with impingement against the dura or periorbita (**Fig. 14.7**). If overt bone destruction or erosion is observed, a neoplasm or an encephalocele should be considered, in which case magnetic resonance imaging (MRI) should also be performed. In the vast majority of cases, however, CT alone is diagnostically sufficient. Modern in-office CT scanners can provide immediate imaging data for diagnostic assessment, patient counseling, and surgical planning, as well as intraoperative navigation.

Allergy and Immunology Evaluation

An atopy workup should be considered in the workup of patients with CRSwNP given that ~50% of patients with polyps will have positive findings. Skin testing is preferred. This may be of particular importance in patients with comorbid asthma or allergic rhinitis symptoms such as itchy, watery eyes, nasal/conjunctival pruritus, sneezing, and seasonal/environmental preponderance of symptoms.

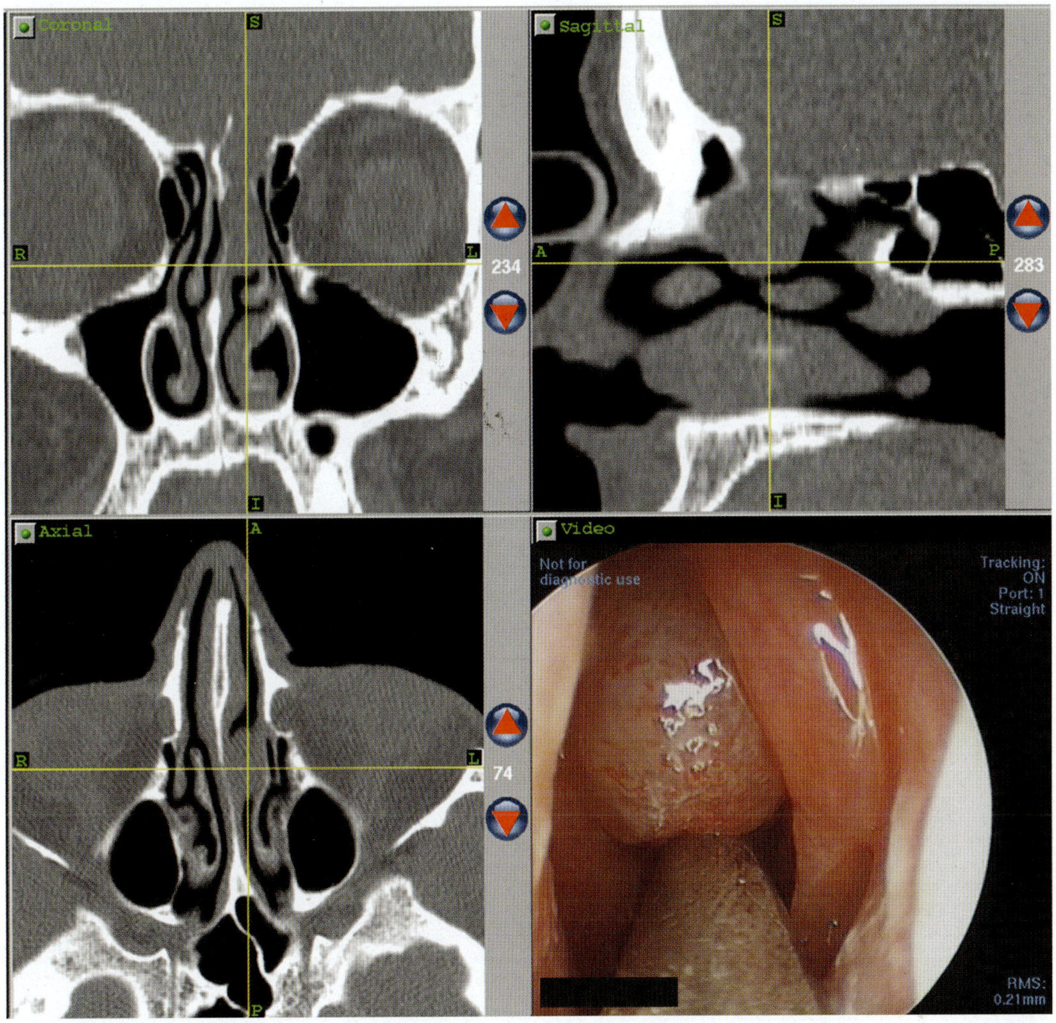

Fig. 14.5 Endoscopy (*right lower panel*) reveals a polyplike mass in the right nasal cavity. Correlation with the coronal computed tomography view (*left upper panel*) reveals an origin medial to the middle turbinate lamella and dehiscence of the cribriform skull base, which is consistent with an encephalocele.

Selected patients, particularly in the pediatric population, should be evaluated for immune deficiencies. Any pediatric patient with nasal polyposis should undergo a workup for CF with a sweat chloride test. If the diagnosis remains in doubt, or if CF is still suspected despite a negative sweat chloride test, genetic testing is available.

Treatment

Management of nasal polyposis typically requires multimodal therapy. In cases of limited polyps, medical therapy alone may be a consideration, using systemic corticosteroid bursts followed by long-term intranasal steroids. However, persistently symptomatic patients and those with advanced diffuse polyposis (especially AFS and AERD patients) often require surgical therapy in concert with a medical regimen that includes steroids. Details of the surgical technique are outlined elsewhere in this text. This section will highlight key management principles and review available evidence for their efficacy.

Steroids and Surgery

Oral Steroids

Oral steroids are typically administered under any of the following clinical scenarios: (1) as part of a regimen of maximal medical therapy prior to considering surgery; (2) use in the perioperative period to reduce the inflammatory burden intraoperatively and to augment optimal healing postoperatively; (3) during exacerbations; (4) management of comorbidities such as asthma or other allergic/inflammatory conditions. Occasionally, intravenous or intramuscular therapy is indicated, but tapering oral doses are preferred. Unfortunately, there is no uniform algorithm regarding exactly when steroids are indicated, and what the appropriate dosage and length of therapy may be.

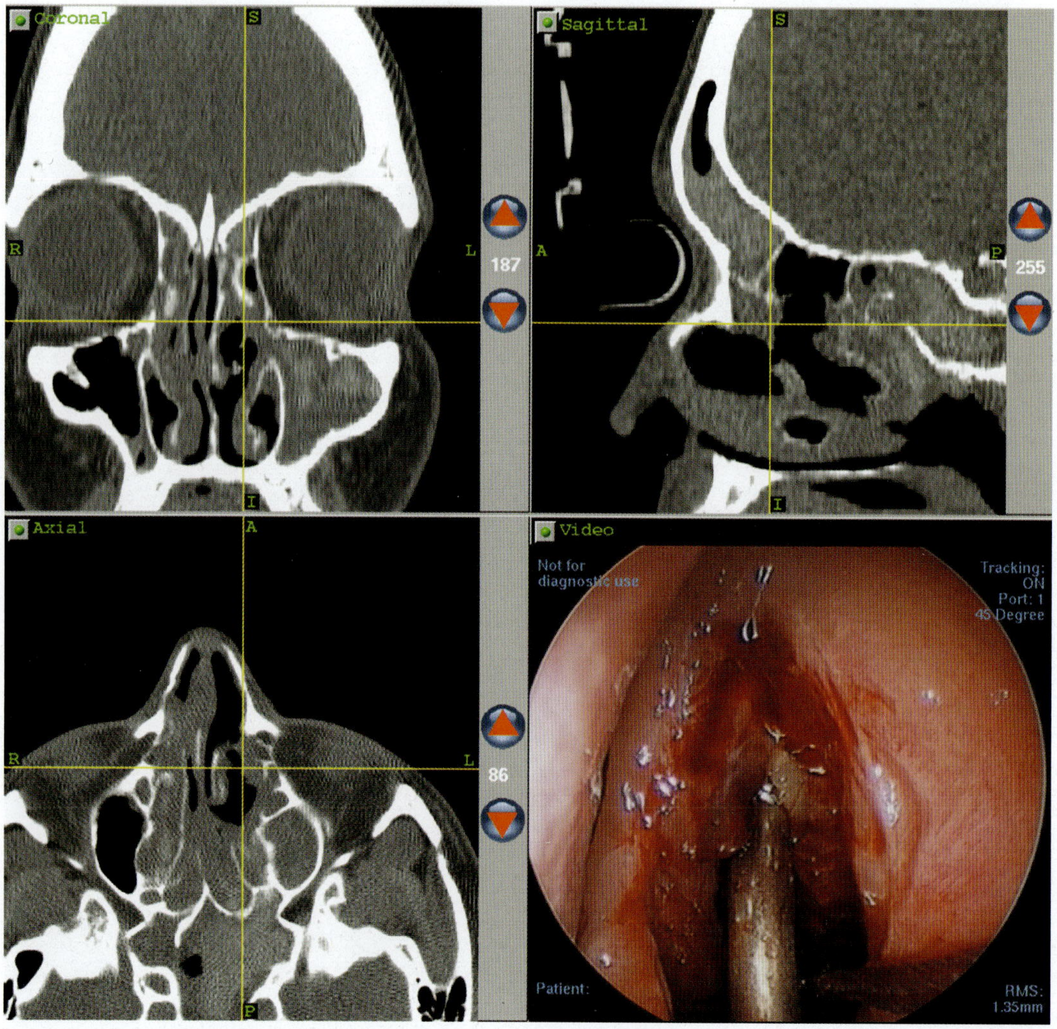

Fig. 14.6 Triplanar computed tomography reconstructions revealing hyperdense material with the opacified maxillary and sphenoid sinuses seen in the coronal (*upper left panel*) and sagittal (*upper right panel*) views, respectively. This is consistent with allergic mucin seen in allergic fungal sinusitis.

This clinical judgment is based on balancing the risks and benefits in any individual patient. Systemic steroids must be used with caution in patients with gastrointestinal ulcers, diabetes, cataracts, glaucoma, and osteoporosis. Nonetheless, oral steroids are considered an integral component in the management of patients with CRSwNP, AFS, and in selected patients with comorbid asthma or allergic conditions.[22] Patients may require tapers that begin in the range of 60 to 80 mg per day. Responses may be significant, and these regimens may avert or delay the need for surgery in some patients. However, it remains unclear why some patients do not respond adequately or else experience rapid recurrence of symptoms after therapy is discontinued. Patients whose symptoms fail to respond to aggressive medical therapy and those with diffuse sinonasal polyposis or AFS are typically considered candidates for surgery. Oral steroids may be initiated from a few days to several weeks preoperatively and then continued postoperatively until a resolution of mucosal inflammatory disease is observed endoscopically. This may require prolonged courses (up to several months) and higher dosages in patients with AERD and AFS. A recent study examining efficacy of oral steroids when used as part of a perioperative treatment regimen has revealed a benefit in improving postoperative endoscopy scores.[23]

Additionally, selected patients will require chronic low-dose steroid therapy, such as prednisone 5 mg daily or 10 mg every other day. Dosages used in chronic low-dose therapies are often below that which induces hypothalamic-pituitary-adrenal axis suppression, and the exact mechanism of action of this treatment is largely unknown. Suggested steroid regimens for various clinical scenarios are described in **Table 14.1**. Additionally, these dosing schemes may require modifications based on the patient's body mass index and medical comorbidities. Patients who require long-term therapy or frequent tapers should undergo frequent monitoring of blood glucose levels, bone density, and ophthalmologic status.

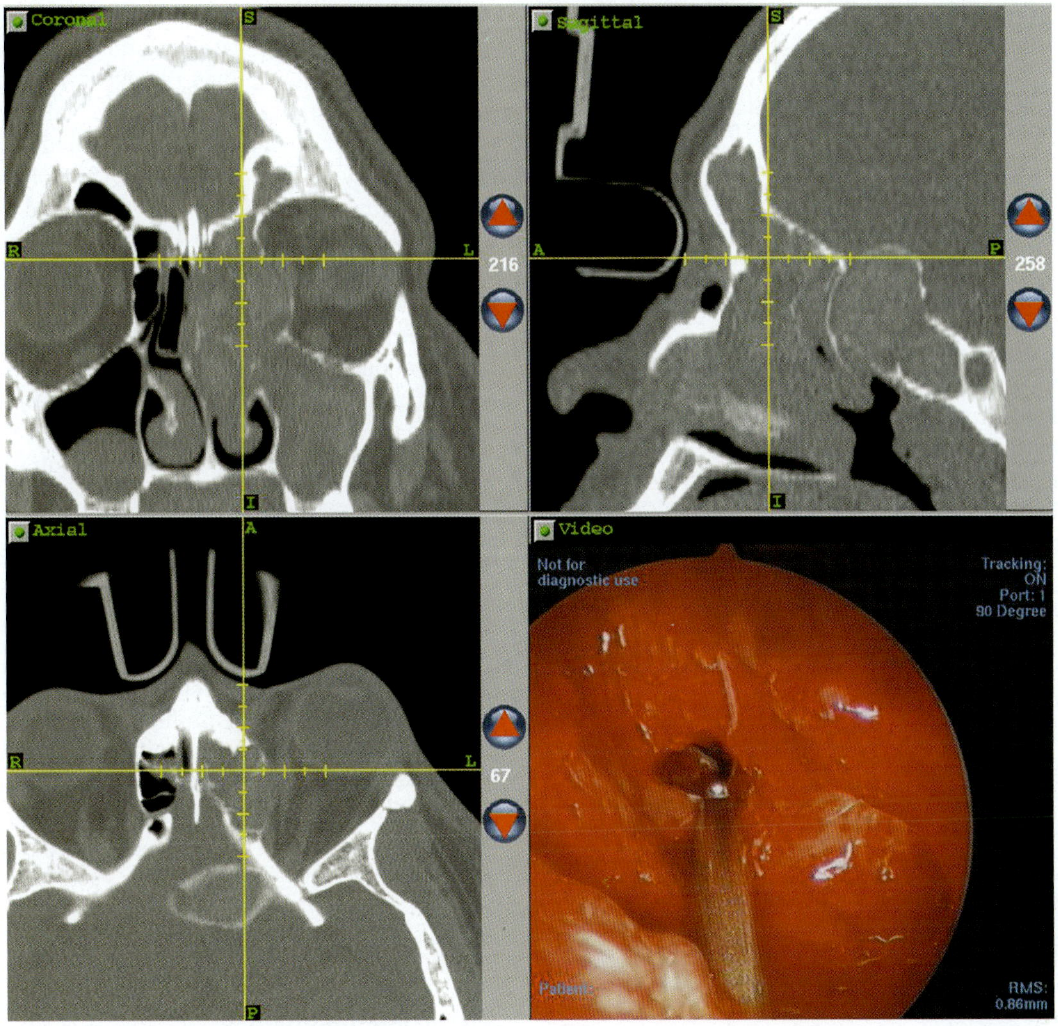

Fig. 14.7 Triplanar computed tomography reconstructions revealing the expansile nature of a chronic hyperplastic pansinusitis secondary to acute fungal sinusitis. Displacement and bowing of the left medial orbital wall is evident in the coronal (*upper left panel*) and axial (*lower left panel*) views. Proptosis of the left eye is also apparent in the axial image. The sagittal image (*upper right panel*) demonstrates bowing of the skull base in a cranial direction.

Table 14.1 Suggested Steroid Regimens for Various Clinical Scenarios

Scenario	CRSwNP	AFS, AERD
Presurgical treatment trial	30 mg po QD × 3 days 20 mg po QD × 3 days 10 mg po QD × 3 days 10 mg po QOD × 3 days	30 mg po BID × 3 days 20 mg po BID × 3 days 10 mg po BID × 3 days 10 mg po QD × 3 days
Perioperative treatment: preoperatively	30 mg po QD × 3 days 20 mg po QD × 3 days Start 6 days preop	30 mg po BID × 7 days 20 mg po BID × 7 days 30 mg po QD × 7 days Start 3 weeks preop
Perioperative treatment: postoperatively	20 mg po QD until endoscopic resolution of disease then tapered off over 1 week	30 mg po QD until endoscopic resolution of disease then tapered off over 1 week
Acute exacerbation	30 mg po QD × 3 days 20 mg po QD × 3 days 10 mg po QD × 3 days 10 mg po QOD × 3 days	30 mg po QD × 3 days 20 mg po QD × 3 days 10 mg po QD × 3 days 10 mg po QOD × 3 days

Abbreviations: AERD, aspirin exacerbated respiratory disease; AFS, acute fungal sinusitis; BID, twice a day; CRSwNP, chronic rhinosinusitis with nasal polyps; po, by mouth; preop, preoperatively; QD, every day; QOD, every other day.

Intranasal Steroids

Intranasal steroids are commonly used in allergic rhinitis and CRS. In many patients without polyps as well as some with mild degrees of polyposis, long-term intranasal steroids may delay or avert the need for surgery. The primary effect of topical steroids is to reduce obstructive symptoms secondary to mucosal inflammatory disease from underlying chronic rhinitis or allergic rhinitis. In addition, nasal steroids have been associated with a decrease in the size of nasal polyps, as well as prevention of polyp recurrence postoperatively.[24] In patients with allergic rhinitis, intranasal corticosteroids have been demonstrated to decrease epithelial and subepithelial eosinophilia based on pre- and posttreatment mucosal biopsies.[25] However, it remains unclear to what degree intranasal steroids may modulate the eosinophilic responses associated with CRS apart from allergic rhinitis. Additionally, studies have shown that penetration into the sinus cavity using a metered dose spray bottle is poor, even in patients who have had prior surgery.[26] In light of this fact, greater interest has been directed towards delivering steroids by more efficacious means. Budesonide dissolved in large volume saline irrigation has become a favored method of topical steroid delivery. Short-term use of less than three months has shown to be safe, although the specific pharmacokinetics of topical budesonide irrigation have not been well characterized. Given an overall favorable risk-benefit profile of intranasal steroids, these medications are considered a mainstay of long-term medical therapy in CRS patients with or without nasal polyps.

Allergy Treatment

Antihistamines

Antihistamines have been shown to decrease activation of eosinophils and mast cells in polyp tissue as measured by decreased production of markers such as eosinophil cationic protein in stimulated ex vivo polyp tissue.[27] Although this might suggest a potential benefit of antihistamines in the management of nasal polyps, clinical studies have revealed no beneficial effect of antihistamines on the number or size of nasal polyps.[28] Current practice is to consider the use of antihistamines in patients with test-proven allergic rhinitis or with hallmark allergic symptoms of itchy watery eyes, nasal/conjunctival pruritus, sneezing, and seasonal/environmental preponderance of symptoms.

Leukotriene Modifiers

Leukotriene modifiers constitute an important class of medications used in allergic rhinitis, and recent investigations have explored a potential role in the management of CRSwNP. Leukotriene modifiers can broadly be classified as either leukotriene receptor antagonists (montelukast, zafirlukast) or 5-lipoxygenase inhibitors (zileuton). One recent investigation examined the effect of montelukast in patients with asthma and polyposis.[29] Montelukast was associated with a subjective improvement of symptoms in patients with and without aspirin tolerance; however, objective parameters of polyp size and nasal airway patency were not improved. Another study demonstrated decreased tissue eosinophilia in polyp patients after treatment with montelukast.[30] This investigation also revealed improvements in symptom scores, and the benefit was most pronounced in patients with perennial allergic rhinitis. In a double-blind randomized controlled trial of zileuton for the treatment of AERD, zileuton was associated with clinically significant improvements in olfaction and rhinorrhea.[31]

In summary, leukotriene inhibitors may provide symptomatic relief for patients with CRS who have comorbid asthma or allergic rhinitis. However, there is no evidence that treatment with leukotriene inhibitors results in the regression of polyps or the elimination of polyp growth in patients with CRSwNP. Leukotriene receptor antagonists have an acceptable safety profile and may be a viable alternative to long-term oral steroid use in selected patients, particularly those with aspirin intolerance, asthma, and/or perennial allergic rhinitis. Patients treated with zileuton, the currently available 5-lipoxygenase inhibitor, must be monitored for hepatoxicity.

Immunomodulatory Treatment

Allergy Immunotherapy

Allergy immunotherapy is a significant consideration in CRSwNP patients who have demonstrable atopy by skin testing. This is an important consideration in light of data suggesting increased postoperative polyp recurrence in allergic patients.[32] It should also be noted that although immunotherapy patients had better postoperative symptomatic outcomes, an effect of immunotherapy in reducing polyp recurrence was not observed.

Aspirin Desensitization

Aspirin desensitization is another consideration in patients with AERD who have persistent/recurrent polyposis or brittle asthma. Patients are treated with successive escalating oral doses of aspirin while under close medical observation. Once the goal dosage is reached, daily maintenance therapy of 650 to 1300 mg per day follows. Protocols for dose escalation vary widely and may be individualized. Outcome studies have revealed that aspirin desensitization can successfully reduce CRS exacerbations, hospitalizations for asthma, and systemic steroid requirements in this difficult subgroup of patients.[33]

Long-Term, Low-Dose Macrolide Therapy

Macrolide antibiotics may manifest anti-inflammatory effects apart from its known antimicrobial properties. Use of this modality in CRS evolved following Japanese reports of efficacy in treating patients with diffuse panbronchiolitis, a condition phenotypically similar to CF.[34] Laboratory analysis has associated macrolide use with a reduction in proinflammatory cytokines (IL-1, IL-6, and IL-8, leukotriene B4), neutrophil recruitment, and proliferation of polyp fibroblasts.[35] Macrolide therapy may decrease the size of nasal polyps in addition to improving subjective symptoms of CRSwNP.[36] Although there is no standardized dosing algorithm, proposed schemes for adults include clarithromycin 500 mg daily or azithromycin 500 mg every other day; children may be treated with azithromycin 250 mg every other day. Low-dose macrolide therapy may be a potential alternative to long-term, low-dose oral steroids in patients with recurrent or persistent polyps.

Antifungals

The observation that some forms of CRSwNP may be secondary to an immune response to fungi has inspired investigation of antifungal therapy in CRS patients outside the setting of classic AFS. Initial studies suggested favorable subjective (patient symptoms) and objective (CT changes) results using amphotericin B irrigations in patients with CRS.[37] However, it was unclear whether the improvement was secondary to a specific fungicidal effect versus the mechanical effects of irrigation, because treatment did not decrease the antigenic load of *Alternaria* within the nose. Additionally, a much larger multicenter double-blind placebo-controlled trial revealed no benefit of topical amphotericin B in any of the subjective or objective parameters studied.[38] Similar findings were observed in a randomized placebo-controlled study with oral terbinafine,[39] where no improvement was seen in any of the subjective or objective (radiologic) parameters after 6 weeks of therapy. Even in patients exhibiting positive fungal cultures, no benefit was demonstrated. The authors hypothesized that either fungi were not a major pathophysiologic force in the development of CRS, or that the drug may have failed to reach therapeutic levels in the mucus. The preponderance of current data does not support a role for antifungals in the routine management of CRS, with or without polyps, and calls into question the exact role of fungi in the pathophysiology of typical CRS. Antifungals may be considered in refractory cases where other conventional therapies have failed, but the use of these medications must be weighted against issues such as cost, drug toxicity (e.g., hepatotoxicity), and the ubiquitous nature of fungi in the environment and the sinonasal tract. It should be noted, however, that some retrospective noncontrolled data suggest that oral antifungal therapy (itraconazole) may reduce the need for revision FESS in patients with classic AFS,[40] and antifungal therapy may be more strongly considered in this setting.

Outcomes

Outcomes assessment can be difficult secondary to several factors,[41] including: (1) the heterogeneous multifactorial nature of CRSwNP; (2) the variability in medical treatments used; and (3) the variation among surgeons regarding the extent of surgery performed. There is evidence to support the observation that CRSwNP patients have a greater disease burden than CRSsNP patients with respect to the extent of disease measured objectively by radiologic or endoscopic scoring.[20,42] Interestingly, some studies have suggested that CRSwNP patients, when compared with CRSsNP patients, actually exhibit lower rhinosinusitis symptom inventory scores and greater quality of life as measured by the chronic sinusitis survey. These findings lend support to current perspectives that CRSwNP and CRSsNP are distinct disease processes, inspiring studies to investigate the effect of endoscopic sinus surgery in each. Data comparing the symptomatic outcomes after surgery suggest that the degree of benefit afforded to CRSwNP patients is similar to that experienced by CRSsNP patients.[42,43] Furthermore, a recent Cochrane Database review revealed symptomatic improvement in 78 to 88% of patients.[41] In terms of specific symptoms, CRSwNP patients tended to have a greater degree of improvement in nasal obstructive symptoms after surgery than did CRSsNP patients. However, symptoms of headache and facial pressure tended to persist in CRSwNP patients after surgery.[44] In addition to these disease-specific measures, other possible benefits of surgery include improvement in asthma and a decrease in oral steroid use.[44] Current outcome studies clearly demonstrate a benefit from endoscopic sinus surgery in the management of nasal polyps. There is need, however, for long-term follow-up (>2 years) data, as well as prospective investigation that controls for confounding variables such as medication usage.

Conclusion

Nasal polyposis is a heterogeneous disorder from an etiologic perspective, in that the pathophysiology is multifactorial or even polyfactorial. The summation of etiologic factors at work in any particular patient results in the phenotypic clinical presentation that is characteristically observed. Diagnostic workup requires a combination of history, physical examination, endoscopy, radiology, and allergy/immunology evaluation. Currently, steroid therapy (oral and topical) and surgery are the mainstays of therapy. However, in light of the evolving body of knowledge regarding the pathophysiology of nasal polyposis, there is a significant potential for novel therapeutic interventions.

References

1. Meltzer EO, Hamilos DL, Hadley JA, et al; Rhinosinusitis Initiative. Rhinosinusitis: developing guidance for clinical trials. J Allergy Clin Immunol 2006;118(5, Suppl)S17–S61
2. Larsen K, Tos M. The estimated incidence of symptomatic nasal polyps. Acta Otolaryngol 2002;122(2):179–182
3. Bellanti JA, Wallerstedt DB. Allergic rhinitis update: Epidemiology and natural history. Allergy Asthma Proc 2000;21(6): 367–370
4. Grigoreas C, Vourdas D, Petalas K, Simeonidis G, Demeroutis I, Tsioulos T. Nasal polyps in patients with rhinitis and asthma. Allergy Asthma Proc 2002;23(3):169–174
5. Lee CH, Rhee CS, Min YG. Cytokine gene expression in nasal polyps. Ann Otol Rhinol Laryngol 1998;107(8):665–670
6. Van Zele T, Claeys S, Gevaert P, et al. Differentiation of chronic sinus diseases by measurement of inflammatory mediators. Allergy 2006;61(11):1280–1289
7. Ferguson BJ, Mabry RL. Laboratory diagnosis. Otolaryngol Head Neck Surg 1997;117(3 Pt 2):S12–S26
8. Swierczynska M, Nizankowska-Mogilnicka E, Zarychta J, Gielicz A, Szczeklik A. Nasal versus bronchial and nasal response to oral aspirin challenge: Clinical and biochemical differences between patients with aspirin-induced asthma/rhinitis. J Allergy Clin Immunol 2003;112(5):995–1001
9. Corrigan C, Mallett K, Ying S, et al. Expression of the cysteinyl leukotriene receptors cysLT(1) and cysLT(2) in aspirin-sensitive and aspirin-tolerant chronic rhinosinusitis. J Allergy Clin Immunol 2005;115(2):316–322
10. Chao SS, Graham SM, Brown CL, Kline JN, Hussain I. Cysteinyl leukotriene 1 receptor expression in nasal polyps. Ann Otol Rhinol Laryngol 2006;115(5):394–397
11. Thivierge M, Doty M, Johnson J, Stanková J, Rola-Pleszczynski M. IL-5 up-regulates cysteinyl leukotriene 1 receptor expression in HL-60 cells differentiated into eosinophils. J Immunol 2000;165(9):5221–5226
12. Sasama J, Sherris DA, Shin SH, Kephart GM, Kern EB, Ponikau JU. New paradigm for the roles of fungi and eosinophils in chronic rhinosinusitis. Curr Opin Otolaryngol Head Neck Surg 2005;13(1):2–8
13. Patou J, Gevaert P, Van Zele T, Holtappels G, van Cauwenberge P, Bachert C. Staphylococcus aureus enterotoxin B, protein A, and lipoteichoic acid stimulations in nasal polyps. J Allergy Clin Immunol 2008;121(1):110–115
14. Conley DB, Tripathi A, Seiberling KA, et al. Superantigens and chronic rhinosinusitis: skewing of T-cell receptor V beta-distributions in polyp-derived CD4+ and CD8+ T cells. Am J Rhinol 2006;20(5):534–539
15. Lane AP, Truong-Tran QA, Schleimer RP. Altered expression of genes associated with innate immunity and inflammation in recalcitrant rhinosinusitis with polyps. Am J Rhinol 2006;20(2):138–144
16. Chen YS, Langhammer T, Westhofen M, Lorenzen J. Relationship between matrix metalloproteinases MMP-2, MMP-9, tissue inhibitor of matrix metalloproteinases-1 and IL-5, IL-8 in nasal polyps. Allergy 2007;62(1):66–72
17. Richer SL, Truong-Tran AQ, Conley DB, et al. Epithelial genes in chronic rhinosinusitis with and without nasal polyps. Am J Rhinol 2008;22(3):228–234
18. Kato A, Truong-Tran AQ, Scott AL, Matsumoto K, Schleimer RP. Airway epithelial cells produce B cell-activating factor of TNF family by an IFN-beta-dependent mechanism. J Immunol 2006;177(10):7164–7172
19. Kato A, Peters A, Suh L, et al. Evidence of a role for B cell-activating factor of the TNF family (BAFF) in the pathogenesis of chronic rhinosinusitis with nasal polyps. J Clin Invest, In press
20. Banerji A, Piccirillo JF, Thawley SE, et al. Chronic rhinosinusitis patients with polyps or polypoid mucosa have a greater burden of illness. Am J Rhinol 2007;21(1):19–26
21. Seybt MW, McMains KC, Kountakis SE. The prevalence and effect of asthma on adults with chronic rhinosinusitis. Ear Nose Throat J 2007;86(7):409–411
22. Landsberg R, Segev Y, DeRowe A, Landau T, Khafif A, Fliss DM. Systemic corticosteroids for allergic fungal rhinosinusitis and chronic rhinosinusitis with nasal polyposis: a comparative study. Otolaryngol Head Neck Surg 2007;136(2):252–257
23. Wright ED, Agrawal S. Impact of perioperative systemic steroids on surgical outcomes in patients with chronic rhinosinusitis with polyposis: evaluation with the novel Perioperative Sinus Endoscopy (POSE) scoring system. Laryngoscope 2007;117(11 Pt 2, Suppl 115)1–28
24. Schleimer RP. Glucocorticoids: their mechanism of action and use in allergic diseases. In: Adkinson NF, Yunginger JW, Busse WW, Bochner BS, Holgate ST, Simons FE, eds. Middleton's Allergy Principles and Practice. St. Louis, MO: Mosby; 2003: 912–914
25. Pullerits T, Praks L, Ristioja V, Lötvall J. Comparison of a nasal glucocorticoid, antileukotriene, and a combination of antileukotriene and antihistamine in the treatment of seasonal allergic rhinitis. J Allergy Clin Immunol 2002;109(6):949–955
26. Hwang PH, Woo RJ, Fong KJ. Intranasal deposition of nebulized saline: a radionuclide distribution study. Am J Rhinol 2006;20(3):255–261
27. Kowalski ML, Lewandowska A, Wozniak J, Makowska J, Jankowski A, DuBuske L. Inhibition of nasal polyp mast cell and eosinophil activation by desloratadine. Allergy 2005;60(1):80–85
28. Haye R, Aanesen JP, Burtin B, Donnelly F, Duby C. The effect of cetirizine on symptoms and signs of nasal polyposis. J Laryngol Otol 1998;112(11):1042–1046
29. Ragab S, Parikh A, Darby YC, Scadding GK. An open audit of montelukast, a leukotriene receptor antagonist, in nasal polyposis associated with asthma. Clin Exp Allergy 2001;31(9):1385–1391
30. Kieff DA, Busaba NY. Efficacy of montelukast in the treatment of nasal polyposis. Ann Otol Rhinol Laryngol 2005;114(12):941–945
31. Dahlén B, Nizankowska E, Szczeklik A, et al. Benefits from adding the 5-lipoxygenase inhibitor zileuton to conventional therapy in aspirin-intolerant asthmatics. Am J Respir Crit Care Med 1998;157(4 Pt 1):1187-1194
32. Nishioka GJ, Cook PR, Davis WE, McKinsey JP. Immunotherapy in patients undergoing functional endoscopic sinus surgery. Otolaryngol Head Neck Surg 1994;110(4):406–412
33. Stevenson DD, Hankammer MA, Mathison DA, Christiansen SC, Simon RA. Aspirin desensitization treatment of aspirin-sensitive patients with rhinosinusitis-asthma: long-term outcomes. J Allergy Clin Immunol 1996;98(4):751–758
34. Kudoh S, Azuma A, Yamamoto M, Izumi T, Ando M. Improvement of survival in patients with diffuse panbronchiolitis treated with low-dose erythromycin. Am J Respir Crit Care Med 1998;157 (6 Pt 1):1829–1832
35. Tamaoki J, Kadota J, Takizawa H. Clinical implications of the immunomodulatory effects of macrolides. Am J Med 2004;117 (Suppl 9A):5S–11S
36. Gotfried MH. Macrolides for the treatment of chronic sinusitis, asthma, and COPD. Chest 2004;125(2, Suppl)52S–60S, quiz 60S–61S
37. Ponikau JU, Sherris DA, Weaver A, Kita H. Treatment of chronic rhinosinusitis with intranasal amphotericin B: a randomized, placebo-controlled, double-blind pilot trial. J Allergy Clin Immunol 2005;115(1):125–131
38. Ebbens FA, Scadding GK, Badia L, et al. Amphotericin B nasal lavages: not a solution for patients with chronic rhinosinusitis. J Allergy Clin Immunol 2006;118(5):1149–1156

39. Kennedy DW, Kuhn FA, Hamilos DL, et al. Treatment of chronic rhinosinusitis with high-dose oral terbinafine: a double blind, placebo-controlled study. Laryngoscope 2005;115(10): 1793–1799
40. Rains BM III, Mineck CW. Treatment of allergic fungal sinusitis with high-dose itraconazole. Am J Rhinol 2003;17(1):1–8
41. Dalziel K, Stein K, Round A, Garside R, Royle P. Endoscopic sinus surgery for the excision of nasal polyps: A systematic review of safety and effectiveness. Am J Rhinol 2006;20(5):506–519
42. Toros SZ, Bölükbasi S, Naiboğlu B, et al. Comparative outcomes of endoscopic sinus surgery in patients with chronic sinusitis and nasal polyps. Eur Arch Otorhinolaryngol 2007;264(9): 1003–1008
43. Bhattacharyya N. Influence of polyps on outcomes after endoscopic sinus surgery. Laryngoscope 2007;117(10):1834–1838
44. Poetker DM, Mendolia-Loffredo S, Smith TL. Outcomes of endoscopic sinus surgery for chronic rhinosinusitis associated with sinonasal polyposis. Am J Rhinol 2007;21(1):84–88

15 Microbiology of Rhinosinusitis and Antimicrobial Resistance

Kevin C. Welch, James N. Palmer, and Alexander G. Chiu

The initial treatment of rhinosinusitis is nearly always medical in nature, with surgery reserved for medical failures or complications associated with rhinosinusitis. In both acute and chronic rhinosinusitis, the identification and treatment of the offending organisms are crucial for efficacious results. Over the past 15 years, the increased incidence of multiple drug-resistant bacteria in rhinosinusitis has made treatment more challenging and has required an alteration in our diagnostic as well as treatment algorithms. This chapter focuses on the most common pathogens (**Table 15.1**) seen within the various stages of rhinosinusitis, and explores their mechanisms for resistance.

Virology

Community-acquired upper respiratory illnesses are common and, although self-limited in nature, contribute to significant morbidity and loss of productivity. In the past, the causes of these upper respiratory illnesses had been difficult to define; however, with current detection techniques, it is well established that the majority of these illnesses are caused by viruses.

Much of the literature focuses on the prevalence of rhinovirus in the etiology of upper respiratory illnesses, especially in viral rhinosinusitis. Rhinovirus, a nonenveloped single-stranded RNA icosahedral-shaped virus, is the

Table 15.1 Most Common Pathogens in Rhinosinusitis

Disease Entity	Pathogen	Reported Frequency
Viral rhinosinusitis	Rhinovirus	55–80%
	Coronavirus	12–15%
	Parainfluenza	7–16%
	Influenza A or B	8–16%
	Respiratory syncytial virus	3–12%
Acute bacterial rhinosinusitis	*Streptococcus pneumoniae*	20–57%
	Haemophilus influenzae	20–60%
	Moraxella catarrhalis	2–10%
	Nonpneumococcus streptococcal species	19–38%
	Anaerobes	13–20%
	Sterile	up to 50%
Nosocomial acquired rhinosinusitis	*Pseudomonas aeruginosa*	16–22%
	Staphylococcus aureus	20–34%
	Coagulase-negative staphylococci	13–15%
	Nonpseudomonal Gram-negative rods	9–12%
	Anaerobes	14–29%
Chronic rhinosinusitis	Coagulase-negative staphylococci	12–44%
	Pseudomonas aeruginosa	7–43%
	Staphylococcus aureus	10–31%
	Nonpseudomonal Gram-negative rods	6–20%
	Haemophilus influenzae	6%
	Streptococcus pneumoniae	6%
	Moraxella catarrhalis	6%

most commonly isolated viral cause of upper respiratory illnesses[1] and has been isolated in close to 60% of patients with the common cold.[2] The virus is highly variable owing to the diversity of its capsid proteins, and there are over 100 known serotypes. This accounts for its commonality in viral upper respiratory illnesses, especially viral rhinosinusitis.

Rhinovirus inoculation occurs primarily through direct contact with the nasal mucosa whereupon it is transported to the nasopharynx.[3,4] There is some indication that rhinovirus is spread via an aerosol as well.[5] When in the nasopharynx, rhinovirus gains entry to the host cell via attachment with intercellular adhesion molecules (ICAM)-1[6] located throughout the stratified squamous epithelium. It is the host immune response that is believed to be the cause of morbidity rather than the direct effect of the virus.[5,7] The identification of interleukin (IL)-1, IL-6, and IL-8 in nasal aspirates of patients with rhinovirus-induced upper respiratory illnesses[5,7] implies a role in the local inflammatory response and recruitment of neutrophils that results in increased vascular permeability and symptomatic nasal obstruction.

Rhinovirus is more successfully isolated by reverse transcriptase polymerase chain reaction (RT-PCR) and less successfully by culture techniques[8] due to the lengthy time to culture and a high rate of false-positive results.[1] RT-PCR has been shown to be sensitive and specific for the detection of rhinovirus.[9,10] Using culture techniques, rhinovirus, parainfluenza, and influenza viruses have been detected in 16% of maxillary sinus puncture cultures.[11,12] Arruda and colleagues[13] isolated rhinovirus in 80% of patients with the common cold during the fall season. Puhakka et al.[8] studied 197 adult patients with symptoms of the common cold (rhinorrhea, sore throat, etc.) and performed radiographic (Water's view) assessments and nasopharyngeal aspirations on days 1, 7, and 21 during the course of the disease. Using RT-PCR techniques, 69.5% of patients had positive cultures, 81.6% of those being viral in nature. Rhinovirus was detected in 55.3% of patients with sinusitis and 48.3% of patients without sinusitis.

Coronavirus, an enveloped single-stranded RNA virus, is also heavily implicated in upper respiratory illnesses and can be seen in 12% of isolates.[8,14] Two major forms of coronavirus have been identified. Coronavirus 229E inoculation occurs through interaction with CD13 receptors on ciliated epithelium[15]; however, the route of infection for coronavirus OC43 is not presently known. Viral proteases appear to play a role in injury to the cell; however, the precise host response to the virus is not presently known well.

Makela et al.[14] used fluoroimmunoassay, enzyme immunoassay (EIA), culture, and RT-PCR to determine the viral etiology in 200 patients with the common cold. Nasopharyngeal aspiration was used to obtain 138 positive cultures: rhinovirus was detected in 76%; coronavirus OC43 or 229E in 12%; influenza A or B in 8.7%; adenovirus in 1.5%; parainfluenza 1, 2, or 3 in 5%; and respiratory syncytial virus (RSV) in 3%. Double viral cultures were positive in 10/138 samples, and both viruses and bacteria were simultaneously cultured in 6/138 subjects. Using RT-PCR techniques of nasal wash specimens, Louie and colleagues[16] identified influenza A or B in 52%, rhinovirus in 23%, and RSV in 12% of patients during the influenza season at a University of California, San Francisco clinic—this study included patients with upper and lower respiratory illnesses.

Bacteriology

Bacterial Carrier Rates

The nasal cavity and nasopharynx become colonized with bacteria early in life and can serve as a reservoir of bacteria that cause otitis media and sinusitis. Colonization begins shortly after birth: Speck et al.[17] demonstrated that by day 14 of life, 44.2% of neonates are colonized by *Staphylococcus aureus* and by day 42 of life, over 50% of infants are colonized by *S. aureus*. Similarly, Bisgaard and colleagues[18] found 61% of neonates at 1 month to be colonized by *S. aureus*. Subsequent studies[19–21] have revealed that the major pathogens classically associated with sinusitis (*Streptococcus pneumoniae*, *Haemophilus influenzae*, and *Moraxella catarrhalis*) colonize nearly 70 to 90% of children during the first 3 years of life. Multiple serotypes and frequent mutation in strains of these species are found as well.[21,22] As the percentage of children with *S. pneumoniae*, *H. influenzae*, and *M. catarrhalis* increases, the percentage of children colonized by *S. aureus* decreases. Vives and colleagues[23] obtained nasopharyngeal cultures in children at 1 month, 3 months, 6 months, and 12 months of age and found that at 1 month of age, children were colonized with *H. influenzae* in 3.9%, *S. pneumoniae* in 3.1%, and *M. catarrhalis* in 6.5%. The proportion of colonization increased substantially over the first year of life such that by 1 year of age, children were colonized with *S. pneumoniae* in 36%, *H. influenzae* in 26%, and *M. catarrhalis* in 28%. Colonization of the nasopharynx appears to peak in the first 3 to 4 years of life: Faden et al.[24] examined 40 healthy children and found a colonization rate of 65% for *H. influenzae*, 52% for *S. pneumoniae*, and 52% for *M. catarrhalis*. Regev-Yochay et al.[25] found a *S. pneumoniae* carriage rate of 41.9% in children <1 year of age, 68.6% in children aged 2 to 3 years, and 46.4% in children aged 4 to 6 years. Colonization becomes more frequent in the daycare setting.[23]

Nasopharyngeal carriage varies depending on geographic location as well as age. Wolf et al.[26] examined nearly 300 nasopharyngeal cultures in children less than 5 years of age in Angolan, Brazilian, and Dutch children and found modest variations in carriage rates among all three nationalities with respect to *S. pneumoniae* (19 to 41%), *H.*

influenzae (41 to 70%), and *M. catarrhalis* (31 to 58%). The highest carrier rates of *S. pneumoniae*, *H. influenzae*, and *M. catarrhalis* were seen in Dutch children. However, nearly 50 to 57% of Angolan and Brazilian children were colonized by enteric and nonfermentative Gram-negative bacilli, compared with only 5% of Dutch children. The authors suggested that environmental and sanitary conditions led to the striking disproportion of enteric and Gram-negative colonization in Angolan and Brazilian children.

The colonization patterns in adults differ from that of children. Jousimies-Somer et al.[27] performed nasal swabs in 286 military recruits and servicemen and found an incidence of *H. influenzae* in 4 to 19%, *S. pneumoniae* in 1 to 13%, and *M. catarrhalis* in 3%. More common isolates were coagulase-negative staphylococci, diphtheroids, and *S. aureus*. Talaat et al.[28] obtained nasopharyngeal cultures in healthy controls and adult patients undergoing adenoidectomy. In control patients, 45% of patients were colonized with diphtheroids, 50% with *Neisseria*, 80% with *Streptococcus viridans*, 35% with coagulase-negative staphylococci, 55% with nonhemolytic streptococci, 35% with *M. catarrhalis*, 10% with *S. pneumoniae*, and 5% with *H. influenzae*. Fairchok et al.[29] found that 29% of military patients were carriers of *S. pneumoniae*. Finally, Regev-Yochay and colleagues[25] screened 1704 adults and children and *S. pneumoniae* carriage was identified in 53% of children but in only 3.7% of adults.

Nasopharyngeal colonization is easily explored; however, colonization of the middle meatus or sinuses may be of more interest to clinicians treating rhinosinusitis. Studies do not agree on whether the middle meatus or sinuses are sterile in the disease-free state. In pediatric patients, cultures of the middle meatus obtained at the time of adenotonsillectomy reveal that the middle meatus is colonized with *S. pneumoniae*, *H. influenzae*, and *M. catarrhalis*—this suggests that middle meatal cultures in children with suspected rhinosinusitis may erroneously lead a clinician to exclude other possible organisms in pediatric sinusitis.[30]

Klossek et al.[31] performed 139 middle meatal cultures in adult patients without evidence of sinusitis within 3 months prior to the culture, and identified aerobic and anaerobic bacteria in 113 of 139 (81%) cases. Commensal organisms were the main finding with only 3.5% of the samples growing either *S. pneumoniae* or *H. influenzae*. Similarly, Nadel et al.[32] endoscopically placed calcium alginate swabs in the middle meatuses of 25 healthy adult volunteers. Eighteen of 41 cultures were sterile; coagulase-negative staphylococci were identified in 18/23; *S. aureus* was identified in 10/23; and diphtheroids in 8/23. In one patient, *Morganella* and *Enterobacter* species were identified. No anaerobic species were identified. These studies suggest that typical organisms responsible for rhinosinusitis do not typically colonize the middle meatus.

Earlier studies of chronic rhinosinusitis used more invasive techniques to sample the maxillary sinus. Bjorkwell[33] performed maxillary sinus antral punctures in 54 healthy patients and was unable to culture any organism. Similarly, Sobin et al.[34] performed 12 antral punctures with sterile saline lavage in asymptomatic patients and identified no organisms. In contrast, Brook[35] examined antral punctures performed with sterile techniques in 12 patients undergoing general anesthesia for nasal reconstructive surgery. In all patients, anaerobic species, chiefly *Bacteroides* and *Fusobacterium*, were identified. Beta-hemolytic (e.g., *Streptococcus pyogenes*) and alpha-hemolytic streptococci were identified in 8 of 12 samples. Less frequently identified were *S. pneumoniae* (2/12), *H. influenzae* (2/12), and *S. aureus* (2/12). These studies suggest that the paranasal sinuses are typically sterile; however, culture techniques may introduce contamination into samples and the correlation between nasal, middle meatal, and direct sinus cultures deserves discussion.

Mechanisms of Culture: Endoscopic Versus Antral Puncture

Much of the literature focuses on invasive cultures (i.e., antral puncture) for the determination of the microbiology in acute bacterial rhinosinusitis. Prior to the introduction of the endoscope, Axelsson et al.[36] and Karma[37] compared intranasal cultures with direct cultures of the maxillary sinus. *S. aureus* (28%) and coagulase-negative staphylococci (35%) were commonly identified from nasal cultures, and cultures of the middle meatus or inferior meatus correlated with direct maxillary sinus cultures in only 41 to 56% of cases.[36] When compared with cultures obtained during Caldwell-Luc procedures for chronic maxillary sinusitis, cultures were positive from the nose in nearly double the cases of the maxillary sinus and showed very poor correlations.[37] Therefore, past studies have relied on invasive techniques to culture the sinuses, as directed nasal cultures appear to have demonstrated contamination and poor correlation with cultures obtained directly from the maxillary sinus.

As techniques in endoscopic evaluation of the sinuses evolved, culture techniques became more precise. Furthermore, our understanding of the clinical significance of the ostiomeatal complex and its relationship to rhinosinusitis improved. In this context, several studies flourished evaluating the sensitivity and specificity of endoscopically obtained cultures (**Fig. 15.1**) compared with "gold standard" antral punctures for the determination of infectious etiologies.

The feasibility of endoscopically directed middle meatal cultures has been shown in several studies.[32,38,39] Various degrees of correlation between endoscopically directed middle meatal cultures and antral puncture cultures have been demonstrated. In a study of 39 children undergoing endoscopic sinus surgery, Orobello et al.[40] compared endoscopic cultures of the middle meatus to cultures of the nasopharynx, maxillary sinus, and ethmoid sinus. Middle meatal cultures correlated with maxillary sinus cultures in 83% of cases and with ethmoid sinus cultures in 80% of cases. Predictably, nasopharyngeal cultures correlated

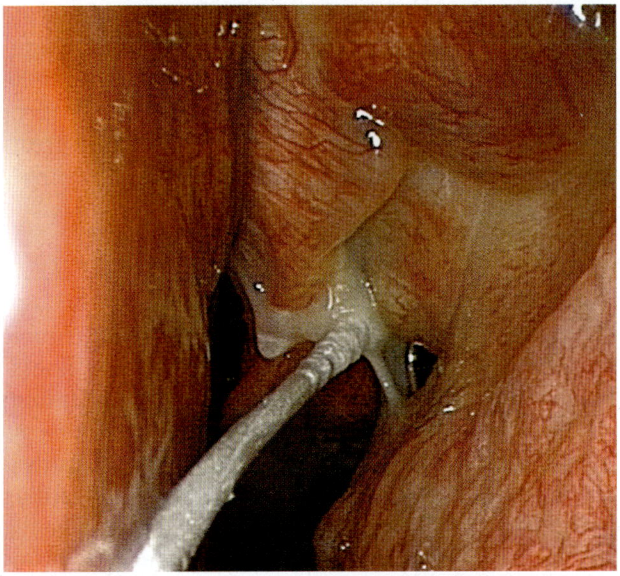

Fig. 15.1 A calcium alginate swab placed into the middle meatus of a patient with chronic rhinosinusitis undergoing endoscopic sinus surgery.

poorly with maxillary sinus cultures (45%) and ethmoid sinus cultures (49%).

Brook et al.[41] obtained 24 cultures in 6 patients undergoing endoscopic maxillary sinusotomies. Middle meatal aerobic cultures correlated with maxillary sinus aspirations in 16/18 cases, and anaerobic cultures correlated in 5/5 cases. In similar studies,[42,43] middle meatal cultures have correlated with direct maxillary sinus cultures in 85 to 90% of cases. When subdivided into aerobic cultures and anaerobic cultures, Vogan at al.[43] found a 93% correlation in aerobic cultures and an 87.4% correlation in anaerobic cultures.

Separate meta-analyses[44,45] have evaluated methods of culture and concluded that middle meatal cultures correlate with direct maxillary sinus cultures (antral tap) in 60 to 87% of cases with an overall sensitivity of 80.9% and a specificity of 90.5% for endoscopically directed middle meatal cultures. Cultures of the nasal cavity did not correlate well with those of the maxillary sinus. These studies establish that when performed in the proper setting and with sterile techniques, endoscopically directed middle meatal cultures correlate well with direct maxillary sinus cultures and can be obtained in a less invasive manner.

Acute Bacterial Rhinosinusitis

The microbiology of acute bacterial rhinosinusitis has been the subject of much research, and the constancy of its bacteriology across multiple studies allows clinicians to empirically treat acute bacterial rhinosinusitis with a fair degree of certainty that the deployed antimicrobial agent will cover the most likely pathogens causing the disease.

Multiple studies[46–48] have confirmed that the major pathogens in community-acquired acute bacterial rhinosinusitis are *S. pneumoniae, H. influenzae,* and *M. catarrhalis*. However, cultures of the purportedly infected sinus are often sterile, viral, or contaminated[49–51] in up to 50% of cases. These unrevealing cultures have led investigators to question whether certain sinuses with radiographic evidence of disease represent true bacterial disease.

Studies[51–54] reveal variations in the pathogenic features of acute bacterial rhinosinusitis; however, they show consistency in the prevalence of recovered organisms. *S. pneumoniae* is isolated in 20 to 57% of cases, *H. influenzae* in 20 to 60% of cases, *M. catarrhalis* in 2 to 10% of cases, group A streptococci in ~5% of cases, and *S. aureus* in ~5% of cases as well. These studies primarily involve an assessment of the maxillary sinus and/or the middle meatus complex. These areas are traditionally accessed more easily. Owing to the relative inaccessibility of the frontal sinus and sphenoid sinus, less is known about the microbiology of these sites. Brook[55,56] cultured multiple sinuses in patients with acute bacterial rhinosinusitis and the most common isolates were *S. pneumoniae* and *H. influenzae*. However, 56% of organisms appeared in only in a single sinus, whereas 44% of which were identified in two or more sinuses, suggesting that different organisms may be isolated from different sinuses. Treatment based on maxillary sinus cultures alone may thus potentially leave pathogens involving other sinuses unaddressed.

Studies involving frontal sinusitis show similar pathogens as in maxillary sinusitis; however, the diversity of pathogens expands. Antila and colleagues[57] evaluated 194 patients with acute frontal sinusitis and treated them with empiric antibiotics. If improvement was not noted within 24 hours, surgery was performed. Trephination of the frontal sinus was performed in 103 patients, and 30 patients produced positive cultures: 37%, *H. influenzae*; 30%, *S. pneumoniae*; 6.6%, *S. aureus*; and 3.3%, *Escherichia coli*. Although the methods of obtaining cultures were unclear, Brook[58] examined 20 isolates in 15 cases of acute frontal sinusitis and results were similar: 30%, *H. influenzae*; 25%, *S. pneumoniae*; 15%, *M. catarrhalis*; and 20%, anaerobes. Herrmann and colleagues[59] examined 16 patients with acute frontal sinusitis (7 of these with pansinusitis). Isolates from surgical cultures included *S. viridans* (38%), *Staphylococcus epidermidis* (38%), *Streptococcus milleri* (19%), *S. pneumoniae* (19%), *H. influenzae* (6%), and *Fusobacterium necrophorum* (13%). Fifty percent of cultures were polymicrobial.

Prior to the era of endoscopy, the sphenoid sinus was a challenge to isolate and culture without the risk of contamination related to varied approaches (external-transethmoidal, trans-septal, intranasal). In an early study, Lew et al.[60] identified streptococci (excluding *S. pneumoniae*) in 41% of cultures, *S. aureus* in 29% of cultures, and *S. pneumoniae* in 17% of cultures. Although not stratified by frequency, Ruoppi[61] found *S. aureus, M. catarrhalis*, and anaerobes to be frequent cultures in isolated sphenoid sinusitis obtained by external and endoscopic approaches. Similarly, external approaches and intranasal endoscopic approaches were used in another study[62] to culture patients with acute and chronic sphenoid sinusitis. Twenty-nine isolates were obtained: *S. aureus* (9), streptococci (8), anaerobes (8), *H. influenzae* (2), *S. pneumoniae* (1), and *P. aeruginosa* (1). Although the usual suspects are present in sphenoid sinusitis, it is difficult to ascertain whether the increased diversity in sphenoid sinusitis cultures reflects the true nature of the disease or contamination of cultures.

Nosocomial Sinusitis

The presence of fever of unknown origin in the critically ill patient is often a frustrating diagnostic dilemma for intensivists, and acute rhinosinusitis is often implicated in the short list of causes. Placement of nasogastric tubes or nasoendotracheal tubes is frequently identified as a causal factor for developing rhinosinusitis. Nasotracheal intubation has been classically associated with a higher likelihood of nosocomial sinusitis than orotracheal intubation[63]; however, orally intubated critically ill patients are commonly treated as well for ventilator-associated sinusitis.

Early studies[64,65] have established that the microbiology of nosocomial sinusitis is different from acute community-acquired rhinosinusitis. The organisms traditionally associated with acute rhinosinusitis (*S. pneumoniae*, *H. influenzae*, *M. catarrhalis*) are isolated less frequently in nosocomial sinusitis. Instead, Gram-positive cocci and Gram-negative bacilli are seen.

Both Caplan[64] and Humphrey[65] demonstrated through intranasal, inferior meatal punctures that *S. aureus* and *P. aeruginosa* were the predominant organisms isolated. Talmor[66] performed a review of the literature regarding the microbiology of acute sinusitis in the critically ill and found that 60% of the episodes were caused by Gram-negative rods: *P. aeruginosa*, 15.9%; *E. coli*, 7.6%; and *Proteus mirabilis*, 7.2%. Approximately 30% of the isolates involved Gram-positive cocci: *S. aureus*, 34%; staphylococci species, 15%; beta-hemolytic streptococci, 4.3%. In a prospective study[67] involving transnasal antral punctures in 103 critically ill patients with fever and rhinosinusitis, 60 Gram-positive organisms and 115 Gram-negative organisms were identified. Included in the Gram-negative samples were *P. aeruginosa* (22.6%), *Klebsiella pneumoniae* (12.2%), *E. coli* (11%), and *P. mirabilis* (9.5%). Gram-positive organisms included *S. aureus* (58%), coagulase-negative staphylococci (13.3%), and *S. pneumoniae* (6.6%). These results compare with that of a study[68] on critically ill pediatric patients. Fifty-eight isolates (30 aerobes and 28 anaerobes) were identified. Aerobic cultures compared with previously stated numbers; however, a higher percentage of anaerobic species were reported: *Peptostreptococcus*, 8/28; *Prevotella*, 6/28; and *Fusobacterium*, 4/28.

The percentages of traditional organisms found in acute bacterial rhinosinusitis are not seen in nosocomial sinusitis, and the greater diversity of organisms that can be associated with acute sinusitis in the critically ill patient warrants prompt identification by means of culture. Treatment should reflect the results of culture and sensitivity testing and rely less on empiric therapy.

Chronic Rhinosinusitis

The precise relationship between bacteria and chronic rhinosinusitis is difficult to define, and studies assessing the bacteriology of chronic rhinosinusitis suffer from all the previously mentioned flaws in methodology. Although the pathophysiology of chronic rhinosinusitis is studied elsewhere in this book, a few aspects regarding it should be highlighted. Inflammation appears to be the root cause of chronic rhinosinusitis, and the mechanisms whereby this inflammation begins or persists is a matter of intense debate. The role of bacteria in chronic rhinosinusitis has been studied extensively, and the prevalence of certain species (e.g., coagulase-negative staphylococci) across multiple studies leads clinicians to question whether bacteria serve as a source of infection, inflammation, or simply become contaminants within the sinuses. Furthermore, comparing patients who have not undergone surgery to those who have undergone surgery becomes difficult, as the microbiology of the sinuses can be different in each group. Several studies combine chronic rhinosinusitis and acute exacerbation of chronic rhinosinusitis together. As with acute bacterial rhinosinusitis, the focus of the literature is on the middle meatus and/or the maxillary sinus. In the era of endoscopy, cultures are obtained endoscopically via the middle meatus with a swab or by aspiration; however, multiple studies reporting microbiology use an inferior nasal antral or canine fossa puncture, introducing the possibility of contamination with *S. aureus* or oral commensal species. All these factors together make an interpretation and a comparison of studies difficult. Nevertheless, despite differences in methodology, and regardless of the role of bacteria in chronic rhinosinusitis, it is clear that the microbiology of chronic rhinosinusitis is different from acute bacterial rhinosinusitis.

Early studies[69–71] demonstrated the polymicrobial nature of chronic rhinosinusitis, and unlike acute bacterial rhinosinusitis, *S. aureus* and *P. aeruginosa* were more frequently isolated organisms than the classic sinusitis organisms (i.e., *S. pneumoniae*, *H. influenzae*, and *M. catarrhalis*). Bolger[72] introduced the concept of Gram-negative sinusitis to highlight the frequency of Gram-negative rods in endoscopic cultures of patients with chronic rhinosinusitis. Anaerobes, when cultured properly, are more common as well and can comprise greater than 50% of culture isolates[73]; however, an abundance of anaerobes may suggest contamination from the oral cavity.

At the time of endoscopic sinus surgery, cultures can be made of the middle meatus, antrostomy, or individual sinuses by using multiple culture techniques. Winther et al.[74] performed endoscopic cultures of 20 patients undergoing endoscopic sinus surgery of the maxillary sinus and found *S. aureus*, Gram-negative rods, *H. influenzae*, and *M. catarrhalis*; however, antrostomy cultures did not necessarily correlate with maxillary sinus aspirates.

Larger studies examining endoscopic cultures highlight not only the polymicrobial nature of chronic rhinosinusitis but also, owing to the multifactorial nature of chronic rhinosinusitis, the relative lack of bacteria. Nadel et al.[75] performed 507 endoscopic cultures in 256 patients—101 cultures revealed no growth. In the remaining 406 cultures, 599 isolates were identified. A predominance of *S. aureus* (31.2%) and coagulase-negative staphylococci (44.2%) was isolated among aerobic bacteria; *H. influenzae*, *S. pneumoniae*, and *M. catarrhalis* accounted for ~18% of aerobic cultures. Gram-negative rods were also prominent (34% of isolates) findings: *P. aeruginosa* (43%), *E. coli* (8%), *Enterobacter* spp. (8%), and *Stenotrophomonas maltophilia* (6%). Higher rates of coagulase-negative staphylococci were obtained intraoperatively when compared with office cultures. Higher rates of pseudomonal cultures were identified intraoperatively in patients recently taking oral corticosteroids and in patients performing nasal irrigations. The prevalence of coagulase-negative staphylococci, traditionally thought of as a contaminant or nonpathogenic, raised the question of its pathogenic relevance or its potential role in inflammation. Similar results (*S. aureus* and coagulase-negative staphylococci) have been confirmed by Schlosser et al.[76] in patients with chronic frontal sinusitis evaluated by trephination.

A multicenter study led by Finegold et al.[77] reported on 134 isolates in cultures performed on patients with chronic rhinosinusitis. Anaerobic bacteria (*Prevotella*, *Fusobacterium*, and anaerobic streptococcal species) were the predominant organisms. Aerobic species showed higher percentages of traditional sinusitis organisms (*S. pneumoniae*, *H. influenzae*, and *M. catarrhalis*); however, *P. aeruginosa* (15%) and *S. aureus* (10%) accounted for equal amounts of aerobic isolates. Canine fossa or nasal antral puncture was the predominant means for culture.

Acute exacerbation of chronic rhinosinusitis is often viewed as a distinct clinical entity within the spectrum of chronic rhinosinusitis. Its microbiology has been studied as well. Cincik and Ferguson[78] found similar ratios of organisms in patients with chronic rhinosinusitis and acute exacerbation of chronic rhinosinusitis. Endoscopic cultures were performed of the middle meatus, sphenoethmoidal recess, maxillary sinus, and ethmoid sinuses via calcium alginate swabs or aspiration in 68 patients (41 patients with chronic rhinosinusitis and 27 patients with acute exacerbation of chronic rhinosinusitis). In both entities, the most common culture finding was no growth. *S. aureus* and *P. aeruginosa* were the most common bacterial isolates in each disease entity, with higher proportions of *S. pneumoniae* and *H. influenzae* in acute exacerbation of chronic rhinosinusitis. Bhattacharyya[79] performed a retrospective review of 290 endoscopic cultures in patients with recurrent rhinosinusitis following endoscopic sinus surgery. Concordant with previous studies, 30% of cultures demonstrated no growth, and predominant organisms were *S. aureus* (18.6%), coagulase-negative staphylococci (12.8%), and *P. aeruginosa* (7.2%). Organisms associated with acute bacterial rhinosinusitis (*S. pneumoniae*, *H. influenzae*, *M. catarrhalis*) comprised 10% of culture results.

Mechanisms of Resistance

Resistance to antimicrobial agents is a growing public health concern.[80,81] As previously mentioned, the vast majority of episodes of acute rhinosinusitis are viral in origin, and the deployment of antibiotics for the treatment of this disease is unsupported and inappropriate. The changing susceptibilities of common pathogens in acute bacterial rhinosinusitis and the conflicting evidence supporting a role of bacteria in chronic rhinosinusitis has prompted multiple groups to establish guidelines[82–85] for the appropriate treatment of rhinosinusitis.

Pathogens involved in rhinosinusitis acquire resistance through multiple mechanisms, primarily through point mutations in DNA or by the acquisition of new genes through the transfer of plasmids or transposons from other resistant species. The major species involved in rhinosinusitis demonstrate resistance to antimicrobial agents through one or more of the following mechanisms: enzymatic inactivation of antibiotics, efflux pump mechanisms, alteration of antibiotic target sites, and/or alteration of antibiotic target enzymes.

A prime example of the use of enzymatic inactivation is penicillin-resistant bacteria. Mainstay therapy for pediatric and adult rhinosinusitis has traditionally been the use of penicillin, penicillin derivatives, or cephalosporin antibiotics.[86,87] These antimicrobial agents contain beta-lactam rings, which are lactone- and amide-containing rings that are involved in the inhibition of bacterial cell wall synthesis. The primary defense against beta-lactam antibiotics is the production of beta-lactamases, which cleave the amide bond of the beta-lactam ring. There are chiefly four classes of beta-lactamases, and they have been demonstrated to affect penicillins and cephalosporins differently. Beta-lactamases have been identified in many Gram-positive and Gram-negative organisms, including *S. aureus*, *S. epidermidis*, *Fusobacterium*, and *H. influenzae*. Transfer of beta-lactamase genes via plasmids has been implicated in the widespread development of resistance to beta-lactam antibiotics. Plasmids can also be responsible for the transfer of aminoglycoside-modifying enzymes as well as macrolide and lincosamide-inactivating enzymes.

Resistance to penicillin can also be achieved through bacteria-induced alteration of the antibiotic target site. Penicillin-binding proteins (PBP) catalyze several reactions that cross-link carbohydrates along the cell wall of replicating bacteria. As such, they are normal components of the cellular wall and are so named because of their affinity for penicillin. Bacterial resistance to penicillins can be achieved through the alteration of the structure of PBP, which can decrease the affinity of PBP to penicillins. Other target enzymes such as DNA gyrase and topoisomerase (involved in DNA replication and are targets of fluoroquinolone drugs) have been shown to undergo point mutations that result in decreased affinity to fluoroquinolone antibiotics. Dihydropteroate synthase and dihydrofolate reductase (targets of sulfonamides and trimethoprim, respectively) also undergo similar point mutations that result in decreased efficacy of antimicrobial agents.

Lastly, efflux pumps are mechanisms whereby bacteria export antimicrobial agents in an active process across cell membranes and are demonstrated in *Pseudomonas* (beta-lactam efflux), *S. aureus*, *S. pneumoniae*, and other streptococcal species.

Major Pathogenic Species

Streptococcus pneumoniae

S. pneumoniae is a Gram-positive alpha-hemolytic facultative anaerobe that is a lancet-shaped coccus that typically forms diplococcic. They are nutritionally fastidious and ferment glucose into lactic acid under anaerobic conditions (5% carbon dioxide; ~20% require absolute anaerobic conditions to culture). There are 90 documented serotypes of *S. pneumoniae*, although only a handful are known to be pathogenic in upper respiratory illnesses. Pneumococcus is encapsulated with polysaccharide bodies that inhibit phagocytosis by preventing C3-mediated opsonization. Resistance patterns among *S. pneumoniae* isolates are increasing,[88,89] chiefly through the mutation in PBP. Approximately 1/3 of *S. pneumoniae* isolates are resistant to penicillin (MIC $\geq$2 μg/mL), and among 16 orally administered antimicrobial agents, the nearly 2400 isolates of *S. pneumoniae* revealed alarming patterns of resistance to the most frequently administered agents. With the exception of fluoroquinolones, vancomycin, ceftriaxone, and linezolid (all >97% in vitro susceptibility), commonly deployed agents (e.g., penicillin, cefuroxime, cefprozil, clindamycin, and sulfamethoxazole/trimethoprim) demonstrate 67 to 88% in vitro susceptibility patterns. Approximately 6.3% of isolates represent multidrug-resistant strains (MDRSP).[88] Recently released data from the PROTEK-US study[89] indicate that in vitro resistance of *S. pneumoniae* to levofloxacin and amoxicillin/clavulanate ranges from 0.8 to 4.4%, whereas resistance to other commonly deployed agents such as cefuroxime, clarithromycin, azithromycin, and sulfamethoxazole/trimethoprim ranges from 20 to 40%. Macrolides such as erythromycin, azithromycin, and clarithromycin inhibit protein synthesis through reversible binding to ribosomal 50S subunits. Mutations in ribosomal encoding genes result in altered pneumococcal 50S subunits, and diminished binding affinities contribute to growing pneumococcal resistance to macrolides.[90,91]

Haemophilus influenzae

Haemophilus influenzae is a nonmotile Gram-negative facultative anaerobe that ferments glucose into lactic acid under anaerobic conditions or uses the electron transport chain under aerobic conditions. This bacterium exhibits complex nutritional needs: hemin (i.e., X factor) and NAD or NADP (V factor) for cultured growth. They are encapsulated (i.e., typeable: a–f) or unencapsulated (i.e., nontypeable), and a decrease in *H. influenzae* type b (Hib) has been noted since the introduction of the Hib vaccine in 1985. Beta-lactam antibiotics easily penetrate the cell membrane of *H. influenzae*.[92] However, antimicrobial resistance has arisen through the elaboration of beta-lactamases and through alteration of PBP. In some cases, *H. influenzae* is capable of exporting antimicrobial agents through efflux mechanisms and have resulted in multidrug resistant strains of *H. influenzae* in recent years.[92,93] Ampicillin-resistant as well as ampicillin-intermediate strains have been identified since the 1970s.[92] During 1997 to 2001, ~5500 North American *H. influenzae* isolates were tested against 18 orally administered antibiotics,[94] and ~28% of strains were resistant to ampicillin, 21% were resistant to sulfamethoxazole/trimethoprim, 19% were resistant to clarithromycin, and 16% were resistant to cefprozil. Strains continue to show strong in vitro susceptibility to other cephalosporins, amoxicillin/clavulanate, and fluoroquinolones, however.

Staphylococcus aureus

S. aureus is a Gram-positive, cluster-forming, catalase-positive, coagulase-positive nonmotile facultative anaerobe that ferments glucose to lactic acid and mannitol, which helps distinguish it from *S. epidermidis*. Tissue invasion occurs through a host of virulence factors that fall into the categories of surface proteins, proteins inhibiting phagocytosis, and exotoxins. Alpha, beta, and delta hemolysin cleave outer cell membranes, and together with the bacterial surface proteins leukocidin, kinases, and hyaluronidase, are significant factors in host cell injury. Bacteria release coagulases, which bind prothrombin and staphylokinases, which lyse fibrin and can result in thrombotic particles as well as local vascular instability. Exotoxins such as SEA-G and TSST act as superantigens, binding to major histocompatibility complex II molecules. As a result, these exotoxins stimulate T-cell responses with massive cytokine release, bypassing traditional antigen presentation/recognition methods.

The greatest problem facing clinicians is the increasing prevalence of methicillin-resistant *S. aureus* (MRSA), not only in the hospital setting, but also now in the community. Antibiotic resistance of *S. aureus* is acquired through penicillinases, and nearly 80% of strains are resistant to penicillin now.[95] Strains producing beta-lactamases were able to overcome penicillinase-resistant forms of antibiotics (e.g., methicillin) within 2 years of the introduction of this case of penicillins[96] via alteration of PBP. Acquisition of altered peptidoglycan structures encoded by *Enterococcus* has resulted in vancomycin-resistant strains of *S. aureus*. Clinically significant MRSA in the hospital setting was apparent in the 1990s; however, increasing community-acquired MRSA has rightfully prompted the attention of the medical community. Renewed interest in clindamycin for the treatment of community-acquired MRSA has been dampened by an increase in strains with inducible resistance to clindamycin. However, sulfamethoxazole/trimethoprim continues to show good activity against MRSA comparable to vancomycin.[97] As isolates of *S. aureus* become more common in chronic rhinosinusitis[74–76] and certain cases of acute bacterial rhinosinusitis,[51,52,55] clinician awareness of susceptibility patterns is imperative.

Pseudomonas aeruginosa

P. aeruginosa is a Gram-negative flagellated aerobic bacillus with relatively few nutritional requirements that grows optimally at 37°C. It is primarily a nosocomial pathogen, and has gained notoriety for its biofilm formation in chronic rhinosinusitis (discussed next). Fimbriae of *P. aeruginosa* permit adherence to upper aerodigestive tract epithelial cells, and pili bind to N-acetylneuraminic acid and N-acetylglucosamine receptors on human respiratory epithelial cells. Invasion occurs through the elaboration of multiple extracellular proteases. *Pseudomonas* has been implicated in multiple studies and cultures of patients with chronic rhinosinusitis, as previously discussed. Multidrug resistant strains of *P. aeruginosa* are emerging, and existing strains susceptible to antimicrobial agents appear to be requiring higher minimum inhibitory concentrations. Recent data[98] from the SENTRY program elaborate the occurrences and susceptibility patterns of nearly 12,000 isolates of *P. aeruginosa*. Orally administered fluoroquinolones are the most frequently prescribed antimicrobial agents used to treat sinonasal cultures with *P. aeruginosa*. The most popular oral agents—ciprofloxacin, gatifloxacin, and levofloxacin—show 73%, 68%, and 71% susceptibility patterns, respectively, with breakpoints between MIC 1 to 2 mg/L. Antimicrobial agents demonstrating the highest susceptibility and breakpoint patterns included amikacin (89%), meropenem (86%), and piperacillin/tazobactam (85%). Multiple strains of *P. aeruginosa* are inherently resistant to beta-lactams due to intrinsic efflux pump mechanisms and the production of beta-lacatamases.[99,100] This occurs both in the periplasmic space and from within the cell membrane. Although the acquisition of plasmids and the alteration of PBPs have been demonstrated in *P. aeruginosa*,[99] these mechanisms are not primarily responsible for emerging resistance patterns.

Biofilms

Bacterial biofilms are not new concepts in the pathogenesis of disease; however, their role in chronic rhinosinusitis has only recently been described. Bacterial biofilms form when aggregates of individual bacterial cells encase themselves in a self-generated polymeric and adherent matrix. Biofilms represent the phenotypic switching of individual bacteria and are marked by the up regulation of a multitude of genes. The result is the amalgamation of living bacteria in nonplanktonic forms. This occurs in stages.

Phenotypic switching from planktonic forms to biofilm forms begins with attachment as a monolayer to an inanimate or animate object by van der Waals forces and ultimately by type IV pili and cell adhesion molecules. A maturation phase proceeds during which cells elaborate a polymeric matrix consisting of exopolysaccharides that protects bacterial cells. The matrix also provides a medium for intracellular communication, and provides a method for cellular contact for cells that are incapable of attaching to the inanimate or animate object themselves. Thus, the mature biofilm forms (**Fig. 15.2**). Both through programmed release or physical disruption, the biofilm ruptures in its last stage of development and planktonic forms are released.[101]

Recent evidence suggests that biofilm formation is important in recurrent acute rhinosinusitis and chronic rhinosinusitis and may be a reason for persistence of the disease despite the administration of culture-directed antibiotics at 100 to 1000 times the minimum inhibitory concentration.[102] There are four proposed mechanisms for biofilm resistance to antibiotics. The surrounding glycocalyx structure of the biofilm can provide a physical barrier to the penetration of antibiotics, protecting deeper layers of the biofilm from the antibiotic. A second mechanism is an alteration in the microenvironment within the biofilm that makes antibiotics less effective. Antibiotic action may be more ineffective in areas that have nutrient depletion or waste product accumulation. Additionally, biofilms are notorious for their slow growth, which makes antibiotics that rely on rapid metabolic activity less effective. Finally, bacteria within a biofilm have been shown to have the ability to differentiate into a protected phenotypic state.

Cryer et al.[103] demonstrated the presence of biofilm formation in patients with chronic rhinosinusitis with culture-positive pseudomonal growth. In rabbit models

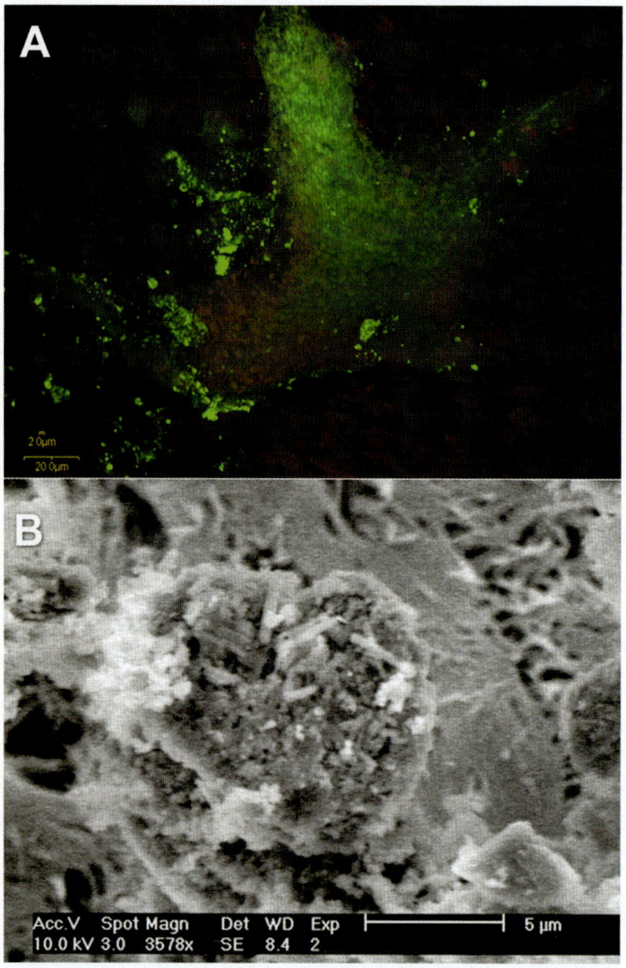

Fig. 15.2 Bacterial biofilm in mucoid-forming *Pseudomonas aeruginosa*.

of chronic sinusitis,[104] maxillary sinuses were inoculated with *P. aeruginosa* to study the biofilm forming effects of this bacterial species. When animals were sacrificed, biofilm formation was seen as early as 5 days after inoculation in 21 of 22 cultures. These species do not seem to form biofilms when type IV pili mutants (surface attachment defective, sad-31) were cultured on silicone sheeting.[105] Biofilm formation of *S. aureus* was also confirmed on silicone frontal sinus stents in six patients after undergoing functional endoscopic sinus surgery.[106]

In addition to *P. aeruginosa* and *S. aureus*, biofilm formation has been identified in multiple other pathogens: *H. influenzae*, various streptococci species, *E. coli*, and *Candida albicans*. Thus, biofilm formation appears to be one mechanism whereby bacteria (or fungi) both perpetuate disease and resist culture-directed antibiotics in chronic rhinosinusitis.

Conclusion

In bacteria commonly seen in rhinosinusitis, the mechanisms behind drug-resistance are multiple and varied. The increasing prevalence of drug resistance has reduced the efficacy of empiric antibiotic therapy and underscores the importance of antibiotic therapy based on endoscopic-directed cultures. The recognition of biofilm-forming bacteria and the increasing incidence of multidrug-resistant staph and Gram-negative organisms have brought about a need for new treatment algorithms and methodology beyond conventional antibiotics.

References

1. Rotbart HA, Hayden FG. Picornavirus infections: a primer for the practitioner. Arch Fam Med 2000;9(9):913–920
2. Rakes G, Arruda E, Ingram J. Human rhinovirus in wheezing children: relationship to serum IgE and nasal eosinophil cationic protein. Am J Respir Crit Care Med. 1995;151:362
3. Winther B, Gwaltney JM Jr, Mygind N, Turner RB, Hendley JO. Sites of rhinovirus recovery after point inoculation of the upper airway. JAMA 1986;256(13):1763–1767
4. Arruda E, Boyle TR, Winther B, Pevear DC, Gwaltney JM Jr, Hayden FG. Localization of human rhinovirus replication in the upper respiratory tract by in situ hybridization. J Infect Dis 1995;171(5):1329–1333
5. Turner RB. The common cold. Pediatr Ann 1998;27(12):790–795
6. Greve JM, Davis G, Meyer AM, et al. The major human rhinovirus receptor is ICAM-1. Cell 1989;56(5):839–847
7. van Kempen M, Bachert C, Van Cauwenberge P. An update on the pathophysiology of rhinovirus upper respiratory tract infections. Rhinology 1999;37(3):97–103
8. Puhakka T, Mäkelä MJ, Alanen A, et al. Sinusitis in the common cold. J Allergy Clin Immunol 1998;102(3):403–408
9. Vuorinen T, Vainionpää R, Hyypiä T. Five years' experience of reverse-transcriptase polymerase chain reaction in daily diagnosis of enterovirus and rhinovirus infections. Clin Infect Dis 2003;37(3):452–455
10. Lee BE, Robinson JL, Khurana V, Pang XL, Preiksaitis JK, Fox JD. Enhanced identification of viral and atypical bacterial pathogens in lower respiratory tract samples with nucleic acid amplification tests. J Med Virol 2006;78(5):702–710
11. Evans FO Jr, Sydnor JB, Moore WE, et al. Sinusitis of the maxillary antrum. N Engl J Med 1975;293(15):735–739
12. Hamory BH, Sande MA, Sydnor A Jr, Seale DL, Gwaltney JM Jr. Etiology and antimicrobial therapy of acute maxillary sinusitis. J Infect Dis 1979;139(2):197–202
13. Arruda E, Pitkäranta A, Witek TJ Jr, Doyle CA, Hayden FG. Frequency and natural history of rhinovirus infections in adults during autumn. J Clin Microbiol 1997;35(11):2864–2868
14. Mäkelä MJ, Puhakka T, Ruuskanen O, et al. Viruses and bacteria in the etiology of the common cold. J Clin Microbiol 1998;36(2):539– 542
15. Yeager CL, Ashmun RA, Williams RK, et al. Human aminopeptidase N is a receptor for human coronavirus 229E. Nature 1992; 357(6377):420–422
16. Louie JK, Hacker JK, Gonzales R, et al. Characterization of viral agents causing acute respiratory infection in a San Francisco University Medical Center Clinic during the influenza season. Clin Infect Dis 2005;41(6):822–828
17. Speck WT, Driscoll JM, Polin RA, Rosenkranz HS. Effect of bacterial flora on staphylococcal colonisation of the newborn. J Clin Pathol 1978;31(2):153–155

18. Bisgaard H, Hermansen MN, Buchvald F, et al. Childhood asthma after bacterial colonization of the airway in neonates. N Engl J Med 2007;357(15):1487–1495
19. Faden H, Duffy L, Wasielewski R, Wolf J, Krystofik D, Tung Y. Relationship between nasopharyngeal colonization and the development of otitis media in children. Tonawanda/Williamsville Pediatrics. J Infect Dis 1997;175(6):1440–1445
20. Faden H, Waz MJ, Bernstein JM, Brodsky L, Stanievich J, Ogra PL. Nasopharyngeal flora in the first three years of life in normal and otitis-prone children. Ann Otol Rhinol Laryngol 1991;100(8): 612–615
21. Faden H, Duffy L, Williams A, Krystofik DA, Wolf J. Epidemiology of nasopharyngeal colonization with nontypeable Haemophilus influenzae in the first 2 years of life. J Infect Dis 1995; 172(1):132–135
22. Faden H, Harabuchi Y, Hong JJ. Epidemiology of Moraxella catarrhalis in children during the first 2 years of life: relationship to otitis media. J Infect Dis 1994;169(6):1312–1317
23. Vives M, Garcia ME, Saenz P, et al. Nasopharyngeal colonization in Costa Rican children during the first year of life. Pediatr Infect Dis J 1997;16(9):852–858
24. Faden H, Stanievich J, Brodsky L, Bernstein J, Ogra PL. Changes in nasopharyngeal flora during otitis media of childhood. Pediatr Infect Dis J 1990;9(9):623–626
25. Regev-Yochay G, Raz M, Dagan R, et al. Nasopharyngeal carriage of Streptococcus pneumoniae by adults and children in community and family settings. Clin Infect Dis 2004;38(5): 632–639
26. Wolf B, Gama A, Rey L, et al. Striking differences in the nasopharyngeal flora of healthy Angolan, Brazilian and Dutch children less than 5 years old. Ann Trop Paediatr 1999;19(3):287–292
27. Jousimies-Somer HR, Savolainen S, Ylikoski JS. Comparison of the nasal bacterial floras in two groups of healthy subjects and in patients with acute maxillary sinusitis. J Clin Microbiol 1989;27(12):2736–2743
28. Talaat AM, Bahgat YS, el-Ghazzawy E, Elwany S. Nasopharyngeal bacterial flora before and after adenoidectomy. J Laryngol Otol 1989;103(4):372–374
29. Fairchok MP, Ashton WS, Fischer GW. Carriage of penicillin-resistant pneumococci in a military population in Washington, DC: risk factors and correlation with clinical isolates. Clin Infect Dis 1996;22(6):966–972
30. Gordts F, Abu Nasser I, Clement PA, Pierard D, Kaufman L. Bacteriology of the middle meatus in children. Int J Pediatr Otorhinolaryngol 1999;48(2):163–167
31. Klossek JM, Dubreuil L, Richet H, Richet B, Sedallian A, Beutter P. Bacteriology of the adult middle meatus. J Laryngol Otol 1996;110(9):847–849
32. Nadel DM, Lanza DC, Kennedy DW. Endoscopically guided sinus cultures in normal subjects. Am J Rhinol 1999;13(2):87–90
33. Bjorkwall T. Bacteriological examinations in maxillary sinusitis. Acta Otolaryngol Suppl 1950;83:9–58
34. Sobin J, Engquist S, Nord CE. Bacteriology of the maxillary sinus in healthy volunteers. Scand J Infect Dis 1992;24(5): 633–635
35. Brook I. Aerobic and anaerobic bacterial flora of normal maxillary sinuses. Laryngoscope 1981;91(3):372–376
36. Axelsson A, Brorson JE. The correlation between bacteriological findings in the nose and maxillary sinus in acute maxillary sinusitis. Laryngoscope 1973;83(12):2003–2011
37. Karma P, Jokipii L, Sipilä P, Luotonen J, Jokipii AM. Bacteria in chronic maxillary sinusitis. Arch Otolaryngol 1979;105(7): 386–390
38. Poole M. Endoscopically guided vs. blind nasal cultures in sinusitis. Otolaryngol Head Neck Surg 1992;107:272
39. Chow J, Hartman J, Stankiewicz J. Endoscopically directed cultures of the maxillary sinus ostium. Oper Tech Otolaryngol—Head Neck Surg 1993;4:86–89
40. Orobello PW Jr, Park RI, Belcher LJ, et al. Microbiology of chronic sinusitis in children. Arch Otolaryngol Head Neck Surg 1991; 117(9):980–983
41. Brook I, Frazier EH, Foote PA. Microbiology of chronic maxillary sinusitis: comparison between specimens obtained by sinus endoscopy and by surgical drainage. J Med Microbiol 1997;46(5): 430–432
42. Gold SM, Tami TA. Role of middle meatus aspiration culture in the diagnosis of chronic sinusitis. Laryngoscope 1997;107 (12 Pt 1):1586–1589
43. Vogan JC, Bolger WE, Keyes AS. Endoscopically guided sinonasal cultures: a direct comparison with maxillary sinus aspirate cultures. Otolaryngol Head Neck Surg 2000;122(3):370–373
44. Dubin MG, Ebert CS, Coffey CS, Melroy CT, Sonnenburg RE, Senior BA. Concordance of middle meatal swab and maxillary sinus aspirate in acute and chronic sinusitis: a meta-analysis. Am J Rhinol 2005;19(5):462–470
45. Benninger MS, Appelbaum PC, Denneny JC, Osguthorpe DJ, Stankiewicz JA. Maxillary sinus puncture and culture in the diagnosis of acute rhinosinusitis: the case for pursuing alternative culture methods. Otolaryngol Head Neck Surg 2002; 127(1):7–12
46. Urdal K, Berdal P. The microbial flora in 81 cases of maxillary sinusitis. Acta Otolaryngol 1949;37:20–25
47. Lystad A, Berdal P, Lund-Iversen L. The bacterial flora of sinusitis with an in vitro study of the bacterial resistance to antibiotics. Acta Otolaryngol Suppl 1964;188(Suppl 188):188, 390
48. Gwaltney JM Jr, Sydnor A Jr, Sande MA. Etiology and antimicrobial treatment of acute sinusitis. Ann Otol Rhinol Laryngol Suppl 1981;90(3 Pt 3):68–71
49. Jousimies-Somer HR, Savolainen S, Ylikoski JS. Macroscopic purulence, leukocyte counts, and bacterial morphotypes in relation to culture findings for sinus secretions in acute maxillary sinusitis. J Clin Microbiol 1988;26(10):1926–1933
50. Jousimies-Somer HR, Savolainen S, Ylikoski JS. Bacteriological findings of acute maxillary sinusitis in young adults. J Clin Microbiol 1988;26(10):1919–1925
51. Gwaltney JM Jr, Scheld WM, Sande MA, Sydnor A. The microbial etiology and antimicrobial therapy of adults with acute community-acquired sinusitis: a fifteen-year experience at the University of Virginia and review of other selected studies. J Allergy Clin Immunol 1992;90(3 Pt 2):457–461, discussion 462
52. Gwaltney JM Jr. Acute community-acquired sinusitis. Clin Infect Dis 1996;23(6):1209–1223, quiz 1224–1225
53. Brook I. Microbiology and management of sinusitis. J Otolaryngol 1996;25(4):249–256
54. Berg O, Carenfelt C, Kronvall G. Bacteriology of maxillary sinusitis in relation to character of inflammation and prior treatment. Scand J Infect Dis 1988;20(5):511–516
55. Brook I. Bacteriology of acute and chronic ethmoid sinusitis. J Clin Microbiol 2005;43(7):3479–3480
56. Brook I. Discrepancies in the recovery of bacteria from multiple sinuses in acute and chronic sinusitis. J Med Microbiol 2004;53 (Pt 9):879–885
57. Antila J, Suonpää J, Lehtonen OP. Bacteriological evaluation of 194 adult patients with acute frontal sinusitis and findings of simultaneous maxillary sinusitis. Acta Otolaryngol Suppl 1997;529:162–164

58. Brook I. Bacteriology of acute and chronic frontal sinusitis. Arch Otolaryngol Head Neck Surg 2002;128(5):583–585
59. Herrmann BW, Chung JC, Eisenbeis JF, Forsen JW Jr. Intracranial complications of pediatric frontal rhinosinusitis. Am J Rhinol 2006;20(3):320–324
60. Lew D, Southwick FS, Montgomery WW, Weber AL, Baker AS. Sphenoid sinusitis. A review of 30 cases. N Engl J Med 1983; 309(19):1149–1154
61. Ruoppi P, Seppä J, Pukkila M, Nuutinen J. Isolated sphenoid sinus diseases: report of 39 cases. Arch Otolaryngol Head Neck Surg 2000;126(6):777–781
62. Brook I. Bacteriology of acute and chronic sphenoid sinusitis. Ann Otol Rhinol Laryngol 2002;111(11):1002–1004
63. Bach A, Boehrer H, Schmidt H, Geiss HK. Nosocomial sinusitis in ventilated patients. Nasotracheal versus orotracheal intubation. Anaesthesia 1992;47(4):335–339
64. Caplan ES, Hoyt NJ. Nosocomial sinusitis. JAMA 1982;247(5): 639–641
65. Humphrey MA, Simpson GT, Grindlinger GA. Clinical characteristics of nosocomial sinusitis. Ann Otol Rhinol Laryngol 1987;96(6):687–690
66. Talmor M, Li P, Barie PS. Acute paranasal sinusitis in critically ill patients: guidelines for prevention, diagnosis, and treatment. Clin Infect Dis 1997;25(6):1441–1446
67. Bert F, Lambert-Zechovsky N. Microbiology of nosocomial sinusitis in intensive care unit patients. J Infect 1995;31(1):5–8
68. Brook I. Microbiology of nosocomial sinusitis in mechanically ventilated children. Arch Otolaryngol Head Neck Surg 1998;124(1):35–38
69. Catlin FI, Cluff LE, Reynolds RC. The bacteriology of acute and chronic sinusitis. South Med J 1965;58(12):1497–1502
70. Su WY, Liu C, Hung SY, Tsai WF. Bacteriological study in chronic maxillary sinusitis. Laryngoscope 1983;93(7):931–934
71. Frederick J, Braude AI. Anaerobic infection of the paranasal sinuses. N Engl J Med 1974;290(3):135–137
72. Bolger WE. Gram negative sinusitis: An emerging clinical entity? Am J Rhinol 1994;8:247–284
73. Nord CE. The role of anaerobic bacteria in recurrent episodes of sinusitis and tonsillitis. Clin Infect Dis 1995;20(6):1512–1524
74. Winther B, Vickery C, Gross C, et al. Microbiology of the maxillary sinus in adults with chronic sinus disease. Am J Rhinol 1996;10:347–350
75. Nadel DM, Lanza DC, Kennedy DW. Endoscopically guided cultures in chronic sinusitis. Am J Rhinol 1998;12(4):233–241
76. Schlosser RJ, London SD, Gwaltney JM Jr, Gross CW. Microbiology of chronic frontal sinusitis. Laryngoscope 2001;111(8): 1330–1332
77. Finegold SM, Flynn MJ, Rose FV, et al. Bacteriologic findings associated with chronic bacterial maxillary sinusitis in adults. Clin Infect Dis 2002;35(4):428–433
78. Cincik H, Ferguson BJ. The impact of endoscopic cultures on care in rhinosinusitis. Laryngoscope 2006;116(9):1562–1568
79. Bhattacharyya N, Kepnes LJ. The microbiology of recurrent rhinosinusitis after endoscopic sinus surgery. Arch Otolaryngol Head Neck Surg 1999;125(10):1117–1120
80. Cohen ML. Epidemiology of drug resistance: implications for a post-antimicrobial era. Science 1992;257(5073):1050–1055
81. Kunin CM. Resistance to antimicrobial drugs—a worldwide calamity. Ann Intern Med 1993;118(7):557–561
82. Benninger MS, Ferguson BJ, Hadley JA, et al. Adult chronic rhinosinusitis: definitions, diagnosis, epidemiology, and pathophysiology. Otolaryngol Head Neck Surg 2003;129(3, Suppl) S1–S32
83. Meltzer EO, Hamilos DL, Hadley JA, et al; Rhinosinusitis Initiative. Rhinosinusitis: developing guidance for clinical trials. J Allergy Clin Immunol 2006;118(5, Suppl)S17–S61
84. Meltzer EO, Hamilos DL, Hadley JA, et al; Rhinosinusitis Initiative. Rhinosinusitis: Developing guidance for clinical trials. Otolaryngol Head Neck Surg 2006;135(5, Suppl)S31–S80
85. Meltzer EO, Hamilos DL, Hadley JA, et al; American Academy of Allergy, Asthma and Immunology (AAAAI); American Academy of Otolaryngic Allergy (AAOA); American Academy of Otolaryngology—Head and Neck Surgery (AAO-HNS); American College of Allergy, Asthma and Immunology (ACAAI); American Rhinologic Society (ARS). Rhinosinusitis: establishing definitions for clinical research and patient care. J Allergy Clin Immunol 2004; 114(6, Suppl)155–212
86. Anon JB, Jacobs MR, Poole MD, et al; Sinus And Allergy Health Partnership. Antimicrobial treatment guidelines for acute bacterial rhinosinusitis. Otolaryngol Head Neck Surg 2004;130(1, Suppl)1–45
87. Rosenfeld RM, Andes D, Bhattacharyya N, et al. Clinical practice guideline: adult sinusitis. Otolaryngol Head Neck Surg 2007;137(3, Suppl)S1–S31
88. Johnson DM, Stilwell MG, Fritsche TR, Jones RN. Emergence of multidrug-resistant Streptococcus pneumoniae: report from the SENTRY Antimicrobial Surveillance Program (1999-2003). Diagn Microbiol Infect Dis 2006;56(1):69–74
89. Jenkins SG, Brown SD, Farrell DJ. Trends in antibacterial resistance among Streptococcus pneumoniae isolated in the USA: update from PROTEKT US Years 1-4. Ann Clin Microbiol Antimicrob 2008;7:1
90. Bozdogan B, Appelbaum PC, Kelly LM, et al. Activity of telithromycin and seven other agents against 1034 pediatric Streptococcus pneumoniae isolates from ten central and eastern European centers. Clin Microbiol Infect 2003;9(7):653–661
91. Nagai K, Davies TA, Ednie LM, et al. Activities of a new fluoroketolide, HMR 3787, and its (des)-fluor derivative RU 64399 compared to those of telithromycin, erythromycin A, azithromycin, clarithromycin, and clindamycin against macrolide-susceptible or -resistant Streptococcus pneumoniae and S. pyogenes. Antimicrob Agents Chemother 2001;45(11): 3242–3245
92. Tristram S, Jacobs MR, Appelbaum PC. Antimicrobial resistance in Haemophilus influenzae. Clin Microbiol Rev 2007;20(2): 368–389
93. Rennie RP, Ibrahim KH. Antimicrobial resistance in Haemophilus influenzae: how can we prevent the inevitable? Commentary on antimicrobial resistance in H. influenzae based on data from the TARGETed surveillance program. Clin Infect Dis 2005;41 (Suppl 4):S234–S238
94. Johnson DM, Sader HS, Fritsche TR, Biedenbach DJ, Jones RN. Susceptibility trends of Haemophilus influenzae and Moraxella catarrhalis against orally administered antimicrobial agents: five-year report from the SENTRY Antimicrobial Surveillance Program. Diagn Microbiol Infect Dis 2003;47(1):373–376
95. Chambers HF. The changing epidemiology of Staphylococcus aureus? Emerg Infect Dis 2001;7(2):178–182
96. Jevons M. 'Celbenin'-resistant staphylococci. BMJ 1961;1: 124–125
97. Markowitz N, Quinn EL, Saravolatz LD. Trimethoprim-sulfamethoxazole compared with vancomycin for the treatment of Staphylococcus aureus infection. Ann Intern Med 1992;117(5): 390–398
98. Jones RN, Sader HS, Beach ML. Contemporary in vitro spectrum of activity summary for antimicrobial agents tested against 18569

strains non-fermentative Gram-negative bacilli isolated in the SENTRY Antimicrobial Surveillance Program (1997-2001). Int J Antimicrob Agents 2003;22(6):551–556

99. Li XZ, Livermore DM, Nikaido H. Role of efflux pump(s) in intrinsic resistance of Pseudomonas aeruginosa: resistance to tetracycline, chloramphenicol, and norfloxacin. Antimicrob Agents Chemother 1994;38(8):1732–1741
100. Li XZ, Ma D, Livermore DM, Nikaido H. Role of efflux pump(s) in intrinsic resistance of Pseudomonas aeruginosa: active efflux as a contributing factor to beta-lactam resistance. Antimicrob Agents Chemother 1994;38(8):1742–1752
101. Palmer J. Bacterial biofilms in chronic rhinosinusitis. Ann Otol Rhinol Laryngol Suppl 2006;196:35–39
102. Stewart PS, Costerton JW. Antibiotic resistance of bacteria in biofilms. Lancet 2001;358(9276):135–138
103. Cryer J, Schipor I, Perloff JR, Palmer JN. Evidence of bacterial biofilms in human chronic sinusitis. ORL J Otorhinolaryngol Relat Spec 2004;66(3):155–158
104. Perloff JR, Palmer JN. Evidence of bacterial biofilms in a rabbit model of sinusitis. Am J Rhinol 2005;19(1):1–6
105. O'Toole GA, Kolter R. Flagellar and twitching motility are necessary for Pseudomonas aeruginosa biofilm development. Mol Microbiol 1998;30(2):295–304
106. Perloff JR, Palmer JN. Evidence of bacterial biofilms on frontal recess stents in patients with chronic rhinosinusitis. Am J Rhinol 2004;18(6):377–380

16 Fungal Rhinosinusitis

Matthew W. Ryan and Bradley F. Marple

Fungal rhinosinusitis has assumed increased importance within otorhinolaryngology–head and neck surgery in the last few decades. Despite the fact that fungal rhinosinusitis has been recognized since the 18th century (Plaignaud reported the first case of fungal rhinosinusitis in 1791), descriptions of fungal sinus disease did not begin to proliferate until the 20th century. Descriptions of fungal rhinosinusitis at first focused on the causative organism; the pathogenic fungus, accordingly, became the criterion for disease classification. This gave rise to the terms "aspergillosis," "mucormycosis," "phaeohyphomycosis," and "zygomycosis"—terms that persist to this day but should probably not be used to describe fungal rhinosinusitis because they are nonspecific. It is now recognized that the causative organism is not the most important feature of fungal rhinosinusitis.

■ Epidemiology and Classification

In the 1960s, Hora[1] described the difference between invasive and noninvasive fungal sinus disease. This distinction is now recognized as being more important than the specific organism in determining the prognosis and treatment of fungal rhinosinusitis. The current classification scheme for fungal rhinosinusitis recognizes four clinically distinct manifestations of fungal rhinosinusitis based primarily on tissue invasiveness and host immunological response to the fungus.[2] This chapter discusses the currently recognized manifestations of fungal sinus disease, describes their clinical and laboratory features, and discusses the role of surgery and medical therapy.

Fungal rhinosinusitis can be broken down into tissue invasive and noninvasive forms. These are further divided based on the host's immune response to the fungus. The two noninvasive forms of fungal rhinosinusitis are a fungus ball and allergic fungal rhinosinusitis. A fungus ball is a dense mat of fungal hyphae—a firm, dark, debris typically filling a solitary obstructed sinus. Mucosal inflammation is minimal to moderate and is confined to the involved sinus. Allergic fungal rhinosinusitis (AFRS) develops in atopic patients and involves multiple sinuses. AFRS may expand and erode the bony sinus anatomy, and is associated with brisk mucosal inflammation and nasal polyposis. The sinuses are filled with thick rubbery debris, which histologically resembles the pulmonary concretions of allergic bronchopulmonary aspergillosis.

Invasive fungal rhinosinusitis is divided into acute, chronic, and granulomatous forms that correlate with the host's immune competence. Patients with acute invasive fungal rhinosinusitis (AIFS) are usually immunocompromised. AIFS develops over days to weeks and is often rapidly fatal, but may become chronic if immunocompromise is reversed or if effective treatment is instituted.[2] Chronic invasive fungal rhinosinusitis (CIFS), as its name implies, develops over a more prolonged period of time, and the disease may progress over months or years. Patients are usually immunocompetent, but may have subtle immune compromise from diabetes or a hematologic malignancy in remission. Granulomatous forms of CIFS have been described and may have a better prognosis.[3]

The epidemiology of fungal rhinosinusitis is unclear, and what we know is based on case series and individual experience. A recent review from one institution found that fungal rhinosinusitis cases made up 7% of all sinus surgical specimens received in the pathology department.[4] Noninvasive fungal rhinosinusitis is certainly more common than invasive fungal rhinosinusitis. Approximately 7% of surgical cases for chronic inflammatory sinonasal disease were for allergic fungal rhinosinusitis in another series.[5] A review by Ferreiro from 1984 to 1994 showed that 3.7% of surgical cases for inflammatory sinus disease were for sinus fungal balls.[6] CIFS is exceedingly rare in the United States with only isolated case reports and a few small series.[7,8] CIFS is much more common in arid regions, and the largest series have come from the Sudan and India. There has been one recent US case report of a "primary paranasal aspergillus granuloma" similar to cases out of Asia.[9] AIFS is rare and its incidence is determined in large part by the prevalence of AIDS and by numbers of patients undergoing chemotherapy and bone marrow transplantation for hematologic malignancy. Incidence rates of AIFS for patients with cancer, leukemia, or bone marrow transplant are between 1 and 2%. Talbot et al. found a 3.4% annual incidence among their population of patients hospitalized for leukemia.[10] Although the exact incidence of fungal rhinosinusitis is uncertain, it is sufficiently common that fungal rhinosinusitis should be considered a possibility in any patient with sinonasal complaints.

Most fungal rhinosinusitis is caused by opportunistic fungi, rather than pathogenic fungi. *Aspergillus* species cause most cases of fungus ball, CIFS, and AIFS. The dematiaceous fungi (*Alternaria, Bipolaris, Drechslera, Curvularia, Exserohilum*) are the most common fungi in AFRS. Identification of the fungi responsible for sinonasal disease may be important to direct appropriate antifungal therapy. Histopathology is important to differentiate invasive from noninvasive disease. Histologic identification of fungus in tissue sections can be difficult and requires special staining techniques. Fungi cannot be reliably identified by the Gram stain or hematoxylin and eosin (H&E) stain, although they may leave "ghosts" where their lack of staining can be seen in the specimen. Silver stains (GMS) and the periodic acid–Schiff stain are more reliable for identifying fungal hyphae. The Fontana-Mason stain is useful to identify dematiaceous fungi. One or more of these special stains should be used by the pathologist to rule out the presence of fungus in suspicious cases. Fungi are best identified by culturing from clinical specimens but in practice can be difficult to culture, and because of delays in obtaining results, empiric treatment is usually begun based on the likely organisms involved. In cases where invasive fungal sinusitis is suspected, frozen section pathologic examination with toluidine blue staining may be diagnostic and may allow for prompt intervention.[11]

Certain fungi tend to be associated with particular manifestations of fungal sinus disease. Overall, the most common fungi are of the genus *Aspergillus*. AIFS is usually caused by the Mucoraceae or *Aspergillus*.[12] Likewise, CIFS is usually due to various *Aspergillus* species.[1] AFRS was initially attributed to *Aspergillus*, but it has become apparent that the dematiaceous fungi are the most common culprits.[13] Fungus balls are almost exclusively due to *Aspergillus*, and the largest series in the literature (Klossek) yielded only *Aspergillus fumigatus*.[14] Despite these general patterns it should be pointed out that a variety of fungi have been described in these conditions.

Immunology and Host-Pathogen Interactions in Fungal Sinus Disease

The pathophysiologic mechanisms of fungal sinus disease are poorly understood. It is unknown why only a small number of individuals suffer from fungal rhinosinusitis, whereas most of us will suffer at some point from viral or bacterial rhinosinusitis. The inoculation of fungal spores into the nose is a daily event, and Ponikau et al.[15] showed that fungi are universally present within the nose. In fact, most humans' nasal cavities become colonized with fungus by 4 months of age.[16]

The pathogenesis of fungal rhinosinusitis must therefore involve rare events. The number and size of inhaled spores, anatomic factors, mucociliary clearance, general mucosal health, and host immune factors are all likely determinants of disease. Fungi may release mycotoxins, which damage the epithelium and disrupt ciliary function, and fungal antigen exposure may trigger local inflammation. Host immune factors determine the manifestations of fungal sinus disease. The fact that AFRS tends to develop in atopic patients, whereas AIFS tends to develop in the immunocompromised, has led to the theory that fungal rhinosinusitis is a spectrum of disease, the manifestations of which depend on the host's response to the fungus.

Fungus Ball

Fungus ball is a term that replaces the misnomer "mycetoma" to denote a dense accumulation of fungus and the associated debris presenting as a noninvasive mass in the sinuses. A true mycetoma is a suppurative, granulomatous subcutaneous fungal infection with draining sinus tracts. Other terms have been used to describe sinus fungus balls, such as "aspergilloma" or simply "sinus aspergillosis." Because these terms are nonspecific, they should probably be avoided.

The diagnosis of a fungus ball is usually stumbled on when treating patients for chronic rhinosinusitis. Fungus balls of the paranasal sinuses tend to develop in older (60+ years of age) patients and cause nonspecific chronic rhinosinusitis symptoms such as nasal obstruction and postnasal drainage.[14] Some patients may be asymptomatic, and the diagnosis made only after imaging for some other condition. There is no evidence of immunocompromise in these patients; Jiang and Hsu found no evidence of humoral immunodeficiency in a series of 30 patients with fungus balls.[17] Zinc may be a growth factor, which facilitates the survival of fungi within the maxillary sinus and promotes fungus ball formation. About 50% of patients with fungus balls have had prior endodontic treatment, and there is some experimental evidence that the zinc within root canal fillings may stimulate fungal growth within the maxillary sinus.[14] In a case-control study, 89% of patients with maxillary sinus fungus balls had a history of endodontic treatment versus 37% in a matched control group.[18]

On physical examination, up to 40% of patients have purulent discharge from the involved sinus and 10% have polyps.[14] The remainder of patients, though, may have a generally normal physical examination. In over 90% of cases a single sinus is involved, and occasionally two contiguous sinuses will be involved. Single sinus involvement and the absence of polyps help to distinguish a fungus ball from AFRS. The majority of fungus balls involve a solitary maxillary sinus or sphenoid sinus; however, frontal and ethmoid fungus balls have been described. Radiologic, endoscopic, and histopathologic examination are needed to confirm the diagnosis.

Sinus fungus balls have characteristic imaging findings. The computed tomographic (CT) appearance of a single opacified sinus with a central area of high attenuation is highly suggestive of fungus ball (**Fig. 16.1**). Centrally within the involved sinus are areas of hyperattenuation that correspond to fungal debris and punctate calcifications. There is usually minimal or no sinus expansion, but there may be a thick osteitic bone reaction from the chronic disease process. Bone erosion is possible, but less

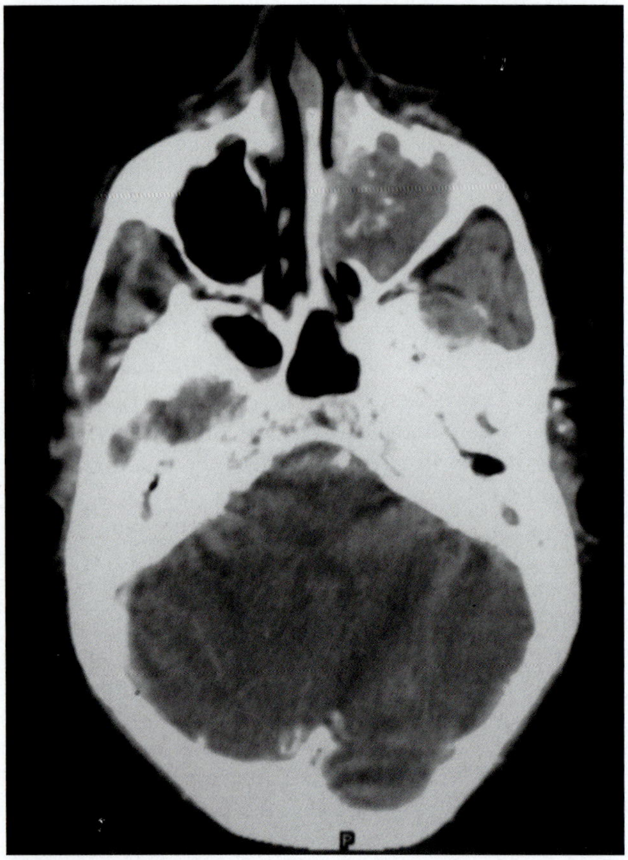

Fig. 16.1 Axial computed tomography scan in soft tissue windows demonstrates opacification of the left maxillary sinus with central hyperattenuation within the sinus, medial bulging of the lateral nasal wall, and bony thickening of the posterolateral maxillary sinus wall. At the operation, an isolated fungus ball was noted.

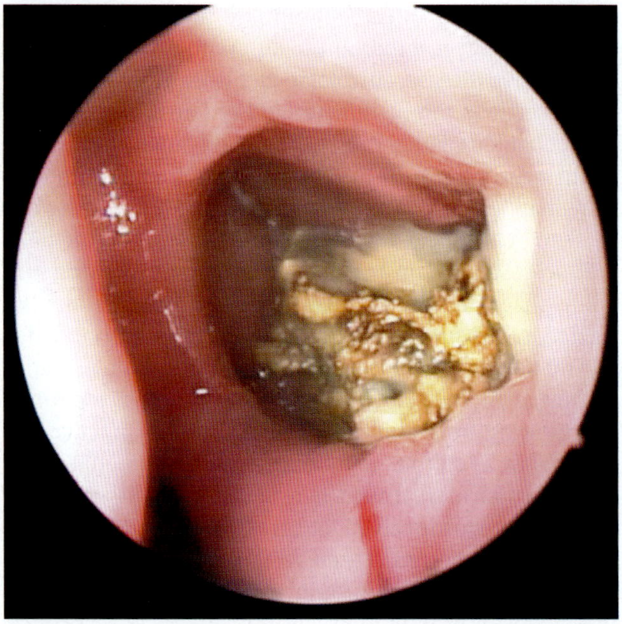

Fig. 16.2 An endoscopic view of the left maxillary sinus demonstrates a fungus ball filling the maxillary antrum.

common. On magnetic resonance imaging (MRI), sinus contents are hypointense on T1- and T2-weighted images. The surrounding mucosa may be hyperintense on T2 or contrasted images.[19]

The diagnosis of a sinus fungus ball is typically made by endoscopic examination at the time of surgical debridement and confirmed by histopathologic exam of sinus contents. Grossly, fungus balls have a characteristic endoscopic appearance, consisting of matted, inspissated debris that forms a dense mass that partially or completely fills the sinus cavity (**Fig. 16.2**). When examined microscopically, the debris found in fungus balls consists of dense tangles of hyphae with calcifications and oxalate crystals.[6] By definition there is no tissue invasion by the fungi. Although acute or chronic inflammatory infiltrates may be present in the adjacent mucosa, granulomas typically are absent.[6] The usual pathogen is one of the *Aspergillus* species. In Klossek's series, surprisingly, only 30% of cases grew fungus and all of these were *Aspergillus fumigatus*.

The treatment of paranasal sinus fungus ball is surgical. Oral and topical antifungal therapies are ineffective against fungus balls. The primary goal of treatment is to remove the hyphal mass and a secondary goal is to reestablish drainage from the involved sinus. Because a paranasal sinus fungus ball is a noninvasive and non-life-threatening disease, conservative surgical treatment is indicated. For almost all cases of fungus balls, this can be accomplished with an endoscopic, mucosal-preserving approach. The thick tenacious debris may be difficult to remove and require a combination of curetting and repeated irrigation. The surrounding sinus mucosa, although edematous, should be preserved and is expected to regain normal morphology and function. Postoperatively, a regimen of saline irrigations and endoscopic debridements are indicated until complete healing has occurred. Assuming the complete removal of the fungus ball, a surgical cure can be expected with conservative endoscopic surgery, and recurrences are uncommon (<4 to 7%).

Allergic Fungal Rhinosinusitis

AFRS is the most common form of fungal rhinosinusitis. AFRS accounts for ~4 to 7% of cases of chronic rhinosinusitis taken to surgery in the United States.[4,5] Perhaps because climatic factors determine exposure to fungi, the highest incidence in the United States is in the south and along the Mississippi basin. AFRS tends to develop in young adults and adolescents.[20] By definition, AFRS patients have allergy that should be evident by skin or in vitro testing, but only about two-thirds of patients will give a history of allergic rhinitis.[20] It appears that AFRS has been overdiagnosed in some instances because of clinical similarity to other forms of chronic rhinosinusitis, and this problem has fueled further interest in the appropriate classification of polypoid rhinosinusitis.

Symptoms of AFRS are insidious in onset and slowly progressive. Patients with AFRS present with a history of rhinosinusitis symptoms lasting months or years typical of other forms of chronic polypoid rhinosinusitis. Some patients will report blowing dark chunks or rubbery mucus from their nose. In rare cases, patients may complain of diplopia or visual loss. The disease process is often well advanced before a diagnosis is made, and physical exam findings in AFRS often reflect the advanced nature of disease at presentation. Up to 20% of patients will have proptosis or telecanthus due to sinus expansion and mucocele formation.[20] Intranasal examination will reveal polyposis that is unilateral in up to 50% of cases. Inspissated yellowish mucus (allergic mucin) may be seen within the nasal cavities.

Testing is important to establish evidence of atopy, because demonstration of type 1 hypersensitivity is required for diagnosis. Possible laboratory abnormalities in AFRS patients include peripheral eosinophilia and elevated total immunoglobulin (Ig)E levels. Total IgE can exceed 1,000 IU/mL (<180 is normal). Skin testing or RAST testing will usually demonstrate IgE-mediated hypersensitivity to multiple fungal and nonfungal antigens.[20]

Radiologic Features

AFRS has characteristic features on CT or MRI and radiologic findings alone may strongly suggest the diagnosis. CT is the initial study of choice for evaluating these patients. CT imaging reveals multiple opacified sinuses that may be unilateral or bilateral, but with a unilateral predominance. CT imaging commonly shows central hyperattenuation, individual sinus mucocele formation, and erosion of the lamina papyracea or skull base with a pushing border (**Fig. 16.3**). The pronounced remodeling of the bony architecture of the paranasal sinuses and their confines has long been a recognized characteristic of the disease. MRI is not usually required, but may be indicated if central nervous system (CNS) or orbital complications are suspected. On MRI, the sinus contents have a low T2 and isointense or hypointense T1 signal. The peripheral mucosa is hyperintense on both T1 and T2 images consistent with inflamed mucosa (**Fig. 16.4**).

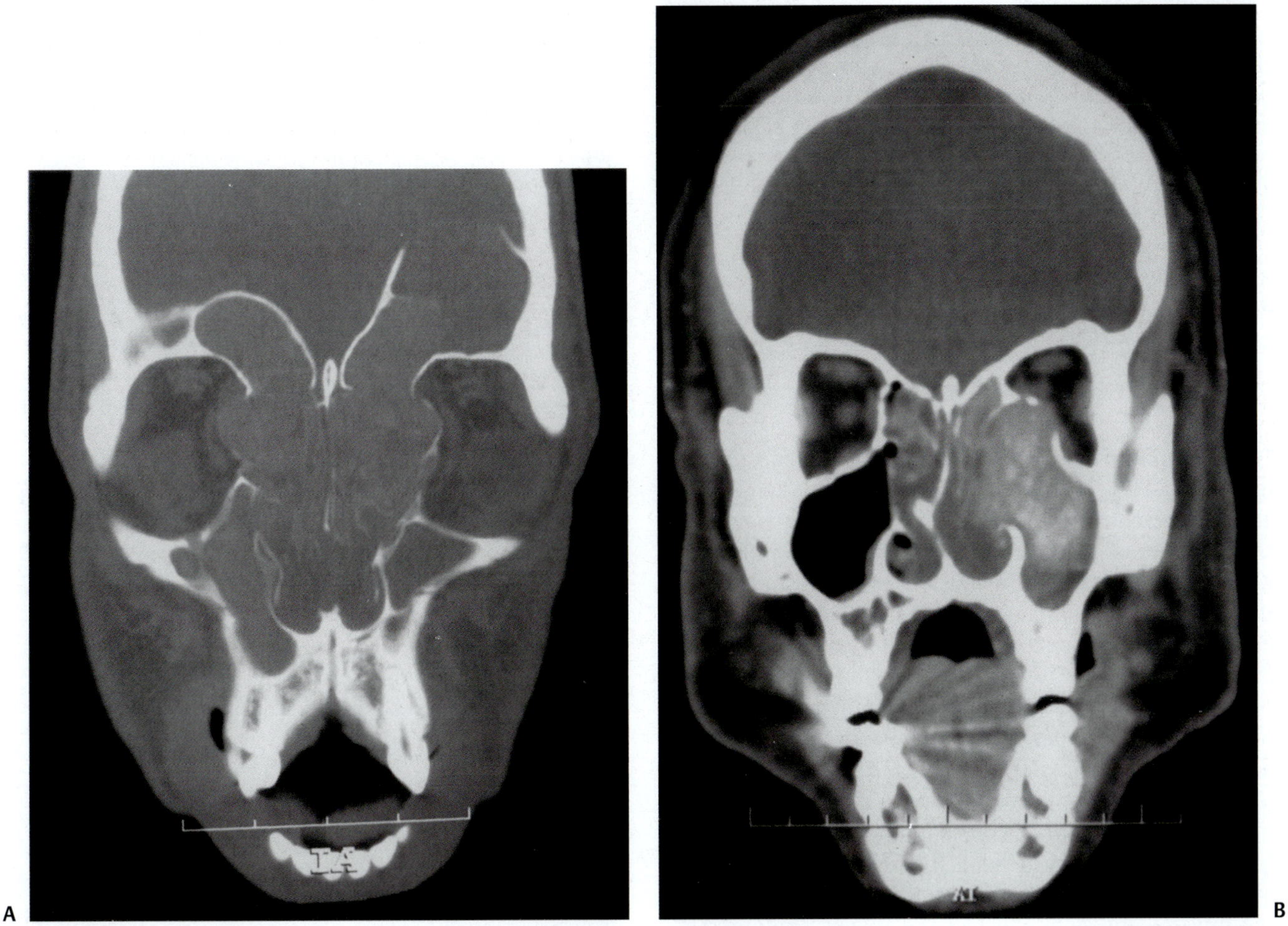

Fig. 16.3 **(A)** Coronal computed tomography (CT) scan in bone windows showing multiple opacified sinuses, frontal and ethmoid mucoceles, and erosion/deformity of the lamina papyracea in a patient with allergic fungal rhinosinusitis. **(B)** Coronal CT scan in soft tissue windows that shows hyperattenuation in the left maxillary sinus with remodeling and erosion of the lamina papyracea/orbital floor. There is associated bilateral ethmoid sinus opacification with hyperdense secretions. This is a classic appearance in allergic fungal rhinosinusitis.

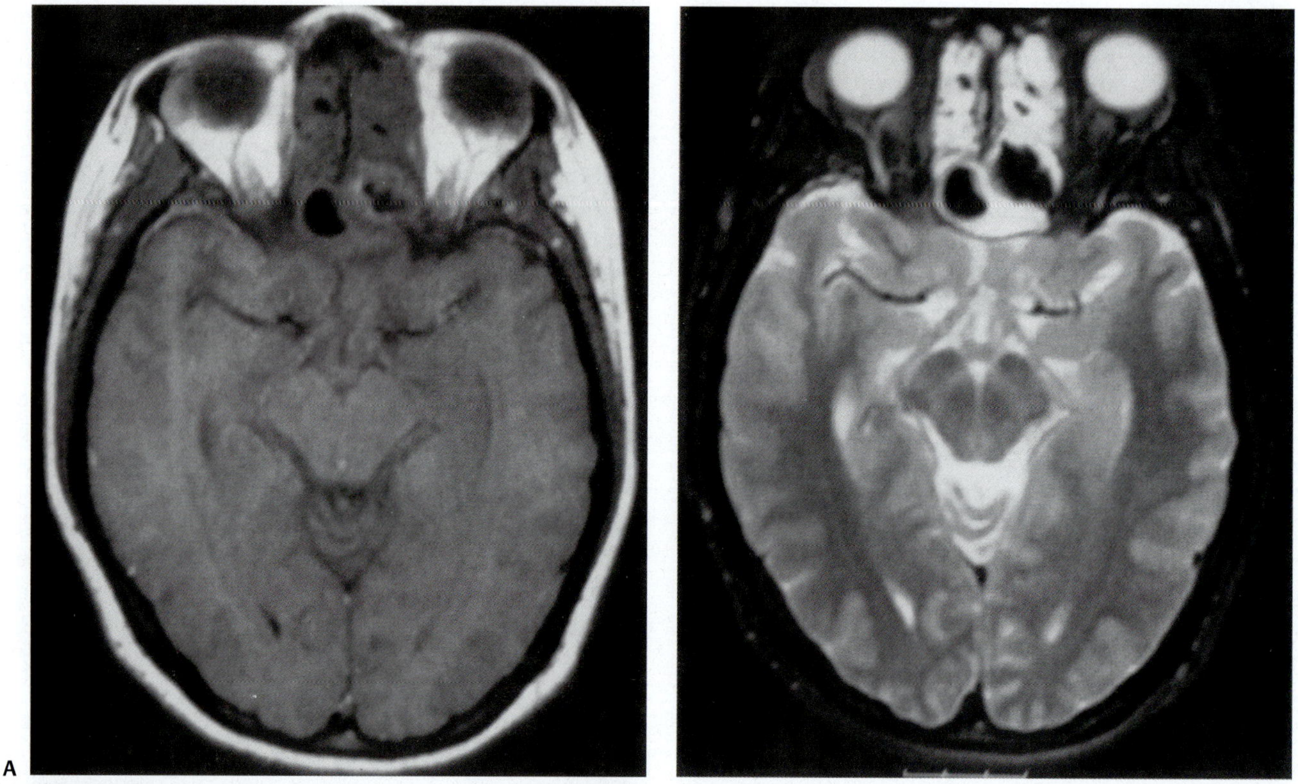

Fig. 16.4 (A) Axial T1-weighted magnetic resonance image (MRI) shows mucosal thickening in bilateral ethmoid sinuses and low-signal intensity in posterior ethmoid cells. At operation, these posterior ethmoid cells were noted to be filled with claylike debris (allergic mucin), and the patient was ultimately diagnosed with allergic fungal rhinosinusitis. Note the bright signal of polypoid mucosa in the bilateral ethmoid sinuses, and the absent signal in the posterior ethmoid sinuses that were found to be filled with allergic mucin. **(B)** T2-weighted axial MRI from the same patient and the same level as image A.

Although definitive diagnosis requires histologic verification, the imaging findings facilitate preoperative planning and patient counseling.

Diagnostic Criteria

There is no universally recognized set of diagnostic criteria for AFRS, although there is general agreement about what constitutes AFRS. An important criterion is the presence of "allergic mucin." Grossly, this thick yellow, brown, or green debris fills the involved sinuses. Although the "allergic mucin" found in allergic fungal rhinosinusitis may appear grossly similar to a fungus ball, microscopically the two are quite different. Within the "allergic mucin" of AFRS, "onionskin laminations" or clusters of necrotic and degranulating eosinophils are prominent (**Fig. 16.5**).[20] Small hexagonal and bipyramidal crystals (Charcot-Leyden) can be found scattered within this mucin. Fungal hyphae are present but scarce, and special fungal stains may be needed for identification. Fungal hyphae are present within the mucin but do not invade the mucosa. Adjacent mucosa and polyps demonstrate a prominent eosinophilic inflammatory infiltrate. The presence of fungal tissue invasion is not compatible with a diagnosis of AFRS. It is also now apparent that many patients with polypoid chronic rhinosinusitis and allergic mucin lack other important clinical characteristics of AFRS. These cases have been variously labeled eosinophilic mucin rhinosinusitis or eosinophilic mucin chronic rhinosinusitis. Finally, the combination of fungal hyphae

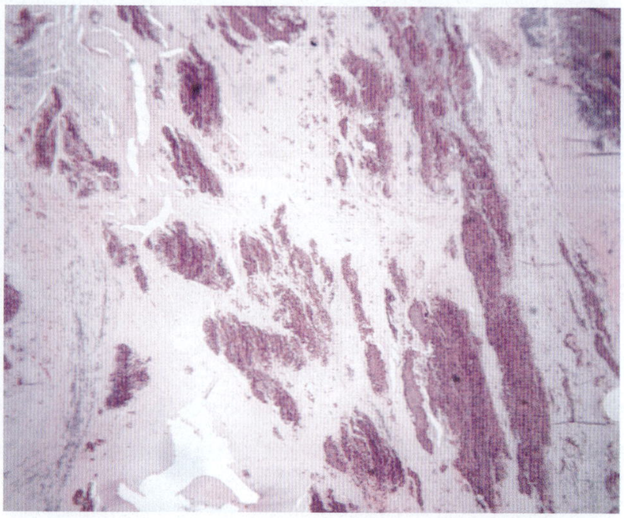

Fig. 16.5 Photomicrograph of allergic mucin showing clusters and sheets of eosinophils in a mucinous background (original magnification 40×).

and eosinophilic mucin has led to the hypothesis that many patients with chronic rhinosinusitis have eosinophilic fungal sinusitis. Further discussion of these issues can be found in Chapters 11 and 12.

The most commonly referenced criteria for AFRS were proposed by Bent and Kuhn,[21] and these criteria have been further refined by the definitions laid out in a recent consensus conference on definitions of rhinosinusitis, as follows.

Diagnostic Criteria for Allergic Fungal Rhinosinusitis

Bent and Kuhn Diagnostic Criteria for Allergic Fungal Rhinosinusitis

Type 1 hypersensitivity confirmed by history, skin test, or serology
Nasal polyposis
Characteristic CT scan findings
Positive fungal stain of sinus contents
Eosinophilic mucus without fungal invasion of sinus mucosa

Consensus Conference Criteria for Allergic Fungal Rhinosinusitis[22]

Symptoms: ≥1 of the following: nasal drainage, nasal obstruction, decreased sense of smell, facial pain/pressure/fullness
Objective findings (all required):
- Endoscopic evidence of rhinosinusitis (polyps, edema)
- Histopathology of allergic mucin showing fungal hyphae and eosinophils
- CT or MRI evidence of rhinosinusitis
- Evidence of fungal-specific IgE (skin test or in vitro test)
- No histologic evidence of invasive fungal disease

These criteria rely on clinical, radiologic, and laboratory features. These include symptoms of rhinosinusitis; endoscopic and radiographic evidence of rhinosinusitis; histologic findings of allergic mucin with fungal hyphae and eosinophils; and fungal-specific allergy. Cases lacking all of the diagnostic criteria should not be considered AFRS. For example, Allphin was the first to recognize that in some cases of presumed AFRS, no fungi could be seen in fungal smears or isolated in culture.[23] Several authors reported similar cases of this AFRS-like syndrome and this condition has been labeled eosinophilic mucin rhinosinusitis (EMRS) by Ferguson. It appears that both fungi and eosinophilic mucin can be isolated from the noses of individuals with a variety of conditions. Their use as sole diagnostic criteria for a particular disease is therefore suspect. There will undoubtedly be more controversy as the fuzzy interface between AFRS and AFRS-like chronic polypoid rhinosinusitis is explored.

Pathophysiology and Natural Course

An immune hypersensitivity to fungi is believed to underlie the pathogenesis of AFRS. The nature of this hypersensitivity to fungi is a matter of great debate today. The predominant theory to explain the pathogenesis of AFRS was adopted from current understanding of allergic bronchopulmonary aspergillosis.[20] AFRS develops in selected patients with a convergence of local, environmental, and genetic factors.[20] Fungi enter the nose and sinuses and trigger a Gell and Coombs type I and III response. This inflammation produces allergic mucin, stasis of secretions, and obstruction of sinus ostia. The trapped fungi continue to stimulate the adaptive immune system in a vicious cycle.[20] Over time, massive polyposis develops and fungal mucoceles distort the sinonasal anatomy. Manning showed powerful evidence for this theory in a series of Bipolaris AFRS cases. He demonstrated elevated specific IgE and IgG by RAST and ELISA testing as well as positive immediate skin reactivity to Bipolaris extract in these patients.[13] Others have also shown elevations of specific IgE and IgG to lend support to the hypothesis that Gell and Coombs types I and III hypersensitivity are involved in the pathophysiology of the disease. A recent study of patients with eosinophilic mucin chronic rhinosinusitis (i.e., patients with polypoid rhinosinusitis and eosinophilic mucin, with or without identified fungal elements), including AFRS cases, found that elevated fungal-specific IgG3 was a distinguishing serologic feature of both eosinophilic mucus chronic rhinosinusitis (EMCRS) and AFRS patients, and IgE levels could be used to distinguish EMCRS from AFRS.

These findings support the concept that IgE- and IgG-dependent mechanisms mediate a hypersensitivity response to fungal antigens in patients with AFRS and EMCRS.[24] In addition to the clinical criteria currently used to diagnose AFRS, perhaps in the future other immunologic parameters such as fungal-specific IgE or IgG could be used clinically to delineate patients with AFRS from other subtypes of "eosinophilic mucin chronic rhinosinusitis" and help direct the most appropriate treatment.

After AFRS was distinguished as a clinicopathologic entity, clinical experience soon revealed that recurrence of this disease following surgical treatment was extremely common. Kupferberg et al. noted universal recurrence in patients treated surgically without vigorous postoperative medical treatment.[25] Reported recurrence rates range from 10 to 100%.[20] Regardless of how they are treated, patients are prone to recurrence for many years. One longitudinal study showed that over a period averaging almost 7 years of follow-up, patients required an average of two surgical procedures, three courses of systemic steroids per year, and many had persistent polypoid mucosal edema and elevated total IgE.[26] This study showed that years after initial treatment a significant number of patients still have objective evidence of inflammatory sinus disease. The chronic and recurring nature of this condition warrants extended follow-up.

Treatment

Surgery is required initially in almost all cases of AFRS. The goals of surgery are to remove allergic mucin and widely marsupialize the involved sinuses.[20] Today, endoscopic surgery is widely employed with excellent results. External surgeries are not necessary to achieve these goals except in rare circumstances where augmented surgical exposure is necessary. For example, a frontal trephination may be used to achieve complete removal of frontal cells and mucus. The sinonasal expansion from massive polyposis and fungal mucoceles actually facilitates surgery by improving surgical access because the middle meatus and frontal recess are frequently enlarged by polyps. Frontal obliteration is to be avoided in AFRS. Disease may distort the normal intranasal landmarks and erode the important bony barriers to the orbit or brain, potentially increasing the risk of surgery. Image guidance is helpful for orientation and facilitates more complete surgery. Surgery alone is not sufficient treatment for AFRS, but is the crucial first step in management.

Postoperatively, patients must be monitored carefully for recurrent disease. Incomplete surgery, with retention of cells filled with allergic mucin, appears to be a risk factor for early recurrence. If a recurrence is recognized at an early stage, management with aggressive medical therapy may suffice. However, surgical treatment for recurrences is indicated when intense medical management fails to clear an exacerbation. Intense medical therapy can reduce polyp volume, but massive polyposis and outflow tract obstruction may not respond to medical management if there is a significant polyp burden or allergic mucin within the sinuses. The goals of surgical treatment for recurrence are the same as for primary surgery—nasal polyps and other sinus obstructions should be removed and allergic mucin should be thoroughly extirpated from the sinonasal cavities.

Ongoing medical treatment for AFRS is absolutely essential to prevent or delay the recurrence of disease. Medical therapy should be directed toward suppressing inflammation, preventing reaccumulation of allergic mucin, and maintaining sinus drainage. Saline irrigations and topical steroid sprays are mainstays of treatment. Nasal steroids have a minimal side effect profile, and are effective at decreasing sinonasal inflammation or even shrinking nasal polyps. Some authors have recommended that nasal steroid sprays be used at up to three times the usual dosage to boost their efficacy. Local treatments, however, are unfortunately often not sufficient to dampen the brisk inflammatory reaction of AFRS and prevent recurrence.

Systemic anti-inflammatory agents are usually required in the treatment of AFRS. A brief course of preoperative systemic corticosteroids will shrink polyps and decrease bleeding during surgery.[20] Systemic corticosteroids given in the immediate postoperative period will prevent early recurrence of polypoid inflammation. Prolonged courses of systemic corticosteroids may delay or obviate any future surgery as long as they are taken. Kuhn's work has shown that prolonged systemic steroid treatment can induce disease remission as long as the steroids are used, and that remission can be sustained after steroids are stopped. Prolonged treatment with systemic steroids may abrogate the vicious cycle of mucosal inflammation in AFRS, but the ideal dosing and treatment course have yet to be defined.

Leukotriene receptor antagonists, anti-inflammatory macrolide antibiotics, and itraconazole may be employed, but these have not been systematically studied in AFRS. Unfortunately, there is no regimen of systemic anti-inflammatory medication that has proven superior for improving patient outcome or reducing the need for revision surgery. In summary, the ideal medical regimen for AFRS is unknown and clinical decisions must be made based on a patient's age, concomitant medical conditions, and response to treatment.

Despite the fact that the fungi in AFRS are not invasive and are present in scant numbers, antifungal therapy for AFRS has been explored in an attempt to decrease the reliance on systemic steroids. However, antifungal therapy has not been widely adopted because structured controlled clinical trials have failed to demonstrate that it adds benefit beyond that achieved with corticosteroids, or that it decreases reliance on systemic steroids. Antifungal drugs have potentially serious toxicities (primarily hepatic) that may limit their usefulness in noninvasive fungal rhinosinusitis. Though newer antifungal agents have an appropriate spectrum and a lower incidence of significant toxicities, prolonged treatment is extremely expensive and may not be justified in the absence of data that demonstrates benefit. The anecdotally observed efficacy of agents like itraconazole may be attributable not to a reduced fungal burden in the nose, but instead possibly to the intrinsic anti-inflammatory properties of the drug molecule.

Topical delivery of antifungals offers the potential for delivering higher doses of medication directly to the site of disease with minimal systemic side effects. Agents like amphotericin B, which has excellent activity against *Aspergillus*, have been evaluated as a topical irrigation (soluble in water rather than saline). However, an evidence-based review of the literature suggests that topical amphotericin B does not demonstrate appreciable benefits for patients with CRS. Further investigation is necessary to establish the efficacy of topical antifungal treatment. Currently, there is no US Food and Drug Administration (FDA)-approved antifungal agent for intranasal use.

Immunotherapy (IT) is another treatment modality that has been proposed to decrease the reliance on systemic steroids in the treatment of AFRS. The rationale for IT presupposes that AFRS is an IgE-mediated process. If it is used as an adjunct to medical therapy, IT should start about 1 month after surgery and continue for a 3- to 5-year period. Folker et al. reported their experience with IT in AFRS patients and compared outcomes to nonimmunotherapy-treated historical controls. After an average 33 months of follow-up, the IT-treated patients had better endoscopic mucosal appearance and had lower chronic rhinosinusitis survey scores. IT patients also required fewer courses of oral steroids (2 vs. 0), and showed less reliance on nasal steroids (73% vs. 27%).[27] Although this was not a randomized double- blind study, these results suggest an important role for IT in the management of cases of AFRS.

AFRS is notorious in its propensity for recurrence. Recurrent disease may silently progress, and allergic mucin may reaccumulate without causing pronounced symptoms. Patients may not seek medical attention until massive intranasal polyposis again creates significant nasal obstruction. If discovered at this point, revision surgery may be required. Therefore, patients should be followed closely for endoscopic evidence of disease recurrence. Endoscopy is the best way to follow the activity of disease, but some have found IgE levels helpful in monitoring patients for recurrence. Marple showed disease quiescence in the majority of patients after several years of follow-up, but some patients continue to develop exacerbations many years after their original diagnosis.[26]

Chronic Invasive Fungal Rhinosinusitis

Diagnosis

CIFS is a rare condition in most parts of the world. Typically, CIFS develops in healthy adults, although some have diabetes. Most patients seem to be immunocompetent.[8] Patients will usually present with rhinosinusitis symptoms and additional findings that suggest an ominous diagnosis. Common presenting features include unilateral proptosis, eye irritation, diplopia, or decreased visual acuity.[7] Cranial nerve deficits, cavernous sinus syndrome, orbital apex syndrome, seizures, or mental status changes may develop before the diagnosis.[7]

Physical examination frequently reveals cranial nerve deficits, palatal erosions, or an intranasal mass. An endoscopic nasal examination may show severe congestion, an intranasal mass of variable color, polypoid mucosa, or fungal debris (grossly not unlike allergic mucin).[7] Taken together, the history and physical exam may suggest a wide variety of possible inflammatory and neoplastic conditions. Frequently, this disease is mistaken for a sinonasal tumor. The diagnosis may only be revealed after a surgical biopsy is obtained.

The diagnosis of CIFS is made by a combination of the clinical presentation and histopathologic examination. The diagnosis of CIFS is made in patients with a prolonged clinical course (symptoms greater than 4 weeks at presentation), radiologic evidence of rhinosinusitis, and the presence of hyphal forms within tissue.[2] Fungal hyphae invade tissue, but vascular invasion is rarely present. A foreign body reaction may be seen with Langerhans-type giant cells, and this characterizes the granulomatous form of CIFS. Necrosis may be present but is not as prominent as in AIFS. Variability in the histology includes proliferative, exudative, necrotizing, and mixed variants. deShazo made the distinction between granulomatous and nongranulomatous forms.[3] In deShazo's series, nongranulomatous CIFS developed in patients with diabetes, and these patients had a worse prognosis than those with granulomatous inflammation.[3] In all cases, special fungal stains are required to demonstrate fungal hyphae within tissue (**Fig. 16.6**). The important diagnostic features of CIFS are a tissue invasive fungus and an indolent clinical course.

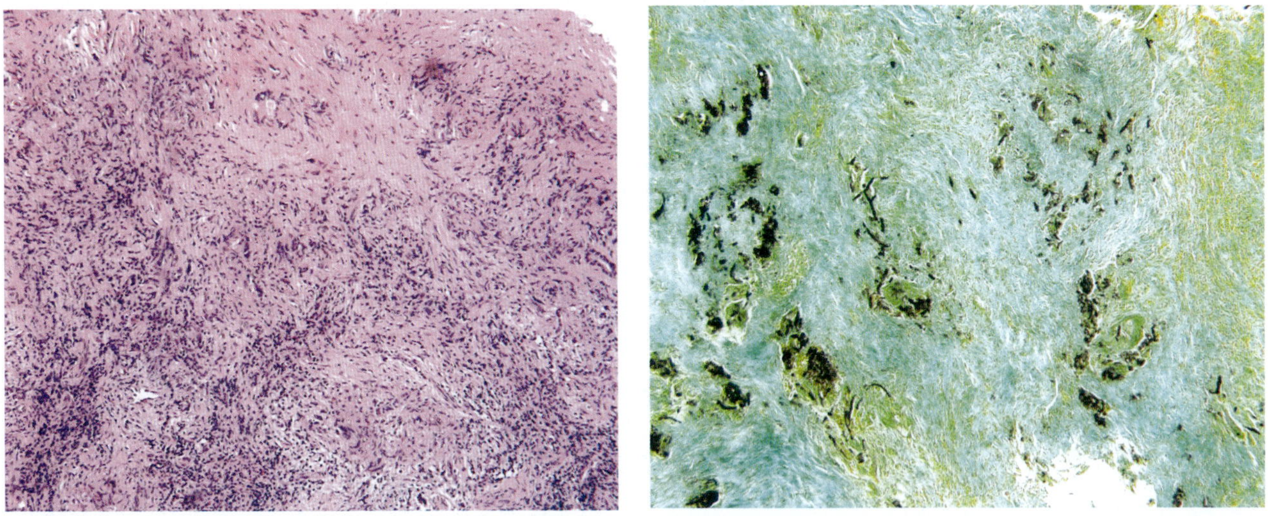

A B

Fig. 16.6 (A) Photomicrograph of sinus tissue specimen stained with hematoxylin and eosin (H&E) shows mixed chronic and granulomatous inflammation. Fungal hyphae cannot be discerned (original magnification 100×). **(B)** Photomicrograph of the same tissue shown in **(A)**, but stained with Gomori methenamine silver stain. This stain shows clusters of necrotic and viable fungal hyphae. This patient was diagnosed with chronic invasive fungal sinusitis (original magnification 100×).

Pathophysiology and Natural Course

The basis for fungal invasion and incomplete host resistance in CIFS disease is incompletely understood. Most cases of CIFS have been reported from arid regions such as the Sudan, and local climatic factors (causing mucosal disease, which leads to fungus trapping) may be extremely important. Also, certain fungal species, like *A. fumigatus*, make toxins that inhibit macrophage phagocytosis and complement activation.[28] These toxins may modulate the host's immune response and explain some breaches of host defense in seemingly immunocompetent individuals. Most likely, a combination of local tissue factors, host systemic factors, and fungal virulence factors interact in the pathogenesis of CIFS.

Patients with CIFS usually do not require emergency treatment. CIFS appears to develop over a period of many months to years. But the disease can be fatal, and there is currently no reliable means to assess prognosis. Some patients eventually die despite aggressive treatment, whereas others are easily cured. To further complicate matters, the clinical distinction between acute and chronic invasive fungal disease becomes murky in patients who are undergoing intermittent immunosuppressive treatments (e.g., chemotherapy cycles). Although the host is immunocompromised, the invasive fungal disease may progress in a rapid and dramatic fashion only to become quiescent with the return of normal immune function.[2]

Radiologic Features

Just as the clinical presentation of CIFS may not suggest the correct diagnosis, imaging findings in CIFS may also be nonspecific. With CT an intranasal soft tissue mass is frequently noted and may be mistaken for a tumor. The CT scan may also show areas of mucosal thickening, sinus opacification with areas of hyperattenuation, bone erosion, or sinus expansion. These findings may suggest fungal rhinosinusitis (particularly AFRS), but cannot distinguish an invasive process. MRI scanning is useful in cases with suspected intracranial extension.[8] The addition of MRI may also help refine an extremely broad radiologic differential diagnosis that includes a variety of inflammatory and neoplastic processes. The ultimate distinction between CIFS and other disease processes is made histologically.

Treatment

Most cases of CIFS have been treated with a combination of surgery and antifungal agents. Unfortunately, treatment recommendations made based on the experience of case reports and small series is not helpful in defining ideal treatment. There seems to be general agreement that surgery is an important part of the treatment of CIFS. The first goal of surgery for suspected CIFS is to secure a diagnosis. Surgical endoscopy permits a thorough intranasal examination, and biopsy alone may suffice as an initial procedure. Cultures of tissue and exudate should also be obtained to facilitate antifungal therapy, should it be warranted.

There is no consensus regarding the extent of surgery required for adequate treatment of CIFS. Options range from endoscopic biopsy to radical exenteration.[7,8] It is also uncertain if the granulomatous form should be treated differently from the nongranulomatous form. deShazo et al. have recommended more aggressive surgery, akin to that for AIFS, for the nongranulomatous form of CIFS after their experience with two fatal cases.[3] On the opposite end of the spectrum, Stringer and Ryan reported a case with orbital invasion, visual loss, telecanthus, and diplopia treated only with biopsy followed by prolonged medical therapy with amphotericin B and itraconazole. After a period of months, the orbital and visual symptoms completely resolved, and CT showed resolution of intraorbital disease.[7] There are reported cures of cases from the Sudan with only incomplete resection. It seems rational to surgically remove all grossly involved tissue, without violating protective tissue planes such as the periorbita and dura that may act as barriers to the further spread of disease, and without sacrificing important structures. Radical surgery should be reserved for the most aggressive cases. Initial conservative surgical treatment is appropriate given the chronic nature of this disease, the ability to follow it clinically and radiologically, and the availability of specific antifungal medical therapy.

The extent and necessity of medical therapy after surgery for CIFS is uncertain. Most patients with CIFS are treated with a combination of surgery and postoperative antifungal therapy.[3,7] Granulomatous CIFS may respond well to surgery alone without antifungal treatment.[3] A postoperative course of antifungal therapy for most patients seems appropriate considering that some cases will recur after surgery, and that the clinical course of an individual patient is difficult to predict.

Most cases of CIFS are due to the *Aspergillus* spp. and appropriate empiric or culture-directed antifungal therapy should be employed. Fungal cultures of biopsied tissue should be obtained to speciate the fungi and to determine antimicrobial susceptibility. During the waiting period for culture results, speciation of fungi can often be differentiated by branching and septation patterns observed on histologic evaluation. In general, antifungal medical therapy for CIFS should be continued until all objective signs of the disease resolve. Amphotericin B and oral antifungal agents such as itraconazole, voriconazole, posaconazole, or caspofungin may be used. Antifungal therapy for CIFS should be tailored to the patient's extent of disease, the response to therapy, and tolerance of antifungal agents. As previously emphasized, the prognosis of CIFS is uncertain. Repeated endoscopy and CT scanning is recommended after surgery at regular intervals to follow the progress of the disease.[7]

Acute Invasive Fungal Rhinosinusitis

Diagnosis

AIFS is a medical emergency. The challenge for the clinician is to catch the disease early before extension into the cranial cavity or other extrasinus tissues. The diagnosis of AIFS must be considered in any immunocompromised patient with rhinosinusitis symptoms. Patients who develop AIFS are usually, but not always, immunocompromised or have diabetic ketoacidosis. An important risk factor for developing AIFS is prolonged neutropenia. Other risk factors include prolonged treatment with systemic corticosteroids. Patients with AIFS develop acute symptoms that initially seem benign, such as clear rhinorrhea or nasal congestion. As the disease progresses, fever, headache, facial pain, and swelling are rapidly followed by decreased visual acuity, other cranial nerve deficits, and facial or palatal necrosis. Extension into the cranial vault may cause seizures, altered mental status, and then death in a matter of days. Unfortunately, AIFS may not be recognized until the diagnosis is all but confirmed.

Physical exam, especially nasal endoscopy, is extremely helpful for making the diagnosis in the early stages of disease. The middle turbinate is the most commonly involved intranasal site of disease, but the entire mucosa of the nasal cavity should be inspected. Nasal endoscopy will reveal areas of pallor and nonbleeding, insensate mucosa. As the disease progresses, the nasal tissues will take on a gray to black appearance with areas of ulceration (**Fig. 16.7**). Perineural or vascular invasion leads to areas of anesthesia, mycotic thrombosis, and ischemic coagulative necrosis of tissue.

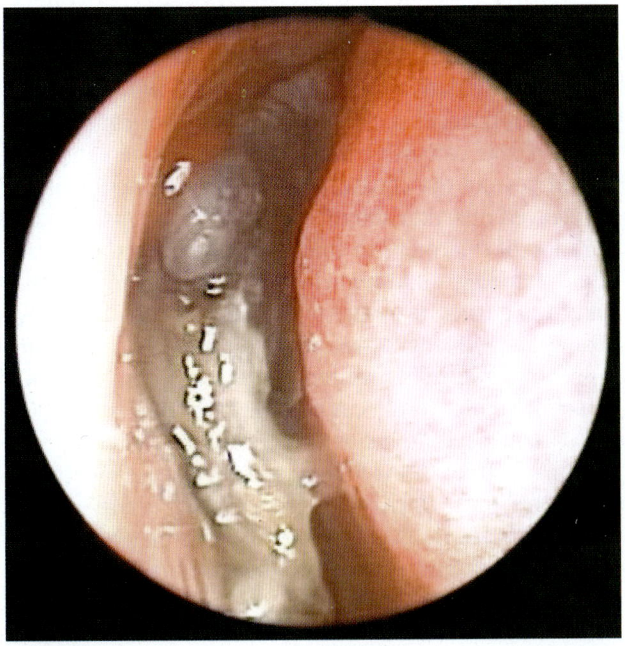

Fig. 16.7 Endoscopic view of the right nasal cavity showing necrotic middle turbinate due to invasive fungal sinusitis.

The diagnosis of AIFS is made by histologic identification of fungal hyphae within tissue. The middle turbinate should be biopsied in all patients suspected of AIFS because tissue invasion and symptoms will precede the appearance of visible anomalies. Any other area of abnormal mucosa should be similarly biopsied. Acute invasive fungal rhinosinusitis is characterized by an invasion of fungal hyphae into the soft tissues with a variable amount of reactive inflammation depending on the patient's underlying disease state. The histologic diagnosis must be sought emergently and may require multiple biopsies and special fungal stains. Given the time-sensitive nature of diagnosing AIFS, a frozen section evaluation of tissue biopsies may be useful in promptly detecting the presence of fungi.

Pathophysiology and Natural Course

Neutropenia is the single most important permissive immune defect in most cases of acute invasive fungal rhinosinusitis. Diabetic ketoacidosis has also long been recognized as a risk factor for acute invasive fungal rhinosinusitis caused by *Mucoraceae*. The hyperglycemia and acidosis create a favorable environment for the proliferation of these fungi and cause qualitative neutrophil defects (impaired phagocytosis, reactive oxygen species generation). This puts patients with diabetic ketoacidosis at significant risk for AIFS. There is some evidence from animal studies that prior viral infection within the nose enhances airway susceptibility to invasive *Aspergillus* rhinosinusitis.[29] And an antecedent upper respiratory infection (URI) may cause perturbations of mucosal immunity that facilitate the development of invasive fungal disease.[10] Basic research into the defense mechanisms against invasive *Aspergillus* infection has shown that innate immunity is crucial to defend against invasive fungal disease. In an *Aspergillus* infection, macrophages are the first-line defense and are responsible for phagocytosis of inhaled conidia (spores). Hyphae are targeted by granulocytes (e.g., neutrophils), which degranulate around the fungus, killing it by a myeloperoxidase-dependent mechanism (through generation of reactive oxygen species). Thus, profound or prolonged neutropenia is a significant risk factor for the development of invasive fungal rhinosinusitis.[30] Furthermore, the administration of systemic steroids may increase the risk of fungal invasion by impairing macrophage function and inhibiting the synthesis of reactive oxygen species. The role of T cells and humoral immunity in resisting fungal tissue invasion is uncertain. Significant T-cell depletion in AIDS patients is rarely associated with invasive fungal rhinosinusitis, although patients with AIDS frequently develop other fungal infections. Cell-mediated immune defects typified by HIV infection may be important in some cases of AIFS, but these become more important with concomitant neutropenia.

A critical distinction between AIFS and the other forms of fungal rhinosinusitis is that the patient with AIFS will die from the disease (in a matter of days) without appropriate treatment. This aggressive course necessitates a high index of suspicion for the disease, a rapid pursuit of the diagnosis, and an emergent administration of appropriate treatment. Even with appropriate treatment, mortality is significant and in some series approaches 90%. The most important factor in determining prognosis is the reversibility of the underlying immunocompromised state. Patients with diabetic ketoacidosis (DKA) have a better prognosis, whereas patients with a failed bone marrow transplant or those who are undergoing chemotherapy for leukemia relapse seem to have the worst prognosis. Without normalization of immune function, most patients will succumb to disease.

Radiologic Features

Radiologic imaging in AIFS is primarily useful to confirm the presence of rhinosinusitis and to localize the disease. CT scanning is the most appropriate initial imaging study. Imaging findings range from mucosal thickening or air/fluid levels or severe unilateral nasal soft tissue swelling, to bone erosion or soft tissue infiltration (**Fig. 16.8**). Imaging findings may not show evidence of invasive disease until late in the course of illness. If intracranial involvement is suspected, an MRI may be helpful in ascertaining the extent of disease. Imaging findings may not correlate with endoscopic or pathologic findings in this disease because soft tissue edema and retained secretions do not reliably localize areas of fungal tissue invasion. For similar reasons, CT may not be particularly useful for following patients' disease progression. Thus, a serial nasal endoscopy is an important adjunct to radiologic studies in following patients with AIFS.

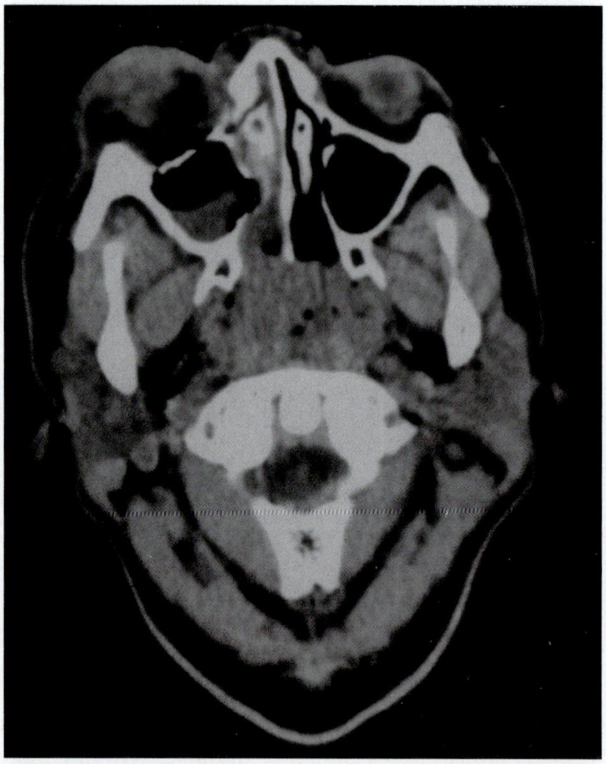

Fig. 16.8 Axial computed tomography scan in soft tissue windows from a patient with acute invasive fungal sinusitis. There is benign-appearing mucosal thickening in the right nasal cavity and maxillary sinus. However, there is severe soft tissue thickening in the nasopharynx and right-sided proptosis.

Treatment

The treatment of AIFS uses a combination of medical and surgical approaches. Endoscopic surgery and newer medications like the lipid formulations of amphotericin B and posaconazole have opened up new avenues of treatment. Medical management of AIFS is directed toward reversing any immunocompromise and retarding the growth of invasive fungi. The most important medical intervention for AIFS is the rapid reversal (if possible) of the underlying responsible disease state. For patients undergoing cytotoxic chemotherapy, this may require adjustments in the treatment schedule, the administration of G-CSF, or even granulocyte transfusions. Some patients may have irreversible immunosuppression, such as those with failed bone marrow transplants or end-stage AIDS; consequently, their prognosis is clearly poorer, which should be considered in making decisions about surgical therapy. The second most important aspect of medical management in AIFS is the use of specific antifungal therapy. Intravenous amphotericin B has been the mainstay for years. It may also be used as a topical agent for irrigation or packing materials postoperatively. The tolerability of amphotericin B is improved by using one of the lipid formulations, which allows for the administration of larger cumulative doses of medication with less renal toxicity. A triazole such as itraconazole, voriconazole, or posaconazole can also be added to the regimen and continued beyond the course of amphotericin treatment. An unresolved question about antifungal therapy is the ideal duration of treatment to control or eliminate the disease while avoiding or minimizing toxicities. In most situations, the desperate nature of the case dictates aggressive dosing and prolonged treatment duration, but once immunocompetence is restored, the disease may take on a behavior similar to CIFS. A good general rule is to follow the patient's symptoms and to perform serial endoscopy and imaging, searching for evidence of disease recurrence or progression. Once objective and subjective disease parameters are resolved, the medications may be stopped with the expectation that they will be restarted should any evidence of disease reactivation present itself.

The importance of surgery for AIFS has long been assumed. The benefits of surgery include tissue biopsy and culture to secure the diagnosis and to direct appropriate medical treatment. Debridement of necrotic tissue also reduces fungal load in areas impenetrable by intravenous antifungals. Widely opening the sinuses also facilitates the application of packings soaked in amphotericin B, or for irrigation of antifungal solutions. A drawback to the surgical treatment of AIFS is the very real risk of hemorrhagic complications. Neutropenic patients are usually anemic and thrombocytopenic. These issues must be considered when planning surgery for AIFS. Available evidence suggests that patients treated with surgery have a better prognosis than those treated with medical therapy alone, although there are cases that have been cured solely with medical therapy.

The types of operations have changed over the years, but the general principle remains: surgery should remove all tissue grossly involved with an invasive fungus. This may be accomplished by open or endoscopic techniques to debride back to healthy bleeding tissue. The endoscopic approach is now recognized as an effective technique, which minimizes the morbidity of surgery, yet frequently allows a complete operation. The external approach may be required, however, if there is extensive disease of the lateral nasal wall, or evidence of orbital, facial, or intracranial extension. These external procedures include medial maxillectomy, total maxillectomy with or without orbital exenteration, or craniofacial resection. Orbital contents should be saved, if at all possible, although the principle of complete resection should prevail. The extent of surgery undertaken should be modified by due consideration of the overall prognosis. Radical surgery in the face of unremitting immunocompromise may be pointless. Patients should be followed closely after surgical debridement and should be prepared for the possibility of staged "second looks" or further operative debridements.

Once immunocompromise is reversed, the fungal rhinosinusitis may resolve completely or take on attributes of CIFS with a chronic, indolent course. Regular, periodic examination should be performed and the patient should be counseled to seek care for any symptoms such as facial pain, rhinorrhea, or congestion, which may signal a recurrence. Once a patient has experienced one episode of invasive fungal rhinosinusitis, they are at risk of recurrence with any immunosuppression, and should be treated prophylactically and monitored accordingly.

Conclusion

Fungal rhinosinusitis can be divided into four distinct types that are determined by the host's response to the fungus. Most cases of fungal rhinosinusitis are due to *Aspergillus*, the dematiaceous fungi, or the Mucoraceae. The different forms of fungal rhinosinusitis can be distinguished by their clinical and radiologic presentations. AIFS is an aggressive, life-threatening condition that requires emergency treatment. The other forms of fungal rhinosinusitis develop slowly, and these do not usually require emergency treatment. Confirmation of the diagnosis of fungal rhinosinusitis requires histopathologic examination. Treatment for fungal rhinosinusitis is both medical and surgical.

References

1. Hora JF. Primary aspergillosis of the paranasal sinuses and associated areas. Laryngoscope 1965;75:768–773
2. Ferguson BJ. Definitions of fungal rhinosinusitis. Otolaryngol Clin North Am 2000;33(2):227–235
3. deShazo RD, O'Brien M, Chapin K, Soto-Aguilar M, Gardner L, Swain R. A new classification and diagnostic criteria for invasive fungal sinusitis. Arch Otolaryngol Head Neck Surg 1997;123(11): 1181–1188
4. Granville L, Chirala M, Cernoch P, Ostrowski M, Truong LD. Fungal sinusitis: histologic spectrum and correlation with culture. Hum Pathol 2004;35(4):474–481
5. Ence BK, Gourley DS, Jorgensen NL, et al. Allergic fungal sinusitis. Am J Rhinol 1990;4:169–178
6. Ferreiro JA, Carlson BA, Cody DT III. Paranasal sinus fungus balls. Head Neck 1997;19(6):481–486
7. Stringer SP, Ryan MW. Chronic invasive fungal rhinosinusitis. Otolaryngol Clin North Am 2000;33(2):375–387
8. Washburn RG, Kennedy DW, Begley MG, Henderson DK, Bennett JE. Chronic fungal sinusitis in apparently normal hosts. Medicine (Baltimore) 1988;67(4):231–247
9. Currens J, Hutcheson PS, Slavin RG, Citardi MJ. Primary paranasal Aspergillus granuloma: case report and review of the literature. Am J Rhinol 2002;16(3):165–168
10. Talbot GH, Huang A, Provencher M. Invasive aspergillus rhinosinusitis in patients with acute leukemia. Rev Infect Dis 1991;13(2):219–232
11. Hofman V, Castillo L, Bétis F, Guevara N, Gari-Toussaint M, Hofman P. Usefulness of frozen section in rhinocerebral mucormycosis diagnosis and management. Pathology 2003;35(3):212–216
12. McGill TJ, Simpson G, Healy GB. Fulminant aspergillosis of the nose and paranasal sinuses: a new clinical entity. Laryngoscope 1980;90(5 Pt 1):748–754
13. Manning SC, Holman M. Further evidence for allergic pathophysiology in allergic fungal sinusitis. Laryngoscope 1998;108(10):1485–1496
14. Klossek JM, Serrano E, Péloquin L, Percodani J, Fontanel JP, Pessey JJ. Functional endoscopic sinus surgery and 109 mycetomas of paranasal sinuses. Laryngoscope 1997;107(1):112–117
15. Ponikau JU, Sherris DA, Kern EB, et al. The diagnosis and incidence of allergic fungal sinusitis. Mayo Clin Proc 1999;74(9):877–884
16. Lackner A, Stammberger H, Buzina W, et al. Fungi: a normal content of human nasal mucus. Am J Rhinol 2005;19(2):125–129
17. Jiang RS, Hsu CY. Serum immunoglobulins and IgG subclass levels in sinus mycetoma. Otolaryngol Head Neck Surg 2004;130(5):563–566
18. Mensi M, Piccioni M, Marsili F, Nicolai P, Sapelli PL, Latronico N. Risk of maxillary fungus ball in patients with endodontic treatment on maxillary teeth: a case-control study. Oral Surg Oral Med Oral Pathol Oral Radiol Endod 2007;103(3):433–436
19. Aribandi M, McCoy VA, Bazan C III. Imaging features of invasive and noninvasive fungal sinusitis: a review. Radiographics 2007;27(5):1283–1296

20. Marple BF. Allergic fungal rhinosinusitis: current theories and management strategies. Laryngoscope 2001;111(6):1006–1019
21. Bent JP III, Kuhn FA. Diagnosis of allergic fungal sinusitis. Otolaryngol Head Neck Surg 1994;111(5):580–588
22. Meltzer EO, Hamilos DL, Hadley JA, et al; American Academy of Allergy, Asthma and Immunology; American Academy of Otolaryngic Allergy; American Academy of Otolaryngology-Head and Neck Surgery; American College of Allergy, Asthma and Immunology; American Rhinologic Society. Rhinosinusitis: Establishing definitions for clinical research and patient care. Otolaryngol Head Neck Surg 2004;131(6, Suppl)S1–S62
23. Allphin AL, Strauss M, Abdul-Karim FW. Allergic fungal sinusitis: problems in diagnosis and treatment. Laryngoscope 1991;101(8):815–820
24. Pant H, Kette FE, Smith WB, Wormald PJ, Macardle PJ. Fungal-specific humoral response in eosinophilic mucus chronic rhinosinusitis. Laryngoscope 2005;115(4):601–606
25. Kupferberg SB, Bent JP III, Kuhn FA. Prognosis for allergic fungal sinusitis. Otolaryngol Head Neck Surg 1997;117(1):35–41
26. Marple B, Newcomer M, Schwade N, Mabry R. Natural history of allergic fungal rhinosinusitis: a 4- to 10-year follow-up. Otolaryngol Head Neck Surg 2002;127(5):361–366
27. Folker RJ, Marple BF, Mabry RL, Mabry CS. Treatment of allergic fungal sinusitis: a comparison trial of postoperative immunotherapy with specific fungal antigens. Laryngoscope 1998;108 (11 Pt 1):1623–1627
28. Rhodes JC. Aspergillosis. In: Murphy JW, Friedman H, Bendinelli M, eds. Fungal Infections and Immune Responses (Infectious Agents and Pathogenesis). New York: Springer; 1993: 366
29. Rehm S, Waalkes MP, Ward JM. Aspergillus rhinitis in Wistar (Crl:(WI)BR) rats. Lab Anim Sci 1988;38(2):162–166
30. Lewis CW, Anderson JG, Smith JE. Health-related aspects of the genus Aspergillus. In: Smith JE, ed. Aspergillus. New York: Plenum Press; 1994: 242

17 Medical Therapies for Rhinosinusitis: Anti-Infective

Howard S. Moskowitz and Berrylin J. Ferguson

Rhinosinusitis refers to a group of heterogeneous disorders characterized by inflammation of the mucosa of the nose and paranasal sinuses and is categorized by a duration of symptoms. The classic chronologic categories of sinusitis are acute rhinosinusitis (ARS), chronic rhinosinusitis (CRS), recurrent acute rhinosinusitis (RARS), and acute exacerbations of chronic rhinosinusitis (AECRS). Rhinosinusitis may be caused by viral, bacterial, or fungal infection or hypersensitivity. The duration of symptoms predicts the most likely pathogen responsible for the symptoms. This chapter outlines a practical approach to either empiric or culture-directed antimicrobial therapy depending on the suspected infectious cause.

General Recommendations

The aims of antibacterial therapy are to shorten the duration of symptoms, eradicate the causative pathogen, reduce the danger of transmitting the infection to others, and prevent the development of permanent mucosal damage, the progression of disease, or serious complications. Current treatment strategies risk being compromised by rapid changes in antibacterial resistance patterns among the most common upper respiratory tract pathogens worldwide. Specific treatment recommendations concerning the choice of antibacterial agent vary among countries, presumably due to differences in antibiotic regulations, disease etiology, and antibacterial resistance patterns. It is important for physicians to understand the local pathogens that predominate in their geographic area as well as trends in resistance to antibiotics among these pathogens. Antibiotic therapy is recommended if a patient's symptoms worsen or persist for more than 7 to 10 days and fail conservative therapy such as analgesics, antipyretics, decongestants, and nasal saline irrigation. If no improvement is observed within 3 days of instituting antibiotic therapy, a nonbacterial cause or infection with drug-resistant bacteria should be considered.

Approximately 70% of cases of ARS are mediated by a viral vector, and in these cases, complete resolution is expected without antimicrobial intervention. In acute bacterial rhinosinusitis (ABRS), up to 50% of cases resolve within 10 days even without the administration of antibiotics. Because spontaneous clearance may occur in approximately half of the patients, a bacteriologic cure rate higher than 80 to 90% should be expected for a 10-day course of antibiotic therapy. Antibiotics with an acute sinusitis indication received this indication through noninferiority trials. An analysis of antibiotic use in patients with ARS indicates that antibiotics generally reduce the rate of treatment failure by ~50%. Since 2006, the U.S. Food and Drug Administration (FDA) has required placebo-controlled or superiority trials, and there have been no antibiotics approved for acute sinusitis since these regulations have been in place. The selection of proper antibiotic choices for ARS is dependent on the spectrum of activity and rates of resistance. The recommended length of therapy for ABRS varies by the antibiotic used and is generally 5 to 10 days. There are no placebo-controlled studies regarding the optimal duration of therapy, which probably varies with individual patients.

In contrast to ABRS, for CRS there are no indicated antibiotics approved by the FDA. However, general consensus dictates that oral antibiotics are helpful in treating the infectious aspects of CRS. Recommendations for duration of therapy for CRS are generally to give the antibiotic for a longer period, often 3 to 6 weeks, as long as symptoms are improving and 1 week beyond symptom plateau.

Antibiotics

Beta-Lactams

The β-lactam nucleus is the biologically active moiety of a large group of antibiotics, including penicillins and their related chemical compounds that extend or change their microbial range. These drugs work by binding to penicillin-binding proteins on the bacterial cell wall and inhibiting peptidoglycan synthesis. Among the penicillins, amoxicillin is generally active against *Streptococcus pyogenes*, *Streptococcus pneumoniae* (including penicillin intermediate sensitivity, MIC ≤ 2), and *Haemophilus influenzae*, and is relatively inexpensive. The clinical use of amoxicillin has been limited by the increasing prevalence of resistance to β-lactams among *H. influenzae* and *Moraxella catarrhalis*. Expression of β-lactamase can be overcome with a β-lactamase inhibitor, such as clavulanic acid. β-lactamase inhibitors do not provide activity against *S. pneumoniae* resistance to penicillin because this is mediated by alterations in penicillin-binding proteins. Second- and third-generation cephalosporins are active against *S. pneumoniae* and *H. influenzae*, but have less activity against penicillin-intermediate sensitive *S. pneumoniae* than high-dose penicillin or amoxicillin. Seven to 8% of patients with a true penicillin allergy have an allergic reaction to a first-generation cephalosporin. However, in penicillin-allergic patients, second- and third-generation cephalosporins are generally tolerated and recommended.

Macrolides

Macrolides, which include erythromycin, azithromycin, and clarithromycin, inhibit protein synthesis of bacteria by binding to the 50S ribosomal subunit. In vitro data suggest that macrolides provide an additional anti-inflammatory effect via changes in cytokine production. These antibiotics are generally active against atypical bacteria, such as *Mycoplasma pneumoniae*, Gram-positive, and some Gram-negative bacteria, although resistance to macrolides among key respiratory pathogens is increasing worldwide. Clarithromycin has slightly more activity against Gram-positive bacteria than other macrolides. Erythromycin has a slightly higher rate of gastrointestinal side effects compared with azithromycin or clarithromycin. Over 20% of patients experience a metallic taste while taking clarithromycin.

Ketolides

Ketolides such as telithromycin are semisynthetic derivatives of erythromycin. They possess structural alterations of the macronolactone ring through the modification and addition of side chain substrates. These structural changes confer additional antibacterial properties against macrolide-resistant pathogens. Ketolides inhibit bacterial synthesis by binding to two sites on the 50S bacterial ribosome. They have activity against macrolide-resistant and penicillin-resistant *S. pneumoniae*. Telithromycin is the most active and potent antibiotic in vitro against *S. pneumoniae* isolates and 99.5% of *S. pneumoniae* isolates were susceptible to telithromycin compared with penicillin (58.0%), amoxicillin-clavulanate (95.5%), cefuroxime (66.1%), trimethoprim-sulfamethoxazole (56.3%), and clarithromycin (55.8%).[1]

Concern for the risk of hepatotoxicity and its adverse effect in patients who have myasthenia gravis have been raised against telithromycin. In 2006, the FDA removed telithromycin's indication for the treatment of ARS and acute exacerbation of chronic bronchitis but retained its indication for the treatment of moderate-to-severe community-acquired pneumonia. Telithromycin is the first antibiotic to have its indication for sinusitis removed after obtaining it.

Fluoroquinolones

Quinolones inhibit bacterial DNA synthesis by blocking the action of the enzyme DNA gyrase. The newer fluorinated derivatives of the quinolones include ciprofloxacin, levofloxacin, and moxifloxacin. In general, these antibiotics offer a broad spectrum of activity with strong potency against *S. pneumoniae*, *H. influenzae*, and *M. catarrhalis*. The most active of the fluoroquinolones against Gram-positive organisms, especially *S. pneumoniae*, is gemifloxacin, which has an indication only for treatment of pneumonia, followed by moxifloxacin and levofloxacin. The activity of ciprofloxacin against Gram-positive bacteria is relatively low. Ciprofloxacin should hence be reserved for culture-directed therapy of Gram-negative bacterial infections (i.e., *Pseudomonas aeruginosa*), for which its efficacy is superior to other fluoroquinolones. The broad spectrum of fluoroquinolone activity raises concerns regarding the selection of class resistance in important pathogens, such as nonrespiratory Gram-negative enteric pathogens, staphylococci, and pneumococci. Thus, fluoroquinolones are only recommended for first-line use in patients at high risk for severe complications, or as second-line therapy in cases of treatment failure, for patients with moderate disease, or those with a history of prior antibiotic use.

Sulfonamides and Antifolate Drugs

Sulfonamides are structural analogues of para-aminobenzoic acid (PABA) and compete with PABA to block its conversion to dihydrofolic acid. Most bacteria that use PABA to synthesize folates and pyrimidines are inhibited by these agents. Antifolate drugs such as trimethoprim inhibit the conversion of dihydrofolic acid to tetrahydrofolic acid by inhibiting the enzyme dihydrofolate reductase. The synergistic effect of combining these agents (trimethoprim/sulfamethoxazole [TMP-SMX]) has proven useful in acute sinusitis, although resistant *S. pneumoniae* is limiting its use. Community-acquired methicillin-resistant *Staphylococcus aureus* (MRSA) is often sensitive to TMP-SMX. In addition, Stevens-Johnson syndrome, a potentially life-threatening desquamating event, is a rare complication of the sulfa class.

Doxycycline

Doxycycline is a tetracycline and inhibits protein synthesis. Overall, doxycycline exerts a clinical spectrum similar to that of macrolides, covering atypicals such as *Chlamydia*, *Mycoplasma*, and *Legionella*. Of particular importance, MRSA is often sensitive to doxycycline, but sensitivity to this agent is generally not routinely tested.

Rifampicin (Rifampin)

Rifampicin was first introduced as a major addition to the cocktail-drug treatment of tuberculosis and inactive meningitis. Rifampicin inhibits DNA-dependent RNA polymerase in bacterial cells, thus preventing transcription to RNA and subsequent translation to proteins. Rifampicin is typically used to treat *Mycobacterium* infections, but it also has a role in the treatment of MRSA. Adverse effects from the administration of rifampin are chiefly related to hepatotoxicity, and it is a potent inducer of hepatic cytochrome P450 enzymes and will increase the metabolism of many other drugs that are cleared by the liver through this enzyme system.

Clindamycin

Clindamycin is a lincosamide antibiotic and interferes with bacterial protein synthesis by binding preferentially to the 50S subunit of the bacterial ribosome. It is most effective against aerobic Gram-positive cocci, including most *Staphylococcus* and *Streptococcus* as well as anaerobic Gram-negative rods, including some *Bacteroides* and *Fusobacterium*. It can be used to treat some MRSA infections. The most notable adverse effect of clindamycin is *Clostridium difficile*-associated colitis and diarrhea.

Acute Rhinosinusitis

Rhinosinusitis is often caused by viruses, such as rhinovirus, influenza virus, parainfluenza virus, and adenovirus, or triggered by allergies. However, in a subset of patients, a secondary bacterial infection may evolve. In children, viral sinusitis may be complicated by bacterial infection in 5 to 13% of cases, whereas in adults, the same is true in only 0.5 to 2% of cases.[2] Numerous studies have used a variety of techniques including sinus puncture, nasal cultures, or surgical procedures to obtain aspirates to identify the most common pathogenic bacteria in ARS. The species most commonly isolated in ARS include *S. pneumoniae*, *H. influenzae*, and *M. catarrhalis*.

The current antimicrobial recommendations are based on empiric therapy, likely microbiology, and resistance patterns present in the community. Antimicrobial therapy is important and can speed the resolution of a disease in acute bacterial sinusitis. Endoscopically guided culture (EGC) of the middle meatus allows for the institution of the most appropriate antibiotic based on culture and sensitivities and should be sent for aerobic culture and Gram stain. EGC allows the clinician to better select targeted antimicrobial therapy according to antibiotic sensitivities without resorting to broad-spectrum nontargeted antibiotics. If the patient is not severely ill, administration of antibiotics can be delayed until the culture results are available. Appropriate antibiotic use is an important step toward decreasing the emergence of antimicrobial resistance.

EGC, although not currently the standard of care in the diagnosis and management of patients with rhinosinusitis, has an acceptable correlation of between 58 and 93% with antral tap, the gold standard method of culture in ARS. EGC represents a good alternative to sinus puncture even in acute cases.[3] EGC of the middle meatus correlates with direct antral cultures taken during sinus surgery in CRS in 86% of cases.[4] Furthermore, the results of EGC were responsible for a change in antimicrobial therapy in half of patients with CRS or AECRS.[5]

Although endoscopic cultures are always preferable to "blind" culture techniques, there may be usefulness in obtaining a nasopharyngeal culture even if endoscopes are not available. Nasopharyngeal cultures must be pursued meticulously so as to avoid inadvertent contamination of the culture swab by colonizing bacteria of the nasal vestibule. In 91% of cases of acute purulent sinusitis, the same pathogen was cultured from both the nasopharynx and the maxillary sinus (by antral tap).[6] There is also evidence that in subjects with pathogenic bacteria in the nasopharynx, some symptoms of the common cold are significantly more severe. Furthermore, in two randomized placebo-controlled trials, adults whose nasopharyngeal secretions contained typical pathogens associated with ARS showed a clear benefit from antibiotics, whereas in the culture-negative patients, outcomes were no different between the placebo and antibiotic groups.[7] These results are not applicable to children who are generally heavily colonized with typical bacterial pathogens even when asymptomatic.

Antibiotic Recommendations

Acute Rhinosinusitis

Most guidelines make no specific antibiotic recommendations beyond recommending amoxicillin as first-line therapy. The Sinus and Allergy Health Partnership (SAHP) in 2006 made extensive recommendations based on suspected or confirmed bacteriology, medical history, and local patterns of antibacterial resistance. The guidelines recommend the stratification of patients prior to selection of a first-line antibiotic based on disease severity at presentation and prior history of antibiotic use (**Table 17.1**). Patients with moderate or severe disease are more likely to require antibiotics to achieve symptom resolution, and they are more likely to experience complications or persistent illness in the absence of effective antimicrobial therapy (**Table 17.2**). Differences in disease severity do not imply the presence or absence of resistant bacteria. In the more severely ill patient, broader spectrum antibiotics may be indicated as first-line therapy because the risk of failure in this population is less acceptable.

In general, the SAHP guidelines recommend the use of amoxicillin, amoxicillin–clavulanate, or second- and third-generation cephalosporins as first-line treatment for ABRS. If the subject is penicillin-allergic, then trimethoprim–sulfamethoxazole, doxycycline, or macrolides are recommended. Penicillin-allergic patients may also tolerate second- or third-generation cephalosporins. If no clinical improvement is noted within 3 days of initiation of treatment, second-line agents such as fluoroquinolones, ceftriaxone, or rifampin plus clindamycin can be implemented.

The response to antibiotic selection is confounded by the high rate of spontaneous resolution as well as the possibility of a new infection with a second organism. The current FDA draft recommendations for ABRS advocate the usage of placebo-controlled and superiority trials. In the future, studies done under such regulations will provide more

Table 17.1 Recommended Antibiotic Therapy for Mild Acute Rhinosinusitis with No Recent Antibiotic Use

Antibiotic	Dosage/Frequency	Activity	Comments
Amoxicillin	1.5–4 g per day, usually given BID or TID depending on formulation	Active against most streptococci and ~70% of *H. influenzae*	Increasing resistance among *H. influenzae* and almost complete resistance amongst *M. catarrhalis*
Amoxicillin/Clavulanate	1.75–4 g/250 mg per day	Beta-lactamase inhibiting compound restores antimicrobial activity of amoxicillin to otherwise resistant bacteria such as *H. influenzae*	
Cefuroxime	250–500 mg per day	Effective against pneumococcus, *H. influenzae*, and *M. catarrhalis*	
Cefpodoxime	100–400 mg per day BID	Antimicrobial activity similar to cefuroxime	
Cefdinir	600 mg per day	Antimicrobial activity similar to cefuroxime	
If β-lactam allergic:			
Trimethoprim/ sulfamethoxazole	80 mg/400 mg per day	Effective against β-lactamase producing *M. catarrhalis* and *H. influenzae*	Skin eruptions (rash, hives, etc.) as well as erythema multiforme, Stevens-Johnson syndrome and aplastic anemia are rare complications
Doxycycline	100 mg BID for first day, followed by 100 mg daily	Increasing resistance among pneumococcus and hemophilus strains; usually effective against community-acquired MRSA	Less expensive penicillin alternative; acidic and can lead to esophagitis
Erythromycin	250–500 mg QID	Effective against atypicals and *M. catarrhalis* but most strains of *H. influenzae* are resistant	Less expensive penicillin alternative, but interacts with cytochrome P-450
Azithromycin	500 mg for one day followed by 250 mg daily for 4 days	Similar activity as erythromycin, although somewhat more active against Gram-negative bacteria	No interaction with cytochrome P-450 and needs once daily dosing
Clarithromycin	500 mg BID or 1000 mg daily	Increased Gram-positive bacteria activity and anaerobic activity	Interacts with P-450 system and should not be used if patient is currently on statins; increased risk of *C. difficile* complication

Abbreviations: BID, twice a day; *C. difficile*, *Clostridium difficile*; *H. influenzae*, *Haemophilus influenzae*; M. catarrhalis, *Moraxella catarrhalis*; MRSA, methicillin-resistant *Staphylococcus aureus*; TID, three times a day; QID, four times a day.

specific outcome differences between agents, such as the speed of recovery, healthcare resource use, and quality-of-life measures. To date, there is not a single placebo-controlled antibiotic trial in bacteriologically positive acute sinusitis diagnosed by antral tap, and few that assess the speed of recovery or quality-of-life impact of antimicrobial therapy in ARS.

The 2004 SAHP guidelines used a mathematical therapeutic outcome model to rank and evaluate antibiotic efficacy, which took into account the pathogen distribution, the rate of spontaneous resolution, and the in vitro susceptibility values of pathogens to antibiotics.[8] As with any modeling, it requires the availability of accurate data for each variable and suffers from the lack of clinical validation. Therefore, the predicted resolution rates generated using in vitro microbiologic efficacy data cannot guarantee correlation with clinical outcomes.

The use of antibiotic cycling—withdrawing and reintroducing antibiotics as resistance rates dictate—could deter the emergence or progression of resistance. A recent Cochrane literature review identified three studies that demonstrated a reduced incidence of resistant bacterial isolates when the antibiotic believed to be inducing the resistance was withdrawn. However, in these studies, the resistance rates rose again on the reintroduction of the agent. A fourth study did not demonstrate any benefits for antibiotic cycling.[9]

Chronic Rhinosinusitis

There are no specific antimicrobials formally indicated for the treatment of chronic bacterial rhinosinusitis. Given the heterogeneity of the disease, it is unlikely that any antimicrobial will receive this indication. Many etiologic factors are implicated in CRS, including anatomic factors

Table 17.2 Recommended Antibiotic Therapy for Mild Acute Rhinosinusitis with Recent Antibiotic Use, or for Moderate Disease

Antibiotic	Dosage	Activity	Comments
Amoxicillin/Clavulanate	4 g/250 mg PO per day	Higher dose of β-lactamase inhibiting compound; amoxicillin provides coverage of penicillin resistant *S. pneumoniae*	
Ceftriaxone	1–2 g per day IV or IM	Effective against intermediate and most highly penicillin-resistant pneumococci, and *H. influenzae*	Only intramuscular or intravenous
Ciprofloxacin, levofloxacin, moxifloxacin	500–750 mg BID (cipro) 500–750 mg per day (levo) 400 mg per day (moxi)	Broad-spectrum antibiotics effective against Gram-negative organisms	Indiscriminate usage promotes resistance; tendinitis or Achilles tendon rupture is uncommon class side effect
If β-lactam allergic:			
Levofloxacin, moxifloxacin	500–750 mg per day (levo) 400 mg per day (moxi)	Broad-spectrum antibiotics effective against Gram-negative organisms	Indiscriminate usage promotes *Pseudomonas* resistance
Clindamycin and rifampin	150 mg QID (clinda) 600 mg per day (rifampin)	Clindamycin is effective against Gram-positive organisms and anaerobes and has good bone penetration; rifampin is effective against Gram-negative organisms; because of high rates of inducible resistance, rifampin should be used concurrently with another antibiotic	Clindamycin is associated with higher rates of *C. difficile* and rifampin potentiates the cystochrome P-450 system and has multiple drug interactions

Abbreviations: BID, twice a day; *C. difficile*, *Clostridium difficile*; *H. influenzae*, *Haemophilus influenzae*; IM, intramuscular; IV, intravenous; PO, by mouth; *S. pneumoniae*, *Streptococcus pneumoniae*; QID, four times a day.

and immunological state. However, a subset of patients responds to antimicrobial treatment.

The bacteria most commonly identified in ARS are found less frequently in patients with CRS. *S. aureus*, *Staphylococcus epidermidis*, and anaerobic Gram-negative bacilli predominate in CRS. *S. aureus* may represent a colonizer or a true pathogen in patients with CRS, whereas most investigators discount *S. epidermidis* as a pathogen because it is found in high levels in normal patients. MRSA is a growing concern and is considered endemic throughout the United States, representing >40% of all *S. aureus* cultures.[10] The incidence of MRSA in patients with sinusitis has been reported to be 2 to 15% of all *S. aureus* cultures. Approximately 5% of patients undergoing functional endoscopic sinus surgery and 10% of patients with CRS overall have been shown to harbor MRSA. *Pseudomonas aeruginosa*, *Proteus mirabilis*, *Escherichia coli*, *Klebsiella pneumoniae*, and other Gram-negative enteric rods are also commonly cultured from cases of CRS, especially in patients who have undergone endoscopic sinus surgery.

The differences in bacterial isolates between patients with ARS and CRS may relate to differences in the pathogenetic significance of bacteria in each disease process. In contrast to ARS, where bacterial pathogens are common and are presumed to be the primary etiology (in ABRS), in CRS, bacteria may be one of multiple factors leading to hyperplastic mucosal disease. The significance of bacterial infection in CRS is more complex and less well understood than in ARS. For example, pathogenic bacteria residing in the form of biofilms may fail to grow vigorously in culture and thus may be difficult to isolate using traditional culture techniques.[11] In addition, colonizing bacteria may actually participate in the pathogenesis of CRS. Regardless of antibiotic resistance patterns, *S. aureus* may secrete exotoxins, which have been implicated in the pathogenesis of CRS with nasal polyps. In fact, *S. aureus* carriage is present in over 50% of patients with nasal polyps.[12] Antistaphylococcal treatments may exert their benefits through reduction of local exotoxin levels, rather than through their bactericidal effects.[13]

Acute exacerbation of chronic rhinosinusitis (AECRS) represents a sudden worsening of the baseline manifestation of CRS with either the worsening of existing symptoms or onset of new symptoms. In AECRS, *S. pneumoniae* and *H. influenza* are more commonly isolated than in CRS but *S. aureus and P. aeruginosa* still predominate.[5] Repeated cultures from individual patients over time may reveal the emergence of different organisms, the disappearance of previously isolated bacteria, or an increase in antimicrobial resistance. Furthermore, AECRS more commonly exhibits a polymicrobial state and more cases of aerobic bacterial growth as compared with CRS.[14] The role of anaerobes in CRS is also controversial, with studies indicating anaerobic incidence ranging from zero to 100%.

Antibiotic Recommendations

Patients who present with CRS should have a culture obtained to guide antibiotic therapy. Retrospective studies suggest the superiority of therapy targeting both aerobic and anaerobic β-lactamase producing bacteria in CRS. The role of *S. aureus* and *P. aeruginosa* in perpetuating disease is unclear and generally, only cultures that show moderate-to-heavy growth are treated. The oral agents recommended as effective in CRS (based solely on expert opinion) include the combination of a penicillin and a β-lactamase inhibitor (amoxicillin-clavulanate); clindamycin; the fluoroquinolones; or the combination of metronidazole and a macrolide. There is some evidence for the therapeutic value of macrolide antibiotics in CRS based on their intrinsic anti-inflammatory properties, which is manifested as a reduction in the expression of proinflammatory cytokines. Overall, there is a considerable lack of randomized controlled trials in the literature for the treatment of CRS. Both Legent et al. and Subramanian et al. studied the efficacy of widely used antibiotics in CRS (without a placebo control) and found overall improvement with active treatment using antibiotics.[15,16] However, both studies failed to show an advantage of one particular antibiotic regimen over another.

Notably, the recommended duration of therapy is longer in CRS than in ARS, but recommendations vary widely between 2 to 12 weeks. We recommend that therapy should be continued as long as there is continuing symptomatic improvement and should be extended 5 to 7 days beyond resolution of the symptoms or the symptom plateau. Ragab et al. revealed no difference in clinical outcomes between medical therapy with macrolides for 12 weeks as compared with endoscopic sinus surgery in patients with CRS.[17] For those patients who fail oral antibiotics and have persistently positive bacterial cultures, alternative regimens may include the use of intravenous or topically applied antibiotics.

Intravenous Antibiotics

Intravenous antibiotics may be clinically beneficial in a very small subset of patients with CRS. Indications for intravenous therapy include the presence of resistant organisms, intracranial or orbital complications, intolerance to oral medications, and bacterial CRS that is refractory to oral therapy. Many intravenous antibiotic regimens can be administered conveniently on an outpatient basis through peripherally inserted central catheters. However, intravenous antibiotics are also associated with a variety of limiting factors and complications. First, intravenous antibiotics are more expensive than oral antibiotics and carry additional expenses related to catheter placement and associated nursing care. Second, there may be significant catheter-related morbidity such as infusion site infections, catheter dislodgement, thrombophlebitis, and thrombosis. Finally, there may be a range of systemic side effects of the antibiotics themselves, including leukopenia, systemic drug reaction, serum sickness, and hepatic failure.

Three uncontrolled retrospective studies describe the use of outpatient antibiotic therapy for CRS. Gross et al. reported that half of adult patients showed complete response and recovery, and concluded that the intravenous delivery of outpatient antibiotics can be a well tolerated adjunct to surgical therapy for CRS.[18] Don et al. performed a retrospective, nonrandomized study of pediatric patients with CRS treated with maxillary sinus aspiration and irrigation and intravenous antibiotics. They reported a 14% complication rate but a resolution rate of 89%, which was similar to the clinical response achieved with endoscopic sinus surgery in this pediatric population. The mean age of the patients responding to intravenous antibiotic therapy was younger than those patients who did not respond to the therapy. Furthermore, a longer history of chronic symptoms was predictive of treatment failure.[19]

Finally, Fowler et al. studied adults with CRS, most of whom had a prior history of endoscopic sinus surgery. These patients had positive sinus cultures obtained by a sterile swab method or a suction trap to determine antibiotic choice. However, significant side effects of intravenous therapy were found and the resolution of CRS occurred in only 29% of patients as defined by a computed tomography (CT) scan, a nasal and sinus endoscopy, or both. Of particular note, the analysis of age, gender, length of treatment, culture results, antibiotic used, asthma or allergic rhinitis, previous surgery, or the concomitant use of systemic glucocorticoids did not predict clinical resolution or an increased time to relapse.[20]

Overall, complication rates from outpatient antibiotic therapy range from 14 to 26%, and often require cessation of therapy. Success rates range from 29 to 89%, with a relapse rate as high as 89% at 12 weeks following the cessation of intravenous antibiotics. Adults with prior endoscopic sinus surgery (ESS) are the least likely group to respond to intravenous antibiotics. Studies to date of outpatient intravenous antibiotics for CRS have all been in retrospective, uncontrolled studies and support only a limited role for the use of intravenous antibiotics. In pediatric patients, intravenous antibiotics may be an alternative to sinus surgery in younger patients who present with a shorter duration of disease.

Topical Antibiotics

Topical antimicrobial therapy is attractive because it limits the adverse effects of systemic antimicrobial therapy and may theoretically be more effective. The bulb syringe, squeeze bottle, nebulizer, aerosol spray bottle, and dental pulse irrigator are all devices that can deliver substances intranasally. However, these devices may vary significantly in their efficacy of delivering the drug to the sinonasal mucosa. Topical administration of antibiotics is generally well tolerated, but side effects of topical therapy may include sore throat, nasal irritation, otalgia, and postnasal drainage. Topical antibiotic therapy permits the delivery of a high local concentration without increased serum concentrations. Topical application can provide a dose that exceeds the minimum inhibitory concentration (MIC) of the targeted organisms, which may not be achievable via systemic therapy. This approach has been applied successfully with pulmonary, ophthalmologic, otologic, urologic, and oral infections.

Aerosolized tobramycin can create levels of antibiotic 10 times greater than the minimal inhibitory concentration of most *P. aeruginosa* isolates while maintaining low serum concentrations.[21] The addition of ceftazidime to nasal irrigation at a dose comparable with commercial otologic and ophthalmic preparations has been reported to lead to good outcomes in uncontrolled studies of CRS.[22] Topical tobramycin lavage after ESS in cystic fibrosis patients led to a significant decrease in revision surgeries.[23] In uncontrolled trials, nebulized antibiotics for patients with prior ESS resulted in a greater than 75% reduction in symptoms such as facial pain and mucopurulent rhinorrhea.[24] A recent larger randomized placebo-controlled trial of nebulized tobramycin in postoperative patients with purulence failed to show efficacy, although a smaller pilot study showed symptomatic improvement at some secondary end points.

One topical antibiotic that has been used extensively is mupirocin, which is produced by submerged fermentation of *Pseudomonas fluorescens*. Mupirocin is an anti-staphylococcal agent that inhibits RNA and protein synthesis. It demonstrates in vitro activity against *H. influenzae, M. catarrhalis,* and *S. pyogenes* and its nasal formulation is effective for the eradication of nasal colonization with MRSA. Mupirocin can either be applied as an ointment or resuspended in nasal saline. Application of mupirocin for MRSA has revealed a 90% negative culture rate at the end of a 5-day therapeutic trial. Additionally, mupirocin has been shown to be active against *S. aureus* biofilm.[25] Resistance to mupirocin is growing and is currently between 3 and 4% for *S. aureus*. Reported side effects have generally been mild including burning, pruritus, and dryness.

A newer alternative for topical administration is retapamulin, a semisynthetic derivative that is the first of a new class of antibacterial agents designated as pleuromutilins. It is indicated for methicillin-sensitive *S. aureus* skin infections and *S. pyogenes*. In vitro studies of retapamulin indicate activity against both methicillin-susceptible and -resistant isolates; however, the MRSA susceptibility to retapamulin in vitro did not correlate with clinical success rates. Retapamulin is indicated for skin infections caused by methicillin-sensitive *S. aureus* or *S. pyogenes* but not MRSA.

Current recommendations for topical antibiotic therapy in the management of CRS are not supported by randomized controlled trials. Nevertheless, individual patients may benefit from the use of topical antibiotics. It is important that antibiotic choice be based on culture results or target the known pathogens in CRS. The culture can guide therapy to the narrowest spectrum antibiotic. If the patient is improving, then the antibiotics may be given as long as the patient is improving, or for 4 to 6 weeks. Topical antibiotic irrigation appears to be a reasonable treatment option for patients who have failed standard medical and surgical therapies but this remains unproven (**Table 17.3**).

Special Considerations: MRSA

Resistance to methicillin confers resistance to all penicillinase-resistant penicillins and cephalosporins. However, community-acquired MRSA is usually sensitive to minocycline, doxycycline, and TMP-SMX. Cultures allow precise targeting of antibiotics to MRSA. Eradication of MRSA by topical antibiotics offers the advantages of high local drug concentrations, minimal systemic absorption, lower costs, and fewer side effects. Mupirocin ointment or nasal irrigations for MRSA exacerbations of CRS, either alone or in combination with either TMP-SMX or doxycycline plus rifampin (agents that penetrate well into nasal secretions), provide an alternative to intravenous antibiotics in the management of these complex patients. Rifampin should not be used alone to treat MRSA infections because MRSA strains easily develop resistance to this agent. An EGC should be obtained to make sure the MRSA is sensitive by culture before committing patients to a course of therapy.

Table 17.3 Recommended Topical Antibiotic Therapy

Antibiotic	Dosage	Activity	Comments
Mupirocin	Apply as ointment, or resuspend as 5 g of ointment in 45 mL normal saline; irrigate each side of the nose with 10 mL BID	Gram-positive organisms, including *S. aureus* and *S. pyogenes*, in vitro activity against *H. influenza* and *M. catarrhalis*	Ointment is water soluble and commonly used in an irrigation or spray
Retapamulin	Apply as ointment BID	*S. aureus* and *S. pyogenes*	
Gentamicin	80 mg mixed in 500 mL normal saline; irrigate each side of nose with 10–60 mL BID	Gram-negative organisms, including most *P. aeruginosa*	

Abbreviations: BID, twice a day; *H. influenzae, Haemophilus influenzae*; *M. catarrhalis, Moraxella catarrhalis*; *P. aeruginosa, Pseudomonas aeruginosa*; *S. aureus, Staphylococcus aureus*; *S. pyogenes, Streptococcus pyogenes*.

Antifungals

Systemic and topical antifungals are the standard of care for invasive fungal sinusitis, despite the absence of placebo-controlled trials demonstrating efficacy (**Table 17.4**).

Management of invasive fungal sinusitis includes endoscopic debridement, often on multiple occasions, combined with both systemic and topical antifungal therapy targeted toward the sensitivities of the fungus isolated. The majority of patients with invasive fungal sinusitis are treated with systemic amphotericin B at intravenous doses of 0.8 to 1.5 mg/kg/day to a total dose of up to 3 g. Fever, chills, nausea, and hypotension are frequent side effects that accompany the first few doses, but nephrotoxicity is the major dose-limiting toxicity and can be reduced with sodium loading. These toxicities can generally be reduced or eliminated with the use of amphotericin B lipid complex, which is amphotericin B delivered through liposomes. These liposomes have an affinity for the reticuloendothelial system and so bypass toxicities otherwise imparted to other tissues by amphotericin B.

Certain fungi also respond to other antifungal agents, and occasionally other antifungal agents are the drug of choice. Approximately half the cases of invasive *Aspergillus* infections in one series were salvaged with itraconazole. Voriconazole is not approved for invasive fungal sinusitis; however, success has been reported in chronic invasive fungal sinusitis and its in vitro activity is greater than itraconazole.[26] Posaconazole is also not approved for fungal sinusitis, but efficacy in Zygomycosis (*Mucor*) sinusitis and *Aspergillus* sinusitis has been reported.[27] Posaconazole may well emerge as the drug of choice for *Mucor* in the future.

The use of oral antifungal agents in CRS is extrapolated from studies of invasive fungal disease in other sites and knowledge of in vitro efficacy. Several placebo-controlled studies have been performed in patients with noninvasive presumed fungal sinusitis. The efficacy of antifungals in this population has thus far been disappointing. No benefit of high-dose oral terbinafine was shown in a randomized placebo-controlled multicenter study of patients with CRS not restricted to AFS.[28] To date, no randomized controlled trials of antifungal therapy in patients with classic allergic fungal sinusitis have been performed. In the pulmonary equivalent of the disease, allergic bronchopulmonary aspergillosis (ABPA), the antifungal itraconazole, at a dose of 200 mg twice a day for 16 weeks, was shown to significantly improve the disease in a randomized placebo-controlled multicenter study.[29] Antibiotics have, on occasion, been reported to improve allergic fungal sinusitis (AFS), but there are no trials to support their use for this indication. If AFS does require the presence of a bacterial superantigen,

Table 17.4 Selected Antifungal Agents

Antifungal	Dosage	Activity	Comments
Amphotericin B IV lipid and non lipid	0.25 up to 1.0 mg/kg QD IV in 5% dextrose; dose varies with lipid formulation	Active against most pathogenic fungi; variable against some *Aspergillus* species and *Zygomycetes; Pseudallescheria boydii* and *Fusarium* species are resistant	Nephrotoxicity reduced with more expensive lipid formulations
Amphotericin B topical	100 μg/mL, 20 mL BID	As previous	Not absorbed via oral route; unproven efficacy in noninvasive fungal sinusitis
Ketoconazole	400 mg po QD	*Candidiasis* and *Pseudallescheria boydii*	Hepatotoxic; monitor liver function
Itraconazole	100 mg 1–2 po BID with meals	Dematiaceous fungi and variable activity against *Aspergillus* species; not active against *Zygomycetes*	Best absorbed in acidic stomach; coadminister with cola or cranberry juice; if used long term, monitor liver function
Posaconazole	Oral suspension of 40 mg/mL; dosage is 400 mg BID	Indicated for the treatment of a broad range of invasive fungal infections including *Zygomycetes*, *Fusarium*, and *Aspergillus* in patients refractory or intolerant of other antifungal therapies	Safety under age 18 not assessed; use with caution with other drugs metabolized through the CYP3A4 system
Terbinafine	250 mg po QD	Variable in vitro antifungal activity; used chiefly for dermatophytosis	Not effective in a randomized controlled trial of noninvasive CRS
Voriconazole	200 mg BID po 1 hour before or following meals; IV formulation given as loading dose, followed by 4 mg/kg BID	Indicated for treatment of a broad range of fungal pathogens	Monitor liver functions; unusual adverse effect is visual disturbance

Abbreviations: BID, twice a day; CRS, chronic rhinosinusitis; IV, intravenous; po, by mouth; QD, every day.

then perhaps antibacterial therapies may have a role, but that role remains to be elucidated.

Given the suggestion for a broader role for fungi in chronic rhinosinusitis patients, intranasal topical antifungal therapy could potentially reduce inflammation. Early nonrandomized, noncontrolled studies reported 70% improvement in symptoms and CT scans after irrigation of the nose with 20 mL of amphotericin B twice a day for 4 months. In a nonrandomized nonblinded study, intranasal amphotericin B applied as a suspension per nostril twice a day eliminated polyposis on endoscopy in 62% of patients with mild nasal polyps and 42% of patients with moderate nasal polyps CRS, whereas patients with severe CRS and completely occlusive polyps showed no improvement.[30] A pilot study by Ponikau conducted in a double-blind, placebo-controlled fashion using a bulb syringe for intranasal amphotericin B in CRS patients showed slightly reduced mucosal thickening on CT scans by 8% (statistically significant compared with controls), but no significant changes in symptom scores, nasal endoscopy scores, intranasal cytokines, or markers for eosinophilic inflammation.[31]

Subsequent studies to assess the effect of intranasal antifungals have been more rigorous. In the best designed study to date, a double-blind randomized placebo-controlled multicenter study showed no objective or subjective benefit from the use of amphotericin irrigation in CRS, specifically excluding patients with AFS.[32] Furthermore, the results of a phase 3 study of a commercial form of topical amphotericin B (SinuNase) were reported, and there was no significant difference in symptoms between patients receiving amphotericin B and patients receiving a placebo. To date, intranasal antifungal therapy shows no efficacy for CRS; however, studies restricting oral or topical antifungals to patients with AFS have not been performed.

Conclusion

Knowledge of the current epidemiologic state of bacterial resistance is mandatory if the continuing rates of increasing resistance are to be halted. The responsible use of antimicrobial agents is crucial for the development of satisfactory patient outcomes and to the future viability of antimicrobial therapy. Antibiotics should not be used for nonbacterial sinus infections. The difficulty is identifying these patients and distinguishing between colonization and infection. A similar difficulty is present in patients with a possible noninvasive fungal etiology of CRS. Increased use of endoscopically guided cultures is strongly recommended for all patients whether their symptoms are acute or chronic in duration. Further research is required to help the clinician identify patients who clearly have an infectious agent underlying their CRS.

References

1. Dohar J, Cantón R, Cohen R, Farrell DJ, Felmingham D. Activity of telithromycin and comparators against bacterial pathogens isolated from 1,336 patients with clinically diagnosed acute sinusitis. Ann Clin Microbiol Antimicrob 2004;3:15
2. Sande MA, Gwaltney JM. Acute community-acquired bacterial sinusitis: continuing challenges and current management. Clin Infect Dis 2004;39(Suppl 3):S151–S158
3. Benninger MS, Payne SC, Ferguson BJ, Hadley JA, Ahmad N. Endoscopically directed middle meatal cultures versus maxillary sinus taps in acute bacterial maxillary rhinosinusitis: a meta-analysis. Otolaryngol Head Neck Surg 2006;134(1):3–9
4. Gold SM, Tami TA. Role of middle meatus aspiration culture in the diagnosis of chronic sinusitis. Laryngoscope 1997;107(12 Pt 1): 1586–1589
5. Cincik H, Ferguson BJ. The impact of endoscopic cultures on care in rhinosinusitis. Laryngoscope 2006;116(9):1562–1568
6. Savolainen S, Ylikoski J, Jousimes-Somer H. Predictive value of nasal bacterial culture for etiological agents in acute maxillary sinusitis. Rhinology 1987;25(1):49–55
7. Kaiser L, Morabia A, Stalder H, et al. Role of nasopharyngeal culture in antibiotic prescription for patients with common cold or acute sinusitis. Eur J Clin Microbiol Infect Dis 2001;20(7):445–451
8. Poole MD. A mathematical therapeutic outcomes model for sinusitis. Otolaryngol Head Neck Surg 2004;130(1, Suppl)46–50
9. Brown EM, Nathwani D. Antibiotic cycling or rotation: a systematic review of the evidence of efficacy. J Antimicrob Chemother 2005;55(1):6–9
10. National Nosocomial Infections Surveillance System. National Nosocomial Infections Surveillance (NNIS) System Report, data summary from January 1992 through June 2004, issued October 2004. Am J Infect Control 2004;32(8):470–485
11. Ferguson BJ, Stolz DB. Demonstration of biofilm in human bacterial chronic rhinosinusitis. Am J Rhinol 2005;19(5):452–457
12. Bernstein JM, Ballow M, Schlievert PM, Rich G, Allen C, Dryja D. A superantigen hypothesis for the pathogenesis of chronic hyperplastic sinusitis with massive nasal polyposis. Am J Rhinol 2003;17(6):321–326
13. Solares CA, Batra PS, Hall GS, Citardi MJ. Treatment of chronic rhinosinusitis exacerbations due to methicillin-resistant Staphylococcus aureus with mupirocin irrigations. Am J Otolaryngol 2006;27(3):161–165
14. Brook I. Acute and chronic bacterial sinusitis. Infect Dis Clin North Am 2007;21(2):427–448
15. Legent F, Bordure P, Beauvillain C, Berche P. A double-blind comparison of ciprofloxacin and amoxycillin/clavulanic acid in the treatment of chronic sinusitis. Chemotherapy 1994;40(Suppl 1):8–15
16. Subramanian HN, Schechtman KB, Hamilos DL. A retrospective analysis of treatment outcomes and time to relapse after intensive medical treatment for chronic sinusitis. Am J Rhinol 2002;16(6):303–312
17. Ragab SM, Lund VJ, Scadding G. Evaluation of the medical and surgical treatment of chronic rhinosinusitis: a prospective, randomised, controlled trial. Laryngoscope 2004;114(5):923–930
18. Gross ND, McInnes RJ, Hwang PH. Outpatient intravenous antibiotics for chronic rhinosinusitis. Laryngoscope 2002;112(10):1758–1761
19. Don DM, Yellon RF, Casselbrant ML, Bluestone CD. Efficacy of a stepwise protocol that includes intravenous antibiotic therapy for the management of chronic sinusitis in children and adolescents. Arch Otolaryngol Head Neck Surg 2001;127(9):1093–1098
20. Fowler KC, Duncavage JA, Murray JJ, Tanner S. Chronic sinusitis and intravenous antibiotic therapy: resolution, recurrence, and adverse events. J Allergy Clin Immunol 2003;111:s85

21. Rosenfeld M, Gibson R, McNamara S, et al. Serum and lower respiratory tract drug concentrations after tobramycin inhalation in young children with cystic fibrosis. J Pediatr 2001;139(4):572–577
22. Leonard DW, Bolger WE. Topical antibiotic therapy for recalcitrant sinusitis. Laryngoscope 1999;109(4):668–670
23. Moss RB, King VV. Management of sinusitis in cystic fibrosis by endoscopic surgery and serial antimicrobial lavage. Reduction in recurrence requiring surgery. Arch Otolaryngol Head Neck Surg 1995;121(5):566–572
24. Vaughan WC, Carvalho G. Use of nebulized antibiotics for acute infections in chronic sinusitis. Otolaryngol Head Neck Surg 2002;127(6):558–568
25. Ha KR, Psaltis AJ, Butcher AR, Wormald PJ, Tan LW. In vitro activity of mupirocin on clinical isolates of Staphylococcus aureus and its potential implications in chronic rhinosinusitis. Laryngoscope 2008;118(3):535–540
26. Baumann A, Zimmerli S, Hausler R, Caversaccio M. Invasive sphenoidal aspergillosis: successful treatment with sphenoidotomy and voriconazole. ORL J Otorhinolaryngol Relat Spec 2007;69(2):121–126
27. Notheis G, Tarani L, Costantino F, et al. Posaconazole for treatment of refractory invasive fungal disease. Mycoses 2006;49 (Suppl 1):37–41
28. Kennedy DW, Kuhn FA, Hamilos DL, et al. Treatment of chronic rhinosinusitis with high-dose oral terbinafine: a double blind, placebo-controlled study. Laryngoscope 2005;115(10): 1793–1799
29. Stevens DA, Schwartz HJ, Lee JY, et al. A randomized trial of itraconazole in allergic bronchopulmonary aspergillosis. N Engl J Med 2000;342(11):756–762
30. Ricchetti A, Landis BN, Maffioli A, Giger R, Zeng C, Lacroix JS. Effect of anti-fungal nasal lavage with amphotericin B on nasal polyposis. J Laryngol Otol 2002;116(4):261–263
31. Ponikau JU, Sherris DA, Weaver A, Kita H. Treatment of chronic rhinosinusitis with intranasal amphotericin B: a randomized, placebo-controlled, double-blind pilot trial. J Allergy Clin Immunol 2005;115(1):125–131
32. Ebbens FA, Scadding GK, Badia L, et al. Amphotericin B nasal lavages: not a solution for patients with chronic rhinosinusitis. J Allergy Clin Immunol 2006;118(5):1149–1156

18 Medical Therapies for Rhinosinusitis: Anti-Inflammatory

Rajiv K. Bhalla and Erin D. Wright

Inflammation is inherent in the very definition and is the sine qua non of rhinosinusitis. As a result, anti-inflammation is thought by most to be the primary target of therapies of this disease, particularly in chronic rhinosinusitis. This chapter discusses techniques that the authors find useful in their daily practice as a means of either reducing or controlling inflammation of the nasal and sinus mucosa. Not only do we emphasize the importance of anti-inflammatory therapy as the sole or primary treatment modality for sinusitis, but also the perioperative and postoperative care that we believe enhances disease control for which surgical therapy is undertaken. In addition, the definition of medical therapy used in this chapter implies more than simply pharmacotherapy, and discusses anti-inflammation on a broader scope.

Mucosal Inflammation and Mucociliary Function in Chronic Rhinosinusitis

In this chapter the discussion of anti-inflammation centers primarily on the management of chronic rhinosinusitis (CRS) and CRS with polyposis (CRSwP). CRS is an inflammatory disease of the sinonasal tract that is of multifactorial etiology and complex classification. However, the process can be generally summarized to involve a complex, overlapping, and often redundant cascade of inflammatory mediators including, but not limited, to a variety of inflammatory cells, cytokines, chemokines, arachidonic acid metabolites, and a variety of proteins released by eosinophils.[1] The eosinophil and eosinophilia of the tissues are considered by many to be key common denominators to sinonasal inflammation.

Sinonasal inflammation generally results in a radiologically and endoscopically detectable hypertrophy of the sinonasal mucosa with associated tissue congestion and edema, excess mucus production, and increased mucus viscosity, all of which will lead to impaired mucociliary clearance. The phenotypic or physical manifestation of this chronic inflammatory response often includes epithelial hyperplasia and subepithelial fibrosis, a process often termed remodeling when well entrenched. Reversal of this complex process is the primary goal of most therapies for CRS and, with diligent therapy targeting inflammation, the chronic histologic and morphologic changes associated with impaired mucociliary function can be reversed.[2]

It is clear, therefore, that CRS is a complex disease with multiple proposed etiologies. Significant progress has been made with respect to our understanding of the molecular and immunopathologic mechanisms that underlie this disease, the common denominator of which is an intense, perpetuated inflammatory process. This drives the formation of polyps and hyperplastic mucosa. It is this inflammatory process that is also the target of virtually all forms of therapy currently available to clinicians involved in the treatment of patients with CRS. Paramount among the therapeutic options in CRS is corticosteroids (steroidal anti-inflammatory agents). Prior to a broader presentation of anti-inflammatory therapies, we present an overview of corticosteroids, including mechanism of action and deleterious effects.

Corticosteroids and Mechanism of Action in Sinonasal Disease

Historical Perspective

The first partial synthesis of cortisone was the culmination of a worldwide chemical effort toward the end of the 1940s. This concluded in a 37-step conversion of deoxycholic acid to cortisone at the Merck Laboratories. The first systemic application of cortisone was in 1948, when Hench and his coworkers treated patients with severe rheumatoid arthritis at the Mayo Clinic.[3] Scientists from the United States, Mexico, and Europe collaborated to discover new synthetic routes to cortisone and to cortisol, the active hormone. This work continued in an intensive effort to discover analogues of cortisol with an improved therapeutic index, but with fewer of the systemic side effects. Hence the discovery of prednisone, prednisolone, and betamethasone at the Schering Corporation (Bloomfield, NJ) in the early 1950s, all of which combined high levels of anti-inflammatory activity with reduced salt retention.[4]

Unfortunately, the systemic side effects of oral corticosteroids made them less than optimal agents when used for the long-term management of airway disease. A major advance in therapy occurred with the introduction of beclomethasone dipropionate (BDP). This was the first corticosteroid found to be of clinical use when delivered by aerosol. Although BDP and subsequent topical corticosteroids have been found to possess increased intrinsic potency when delivered by aerosol, they have considerably lower systemic effects than corticosteroids such as hydrocortisone and dexamethasone when administered similarly. This is a result of the rapid first-pass metabolism in the liver of the swallowed fraction of drug. The remaining systemic effects of topical corticosteroids occur as a consequence of absorption of the unmetabolized drug through the sinonasal vasculature. That corticosteroids can be delivered intranasally by a variety of means, including sprays and drops, facilitates their use and reduces the risk of systemic side effects (especially if used in low doses and for short periods of time). Topical treatment favors improved patient compliance; however, it is worth noting that the topical preparations may still produce unfavorable local side effects.[5,6]

The Cellular Action of Corticosteroids

The mode of action of glucocorticoids in suppressing inflammation in CRS is not completely understood, but is thought to occur because glucocorticoids suppress the many inflammatory genes that are activated in chronic inflammatory disease. Glucocorticoids act by reversing histone acetylation of activated inflammatory genes by two mechanisms: through binding of liganded glucocorticoid receptors to coactivator molecules and through recruitment of histone deacetylase-2 to the activated transcription complex.[7]

Activated glucocorticoid receptors also bind to recognition sites in the promoters of certain genes to activate their transcription. This results in the secretion of anti-inflammatory proteins, such as mitogen-activated protein kinase phosphatase-1, which inhibits mitogen-activated protein kinase signaling pathways.[8]

Overall, corticosteroids also help to reduce sinonasal mucosal edema and thickening. The late response to allergen exposure is prevented by an inhibitory action on monocytes and granulocytes. Corticosteroids also inhibit the presentation of antigens by macrophages to lymphocytes, lymphocyte proliferation, activation and differentiation, and cytokine production and action.[9] Virtually all species of lymphocytes appear to be sensitive to these inhibitory effects, including the T-lymphocyte subsets that appear to be predominant in CRS. Corticosteroids are also potent inhibitors of eosinophils and have been used clinically to treat a variety of related chronic inflammatory disorders associated with eosinophilia including asthma, Churg-Strauss syndrome, hypereosinophilic syndrome, and chronic eosinophilic pneumonia.

The Mechanisms by Which Intranasal Corticosteroids Produce Systemic Activity

The systemic bioavailability of intranasal steroids (INSs), and thus systemic activity, is a consequence of direct absorption from the mucosa of the nose and sinuses, where there is no first-pass metabolism. The availability of more potent and lipophilic corticosteroids necessitates a continuous reevaluation of safety issues and, in particular, systemic adverse effects. The systemic bioavailability of INS is greatly influenced by the pharmacokinetic profile. Highly lipophilic drugs, such as fluticasone propionate or mometasone furoate, are preferentially partitioned into the systemic tissue compartment. Consequently, there is a large volume of distribution at a steady state. On the contrary, drugs with lower lipophilicity, such as triamcinolone acetonide or budesonide, have a smaller volume of distribution. The implication of this is that the systemic tissue compartment may act as a slow release reservoir, which results in a longer elimination half-life for the lipophilic drugs. The systemic complications of INSs are extensively studied and well documented in the literature[10] and will be discussed further, along with the complications of systemic therapy.

Deleterious Effects of Corticosteroids

For all their many uses and potentially lifesaving effects, few drugs inspire more trepidation than corticosteroids, and justifiably so. The list of potential corticosteroid-related side effects is long and concerning (**Table 18.1**). In the treatment of CRS, there are two general forms of corticosteroid therapy, topical and systemic, which are both discussed in the context of some of the more relevant or common side effects.

In the context of short-duration therapy, the side effect profile of topical nasal steroids is more favorable than oral/systemic therapy. Topical INS use is generally well tolerated but may be associated with epistaxis, headache, or localized nasal/throat irritation. For oral steroid therapy, the short-term side effects of greatest relevance are gastric irritation, fluid retention, increased appetite, hyperglycemia, insomia, and psychiatric disturbances. Psychiatric side effects may range from increased irritability to, rarely, frank psychosis. These side effects are all, fortunately, reversible with cessation of the therapy.

Table 18.1 Systemic Side Effects of Corticosteroid Therapy

- Cushing syndrome
- Weight gain
- Truncal obesity
- Hypertension
- Disfiguring skin lesions
- Diabetes mellitus
- Immunosuppression, leading to an increased susceptibility to infections
- Opportunistic infections
- Myopathy
- Osteoporosis
- Peptic ulcer disease
- Hyperlipoproteinemia
- Atherosclerosis
- Mood and mental changes
- Pancreatitis
- Osteonecrosis
- Cataracts
- Adrenal suppression
- Easy bruising

Avascular necrosis of the hip is one of the classic, acute, and catastrophic consequences of oral corticosteroid use, most commonly at higher doses.[11] Unlike osteoporosis, which only develops after at least 3 months of continuous therapy, osteonecrosis has been observed as early as 7 days after an initiation of steroid therapy, albeit only very rarely and generally only with higher doses. Moreover, steroid-induced osteonecrosis may involve both hips and several other joints as well, with involvement particularly in the femoral heads and condyles, the humeral heads, and the tali. To date, there are no data on the risk of osteonecrosis with INS.

Despite the general association between systemic corticosteroid use and impaired wound healing, few studies have addressed the potential effects of systemic corticosteroids on wound healing in endoscopic sinus surgery (ESS). One recent randomized clinical study where patients were treated post-ESS with mometasone furoate topical nasal steroid for 6 months demonstrated a nonstatistically significant trend toward improved wound healing as measured endoscopically.[12] As illustrated by this finding, there are theoretical advantages to some impairment in wound healing with respect to the common dilemma of synechiae formation post-ESS.

Immunosuppression with oral steroid therapy is a well documented and often intentional effect. In general, lower doses of corticosteroids do not appear to increase systemic infection risk, and the short-term use of these medications in an otherwise immunocompetent individual does not appear to be a risky maneuver. Even if the corticosteroids are unlikely to precipitate systemic or peripheral infections, the risk of local infection and its effect on clinical outcomes cannot be completely ignored. However, the potential for negative effects on local infections are offset by the favorable impact of the anti-inflammatory effect on resolution of sinusitis. In contrast to oral corticosteroid therapy, INSs are likely to have a negligible risk of immune suppression.

The suppression of hypothalamic-pituitary-adrenal (HPA) function after prolonged oral corticosteroid therapy is well documented. However, clinically significant suppression of the HPA axis with INS is unlikely to occur.[13] Nevertheless, high doses of INS delivered over long periods of time have the theoretical potential to cause clinically important suppression, manifesting as an abnormal response to physiological stress. With many INSs, the associated reduction in oral corticosteroid use is accompanied by recovery of the HPA axis function. Nonetheless, to diminish the risk of clinically significant HPA suppression, it is probably prudent that the dose of INS is titrated to the lowest dose needed to maintain effective control of CRS.

Clearly, systemic steroids have significant advantages in many disease states, including CRS, but this is counterbalanced by the not insignificant potential side effects. Systemic corticosteroids should only be used in situations where the indications are solid, the evidence for their efficacy is accepted if not proven, and the medical comorbidities are taken into account. From the perspective of INS, it can safely be said that aside from the local irritative effects of the aqueous delivery systems in the anterior portion of the nose, systemic side effects are negligible or unproven even with long-term use. In addition, diligent use of INS can be viewed as enhancing the safety of CRS therapy by limiting the need for oral corticosteroid use.

Management of Sinonasal Inflammation

Most patients with CRS respond to one or a combination of treatments that may include antihistamines, nasal decongestants, antibiotics, and corticosteroids. Of the medical anti-inflammatory therapies, antibiotics and corticosteroids have warranted the greatest research interest, and are elaborated on in the following discussion. This discussion not only focuses on anti-inflammation as a primary modality for therapy but also on the value of these therapies in the perioperative and postoperative time frames, recognizing that, generally, ESS is reserved for patients with CRS, with or without nasal polyposis, who are refractory to maximal medical management.

Included in tabular form are specific therapies targeted at inflammation in CRS including: details of therapy, the specific reference that supports the therapy, as well as the level of evidence in the reference (**Table 18.2**). It is worth reiterating, as outlined in this chapter and others, that CRS is a complex disease and that therapeutic options will be selected by the clinician in such a way as to address the underlying etiology or disease process of an individual patient against the severity of the disease and the potential side effects of the therapy.

Nonsteroidal Pharmacologic Therapy

After educating the patient regarding the extrinsic causes of rhinosinusitis and on the avoidance of allergens/irritants, the clinician should recommend pharmacological medications to control persistent daytime and nighttime symptoms. The aim of pharmacological intervention is to promptly alleviate symptoms and to optimize nasal airflow.

Currently, nonsteroid pharmacological therapy is most appropriate where an allergic/nonallergic rhinitis contribution for CRS is suspected. This usually entails therapy with cromoglycate, topical or systemic antihistamines, or ipratropium bromide. Decongestants, whether topical or systemic, are advocated only during the acute phase (first 3 to 4 days) of a viral or bacterial illness, where they may provide a role in reducing mucosal edema and enabling the sinuses to drain.

Antibiotics for Anti-Inflammation

From the perspective of anti-inflammation, antibiotics have been thought to play two potential roles. The first is in the context of acute infectious exacerbation (or perpetuation) of seemingly inflammatory CRS. In this context, endoscopically guided cultures and culture-directed antibiotics are

Table 18.2 Evidence-based Recommendations for Primary Disease Therapy in Chronic Rhinosinusitis

Therapy	Goal/Effect	Dosing Regimen	Reference	Evidence Level
Topical intranasal steroid	Reduce edema, congestion, and discharge; encourage drainage of secretions along natural pathways; enhance nasal airflow	1 to 2 puffs each nostril, once or twice daily, for at least 4 uninterrupted weeks	Fokkens et al.[40]	Ib
Systemic steroid	Reduce proinflammatory cytokines in the sinonasal mucosa of patients with chronic rhinosinusitis; reduce edema and congestion	Prednisone 0.5 mg/kg by mouth every day, tapered over 10 days	Lennard et al.[41]	III
Saline irrigation	Reduce inflammation and thin secretions; pH restoration; humidification	Normal/isotonic saline 60 mL each nostril BID	Taccariello et al.[42] Lund[43]	III
Macrolide antibiotic	Anti-inflammatory effect on sinonasal mucosa	Erythromycin 500 mg twice a day by mouth for 2 weeks, followed by 250 mg BID for 10 weeks Clarithromycin 400 mg every day for 8 to 12 weeks	Ragab et al.[15] Hashiba and Baba[44]	Ib III
Selective sinus medication	Selective treatment of congested and/or infected mucosa and edema within individual sinuses	Budesonide 256 μg every day for 3 weeks, administered via selective intubation of maxillary or ethmoid sinuses	Lavigne et al.[34]	IV
Mucolytic	Reduce viscosity of thick, tenacious secretions to encourage drainage from sinuses	Guaifenesin 2400 mg by mouth every day for 3 weeks	Szmeja et al.[45]	III

Abbreviations: BID, twice a day.

appropriate and can be viewed as reducing the acute exacerbation of the chronic inflammatory response.

Perhaps the most interesting and novel evidence supporting the benefit of antibiotics involved a study of mucociliary clearance in patients treated with antibiotics for CRS.[14] In this study, 10 patients with CRS underwent nasal brushings for the assessment of ciliary beat frequency and then received 3 months of continuous oral antibiotic therapy, after which repeat nasal brushings demonstrated increased ciliary beat frequencies in all patients. The authors concluded that depression of mucociliary clearance was a result of chronic sinonasal infection and that prolonged antibiotic use helped to restore mucociliary function.

Although antibiotics are generally thought to be of benefit through their antimicrobial properties, considerable work has examined the anti-inflammatory/immunomodulatory effects of the macrolides, an effect that may be more important in CRS than the antimicrobial effect. Clarithromycin, in particular, possesses immunosuppressive effects, including in vitro reduction in the cellular production of transforming growth factor-β, nuclear factor κ-β, and of interleukin (IL)-5, IL-8, and granulocyte-macrophage colony-stimulating factor. This has led some authors to routinely prescribe macrolide therapy in their medical management prior to considering a patient as a candidate for ESS.[15] Because the anti-inflammatory effects of macrolides are manifest at doses below what is normally prescribed for bacterial infection, low-dose macrolide therapy has been described for CRS. Typically, half-dosing clarithromycin, erythromycin, or roxithromycin can be considered with an assessment of response after 90 days of treatment. Given concerns around microbial resistance, the routine use of antibiotic therapy for the purposes of anti-inflammation in the primary management of CRS remains justifiably controversial, especially when considering long-term, low-dose regimens.

Saline Irrigations

The value of topical saline irrigations cannot be overstated in the context of reducing inflammation and optimizing mucociliary function. These may be isotonic, hypertonic, nonbuffered, or buffered. Mucociliary function is enhanced due to the beneficial effects of humidification, pH restoration, and the thinning of secretions. There will likely be an improvement in symptoms of rhinosinusitis and, quite possibly, a reduction in the use of medication in those individuals that use a saline irrigation compliantly and on a regular basis.[16] Hypertonicity and buffering do not appear to confer any additional benefit with regard to the symptoms of rhinosinusitis, although marginal improvements in mucociliary function may be observed.

Intranasal Corticosteroids

The evidence that topical corticosteroids have a beneficial effect in CRS and nasal polyposis is quite compelling. Eosinophilia, CD3, CD4, and CD8 T lymphocytes are significantly reduced in treated mucosa. Subsequently, the benefit of various preparations of topical corticosteroids for CRS and nasal polyposis—such as betamethasone sodium phosphate nose drops and beclomethasone dipropionate, fluticasone propionate, and budesonide nasal sprays—has been demonstrated in several randomized, placebo-controlled trials.[17] Steroid may effectively be delivered in a droplet preparation, more commonly as a spray of aerosolized medication, or, as is increasingly the case, especially in cases of refractory CRS, as part of a saline irrigation.[18]

In examining the different delivery methods, there are several factors worth considering. The first is the effectiveness of the delivery method. It has been shown in two recent, well conducted studies that the penetration of nebulized or irrigated medication into nonoperated paranasal sinuses is limited at best. Even after surgery, penetration of the sprays and nebulizers was limited.[19,20] A second, perhaps more important factor to consider is the actual evidence for these delivery methods in terms of clinical efficacy as primary therapy. In fact, the limited evidence available is not strongly supportive of the efficacy of nasal sprays, showing nonsignificant trends with small population sizes.[21,22]

The liquid formulations are associated with a higher topical dose of corticosteroid and remain the one delivery method that has been scientifically demonstrated to be effective in primary therapeutic use.[23,24] These steroid drop formulations are generally of use in situations where inflammatory disease is to be brought under control rapidly or to avoid the need for surgery[24]; however, they are not available in all areas (e.g., North America) but are available in many parts of Europe. The spray formulations may be more appropriate for the maintenance of disease control and the treatment of rhinitis symptoms, and the dosing regimen can be tailored to the individual requirements.

The past few years have seen the emerging popularity of off-label liquid steroid delivery into the nose by using saline irrigations as the delivery vehicle for a concentrated form of topical steroid. The use of budesonide ampules dissolved in normal saline is commonly used in Canada and now more so in the United States and United Kingdom. However, the only scientific studies to date are small series that have looked at side effect profiles,[18,25] although one of these studies had as a secondary objective: the measurement of subjective outcomes. In this small series, there was a small but significant improvement in Sino-Nasal Outcome Test (SNOT)-20 scores.[26]

Despite some evidence that topical corticosteroids have efficacy in the primary medical management of rhinosinusitis, only recently have investigators examined the potential benefit of INS postoperatively.[27] The investigators concluded that there was no significant beneficial effect of topical steroids in patients who have undergone ESS and this is, again, evidence to support the contention that topical steroid sprays, despite their widespread use, have not been proven terribly effective in treating CRS.

Systemic Corticosteroids

The impact of oral corticosteroids at alleviating symptoms of rhinosinusitis is undeniable, with significant symptomatic improvement in all but a small subset of patients. However, the large majority of reported complications of corticosteroid use are attributable to their systemic use, either at high doses or for prolonged periods of time. Retardation of growth in children, osteoporosis, HPA axis suppression, altered glucose metabolism, and fluid retention are among some of the major side effects of systemic steroid therapy. As clinicians, we are also aware that the benefit that systemic steroids provide in CRS, and particularly CRSwP, is often short-lived unless longer term therapy is used. In patients with severe CRSwP, oral steroid therapy will often postpone but will generally not avoid the need for surgery combined with intensive, diligent postoperative medical therapy. Where oral corticosteroids may be more useful, however, is in the preoperative preparation of patients[28] or in a situation where significant congestive or obstructive symptoms warrant amelioration while awaiting more definitive therapy.

Leukotriene Inhibitors

Cysteinyl-leukotrienes are potent endogenous mediators of inflammation. They have a significant role in contributing to airway inflammation due to their effects of stimulating mucosal edema, mucus hypersecretion, neutrophil-endothelial interactions, ingress of eosinophils, and dendritic cell maturation—a prerequisite for future allergic response. Leukotriene inhibitors block type-1 cysteinyl-leukotriene receptors in the smooth muscle and endothelium of respiratory mucosa and in those found on immunocytes. Consequently, leukotriene-receptor antagonists may offer a useful adjunct in the management of rhinosinusitis with a strong allergic pathoetiology. Their efficacy in reducing the symptoms of allergic rhinosinusitis appears to lie somewhere between systemic antihistamines and topical INS. They may also enhance the efficacy of antihistamines when used as combination therapy. Undoubtedly, those with asthma and allergic rhinosinusitis are most likely to benefit from the addition of a leukotriene inhibitor. However, they should not be given in preference to a topical INS, which is generally considered to furnish the most significant relief of adverse allergic symptoms.

Immunotherapy and Vaccination

Given that inflammation is paramount in the development and perpetuation of CRS and nasal polyposis, and that the benefits of corticosteroids in the treatment of both conditions is unquestionable, the role for alternative immunomodulating therapy has attracted greater interest. In patients suspected of having dysregulated interferon-gamma (IFN-γ) production, where the treatment of their CRS becomes resistant to the usual medical interventions, exogenous IFN-γ therapy (50 μg/m²) for longer than 3 months may offer enhanced symptom control.[29] Therefore, exogenous IFN-γ may be a therapeutic option in a subset of patients with treatment-resistant CRS and with evidence of dysregulated IFN-γ production.

Traditional immunotherapy has focused on desensitization, where increasing aliquots of purified allergen proteins are injected into sensitive individuals with the intention of modulating and reducing the severity of their allergic response over a period of time. The therapy is believed to exert its effects by the induction of blocking antibodies, the switching of T helper (Th)2 to a more Th1 allergen-specific immune response, and the induction of anergy, probably via the development of allergen-specific regulatory T cells. The vaccines themselves are now far better characterized and standardized, with new allergen forms and formulations being designed with these specific T-cell targets in mind. In addition, allergoids are being employed more frequently, which are allergens modified chemically to reduce allergenicity but to retain immunogenicity. More modern depot forms, such as those containing tyrosine or calcium phosphate, are replacing aqueous extracts and older depot adjuvants such as alum. T-cell reactive peptides and recombinant allergens or their muteins are also being studied as replacements for whole extracts and have shown some potential. Immunomodulators, such as monophosphoryl lipid A, designed with defined targets in mind, are now included in some vaccines and help to accelerate the process.[30] All these measures have led to a reduction in the need for the traditional long injection schedules.

More recently, tablet-based immunotherapy, delivered via a sublingual route, has become available. Its use is currently limited to the management of grass pollen and house dust mite allergies. Results, in terms of quality of life and cost-effectiveness, have shown promise. In recent years, anti-immunoglobulin (Ig)E antibody (omalizumab) has become a treatment option for atopic asthma, leading some clinicians to consider its applicability in the treatment of CRS.[31] Preliminary data are, however, limited, and the high cost and potential adverse side effects remain significant considerations. Future developments in novel allergic therapies (perhaps specifically targeting IL-5 secretion and staphylococcal superantigens) will undoubtedly complement the management of the atopic aspects of both acute and chronic rhinosinusitis, and airway disease in general.[32]

Selective Sinus Therapy

Traditional vehicles for the delivery of corticosteroids to the sinonasal mucosa are spray or drops. Alternative modalities of delivering the drug to individual sinuses have also been explored. Patients with an allergy to house dust mites and a prior history of ESS, but with persistent disabling symptoms of rhinorrhea or pressure, have had the affected sinus selectively medicated. Their management was otherwise resistant to oral antibiotics and intranasal corticosteroids. Under these circumstances, 256 μg of budesonide was administered daily through a maxillary antrum sinusotomy tube into one of the maxillary sinuses for 3 weeks. The intervention was found to be superior to placebo.[33] Selective irrigation of the sinuses with a solution containing antibiotics and corticosteroids has also shown potential, such as in refractory CRS associated with chronic purulence.[34]

Perioperative Corticosteroids in CRS and CRSwP

Perioperative corticosteroid therapy (systemic, topical, or both) in patients undergoing ESS was, until recently, believed by many to be important, although there was considerable variability in actual practice based on published data (**Table 18.3**).

Table 18.3 Evidence-based Recommendations for the Management of Perioperative Inflammation in Chronic Rhinosinusitis

Therapy	Goal/Effect	Dosing Regimen	Reference	Evidence Level
Topical intranasal steroid	Reduce edema, congestion, and discharge; encourage drainage of secretions along natural pathways; enhance nasal airflow	2 puffs each nostril twice a day, for at least 4 uninterrupted weeks	Fokkens et al.[40]	Ib
Saline irrigation	Reduce inflammation and thin secretions; pH restoration; humidification	Normal/isotonic saline 60 mL each nostril bid	Taccariello et al.[42] Lund[43]	III
Higher dose topical intranasal steroid	Beneficial in refractory and recurrent CRS, and polyposis; reduce edema, congestion, and discharge	Budesonide 1 mg in 240 mL normal saline—irrigate 60 mL in each nostril bid	Bhalla et al.[18]	IV
		Fluticasone propionate 200 μg each nostril once or twice daily	Aukema et al.[24]	Ib
Systemic steroid	Reduce mucosal inflammation and edema; improve operative field and surgical outcome	Prednisone 30 mg by mouth every day for 5 days prior to surgery followed by 9 days postoperatively	Wright and Agrawal[28]	Ib
Macrolide antibiotic	Anti-inflammatory effect on sinonasal mucosa	Erythromycin 500 mg twice a day by mouth for 2 weeks postoperatively	Ragab et al.[15]	Ib

Abbreviations: CRS, chronic rhinosinusitis.

The rationale for the use of corticosteroids in the preoperative period is to reduce inflammation in the operative field. Indeed, in a recent randomized, placebo-controlled study, systemic corticosteroids in the perioperative period have been shown to furnish benefit, both in terms of an improved surgical field and improved healing of sinus cavities in the short and medium term, presumably by stabilizing or reducing inflammation and impairing formation of synechiae while the cavities are healing.[28]

Drug-Eluting Nasal Dressings

In a logical follow-up to the study examining perioperative systemic steroids, a more prolonged and direct delivery of topical steroids in the immediate postoperative time frame was demonstrated to improve wound healing and objective surgical outcomes. Using a fragmentable nasal stent/dressing impregnated with triamcinolone, which was left in place for 1 week and subsequently debrided away, the authors identified significantly healthier cavities in the short and medium term[35] as evidenced by improved Lund-Kennedy and Perioperative Sinus Endoscopy (POSE) scores.[35]

A novel mometasone-eluting bioabsorbable stent designed to be placed in the ethmoid cavity has been recently approved for clinical use. In a pilot study, use of the device was associated with improved endoscopic inflammation scores versus placebo after ESS for CRS.[36] However, the device's efficacy in broader clinical practice remains to be seen.

Nonmedical Interventions as a Means of Anti-Inflammation

The Role of Endoscopic Sinus Surgery

Artificially divorcing surgical and medical therapies may not reflect the current approach to CRS, because ESS can also be considered a form of anti-inflammatory therapy. Although discussed in detail in other chapters, ESS is a technique that serves to remove chronically inflamed tissue and perhaps, just as importantly, bone, which can thus remove a source for ongoing inflammation.[37] In addition, ESS can serve to render medical anti-inflammatory therapy more effective both by reducing disease load and by providing better access for topical therapies.

In cases of recurrent disease, revision ESS can be a useful adjunct to medical therapy by debulking inflammatory tissue, removing an infective nidus, and clearing bony partitions and fragments left behind after earlier surgical intervention. In either case, the aim of surgical intervention should be the attainment of reventilated sinus cavities with a low volume of residual disease, which should be more accessible to topical anti-inflammatory medications (**Table 18.4**).

Debridement

Although many surgeons believe that routine postoperative care, including endoscopic debridement, optimizes surgical outcomes, the evidence is conflicting. However, studies dismissive of postoperative debridement have, in general, been poorly conducted with patients lost to follow-up. The general consensus appears to be that some perioperative management is indicated.

During the period of postoperative mucosal recovery and regeneration, the authors provide judicious care to the sinus cavities by removing retained secretions, devitalized soft tissue, and bone under endoscopic guidance. We request of the patient a similar level of devotion with regard to regular and compliant, gentle sinonasal lavage using isotonic saline. Topical steroid therapy in the postoperative period is unproven to furnish any additional benefit in the healing cascade. However, where we find that cavities are very inflamed following surgery, the use of topical INS dissolved in saline and used as an irrigation, particularly at a higher dose, may provide a useful adjunct in the postoperative management of these patients.[17]

Table 18.4 Evidence-based Recommendations for the Management of Recurrent or Refractory Chronic Rhinosinusitis

Therapy	Goal/Effect	Dosing Regimen	Reference	Evidence Level
Saline irrigation	Reduce inflammation and thin secretions; pH restoration; humidification	Normal/isotonic saline 60 mL each nostril BID	Taccariello et al.[42] Lund[43]	III
Topical intranasal steroid	Reduce edema, congestion, and discharge; encourage drainage of secretions along natural pathways; enhance nasal airflow	2 puffs each nostril BID for at least 4 uninterrupted weeks	Dijkstra et al.[27]	Ib (negative)
Higher dose topical intranasal steroid	Reduce edema, congestion, and discharge; encourage drainage of secretions along natural pathways; enhance nasal airflow	Budesonide 1 mg in 240 mL normal saline—irrigate 60 mL in each nostril BID	Bhalla et al.[18]	IV
		Fluticasone propionate 200 μg each nostril once or twice daily	Aukema et al.[24]	Ib
Selective sinus medication	Selective treatment of congested and/or infected mucosa and edema within maxillary sinuses	Budesonide 256 μg every day for 3 weeks, administered through a maxillary antrum sinusotomy tube	Lavigne et al.[34]	Ib

Abbreviations: BID, twice a day.

Future Developments

Postsurgical dressing of the sinonasal cavity has now been demonstrated as an effective method for anti-inflammatory therapy.[35] Recent years have seen increasing use of biocompatible materials such as hyaluronic acid and rapidly degradable oxidized cellulose products.[38] Future developments, which may not be long off, are likely to include bioengineered dressings and stents that are impregnated with medications delivered locally such as steroids, antibiotics, or more targeted agents of anti-inflammation, or those that promote optimal wound healing.[39]

The Importance of the Care Pathway

At the outset of this chapter, it was our stated goal to discuss the current modalities available for the purposes of medical anti-inflammation of the mucosa of the nose and paranasal sinuses. In doing so, we have touched upon the importance of primary medical therapy, as well as perioperative and postsurgical anti-inflammatory therapies to optimize the outcomes in patients with CRS and CRSwP (**Fig. 18.1**).

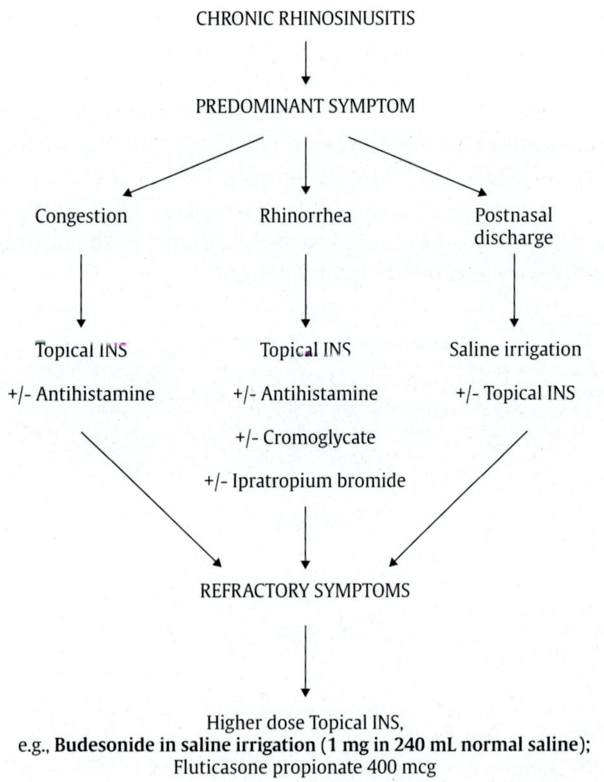

Fig. 18.1 A systematic, symptom-based approach to the management of sinonasal inflammation. *INS*, intranasal steroid.

We believe that the patient with CRS requires an investment of not only expertise, but also of time and effort, and a similar level of commitment on the part of the individual patient. Successful control of symptoms begins with an accurate and early diagnosis, followed by a prompt initiation of therapy at a dose that is likely to control adverse symptoms. Doses can ultimately be titrated to the level of response, always with the option of increasing them for short periods of time until symptom control is achieved. In the perioperative period, systemic steroids enhance the visual field during surgery and, ultimately, the quality of the surgical outcome. In the postoperative period, meticulous care of the sinus cavities combined with the anti-inflammatory interventions alluded to previously will promote early epithelialization, minimal troublesome scarring, and the restoration of mucociliary functions.

Careful consideration of the patient, the disease, and its supervision is an ongoing process that necessitates re-evaluation at all stages of the care pathway if successful results are to be achieved and maintained in the management of CRS.

Conclusion

CRS and CRSwP are complex morbidities that have a detrimental bearing on quality of life and, although not life-threatening, place a huge burden on our health care economies. This chapter reaffirms the eosinophil as the important exponent and catalyst for inflammation in the sinonasal tract and lower airways, and although corticosteroids remain the mainstay of treatment, in an effort to reduce steroid-related systemic side effects, more novel delivery modalities are being extensively explored. The aims of effective anti-inflammatory therapy remain the relief of adverse symptoms and the prevention of long-term mucosal and submucosal changes, such as remodeling. Central to disease control using pharmacotherapy is patient compliance, and it is essential that specialists educate not only sufferers on the potential benefits of compliant self-medication, but also primary care physicians on optimum dosing, delivery methods, characteristics, and safety of new drugs or formulations, advances in surgical management, and maintenance of therapy over a long period of time. It is unreasonable to ask our patients to use medication compliantly that requires multiple, inconvenient, daily doses of a foul-tasting and ineffective medication that produces troublesome side effects simply because it is the cheapest option. The advancement of medical anti-inflammation possibly depends on more potent but highly selective pharmacotherapy, such as antihistamines, antieosinophils, and highly selective oral immunotherapy. The authors have also subtly emphasized the necessary skill with the endoscope, particularly angled endoscopes, which is invaluable and perhaps essential in the management of sinonasal inflammation. This has an obvious implication for training, where it is critical that our specialists of the future be familiarized with the technical nuances and benefits of the angled endoscope, particularly in the outpatient setting. Ultimately, endoscopic surgical management is a necessary adjunct to topical anti-inflammation due to otherwise poor penetration of agents into unoperated sinus chambers and also its role in the reduction of disease burden. Thus, this chapter accentuates anti-inflammation in sinonasal disease as an important concept in the overall management of CRS and CRSwP, and perhaps the area in which the most intensive research is ongoing and necessary to ensure satisfactory outcomes and long-term results.

References

1. Szucs E, Ravandi S, Goossens A, Beel M, Clement PA. Eosinophilia in the ethmoid mucosa and its relationship to the severity of inflammation in chronic rhinosinusitis. Am J Rhinol 2002; 16(3):131–134
2. Chen B, Antunes MB, Claire SE, et al. Reversal of chronic rhinosinusitis-associated sinonasal ciliary dysfunction. Am J Rhinol 2007;21(3):346–353
3. Lundberg IE, Grundtman C, Larsson E, Klareskog L. Corticosteroids—from an idea to clinical use. Best Pract Res Clin Rheumatol 2004;18(1):7–19
4. Herzog H, Oliveto EP. A history of significant steroid discoveries and developments originating at the Schering Corporation (USA) since 1948. Steroids 1992;57(12):617–623
5. Bhalla RK, Jones AS, Roland NJ. Prevalence of pharyngeal and laryngeal complications in adult asthmatics using inhaled corticosteroids. J Laryngol Otol 2008;122(10):1078–1083
6. Bhalla RK, Watson G, Taylor W, Jones AS, Roland NJ. Acoustic analysis in asthmatics and the influence of inhaled corticosteroid therapy. J Voice 2009;23(4):505–511
7. Barnes PJ. Mechanisms and resistance in glucocorticoid control of inflammation. J Steroid Biochem Mol Biol 2010;120(2-3): 76–85
8. Barnes PJ. Corticosteroid effects on cell signalling. Eur Respir J 2006;27(2):413–426
9. Boumpas DT, Chrousos GP, Wilder RL, Cupps TR, Balow JE. Glucocorticoid therapy for immune-mediated diseases: basic and clinical correlates. Ann Intern Med 1993;119(12):1198–1208
10. Blaiss MS. Safety considerations of intranasal corticosteroids for the treatment of allergic rhinitis. Allergy Asthma Proc 2007; 28(2):145–152
11. Mirzai R, Chang C, Greenspan A, Gershwin ME. The pathogenesis of osteonecrosis and the relationships to corticosteroids. J Asthma 1999;36(1):77–95
12. Jorissen M, Bachert C. Effect of corticosteroids on wound healing after endoscopic sinus surgery. Rhinology 2009;47(3):280–28
13. Wilson AM, Sims EJ, McFarlane LC, Lipworth BJ. Effects of intranasal corticosteroids on adrenal, bone, and blood markers of systemic activity in allergic rhinitis. J Allergy Clin Immunol 1998;102(4 Pt 1):598–604
14. Scadding GK, Lund VJ, Darby YC. The effect of long-term antibiotic therapy upon ciliary beat frequency in chronic rhinosinusitis. J Laryngol Otol 1995;109(1):24–26
15. Ragab SM, Lund VJ, Scadding G. Evaluation of the medical and surgical treatment of chronic rhinosinusitis: a prospective, randomised, controlled trial. Laryngoscope 2004;114(5):923–930
16. Papsin B, McTavish A. Saline nasal irrigation: Its role as an adjunct treatment. Can Fam Physician 2003;49:168–173
17. Badia L, Lund V. Topical corticosteroids in nasal polyposis. Drugs 2001;61(5):573–578
18. Bhalla RK, Payton K, Wright ED. Safety of budesonide in saline sinonasal irrigations in the management of chronic rhinosinusitis with polyposis: lack of significant adrenal suppression. J Otolaryngol Head Neck Surg 2008;37(6):821–825
19. Harvey RJ, Goddard JC, Wise SK, Schlosser RJ. Effects of endoscopic sinus surgery and delivery device on cadaver sinus irrigation. Otolaryngol Head Neck Surg 2008;139(1):137–142
20. Hwang PH, Woo RJ, Fong KJ. Intranasal deposition of nebulized saline: a radionuclide distribution study. Am J Rhinol 2006;20(3):255–261
21. Parikh A, Scadding GK, Darby Y, Baker RC. Topical corticosteroids in chronic rhinosinusitis: a randomized, double-blind, placebo-controlled trial using fluticasone propionate aqueous nasal spray. Rhinology 2001;39(2):75–79
22. Qvarnberg Y, Kantola O, Salo J, Toivanen M, Valtonen H, Vuori E. Influence of topical steroid treatment on maxillary sinusitis. Rhinology 1992;30(2):103–112
23. Keith P, Nieminen J, Hollingworth K, Dolovich J. Efficacy and tolerability of fluticasone propionate nasal drops 400 microgram once daily compared with placebo for the treatment of bilateral polyposis in adults. Clin Exp Allergy 2000;30(10):1460–1468
24. Aukema AA, Mulder PG, Fokkens WJ. Treatment of nasal polyposis and chronic rhinosinusitis with fluticasone propionate nasal drops reduces need for sinus surgery. J Allergy Clin Immunol 2005;115(5):1017–1023
25. Welch KC, Thaler ER, Doghramji LL, Palmer JN, Chiu AG. The effects of serum and urinary cortisol levels of topical intranasal irrigations with budesonide added to saline in patients with recurrent polyposis after endoscopic sinus surgery. Am J Rhinol Allergy 2010;24(1):26–28
26. Sachanandani NS, Piccirillo JF, Kramper MA, Thawley SE, Vlahiotis A. The effect of nasally administered budesonide respules on adrenal cortex function in patients with chronic rhinosinusitis. Arch Otolaryngol Head Neck Surg 2009;135(3):303–307
27. Dijkstra MD, Ebbens FA, Poublon RM, Fokkens WJ. Fluticasone propionate aqueous nasal spray does not influence the recurrence rate of chronic rhinosinusitis and nasal polyps 1 year after functional endoscopic sinus surgery. Clin Exp Allergy 2004;34(9): 1395–1400
28. Wright ED, Agrawal S. Impact of perioperative systemic steroids on surgical outcomes in patients with chronic rhinosinusitis with polyposis: evaluation with the novel Perioperative Sinus Endoscopy (POSE) scoring system. Laryngoscope 2007;117(11 Pt 2, Suppl 115)1–28
29. Jyonouchi H, Sun S, Kelly A, Rimell FL. Effects of exogenous interferon gamma on patients with treatment-resistant chronic rhinosinusitis and dysregulated interferon gamma production: a pilot study. Arch Otolaryngol Head Neck Surg 2003;129(5):563–569
30. Wheeler AW, Woroniecki SR. Allergy vaccines—new approaches to an old concept. Expert Opin Biol Ther 2004;4(9):1473–1481
31. Pinto JM, Mehta N, DiTineo M, Wang J, Baroody FM, Naclerio RM. A randomized, double-blind, placebo-controlled trial of anti-IgE for chronic rhinosinusitis. Rhinology 2010;48(3): 318–324
32. Bachert C, Claeys SE, Tomassen P, van Zele T, Zhang N. Rhinosinusitis and asthma: a link for asthma severity. Curr Allergy Asthma Rep 2010;10(3):194–201

33. Lavigne F, Cameron L, Renzi PM, et al. Intrasinus administration of topical budesonide to allergic patients with chronic rhinosinusitis following surgery. Laryngoscope 2002;112(5):858–864
34. Lavigne F, Tulic MK, Gagnon J, Hamid Q. Selective irrigation of the sinuses in the management of chronic rhinosinusitis refractory to medical therapy: a promising start. J Otolaryngol 2004;33(1):10–16
35. Côté DW, Wright ED. Triamcinolone-impregnated nasal dressing following endoscopic sinus surgery: a randomized, double-blind, placebo-controlled study. Laryngoscope 2010;120(6):1269–1273
36. Murr AH, Smith TL, Hwang PH, et al. Safety and efficacy of a novel bioabsorbable, steroid-eluting sinus stent. Int Forum Allergy Rhinol 2011;1:23–32
37. Khalid AN, Hunt J, Perloff JR, Kennedy DW. The role of bone in chronic rhinosinusitis. Laryngoscope 2002;112(11):1951–1957
38. Franklin JH, Wright ED. Randomized, controlled, study of absorbable nasal packing on outcomes of surgical treatment of rhinosinusitis with polyposis. Am J Rhinol 2007;21(2):214–217
39. Li PM, Downie D, Hwang PH. Controlled steroid delivery via bioabsorbable stent: safety and performance in a rabbit model. Am J Rhinol Allergy 2009;23(6):591–596
40. Fokkens W, Lund V, Bachert C, et al; EAACI. EAACI position paper on rhinosinusitis and nasal polyps executive summary. Allergy 2005;60(5):583–601
41. Lennard CM, Mann EA, Sun LL, Chang AS, Bolger WE. Interleukin-1 beta, interleukin-5, interleukin-6, interleukin-8, and tumor necrosis factor-alpha in chronic sinusitis: response to systemic corticosteroids. Am J Rhinol 2000;14(6): 367–373
42. Taccariello M, Parikh A, Darby Y, Scadding G. Nasal douching as a valuable adjunct in the management of chronic rhinosinusitis. Rhinology 1999;37(1):29–32
43. Lund VJ. Maximal medical therapy for chronic rhinosinusitis. Otolaryngol Clin North Am 2005;38(6):1301–1310, x
44. Hashiba M, Baba S. Efficacy of long-term administration of clarithromycin in the treatment of intractable chronic sinusitis. Acta Otolaryngol Suppl 1996;525:73–78
45. Szmeja Z, Golusiński W, Mielcarek-Kuchta D, Laczkowska-Przybylska J. Use of mucolytic preparations (Mucosolvan) in selected diseases of the upper respiratory tract. Part II. Otolaryngol Pol 1997;51(5):480–486

19 Management of Recalcitrant Chronic Rhinosinusitis Following Endoscopic Sinus Surgery

Nathan B. Sautter and Timothy L. Smith

Chronic rhinosinusitis (CRS) is a chronic sinonasal inflammatory mucosal disease that responds well to both medical and surgical management in the majority of patients. It is one of the most common chronic diseases in the US population, affecting up to 14% of the adult population. Patients with CRS who fail maximal medical therapy are candidates for endoscopic sinus surgery (ESS). Patients undergoing ESS should be counseled that surgery is not a panacea, and continued long-term medical therapy in the form of both topical and systemic anti-inflammatory and/or antimicrobial medications is likely necessary. Many otorhinolaryngologists, however, have encountered patients who continue to suffer from severe symptoms of CRS following appropriate ESS despite continued "standard" maximal medical therapy in the form of routine nasal saline irrigations, topical nasal steroids, leukotriene inhibitors, allergy therapy, and appropriate courses of systemic steroids and antibiotics, when indicated.[1] This subset of patients may relapse quickly with frequent exacerbations despite optimal ESS and optimal standard medical therapy. This relatively small, yet challenging, patient population poses a significant and often frustrating dilemma to the rhinologic surgeon. To date, there is no consensus regarding the optimal treatment of this subset of patients suffering from recalcitrant CRS.

CRS is widely accepted to be a multifactorial disease with no definitively proven single etiology. A common underlying factor in all cases of CRS, however, is chronic sinonasal mucosal inflammation. Several etiologies for chronic mucosal inflammation have been proposed, including chronic bacterial infection, allergy, immune dysregulation, biofilms, fungus, superantigen production, ciliary dysfunction, and immunoglobulin deficiency, among others. Therapies for CRS are directed at reducing sinonasal inflammation at various points along the inflammatory cascade while simultaneously eliminating or controlling the underlying source of the inflammation. Inflammation and edema of the sinonasal mucosa leads to ostial occlusion and subsequent hypoxia within the occluded sinus. This leads to goblet cell hyperplasia, increased mucus viscosity, and the accumulation of thick, sticky mucus within the sinus resulting from impaired mucociliary clearance. Mycostasis provides an opportunity for bacterial overgrowth and chronic bacterial infection within the sinonasal cavities, which summons further inflammation due to intrinsic host defense factors.

The ultimate goal of primary ESS is to optimize sinus drainage and ventilation by surgically enlarging the natural sinus ostia while simultaneously preserving a maximum amount of normal and healthy mucosa. Consequently, normal sinonasal mucociliary clearance resumes and is maintained in a majority of patients with CRS following ESS. An additional benefit following ESS is an improved delivery of topical therapies to the sinonasal mucosa. Some patients with CRS require revision ESS due to inadequate or incomplete initial surgery. However, even after optimal surgery resulting in a widely patent sinus ostia, a subset of patients continues to suffer from severe mucosal inflammation with associated symptoms of CRS. These symptoms are often debilitating and may impact significantly on the patient's quality of life. Common complaints in this patient population include thick nasal discharge, postnasal drainage, facial pain, pressure, and nasal congestion. Treatments should be tailored to the individual patient with a focus on his or her specific symptoms.

The purpose of this chapter is to review some of the common reasons or theories for refractory CRS following ESS. Subsequently, we provide methods to evaluate and manage patients with difficult to control sinonasal disease despite optimal ESS and standard medical therapies.

General Management of the Recalcitrant Chronic Rhinosinusitis Patient

The nose functions as a filter and the first line of defense against inspired pathogens and particulate matter. Often, the environment is a contributing factor to recalcitrant disease, and patients should be questioned regarding environmental or seasonal triggers. All patients with a history or presentation typical of allergic rhinitis should be counseled regarding environmental control, and allergen avoidance is indicated in all allergic patients, according to expert panel guidelines.[2–4] The home environment may be rid of dust, mold, and animal dander with the use of environmental control and avoidance measures.

The first randomized controlled trial demonstrating improvement in allergic symptoms following environmental control was published in 2007.[5] Asthmatic and allergic patients followed a home mold reduction protocol, which included removal of all visible mold and house cleaning with detergents and fungicides. Patients following the protocol experienced significant reductions in allergic symptoms and medication use. Other measures, such as removal of household plants, avoiding wet areas on the walls and floors, and appraisal for water damage may be helpful as well. High-efficiency particulate air (HEPA) filters, which are capable of filtering particulate matter larger than 0.3 µm, may be installed in the bedroom and living areas, although there is little evidence currently to support their use. Measures to reduce dust mite exposure include use of dust mite impermeable pillow and mattress covers, washing all bedding in hot water, and deep cleaning of all carpeting and upholstery.

Medical management of recalcitrant CRS begins with careful counseling of the patient regarding the nature of their disease. Patients should be counseled regarding the need for daily maintenance therapies in the form of topical nasal steroid sprays, nasal saline lavages, and medical control of allergy in the form of antihistamines and leukotriene inhibitors, when indicated. The unified airway theory posits that mucosal inflammation may be triggered by factors affecting both the upper and lower airways. Asthmatic patients should be questioned regarding the frequency of use of albuterol "rescue" inhalers, and close follow-up with pulmonary colleagues to ensure proper asthma control is de rigueur.

Patients with recalcitrant CRS experience frequent exacerbations due to upper respiratory viral infections, environmental factors, and fluctuations in disease, among other factors. In addition to appropriate environmental and allergy control, management of acute exacerbations in recalcitrant CRS begins with appropriate courses of antibiotics and steroids. Increasing frequency of saline irrigations during acute exacerbations helps to promote mucociliary clearance and prevents buildup of crusting and thick mucus. Long-term topical nasal steroid use is indicated in the majority of patients, and addition of steroids, surfactants, and antimicrobial agents to irrigations may be helpful in some cases. Often, creative solutions tailored to the individual patient are most successful. Frequent follow-up and coaching is often necessary to ensure proper compliance with a long-term medical maintenance regimen. Comprehensive medical management of CRS is beyond the scope of this chapter, and is covered in greater depth in prior chapters.

Diagnostic Approach in Recalcitrant Chronic Rhinosinusitis

Multiple etiologic factors may be at play in the recalcitrant patient, and the diagnostic approach should begin with broad measures such as computed tomography (CT) and nasal endoscopy. The clinician may be clued in to more specific approaches through a careful history and review of previous therapeutics. Nasal endoscopy may reveal the presence of scarring, localized inflammation, synechiae and accessory ostia, which may in turn provide clues to the presence of recirculation and other disorders of mucociliary clearance. Complete allergy and immunologic testing should be updated in cases where severity of symptoms is increasing, or when prior testing is remote or inconclusive. CT scanning should be considered when the endoscopic exam is unable to provide information regarding the status of distal sinus mucosa. In some instances, mucosal biopsy may be indicated for ciliary analysis.

Allergy

Although inhalant allergy is not necessarily the sole inciting factor in CRS, allergic rhinitis (AR) is a common problem that may contribute to the inflammatory disease process in patients with CRS. AR is known to be present in ~20% of the US population, and in 40 to 84% of US adults with CRS.[6,7] Following nasal allergen exposure and sensitization, patients with AR experience IgE-mediated mast cell degranulation (Coombs type I reaction), resulting in the release of various inflammatory mediators as well as vasodilation, inflammatory cell chemotaxis, mucosal edema, and, in some cases, bronchospasm. Peripheral eosinophilia is a common finding.

Evaluation

Classic presenting symptoms of AR include nasal congestion; itchy, watery eyes; turbinate hypertrophy; a skin rash; and watery rhinorrhea. Common signs include a supratip crease and "allergic shiners" (i.e., dark circles under the eyes due to venous congestion within the sinonasal cavity). Symptoms may be either seasonal or perennial.

Any patient presenting with these symptoms should be considered for allergy testing. Several methods are available, including serum testing for antibodies to common allergens (radioallergosorbent [RAST] test), skin prick testing, and intradermal testing. Intradermal testing is slightly more sensitive than skin prick testing, which is in turn more sensitive than RAST testing. Other less specific tests that may help bolster the diagnosis of AR include elevated serum IgE levels and a complete blood count (CBC) with differential with attention to elevated eosinophil counts. Testing for common allergens should be tailored to the patient's geographic location. Therefore, a practitioner with knowledge of common regional allergens and their seasonal cycles should administer and oversee this testing.

Treatment

Patients with proven AR should first be treated medically. The first line of treatment is avoidance of the allergen, if possible. Initial medical therapy consists of administration of topical steroid sprays and antihistamines. Second- and third-generation antihistamines tend to be less sedating and equally effective as first-generation antihistamines. Saline nasal irrigations are useful for removing allergens and inflammatory mediators from the sinonasal mucosa. Intranasal antihistamines (azelastine, olopatadine) and topical mast cell stabilizers (cromolyn) may also be useful. For more refractory cases, systemic agents designed to inhibit the leukotriene pathway such as montelukast (leukotriene receptor antagonist) or zileuton (5-lipoxygenase inhibitor) may be useful. Liver enzymes should be checked on a regular basis during zileuton therapy due to the risk of liver toxicity with this treatment. Zileuton should be immediately discontinued at the first sign of liver toxicity.

Immunotherapy, or desensitization to the offending environmental allergens via serial injections of decreasing dilution of the allergen in a subcutaneous fashion, may be an effective therapy in alleviating AR in patients who do not tolerate avoidance measures or medical therapy. Many patients respond well to this mode of therapy, but the risk of anaphylaxis and the importance of regular follow-up should be stressed prior to initiating therapy. Immunotherapy should be performed under direct clinician supervision due to the risk of anaphylaxis. A newer form of administration, sublingual immunotherapy (SLIT), may offer efficacy with lower risks of adverse reactions.[8]

Patients with AR who fail these therapies may become candidates for more aggressive modes of treatment. Omalizumab is an intravenous anti-IgE antibody that binds to mast cell IgE molecules, preventing antibody cross-linking and subsequent mast cell degranulation. Further study is required before any conclusions can be made regarding the efficacy of omalizumab therapy in patients with both CRS and AR.

Clinical studies have demonstrated the importance of allergy management in the treatment of CRS. Nishioka et al. demonstrated improved postoperative outcomes in patients with AR and CRS undergoing ESS. Patients who underwent desensitization prior to ESS were noted to have less scarring and an improved endoscopic appearance of the sinonasal mucosa following surgery.[9] Similar findings were described by Krouse, who noted a higher surgical failure rate in CRS patients with untreated AR.[10]

Fungal Rhinosinusitis (Noninvasive)

Fungal involvement in rhinosinusitis is a controversial topic. In the early 1980s, Millar and Katzenstein proposed that fungi may play a role in CRS.[11,12] Since that time, the role of fungi in CRS has undergone significant exploration but requires more investigation.

A select population of patients have been described as having allergic fungal sinusitis (AFS), as defined by Kuhn and Javer. This includes five major criteria: (1) evidence of type I hypersensitivity (immunoglobulin E [IgE] mediated) to fungi; (2) nasal polyposis; (3) characteristic CT findings; (4) eosinophilic mucus; and (5) a positive fungal smear.[13] AFS is a noninvasive form of fungal sinusitis and is associated with *Aspergillus* species and members of the Dematiaceous genera such as *Alternaria, Fusarium,* and *Helminthosporium.*[14]

Others have proposed that fungi play a role in most, if not all, cases of CRS. In a controversial study, Ponikau noted that fungi were present in 93% of patients undergoing ESS for CRS using meticulous culture techniques, which is a much higher percentage than previously reported (commonly ~10%). Most of these patients, however, did not exhibit type I IgE hypersensitivity to fungi, and therefore the name eosinophilic fungal rhinosinusitis was suggested.[15] Therefore, many of these patients did not meet the true criteria for AFS as defined by Kuhn and Javer.[13] The theory that fungi are involved in most cases of CRS has been criticized due to the fact that fungus has been detected in equal amounts in the noses of both normal subjects and patients with CRS using identical quantitative techniques.[16] This finding is not surprising due to the ubiquitous presence of fungal spores in the atmosphere. Therefore, the role of fungi in initiating and potentiating CRS remains poorly defined.

Treatment

In patients where inflammation is particularly recalcitrant, some clinicians consider the possibility of fungal involvement and propagation of the inflammation and consider a trial of empiric treatment with antifungal therapy. Sinonasal polyposis, severe mucosal inflammation, and thick eosinophilic mucin can be seen in these patients (**Fig. 19.1**). Antifungal therapy is available in several formulations, including oral and topical treatments, but antifungal treatment remains controversial due to the potentially toxic nature of these medications.

Topical amphotericin B has been one form of therapy proposed for CRS patients thought to have fungal involvement. Ponikau et al. noted a decrease in CRS symptoms in 75% of patients following every other day amphotericin B nasal lavages for at least 3 months.[17] In a similar study, Ricchetti et al. demonstrated significant improvement in nasal polyposis following 1 month of amphotericin B irrigations.[18] Subsequent studies have failed to show any clinical benefit with intranasal amphotericin B treatments.[19,20] Ebbens et al. conducted a multicenter placebo-controlled trial showing no clinical benefit of topical intranasal amphotericin in patients with CRS.[21] In addition, placebo-controlled trials have shown no reduction in inflammatory biomarkers in CRS patients with and without nasal polyposis.[22,23] Therefore, the indication for use of amphotericin B nasal irrigations in CRS remains controversial.

Both the patient and practitioner must be aware that topical sinonasal amphotericin B is not a benign or simple treatment. Amphotericin requires compounding in sterile water, resulting in a hypotonic solution that may be irritating to the sinonasal mucosa in a significant proportion of patients. The solution cannot be exposed to light and the formulation has a short half-life. For these reasons, many patients have difficulty complying with amphotericin B irrigations, and this therapy is not used routinely

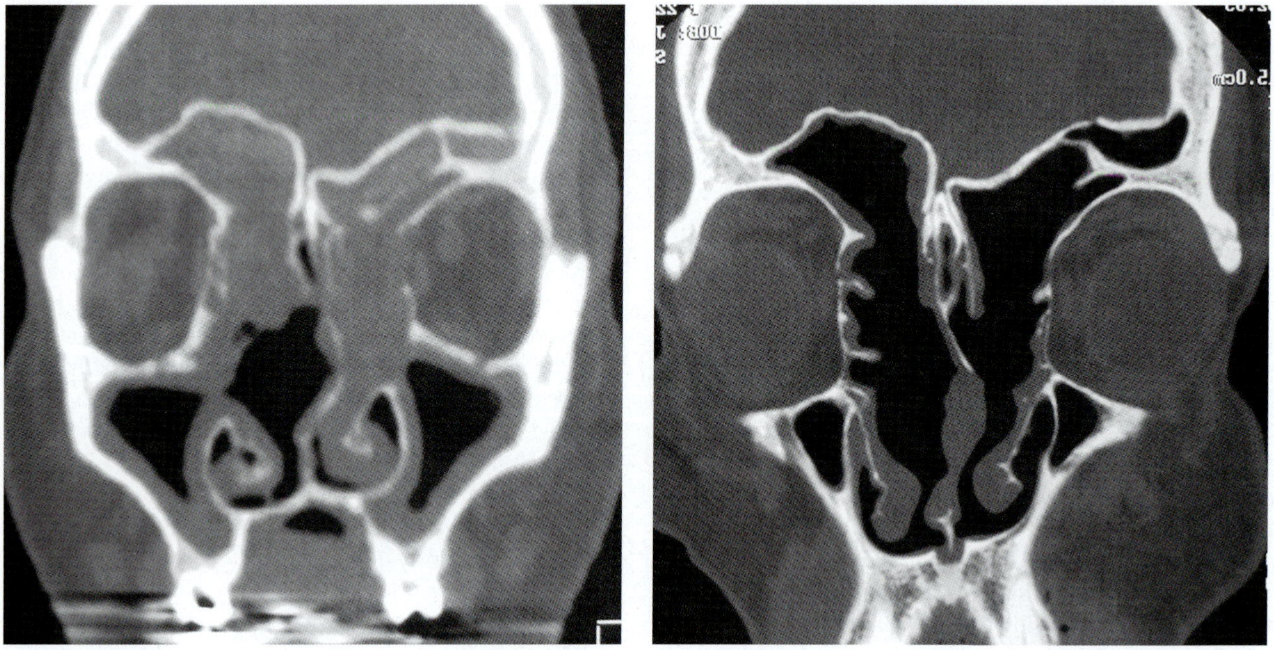

A B

Fig. 19.1 (A) Coronal computed tomography (CT) scan of a patient with characteristic fungal rhinosinusitis. Note the bony expansion and remodeling, polyposis, and osteoneogenesis. **(B)** Coronal CT of same patient in **(A)** following functional endoscopic sinus surgery.

at most centers. Prefabricated formulations of amphotericin B spray and nasal irrigations have recently been marketed.

Oral itraconazole (Sporanox) is an option for treatment in some patients with presumed fungal rhinosinusitis who fail other therapies. Rains et al. demonstrated a significantly lower relapse rate (50%) in 139 patients with AFS using a regimen consisting of itraconazole, low-dose oral steroids, and topical nasal steroid sprays.[24] None of the patients in the study suffered any adverse effects from long-term itraconazole therapy.

Patients should be counseled carefully regarding the side effects of antifungal treatment prior to initiating itraconazole. Compromised liver function is a reported complication of itraconazole treatment; therefore, these patients must be followed closely for any signs of liver toxicity. A baseline liver function panel should be drawn at the onset of therapy and repeated at regular intervals for the duration of therapy. The duration of therapy varies widely and should be individually tailored to the patient's response to the treatment. Limited data are available to further direct treatment.

Biofilms

Biofilms represent a quiescent form of bacterial community capable of forming a polymeric matrix adherent to an inert or living surface, such as the sinonasal mucosa (**Fig. 19.2**).[25] Biofilms are particularly resistant to host defenses and standard oral antibiotic therapy. Biofilms have been proven to play a role in CRS[25–28] and may be associated with common sinonasal pathogens such as *Staphylococcus aureus* and *Pseudomonas aeruginosa*. Direct detection of biofilms on the mucosal surface requires electron microscopy or confocal scanning laser microscopy.[29] Due to the high degree of resistance to standard therapies, mechanical debridement remains the only reliable method of biofilm eradication at this time.

Although biofilms have been shown to be present within the sinonasal mucosa of patients both with and without CRS, increasing evidence suggests that biofilms may play a significant role in recalcitrant CRS. In a recent prospective study, Psaltis et al. found that patients with biofilms present

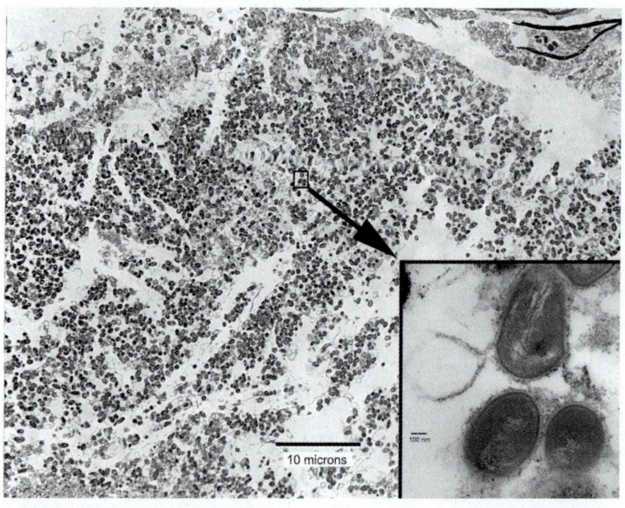

Fig. 19.2 Transmission electron micrograph of a biofilm. Numerous bacterial cells are seen residing in a polymeric matrix. (Courtesy of Richard A. Chole, MD, PhD.)

on their sinonasal mucosa following ESS had significantly worse postoperative symptoms and mucosal outcomes.[30] In a separate study, patients with biofilm-forming *S. aureus* and *P. aeruginosa* infections were noted to have worse symptomatic outcomes following ESS.[31]

Treatment

Topical antibiotic irrigations have been proposed in the treatment of biofilms. The goal of topical antibiotics therapy is the delivery of a higher concentration of antibiotics to the mucosal surface while avoiding the systemic side effects associated with equivalent doses of oral or parenteral antibiotics. Topical sinonasal aminoglycoside therapy has been shown to decrease the rate of pulmonary complications in cystic fibrosis (CF) patients following a lung transplantation.[32] In a separate study using a rabbit model, tobramycin nasal irrigations were not shown to be effective at eradicating *Pseudomonas* spp. biofilms from the mucosal surface.[33] Despite anecdotal reports of success with this treatment, the efficacy of topical antibiotic irrigations remains a controversial topic. In addition, the formulation of these treatments requires a compounding pharmacy, and the systemic absorption of antibiotics with such treatments has not yet been fully assessed.

A novel therapy was suggested by Chiu et al. in the form of 1% baby shampoo in normal saline nasal irrigations.[34] This was the optimal concentration shown to inhibit growth of biofilm-forming *P. aeruginosa* bacteria. Because this is a low concentration of a nonirritating substance, the baby shampoo irrigations are tolerated well. The solution works as a chemical surfactant by preventing the formation of new biofilms. Symptomatic improvement was noted in 60% of patients with this treatment in this study, particularly in patients with a thick nasal discharge and postnasal drainage.

Other novel surfactants have been studied as possible therapeutic agents. A combination of citric acid and caprylyl sulfobetaine, a zwitterionic surfactant, demonstrated promise in its ability to eradicate biofilms when applied topically in vitro.[35] However, when applied to a rabbit sinus model, the topical agent was noted to be ciliotoxic.[36] No human trials have been conducted at this time.

Further research is ongoing in the understanding of the underlying pathophysiology and treatment of biofilms, including their role in CRS. The use of topical chemical surfactants, enzymes, and other novel therapies aimed at eradicating or inhibiting the growth of sinonasal biofilms will likely play a role in the future treatment of recalcitrant CRS.

Bacterial Resistance

Bacterial resistance to antibiotics is a burgeoning problem that continues to complicate the treatment of many infectious disorders.[37] Patients with CRS may be susceptible to infections with resistant organisms, such as methicillin-resistant *Staphylococcus aureus* (MRSA). Additionally, patients with CRS who have previously undergone ESS exhibit altered sinonasal bacteriology compared with CRS patients who have not undergone sinus surgery. Following ESS, patients are more prone to polymicrobial infections, including Gram-negative enteric rods, staphylococci, and anaerobes. Post-ESS patients also tend to have higher rates of colonization and infection with antibiotic-resistant bacteria.[38] In one study, 43% of patients with CRS developed colonization with beta-lactam resistant Gram-positive cocci following ESS.[39]

Evaluation and Treatment

Broad-spectrum antibiotics, such as penicillinase-resistant beta-lactams, cephalosporins, fluoroquinolones, and macrolides, are a mainstay of therapy for acute exacerbations of CRS. There is no consensus regarding a proper duration of treatment, but most studies describe 2 or more weeks of therapy. In certain cases, however, the chosen antibiotic may not cover the offending organism or organisms. Consequently, endoscopically guided cultures with culture-directed antibiotics have been proposed to ensure proper antimicrobial coverage.[40] Contamination with normal nasal flora while taking the culture may be avoided by a careful use of calcium alginate swabs or a Lukens trap attached to suction. The clinician should take care to send the specimen to the microbiology laboratory for both culture and antibiotic sensitivities, including both aerobes and anaerobes.

When resistant organisms are suspected, grossly purulent material within the nose and sinuses should be cultured. Sterile cultures are not uncommon in patients who have been on recent antimicrobial therapy. Patients may be maintained on a broad-spectrum antibiotic until culture results are available, then switched to a separate, more appropriate antibiotic if necessary once the culture results and sensitivities are available.

Long-Term Macrolide Therapy

Macrolides are a commonly used class of antibiotics that exert their antimicrobial effects via binding of the 50s bacterial ribosomal subunit leading to inhibition of bacterial DNA synthesis. Commonly used macrolides include erythromycin, clarithromycin, and azithromycin. In 1991, Kikuchi et al. produced the first report in the English literature on the immunomodulatory effects of long-term, low-dose macrolide therapy in patients with CRS.[41] Since this time, further research has confirmed that macrolides do indeed exert several immunomodulatory effects in addition to their antimicrobial actions. Although many of these mechanisms remain poorly defined, several studies have demonstrated decreased cytokine production, improved mucociliary clearance, and alterations in biofilm structure, among others. Clinical studies in patients with CRS undergoing long-term, low-dose macrolide therapy have demonstrated symptomatic improvement in up to 50 to 88% of patients.[42]

Mechanisms of Action

Several studies have demonstrated a decrease in cytokines following long-term macrolide therapy, including interleukin (IL)-5, IL-6, IL-8, tumor necrosis factor (TNF)-α, and transforming growth factor (TGF)-α.[43–45] It is thought that macrolides decrease IL production in neutrophils and decrease inflammatory cell recruitment. Other studies have demonstrated alterations in biofilm formation,[46] as well as improved mucociliary clearance in patients with CRS following long-term, low-dose macrolide therarpy.[47,48]

Treatment

Most of the commonly used macrolide antibiotics, including clarithromycin, azithromycin, erythromycin, and roxithromycin, have been shown to be effective in clinical studies. Most investigators use half the standard dose for a bacterial infection. Some investigators have suggested starting with a full dose, then decreasing to half the dose after 2 to 4 weeks. The minimum treatment period is 10 to 12 weeks.[42] If, at that time, the patient has responded favorably, the treatment may be continued for another 3 to 9 months as further improvement is possible.[49,50] Once off therapy, patients should be monitored for recurrence. Additional courses of long-term macrolide therapy may be used; however, there is a theoretical concern for bacterial resistance although there are no data suggesting that this treatment contributes to bacterial resistance.[42] In general, these medications are well tolerated and are associated with few side effects. Further research is needed to determine efficacy, optimum dosage, and length of treatment with long-term macrolide therapy.

Aspirin-Exacerbated Respiratory Disease

Aspirin-exacerbated respiratory disease (AERD), also known as aspirin triad or Samter's triad, is defined by three primary clinical features: the development of anaphylactoid response upon exposure to acetylsalicylic acid (ASA, or aspirin) or nonsteroidal antiinflammatory drugs; nasal polyposis; and asthma. AERD is not an IgE-mediated illness but is rather due to an overproduction of leukotrienes and other proinflammatory arachidonic acid products. Thus, the terminology "aspirin allergy" is a misnomer; "aspirin intolerance" or AERD is preferred. Patients with AERD tend to harbor a more challenging disease than sinonasal polyposis patients without ASA sensitivity. They often require multiple surgical polypectomies, and regrowth of polyps tends to be more difficult to control medically than in patients without ASA sensitivity (**Fig. 19.3**). It is estimated that up to 40% of CRS patients with nasal polyposis present with or will develop aspirin sensitivity during the course of their disease.[51]

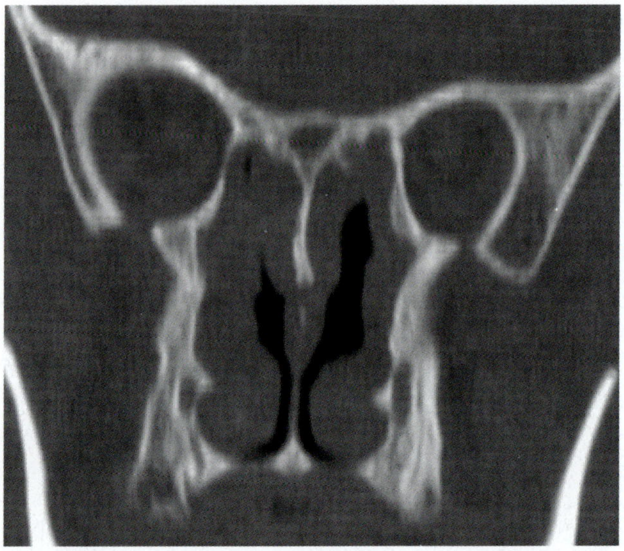

Fig. 19.3 Coronal computed tomography of a patient with acetylsalicylic acid sensitivity demonstrating diffuse mucosal thickening.

Patients with ASA sensitivity who do not respond favorably to standard medical therapy or ESS should be considered for ASA desensitization. This treatment consists of a sequential administration of oral challenges of escalating doses of aspirin. Patients require close clinical supervision, often in an inpatient setting, due to the risk of severe anaphylactoid reactions. The diagnosis may be confirmed with oral, intranasal, or inhaled ASA provocation testing. Desensitization is accomplished with initial low-dose ASA followed by increasing doses until 650 mg twice daily is tolerated. Following desensitization, patients are maintained on daily ASA indefinitely to prevent relapse.[52] Many patients with otherwise difficult to control mucosal disease and an associated ASA triad respond favorably to this treatment with resolution or improvement of many sinonasal symptoms. In a large clinical trial, ASA desensitization followed by daily low-dose therapy in ASA-sensitive CRS patients significantly reduced the number of sinus infections, the need for steroids, and the need for revision ESS. Additionally, symptom scores for anosmia, rhinitis, and asthma were significantly reduced. Overall, 87% of patients noted a favorable response to this therapy.[51]

Laryngopharyngeal Reflux

Laryngopharyngeal reflux (LPR) has been implicated in several head and neck disorders since Koufman described this phenomenon in the early 1990s.[53] In 1950, Holmes et al.

were the first to suggest a connection between gastric hypersecretion and sinonasal pathophysiology.[54] Recently, further evidence has mounted that LPR may contribute to refractory CRS. Wise et al. detected nasopharyngeal reflux with a pH of 5 or less using 24-hour pH probes with nasopharyngeal sensors in 71% of patients with persistent mucosal disease following ESS.[55] Loehrl et al. demonstrated that patients with chronic postnasal drip exhibited a statistically greater degree of pharyngeal acid exposure than control subjects.[56] Other authors have demonstrated a higher incidence of pH probe-proven gastroesophageal reflux in patients with refractory CRS.[57,58]

This topic, however, remains controversial. In a study using a four-channel nasopharyngeal probe, only two discrete episodes of acid reflux were recorded in 40 patients with CRS. The authors concluded that nasopharyngeal reflux was not a significant contributing factor in CRS.[59]

Evaluation and Treatment

Patients with refractory CRS should be questioned regarding their symptoms of LPR, such as chronic dry cough, globus, hoarseness, and sore throat. Twenty-four-hour pH probe testing is the gold standard for the diagnosis of LPR but is time consuming and sometimes challenging to interpret. Many patients may be treated empirically with antireflux medications simply on the basis of their clinical presentation. Proton pump inhibitors (PPI) such as omeprazole and esomeprazole are effective medical treatments for reflux and may be taken once or twice daily. Patients should be counseled that months of daily therapy may be required before any symptomatic relief is noted. Little evidence exists to further direct therapy. Although PPI dosing over extended periods of time is usually well tolerated with few adverse effects, recent reports suggest that long-term PPI use may occasionally be associated with abnormal calcium and bone homeostasis, as well as hypomagnesemia.[60–62]

Ciliary Dysmotility

Functional ciliary dysmotility is a reversible phenomenon associated with CRS. Viral infection and certain environmental irritants, such as cigarette smoke, are also known to cause temporary mucociliary dysfunction. However, there are several disorders associated with permanent ciliary dysmotility that should be considered in recalcitrant rhinosinusitis.

Kartagener syndrome is a form of primary ciliary dyskinesia due to an absence or a malformation of the dynein arm. It is inherited in an autosomal recessive fashion. Situs inversus and dextrocardia on chest X-ray raises suspicion. Classically, these patients will present early in childhood with recurrent sinonasal and pulmonary infections. Diagnosis is made by an electron microscopy (EM) analysis of the ciliary dynein arm. A careful family history is also particularly important in these patients.[63]

CF is another inherited disorder resulting in secondary ciliary dysmotility. CF is associated with childhood CRS, bronchiectasis, and recurrent pulmonary infections. It is inherited in an autosomal recessive fashion. There are several known genetic mutations that occur in CF, all affecting the transmembrane transport of chloride ions, which ultimately results in thick, sticky mucus that is unable to be cleared by standard mucociliary mechanisms. Again, a careful family history is paramount in these patients. Although unusual, less severe phenotypes of CF may not present until later in life. Wang et al. have demonstrated that carriers of mutations in the cystic fibrosis transmembrane conductance regulator (CFTR) gene are more likely to meet the diagnostic criteria for CRS than noncarriers.[64] In a subsequent study, 36% of obligate carriers (i.e., parents of CF patients) self-reported a history of CRS.[65]

Although the majority of these genetic disorders of ciliary function are diagnosed in childhood, the clinician should consider a nasal biopsy with EM analysis, sweat chloride testing, or referral for genetic testing in any patient who exhibits these characteristics to rule out occult CF or primary ciliary dyskinesia.

Immunoglobulin Deficiencies

Deficiencies in immunoglobulin should be considered in patients with refractory sinusitis and recurrent pulmonary infections. These deficiencies may be inherited or acquired. IgA deficiency is the most common intrinsic Ig deficiency, followed by IgG and IgM. A deficiency in more than one subtype is termed common variable immunodeficiency (CVID). Assays for all IgG subtypes are available; however, the clinical implications of a single IgG subset deficiency remain largely unknown. Regardless, total serum IgG is an important indicator of Ig deficiency associated with refractory sinopulmonary disease.

Chee et al. obtained Ig testing on 79 patients with medically and surgically refractory CRS: 10% of patients were found to have CVID and 6% were diagnosed with IgA deficiency.[66] Any patient presenting with recurrent, refractory sinonasal infection should be tested for Ig deficiencies. Intravenous forms of Ig are available and may be useful in improving sinonasal symptoms in patients with a proven Ig deficiency.[66]

Recirculation

In cases where a surgically created maxillary antrostomy is not in continuity with the natural maxillary ostium, or when a posterior accessory ostium is present,

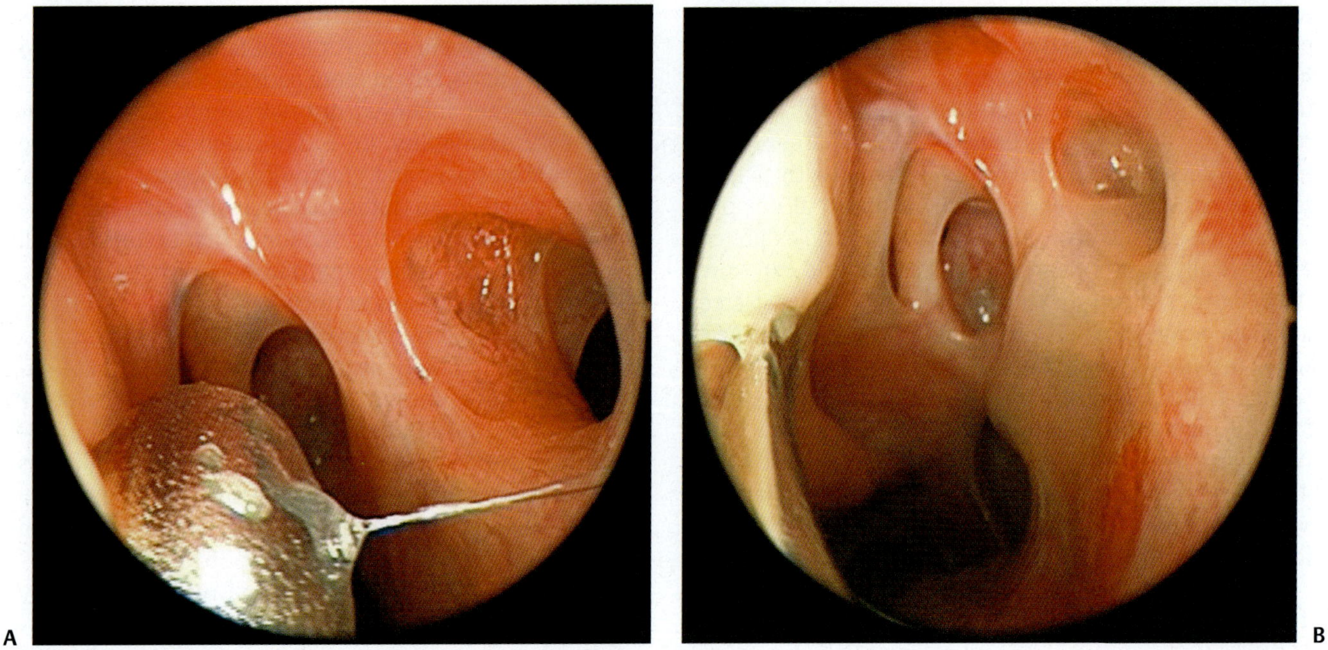

Fig. 19.4 **(A)** Endoscopic view of the left maxillary ostium with mucus seen recirculating around a bridge of scar tissue. **(B)** Endoscopic view in the same patient following suctioning of the recirculating mucus.

natural mucociliary clearance mechanisms may result in the recirculation of mucus around the bridge of tissue present between the two ostia in a circular manner (**Fig. 19.4**). This often results in mycostasis with an opportunity for bacterial overgrowth and chronic infection and/or local mucosal irritation and inflammation.[67] Because this is a structural issue, surgical removal of the bridge of tissue is sometimes required to eliminate the circulatory cycle. Any patient with persistent maxillary sinus disease should be carefully inspected for evidence of recirculation. The most common cause of recirculation is the creation of a maxillary antrostomy that is not in continuity with the natural maxillary sinus os. Recirculation may not be apparent on imaging studies, thus a careful endoscopic exam is paramount to making the appropriate diagnosis. In addition, it is important to note that some patients will have evidence of asymptomatic recirculation that is noted on a postoperative evaluation. It does not appear that this recirculation requires any further treatment.

Odontogenic Infection

Infections arising from the maxillary dentition are an overlooked etiology of maxillary sinusitis. Although dental infections rarely result in sinusitis, some authors have stated that ~10% of all cases of maxillary sinusitis arise from an odontogenic origin.[68] Maxillary sinusitis may arise from infections involving a maxillary tooth root, or may result from dental trauma, extractions, or implants. If untreated, infection and inflammation may spread to involve the remainder of the sinuses on that side of the nose, resulting in unilateral pansinusitis. Management in these cases should focus primarily on addressing the underlying etiology while concomitantly treating the sinusitis.

Evaluation and Treatment

Patients with unilateral sinusitis should be questioned regarding their dental health. The maxillary dentition should be carefully inspected. The presence of loose maxillary molars and gingival inflammation and swelling should raise suspicion. Apical root abscesses of the maxillary dentition may be detected on CT, although Panorex remains the imaging study of choice for a radiographic assessment of the dentition. Patients with a history of dental extraction or with a removal of a dental implant may have an oroantral fistula visible on the exam. In these cases, excision and closure of the fistula should be considered if spontaneous closure does not occur with standard treatment. If the patient has not undergone ESS, a maxillary antrostomy with uncinectomy is often necessary to allow for adequate sinus drainage and aeration while the fistula closure site heals.

Conclusion

CRS is a multifactorial disease. Nearly all rhinologists have encountered a subset of patients with CRS who do not respond favorably to standard medical and optimal surgical therapy. In these patients, medical management of sinonasal mucosal inflammation is difficult. A careful history in conjunction with an endoscopic nasal examination may reveal one or more underlying factors that are not treated adequately with either surgical or "standard" medical therapy. Several considerations arise in this patient population. These patients should be approached with an open mind and a broad view of the various causes of sinonasal disease. A trial and error approach is often required. However, with persistence and close follow-up, the majority of these patients will respond favorably to some of the unconventional treatments described in this chapter.

References

1. Lund VJ. Maximal medical therapy for chronic rhinosinusitis. Otolaryngol Clin North Am 2005;38(6):1301–1310
2. Bousquet J, Van Cauwenberge P, Khaltaev N. Allergic rhinitis and its impact on asthma. J Allergy Clin Immunol 2001;108(Suppl 5):S147–334
3. Dykewicz MS, Fineman S, Skoner DP, et al. Diagnosis and management of rhinitis: complete guidelines of the Joint Task Force on Practice Parameters in Allergy, Asthma, and Immunology. Ann Allergy Asthma Immunol 1998;81:478–518
4. van Cauwenberge P, Bachert C, Passalacqua G, et al. Consensus statement on the treatment of allergic rhinitis. European Academy of Allergology and Clinical Immunology. Allergy 2000;55:116–134
5. Burr ML, Matthews IP, Arthur RA, et al. Effects on patients with asthma of eradicating visible indoor mold: a randomized controlled trial. Thorax 2007;62:766–771
6. Van Dishoeck HA, Franssen MGC. The incidence and correlation of allergy and chronic maxillary sinusitis. Pract Otorhinolaryngol (Basel) 1957;19(6):502–506
7. Emanuel IA, Shah SB. Chronic rhinosinusitis: allergy and sinus computed tomography relationships. Otolaryngol Head Neck Surg 2000;123(6):687–691
8. Wilson DR, Lima MT, Durham SR. Sublingual immunotherapy for allergic rhinitis: systematic review and meta-analysis. Allergy 2005;60(1):4–12
9. Nishioka GJ, Cook PR, Davis WE, McKinsey JP. Immunotherapy in patients undergoing functional endoscopic sinus surgery. Otolaryngol Head Neck Surg 1994;110(4):406–412
10. Krouse JH, Krouse HJ. Patient use of traditional and complementary therapies in treating rhinosinusitis before consulting an otolaryngologist. Laryngoscope 1999;109(8):1223–1227
11. Millar JW, Johnston A, Lamb D. Allergic aspergillosis of the maxillary sinus. Proc Scot Thor Soc 1981;36:710
12. Katzenstein AL, Sale SR, Greenberger PA. Allergic Aspergillus sinusitis: a newly recognized form of sinusitis. J Allergy Clin Immunol 1983;72(1):89–93
13. Kuhn FA, Javer AR. Allergic fungal rhinosinusitis: perioperative management, prevention of recurrence, and role of steroids and antifungal agents. Otolaryngol Clin North Am 2000;33(2):419–433
14. Marple BF. Allergic fungal rhinosinusitis: current theories and management strategies. Laryngoscope 2001;111(6):1006–1019
15. Ponikau JU, Sherris DA, Kern EB, et al. The diagnosis and incidence of allergic fungal sinusitis. Mayo Clin Proc 1999;74(9):877–884
16. Catten MD, Murr AH, Goldstein JA, Mhatre AN, Lalwani AK. Detection of fungi in the nasal mucosa using polymerase chain reaction. Laryngoscope 2001;111(3):399–403
17. Ponikau JU, Sherris DA, Kita H, Kern EB. Intranasal antifungal treatment in 51 patients with chronic rhinosinusitis. J Allergy Clin Immunol 2002;110(6):862–866
18. Ricchetti A, Landis BN, Maffioli A, Giger R, Zeng C, Lacroix JS. Effect of anti-fungal nasal lavage with amphotericin B on nasal polyposis. J Laryngol Otol 2002;116(4):261–263
19. Weschta M, Rimek D, Formanek M, Polzehl D, Podbielski A, Riechelmann H. Topical antifungal treatment of chronic rhinosinusitis with nasal polyps: a randomized, double-blind clinical trial. J Allergy Clin Immunol 2004;113(6):1122–1128
20. Helbling A, Baumann A, Hänni C, Caversaccio M. Amphotericin B nasal spray has no effect on nasal polyps. J Laryngol Otol 2006;120(12):1023–1025
21. Ebbens FA, Scadding GK, Badia L, et al. Amphotericin B nasal lavages: not a solution for patients with chronic rhinosinusitis. J Allergy Clin Immunol 2006;118(5):1149–1156
22. Weschta M, Rimek D, Formanek M, Podbielski A, Riechelmann H. Effect of nasal antifungal therapy on nasal cell activation markers in chronic rhinosinusitis. Arch Otolaryngol Head Neck Surg 2006;132(7):743–747
23. Ebbens FA, Georgalas C, Luiten S, et al. The effect of topical amphotericin B on inflammatory markers in patients with chronic rhinosinusitis: a multicenter randomized controlled study. Laryngoscope 2009;119(2):401–408
24. Rains BM III, Mineck CW. Treatment of allergic fungal sinusitis with high-dose itraconazole. Am J Rhinol 2003;17(1):1–8
25. Palmer J. Bacterial biofilms in chronic rhinosinusitis. Ann Otol Rhinol Laryngol Suppl 2006;196:35–39
26. Ferguson BJ, Stolz DB. Demonstration of biofilm in human bacterial chronic rhinosinusitis. Am J Rhinol 2005;19(5):452–457
27. Ha KR, Psaltis AJ, Tan L, Wormald PJ. A sheep model for the study of biofilms in rhinosinusitis. Am J Rhinol 2007;21(3):339–345
28. Post JC, Hiller NL, Nistico L, Stoodley P, Ehrlich GD. The role of biofilms in otolaryngologic infections: update 2007. Curr Opin Otolaryngol Head Neck Surg 2007;15(5):347–351
29. Psaltis AJ, Ha KR, Beule AG, Tan LW, Wormald PJ. Confocal scanning laser microscopy evidence of biofilms in patients with chronic rhinosinusitis. Laryngoscope 2007;117(7):1302–1306
30. Psaltis AJ, Weitzel EK, Ha KR, Wormald PJ. The effect of bacterial biofilms on post-sinus surgical outcomes. Am J Rhinol 2008;22(1):1–6
31. Bendouah Z, Barbeau J, Hamad WA, Desrosiers M. Biofilm formation by Staphylococcus aureus and Pseudomonas aeruginosa is associated with an unfavorable evolution after surgery for chronic sinusitis and nasal polyposis. Otolaryngol Head Neck Surg 2006;134(6):991–996
32. Davidson TM, Murphy C, Mitchell M, Smith C, Light M. Management of chronic sinusitis in cystic fibrosis. Laryngoscope 1995;105(4 Pt 1):354–358
33. Chiu AG, Antunes MB, Palmer JN, Cohen NA. Evaluation of the in vivo efficacy of topical tobramycin against Pseudomonas sinonasal biofilms. J Antimicrob Chemother 2007;59(6):1130–1134
34. Chiu AG, Palmer JN, Woodworth BA, et al. Baby shampoo nasal irrigations for the symptomatic post-functional endoscopic sinus surgery patient. Am J Rhinol 2008;22(1):34–37
35. Desrosiers M, Myntti M, James G. Methods for removing bacterial biofilms: in vitro study using clinical chronic rhinosinusitis specimens. Am J Rhinol 2007;21(5):527–532
36. Tamashiro E, Banks CA, Chen B, et al. In vivo effects of citric acid/zwitterionic surfactant cleansing solution on rabbit sinus mucosa. Am J Rhinol Allergy 2009;23(6):597–601
37. Moellering RC Jr, Graybill JR, McGowan JE Jr, Corey L; American Society for Microbiology. Antimicrobial resistance prevention initiative—an update: proceedings of an expert panel on resistance. Am J Infect Control 2007;35(9):S1–S23, quiz S24–S26

38. Zacharek MA, Hwang PH, Fong KJ. The office management of recalcitrant rhinosinusitis. Otolaryngol Clin North Am 2004;37(2):365–379
39. Bhattacharyya N, Kepnes LJ. The microbiology of recurrent rhinosinusitis after endoscopic sinus surgery. Arch Otolaryngol Head Neck Surg 1999;125(10):1117–1120
40. Nadel DM, Lanza DC, Kennedy DW. Endoscopically guided cultures in chronic sinusitis. Am J Rhinol 1998;12(4):233–241
41. Kikuchi S, Susaki H, Aoki A, et al. Clinic effect of long-term low-dose erythromycin therapy for chronic sinusitis. Pract Otorhinolaryngol 1991;84:41–47
42. Cervin AC, Wallwork B. Anti-inflammatory effects of macrolide antibiotics in the treatment of chronic rhinosinusitis. Otolaryngol Clin North Am 2005;38(6):1339–1350
43. Wallwork B, Coman W, Feron F, Mackay-Sim A, Cervin A. Clarithromycin and prednisolone inhibit cytokine production in chronic rhinosinusitis. Laryngoscope 2002;112(10):1827–1830
44. Wallwork B, Coman W, Mackay-Sim A, Cervin A. Effect of clarithromycin on nuclear factor-kappa B and transforming growth factor-beta in chronic rhinosinusitis. Laryngoscope 2004;114(2):286–290
45. Suzuki H, Shimomura A, Ikeda K, Furukawa M, Oshima T, Takasaka T. Inhibitory effect of macrolides on interleukin-8 secretion from cultured human nasal epithelial cells. Laryngoscope 1997;107(12 Pt 1):1661–1666
46. Wozniak DJ, Keyser R. Effects of subinhibitory concentrations of macrolide antibiotics on Pseudomonas aeruginosa. Chest 2004;125(2, Suppl)62S–69S, quiz 69S
47. Nishi K, Mizuguchi M, Tachibana H, et al. Effect of clarithromycin on symptoms and mucociliary transport in patients with sino-bronchial syndrome. Nihon Kyobu Shikkan Gakkai Zasshi 1995;33(12):1392–1400
48. Rubin BK, Druce H, Ramirez OE, Palmer R. Effect of clarithromycin on nasal mucus properties in healthy subjects and in patients with purulent rhinitis. Am J Respir Crit Care Med 1997;155(6): 2018–2023
49. Hashiba M, Baba S. Efficacy of long-term administration of clarithromycin in the treatment of intractable chronic sinusitis. Acta Otolaryngol Suppl 1996;525:73–78
50. Cervin A, Kalm O, Sandkull P, Lindberg S. One-year low-dose erythromycin treatment of persistent chronic sinusitis after sinus surgery: clinical outcome and effects on mucociliary parameters and nasal nitric oxide. Otolaryngol Head Neck Surg 2002;126(5):481–489
51. Lee JY, Simon RA. Does it make sense to "desens"? Aspirin desensitization in the treatment of chronic rhinosinusitis. Curr Allergy Asthma Rep 2006;6(3).183–184
52. Jenneck C, Juergens U, Buecheler M, Novak N. Pathogenesis, diagnosis, and treatment of aspirin intolerance. Ann Allergy Asthma Immunol 2007;99(1):13–21
53. Koufman JA. The otolaryngologic manifestations of gastroesophageal reflux disease (GERD): a clinical investigation of 225 patients using ambulatory 24-hour pH monitoring and an experimental investigation of the role of acid and pepsin in the development of laryngeal injury. Laryngoscope 1991;101(4 Pt 2, Suppl 53)1–78
54. Holmes TH, Goodell H, Wolf S, et al. The Nose: An Experimental Study of Reactions within the Nose in Human Subjects During Various Life Experiences. Springfield, IL: Charles C Thomas; 1950: 1–54
55. Wise SK, Wise JC, DelGaudio JM. Association of nasopharyngeal and laryngopharyngeal reflux with postnasal drip symptomatology in patients with and without rhinosinusitis. Am J Rhinol 2006;20(3):283–289
56. Loehrl TA, Smith TL, Merati A, Torrico-Brusky L, Hoffman RG, Toohill RJ. Pharyngeal pH probe findings in patients with postnasal drainage. Am J Rhinol 2005;19(4):340–343
57. DiBaise JK, Huerter JV, Quigley EM. Sinusitis and gastroesophageal reflux disease. Ann Intern Med 1998;129(12):1078
58. Ulualp SO, Toohill RJ, Hoffmann R, Shaker R. Possible relationship of gastroesophagopharyngeal acid reflux with pathogenesis of chronic sinusitis. Am J Rhinol 1999;13(3):197–202
59. Wong IWY, Omari TI, Myers JC, et al. Nasopharyngeal pH monitoring in chronic sinusitis patients using a novel four channel probe. Laryngoscope 2004;114(9):1582–1585
60. Schinke T, Schilling AF, Baranowsky A, et al. Impaired gastric acidification negatively affects calcium homeostasis and bone mass. Nat Med 2009;15(6):674–681
61. Gray SL, LaCroix AZ, Larson J, et al. Proton pump inhibitor use, hip fracture, and change in bone mineral density in postmenopausal women: results from the Women's Health Initiative. Arch Intern Med 2010;170(9):765–771
62. Hoorn EJ, van der Hoek J, de Man RA, Kuipers EJ, Bolwerk C, Zietse R. A case series of proton pump inhibitor-induced hypomagnesemia. Am J Kidney Dis 2010;56(1):112–116
63. Bush A, Chodhari R, Collins N, et al. Primary ciliary dyskinesia: current state of the art. Arch Dis Child 2007;92(12):1136–1140
64. Wang X, Moylan B, Leopold DA, et al. Mutation in the gene responsible for cystic fibrosis and predisposition to chronic rhinosinusitis in the general population. JAMA 2000;284(14):1814–1819
65. Wang X, Kim J, McWilliams R, Cutting GR. Increased prevalence of chronic rhinosinusitis in carriers of a cystic fibrosis mutation. Arch Otolaryngol Head Neck Surg 2005;131(3):237–240
66. Chee L, Graham SM, Carothers DG, Ballas ZK. Immune dysfunction in refractory sinusitis in a tertiary care setting. Laryngoscope 2001;111(2):233–235
67. Matthews BL, Burke AJ. Recirculation of mucus via accessory ostia causing chronic maxillary sinus disease. Otolaryngol Head Neck Surg 1997;117(4):422–423
68. Mehra P, Murad H. Maxillary sinus disease of odontogenic origin. Otolaryngol Clin North Am 2004;37(2):347–364

20 Pediatric Rhinosinusitis

Janaki Emani, Dana L. Suskind, and Fuad M. Baroody

Rhinosinusitis is a commonly encountered problem in both pediatric and otorhinolaryngologic practices. The exact prevalence of the disease is difficult to determine as only a small percentage of cases present to the physician's office. However, in both adult and pediatric populations, there has been a recent increase in the diagnosis of both acute and chronic rhinosinusitis (CRS), likely a consequence of an improved understanding of the etiology, pathophysiology, and microbiology of the disease. Significant controversy still surrounds medical and surgical management of this disease in children.

The clinical diagnosis of rhinosinusitis in children is challenging related to the overlap of symptoms with other common childhood nasal diseases such as viral upper respiratory tract infections as well as the challenges related to the physical examination. Symptoms consistent with the diagnosis of rhinosinusitis such as cough and purulent rhinorrhea may affect as many as 40% of the pediatric population at some point in childhood. Furthermore, the symptoms of acute and CRS are often subtle, and the history is limited to the observations and subjective evaluation of the child's parent. Because most children do not tolerate nasal endoscopy, clinicians are often hindered in their physical examination and have to rely on history and or imaging studies for an appropriate diagnosis.

Chronic and recurrent rhinosinusitis in children, as well as in adults, leads to an impaired quality of life. In a study of children with recurrent and CRS failing medical treatment and requiring surgical intervention, Cunningham and colleagues administered parental and childhood quality of life questionnaires.[1] The results showed significant impairment of the quality of life of these children and, surprisingly, significantly lower quality of life scores than that of children with other common chronic childhood diseases such as asthma, attention deficit hyperactivity disorder, juvenile rheumatoid arthritis, and epilepsy.

Rhinosinusitis is a common disorder often preceded by a viral upper respiratory tract infection (URI). Children can suffer up to eight viral URIs per year, with acute bacterial rhinosinusitis complicating 0.5 to 2% of these cases. Approximately 20 million cases of acute bacterial rhinosinusitis are diagnosed every year. The disease results in more than 1.5 million ambulatory care visits annually and $5.3 billion in health-care expenditures for physician office visits, diagnostic procedures, and antibiotics. In children under 12 years, expenditures in 1996 were estimated to be $1.8 billion. An additional $1.6 billion are expended on the indirect costs of rhinosinusitis.[2–5]

Thus, because of the significant health impact of pediatric rhinosinusitis, its negative effect on quality of life of children, and the substantial treatment expenditures incurred, it is of clinical and practical importance to be able to accurately diagnose the disease. The goal of this chapter is to review the recent literature and outline the most current diagnostic and treatment algorithms in the management of acute and chronic pediatric rhinosinusitis.

Development of the Paranasal Sinuses

Not all sinuses are well developed at birth. The frontal sinuses are indistinguishable from the anterior ethmoid cells and they grow slowly after birth so that they are barely seen anatomically at 1 year of age. After the 4th year, the frontal sinuses begin to enlarge and can usually be demonstrated radiographically in children over 6 years of age. Their size continues to increase into the late teens. At birth, the ethmoid and maxillary sinuses are the only sinuses that are large enough to be clinically significant as a cause of rhinosinusitis. By the age of 12 years, the ethmoid air cells have almost reached their adult size. The volume of the maxillary sinus is estimated to be 6 to 8 cm^3 at birth. The sinus then grows rapidly until 3 years of age and then more slowly until the 7th year. At this point, another growth acceleration occurs through age 12 years. By then, pneumatization has extended laterally as far as the lateral wall of the orbit and inferiorly so that the floor of the sinus is even with the floor of the nasal cavity. Much of the growth that occurs after the 12th year is in the inferior direction with pneumatization of the alveolar process after eruption of the secondary dentition. By adulthood, the floor of the maxillary sinus is usually 4 to 5 mm inferior to the floor of the nasal cavity.

At birth, the size of the sphenoid sinus is small and is little more than an evagination of the sphenoethmoid recess. By the age of 7 years, the sphenoid sinuses have extended posteriorly to the level of the sella turcica. By the late teens, most of the sinuses have aerated to the dorsum sellae, and some further enlargement may occur in adults. Thus, although the ethmoid and the maxillary sinuses are responsible for most occurrences of rhinosinusitis in the first several years of life, the frontal and sphenoid sinuses play a more clinically significantly role by 6 or 7 years of age.

Pathophysiology

The pathophysiology of rhinosinusitis is multifactorial and still poorly understood. Similar to adults, the ostiomeatal complex (OMC) is believed to be the critical anatomic structure in rhinosinusitis and is entirely present, although not at full size, in newborns. Changes occurring in the anterior ethmoids are known to impair drainage through the OMC, resulting in chronic maxillary sinusitis and, occasionally, frontal sinusitis. Sivalsi et al. studied the anatomical variations of the paranasal sinuses in pediatric patients with CRS.[6] A pneumatized middle concha was the most common anatomic variation, followed by pneumatization of the superior concha, Haller cell, and agger nasi cell. Compared with adults, nasal septal deformities tended to be less common.

The normal movement of mucus by mucociliary transport toward the natural ostia of the sinuses and eventually to the nasopharynx can be disrupted by any ciliary dysfunction or mucosal inflammation. This, in addition to edema of the ostiomeatal area, is thought to be the primary mechanism leading to the progression of viral upper respiratory tract infections to rhinosinusitis. Other predisposing factors for CRS include bacterial superinfection, chronic pathogen reservoirs such as biofilms and adenoids, fungal infections, allergic rhinitis, gastroesophageal reflux (GER), immune deficiency, cystic fibrosis (CF), and disorders of ciliary function as seen in CF and Kartagener syndrome. Of note, Gwaltney et al. in 1994 obtained computed tomography (CT) scans in adults during community-acquired viral URIs and found that over 50% of these scans showed ostiomeatal unit and sinus abnormalities.[7] Follow-up CT scans were obtained 2 weeks later after conservative and supportive therapy, and the majority of the radiologic abnormalities had resolved. This supports the notion that the nose and the sinuses are intimately related cavities and that there is a transient viral sinusitis during the course of viral rhinitis in a large proportion of patients—thus, the term rhinosinusitis.

The bacteriology of acute rhinosinusitis was studied by Wald et al. in 1981. They obtained cultures from children with maxillary sinus opacification documented by Water's X-ray and found that *Streptococcus pneumoniae*, *Haemophilus influenzae*, and *Moraxella catarrhalis* were the organisms most frequently isolated from maxillary sinus aspirates in these children.[8] Several studies since then have confirmed that the most common organisms responsible for acute bacterial rhinosinusitis in children are *S. pneumoniae* (35 to 40%), *H. influenzae* (21 to 28%), *M. catarrhalis* (21 to 28%), *Streptococcus pyogenes* (3 to 7%), and anaerobes. Recently, Hwang et al. performed a retrospective review of all pediatric patients requiring intervention for acute rhinosinusitis over a 7-year period.[9] They reported that instead of the common triad of bacteria noted previously, *Streptococcus viridans* was the major culprit in sinus cultures. Brook et al. found anaerobic bacteria in acute infections as well; however, these organisms are most frequently seen in chronic maxillary rhinosinusitis due to odontogenic causes. The predominant anaerobic bacteria were Gram-negative bacilli such as *Peptostreptococcus* and *Fusobacterium*.[10,11]

The pathogens involved in CRS are difficult to identify due to low bacterial concentration rates, inconsistent data, and because most cultures are obtained at the time of surgery after patients have been treated with antibiotic therapy. Muntz and Lusk reported bacteriologic findings in 105 children with CRS when they obtained cultures from the anterior ethmoid cell at the time of endoscopic sinus surgery.[12] The most common bacterial species recovered were alpha-hemolytic streptococci and *Staphylococcus aureus*, followed by *S. pneumoniae*, *H. influenzae*, and *M. catarrhalis*. Anaerobic organisms were grown from 6% of specimens. Brook et al. also reported that the incidence of anaerobic organisms recovered increased with chronic infections.[10] In 1981, his group obtained sinus cultures from 37 of 40 children with CRS and isolated anaerobic organisms from all specimens.[13] The most common organisms were anaerobic Gram-positive cocci, followed by other anaerobic organisms including *Bacteroides* species and *Fusobacteria*. Aerobes were recovered in 38% of these cultures and included streptococci, staphylococci, and few *Haemophilus* species. One hypothesis to explain the high prevalence of anaerobic bacteria is that obstruction of sinus ostia decreases the oxygen tension, increases the acidity of secretions, and thus creates an environment conducive to anaerobic growth.

Biofilms

Biofilms are complex aggregations of bacteria distinguished by a protective and adhesive matrix, and have recently been implicated in CRS. Biofilms are also characterized by surface attachment, structural heterogeneity, genetic diversity, and complex community interactions, which all contribute to their resistance to antibiotic treatment.[14] (For additional information on biofilms, please see Chapter 15.)

It is hypothesized that biofilms may provide a chronic reservoir for bacteria and may be responsible for the resistance to antibiotics seen in pediatric patients with CRS. Zuliani et al. collected adenoid specimens obtained from children with chronic rhinosinusitis and obstructive sleep apnea and examined them for the presence of biofilms using electron microscopy.[15] They found that a large percentage (88 to 99%) of the mucosal surface area of all the specimens from children with CRS was covered with a dense biofilm. This was in contrast with the adenoids obtained from patients with sleep apnea where modest percentages (0 to 6.5%) of the surface area were found to be covered by biofilm. Although the number of specimens in this study was small, the work provides a potential explanation for the improvement seen with an adenoidectomy in antibiotic-resistant CRS. Furthermore, Sanclement and colleagues evaluated sinus mucosa obtained at the time of surgery for CRS for the presence of biofilms and, in a mixed adult and pediatric population, demonstrated the presence of biofilms in 24 out of 30 (80%) specimens.[16] Although the existence of biofilms is now well documented in rhinosinusitis, more research is needed to clearly characterize their contribution to the pathophysiology of CRS in children.

Allergic Fungal Rhinosinusitis

In addition to bacteria, other pathogens such as fungi have been implicated in the disease process. Allergic fungal rhinosinusitis (AFS) is thought to be an allergic inflammatory reaction to environmental fungi in immunocompetent patients. This causes a significantly severe form of rhinosinusitis with significant opacification of one or more paranasal sinuses and pressure on surrounding organs leading to findings such as proptosis. The fungi responsible for AFS are uniform in adult and pediatric populations and include *Bipolaris* species, followed by *Curvularia*.[17,18] The exact incidence of AFS in the pediatric population is not well-known but it tends to occur in older children. Some investigators have suggested that CRS, distinct from typical AFS, may also result from fungal-induced eosinophilic inflammation.[19] Most of these data have been derived from studies in adults, and there are no data to support the existence of such an etiology in children. Furthermore, treatment with antifungals in adult CRS populations has yielded disappointing results, casting doubt on the importance of this pathway in CRS.[20]

Studies of the cellular response in pediatric CRS indicate that eosinophils and CD4+ lymphocytes play a significant role in tissue inflammation. Baroody et al. found higher numbers of eosinophils in the sinus mucosa of children obtained at the time of surgery for CRS as compared with sphenoid sinus mucosal specimens of adults with no previous history of sinusitis.[21] Lymphocytes, particularly the CD4+ population, are also increased in the sinus mucosa of children with CRS regardless of allergic status.[22] Studies in adult patients suggest that these CD4+ cells follow either a T helper (Th)1 or Th2 cytokine expression pattern, which tends to differ depending on allergy status or the presence of eosinophils in the tissue. With allergic rhinitis and chronic rhinosinusitis, a Th2 cytokine profile was observed: interleukin (IL)-4, IL-5, and IL-13, with little interferon (IFN)-γ. In contrast, nonallergic patients with chronic rhinosinusitis demonstrated a Th1 cytokine profile: IL-3, IFN-γ, and granulocyte macrophage–colony stimulating factor with less IL-5 and virtually no IL-4.[23] Thus, there is mounting evidence that chronic inflammation of the sinus mucosa is an important pathophysiologic factor in CRS and, indeed, might be as important as our conventional appreciation of the role of bacteria in this entity. This has obvious implications when choosing treatment options.

Comorbid Diseases

Allergic Rhinitis

Allergic rhinitis is a common coexisting disease in pediatric patients with rhinosinusitis.[24–27] A recent study showed positive allergy tests in 30% of 351 Italian children with CRS, a prevalence that was not much different than that of allergy in the general population (32%).[28] When age was examined, the incidence of positive allergy testing was significantly higher in children older than 6 years as compared with those younger than 3 years of age. Possible explanations for the close relationship between allergic rhinitis and CRS include: allergen-induced edema could obstruct sinus drainage; mucociliary clearance could be impaired by allergic inflammation; inflammatory mediators released by eosinophils during an allergic reaction could disrupt the epithelial defensive barrier; allergic inflammation could “prime” circulating leukocytes which, when recruited to the sinus mucosa, propagate the inflammatory response; local mucosal response to allergens involving Th2 cells could impair the Th1 response to infection; and, finally, nasal allergic inflammation could induce neurogenic inflammation within the sinuses via neural reflexes. Evidence for most of these hypotheses is available from human and animal studies, and it is likely that most of these mechanisms contribute, in part, to the relationship between allergic rhinitis and CRS in children.

Asthma

Asthma is another disease that is commonly associated with CRS in the pediatric age group. Rachelefsky and colleagues reported on treatment outcomes in 48 nonrandomized children with moderate-to-severe asthma and comorbid CRS.[29] After pharmacologic or surgical intervention for sinusitis, 80% of these children were able to discontinue asthma medications. Furthermore, asthma recurred when sinusitis subsequently relapsed. In another study, Tosca and colleagues identified 18 children, 5 to 12 years of age, with poorly controlled asthma and comorbid CRS.[30] The patients were treated for 14 days with antibiotics and intranasal and systemic steroids, and were evaluated at baseline, after treatment, and 1 month later. Patients showed not only improvement in their nasal symptoms, but also significant improvement in spirometry, wheezing, and inflammatory markers in nasal lavage. These and other studies support the concept that clinical control of CRS may be important in optimizing the control of difficult-to-treat asthma.

Gastroesophageal Reflux Disease

Gastroesophageal reflux disease (GERD) has also been associated with rhinosinusitis in several studies.[31–33] Phipps et al. conducted a prospective study of 30 pediatric patients with CRS who underwent a 24-hour pH probe and found that 63% of children with CRS had GERD. In addition, 79% of children experienced improvement in rhinosinusitis symptoms after a medical treatment of GERD.[31] Another retrospective study by Bothwell showed that treatment for GERD in patients with CRS allowed many patients to improve and to obviate planned surgical procedures.[34]

Clinical Presentation

The symptoms of rhinosinusitis may be easily confused with those of other upper airway illnesses such as allergic rhinitis and viral URIs. Adding to the difficulty of making an accurate diagnosis in children is the fact that younger children are not capable of communicating and localizing their symptoms. Furthermore, nasal endoscopy, an important diagnostic procedure, is often not well tolerated in children. The American Academy of Otolaryngology-Head and Neck Surgery (AAO-HNS) symptom profiles of acute and chronic rhinosinusitis are divided into major symptoms (facial pain/pressure, facial congestion/fullness, nasal obstruction/blockage, nasal discharge/purulence/ discolored postnasal drainage, hyposmia/anosmia, and fever [acute rhinosinusitis only]) and minor symptoms (headache, halitosis, fatigue, dental pain, cough, and ear pain/ pressure/fullness). Furthermore, basing a diagnosis of rhinosinusitis on symptoms alone has been shown to be unreliable in adults, thus the most recent guidelines suggest coupling that to signs of nasal infection/inflammation on endoscopy or evidence of disease on radiologic tests.[35,36]

In children, acute rhinosinusitis most often presents as either a severe upper respiratory tract illness with fever >39°C, purulent rhinorrhea, and facial pain or, more commonly, as a prolonged URI with chronic cough and nasal discharge. Studies examining clinical characteristics of pediatric patients with CRS suggest that the four most common clinical symptoms are cough, rhinorrhea, nasal congestion, and postnasal drip with a slightly higher predominance of chronic cough.[37,38] Tatli et al. found that 66% of children undergoing an evaluation for chronic cough had CT scan abnormalities suggestive of CRS.[39] In those children, the most frequent symptoms reported, other than cough, included rhinorrhea, sniffling, and halitosis.

Distinguishing between acute and chronic rhinosinusitis is based on the duration of illness in both children and adults. Acute rhinosinusitis is defined by symptoms lasting up to 4 weeks preceded by a viral URI that lasts more than 10 days. Furthermore, URIs that worsen after 5 days or have severe, atypical symptoms are also suggestive of acute superimposed bacterial rhinosinusitis. Recurrent acute rhinosinusitis is defined as four or more episodes each year with interim complete resolution of symptoms. Symptoms lasting at least 12 weeks despite the initiation of medical therapy are considered to be consistent with CRS. A thorough history of the timing of symptoms is critical to attempt to understand the category of disease that best applies to each patient. A very common clinical scenario in children presenting to the otorhinolaryngologist's office is that of CRS with URI-induced acute exacerbations.

In the setting of recurrent acute or chronic cases, an investigation of underlying causes such as CF, immunodeficiency, ciliary dyskinesia, allergic rhinitis, or GERD must be considered. Inquiring about the seasonal nature of exacerbations may help establish if allergic rhinitis plays a role in the disease course. As some of these diseases are genetically based, obtaining a family history is also important. Upper airway symptoms such as snoring, apnea, and mouth breathing can alert the clinician to anatomical abnormalities such as adenotonsillar hypertrophy.

Pediatric allergic fungal rhinosinusitis has a unique set of symptoms that distinguish it from the adult disease. Most notably, children with this disease tend to present with obvious abnormalities of the facial skeleton. This is presumed to occur because the growing facial bones are more pliable and deform easily under the mass effect of fungal disease.

Diagnostic Workup

A complete physical exam should follow a carefully obtained medical and family history. The physical examination should include the otorhinolaryngologic as well as the integumentary, cardiovascular, pulmonary, gastroenterologic, and neurologic exams. The nasal exam in children should begin with an anterior rhinoscopy to examine the middle meatus, inferior turbinates, mucosal character, and presence of purulent drainage. Topical decongestion may improve visualization but may not always be tolerated in younger children. Nasal endoscopy, which will allow for a superior visualization of the middle meatus, adenoid bed, and nasopharynx, is strongly recommended in children who are able to tolerate the examination. An oral cavity exam may reveal purulent drainage, cobblestoning of the posterior pharyngeal wall, or tonsillar hypertrophy.

Following the history and physical examination, appropriate diagnostic tests should be considered. Allergy skin testing or serologic testing should be considered in those children with other atopic diseases, a family history of atopy, and seasonal predilection of symptoms. Immunodeficiency testing should be pursued in children with recurrent or chronic disease, a poor response to medical and surgical treatment, a history of other infectious diseases (such as recurrent pneumonia), or when unusual organisms are cultured from the sinus contents. Shapiro et al. found that up to one-third of patients referred by primary care physicians and pediatricians with recurrent rhinosinusitis also had concomitant immune deficiencies.[40] Several types of immunological deficiencies can be associated with recurrent/chronic rhinosinusitis including common variable immunodeficiency, IgG subclass deficiency, selective antibody deficiency, and IgA deficiency. Sethi and colleagues reported the following immune deficits in 20 patients (ranging from 3 to 51 years) with recurrent/chronic rhinosinusitis: isolated IgA and IgG1 deficiency, low immunoglobulin levels with a poor response to the pneumococcal vaccine, and low immunoglobulin levels with normal vaccine responses.[41] Based on their findings, they suggested that the minimum evaluation should include quantitative immunoglobulins and IgG subclass levels, a complete blood count (CBC) with differential, pre- and post-pneumococcal vaccine titers, and tetanus and diphtheria titers. The approximate cost of these tests was estimated at $300. Other immunological tests such as HIV, complement deficiencies, or other genetic tests should be undertaken if the history is suggestive.

In patients who have not responded to conventional medical treatment, obtaining a culture may be useful in directing further therapy. In adults, middle meatal cultures seem to correlate relatively well with cultures obtained from punctures or aspirates of the maxillary sinuses.[42] In children, data regarding the usefulness of this approach are limited. Orobello and colleagues cultured the middle meatus at the time of endoscopic sinus surgery in children with CRS and then obtained cultures from the maxillary antrum and the ethmoids during the procedure.[43] They reported a strong association between cultures of the middle meatus and cultures of the maxillary (83%) and ethmoid sinuses (80%). In a recent study, Hsin and colleagues obtained middle meatal cultures and maxillary sinus aspirates under general anesthesia from children with rhinosinusitis who were unresponsive to medical treatment.[44] Endoscopic sampling provided a sensitivity of 75%, a specificity of 88.9%, a positive predictive value of 96%, a negative predictive value of 50%, and an accuracy of 50%, making it a little less favorable compared with results from the adult studies. We reserve this technique for older children who have a complicated course and who are likely to tolerate a rigid endoscopy in the office setting. If general anesthesia is needed, one should revert to the gold standard, which is obtaining a culture from the maxillary sinus itself by antral puncture, a technique that also allows the potential benefit of sinus irrigation.

Interdisciplinary consultations are useful in evaluating the pediatric patient with medically refractory disease. Consultants may include those in the disciplines of allergy-immunology, infectious disease, pulmonary, or genetics to aid in a further workup. Although it is widely agreed that children with an unremitting cough warrant an investigation for recurrent or CRS, other etiologies, including asthma and GERD, must be considered. Other sinus diseases with a related pulmonary component include CF, an autosomal recessive disease that adversely affects the respiratory and digestive system due to an increased viscosity of mucosal secretions. The primary manifestations of CF in the otorhinolaryngology–head and neck surgery practice are the development of nasal polyposis and/or CRS. The finding of nasal polyps in children is extremely unusual and, if seen on exam, should immediately raise the suspicion for CF. The evaluation for CF includes sweat chloride testing and genetic testing for mutations associated with the disease and is most effective when done in collaboration with a pulmonologist.[45]

Although the diagnosis of both acute and chronic rhinosinusitis in the pediatric population is generally made on clinical grounds, CT is the imaging modality of choice.[46] Luckily, the fast acquisition times of newer scanners and the fact that contrast injection is not needed have made it easier for many children to have the test done without sedation. Imaging remains challenging in younger and in some older children, requiring sedation in these cases to prevent motion artifact. The recommendations of the American Academy of Pediatrics, published in 2001, state that CT should be reserved for those patients with symptoms persisting after 10 days of appropriate therapy and in patients with suspected complications (especially in the brain and in the orbit).[47] In the context of uncomplicated CRS, we reserve scanning to evaluate for residual disease and anatomic abnormalities after maximal medical therapy. In children with the clinical diagnosis of rhinosinusitis, the most commonly involved sinus is the maxillary sinus (99%), followed by the ethmoid sinus (91%).[39] Magnetic resonance imaging (MRI) of the sinuses, orbits, and brain should be performed whenever complications of rhinosinusitis are suspected.

CT scans provide an anatomic road map for surgical treatment and are also useful for identifying areas of bony erosion or attenuation.[48] Two examples of sinonasal diseases with characteristic radiologic appearances are allergic fungal sinusitis and cystic fibrosis. In AFS, expansile disease may attenuate the bony skull base or orbital wall on CT. In addition, a speckled pattern of high attenuation ("starry sky") on both soft tissue and bone window settings correlates with the presence of thick allergic mucin and associated calcifications that may be noted intraoperatively (**Fig. 20.1**). MRI T1 images show low signal in areas of fungal mucin, and T2 images show central signal void in areas of fungal mucin, with high signal in peripheral inflamed mucosa.[49] In patients with CF, CT scans characteristically demonstrate panopacification of the sinuses and medial displacement of the lateral nasal wall, which may obstruct the nasal passages (**Fig. 20.2**).[50]

Treatment of Rhinosinusitis

Medical Treatments

Medical therapy comprises the mainstay of management of acute and chronic rhinosinusitis. Antibiotics are the most frequent single treatment administered to children with acute and chronic rhinosinusitis. Topical steroids have become an important aspect of the treatment algorithm in light of increasing recognition of inflammation in the etiology of CRS. In 1995, Sobol et al. reported that pediatric otorhinolaryngologists treated 95% of patients with antibiotics, 90% with topical steroids, and 68% with saline sprays.[51]

For a child with symptoms of acute rhinosinusitis that have persisted beyond 10 days of a viral URI, most practitioners will treat with a 10- to 14-day course of antibiotics. Although acute rhinosinusitis is a benign and typically self-limited illness, the clinical impression of most physicians suggests that a course of antibiotics when given for

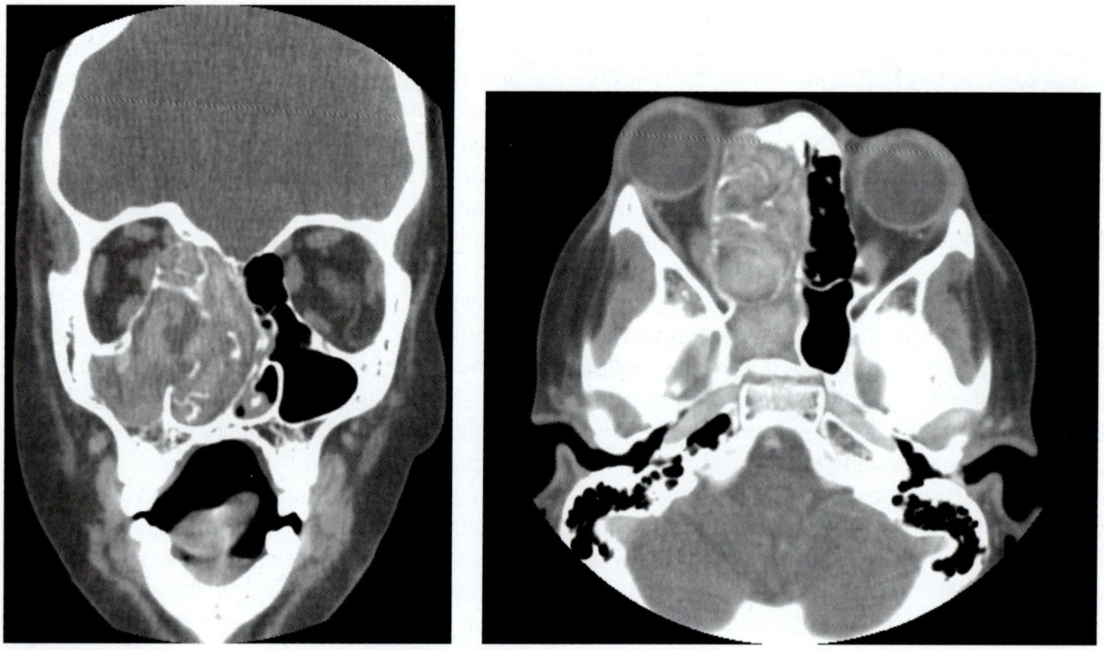

Fig. 20.1 (A) Coronal and **(B)** axial views on a computed tomography scan of a patient with allergic fungal sinusitis. These soft tissue windows show the typical expansile disease displacing the nasal septum to the left on the coronal view and the speckled pattern of high attenuation within the sinuses, which usually corresponds to the thick allergic mucin.

appropriately diagnosed patients will lead to a more rapid resolution of symptoms and thus a more rapid return to regular, everyday activities. This clinical impression is indeed supported by the results of a recent meta-analysis of randomized controlled trials evaluating antibiotic treatments for acute rhinosinusitis in which 3 of the 17 evaluated studies were performed in the pediatric age group.[52] The results suggest that, as compared with placebo, antibiotics were associated with a higher rate of cure or improvement, with the rate of resolution of symptoms being faster with antibiotics in most randomized controlled trials. Interestingly, a 2005 study compared the use of cefuroxime to placebo in children with clinical and radiologic evidence of rhinosinusitis and the results showed that both groups improved on treatment with no significant difference between the treatments.[53] In another study, children with persistent upper respiratory symptoms for 10 to 28 days and a clinical diagnosis of acute sinusitis were randomized to receive amoxicillin, amoxicillin-clavulanate, or placebo for 14 days.[54] All children improved compared with baseline but there was no significant difference between the treatment groups. These studies could be criticized for potentially including patients with ongoing viral URIs in the first study and selecting patients on the basis of clinical symptoms and exam only without radiologic documentation in the second. These results and others, however, suggest that most cases of uncomplicated acute sinusitis will improve regardless of the treatment used. Because of the detrimental effects of these infections on the quality of life of children as well as concern about the rare, but potentially serious complications, most practitioners will treat acute rhinosinusitis with antibiotics.

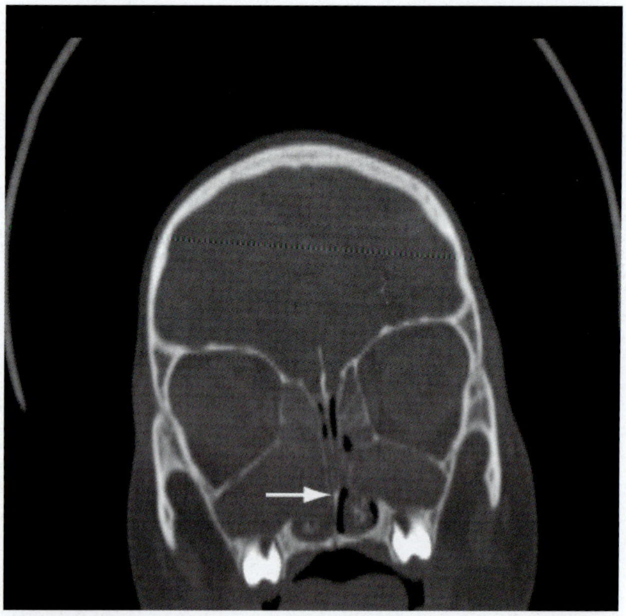

Fig. 20.2 Pansinusitis in a 4-year-old girl with cystic fibrosis and chronic nasal obstruction. Notice the medial displacement of the medial wall of the maxillary sinus (*arrow*), which completely obstructs the right nasal cavity.

When considering antibiotic choices, one should keep in mind that over the past one to two decades, increasing resistance to antimicrobials has emerged among the organisms that are encountered in common upper respiratory infections in the pediatric age group. Increased resistance via beta-lactamase production is found in 50% of *Haemophilus influenzae* and in 90 to 100% of *Moraxella catarrhalis* strains. Alteration of penicillin-binding proteins is also responsible for intermediate and high resistance to penicillin in 50% of *Streptococcus pneumoniae*.[55] With that in mind, uncomplicated acute rhinosinusitis in a child who has not received multiple previous courses of antibiotics can still be treated with amoxicillin (40 mg/kg/day). Another reasonable and safe choice is high-dose amoxicillin (80 mg/kg/day), which can overcome penicillin resistance in *S. pneumoniae*. Amoxicillin/clavulanate (comes in two preparations, one that allows the administration of 40 mg/kg/day of amoxicillin and an extra strength formulation that allows the administration of double the dose of amoxicillin without increasing the dose of clavulanate) and cephalosporins provide good coverage of typical organisms, especially those producing betalactamase. If hypersensitivity to any of these antimicrobials is suspected, alternative choices include trimethoprim/sulfamethoxazole, azithromycin, clarithromycin, or erythromycin, although treatment failure rates may range from 20 to 25%. Clindamycin is useful if anaerobic organisms are suspected, but it provides no coverage against Gram-negative organisms. CRS is treated with the same antibiotics listed here but typically for longer periods of time, which may vary between 3 and 6 weeks. It is noteworthy to mention that no good data support these prolonged treatment trends, so their usefulness must be weighed against the increasing risks of inducing antimicrobial resistance.

In adults, fluoroquinolones are used as second-line agents and have yielded good results. However, no oral quinolones are approved by the US Food and Drug Administration (FDA) for use in children in the United States. Physicians have been reluctant to use these medications in children because animal studies done in the late 1990s raised the concern for cartilage damage. However, these findings have been refuted by more recent animal studies using a lamb model in which no quinolone-associated chondrotoxicity was observed.[56] Yee et al. compared the incidence of tendon and joint disorders in children who received a fluoroquinolone (ciprofloxacin or ofloxacin) with the incidence in those who received azithromycin. They found no significant effect in children who had received the fluoroquinolones.[57] Many pulmonologists have broad experience using quinolone agents for pediatric patients with CF whose lungs and paranasal sinuses are colonized with *Pseudomonas*. Selective use of quinolone therapy in pediatric patients appears to be justified for difficult-to-treat patients.[58]

Intravenous antibiotic therapy for resistant CRS has been advocated as an alternative to surgical intervention. In a retrospective analysis of 70 children aged 10 months to 15 years with CRS, Don et al. found that 89% had complete resolution of symptoms after maxillary sinus irrigation and selective adenoidectomy followed by 1 to 4 weeks of culture-directed intravenous antibiotics.[59] Only eight patients required subsequent functional endoscopic sinus surgery (FESS). Cefuroxime IV was most frequently used, followed by ampicillin-sulbactam, ticarcillin, clavulanate, and vancomycin. Major complications of intravenous therapy included superficial thrombophlebitis (9%) and dislodgment of the wire during placement, which necessitated a venotomy (1%). Antibiotic-related complications included serum sickness, pseudomembranous colitis, and drug fevers. The potential benefits of intravenous therapy must be weighed against the potential for significant complications and morbidities. Studies in adult populations support the use of intravenous antibiotics in highly selected cases, but evidence for the routine use of intravenous antibiotics for CRS is extremely limited.[60,61]

The use of intranasal steroids has been widely studied, proving useful in the treatment of allergic rhinitis and rhinosinusitis. The efficacy of these agents and their superiority over H1 antihistamines in the setting of allergic rhinitis is well established.[62,63] The evidence for using intranasal steroids in acute rhinosinusitis is developing. Studies in adults with acute sinusitis suggest that intranasal steroids may provide an additive benefit (versus placebo) when used in addition to antibiotic therapy.[64,65] Barlan et al. conducted a double-blind placebo-controlled trial in 89 children with acute rhinosinusitis.[66] All were treated with oral antibiotics; 43 also received intranasal budesonide (50 μg), whereas 46 received a placebo saline spray. Budesonide was associated with greater improvements in nasal discharge and cough by the 2nd week of treatment, but by the end of 4 weeks, both groups had a comparable improvement in symptom scores.

Nasal irrigations and decongestants have also been thought to help in decreasing the frequency of rhinosinusitis episodes. Michel et al. in 2005 performed a randomized, prospective, double-blind, controlled study looking at the effect of a 14-day treatment (1 to 2 sprays) with either isotonic saline solution or a nasal decongestant in children 2 to 6 years of age.[67] Outcomes evaluated included the degree of mucosal inflammation and nasal patency. They found that both groups experienced improvement in outcomes measured with no significant differences between the groups. There were no side effects observed with the saline spray. The decongestant group used 120% more drug than prescribed, demonstrating the potential for these medications to be overused. No cases of rhinitis medicamentosa were reported.

Clinicians have certainly tried other treatments for chronic rhinosinusitis, including antihistamines and leukotriene modifiers, especially in light of their effectiveness in treating allergic rhinitis. However, no data exist about their potential efficacy and thus usefulness in the context of acute and chronic rhinosinusitis. We reserve the use of these agents for children with documented allergic rhinitis.

Surgical Treatments

Surgical intervention for rhinosinusitis is considered for patients with CRS who have failed maximal medical therapy (and, less commonly, in complicated acute sinusitis).

Adenoidectomy with or without antral irrigation and FESS are the most commonly used modalities.

Adenoidectomy is often the first-line surgical option in children with CRS, with success rates ranging between 47 and 58% of cases.[68] Anatomic obstruction and/or biofilm formation and the notion of the adenoids as a bacterial reservoir are the primary underlying rationale for adenoidectomy. Tuncer and colleagues investigated the relationship of adenoid hypertrophy and CRS in 30 children diagnosed with CRS clinically and radiologically.[69] Their data were inconclusive in establishing a direct relation between size and severity of disease, but they postulated that medium-sized adenoids cause partial obstruction, possibly leading to changes in the bacterial milieu. Ramadan and Tiu reported on the failures of adenoidectomy over a 10-year period and found that children younger than 7 years of age and those with asthma were more likely to fail after an adenoidectomy and go on to require salvage FESS.[70]

Maxillary antral irrigation is frequently performed in conjunction with an adenoidectomy. To evaluate the efficacy of this added intervention, Ramadan and colleagues analyzed 60 children who underwent an adenoidectomy for CRS, 32 of which also had a sinus wash and culture via the middle meatus.[71] All children received postoperative antibiotics for 2 weeks and outcomes were assessed at least 12 months postoperatively. Patients who underwent an adenoidectomy alone had a 61% success rate at 12 months compared with children who underwent an adenoidectomy with a sinus wash, who had a higher success rate of 88%. Children with a high Lund-Mackay CT score and asthma had better success with an adenoidectomy with a wash compared with an adenoidectomy alone. These data suggest that antral irrigation should be considered in addition to an adenoidectomy in children with asthma who have more severe disease on preoperative CT scans.

FESS has been shown to be superior to medical management alone in CRS. Surgical indications in acute rhinosinusitis are generally limited to complications (e.g., a subperiosteal or epidural abscess in an immunocompromised host) because most uncomplicated cases resolve spontaneously or with targeted antibiotic therapy. In a 10-year follow-up of patients who underwent FESS versus medical management alone, surgery resulted in a greater relief of nasal obstruction and purulent discharge, as well as a higher parent satisfaction.[72] A prospective study by Ramadan et al. examined the outcome differences between FESS and adenoidectomies, and found that FESS resulted in improved symptom status 6 months postintervention.[73] Furthermore, retrospective questionnaires to the parents of children having undergone FESS for the treatment of CRS indicated a success rate that varied between 70 and 80%.[74] A recent meta-analysis of FESS results has shown that surgery is effective at reducing symptoms, with an 88% success rate.[75] Initial concerns about possible adverse effects of FESS on facial growth have been allayed by a long-term follow-up study by Bothwell and colleagues that showed no impact of FESS on qualitative and quantitative parameters of pediatric facial growth, as evaluated up to 10 years postoperatively.[76]

Current literature supports the use of FESS in children, with CRS who have failed maximal medical treatment and possibly an earlier adenoidectomy, or when anatomic variations are clearly obstructing normal drainage pathways. Other indications include orbital and intracranial complications of acute rhinosinusitis and obstructing nasal polyposis in cases of CF.

Many advocate a limited approach to FESS in children, consisting of the removal of any obvious obstruction (such as polyps and concha bullosa), as well as an anterior bulla ethmoidectomy, and a maxillary antrostomy. This approach typically yields significant improvements in nasal obstruction (91%), rhinorrhea (90%), PND (90%), headache (97%), hyposmia (89%), and chronic cough (96%).[77]

Whereas second look procedures were common after FESS to clean the cavities, the advent of absorbable packing has made it possible to avoid a second look procedure. Walner et al. found comparable rates of revision sinus surgery in children with and without a second look procedure, suggesting that it may not be necessary.[78] Ramadan and colleagues observed that the use of corticosteroids during an initial FESS might obviate a second look procedure.[79] Younis, in a review of available data, suggested that a second look is not necessary in most children after FESS.[80]

Most recently, balloon sinuplasty has been investigated as an alternative to FESS in adults, with evidence that sinus ostia maintain their patency in 80% of cases 1 year after intervention.[81] The technology was approved by the FDA for use in children in 2006, and a preliminary study in children has shown the procedure to be safe and feasible.[82] In this study, the cannulation success rate was 91% and the majority of the sinuses addressed were maxillaries. The most common cause of failure of cannulation with the balloon catheter was the presence of a hypoplastic maxillary sinus. Most surgeons now use the illuminated catheter to confirm cannulation of the sinus, thus avoiding fluoroscopy and its inherent risks. In a recent nonrandomized, prospective evaluation of children with CRS failing maximal medical therapy, a balloon catheter sinuplasty was performed at the time of the adenoidectomy and was sometimes accompanied by a concomitant irrigation of the maxillary sinus.[83] The children were followed with a sinonasal questionnaire for 52 weeks postoperatively. Ninety-six percent of the sinuses were successfully dilated in 30 children (48 maxillaries, 2 frontals, 5 sphenoids), 17 of 30 children underwent a concomitant adenoidectomy, 9 of 30 had had a previous adenoidectomy, and the number of children who underwent a sinus wash is unclear. The success rate in this study is reported at 80%.

Despite the encouraging preliminary data with the use of balloon sinuplasty and other surgical options for pediatric rhinosinusitis, randomized, prospective trials are lacking. In these trials, the severity of disease on CT scans and the symptom questionnaire should ideally be matched preoperatively and the following interventions would be compared: adenoidectomy alone, adenoidectomy with a wash, adenoidectomy with a wash and balloon maxillary sinuplasty, and endoscopic sinus surgery. In the interim, the authors believe that a balloon sinuplasty with irrigation in conjunction with an adenoidectomy is a reasonable and safe addition to our surgical armamentarium for pediatric CRS failing maximal medical therapy.

Complications

The complications of rhinosinusitis, which may include an orbital and intracranial extension of infection, are quite rare but can be serious medical emergencies. The proximity of the paranasal sinuses to the orbit and the brain allows for the spread of infection via a direct route. Extension to the orbit can occur when there is a dehiscent lamina papyracea through the neurovascular foramina and via thrombophlebitis of the ophthalmic veins. Hematogenous spread is mainly responsible for the development of intracranial complications, although direct extension can occur due to the proximity of the frontal, ethmoid, and sphenoid sinuses to the cranial vault. Bacteria may spread through the diploic veins of the skull and ethmoid sinuses and seed the adjacent meninges. It is paramount to recognize the incipient stages of these complications and initiate an appropriate treatment in a timely fashion. This is especially challenging and critical in the case of intracranial complications in which symptoms may be nonspecific in the early stages but can progress rapidly and have significant ramifications if not recognized and treated promptly. The diagnosis of orbital complications is best achieved by a physical exam that is supplemented by a contrast-enhanced CT scan (**Fig. 20.3**). MRI with or without a venogram is preferred for intracranial evaluation.

Orbital complications, as categorized by the Chandler staging, begin with preseptal cellulitis (stage I), commonly seen with ethmoid rhinosinusitis and which presents as edema, erythema, and tenderness of the upper eyelid. Extraocular movements and visual acuity remain intact. Orbital cellulitis (stage II) can have a similar symptom profile, but can rapidly progress to subperiosteal (stage III) or orbital abscesses (stage IV). Mass effect of an abscess can lead to chemosis, exophthalmos, visual impairment, and ophthalmoplegia. Thrombophlebitis of the orbital vessels can lead to cavernous sinus thrombosis (stage V), which is considered both an orbital and an intracranial complication. Severe retro-orbital pain, high fever, meningitis, ophthalmoplegia, and blindness can all occur if this complication is not treated early and aggressively.

In general, most clinicians treat early preseptal and orbital cellulitis with oral antibiotics targeted to the common pathogens of rhinosinusitis. Advanced preseptal cellulitis (severe lid edema, eye pain, or copious discharge) or a lack of improvement with oral antibiotics should be treated with intravenous antibiotics. The transition from intravenous therapy to oral therapy has not been well studied, but ranges between 24 and 48 hours and hinges on improvement on the physical exam. In 1987, Israele and colleagues published their findings of the successful treatment of postseptal cellulitis with targeted intravenous therapy alone.[84] They noted in their findings that orbital cellulitis

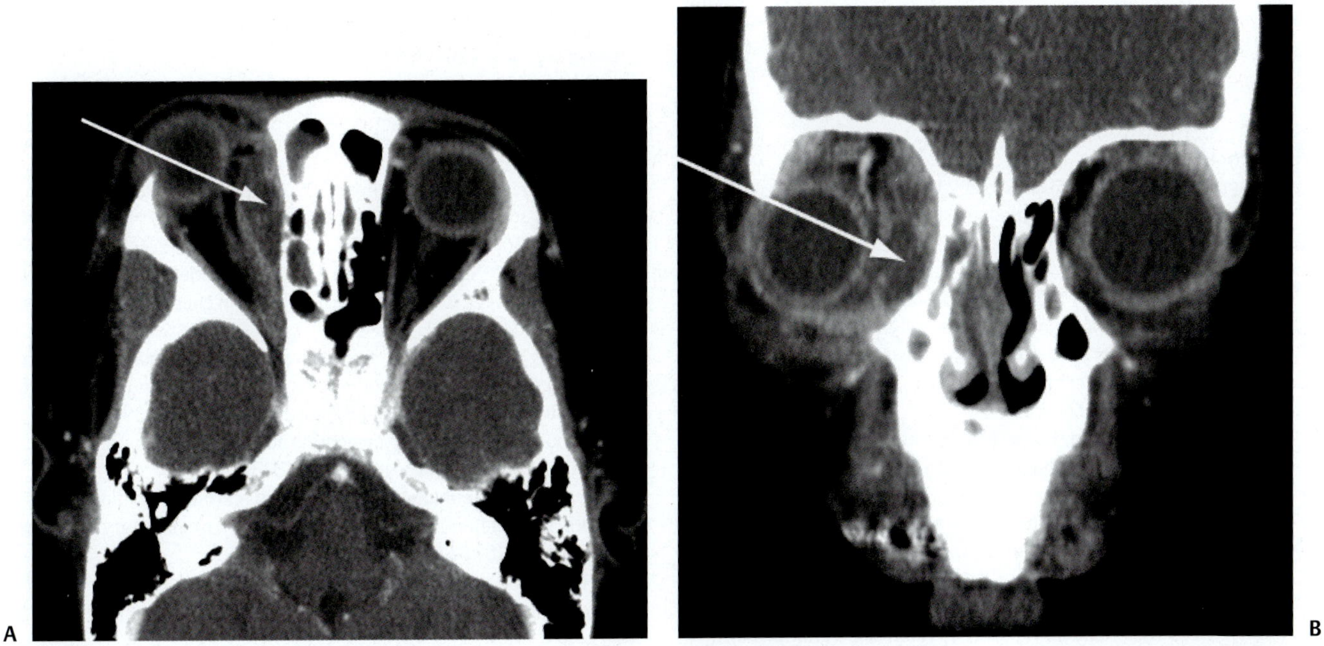

Fig. 20.3 Subperiosteal orbital abscess in a child as seen in **(A)** axial and **(B)** coronal sections in a computed tomography scan performed with intravenous contrast. Notice the enhancing rim seen on the axial view. Arrows denote the abscess cavity.

seems to present more commonly in very young children (under 5 years of age). Similar reports have been published since then in the ophthalmology and otorhinolaryngology–head and neck surgery literatures, suggesting that medical therapy was very effective in this young age group.[85,86]

Historically, the presence of a subperiosteal or orbital abscess was an indication for surgical drainage in addition to intravenous (IV) therapy. However studies have shown that empiric IV antibiotic therapy (ampicillin-sulbactam) for 24 to 48 hours followed by oral therapy is curative in many cases.[87] In communities where there is a high prevalence of methicillin-resistant *Staphylococcus aureus*, antibiotic coverage may be modified accordingly.[86] In the case of a subperiosteal orbital abscess documented by CT scan in a child, we usually initiate IV broad spectrum antibiotics (clindamycin and ceftriaxone) and obtain an ophthalmology consultation. If the eye findings are benign, we will continue IV antibiotics and follow the patient daily, including serial ophthalmology exams. If the clinical exam does not improve or the eye findings deteriorate, we proceed with surgical drainage, which is usually possible endoscopically. In these cases, an ethmoidectomy is performed with opening of the lamina papyracea and drainage of the subperiosteal abscess. The orbital periosteum is usually not violated. In the rare cases where drainage is not feasible endoscopically, an external ethmoidectomy with drainage is performed.

Intracranial complications include meningitis (most common), cavernous sinus thrombosis, and subdural, intracerebral, and epidural abscesses. The incidence of these complications is between 3 and 10%.[88] Altman et al. have noted that adolescent males with frontal rhinosinusitis are at an increased risk of rapidly developing intracranial complications and should be aggressively managed. In their series of seven patients, surgical intervention was required with a combined approach with neurosurgery.[89] In a large review of cases at two institutions (including adult patients), Clayman et al. found that intracerebral abscesses localized to the frontal lobe were the most common manifestation.[90] Headache and eye pain are the most frequently reported symptoms. A prompt neurological evaluation and imaging should be obtained if any suspicion exists because intracranial abscesses can be preceded by a quiescent course. Although CT scanning offers excellent visualization of the orbit and bony limits of the brain, MRI is superior in delineating intracranial suppuration.[88] Antibiotic therapy for intracranial complications is appropriate in the setting of meningitis and cavernous sinus thrombosis, but any evidence of an abscess by MRI evaluation is an indication for neurosurgical consultation for a possible craniotomy in combination with FESS.[91]

Overall, intraorbital and intracranial complications have a good long-term prognosis, although morbidity does increase with lengthened hospital stays. It is important to keep the age predilection of more severe complications in mind when evaluating children with rhinosinusitis. An early diagnosis and appropriate intervention for these complications can limit management to IV antibiotic therapy and circumvent the need for more aggressive treatment modalities.

Conclusion

Pediatric rhinosinusitis is a common problem treated by both pediatricians and otorhinolaryngologists. Over the last several years significant advancements have been made in understanding the pathophysiology, diagnosis, and treatment of both acute and chronic rhinosinusitis. The child who occasionally develops acute bacterial rhinosinusitis as a result of a URI can be managed with a limited course of antibiotics. Yet, the challenge continues in determining how to best diagnose, treat, and follow the young patient with CRS.

References

1. Cunningham JM, Chiu EJ, Landgraf JM, Gliklich RE. The health impact of chronic recurrent rhinosinusitis in children. Arch Otolaryngol Head Neck Surg 2000;126(11):1363–1368
2. Gwaltney JM Jr. Acute community-acquired sinusitis. Clin Infect Dis 1996;23(6):1209–1223, quiz 1224–1225
3. Henry DC, Kapral D, Busman TA, Paris MM. Cefdinir versus levofloxacin in patients with acute rhinosinusitis of presumed bacterial etiology: a multicenter, randomized, double-blind study. Clin Ther 2004;26(12):2026–2033
4. Freid VM, Makuc DM, Rooks RN. Ambulatory health care visits by children: principal diagnosis and place of visit. Vital Health Stat:1–23
5. Ray NF, Baraniuk JN, Thamer M, et al. Healthcare expenditures for sinusitis in 1996: contributions of asthma, rhinitis, and other airway disorders. J Allergy Clin Immunol 1999;103(3 Pt 1):408–414
6. Sivasli E, Sirikçi A, Bayazýt YA, et al. Anatomic variations of the paranasal sinus area in pediatric patients with chronic sinusitis. Surg Radiol Anat 2003;24(6):400–405
7. Gwaltney JM Jr, Phillips CD, Miller RD, Riker DK. Computed tomographic study of the common cold. N Engl J Med 1994;330(1):25–30
8. Wald ER, Milmoe GJ, Bowen AD, Ledesma-Medina J, Salamon N, Bluestone CD. Acute maxillary sinusitis in children. N Engl J Med 1981;304(13):749–754
9. Huang WH, Fang SY. High prevalence of antibiotic resistance in isolates from the middle meatus of children and adults with acute rhinosinusitis. Am J Rhinol 2004;18(6):387–391
10. Brook I. Bacteriology of acute and chronic ethmoid sinusitis. J Clin Microbiol 2005;43(7):3479–3480
11. Brook I. Microbiology of acute and chronic maxillary sinusitis associated with an odontogenic origin. Laryngoscope 2005;115(5):823–825
12. Muntz HR, Lusk RP. Bacteriology of the ethmoid bullae in children with chronic sinusitis. Arch Otolaryngol Head Neck Surg 1991;117(2):179–181
13. Brook I. Bacteriologic features of chronic sinusitis in children. JAMA 1981;246(9):967–969

14. Prasad AS, Tran V, Yun R, Haupert M, Berk R, Coticchia J. Identification of adenoid biofilm in recurrent acute otitis media. Arch Otolaryngol Head Neck Surg 2009;118(7):519–524
15. Zuliani G, Carron M, Gurrola J, et al. Identification of adenoid biofilms in chronic rhinosinusitis. Int J Pediatr Otorhinolaryngol 2006;70(9):1613–1617
16. Sanclement JA, Webster P, Thomas J, Ramadan HH. Bacterial biofilms in surgical specimens of patients with chronic rhinosinusitis. Laryngoscope 2005;115(4):578–582
17. Torres C, Ro JY, el-Naggar AK, Sim SJ, Weber RS, Ayala AG. Allergic fungal sinusitis: a clinicopathologic study of 16 cases. Hum Pathol 1996;27(8):793–799
18. deShazo RD, Swain RE. Diagnostic criteria for allergic fungal sinusitis. J Allergy Clin Immunol 1995;96(1):24–35
19. Ponikau JU, Sherris DA, Kern EB, et al. The diagnosis and incidence of allergic fungal sinusitis. Mayo Clin Proc 1999;74(9):877–884
20. Ebbens FA, Scadding GK, Badia L, et al. Amphotericin B nasal lavages: not a solution for patients with chronic rhinosinusitis. J Allergy Clin Immunol 2006;118(5):1149–1156
21. Baroody FM, Hughes CA, McDowell P, Hruban R, Zinreich SJ, Naclerio RM. Eosinophilia in chronic childhood sinusitis. Arch Otolaryngol Head Neck Surg 1995;121(12):1396–1402
22. Driscoll PV, Naclerio RM, Baroody FM. CD4+ lymphocytes are increased in the sinus mucosa of children with chronic sinusitis. Arch Otolaryngol Head Neck Surg 1996;122(10):1071–1076
23. Hamilos DL, Leung DYM, Wood R, et al. Evidence for distinct cytokine expression in allergic versus nonallergic chronic sinusitis. J Allergy Clin Immunol 1995;96(4):537–544
24. Savolainen S. Allergy in patients with acute maxillary sinusitis. Allergy 1989;44(2):116–122
25. Shapiro GG, Virant FS, Furukawa CT, Pierson WE, Bierman CW. Immunologic defects in patients with refractory sinusitis. Pediatrics 1991;87(3):311–316
26. Furukawa CT. The role of allergy in sinusitis in children. J Allergy Clin Immunol 1992;90(3 Pt 2):515–517
27. Benninger M. Rhinitis, sinusitis and their relationships to allergies. Am J Rhinol 1992;6:37–43
28. Leo G, Piacentini E, Incorvaia C, Consonni D, Frati F. Chronic rhinosinusitis and allergy. Pediatr Allergy Immunol 2007;18(Suppl 18):19–21
29. Rachelefsky GS, Katz RM, Siegel SC. Chronic sinus disease with associated reactive airway disease in children. Pediatrics 1984;73(4):526–529
30. Tosca MA, Cosentino C, Pallestrini E, Caligo G, Milanese M, Ciprandi G. Improvement of clinical and immunopathologic parameters in asthmatic children treated for concomitant chronic rhinosinusitis. Ann Allergy Asthma Immunol 2003;91(1):71–78
31. Phipps CD, Wood WE, Gibson WS, Cochran WJ. Gastroesophageal reflux contributing to chronic sinus disease in children: a prospective analysis. Arch Otolaryngol Head Neck Surg 2000;126(7):831–836
32. Caruso G, Passali FM. ENT manifestations of gastro-oesophageal reflux in children. Acta Otorhinolaryngol Ital 2006;26(5): 252–255
33. El-Serag HB, Gilger M, Kuebeler M, Rabeneck L. Extraesophageal associations of gastroesophageal reflux disease in children without neurologic defects. Gastroenterology 2001;121(6): 1294–1299
34. Bothwell MR, Parsons DS, Talbot A, Barbero GJ, Wilder B. Outcome of reflux therapy on pediatric chronic sinusitis. Otolaryngol Head Neck Surg 1999;121(3):255–262
35. Stankiewicz JA, Chow JM. A diagnostic dilemma for chronic rhinosinusitis: definition accuracy and validity. Am J Rhinol 2002;16(4):199–202
36. Benninger MS, Ferguson BJ, Hadley JA, et al. Adult chronic rhinosinusitis: definitions, diagnosis, epidemiology, and pathophysiology. Otolaryngol Head Neck Surg 2003;129(3, Suppl)S1–S32
37. Rachelefsky GS, Goldberg M, Katz RM, et al. Sinus disease in children with respiratory allergy. J Allergy Clin Immunol 1978;61(5):310–314
38. Rachelefsky GS, Shapiro GG. Diseases of paranasal sinuses in children. In: Bierman W, Pearlman D, eds. Management of Upper Respiratory Tract Disease. Philadelphia: WB Saunders; 1980
39. Tatli MM, San I, Karaoglanoglu M. Paranasal sinus computed tomographic findings of children with chronic cough. Int J Pediatr Otorhinolaryngol 2001;60(3):213–217
40. Shapiro GC, Virant FS, Furukawa CT, Pierson WE, Bierman CW. Immune defects in patients with refractory sinusitis. Pediatrics 1991;89:311
41. Sethi DS, Winkelstein JA, Lederman H, Loury MC. Immunologic defects in patients with chronic recurrent sinusitis: diagnosis and management. Otolaryngol Head Neck Surg 1995;112(2): 242–247
42. Dubin MG, Ebert CS, Coffey CS, Melroy CT, Sonnenburg RE, Senior BA. Concordance of middle meatal swab and maxillary sinus aspirate in acute and chronic sinusitis: a meta-analysis. Am J Rhinol 2005;19(5):462–470
43. Orobello PW Jr, Park RI, Belcher LJ, et al. Microbiology of chronic sinusitis in children. Arch Otolaryngol Head Neck Surg 1991;117(9):980–983
44. Hsin CH, Tsao CH, Su MC, Chou MC, Liu CM. Comparison of maxillary sinus puncture with endoscopic middle meatal culture in pediatric rhinosinusitis. Am J Rhinol 2008;22(3):280–284
45. Brihaye P, Jorissen M, Clement PA. Chronic rhinosinusitis in cystic fibrosis (mucoviscidosis). Acta Otorhinolaryngol Belg 1997;51(4):323–337
46. Triulzi F, Zirpoli S. Imaging techniques in the diagnosis and management of rhinosinusitis in children. Pediatr Allergy Immunol 2007;18(Suppl 18):46–49
47. American Academy of Pediatrics. Subcommittee on Management of Sinusitis and Committee on Quality Improvement. Clinical practice guideline: management of sinusitis. Pediatrics 2001;108(3):798–808
48. Park AH, Muntz HR, Smith ME, Afify Z, Pysher T, Pavia A. Pediatric invasive fungal rhinosinusitis in immunocompromised children with cancer. Otolaryngol Head Neck Surg 2005;133(3):411–416
49. Manning SC, Merkel M, Kriesel K, Vuitch F, Marple B. Computed tomography and magnetic resonance diagnosis of allergic fungal sinusitis. Laryngoscope 1997;107(2):170–176
50. Krzeski A, Kapiszewska-Dzedzej D, Jakubczyk I, Jedrusik A, Held-Ziółkowska M. Extent of pathological changes in the paranasal sinuses of patients with cystic fibrosis: CT analysis. Am J Rhinol 2001;15(3):207–210
51. Sobol SE, Samadi DS, Kazahaya K, Tom LW. Trends in the management of pediatric chronic sinusitis: survey of the American Society of Pediatric Otolaryngology. Laryngoscope 2005;115(1):78–80
52. Falagas ME, Giannopoulou KP, Vardakas KZ, Dimopoulos G, Karageorgopoulos DE. Comparison of antibiotics with placebo for treatment of acute sinusitis: a meta-analysis of randomised controlled trials. Lancet Infect Dis 2008;8(9):543–552
53. Kristo A, Uhari M, Luotonen J, Ilkko E, Koivunen P, Alho OP. Cefuroxime axetil versus placebo for children with acute respiratory infection and imaging evidence of sinusitis: a randomized, controlled trial. Acta Paediatr 2005;94(9):1208–1213
54. Garbutt JM, Goldstein M, Gellman E, Shannon W, Littenberg B. A randomized, placebo-controlled trial of antimicrobial treatment for children with clinically diagnosed acute sinusitis. Pediatrics 2001;107(4):619–625

55. Huang WH, Fang SY. High prevalence of antibiotic resistance in isolates from the middle meatus of children and adults with acute rhinosinusitis. Am J Rhinol 2004;18(6):387–391
56. Sansone JM, Wilsman NJ, Leiferman EM, Conway J, Hutson P, Noonan KJ. The effect of fluoroquinolone antibiotics on growing cartilage in the lamb model. J Pediatr Orthop 2009;29(2):189–195
57. Yee CL, Duffy C, Gerbino PG, Stryker S, Noel GJ. Tendon or joint disorders in children after treatment with fluoroquinolones or azithromycin. Pediatr Infect Dis J 2002;21(6):525–529
58. Grady R. Safety profile of quinolone antibiotics in the pediatric population. Pediatr Infect Dis J 2003;22(12):1128–1132
59. Don DM, Yellon RF, Casselbrant ML, Bluestone CD. Efficacy of a stepwise protocol that includes intravenous antibiotic therapy for the management of chronic sinusitis in children and adolescents. Arch Otolaryngol Head Neck Surg 2001;127(9):1093–1098
60. Anand V, Levine H, Friedman M, et al. Intravenous antibiotics for refractory rhinosinusitis in nonsurgical patients: preliminary findings of a prospective study. Am J Rhinol 2003;17(6):363–368
61. Gross ND, McInnes RJ, Hwang PH. Outpatient intravenous antibiotics for chronic rhinosinusitis. Laryngoscope 2002;112(10) 1758–1761
62. Weiner JM, Abramson MJ, Puy RM. Intranasal corticosteroids versus oral H1 receptor antagonists in allergic rhinitis: systematic review of randomised controlled trials. BMJ 1998;317(7173):1624–1629
63. Yáñez A, Rodrigo GJ. Intranasal corticosteroids versus topical H1 receptor antagonists for the treatment of allergic rhinitis: a systematic review with meta-analysis. Ann Allergy Asthma Immunol 2002;89(5):479–484
64. Meltzer EO, Charous BL, Busse WW, Zinreich SJ, Lorber RR, Danzig MR; The Nasonex Sinusitis Group. Added relief in the treatment of acute recurrent sinusitis with adjunctive mometasone furoate nasal spray. J Allergy Clin Immunol 2000;106(4):630–637
65. Dolor RJ, Witsell DL, Hellkamp AS, Williams JW Jr, Califf RM, Simel DL; Ceftin and Flonase for Sinusitis (CAFFS) Investigators. Comparison of cefuroxime with or without intranasal fluticasone for the treatment of rhinosinusitis. The CAFFS Trial: a randomized controlled trial. JAMA 2001;286(24):3097–3105
66. Barlan IB, Erkan E, Bakir M, Berrak S, Başaran MM. Intranasal budesonide spray as an adjunct to oral antibiotic therapy for acute sinusitis in children. Ann Allergy Asthma Immunol 1997;78(6):598–601
67. Michel O, Essers S, Heppt WJ, Johannssen V, Reuter W, Hommel G. The value of Ems Mineral Salts in the treatment of rhinosinusitis in children. Prospective study on the efficacy of mineral salts versus xylometazoline in the topical nasal treatment of children. Int J Pediatr Otorhinolaryngol 2005;69(10):1359–1365
68. Vandenberg SJ, Heatley DG. Efficacy of adenoidectomy in relieving symptoms of chronic sinusitis in children. Arch Otolaryngol Head Neck Surg 1997;123(7):675–678
69. Tuncer U, Aydogan B, Soylu L, Simsek M, Akcali C, Kucukcan A. Chronic rhinosinusitis and adenoid hypertrophy in children. Am J Otolaryngol 2004;25(1):5–10
70. Ramadan HH, Tiu J. Failures of adenoidectomy for chronic rhinosinusitis in children: for whom and when do they fail? Laryngoscope 2007;117(6):1080–1083
71. Ramadan HH, Cost JL. Outcome of adenoidectomy versus adenoidectomy with maxillary sinus wash for chronic rhinosinusitis in children. Laryngoscope 2008;118(5):871–873
72. Lusk RP, Bothwell MR, Piccirillo J. Long-term follow-up for children treated with surgical intervention for chronic rhinosinusitis. Laryngoscope 2006;116(12):2099–2107
73. Ramadan HH. Adenoidectomy vs endoscopic sinus surgery for the treatment of pediatric sinusitis. Arch Otolaryngol Head Neck Surg 1999;125(11):1208–1211
74. Lusk RP, Muntz HR. Endoscopic sinus surgery in children with chronic sinusitis: a pilot study. Laryngoscope 1990;100(6): 654–658
75. Hebert RL II, Bent JP III. Meta-analysis of outcomes of pediatric functional endoscopic sinus surgery. Laryngoscope 1998;108(6): 796–799
76. Bothwell MR, Piccirillo JF, Lusk RP, Ridenour BD. Long-term outcome of facial growth after functional endoscopic sinus surgery. Otolaryngol Head Neck Surg 2002;126(6):628–634
77. Chang PH, Lee LA, Huang CC, Lai CH, Lee TJ. Functional endoscopic sinus surgery in children using a limited approach. Arch Otolaryngol Head Neck Surg 2004;130(9):1033–1036
78. Walner DL, Falciglia M, Willging JP, Myer CM III. The role of second-look nasal endoscopy after pediatric functional endoscopic sinus surgery. Arch Otolaryngol Head Neck Surg 1998;124(4):425–428
79. Ramadan HH. Corticosteroid therapy during endoscopic sinus surgery in children: is there a need for a second look? Arch Otolaryngol Head Neck Surg 2001;127(2):188–192
80. Younis RT. The pros and cons of second-look sinonasal endoscopy after endoscopic sinus surgery in children. Arch Otolaryngol Head Neck Surg 2005;131(3):267–269
81. Bolger WE, Brown CL, Church CA, et al. Safety and outcomes of balloon catheter sinusotomy: a multicenter 24-week analysis in 115 patients. Otolaryngol Head Neck Surg 2007;137(1):10–20
82. Ramadan HH. Safety and feasibility of balloon sinuplasty for treatment of chronic rhinosinusitis in children. Ann Otol Rhinol Laryngol 2009;118(3):161–165
83. Ramadan HH, Terrell AM. Balloon catheter sinuplasty and adenoidectomy in children with chronic rhinosinusitis. Ann Otol Rhinol Laryngol 2010;119(9):578–582
84. Israele V, Nelson JD. Periorbital and orbital cellulitis. Pediatr Infect Dis J 1987;6(4):404–410
85. Herrmann BW, Forsen JW Jr. Simultaneous intracranial and orbital complications of acute rhinosinusitis in children. Int J Pediatr Otorhinolaryngol 2004;68(5):619–625
86. Wald ER. Periorbital and orbital infection. In: Long SS, Pickering LD, Prober CG, eds. Principles and Practice of Pediatric Infectious Diseases. 2nd ed. New York: Churchill Livingstone; 2003: 508–513
87. Brown CL, Graham SM, Griffin MC, et al. Pediatric medial subperiosteal orbital abscess: medical management where possible. Am J Rhinol 2004;18(5):321–327
88. Lerner DN, Choi SS, Zalzal GH, Johnson DL. Intracranial complications of sinusitis in childhood. Ann Otol Rhinol Laryngol 1995;104(4 Pt 1):288–293
89. Altman KW, Austin MB, Tom LW, Knox GW. Complications of frontal sinusitis in adolescents: case presentations and treatment options. Int J Pediatr Otorhinolaryngol 1997;41(1):9–20
90. Clayman GL, Adams GL, Paugh DR, Koopmann CF Jr. Intracranial complications of paranasal sinusitis: a combined institutional review. Laryngoscope 1991;101(3):234–239
91. Lieser JD, Derkay CS. Pediatric sinusitis: when do we operate? Curr Opin Otolaryngol Head Neck Surg 2005;13(1):60–66

21 Complications of Rhinosinusitis

Ian J. Witterick and Allan D. Vescan

Complications from acute rhinosinusitis commonly involve intracranial structures, but can also involve the orbit and adjacent bone and soft tissues. An evaluation of patients by a thorough history and physical examination, culture of purulent discharge or infected bone, and axial and coronal computed tomography (CT) scanning with contrast is crucial for an optimal diagnosis and treatment planning. Consultations with ophthalmology, neurosurgery, and infectious disease colleagues is often needed. Treatment of complications uniformly involves the use of intravenous antibiotics and appropriate drainage procedures to arrest the infection and to allow for resolution of the inflammatory complication. Early, aggressive intervention has been shown to decrease morbidity and shorten hospital stays, although significant morbidity and mortality from complications can still occur despite aggressive medical and surgical treatment.[1]

The suppurative complications of sinusitis can be divided into two types: orbital infections and intracranial complications; yet, it is not uncommon for a patient to exhibit more than one focus of infection (i.e., intracranial or orbital, or both). Orbital symptoms frequently precede an intracranial extension of the disease.

Epidemiology

Orbital Infections

Sinusitis is one of the main causes of orbital infections. The ethmoid sinuses are the most common site of origin, followed in decreasing order by the frontal, sphenoid, and maxillary sinuses; isolated infection in the sphenoid sinus rarely causes orbital complications. Acute pansinusitis leads to 60 to 80% of orbital complications.[2,3] Approximately 3% of patients with sinusitis experience some form of orbital involvement; indeed, the manifestations of orbital infection may be the first signs of sinus infection. Orbital complications primarily affect children, with a peak incidence between the ages of 5 and 10 years (1 to 2 decades earlier than the peak incidence of frontal sinusitis complications).

Intracranial Complications

Intracranial complications are second to orbital complications in frequency, and sinus disease is the presumed underlying cause of ~10% of intracranial suppuration. The most common source is the frontal sinus, followed by the ethmoid, sphenoid, and maxillary sinuses. Complications occur most frequently in the adolescent male, thought to be related to the continued growth of the frontal bone and the extensive diploic venous system seen in this patient group.[4]

The frontal sinus is the most common sinus involved with osteomyelitis; osteomyelitis of other paranasal sinuses is rare.

Meningitis is among the most common intracranial complications of sinusitis in adults and children—most often secondary to an extension from ethmoid or sphenoid sinusitis and rarely from frontal sinusitis alone.

An epidural abscess is a relatively infrequent complication of sinusitis, but it typically occurs just posterior to the frontal sinus, where free venous communication and loose dura predispose it to abscess formation between the dura and the cranial vault.[5] Most cases of subdural empyema occur in the second decade of life in patients who are otherwise healthy. As with other intracranial complications, males have a marked predisposition. Many subdural empyemas in infants occur when a subdural effusion related to meningitis becomes infected. Compared with other causes of intracranial suppuration, a greater proportion of subdural empyemas (41 to 67%) result from sinusitis.[6] When sinusitis is the cause, the frontal sinuses are most often implicated.

Pathophysiology

Orbital Infections

The orbital septum is a connective tissue extension of the periosteum (or periorbita) that is reflected into the upper and lower eyelids. Infection of tissues anterior to the orbital septum is described as *periorbital* or *preseptal*.

Veins that drain the orbit, ethmoid and maxillary sinuses, and the skin of the eye and periorbital tissues constitute an anastomosing and valveless network. The venous system provides an opportunity for the spread of infection from one anatomical site to another, and predisposes the involvement of the cavernous sinus. Extension of sinusitis into the orbit can occur through either direct extension or retrograde thrombophlebitis. Direct extension occurs through congenital bony dehiscences, open suture lines or foramina, or by erosion through bony barriers (e.g., lamina papyracea). Retrograde thrombophlebitis occurs through the network of orbital veins described here. There are no lymphatics in the orbit, so it is unlikely that they play a significant role in disease propagation.

Orbital inflammation can lead to temporary or permanent loss of vision. Indeed, blindness can occur without any funduscopic abnormalities; thus, it is crucial to monitor visual acuity at frequent intervals. There are several postulations regarding underlying visual loss.[7] The first is ischemic optic neuropathy involving vascular compromise of the optic nerve and retina through compression and subsequent decreased perfusion of the branches of the central and ophthalmic arteries. Central retinal artery occlusion can result and, unless circulation is restored within 100 minutes, permanent blindness will result. The second possible cause is compressive optic neuropathy due to direct pressure on the optic nerve. With this, there is usually an associated ethmoiditis; an afferent pupillary defect is often seen as well. The third possible cause is inflammatory optic neuropathy, which often occurs as a result of optic nerve damage as a reaction to adjacent infection. Unfortunately, even today, a 10% incidence of permanent visual loss has been reported with orbital complications.[7]

Patients with complications of acute rhinosinusitis commonly receive antibiotic treatment before cultures of any purulent material are taken. This makes an accurate description of the primary bacteriology elusive. Whenever possible, middle meatal cultures should be obtained. The organisms most commonly associated with orbital complications are similar to those involved in acute rhinosinusitis and include *Streptococcus pneumoniae*, *Haemophilus influenzae*, *Moraxella catarrhalis*, and *Streptococcus pyogenes*.[8] *S. aureus* and anaerobes are cultured less often. Bacteremia can be seen with orbital complications and is more common in the pediatric population.

Intracranial Complications

The pathogenesis of intracranial complications includes two major mechanisms: direct extension and, more commonly, retrograde thrombophlebitis via the valveless diploic veins. The close anatomic proximity of the sinuses to the intracranial cavity allows for direct extension of infection to bone (i.e., osteomyelitis) and subsequent erosion into the epidural space. On occasion, there is further penetration of purulence through the dura to the subdural space. Retrograde thrombophlebitis is facilitated by the shared venous drainage of the sinuses and the intracranial structures. The pathogenesis of subdural empyema in infants is different than in adults, with most cases resulting from infection of subdural effusions developing from initial meningitis.

If infection reaches the subdural space, it spreads easily over the convexities of the brain, owing to a lack of septations. With progression, subdural pus will cause local inflammation of the leptomeninges and superficial cortex, vasculitis, and septic venous thrombosis, leading to local edema and infarction. Venous infarction, in turn, causes further edema and infarction. Ultimately, death can occur from transtentorial herniation.

A brain abscess most commonly involves the frontal lobe and is usually secondary to frontal sinusitis, with septic retrograde embolization from the diploic veins of the sagittal sinus and cortical veins. Encapsulation of the abscess begins at 10 to 14 days, and may extend to form multiple abscesses. Abscesses tend to form in the white matter, due to its poor vascular supply. The junction of white and gray matter is at highest risk.

Superior sagittal sinus thrombosis consistently occurs secondary to retrograde thrombophlebitis from frontal sinusitis and is often reported in conjunction with epidural, subdural, or brain abscesses.

Cavernous sinus thrombosis (CST) usually presents as a complication of ethmoid and sphenoid sinusitis, by direct extension or through retrograde thrombophlebitis of the ophthalmic veins. It can also result from epidural or subdural abscesses.

Organisms cultured intracranially or from the offending sinuses include *S. aureus*, *Streptococcus*, *H. influenzae*, *Bacteroides*, and other Gram-positive aerobes and anaerobic organisms, including microaerophilic streptococci.[4,9,10] Patients with Pott's puffy tumor of the frontal sinus frequently have polymicrobial infections. In one study, alpha- and beta-hemolytic streptococci, *Bacteroides* species, and less frequently, staphylococci and enterococci were the predominant organisms.[11]

Clinical Presentation

Orbital Infections

Infection of the eye can be periorbital or orbital in origin, and must be distinguished from noninfectious causes of swelling in or around the eye, including tumor, local edema, allergy, or blunt trauma. In cases of the latter, a history provides the key to diagnosis: eyelid swelling continues to increase for 48 hours and then resolves over several days.

Differentiating orbital cellulitis or an abscess from a developing CST may be difficult. The most important clinical signs of a developing cavernous sinus thrombophlebitis include bilateral orbital involvement, rapidly progressive severe chemosis and ophthalmoplegia, severe retinal engorgement, fever to 105°F (40°C), and prostration. Even with rapid recognition and treatment, this condition may progress to loss of vision, meningitis, and even death.

Chandler and colleagues' classic description of orbital complications organizes the typical patterns of secondary orbital involvement into a logical progression,[9] and includes the following: (class I) periorbital cellulitis; (class II) orbital cellulitis; (class III) subperiosteal abscess; (class IV) orbital abscess; and (class V) CST. This classification scheme is somewhat arbitrary, but its anatomical distinctions are important, because they aid in determining a prognosis as well as a treatment plan.

- ***Periorbital cellulitis*** *(Chandler class I)* is the most common and least severe orbital complication of sinusitis, and constitutes 70 to 80% of cases in most

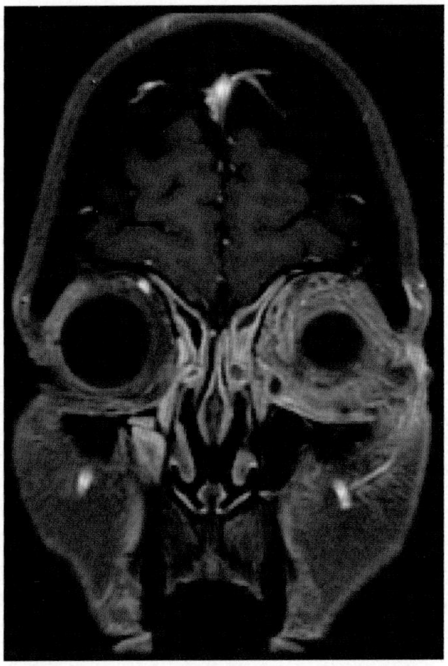

Fig. 21.1 Diffuse enhancement of the left orbit consistent with cellulitis secondary to sinusitis (coronal T1-weighted magnetic resonance post-gadolinium with fat suppression image).

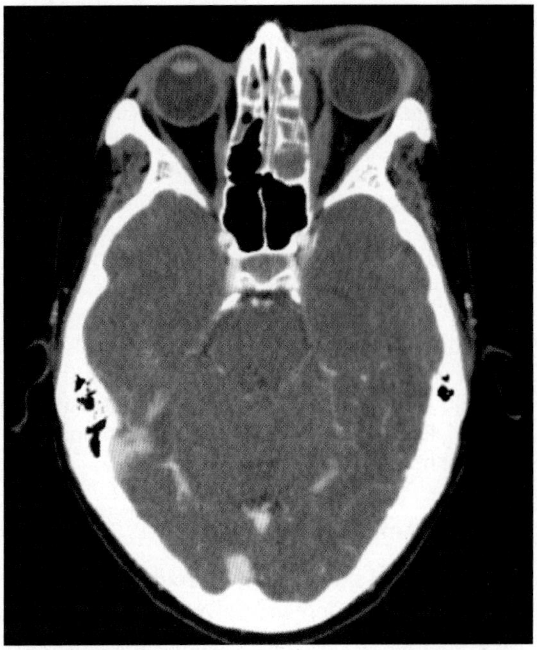

Fig. 21.2 Left subperiosteal abscess secondary to a left ethmoid sinusitis. A mass lesion along the anteromedial orbit is seen. The convex configuration suggests a subperiosteal location. There is also associated left proptosis, enlargement of the left medial rectus muscle, and left ethmoid opacification (axial computed tomography scan soft tissue algorithm).

large series.[2,3] It involves inflammatory edema of the eyelid without evidence of an intraorbital infection and presents with swollen and tender eyelids, sometimes with associated erythema of the eyelid skin. The edema is confined to the periorbital eyelid by the orbital septum. Mild proptosis may be seen, but there is no change in extraocular movement or an impairment of vision.

- ***Orbital cellulitis*** *(Chandler class II)* involves diffuse edema and inflammation of the orbital contents without abscess formation (**Fig. 21.1**). Nearly all patients with orbital cellulitis have periorbital swelling, edema (95%), and proptosis; orbital pain is present in 85 to 89% of cases.[2]
- ***Subperiosteal abscess*** *(Chandler class III)* represents a collection of pus between the orbital periosteum and the bony orbital wall, typically between the lamina papyracea and the medial periorbita (**Fig. 21.2**). The abscess usually collects medially, pushing the orbital contents inferiorly and laterally. Initially, when the abscess is small, extraocular movement and vision are intact. With advancing infection, ocular mobility and visual acuity are affected, and chemosis develops. The abscess may penetrate through the periosteum into the orbit or anteriorly into the eyelid.
- ***Orbital abscess*** *(Chandler class IV)* represents a collection of pus in the orbital tissues. The collection may be extraconal (between the periosteum and the extraocular muscles) or intraconal (located centrally within the muscle cone) (**Fig. 21.3**). The abscess may occur as a result of progression of orbital cellulitis or the spread of infection from a subperiosteal abscess.

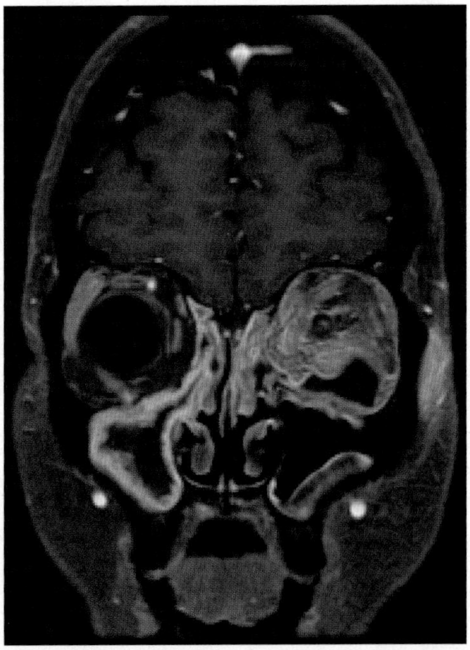

Fig. 21.3 Intraorbital abscess secondary to sinusitis. Note the diffuse enhancement of the left orbit (cellulitis) with a low density area (fluid) within the inferolateral orbit consistent with an intraorbital abscess (coronal T1-weighted magnetic resonance post-gadolinium with fat suppression image).

Patients with orbital abscesses generally present with proptosis, a limitation of extraocular movement, and visual loss.

- ***Cavernous sinus thrombosis, or CST*** *(Chandler class V)* presents with proptosis, chemosis, reduced or absent extraocular motion, and reduced vision, ultimately progressing to complete loss of vision. Early signs and symptoms of CST include fever, headache, photophobia, diplopia, and periorbital edema. Classic findings include ptosis, proptosis, chemosis, ocular palsy, and decreased visual acuity. Pituitary insufficiency can occur if the pituitary gland becomes inflamed. The hallmark of CST is the appearance of bilateral ocular symptoms, but CST should be also suspected in unilateral ocular findings, especially if accompanied by signs of meningitis and cranial neuropathies.

Intracranial Complications

Patients with frontal sinusitis demonstrating persistent fever, forehead swelling, or failure to resolve symptoms warrant radiologic evaluation to investigate silent intracranial involvement, even in the absence of intracranial signs.[5] Presentation can be acute and fulminant with bacterial meningitis, CST, and subdural empyema. Brain abscesses and epidural abscesses typically have a more indolent presentation, although the rupture of a brain abscess into the ventricular system can precipitate an acute neurological deterioration.

- ***Osteomyelitis:*** Headache is a common presenting symptom. A well circumscribed swelling of the forehead with edema of the overlying skin and collection of pus under the periosteum—classically described as Pott's puffy tumor—may be seen (**Fig. 21.4**). This subperiosteal abscess caused by osteomyelitis of the anterior table of the frontal bone was first described in 1775 by Sir Percival Pott and can result from both acute and chronic frontal sinusitis, although it has become decidedly less frequent since the introduction of antibiotics. Pott's puffy tumor can be secondary to frontal osteomyelitis, but an isolated Pott's puffy tumor without associated osteomyelitis can also occur by the deposition of organisms under the cranial periosteum via retrograde thrombophlebitis. When bone erosion is seen on CT, the diagnosis of osteomyelitis can be confirmed with technetium 99-m pertechnetate and gallium-67-citrate bone scans.
- ***Meningitis:*** Symptoms include headache, fever, seizure, and irritability, followed by somnolence, delirium, and coma. Hydrocephalus and subdural collection can result, and postinfection sequelae are especially common in children. Patients with persistent high fever, changes in mental status, photophobia, meningismus, or severe headache should be evaluated for meningitis, and all patients suspected of suffering from meningitis should undergo contrast CT or magnetic resonance imaging (MRI) to assess for other intracranial pathology (**Fig. 21.5**). Lumbar puncture is diagnostic, and shows pleocytosis, elevated protein, low glucose, and infecting organisms.
- ***Epidural abscess:*** This type of abscess may rupture into the subdural space or extend to other intracranial structures through the venous network, and can often

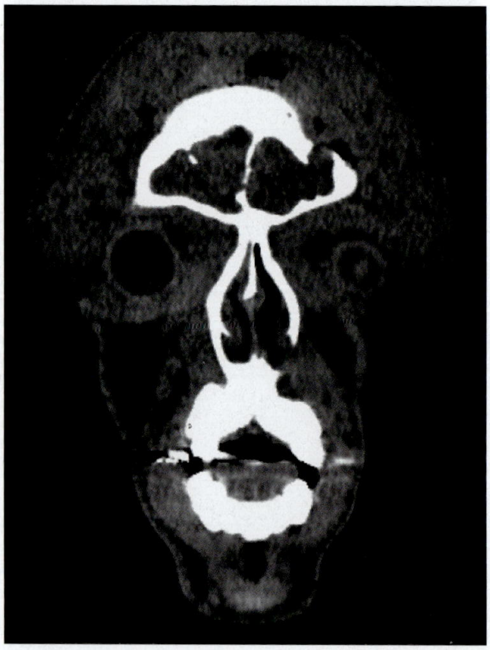

Fig. 21.4 Frontal sinusitis with erosion of bone (left superior frontal sinus) and diffuse edema and air in the adjacent forehead soft tissues consistent with Pott's puffy tumor (coronal computed tomography scan).

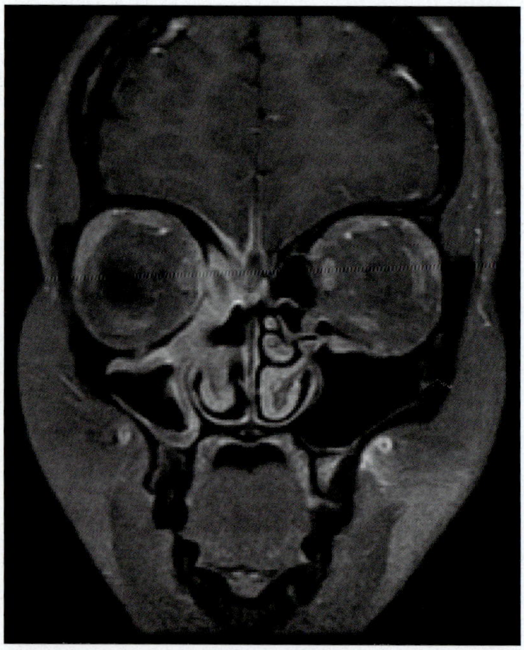

Fig. 21.5 Right ethmoid sinusitis with enhancement of adjacent dura causing meningitis and encephalitis (coronal T1-weighted magnetic resonance post-gadolinium with fat suppression image).

go unrecognized because symptoms are commonly mild and neurologic deficits are absent (**Fig. 21.6**). Orbital inflammation is common, and forehead swelling and tenderness can also occur. Patients typically experience headache and low-grade fever. Progressive enlargement can also cause symptoms of increased intracranial pressure.

- ***Subdural empyema:*** The presenting symptoms of subdural empyema are reflective of increased intracranial pressure, meningeal irritation, and cerebritis, and include increased headache, fever, neck stiffness, leukocytosis, and signs of localized meningeal inflammation. If the empyema is located in the frontal lobe, clinical presentation can be subtle, including changes in personality or mood and focal neurologic symptoms.[12] Patients are frequently febrile, demonstrating meningismus and systemic signs of infection. As the subdural empyema expands, symptoms and signs of cortical ischemia and infarctions develop. Seizures occur in 25 to 80% of cases and are more common in subdural empyema than with other intracranial complications. More ominous findings can evolve rapidly and include depressed level of consciousness, focal neurologic deficits or cranial nerve palsies, hemiparesis, bradycardia, hypertension, papilledema, nausea, vomiting, and septic shock. Rapid progression is a hallmark of subdural empyema and underscores the importance of prompt intervention. Subdural empyema is a true neurosurgical emergency.
- ***Brain abscess:*** A clinical diagnosis of a brain abscess is difficult because of the lack of focal neurologic signs caused by frontal lobe processes. Mental dullness, lethargy, and headache should raise the index of suspicion. In one series, only 57% of patients with a brain abscess had an altered level of consciousness, 26% had cranial nerve palsies, and 19% ultimately died.[5] Death will occur quickly if the abscess ruptures into the ventricular system.

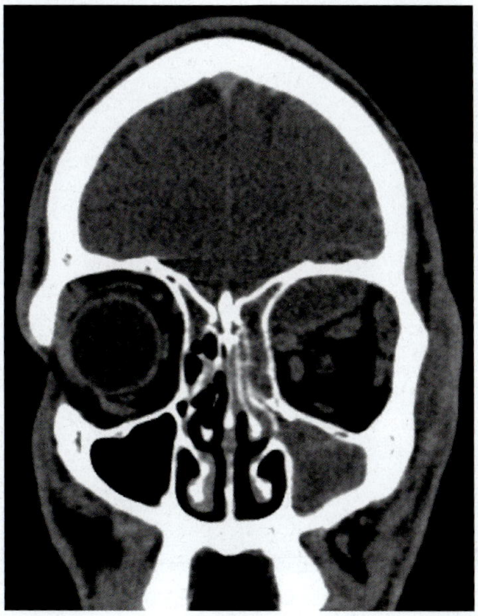

Fig. 21.6 Left superomedial subperiosteal abscess and adjacent left epidural abscess secondary to left-sided acute sinusitis (coronal computed tomography scan).

Diagnostic Workup

Orbital Infections

A clinical examination should test for changes in visual acuity, pupillary reactivity, and extraocular motion. Diminished pupillary reflexes may be not seen until significant visual loss has occurred. The ability to distinguish colors may be used as a guide to disease progression; increasing intraorbital pressure causes loss of red/green perception before visual acuity deteriorates. The ease of examination and certainty of objective clinical findings play a major role in guiding management.

CT can be used to correctly stage orbital complications in most cases; several studies may be necessary to monitor the patient's clinical status. Coronal and axial images with bone and soft tissue windows obtained with and without intravenous contrast are necessary to provide accurate information concerning the extent of infection in and beyond the sinus cavities.

Most authors recommend CT when clinical evidence of periorbital infection is present (i.e., with exophthalmos and limited eye movement) or when there is failure to improve with antibiotics. Because disease can be more aggressive in pediatric patients, CT should be considered when clinical evidence of periorbital inflammation is present (preseptal orbital edema is a common finding in sinusitis, particularly in children).

CT is the single best study for differentiating a subperiosteal abscess from an orbital abscess (**Fig. 21.7**). However, it should not be relied on to determine the need for surgical intervention[7]; clinical examination remains the most important indicator for surgical intervention in patients with orbital complications from sinusitis.

As the infection spreads from the ethmoid sinus to the orbit, the orbital periosteum becomes inflamed, thickened, and elevated, with accumulation of an inflammatory phlegmon. On CT, this appears as an ill-defined, slightly enhanced mass on the sinus and orbital sides of the lamina papyracea. It is limited laterally by the periosteum; however, in more advanced cases, it emerges with a thickened and enhanced medial rectus muscle, which is displaced laterally. CT findings of low-attenuation material surrounded by an enhancing rim suggest an abscess rather than a phlegmon, although the distinction between these two states can be difficult given the continuum existing between them.

On occasion, CT scans can be misleading, suggesting an abscess when in fact inflammatory edema is present. Additionally, CT scans have been found to correlate with surgical findings in only 84% of orbital complications of sinusitis, and can miss up to 50% of intracranial compartment complications.[6,13]

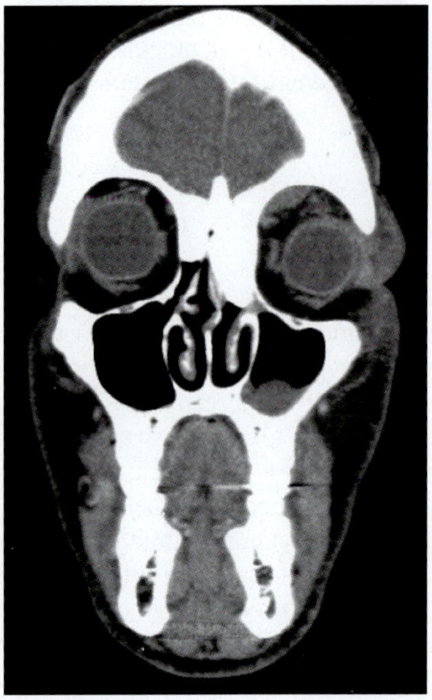

Fig. 21.7 Left superolateral subperiosteal abscess secondary to frontal sinusitis from an outflow obstruction from a large fibro-osseous lesion (coronal computed tomography scan).

Intracranial Complications

Cultures of purulent drainage, abscess fluid, and bone removed in surgery should be sent for Gram stain and anaerobic and aerobic cultures. A histologic examination of specimens for fungal invasion should be obtained urgently in immunocompromised or ketoacidotic patients when invasive fungal sinusitis is suspected.

The risk of brain herniation outweighs the diagnostic benefits of lumbar puncture in most intracranial complications.[4] As such, lumbar puncture is indicated primarily to rule out meningitis. If a lumbar puncture is considered, radiologic studies are mandatory prior to the procedure, and caution must be exercised to prevent uncal herniation.

Radiographic imaging should be done in all patients who are suspected of having subdural empyema. MRI is more sensitive in showing parenchymal abnormalities such as abscess, but cranial CT is often done first because of its widespread availability and the need for a rapid diagnosis. CT is also the test of choice for visualizing the paranasal sinuses and associated bony abnormalities. Some patients may need to be followed up with serial imaging studies to monitor the progression of infection and to determine the timing of surgical intervention.

MRI is superior to CT for identifying marrow-space abnormalities such as edema or osteomyelitis, inflammation of the meninges, extra-axial empyemas, and early cerebritis. However, an MRI study takes longer than CT scanning, is sensitive to motion artifact, and requires either general anesthesia in younger children or sedation in older children. One study found that for patients with intracranial complications, meningitis was the most common diagnosis, and MRI was more accurate (97%) in determining the diagnosis than CT (87%) or clinical findings (82%).[14] CT or MRI may also help in identifying rare vascular complications from sinusitis (**Fig. 21.8**).

In subdural empyema, T1-weighted MRIs show mass effect in hypointense areas of purulence, which are hyperintense on T2-weighted images. The abscess usually has a hyperintense rim on noncontrast T1-weighted images.

MRI and magnetic resonance venogram are very sensitive studies for demonstrating CST. Filling defects may be seen on contrast CT, although false-negative scans can occur until late in the disease. The superior ophthalmic

A

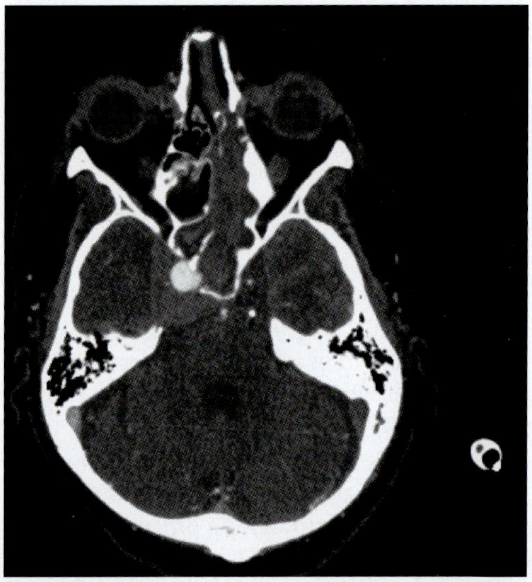

B

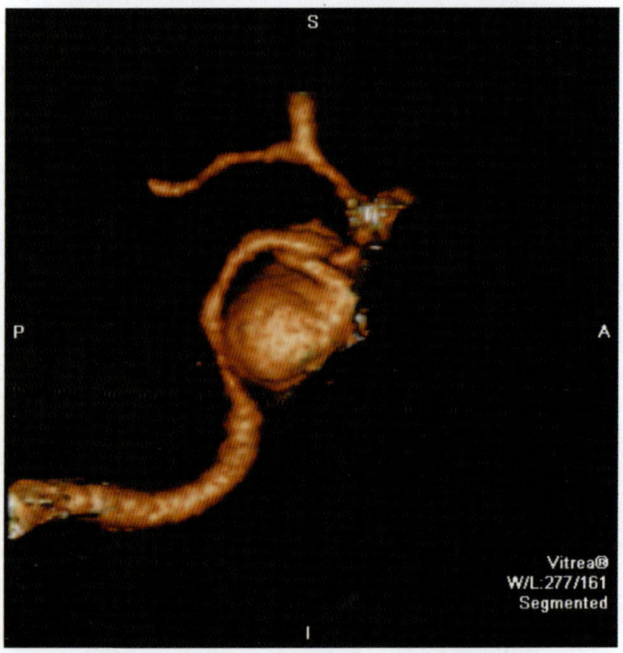

Fig. 21.8 Right carotid pseudoaneurysm secondary to acute sinusitis involving the sphenoid sinus. **(A)** An axial-enhanced computed tomography (CT) scan with dilation of the carotid artery. **(B)** A sagittal CT angiogram of the pseudoaneurysm.

vein is typically enlarged or thrombosed, and extraocular muscles can be markedly larger from venous engorgement. Orbital venogram is the most sensitive study, especially for chronic CST, but is uncommonly performed because of the wide availability of MRI.

Treatment of Complications

Orbital Infections

After admission to the hospital, an evaluation by otorhinolaryngology and ophthalmology should be undertaken, and an antimicrobial agent that crosses the blood-brain barrier and has appropriate coverage for the appropriate organisms (see previous) (including beta-lactamase–producing strains) should be chosen. Antibiotics should be adjusted according to culture results. The most commonly recommended empiric initial parenteral antibiotic choices for severe sinusitis with suspected orbital or intracranial extension are ceftriaxone, a third-generation cephalosporin with good blood-brain penetration, or ampicillin/sulbactam.[15] Aminoglycosides are still considered first-line agents for Gram-negative serious infections, whereas vancomycin may play an increasing role for severe sinusitis with suppurative complications due to resistant *S. aureus* or highly resistant *S. pneumoniae*.

Adjunctive therapy with topical vasoconstrictors may be useful. Corticosteroid therapy is not recommended in patients with orbital infections.

The result of a CT scan should not be the sole factor used to make treatment decisions, as CT scan documentation of sinus complications may be inexact. Rather, CT findings should supplement clinical evaluation in the decision-making process.

In a patient with a large, well-defined abscess, complete ophthalmoplegia, or impairment of vision, prompt operative drainage of the paranasal sinuses and abscess is indicated. The progression of ocular findings—particularly diminishing vision—also deserves prompt surgical exploration. The following criteria for surgery have been suggested in the literature: abscess formation, visual acuity <20/60, progression of disease for more than 24 hours, and lack of resolution on antibiotics for 48 to 72 hours.[3]

When planning surgery, clear communication between the otorhinolaryngologist–head and neck surgeon and the ophthalmologist is critical and often time sensitive. Indeed, the intraoperative availability of an ophthalmology colleague is extremely helpful and is encouraged, particularly when dealing with an orbital abscess.

The objectives of the surgical management of a subperiosteal or orbital abscess include draining the orbital collection, addressing the offending sinuses, and obtaining intraoperative cultures. In addition, decompression of one or more orbital walls may be necessary if intraoperative orbital pressures continue to be elevated despite an adequate drainage procedure. Involved sinuses can be drained by frontal trephination, external or endoscopic ethmoidectomy, sphenoidotomy, or antrostomy. The surgeon should weigh the advantages and disadvantages of the various surgical approaches to achieve the previously-stated objectives.

Subperiosteal Abscess

Most subperiosteal abscesses require surgical drainage. Controversy exists about the optimal initial management of medial subperiosteal abscesses in children. Some favor prompt drainage of the abscess, whereas others recommend a trial of intravenous antibiotics, with surgery reserved for those who do not respond to medical treatment and in whom a medial subperiosteal abscess is confirmed by CT.[16,17]

Conventionally, a subperiosteal abscess is drained via an external Lynch incision; an ethmoidectomy is performed at the same time. More recently, however, successful drainage of a subperiosteal abscess has been accomplished endoscopically with less morbidity and superior outcomes. The main limitation of the endoscopic approach is related to the bleeding potential of acutely inflamed mucosa, which may compromise visualization, especially in the confines of a pediatric nose. Even for experienced endoscopists, significant bleeding and poor visualization may compromise the safety and completeness of the procedure. Measures to improve hemostasis and enhance visualization may not always be successful, and the surgeon should be prepared to convert to an external approach if the need should arise.

Orbital Abscess

Surgical approaches to drain medial orbital abscesses can be divided into open, transnasal endoscopic, or combined approaches. The traditional approach for draining medial orbital collections has been through an external ethmoidectomy incision and orbitotomy. An incision of the periorbita is usually necessary to drain an orbital abscess. This should be done using a sharp sickle knife, with the tip of the knife remaining superficial; the incision is made from posterior to anterior, and usually affords good drainage of most extraconal abscesses. Drainage of intraconal abscesses is best achieved through a combined approach and ideally includes the active participation of an ophthalmologic colleague. The intraoperative measurement of orbital pressures is helpful and often dictates the extent of orbital decompression.

Intracranial Complications

Medical therapy begins with admission to the hospital, where the patient should be placed on high-dose intravenous antibiotics that cross the blood-brain barrier (e.g., third-generation cephalosporin plus metronidazole).[4] As noted previously, culture results should guide antibiotic therapy. Anticonvulsant medications may be started prophylactically in consultation with neurology colleagues, as the incidence of seizures in intracranial complications is high. Neurosurgical consultation is required in patients with intracranial complications to help coordinate the medical and surgical treatment plan.

The use of steroids is controversial; however, they can be used in cases where severe edema of the brain is suspected.[4] Corticosteroids have been advocated by some clinicians for patients with acute clinical deterioration of significant cerebral edema, whereas others do not advocate their use. Steroids may interfere with antibiotic penetration and host immunologic response and inhibit capsule formation around abscesses.[4] The addition of intravenous steroids seemed to show little effect on early or late mortality and the incidence of abscess formation in animal studies of brain abscess.[18]

With few exceptions, once intracranial complications occur and there is an intracranial infection, medical therapy alone is insufficient. Timely surgical intervention should address both the intracranial complication and the underlying sinus infection. The optimal surgical procedure for sinus infection depends on the sinus involved, as well as the neurosurgical approach. Sinuses can be addressed by frontal trephination, external or intranasal ethmoidectomy, sphenoidotomy, or antrostomy. In the past, sinus infection was usually addressed by an external approach. However, with the current understanding of sinusitis, frontal and other sinuses are being approached through endoscopic procedures with increasing frequency.[19,20]

A surgical approach should be chosen that provides egress for the pathogens trapped in the sinus and enhances the likelihood for improved sinus drainage after the acute infection has subsided. Simultaneous performance of neurosurgical and rhinologic procedures decreases the rate of neurosurgical and sinus re-exploration and prevents further seeding of intracranial sites from the infected sinuses. Extensive surgical widening of all affected sinuses, rather than limited drainage procedures, also appears to decrease the need for re-exploration of the sinuses.

If a patient's condition does not permit an extensive procedure, then targeted drainage of the acute infection with treatment of the intracranial complication should be the goal. If craniotomy is performed, the posterior wall of the frontal sinus should be inspected from behind. Cranialization with obliteration of the frontal recess may be indicated where extensive destruction of the posterior table has occurred.

Osteomyelitis

Management of acute osteomyelitis consists of surgical drainage and antimicrobial therapy. Surgical debridement is needed infrequently after a properly extended course of parenteral antimicrobial therapy. Consistent with osteomyelitis in long bones, antibiotic therapy for a minimum of 6 weeks is recommended.[1] Monitoring for further possible intracranial complications is warranted.

Chronic osteomyelitis is most often a result of inadequate treatment of acute osteomyelitis. The symptoms are similar to those of acute osteomyelitis but are more often less severe and sometimes intermittent. CT should be performed and gallium bone scanning may contribute to the diagnosis by indicating the amount of inflammatory activity in the bone. Treatment should consist of aggressive debridement of necrotic bone and long-term culture-directed intravenous antibiotics.

True osteomyelitis with infection, necrosis, and erosion of the frontal bone requires wide debridement to bleeding viable bone margin. In addition, prolonged intravenous antibiotic use, usually for 4 to 8 weeks, is usually recommended. The end point of antibiotic therapy can be determined by serial gallium scans, which become negative with the resolution of active infection. Reconstructive surgery should be delayed until the infection is completely resolved.

Meningitis

Clinical judgment should be used to determine whether the initial treatment of sinusitis in cases of meningitis should be medical or surgical. Intravenous antibiotics with cerebrospinal fluid (CSF) penetration are critical in either situation, and should be started immediately. Most institutions recommend a third-generation intravenous cephalosporin and metronidazole for empiric therapy. The use of vancomycin is controversial because of variable CSF penetration.

Intravenous steroids have been shown to help reduce the incidence of hearing loss from meningitis-related otitis media, especially in the younger population, but the benefits of steroid use in meningitis of sinogenic origin remain unproved and controversial.

If medical therapy fails to improve the patient's condition in 24 to 48 hours, progressive surgical intervention for the sinus disease should be considered.

Epidural Abscess

Treatment is most often successful and consists of drainage of the abscess by craniotomy or the transfrontal route. There is commonly a communication between the abscess cavity and the frontal sinus leading to cranialization of the sinus but, in some cases, sinus drainage can be re-established and the integrity of the sinus can be maintained. Uncomplicated epidural abscess is drained by burr holes. The dura should not be opened, as this will break the protective barrier and allow for further extension of infection.

Subdural Empyema

Surgical management of subdural empyemas is an integral part of therapy and should be undertaken without delay. Isolated medical management has been successful in only a few case reports.[21] The goals of surgical intervention are decompression of the brain and complete evacuation of the purulence. There is controversy in the neurosurgical literature regarding preferred surgical intervention: burr hole versus craniotomy.[6] Several authors have advocated the use of craniotomy, which they contend allows for more complete drainage of the collection.[22–24] Bannister et al. report a mortality rate three times higher with burr holes than with a craniotomy because of undiagnosed extensions of the subdural empyema.[23] In addition, some patients treated with a burr hole require additional surgery or conversion to craniotomy.[6,21,24,25] However, other authors have reported more favorable results with use of burr holes, especially when combined with high-definition CT to help localize the abscess.[21] Currently, both procedures are acceptable, and the choice of procedure should be made in consultation with a neurosurgeon. Multiple burr holes with surgical irrigation and decompression craniectomy are other surgical options.[6]

In addition to drainage of intracranial purulence, definitive management of the infected sinuses should be undertaken, preferably at the same time as the empyema drainage. The choice of surgical approach depends on the involved sinus. The development of endoscopic sinus surgery has made it the most popular otorhinolaryngology intervention in subdural empyema in recent years.[14]

Brain Abscess

Treatment of brain abscess is controversial and depends on the patient's condition, the maturity of the abscess wall, and the location in the brain. Some abscesses may resolve with medical therapy, whereas others require CT-guided or open drainage.[4] Generally, it seems preferable to leave the abscess wall intact and treat by local excision or aspiration and drainage. Some have found no difference between the two techniques; Rosenblum et al. report no difference in mortality rates,[26] but more recently, repeated aspiration has been favored.[27] The desired end result is decompression of the mass effect. Medical treatment alone can be attempted for abscesses that are small, multiple, and located in surgically inaccessible areas or in the cerebritis stage, and if the patient is neurologically stable.[27]

Another option is immediate excision of the abscess via a craniotomy to reduce intracranial pressure and decrease the chance of recurrence from residual abscess. Total excision can be used for a large, well encapsulated abscess that does not involve the primary cortical areas or in cases of failed aspiration.

Cavernous Sinus Thrombosis

Treatment of CST consists of intravenous antibiotics, drainage of the offending sinus, and selective anticoagulation. Early use of an anticoagulant may prevent the spread of thrombosis and decrease the mortality and morbidity associated with CST.[10,28] One retrospective study showed that the use of therapeutic doses of heparin reduces mortality in selected cases of CST.[10] Potential complications of using anticoagulants are bleeding from hemorrhagic venous infarcts and from the intracavernous portion of the carotid artery.[10] Steroids are indicated for pituitary insufficiency. In CST, the infected sinuses should be drained surgically but the optimal timing of the procedure is unknown. The dura should not be opened, as this will open the protective barrier and allow for further extension of infection.[4]

Outcomes

In the preantibiotic era, orbital complications led to meningitis in 17% and blindness in 20% of cases.[29] The advent of antibiotic use has not changed the incidence of sinusitis, but it has resulted in decreased frequency of complications. For example, the incidence of sinogenic brain abscess—which may have accounted for up to 32% of all brain abscesses in the preantibiotic era—has now dropped to ~13%.[5]

With aggressive neurosurgical and otorhinolaryngologic drainage, mortality rates for intracranial complications have dropped.[1] Mortality from intracranial sinusitis-associated infection in the pre-CT era was once as high as 66%,[30] but in recent years has decreased to 2 to 7%.[4,12] Nevertheless, a subdural abscess still confers a particularly poor prognosis. Although the incidence of meningitis has declined over time, mortality remains high; in one large series of patients, mortality was 45% despite aggressive treatment.[5] Before the availability of antibiotics, subdural empyemas were almost always fatal, even with surgical drainage; antimicrobials have since decreased the mortality rate to 5.6 to 41%.[30] Mortality from CST remains greater that 40%.[10]

Conclusion

Despite advances in diagnostic and therapeutic modalities, complications of sinusitis still occur, and mortality from sinogenic intracranial complications remains significant. Awareness of potential complications can lead to early recognition of the disease process, and may in time help lessen the morbidity and mortality associated with these complications.

References

1. Goldberg AN, Oroszlan G, Anderson TD. Complications of frontal sinusitis and their management. Otolaryngol Clin North Am 2001;34(1):211–225
2. Jackson K, Baker SR. Clinical implications of orbital cellulitis. Laryngoscope 1986;96(5):568–574
3. Schramm VL Jr, Curtin HD, Kennerdell JS. Evaluation of orbital cellulitis and results of treatment. Laryngoscope 1982;92(7 Pt 1):732–738
4. Clayman GL, Adams GL, Paugh DR, Koopmann CF Jr. Intracranial complications of paranasal sinusitis: a combined institutional review. Laryngoscope 1991;101(3):234–239
5. Singh B, Van Dellen J, Ramjettan S, Maharaj TJ. Sinogenic intracranial complications. J Laryngol Otol 1995;109(10):945–950
6. Nathoo N, Nadvi SS, van Dellen JR, Gouws E. Intracranial subdural empyemas in the era of computed tomography: a review of 699 cases. Neurosurgery 1999;44(3):529–535, discussion 535–536
7. Patt BS, Manning SC. Blindness resulting from orbital complications of sinusitis. Otolaryngol Head Neck Surg 1991;104(6): 789–795
8. Schramm VL, Myers EN, Kennerdell JS. Orbital complications of acute sinusitis: evaluation, management, and outcome. Otolaryngology 1978;86(2):ORL221–ORL230
9. Chandler JR, Langenbrunner DJ, Stevens ER. The pathogenesis of orbital complications in acute sinusitis. Laryngoscope 1970;80(9):1414–1428
10. Southwick FS, Richardson EP Jr, Swartz MN. Septic thrombosis of the dural venous sinuses. Medicine (Baltimore) 1986;65(2):82–106
11. Feder HM Jr, Cates KL, Cementina AM. Pott puffy tumor: a serious occult infection. Pediatrics 1987;79(4):625–629
12. Jones NS, Walker JL, Bassi S, Jones T, Punt J. The intracranial complications of rhinosinusitis: can they be prevented? Laryngoscope 2002;112(1):59–63
13. Clary RA, Cunningham MJ, Eavey RD. Orbital complications of acute sinusitis: comparison of computed tomography scan and surgical findings. Ann Otol Rhinol Laryngol 1992;101(7):598–600
14. Younis RT, Anand VK, Davidson B. The role of computed tomography and magnetic resonance imaging in patients with sinusitis with complications. Laryngoscope 2002;112(2):224–229
15. Manning SC. Medical management of nasosinus infectious and inflammatory disease. In: Cummings CW, Flint PW, Haughey BH, et al., eds. Otolaryngology: Head & Neck Surgery. 4th ed. New York: Mosby; 2003: 52
16. Herrmann BW, Forsen JW Jr. Simultaneous intracranial and orbital complications of acute rhinosinusitis in children. Int J Pediatr Otorhinolaryngol 2004;68(5):619–625
17. Brown CL, Graham SM, Griffin MC, et al. Pediatric medial subperiosteal orbital abscess: medical management where possible. Am J Rhinol 2004;18(5):321–327
18. Schroeder KA, McKeever PE, Schaberg DR, Hoff JT. Effect of dexamethasone on experimental brain abscess. J Neurosurg 1987;66(2):264–269
19. Lusk RP, Tychsen L, Park TS. Complications of sinusitis. In: Lusk RP, ed. Pediatric Sinusitis. New York: Raven Press; 1992: 127–146
20. Manning SC. Endoscopic management of medial subperiosteal orbital abscess. Arch Otolaryngol Head Neck Surg 1993;119(7): 789–791
21. Bok AP, Peter JC. Subdural empyema: burr holes or craniotomy? A retrospective computerized tomography-era analysis of treatment in 90 cases. J Neurosurg 1993;78(4):574–578
22. Feuerman T, Wackym PA, Gade GF, Dubrow T. Craniotomy improves outcome in subdural empyema. Surg Neurol 1989;32(2): 105–110
23. Bannister G, Williams B, Smith S. Treatment of subdural empyema. J Neurosurg 1981;55(1):82–88
24. Wackym PA, Canalis RF, Feuerman T. Subdural empyema of otorhinological origin. J Laryngol Otol 1990;104(2):118–122
25. Tsai YD, Chang WN, Shen CC, et al. Intracranial suppuration: a clinical comparison of subdural empyemas and epidural abscesses. Surg Neurol 2003;59(3):191–196, discussion 196
26. Rosenblum ML, Hoff JT, Norman D, Weinstein PR, Pitts L. Decreased mortality from brain abscesses since advent of computerized tomography. J Neurosurg 1978;49(5):658–668
27. Yang SY, Zhao CS. Review of 140 patients with brain abscess. Surg Neurol 1993;39(4):290–296
28. Levine SR, Twyman RE, Gilman S. The role of anticoagulation in cavernous sinus thrombosis. Neurology 1988;38(4):517–522
29. Gamble RC. Acute inflammation of the orbit in children. Arch Ophthalmol 1933;10:483–497
30. Small M, Dale BA. Intracranial suppuration 1968-1982—a 15 year review. Clin Otolaryngol Allied Sci 1984;9(6):315–321

22 Office Rhinology and Surgical Biomaterials

Richard R. Orlandi and Peter H. Hwang

Much of rhinologic teaching focuses on surgical techniques. Yet the majority of care delivered to patients takes place in the office, not in the operating room. Beyond simple evaluation and medical management of patients with nasal and sinus complaints, several investigations and interventions can be employed in the office. These include diagnostic nasal endoscopy, olfactory assessment, allergy testing and therapy, management of epistaxis, biopsy and culture of the nose and sinuses, endoscopic debridement (including minor revision and polypectomy), and inferior turbinate reduction. More recently, balloon dilation technologies have also been adapted for office use. Pre- and postoperative care for patients undergoing endoscopic sinus surgery is also based in the office and is a critical component in the success of sinus surgery.[1]

The array of equipment available in the office may vary considerably from practice to practice and may include in-office radiologic imaging and an operating suite with general anesthesia capabilities. This chapter nevertheless focuses on practices readily available to the rhinologist with a modest set of instruments and nonspecialized office facilities. A substantial portion of the care performed in the office, such as epistaxis management and postoperative sinus surgery care, involves biomaterials and these are discussed as well.

Anesthesia for Office Procedures

Topical anesthesia and decongestion of the nasal cavity facilitates a thorough and more comfortable examination for both patient and rhinologist. Topical anesthesia is readily available, easy to deliver, and lacks significant side effects. Its use minimizes the patient's discomfort and, by doing so, facilitates the patient's compliance with current and future examinations and therefore improves the thoroughness of care.

Lidocaine or tetracaine may be used topically for anesthesia. Lidocaine has a shorter onset of action whereas tetracaine has a longer duration of anesthesia. Lidocaine is typically delivered in a 4% solution whereas tetracaine is delivered in a 2% solution. To provide vasoconstriction, phenylephrine is typically added to the anesthetic solution. This combination is typically sufficient for diagnostic nasal endoscopy and minor nasal procedures. Where more anesthesia is required, especially in focal areas, the same topical anesthesia and vasoconstrictor combination can be delivered on a cotton-tipped applicator. Lidocaine (1%) with epinephrine (1:100,000 or 1:200,000) can be injected into these areas as well, using a 25- or 27-gauge needle. Benzocaine should be used with caution as a topical anesthetic agent, as its use may be associated with a risk of developing methemoglobinemia, especially in pediatric patients.[2]

Another useful adjunct that delivers a large field of anesthesia and vasoconstriction is a transpalatal injection of the pterygopalatine fossa. This anesthetic block targets the sphenopalatine ganglion as well as the sphenopalatine artery where it emerges from the pterygopalatine fossa to enter the nasal cavity. The greater palatine foramen can typically be found 16 mm lateral to the midsagittal plane of the palate, near the junction between the second and third molars.[3] A 25-gauge needle is bent at 2.5 cm and inserted transorally into the greater palatine foramen to the bend. This measurement places the tip of the needle safely within the pterygopalatine fossa without the risk for violation or infiltration of the orbital apex. After withdrawing slightly to ensure that the needle is not within a vessel, 1.5 mL of a 1% lidocaine solution with 1:100,000 epinephrine is then injected slowly. This injection provides anesthesia and vasoconstriction to the posterior septum, middle turbinate, sphenoid sinus, and posterior ethmoid cavity, areas often poorly reached by topical spray. A transpalatal injection is quite effective in the diagnosis and temporizing of posterior epistaxis as well.[4]

Basic Equipment for Office Rhinology

Nasal endoscopes are the mainstay of an office rhinology practice. Visualization with a nasal speculum is limited to the anterior nasal cavity only, whereas nasal endoscopes enable the rhinologist to visualize the entire nasal cavity for both diagnostic and therapeutic purposes. Rigid endoscopes are available in various diameters and viewing angles. A 4-mm diameter, 30-degree scope is the workhorse of the practice, used in adult diagnostic endoscopies and most procedures. A 0-degree scope allows for the visualization of the nasopharynx and work within the sphenoid sinus and also facilitates procedures where angled visualization is not necessary. The frontal recess and maxillary sinuses can be visualized with the 30-degree scope, but it is often advantageous to use a 45- or even 70-degree scope. For narrower noses, including pediatric patients, 2.7-mm diameter scopes are helpful. Because of the scopes' narrower diameter, the field of view is smaller and less illuminated, and the scopes are less robust. More recently available 3.0-mm endoscopes offer an attractive compromise between scope size and optical quality.

Flexible fiberoptic nasal and nasopharyngeal scopes enable visualization of anatomy posterior and superior to significant septal deviations. They are also helpful in visualizing the interior of the postoperative maxillary sinus and, to a lesser degree, the frontal sinus. Flexible scopes require the use of both hands and therefore are largely limited to diagnostic uses, where no additional instrumentation is required. Specialized flexible scopes with working channels for suction or delivery of topical medications are available and may be useful in specialized situations.

The light source and cord should be sufficiently bright to illuminate the nasal cavity and sinuses. For diagnostic endoscopy, lower powered light sources are acceptable, but for procedures where blood or secretions are often present, 150- or 300-W xenon light sources provide superior illumination. Although video components such as cameras and display screens are not required for performing office rhinologic procedures, their use makes the procedures more comfortable and ergonomic for the rhinologist (**Fig. 22.1**).

Avoiding neck and shoulder problems may provide a propitious future return on investment. Another advantage of video monitors is the ability to display images to patients and family members, which can enhance their understanding of the clinical condition and enhance participation in treatment decision making (**Fig. 22.2**). Furthermore, digital image archiving is now possible, which allows for server-based storage of digital still or movie files. A patient's prior endoscopic exams can be readily accessed for comparison to the current examination. This capability is particularly valuable in longitudinal monitoring of patients treated for sinonasal neoplasms or polyposis.

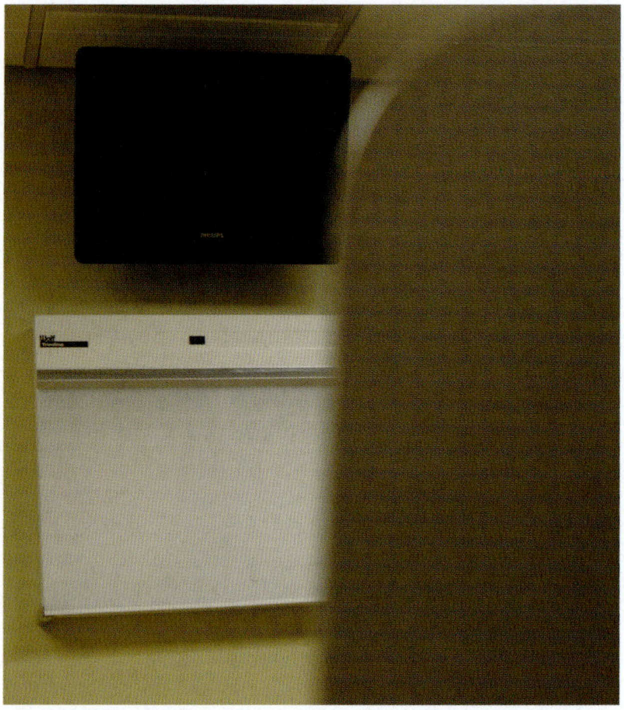

Fig. 22.2 A second video screen in the examination room across from the patient examination chair facilitates understanding and participation.

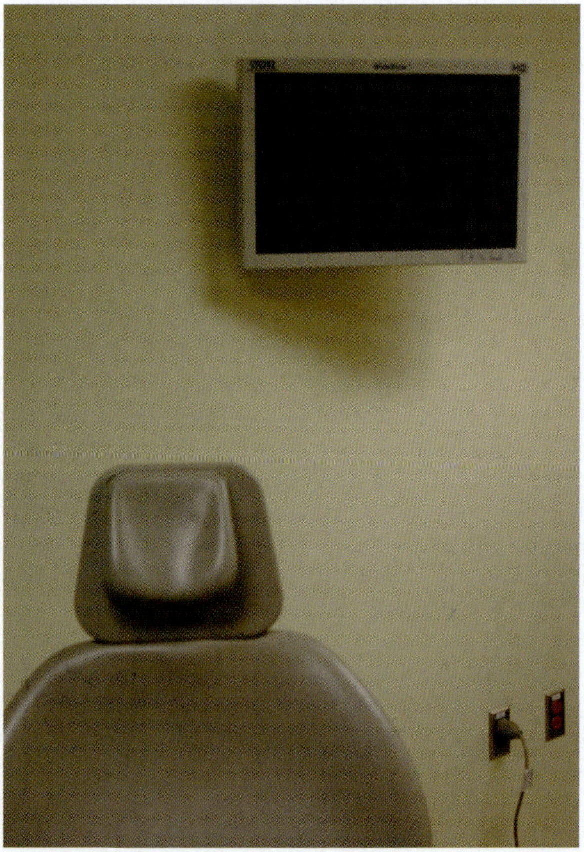

Fig. 22.1 Office examination room video screen ergonomically placed behind the patient for the rhinologist's view.

Suction cannulas with a strong suction source are necessary for removing secretions during examination and for assisting in debridements following surgery. Straight Frazier cannulas and curved olive-tipped cannulas can reach most areas within the nose and sinuses. Malleable suction cannulas may further facilitate removal of secretions and debris from the maxillary, sphenoid, and frontal sinuses.

Common Rhinologic Office Procedures

With a basic set of instruments and topical anesthetics, a diagnostic visualization of the nasal cavity and sinuses is possible. Additions to the basic instrumentation significantly broaden the range of services that the rhinologist can provide to patients in the office, from postoperative care following endoscopic sinus surgery to polypectomy and turbinate reduction. Olfactory and gustatory testing as well as allergy management are other possible additions.

Diagnostic Nasal Endoscopy

Nasal endoscopy for diagnosis and evaluation is the foundation of rhinologic care in the office. A thorough nasal endoscopy provides information about the inflammatory state of the mucosa, the nature and amount of secretions, and the presence of mucosal abnormalities such as polyps or other lesions.

A diagnostic nasal endoscopy is classically described as occurring in three passes (**Fig. 22.3**). The first pass proceeds from anterior to posterior along the floor of the nasal cavity. During this first pass, the external and internal nasal valve is evaluated, the inferior portion of the nasal septum is examined to the posterior choana, and the nasopharynx is visualized, including adenoidal tissue that may contribute to nasal obstruction and the patency of the eustachian tube orifice. Secretions from the sinuses may be seen in the area of the eustachian tube orifice; secretions draining posterosuperior to the orifice typically arise from the posterior ethmoid or sphenoid sinuses, whereas secretions anteroinferior to the orifice usually originate from the anterior ethmoid, maxillary, or frontal sinuses. If an angled scope is used for the endoscopy, the inferior meatus can be visualized during withdrawal of the scope. Here the condition of lacrimal secretions draining through Hasner's valve can be assessed, as well as the presence of an inferior meatal antrostomy.

The second pass of nasal endoscopy proceeds from anterior to posterior between the middle and inferior turbinates. Conditions affecting the middle turbinate, such as paradoxical shape, lateralization, resection, or pneumatization (concha bullosa) are noted. The scope is passed posteriorly, and guided medial and inferior to the middle

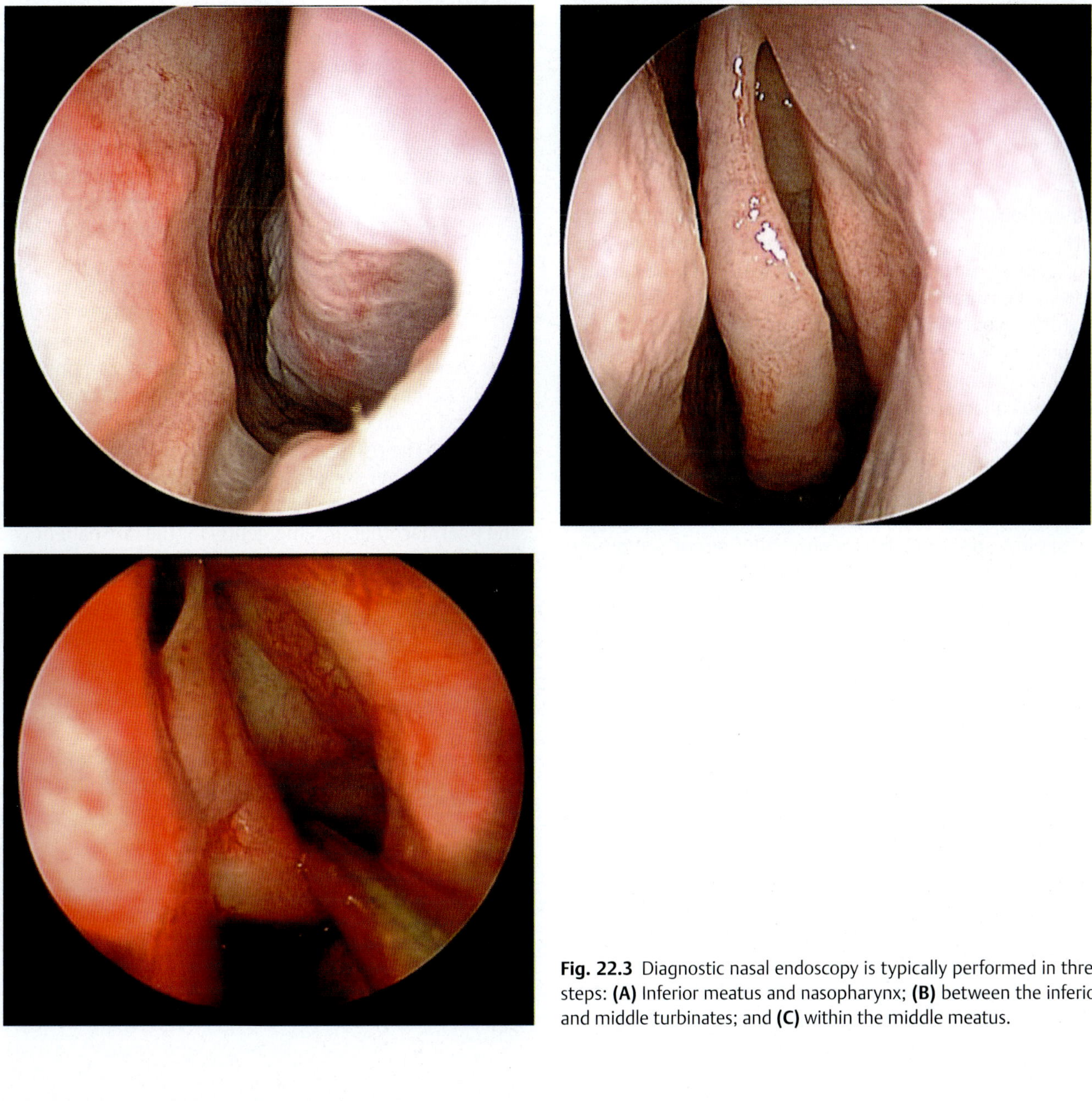

A B C

Fig. 22.3 Diagnostic nasal endoscopy is typically performed in three steps: **(A)** Inferior meatus and nasopharynx; **(B)** between the inferior and middle turbinates; and **(C)** within the middle meatus.

and superior turbinates, to the sphenoethmoidal recess. Within the sphenoethmoidal recess, the sphenoid ostium may be visualized, in addition to the presence of edema, polyps, or abnormal secretions. A thorough evaluation of the sphenoethmoidal recess, as well as the olfactory cleft, may require the use of narrower scopes.

The third pass is performed retrograde, immediately following the second pass, with introduction of the scope into the middle meatus. The scope is rolled under the middle turbinate and withdrawn from posterior to anterior. While passing through the middle meatus, the condition of the mucosa and secretions are noted. In a patient who has not undergone previous surgery, the third pass often does not permit full visualization of the middle meatus, or otherwise requires distraction of the middle turbinate medially, which may be painful. Additional topical or injected anesthesia in the middle meatus and root of the middle turbinate may facilitate examination. In patients who have previously undergone surgery, scarring between the middle turbinate and the lateral nasal wall, retained uncinate process, and the presence of mucus recirculation between the maxillary antrostomy and natural ostium are all assessed.

Olfactory Testing

Diminution of olfaction is a common complaint in patients with nasal and sinus conditions. Hyposmia and anosmia can cause significant impairment of quality of life parameters as measured by objective outcomes instruments, and thus the characterization of olfactory impairment can be an important aspect of the workup.[5] Assessment of these patients is facilitated by an objective measurement of the degree of olfactory impairment. Olfactory testing establishes the diagnosis and allows for an objective measurement of response to treatment. Testing methods include qualitative testing, which assesses the patient's ability to correctly discriminate and identify various odors; and threshold testing, which uses serial dilutions of a common odor, such as phenyl ethyl alcohol or n-butanol.[6] Some testing algorithms use both modalities for comprehensive assessment.[7] Both types of tests are available commercially and have validated norms for age and gender, both of which affect olfactory ability (Smell Identification Test, Sensonics, Inc., Haddon Heights, NJ; Sniffin' Sticks, Burghart Messtechnik, Wedel, Germany) (**Fig. 22.4**). These tests are readily available, are relatively inexpensive, and are well within the scope of the office rhinology practice. Dedicated olfactometers that can measure olfactory-evoked potentials are available in some research centers but are beyond the scope of the normal office practice.

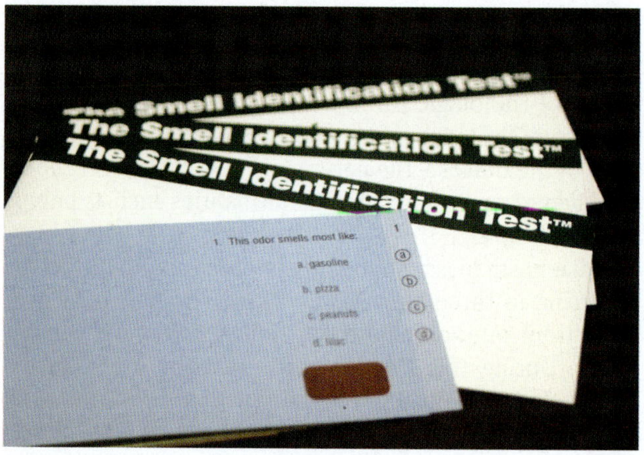

Fig. 22.4 Olfactory testing that uses scents released by scratching a portion of the card.

Allergy Testing and Management

Evaluating patients for inhalant allergies forms an important part of the office rhinology practice. Skin testing can be accomplished using a variety of techniques to identify possible etiologies of chronic nasal and sinus inflammation. Qualitative methods such as skin prick testing can be used to identify inhalant allergens and to assist in planning environmental avoidance and pharmacotherapy while more quantitative measures are used to plan desensitization therapy (**Fig. 22.5**).[8] Subcutaneous immunotherapy can be effective in controlling allergic components of sinonasal inflammation. Selected patients may also be candidates for sublingual immunotherapy, which offers the advantage of home administration.

Allergy testing and desensitization carry the risk of an anaphylactic reaction, and thus the rhinologist practicing the allergy testing must be prepared to manage allergy emergencies in the office. A recent review demonstrated 19 (0.13%) of 14,085 immunotherapy injections resulted in the need for an epinephrine injection, and there were no fatalities.[9] The risk of an anaphylactic reaction during testing is even lower. Nevertheless, the office providing allergy care must be able to provide oxygen, intravenous access, and pharmacotherapy emergently for the rare patient who

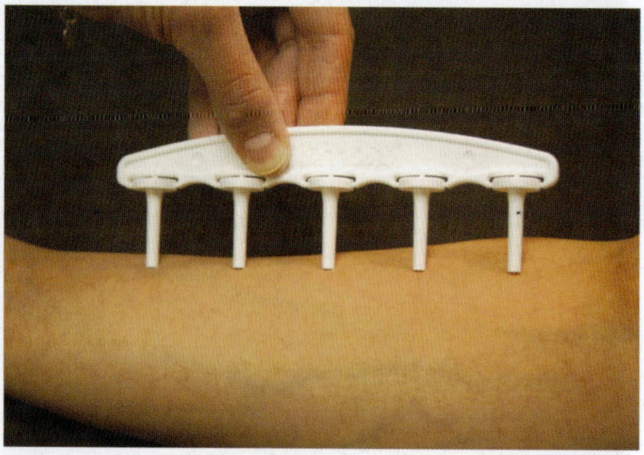

Fig. 22.5 Skin prick testing performed using a multiple-antigen delivery device.

Table 22.1 Basic Equipment and Medications Necessary to Treat Anaphylaxis in the Office

- Sphygmomanometer, stethoscope, and pulse oximeter
- Intravenous catheters and fluids
- Tourniquet to be placed above site of injection
- Oxygen
- Medications:
  - Lidocaine (1%) with epinephrine (1:100,000): injected at injection/testing site
  - Epinephrine (1:1000): injected intramuscularly, subcutaneously, or (slowly) intravenously
  - Diphenhydramine: injected intravenously or intramuscularly
  - Ranitidine: injected intravenously or intramuscularly
  - Hydrocortisone: injected intravenously or intramuscularly
  - Albuterol: inhaled
  - Heparin: injected intravenously or intramuscularly

develops an allergy emergency. **Table 22.1** lists medications and equipment that enable basic resuscitation in the event of an anaphylactic emergency.

Epistaxis Care

Minor nasal bleeding is a common complaint in a rhinologic practice. Several treatments are available for epistaxis and should be available in the rhinology office.[4] Cauterization of nasal bleeding using silver nitrate is readily and commonly performed for anterior epistaxis. Additional remedies usually involve dissolvable biomaterial or removable packing. Severe cases of bleeding may require more intensive or even operative treatment but most cases are effectively resolved in the office.

Endoscopic Biopsy and Culture

Sinonasal biopsy has a limited role outside of the operating room in the diagnosis of inflammatory rhinosinusitis, but it has an important role in determining the nature of focal lesions. Biopsy can typically take place following the sequential application of topical and injected anesthesia. A review of skull base imaging prior to biopsy is essential to rule out the presence of a skull base dehiscence and a possible sinonasal meningoencephalocele. Unilateral polypoid masses may be biopsied in the office to make the diagnosis of a possible inverted papilloma. Submucosal masses in young men with a history of epistaxis should not undergo biopsy in the office as these lesions are likely nasopharyngeal angiofibromas and severe bleeding may ensue. In cases where invasive fungal sinusitis is suspected, biopsy of the middle turbinate or any insensate area within the nasal cavity should be performed.[10]

Ciliary abnormalities can also be detected by tissue sampling in the office. In many cases, a full-thickness mucosal biopsy is not necessary, and instead, epithelial cells can be harvested by brushing the inferior turbinate. A simple cerumen curette may be used instead of a cytology brush to gently scrape the surface of the turbinate. Cells collected for ciliary ultrastructural analysis are typically fixed in a glutaraldehyde solution rather than the usual formalin solution used for conventional histology. The ciliary ultrastructure can then be examined by electron microscopy. Functional studies, such as ciliary beat frequency, require specialized stroboscopic imaging equipment that may not be as widely available.

An assessment of bacterial conditions within the sinuses can be difficult in patients who have not undergone previous surgery. Because of the bacterial colonization within the nasal cavity, swabbing the nasal vestibule or nasal cavity likely does not accurately reflect bacterial conditions within the sinuses. Aspiration of the maxillary sinus via an inferior meatal or canine fossa puncture (also known as a maxillary sinus "tap") accurately identifies pathogenic organisms within the sinus itself but is painful and poorly tolerated by patients. An ideal culture method would mimic the accuracy of a maxillary sinus tap but would minimize the discomfort and the risk of contamination from the oral or nasal cavities. Endoscopically directed cultures of the middle meatus appear to correlate well with maxillary sinus aspirates, especially in adults and when visibly purulent secretions are sampled. Correlation of middle meatal cultures with maxillary aspirates in children does not appear to be as robust as in adults.[11]

Following topical anesthesia and decongestion of the nasal cavity, a small swab on a wire (e.g., Calgiswab; Hardwood Products Company, Guilford, ME) or a sinus aspirator (e.g., Medtronic Tami Sinus Secretion Collector; Medtronic, Inc., Minneapolis, MN) is used to collect secretions. Use of sterile suction tubing allows for swabbing of the lumen of the tubing to obtain a specimen as well. Great care is taken to avoid contamination with nasal cavity or nasal vestibule secretions. Gentle retraction of the nasal ala with the endoscope allows for passage of a culture swab or suction with minimal risk of contamination by the nasal vestibule. The specimen is placed in an appropriate transport medium for aerobic and, if desired, anaerobic culture and delivered promptly to the microbiology laboratory. If fungal secretions are desired, yields will be higher if the secretions can be submitted in toto versus simply swabbed.

Care Before and Following Endoscopic Sinus Surgery

Success in surgically managing inflammatory sinus disease not only requires meticulous techniques in the operating room, but also careful and thorough endoscopic intervention both before and after surgery in the office setting.

One of the most important aspects of preoperative care is counseling and education of the patient regarding risks and benefits of endoscopic sinus surgery. For most patients, even those who are seeking revision surgery, the sinuses are a "black box." Their structure and function is poorly understood and a brief explanation of their anatomy and physiology will assist in the patient's understanding of their sinus disease and the upcoming surgery. Individuals have different methods of learning so the office should be able to provide verbal as well as visual or conceptual explanations of the sinuses. Written descriptions of the sinuses or simple verbal analogies ("the sinuses are like rooms off of a hallway. . .") complement information from pictures and models. Review of imaging with the patients also facilitates their understanding of the goals of the surgery and its risks due to the proximity of the orbit and brain. Realistic expectations of clinical outcome should be articulated by the surgeon, and a detailed discussion of concerns and questions should ensue.

Preoperative office care also includes minimizing mucosal inflammation prior to surgery. Failure to address infection and inflammation leads to increased bleeding from vasodilation that can hamper visualization during surgery. Preoperative diagnostic endoscopy guides preoperative anti-inflammatory and antimicrobial medical therapy. Antibiotics are typically indicated when infection is present preoperatively and are preferably culture-directed. Topical corticosteroids usually help reduce inflammation and in cases of significant preoperative inflammation such as nasal polyposis, systemic corticosteroids may be indicated as well. Optimizing surgical conditions with preoperative medical therapy can help to ensure that the surgeon is able to perform as thorough and safe a surgery as possible.

Postoperative examination and debridement are critical to manage the inflammation, blood deposits, and impaired mucus clearance immediately following sinus surgery. Postoperative care continues to manage mucosal inflammation, which is typically exacerbated by the traumatic insult of the surgery, and the appearance of the healing sinus cavity guides further medical management. Postoperative care can rarely fully compensate for a poor surgical technique but instead is intended to preserve the gains made intraoperatively from using meticulous surgical technique.

Prior to the examination and debridement, topical anesthesia and vasoconstriction are delivered by spraying, as described previously. As debris covering the mucosal surface is removed, it may be necessary to reapply the spray or to topically deliver additional medicine with a cotton applicator. An injection of anesthetics is rarely necessary but may be helpful when topical delivery is not sufficiently effective. Rarely, a patient cannot tolerate debridement under local anesthesia in the office. In these cases where the inability to debride and examine the cavity may put the success of the surgery at risk, debridement can be done in the operating room.

Aggressive debridement likely slows healing but gentle debridement throughout the sinuses can remove potential media for bacterial growth and also enhance access of topical medications. The authors' experience with saline nasal irrigation following endoscopic sinus surgery indicates that it reduces the time needed to debride the cavity. Nasal endoscopy during the postoperative period provides the opportunity to remove mucus and old blood from the cavity, remove fibrinous debris to prevent scarring and ostial narrowing, and tailor medical therapy. This is especially important in the narrow confines of the frontal recess where mucosal disruption and fibrin bridges more easily lead to scarring and stenosis.

Proper instrumentation is essential for adequate postoperative care. Additional instruments beyond nasal telescopes and suction are necessary to effectively debride the sinus and nasal cavity (**Fig. 22.6**). Straight and upbiting grasping

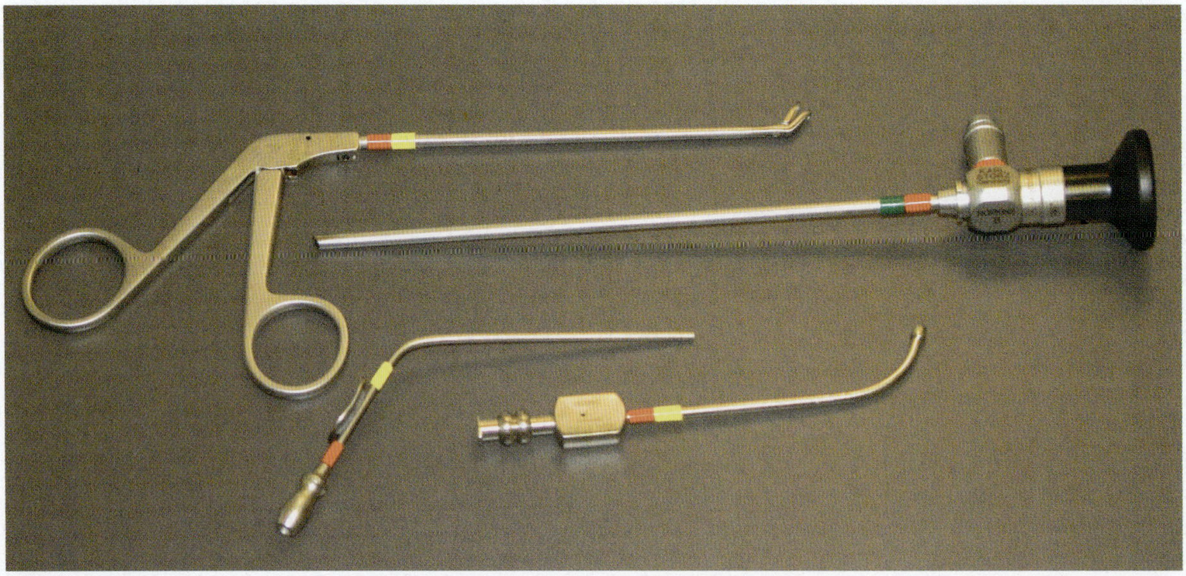

Fig. 22.6 Basic set of instruments for office rhinology, including nasal endoscopy (with a 30-degree nasal telescope), and simple debridement following sinus surgery.

forceps are the main instruments that facilitate crust removal in the ethmoid cavity. Although bayonet-shaped forceps can also be used, the nasal aperture's tendency to force the forceps together when placed farther posteriorly limits their use in the sinuses. Blakesley-type forceps are more precise and more easily manipulated alongside a nasal telescope. Through-cutting forceps and a sickle knife are also necessary to sharply cut or resect scar bands.

Debridement following frontal sinus surgery requires specialized curved-neck instruments. A 90-degree angled curette or probe can gently free crusts within the frontal recess, which can then be removed with grasping forceps, with an either vertical or horizontal opening. Through-cutting frontal sinus "giraffe"-type forceps are necessary to resect scar bands that may form in the frontal recess (**Fig. 22.7**).

The frequency of nasal endoscopy and debridement following endoscopic sinus surgery is individualized, depending on the control of the patient's perioperative inflammation and the predisposition to scarring.[1] There is no "cookbook" approach or schedule for patients postoperatively. Given the relatively poor quality of available evidence in debridement-related clinical outcomes, general guidelines and principles dictate the appropriate care.[12] As mentioned earlier, in our practices, saline irrigation is started on the first postoperative day and continued through the perioperative period to mechanically debride the nose and sinuses of stagnant mucus and old blood. This practice not only makes office debridement easier for the patient and physician alike, but also diminishes potential sources of infection and inflammatory mediators. Diagnostic nasal endoscopy guides the medical treatment of the patient postoperatively, which may include antibiotics, corticosteroids (topical or systemic), and other immune modulators.

Minor Revision of Endoscopic Sinus Surgery and Polypectomy

Given that the visualization, illumination, and instrumentation available in the office can readily replicate the conditions of the operating room, it is possible to transition to more advanced surgical procedures in the office once basic debridement has been mastered. With properly applied topical anesthesia and directed injections of local anesthetic, a motivated and compliant patient can undergo a straightforward revision of the ethmoid, sphenoid, maxillary, or frontal sinuses in the office. For example, areas of mature scars causing recirculation or sinus obstruction can often be addressed with a local office procedure. Patients who are poor candidates for general anesthesia or sedation, typically due to pulmonary issues, may be acceptable candidates for minor revision of their sinus surgery or polypectomy with local anesthesia. When the office procedure has been executed successfully, these patients are typically discharged after a brief period of postprocedure observation, and they may rapidly return to their normal daily activities.

Hemostasis is a significant component of any sinus surgery but becomes even more important during office revision sinus procedures. Vasoconstriction with topical

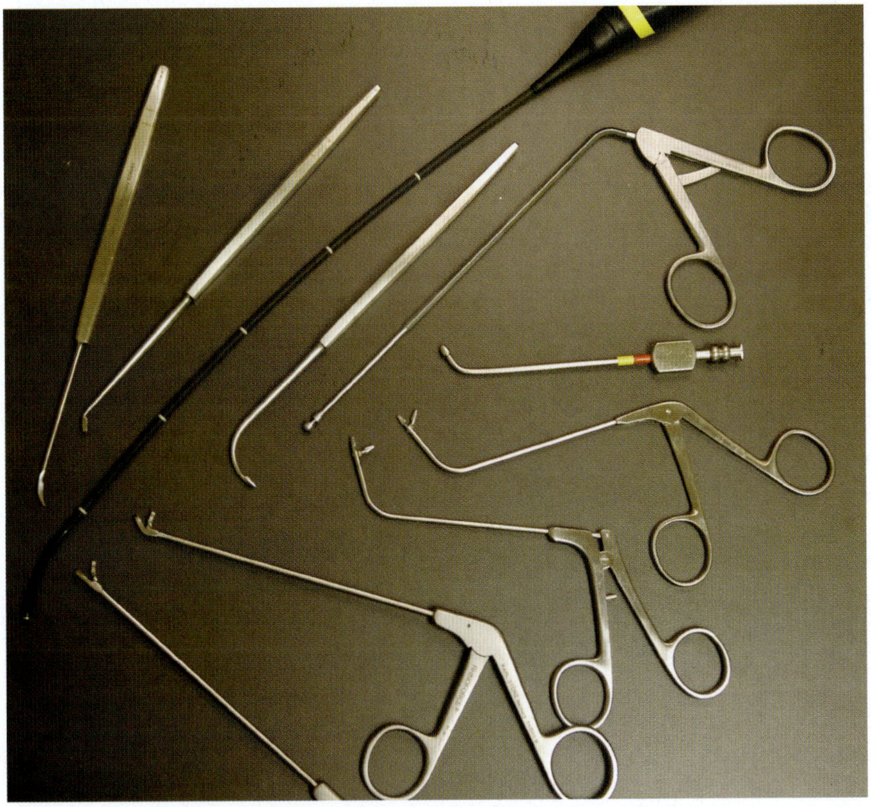

Fig. 22.7 Additional instruments useful for performing more advanced office rhinologic care, including debridements during frontal sinus surgery.

and injected medications is essential to preserve visualization throughout the procedure, ensuring a more meticulous and thorough dissection irrespective of the setting of the procedure. Topical vasoconstriction can be applied repeatedly throughout the procedure as needed, using cottonoids soaked in either oxymetazoline or 1:1,000 epinephrine. The use of topical concentrated epinephrine is avoided in geriatric populations and in patients with poorly controlled hypertension but is otherwise safe.[13,14] As with scar management, cutting instruments should be employed whenever possible to avoid mucosal loss, which can lead to delayed healing with disorganized ciliary function and the perpetuation of inflammation.[15–17]

Polypectomy in the office can be a useful adjunct for patients who have undergone thorough endoscopic ethmoidectomy yet have had significant recurrence of their polyps. When the proposed polyp surgical treatment is limited to soft tissue resection (all bone partitions and ostia have been previously managed), office polypectomy is a viable option. This procedure can be accomplished using hand instruments but may be more effectively and efficiently performed using a microdebrider or other powered tissue dissector. Use of nasal telescopes provides superb visualization for both safety and thoroughness of polyp resection. Preoperative management with systemic corticosteroids reduces the size and vascularity of the polyps, facilitating their removal with minimal blood loss.[14] With the appropriate control of inflammation prior to the procedure and careful control of bleeding during the polypectomy, packing is rarely required. Patients are typically observed for 10 to 30 minutes following the procedure to ensure hemostasis has been achieved, and then discharged from the office with instructions to avoid heavy physical exertion for 3 to 4 days.

During any office procedure, care must be taken to protect the patient's airway from blood and tissue aspiration, and the physician must be prepared to deal with possible excessive bleeding. This procedure nevertheless remains a viable option for patients who need only a soft tissue resection who are motivated to avoid the time and expense of the operating room.

Inferior Turbinate Tissue Reduction

Management of nasal obstruction due to inferior turbinate hypertrophy is another treatment readily performed in the rhinology office. Patients who have not found satisfactory results with medical management of the turbinates yet have no septal deviation or other obstructive conditions may be good candidates for office-based inferior turbinate tissue reduction. Both radiofrequency and microdebrider technologies are amenable to office application and are well tolerated by the patient under local anesthesia. Anesthesia is performed first topically and then using careful injection of local anesthetic with epinephrine into the soft tissue of the inferior turbinate. After anesthesia and vasoconstriction have taken effect (usually 10 to 15 minutes after injection), the microdebrider blade or radiofrequency apparatus is introduced submucosally and then activated, ablating or removing the submucosal tissue. Direct visualization using a nasal speculum or nasal telescope anteriorly allows precise control of tissue removal. With either device, bleeding is typically minimal and packing is rarely needed. The patient can typically leave the office within 15 minutes of terminating the procedure and return to normal activities immediately.

Balloon Dilation

Balloon dilation technology offers a tissue-preserving approach to enlargement of the sinus ostia. First introduced as a surgical tool for rhinologic procedures in the operating room, balloon catheters were used both in conjunction with traditional endoscopic sinus surgery (ESS) and as a standalone procedure. Initial procedures were performed under general anesthesia or monitored anesthesia care with sedation. In recognition of the excellent patient tolerance for these procedures, balloon dilation procedures have evolved toward increasing use in an office setting under local anesthesia without sedation. Current literature suggests that both transnasal and transantral approaches are well tolerated by patients.[18] The maxillary, frontal, and sphenoid sinuses have been successfully treated in limited case series reports. Selected post-ESS patients with evidence of sinus ostial stenosis may be candidates for balloon dilation as an alternative to formal revision surgery.[19] Although early experiences with office-based balloon dilation are promising, long-term outcomes assessment is necessary to understand the durability of the procedure and the optimal candidates for office-based treatment.[20]

■ Biomaterials in Rhinology

As the techniques of ESS have evolved and expanded since their introduction, the use and scope of biomaterials have also grown significantly, reflecting ongoing biotechnical innovations. The use of biomaterials during surgery and postoperatively can have a significant impact on the clinical course of patients undergoing rhinologic surgery. An understanding of the current issues in biomaterial development and usage is therefore relevant to the office-based management of the rhinology patient.

Biomaterials are substances that interface with the body to evaluate, treat, augment, or replace tissues or functions of the body.[21] They may be either synthetic or natural, including materials processed from naturally occurring sources. Originally derived from either plant or animal sources, they are typically designed to be broken down and absorbed by the body. Processed cellulose products are examples of plant-derived materials, which are used to control bleeding by acting as a scaffold for platelet aggregation. Gelatin products derive from animal connective tissues and also act as a platelet scaffold. Hyaluronan-based products may be obtained from animal sources or, more recently, genetically engineered bacteria, and have been used in rhinology as space-fillers to prevent surgical adhesions. These products also have the potential for enhancing wound healing and providing sustained delivery of pharmacotherapeutics. Hydroxyapatite cements have been used in many applications for bone reconstruction, including frontal sinus and skull base defects.

Biomaterials interact with the implanted host and affect inflammation and healing, which may have intentional salutary or unintentional deleterious effects. Many of the biomaterials used in rhinology are adapted from nonrhinologic applications and these "off-label" adaptations have not always been prospectively studied. Occasionally, they have been found to have unanticipated troublesome effects. Even products that have regulatory approval for rhinologic use may represent a compromise, excelling in one goal (e.g., controlling bleeding, filling a defect) while possibly worsening another (e.g., inducing scarring or infection). An understanding of sinus wound healing and a careful evaluation of these materials is necessary to understand their potential benefits and risks.

Mucosal Wound Healing

Despite the fact that sinus surgery is performed nearly half a million times a year in the United States and more worldwide, little is known about rhinologic wound healing, and most current information on mucosal wound healing comes from epidermal studies.[22] Although general principles may be similar, caution should be used in applying findings in skin to nasal and sinus wound healing.

Wound healing is a complex yet orderly sequence of events that involves a variety of cell types and subcellular signals. Inflammation is the first of the three phases of wound healing, followed by proliferation and remodeling. The inflammatory phase involves the influx of macrophages and other cells from the circulation and the subsequent release of modulators such as cytokines.[23,24] Reactive oxygen species are generated in the early phases of wounding and may cause further tissue damage. Following the inflammatory phase, proliferation of new tissue takes place. Within a few days of the injury, a loose connective tissue matrix containing hyaluronan, fibronectin, and collagen is present. Inflammatory cells continue to provide signals that regulate the healing processes at this stage, such as angiogenesis, fibroplasia, and reepithelialization. As inflammation and proliferation subside, remodeling of the wound takes place. The extracellular matrix changes, with hyaluronan and other glycosaminoglycans diminishing while elastin and proteoglycan deposition increases. These remodeling changes evolve over months.

Unlike epidermal injuries, where skin appendages provide the primary source for new epithelial cells, respiratory epithelium appears to regenerate mostly from undifferentiated basal cells from adjacent noninjured areas. Although healed sinus mucosa may appear identical to nontraumatized mucosa grossly, marked fibrosis, decreased glands, and cilial abnormalities are seen at a microscopic level.[15,25] Ciliary function is also impaired following mucosal regeneration, with slowed and disorganized mucus transport.[16] These facts underscore the importance of minimizing mucosal injury during surgery, which in turn decreases the risk of scarring and mucosal dysfunction.

Modulation of inflammation, wound healing, and tissue regeneration are areas of active work in biomaterials. These potential uses of biomaterials also impact rhinology and a large number of biomaterials have been used in the nose and sinuses. They have been used to repair frontal sinus and skull base defects, control epistaxis, and prevent scarring and adhesions following sinus surgery.

Biomaterials and Endoscopic Sinus Surgery

As discussed previously, endoscopic examination and debridement form an important part of the care of endoscopic sinus patients to prevent scarring and stenosis. Biomaterials have the potential to address many of the scarring problems that complicate ESS. An ideal biomaterial would prevent scarring and middle turbinate adhesions, inhibit ostial stenosis, promote epithelial healing and return to normal functioning, and diminish inflammation. Reduction of perioperative bleeding through platelet scaffolding or coagulation activation would be an added advantage. Sustained delivery of pharmacotherapeutic agents would further enhance the effectiveness of a rhinologic biomaterial.

Gelatin is a common hemostatic that consists primarily of hydrolyzed collagen, produced by treating animal connective tissues with strong acids and bases at high temperatures. Derived from either bovine or porcine sources, it typically generates a foreign-body reaction when implanted in humans. Thrombin may be added to gelatin to improve conversion of fibrinogen to fibrin, thus combining the terminal effects of the clotting cascade with the platelet aggregating effect of the gelatin particles.

Gelatin has been studied as a spacer and thrombin-gelatin paste has been studied in sinus surgery. Although there is little doubt about the efficacy of thrombin-gelatin paste in treating bleeding, its potential to promote scarring is more in question. The gelatin appears to enter the submucosal space and provokes a foreign body reaction or acts as a collagen bridge for scarring.[26–29] Long-term follow-up has been mixed in the presence of scarring with thrombin-gelatin paste. More studies are needed to resolve these conflicting data and determine gelatin's most appropriate role in ESS.

Hyaluronan (HA)-based biomaterials may potentially address scarring issues following ESS. HA, a ubiquitous glycosaminoglycan related to heparin and chondroitin, has crucial functions in normal wound healing, such as scavenging reactive oxygen species and enhancing re-epithelialization. Human fetal skin, rich in HA, heals with markedly reduced fibrosis, and it appears that fetal wounds heal by regeneration rather than by scarring.[30] HA appears to modulate the inflammatory response by inhibiting key cytokines involved in fibrosis.[31] HA may therefore have great potential as a promoter of improved wound healing.

HA as a starting molecule is ubiquitous and is nonimmunogenic, but because it is rapidly degraded in vivo and continually turned over, therapeutic HA preparations involve modifications that will slow the degradation. Such modifications, however, may alter the desired wound-healing effects of these HA products, such as their ability to scavenge reactive oxygen species or regulate cell signals. Furthermore, commercial preparations may include contaminants, or the modified HA material itself may provoke an inflammatory reaction. Some modified HA materials have indeed failed to show improvements in wound healing and, in fact, have shown some deleterious effects, whereas others with different chemical modifications appear to inhibit scarring while showing much less inflammatory provocation.[32–34] The chemical composition of modified HA biomaterials appears to have profound effects on their biocompatibility and efficacy in preventing scarring. In essence, all biomaterials, even two compositions derived from the same starting material, are not created equal. Careful evaluation is therefore necessary prior to use in patients.

Chitosan has emerged as a material with promise both in diminishing mucosal scarring and as a platform for drug delivery in the sinuses. It also offers hemostatic properties. Chitosan appears to have little proinflammatory effect in early investigations.

Biomaterials and Frontal Sinus Obliteration

Biomaterials have a rich history in frontal sinus surgery, particularly frontal sinus obliteration. Numerous autologous and heterologous materials have been used to fill the frontal sinus, including fat, blood, plasma, fibrin, synthetic collagen, gelatin, cancellous bone chips, plaster of Paris, Silastic, Teflon paste, methylmethacrylate, aluminum plates, Vitallium, paraffin, gold, zirconium, tantalum, polyvinyl sponge, stainless steel, glass wool, celluloid, acrylic plates, and bioactive glass.[35] None of these has proven superior to autologous fat, which remains the gold standard for this surgery.

Hydroxyapatite cement (HAC) has been used to obliterate the frontal sinus to avoid a harvest wound and to promote ossification of the obliterated cavity. Theoretically, this replacement with bone would make radiologic detection of mucoceles much easier. In practice, however, the cement rarely ossifies, and the use of HAC in the frontal sinus has been called into question. Several surgeons have found late complications with HAC, particularly infection, which occurs on average 2 years following implantation.[36] The ability of HAC to induce vascular ingrowth and ossification appears to be limited to the periphery of the implant only so that a large portion of the biomaterial remains devascularized. With implantation often occurring in an infected/inflamed sinus, and the possibility of the material becoming exposed within the frontal recess, infection becomes a significant risk. Biomaterials, which can provide a sustained delivery of provascularization growth factors and defined porosity for vascular ingrowth, may prove to be a significant advantage in the future.

Conclusion

Office care forms the heart of the rhinology practice. Beyond diagnostic procedures, with modest equipment and supplies many interventions can take place in the office. These interventions include olfactory testing, allergy testing and management, epistaxis care, endoscopic biopsy and culture, preoperative and postoperative sinus care, inferior turbinate submucous resection, and even revision sinus surgery, balloon dilation, and polypectomy. Biomaterials have been used during and following sinus surgery to enhance hemostasis and prevent scarring. Their effects depend greatly on individual chemistry and may be quite variable with subtle changes in their composition. Surgeons should be familiar with biomaterials' effects before employing them in their patients.

References

1. Orlandi RR, Hwang PH. Perioperative care for advanced rhinology procedures. Otolaryngol Clin North Am 2006;39(3):463–473
2. U.S. Food and Drug Administration. FDA Drug Safety Communication: FDA continues to receive reports of a rare, but serious and potentially fatal adverse effect with the use of benzocaine sprays for medical procedures. http://www.fda.gov/Drugs/DrugSafety/ucm250040.htm#safety. Accessed April 30, 2011
3. Hwang SH, Seo JH, Joo YH, Kim BG, Cho JH, Kang JM. An anatomic study using three-dimensional reconstruction for pterygopalatine fossa infiltration via the greater palatine canal. Clin Anat 2011;24(5):576–582
4. Gifford TO, Orlandi RR. Epistaxis. Otolaryngol Clin North Am 2008;41(3):525–536, viii
5. Neuland C, Bitter T, Marschner H, Gudziol H, Guntinas-Lichius O. Health-related and specific olfaction-related quality of life in patients with chronic functional anosmia or severe hyposmia. Laryngoscope 2011;121(4):867–872
6. Doty RL. Office procedures for quantitative assessment of olfactory function. Am J Rhinol 2007;21(4):460–473
7. Hummel T, Sekinger B, Wolf SR, Pauli E, Kobal G. 'Sniffin' sticks': olfactory performance assessed by the combined testing of odor identification, odor discrimination and olfactory threshold. Chem Senses 1997;22(1):39–52
8. Krouse JH, Mabry RL. Skin testing for inhalant allergy 2003: current strategies. Otolaryngol Head Neck Surg 2003;129(4, Suppl) S33–S49

9. Calderon MA, Alves B, Jacobson M, Hurwitz B, Sheikh A, Durham S. Allergen injection immunotherapy for seasonal allergic rhinitis. Cochrane Database Syst Rev 2007;1(1):CD001936
10. Gillespie MB, O'Malley BW Jr, Francis HW. An approach to fulminant invasive fungal rhinosinusitis in the immunocompromised host. Arch Otolaryngol Head Neck Surg 1998;124(5): 520–526
11. Meltzer EO, Hamilos DL, Hadley JA, et al; American Academy of Allergy, Asthma and Immunology; American Academy of Otolaryngic Allergy; American Academy of Otolaryngology-Head and Neck Surgery; American College of Allergy, Asthma and Immunology; American Rhinologic Society. Rhinosinusitis: Establishing definitions for clinical research and patient care. Otolaryngol Head Neck Surg 2004;131(6, Suppl)S1–S62
12. Ramakrishnan VR, Suh JD. How necessary are postoperative debridements after endoscopic sinus surgery?1. Laryngoscope 2011; 121(1):8–9
13. Higgins TS, Hwang PH, Kingdom TT, Orlandi RR, Stammberger H, Han JK. Systematic review of topical vasoconstrictors in endoscopic sinus surgery. Laryngoscope 2011;121(2):422–432
14. Orlandi RR, Lanza DC. Is nasal packing necessary following endoscopic sinus surgery? Laryngoscope 2004;114(9):1541–1544
15. Benninger MS, Schmidt JL, Crissman JD, Gottlieb C. Mucociliary function following sinus mucosal regeneration. Otolaryngol Head Neck Surg 1991;105(5):641–648
16. Min YG, Kim IT, Park SH. Mucociliary activity and ultrastructural abnormalities of regenerated sinus mucosa in rabbits. Laryngoscope 1994;104(12):1482–1486
17. Perloff JR, Gannon FH, Bolger WE, Montone KT, Orlandi R, Kennedy DW. Bone involvement in sinusitis: an apparent pathway for the spread of disease. Laryngoscope 2000;110(12): 2095–2099
18. Stankiewicz J, Tami T, Truitt T, Atkins J, Liepert D, Winegar B. Transantral, endoscopically guided balloon dilatation of the ostiomeatal complex for chronic rhinosinusitis under local anesthesia. Am J Rhinol Allergy 2009;23(3):321–327
19. Luong A, Batra PS, Fakhri S, Citardi MJ. Balloon catheter dilatation for frontal sinus ostium stenosis in the office setting. Am J Rhinol 2008;22(6):621–624
20. Batra PS, Ryan MW, Sindwani R, Marple BF. Balloon catheter technology in rhinology: Reviewing the evidence. Laryngoscope 2011;121(1):226–232
21. Orlandi RR. Biomaterials for sinus implantation. Curr Opin Otolaryngol Head Neck Surg 2007;15(1):44–47
22. Watelet JB, Bachert C, Gevaert P, Van Cauwenberge P. Wound healing of the nasal and paranasal mucosa: a review. Am J Rhinol 2002;16(2):77–84
23. Branski RC, Rosen CA, Verdolini K, Hebda PA. Markers of wound healing in vocal fold secretions from patients with laryngeal pathology. Ann Otol Rhinol Laryngol 2004;113(1):23–29
24. Kenyon NJ, Ward RW, McGrew G, Last JA. TGF-beta1 causes airway fibrosis and increased collagen I and III mRNA in mice. Thorax 2003;58(9):772–777
25. Toskala E, Rautiainen M. Electron microscopy assessment of the recovery of sinus mucosa after sinus surgery. Acta Otolaryngol 2003;123(8):954–959
26. Chandra RK, Conley DB, Haines GK III, Kern RC. Long-term effects of FloSeal packing after endoscopic sinus surgery. Am J Rhinol 2005;19(3):240–243
27. Jameson M, Gross CW, Kountakis SE. FloSeal use in endoscopic sinus surgery: effect on postoperative bleeding and synechiae formation. Am J Otolaryngol 2006;27(2):86–90
28. Maccabee MS, Trune DR, Hwang PH. Effects of topically applied biomaterials on paranasal sinus mucosal healing. Am J Rhinol 2003;17(4):203–207
29. Tom LW, Palasti S, Potsic WP, Handler SD, Wetmore RF. The effects of gelatin film stents in the middle meatus. Am J Rhinol 1997;11(3):229–232
30. Colwell AS, Longaker MT, Lorenz HP. Fetal wound healing. Front Biosci 2003;8:s1240–s1248
31. Border WA, Noble NA. Transforming growth factor beta in tissue fibrosis. N Engl J Med 1994;331(19):1286–1292
32. Proctor M, Proctor K, Shu XZ, McGill LD, Prestwich GD, Orlandi RR. Composition of hyaluronan affects wound healing in the rabbit maxillary sinus. Am J Rhinol 2006;20(2):206–211
33. Rajapaksa SP, Cowin A, Adams D, Wormald PJ. The effect of a hyaluronic acid-based nasal pack on mucosal healing in a sheep model of sinusitis. Am J Rhinol 2005;19(6):572–576
34. Wormald PJ, Boustred RN, Le T, Hawke L, Sacks R. A prospective single-blind randomized controlled study of use of hyaluronic acid nasal packs in patients after endoscopic sinus surgery. Am J Rhinol 2006;20(1):7–10
35. Donald PJ. (1995). Surgical management of frontal sinus infections. In: Donald PJ, Gluckman JL, Rice DH, eds. The Sinuses. New York: Raven Press; 1995: 201–232
36. Verret DJ, Ducic Y, Oxford L, Smith J. Hydroxyapatite cement in craniofacial reconstruction. Otolaryngol Head Neck Surg 2005;133(6):897–899

23 Surgical Navigation and Intraoperative Imaging

Martin J. Citardi

The era of endoscopic sinus surgery (ESS) has been marked by dramatic advances in the diagnosis and treatment of a wide variety of diseases and disorders of the nose, paranasal sinuses, and skull base. The nasal telescope, which has been the key instrument throughout this time, provides excellent visualization and brilliant illumination, but the resultant images are only two-dimensional (2D) representations of a complex three-dimensional (3D) space. Because the telescope provides a wide-angle perspective, there is also a fish-eye effect (similar to spherical aberration). Rhinologists have recognized that these perceptual issues may produce surgical errors that carry potentially catastrophic consequences. Thus, interest in image-guided surgery (IGS) had been considerable even it is early relatively primitive iteration, because IGS represented a potential solution for the intrinsic limitations of surgical nasal endoscopy. Subsequent enhancements greatly improved IGS technology and, over the past decade, advances in IGS have made the technology indispensable for most complex rhinologic procedures at most centers.

Terminology

Since the early 1990s, the International Society for Computer-Aided Surgery has advanced a broad agenda for semiconductor-based technologies:

> The scope of Computer Aided Surgery encompasses all fields within surgery, as well as biomedical imaging and instrumentation, and digital technology employed as an adjunct to imaging in diagnosis, therapeutics, and surgery. Topics featured include frameless as well as conventional stereotaxic procedures, surgery guided by ultrasound, image guided focal irradiation, robotic surgery, and other therapeutic interventions that are performed with the use of digital imaging technology.[1]

Thus, the domain of computer-aided surgery (CAS) encompasses digital technologies for both diagnostics and therapeutics; CAS includes computer-enabled image review, surgical navigation, robotic surgery, telemedicine, and electronic medical records. This chapter should be placed within this much broader context of these technologies that are shaping surgery.

Surgical navigation (SN) refers to a specific technology that integrates 3D digitizers that can track instrument position with imaging data; through this technology, the surgeon can see the position of an instrument tip relative to imaging data projected in the three orthogonal planes (and sometimes relative to reformatted 3D reconstructions). IGS incorporates both surgical navigation and computer-enabled review of imaging (or surgical planning). Until recently, IGS and SN relied on preoperative imaging; now, intraoperative imaging (II), which is most commonly computed tomography (CT), but also may be magnetic resonance imaging (MRI), has been introduced and is being used for IGS and SN.

Numerous other terms are in use. "Computer-assisted surgery," "computer navigation," etc. are commonly used interchangeably with terms for CAS, SN, and IGS. Because these terms are relatively imprecise, their usage should be avoided.

Equipment

Although vendors for surgical equipment will highlight differences among various product lines, all equipment for IGS (**Figs. 23.1 and 23.2**) and II (**Fig. 23.3**) is remarkably similar, because similar underlying principles govern all of the systems. Thus, in the operating room, equipment from different vendors will function in remarkably similar ways.

Equipment for Image-Guided Surgery

The computer workstation functions as the central component of all IGS systems because it calculates the registration (defined later) and integrates positional information from the tracking system with the imaging data.[2,3] When the tracking system is inactivated, or if it is not present with the computer workstation, this computer provides a platform for the review of triplanar images and surgical planning. IGS system software typically includes a variety of software tools that permit the viewing and manipulation of imaging data.

The tracking system drives a digitizer that transmits positional information about surgical instruments that carry intraoperative localization devices (ILDs) (**Fig. 23.4**). Both electromagnetic (EM) and optical tracking systems are commercially available for IGS. In EM tracking, an EM field emitter creates an EM field that is detected by an EM sensor that sends positional information to the computer for processing. Traditionally, the EM field emitter is attached to the patient and the EM sensor is attached to an instrument, although in theory, the EM field emitter does not need to be attached to the patient if an EM sensor is attached to the

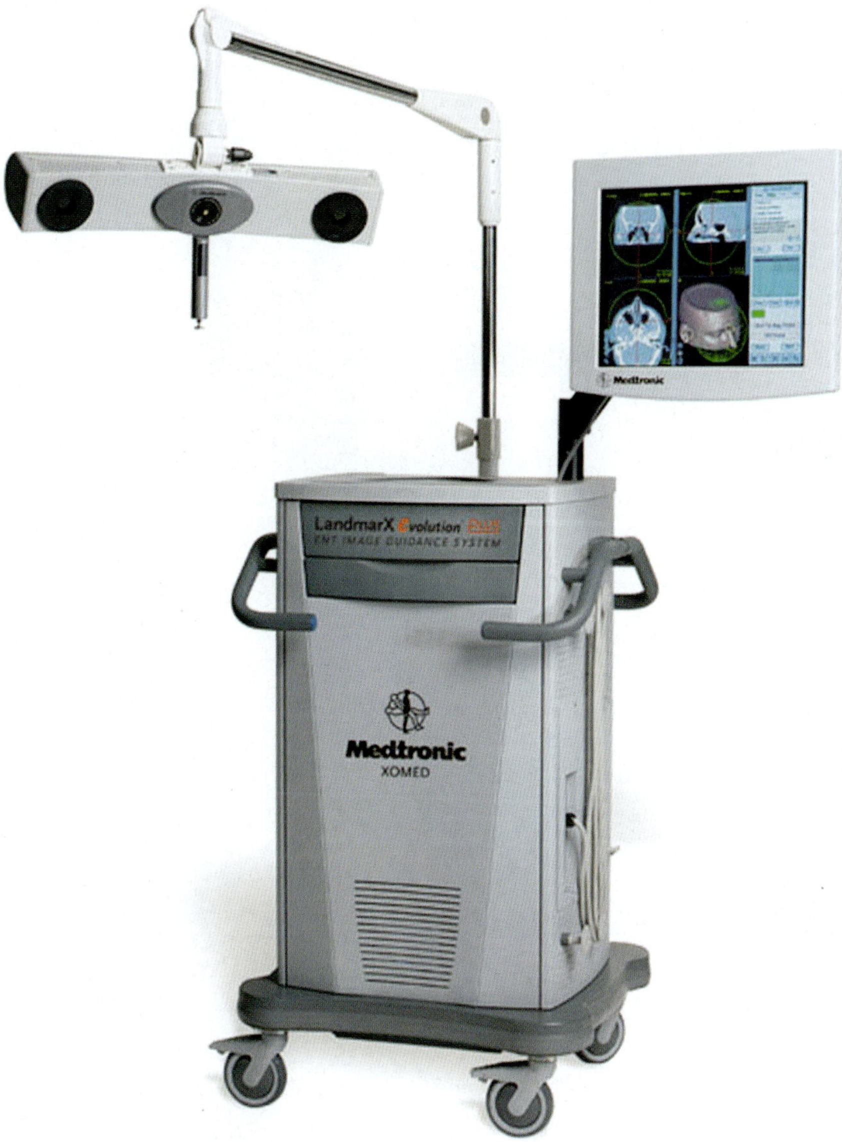

Fig. 23.1 Surgical navigation systems with optical instrument tracking include an overhead camera array (known as a digitizer), which is attached to the cart for the image-guided surgery equipment, as in this example of the LandmarX Evolution Plus (Medtronic ENT, Jacksonville, FL). (Courtesy of Medtronic ENT, Minneapolis, MN.)

patient (**Fig. 23.5**). For active optical tracking, an overhead camera array can "see" the position of ILDs composed of light-emitting diodes (LEDs). Such ILDs are attached both to the patient and to instruments. In passive optical tracking, highly reflective spheres are substituted for the LEDs, and an infrared emitter, which is incorporated into the camera array, bathes the LEDs with infrared light, which is then reflected and detected by the camera array.

The IGS software coordinates all of the various functions of the IGS system. The software must be robust for the storage and retrieval of large image files. In addition, software tools facilitate the review of imaging data and, thus, surgical planning. Commonly, scrolling through the triplanar images is emphasized, but other software features, including window width/level adjustments, trajectory views, and 3D cut views should not be discounted. In certain applications, surgical planning involves the marking of specific surgical targets, and during SN, the software calculates positional information relative to these targets. (Currently, this application is rarely used in otorhinolaryngology, but neurosurgeons do find it much more helpful.)

Equipment for Intraoperative Imaging

Obviously, II requires the presence of the hardware for image acquisition within the operating room. The specific imaging modality determines adjustments to operating room setup and function. For all systems, adjustments in patient position are typically required, and in many instances, specific equipment for patient positioning must be used. For intraoperative CT and fluoroscopy, precautions against the effects of ionizing radiation exposure must be undertaken. Although an intraoperative CT scanner and a fluoroscopy unit are both mobile pieces of equipment that can be rolled into almost any operating room, an intraoperative MRI scanner requires a dedicated

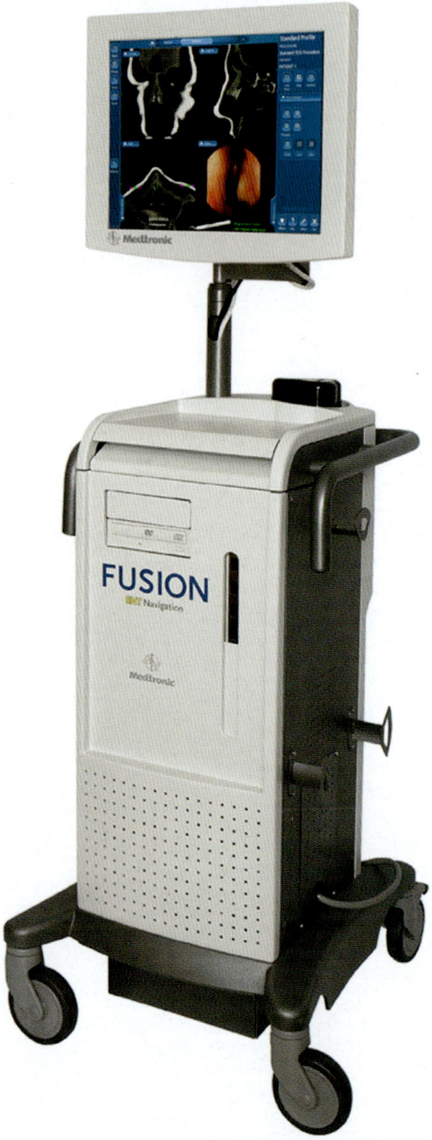

Fig. 23.2 A surgical navigation system based upon electromagnetic tracking offers a more compact footprint due to the absence of digitizer array. The Fusion IGS system (Medtronic ENT, Jacksonville, FL) is a representative electromagnetic surgical navigation platform. (Courtesy of Medtronic ENT, Minneapolis, MN.)

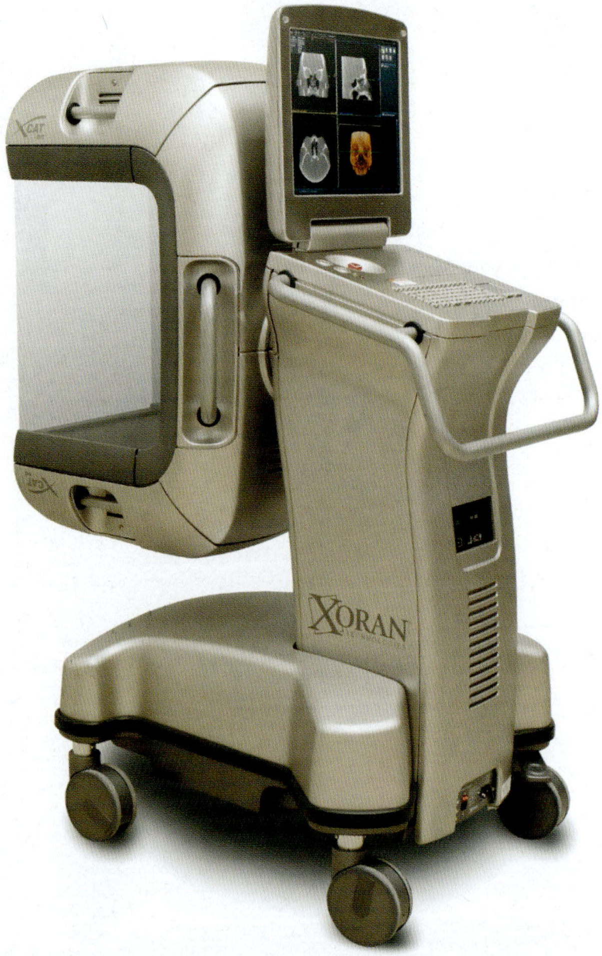

Fig. 23.3 This portable volume computed tomography scanner (xCAT, Xoran Technologies, Ann Arbor, MI) has been optimized for easy usage in the operating room. The device has a relatively small footprint, and produces images with excellent bony detail.

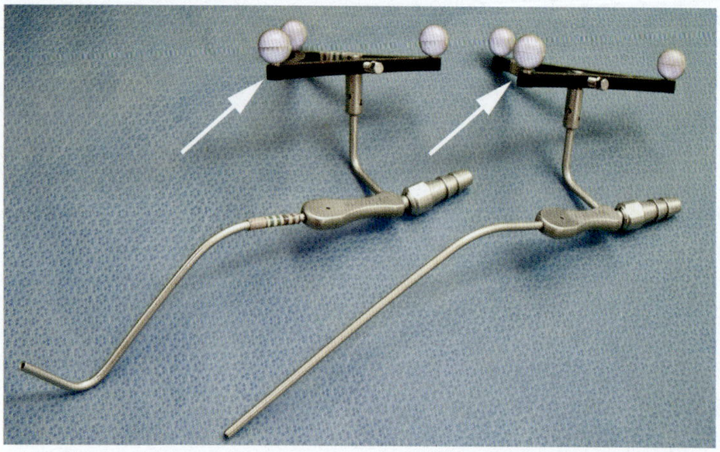

Fig. 23.4 Intraoperative localization devices (ILDs) are recognized by the image-guided surgery system tracking system. These suctions carry ILDs (*arrows*) with reflective spheres, which will reflect infrared light from the overhead digitizer array. The digitizer can "see" the ILDs and track their positions.

room and instrumentation—all equipment must be compatible with the strong magnetic fields generated by the MRI scanner.

Images from II may be reviewed at the computer workstation for assessment of the impact of the surgical manipulations. In addition, the imaging dataset may be uploaded to the IGS system for SN with updated imaging information.

Registration

Registration is the process of establishing a one-to-one mapping relationship between corresponding points (known as fiducial points) in the operating field volume and in the imaging dataset volume. Each point in each volume has a unique *xyz* coordinate. Registration aligns corresponding *xyz* coordinates. Regardless of the specific registration protocol, successful registration hinges on defining and correlating the corresponding fiducial points in the operating field volume and in the imaging dataset.

Registration is not the same concept as calibration. Calibration refers to the process of defining the relationship between an instrument tip and the attached ILD. In some systems, calibration is merely a confirmatory step for the predefined relationship between instrument tip and ILD.

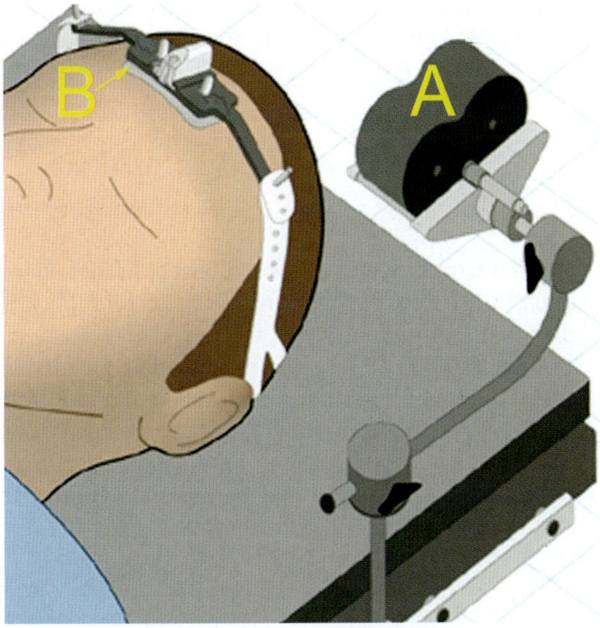

Fig. 23.5 This schematic representation of equipment setup for the Fusion IGS (Medtronic ENT, Jacksonville, FL) shows the electromagnetic field generator **(A)** in close proximity to the patient. An intraoperative localization device **(B)** is attached to the patient and monitors patient movement so that such movement does not significantly reduce surgical navigation accuracy after registration. (Courtesy of Medtronic ENT, Minneapolis, MN.)

Paired Point Registration

As its name implies, paired point registration (PPR) is a manual process of mapping out corresponding points in a three-step process. First, the fiducial points must be marked in the imaging dataset. In the next step, the surgeon identifies corresponding points in the surgical volume by localizing against each fiducial point. Finally, the computer calculates the registration.

In the early era of SN, bone-anchored screws were used as fiducial markers. Later, taped-on skin markers were introduced. When PPR is employed for rhinology, typically, anatomic fiducial points are used.

Automatic Registration

The central feature in automatic registration (AR) is a fiducial headset, which is designed such that its positioning on the patient's head is reproducible. The headset contains fiducial markers and, thus, each time the headset is placed on the patient, the relationship between those fiducial markers and the operating field volume is functionally identical (**Fig. 23.6**). The patient must wear the same, or a functionally similar headset both during scan acquisition and in the operating room. During registration, software identifies the fiducial markers in the imaging dataset, and then calculates the registration.

Contour-Based Registration

Contour-based registration (CBR) is closely related to PPR. In CBR, the IGS software creates a 3D model that defines the patient's surface contour, and then the surgeon defines that contour in the operating field volume. That process is

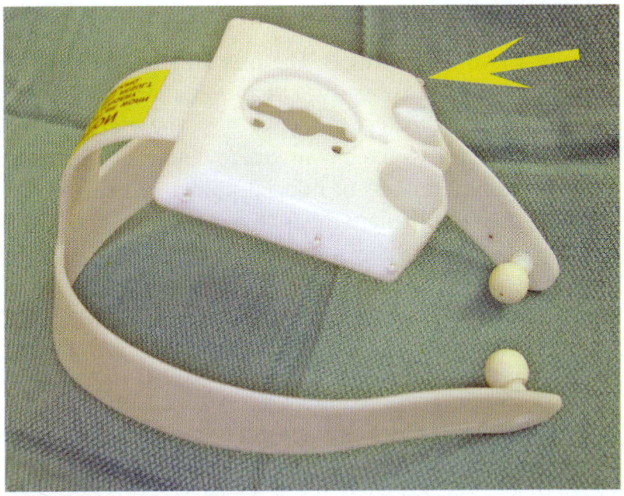

Fig. 23.6 For automatic registration, the patient wears a headset that carries a fiducial array (*arrow*); the headset is designed so that its position on the patient is reproducible (i.e., the relationship between the fiducial array and the patient is functionally identical with each placement on the patient). This headset is for the InstaTrak (GE Navigation & Visualization, Lawrence, MA).

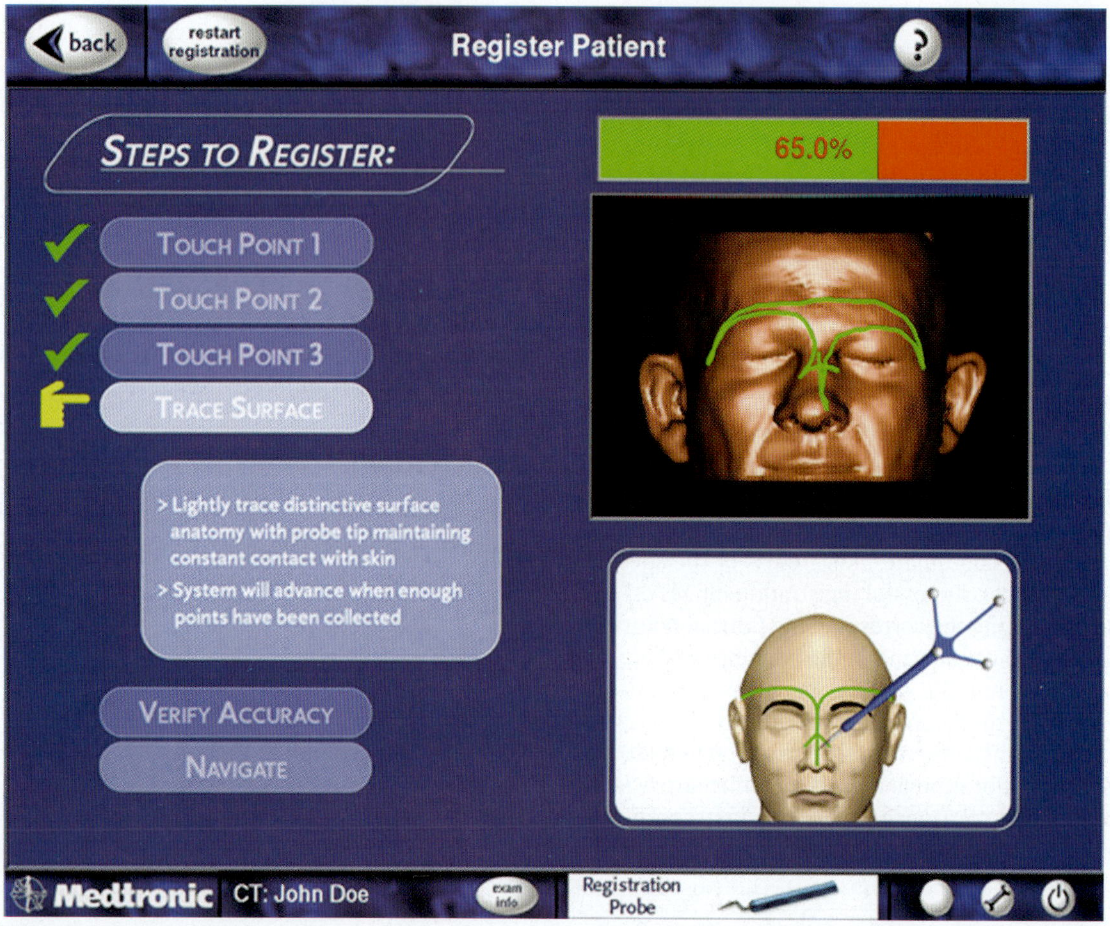

Fig. 23.7 During contour-based registration, the surgeon runs a tracked probe along curvilinear, relatively fixed surfaces to collect a large number of points that form the registration. This screen capture, obtained during contour-based registration using LandmarX (Medtronic ENT, Jacksonville, FL), shows the stylized ideal distribution of points (*lower right panel*) as well as the distribution of collected points (*upper right panel*). The left side of the screen serves as a guide to the user. The horizontal bar (*upper right*) represents the degree to which point acquisition is complete. (Courtesy of Medtronic ENT.)

actually a two-step process. The first step is a rough PPR with 3 to 4 points—this serves as an initial orientation for the second step. During the second step, the user runs the tracked probe across fixed contours to define a large number (100 to 500 points) of fiducial points, which the IGS software uses to calculate the final registration (**Fig. 23.7**). In place of a fixed probe, a handheld laser device may be used to define the contour.

Surgical Navigation Accuracy

Even under nearly ideal circumstances, registration may be an imprecise process. Errors in registration occur in all cases; that is, there is never an exact relationship between the indicated position of an instrument and its actual position. In most circumstances, this difference is below what is clinically meaningful, but in other cases, it may be a major issue. Thus, the surgeon must monitor SN accuracy throughout each case.

Registration Error Concepts

Registration error theory provides a robust basis for understanding the accuracy of SN.[4] Although these concepts are complex and seem remote from the day-to-day usage of SN, it is important for all surgeons to appreciate the fundamental principles of registration error theory. Registration error theory was developed for PPR, but the concepts may be extrapolated to both CBR and automatic registration paradigms. Registration error may be classified as fiducial localization error (FLE), fiducial registration error (FRE), and target registration error (TRE).

Fiducial Localization Error

FLE is the difference between the actual position of a fiducial marker in the operating room space and its measured position in the imaging space. FLE, which cannot be measured directly, is typically derived from Sibson's relationship.[5] FLE is reported as the root mean square (RMS) average, or the square root of the squared value (RMS=√([FLE]).[2] FLE is influenced by various factors related to the image space, including the shape and size of the fiducial marker, the image's voxel dimensions, the image's digital intensity, contrast of the fiducial marker relative to background, and any geometrical distortion of the image.[4,6] Furthermore, FLE is also a function of the number, configuration, and type of fiducial markers used.[7]

Fiducial Registration Error

FRE is the residual error between fiducial points that are employed for SN after registration (or the distance, after registration, between the measured position of a fiducial marker in the physical space and its measured position in the image space). Although FRE may refer to a specific fiducial marker, commonly, FRE is presented as the RMS of the individual registration errors of each fiducial marker. IGS platforms can directly measure FRE. In general, lower FRE values are correlated with better overall accuracy, but this relationship may not hold for each individual case.

Target Registration Error

TRE represents the real world accuracy of SN, because it alone is the distance, after registration, of the true position of a surgical target in the operating field volume and its measured position in the imaging space. TRE represents how well the IGS system is tracking instrument tip position relative to the preoperative imaging. Clinically, the surgeon estimates TRE by localizing against known landmarks, although in dry laboratory conditions, other more precise methods may be used. TRE is a vector quantity; that is, it has both an absolute magnitude and a direction. For this reason, the surgeon may compensate for suboptimal TRE by noting both its apparent magnitude and direction.

Factors That Influence Surgical Navigation Accuracy

Each step in the registration process introduces additional errors; thus, attention must be directed at reducing errors at each step. In general, fiducial marker selection is a key variable, even for automatic registration and CBR.

Fiducial Marker Selection

As outlined previously, each fiducial marker has its own FLE (or error associated with localization of the marker). Inclusion of fiducial markers with high FLE will degrade subsequent accuracy.[8] Some SN systems will automatically exclude fiducial points with high FLE values. Steps to reduce FLE include a scan acquisition with as thin of a slice as feasible. Operator error may also introduce high FLE; this is an important consideration, because commonly, registration is left to the least experienced member of the operating room team. Appropriate training and experience is likely to reduce FLE.

Fiducial Marker Number

At least three points are necessary to generate a 3-D registration. General practice dictates the inclusion of as many fiducial points as possible. But, there are caveats. A registration based on a lower number of well localized points is likely to generate a better TRE than a registration from a higher number of poorly localized points. In a dry laboratory simulation of CBR, optimal TRE was noted for registrations based upon as few as 50 or 125 points, rather than 250 or 500 points.[9]

Fiducial Marker Configuration

In general, TRE will be lowest at the centroid (mean *xyz* coordinate of each fiducial point) or the center of the fiducial marker configuration. When fiducial points are collinear (or nearly collinear), TRE will decrease as the distance from the centroid increases.[10,11] An often observed reduction in TRE at the posterior ethmoid and sphenoid is a reflection of greater TRE with greater distance from the centroid achieved with most commercially available SN platforms for rhinologic surgery. Ideally, fiducial points should be distributed around the area of surgical interest so that the centroid is close to this region.[12]

Image Acquisition

Current IGS systems accept axial imaging data that are then processed to create coronal and sagittal images as well as 3D models. Thinner slice thicknesses will yield imaging datasets with more anatomic information. Imaging datasets are "granular"; that is, they are composed of a stack of image slices. The thickness of each slice will determine the best case scenario for TRE. In addition, thinner slices will facilitate better fiducial marker localization, further reducing the resultant TRE after registration.

Practical Approach to Surgical Navigation Accuracy

During actual surgery, estimates of SN accuracy (TRE) must be done via visual estimates. TRE should be assessed by considering each of the positional vectors (that is, *x*-axis, *y*-axis, and *z*-axis) of the error individually. Although TRE is often considered to be an absolute value, in reality it has both a magnitude and a direction. Furthermore, the surgeon's ability to estimate positions and distances under endoscopic visualization is not as great as many believe. Thus, the approach to TRE must be systematic, thoughtful, and comprehensive.

From a practical standpoint, the superomedial part of the posterior maxillary wall is a nearly ideal reference point for assessing TRE. This position is relatively easy to identify after maxillary antrostomy and, in most cases, it is not disturbed by surgical manipulation. The posterior maxillary wall provides information about the *z*-axis error, whereas the medial maxillary wall gives a reference for assessing the *x*-axis error. The inferior orbital wall gives information about the *y*-axis error. Of course, other points may be used for assessing TRE, but rarely do they provide as much reliable information as this superomedial aspect of the posterior maxillary wall.

When assessing TRE, it is important to remember a few practical considerations. First, TRE may vary in different parts of the surgical volume due to rotational and translational misalignments in the registration of the real world with the imaging dataset. In addition, TRE may change during surgery for a wide variety of technical reasons, including bent instruments, hardware failures, and headset slippage. Thus, the surgeon must monitor TRE actively throughout the entire case.

Some surgeons have proposed assessing TRE against external landmarks; however, this approach may lead to false conclusions about TRE at the actual site of surgery. These external landmarks are relatively far from the area of surgical interest, and thus there is considerable potential for differences between TRE at the external landmark and TRE within the operating field volume.

Reports of Surgical Navigation Accuracy

The published reports of TRE for otorhinolaryngology are difficult to assess due to inconsistent metholology.[13] Early publications highlight TRE values of ~2 mm for dry laboratory conditions that used acrylic or plastic models. Subsequent clinical reports note TRE values of 1.5 to 2.4 mm.[14–16] Most clinicians feel that TRE levels of 1.5 to 2.0 mm can be routinely achieved.[8,9,17–20] Under certain circumstances, even better TRE values may be achieved, but this is an inconsistent event, and thus one cannot rely on it. From a practical standpoint, TRE values of 1.5 to 2.0 mm are deemed sufficient for most intraoperative decision making, although even lower TRE values may be desirable for certain procedures.

Indications for Guided Surgery

The policy statement on CAS/IGS/SN issued by the American Academy of Otolaryngology–Head and Neck Surgery (AAO-HNS) summarizes well the current accepted role of this technology among otorhinolaryngologists[21]:

> The American Academy of Otolaryngology–Head and Neck Surgery endorses the intraoperative use of computer-aided surgery in appropriately select cases to assist the surgeon in clarifying complex anatomy during sinus and skull base surgery. There is sufficient expert consensus opinion and literature evidence base to support this position. This technology is used at the discretion of the operating surgeon and is not experimental or investigational. Furthermore, the American Academy of Otolaryngology—Head and Neck Surgery is of the opinion that it is impossible to corroborate this with Level 1 evidence. These appropriate, specialty specific, and surgically indicated procedural services should be reimbursed whether used by neurosurgeons or other qualified physicians regardless of the specialty. Examples of indications in which use of computer-aided surgery may be deemed appropriate include:
>
> 1. Revision sinus surgery.
> 2. Distorted sinus anatomy of development, postoperative, or traumatic origin.
> 3. Extensive sinonasal polyposis.
> 4. Pathology involving the frontal, posterior ethmoid and sphenoid sinuses.
> 5. Disease abutting the skull base, orbit, optic nerve, or carotid artery.
> 6. CSF rhinorrhea or conditions where there is a skull base defect.
> 7. Benign and malignant sinonasal neoplasms.

Current practices among otorhinolaryngologists in the United States seem to reflect the approach outlined in the AAO position statement. In a survey of American Rhinologic Society members, revision endoscopic ethmoidectomy and revision endoscopic frontal sinusotomy were both felt to be indications for IGS by 90% or greater of all respondents, whereas primary anterior ethmoidectomy was noted not to be an indication for IGS by 90% of respondents.[22]

Indications for Intraoperative Imaging

The indications for II are less developed than those for IGS, because II applications have not been widely explored. Although II technology has been available for many years, it has been cumbersome and costly. Recent advances have reduced the complexity and costs, but even with these changes, barriers for the adoption of II are still considerable. Thus, it is difficult to anticipate the final consensus for II indications.

Centers that are employing II tend to use it for the same cases in which IGS is commonly used. It seems likely that II will be reserved for the most complex cases in which IGS is currently employed as a standalone technology.

Clinical Reports of Image-Guided Surgery

In a comprehensive review using evidence-based medicine (EBM) principles, Smith et al. tried to assess the evidence for IGS in reducing complications and improving outcomes.[23] They noted that the current evidence supporting the use of IGS is level 4 (case series) and level 5 (expert opinion), and they emphasize that the demands of sample size and study design preclude randomized trials for this technology. Although EBM concepts can be powerfully informative, rigid reliance on them may adversely impact the acceptance of new technologies. Under certain circumstances, a critical approach that relies on common sense may be appropriate for certain interventions, as implied in a 2005 tongue-in-cheek review of randomized trials of parachute effectiveness and safety.[24] A common theme throughout the literature is that IGS enhances the surgeon's "comfort" and thus facilitates complex procedures—capturing that impact through retrospective and prospective studies may be nearly impossible.

Numerous reports describe IGS applications in endoscopic sinus surgery. Early reports were mostly descriptive and noted that barriers to IGS usage were manageable and that IGS seemed to improve surgical outcomes (although data to support that conclusion were sparse).[25–32] Later reports have emphasized more specific information. In a review of 1000 cases done at an academic medical center by 42 surgeons, Metson noted trends for greater use; this observation was felt to reflect the consensus that IGS offered potential improvements in surgical effectiveness and safety.[33] IGS for revision sinus surgery has been emphasized in other reports.[34]

The role of IGS for osteoplastic frontal sinusotomy has been described. A cadaveric study has reported that measurements provided through IGS were statistically superior to those provided by conventional 6-foot Caldwell films and simple transillumination.[35] A report of the cases confirmed the feasibility of IGS for planning the osteoplastic flap in the operating room.[36] IGS seems to reduce complications associated with osteoplastic flap surgery.[37]

The use of IGS in endoscopic cerebrospinal fluid (CSF) leak repair is common because, intuitively, the technology should enhance recognition of the skull base defect and should facilitate surgical dissection, especially in the setting of previous surgery, trauma, or congenital anomaly. Nonetheless, in a comparison of endoscopic CSF leak repair cases performed with and without IGS, Tabaee et al. did not show differences in success rates related to this technology.[38]

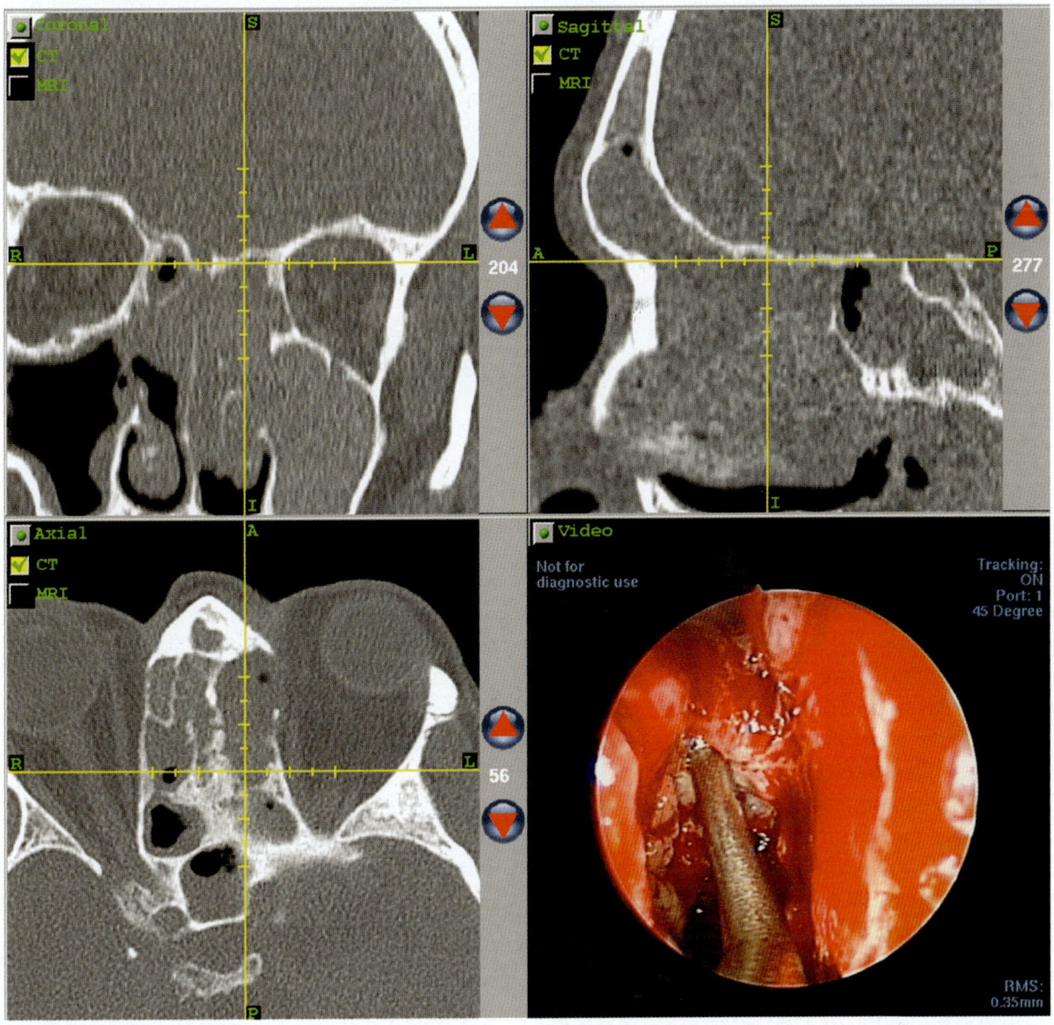

Fig. 23.8 This screen capture, obtained on the InstaTrak 3500 Plus (GE Navigation & Visualization, Lawrence, MA), illustrates the use of surgical navigation during revision functional endoscopic sinus surgery. The lower right endoscopic image shows the tracked instrument tip, whose position is depicted by the cross-hairs on the orthogonal computed tomography images. In this revision case, previous surgery and extensive inflammatory disease had altered standard surgical landmarks; surgical navigation provided key anatomic information for successful and safe completion of the procedure.

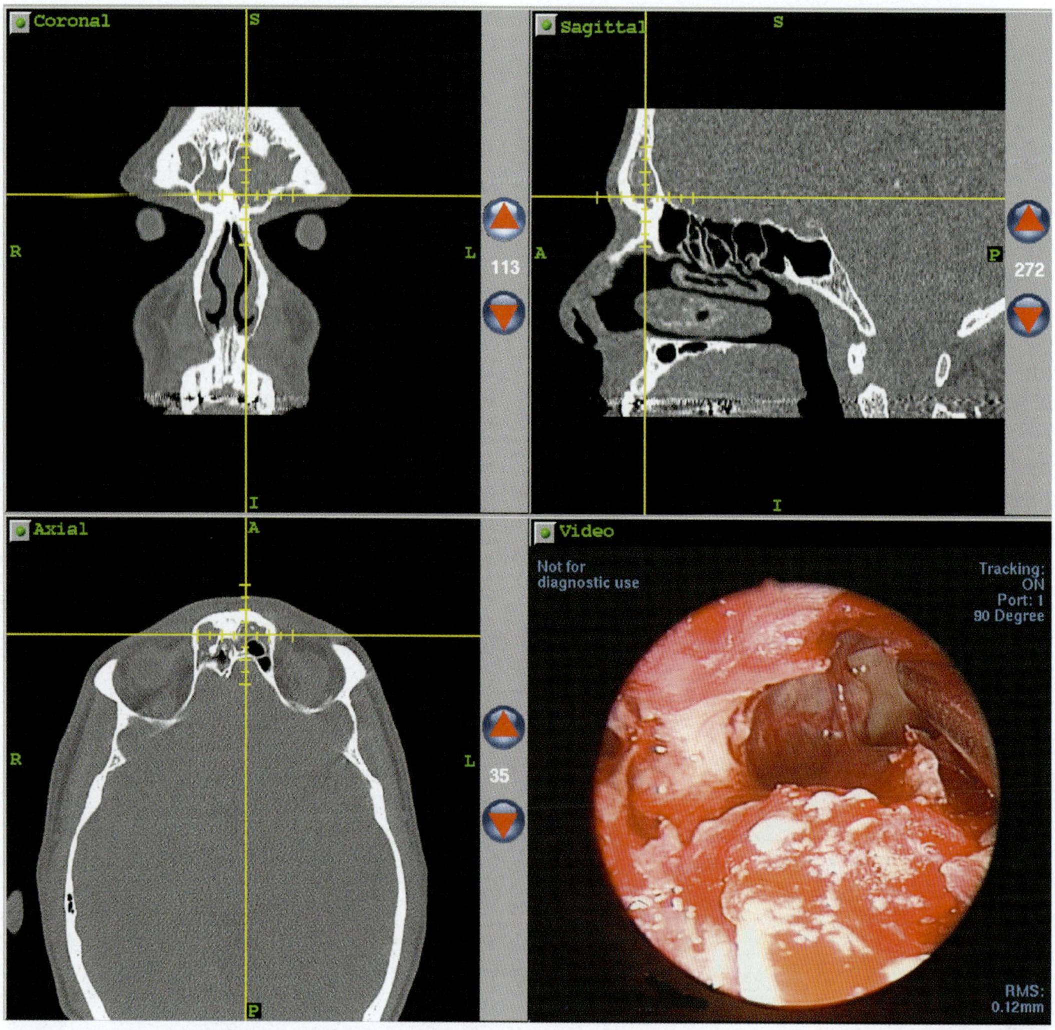

Fig. 23.9 This screen capture, obtained on InstaTrak 3500 Plus (GE Navigation & Visualization, Lawrence, MA) during a modified endoscopic Lothrop procedure, shows the instrument tip within the frontal sinus proper. In this case, the navigation system was used to gauge the completeness of bone removal at the frontal sinus floor.

Because of the proximity of the internal carotid artery, the cavernous sinus, the optic nerve, and other cranial nerves and brain parenchyma, IGS is appealing for transsphenoidal hypophysectomy procedures. Jagannathan et al., in a series of 176 cases, noted that IGS seemed to yield a reduction in operative time and that IGS was especially useful after previous failed pituitary procedures.[39]

Although the consensus among otorhinolaryngologists strongly favors IGS for more complex cases (for the indications outlined in the AAO consensus statement), data demonstrating a positive impact from IGS are rare. In a retrospective review in which IGS cases were compared with a historical control group of cases completed before the availability of IGS, Fried et al. reported a lower complication rate in cases performed with IGS.[19] A more sophisticated approach to assessing the impact of IGS was proposed by Strauss et al., who developed a measure of the information before and after each IGS application in actual surgery.[40] In almost 50% of uses, IGS resulted in a change in surgical strategy, and less experienced surgeons more frequently adjusted their surgical strategies based upon IGS information. Finally, in only 3 out of 792 localizations, information was considered "detrimental," and in these 3 instances, no adverse outcomes were noted. This report confirms that IGS commonly impacts surgery (in almost 50% of localizations), and this impact is almost uniformly constructive.

These case series attempt to formally assess the specific clinical use of IGS and SN. Specific case examples serve to illustrate the impact of this technology for practicing rhinologic surgeons (**Figs. 23.8, 23.9, 23.10, 23.11, and 23.12**).

Clinical Reports of Intraoperative Imaging

Conventional SN relies on preoperative imaging and intrinsically does not incorporate changes rendered by the surgery itself. The ability to update the imaging through repeat

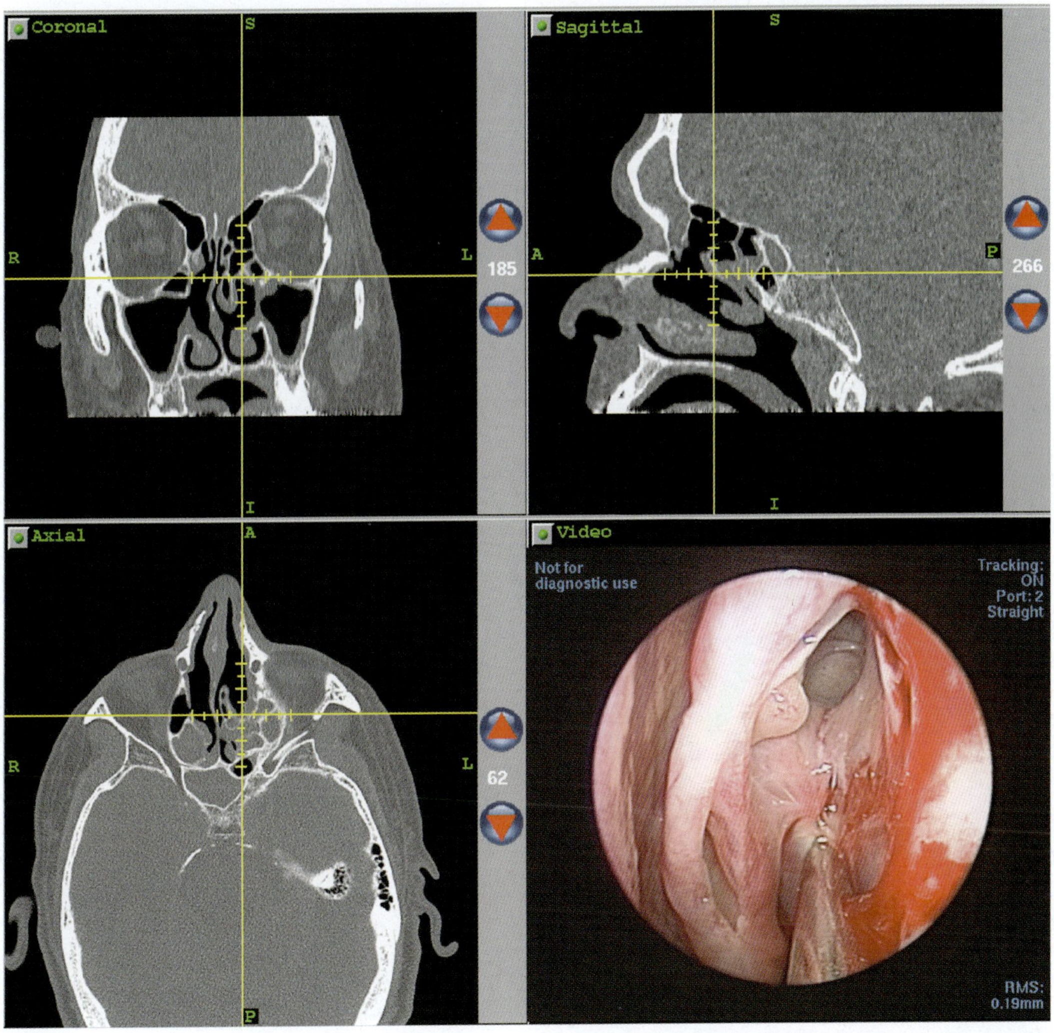

Fig. 23.10 In this screen capture, obtained on an InstaTrak 3500 Plus (GE Navigation & Visualization, Lawrence, MA) during a revision endoscopic sinus surgery, the instrument tip, shown in the lower right panel, rests on the residual basal lamella. During the previous surgery, the middle turbinate had been partially resected. As a result, an important cue for dissection was lost. With surgical navigation, it was possible to assess the residual ethmoid partitions and their positions relative to skull base and orbit.

II has a natural appeal because it would minimize this obvious limitation. Intraoperative MRI has been available for more than a decade, and it has been used for sinus surgery. Unfortunately, high costs and challenges in implementation (i.e., all equipment must be MRI-compatible—a very difficult and expensive proposition) preclude wide adoption of intraoperative MRI for most rhinologic procedures.[41,42] Nonetheless, II with MRI may have a role in certain specific instances, such as endoscopic hypophysectomy[43] and other endoscopic procedures of the skull base.

Recently, II with CT-based modalities has gathered much more interest. Rafferty et al. described cone-based CT for frontal recess surgery in a cadaveric model and reported that the use of cone beam CT (CBCT) facilitated the surgical dissection and was a valuable teaching tool.[44] Intraoperative fluoroscopic CT (FluoroCAT, GE Healthcare Surgical Navigation, Lawrence, MA) has also been reported in a series of 14 cases, of which image quality was deemed satisfactory in only 6 instances.[45] These authors note that the large size of the equipment requires a large operating room and that a dedicated technician is necessary to operate the fluoro-CT equipment.

Volume CT scanner technology has also been adapted for intraoperative use. In a pilot cadaveric study, repeat imaging with a volume CT scanner (xCAT, Xoran Technologies, Ann Arbor, MI) after an endoscopic dissection was performed and then uploaded to three different IGS systems, the apparent "accuracy" of the IGS system improved.[46] The methodology for the determination of surgical navigation accuracy was not specified, and both the predissection and postdissection imaging was done on the same machine. Thus, the reasons for the apparent increased "accuracy" are unclear. Because the investigators were not blinded, bias cannot be excluded. Jackman et al. applied the same technology in the operating room, where volume CTs were performed after functional endoscopic sinus surgery in 30 patients.[47] Information from the repeat CTs led to a change in surgical plan in 30% of cases. In another report of 25 patients in whom II with a volume CT

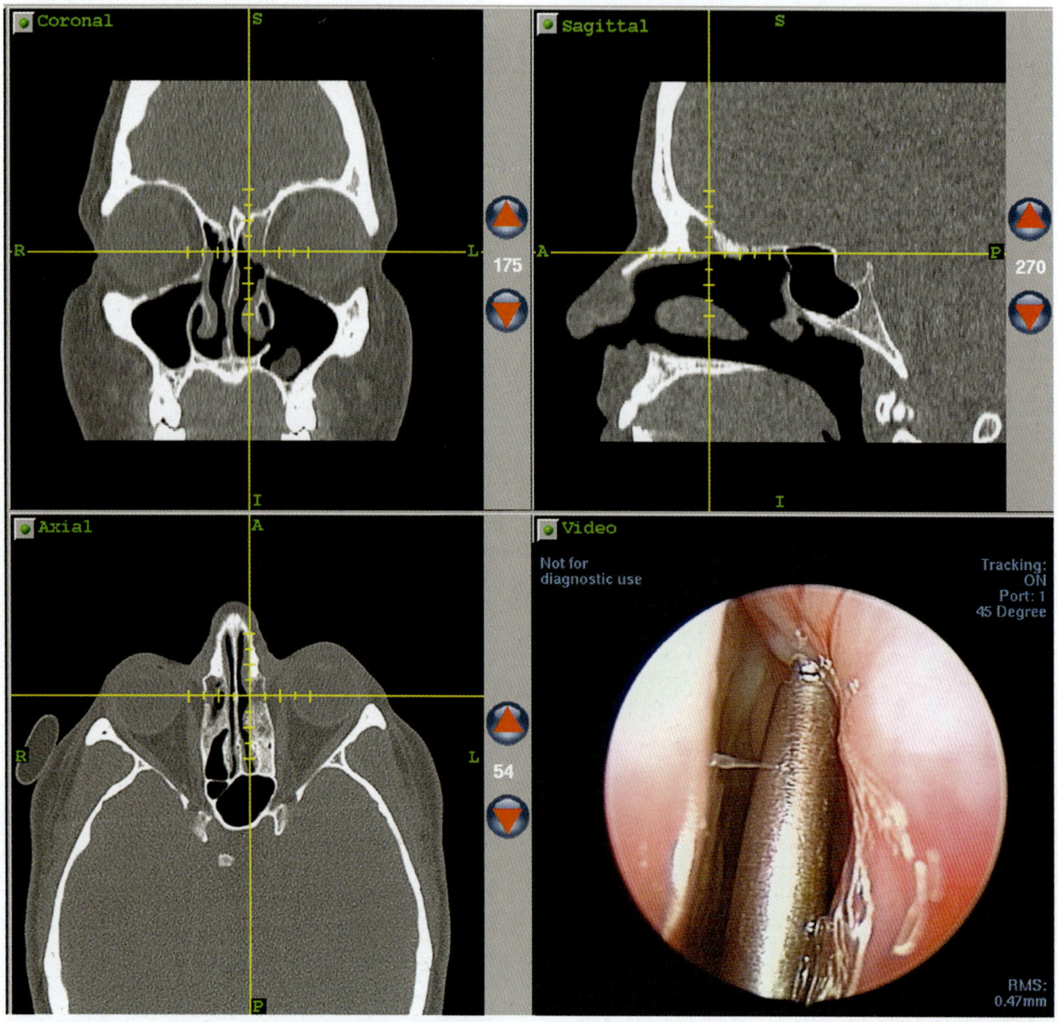

Fig. 23.11 Scarring after a middle turbinate resection can lead to closure of the frontal recess; when this occurs, the blocked frontal recess has a smooth surface that is seen during a transnasal endoscopy. In this screen capture, obtained on InstaTrak 3500 Plus (GE Navigation & Visualization, Lawrence, MA), the tracked aspirator tip (*lower right panel*) rests on the frontal recess that is scarred shut. With surgical navigation, it is possible to assess the anatomic configuration of this obstruction and then implement the surgical plan accordingly. Surgical navigation is also important for avoiding inadvertent injury to the skull base.

scanner (xCAT, Xoran Technologies) was performed during endoscopic sinus surgery, additional surgical interventions were performed in six patients.[48] It should be noted that this report highlights a complex group of procedures performed at a tertiary rhinology center and, thus, extrapolations from these data may not be applicable to general otorhinolaryngology practice. Nonetheless, II influenced surgical decision making in a distinct subgroup of patients (**Fig. 23.13**).

Limitations of Image-Guided Surgery

Although it is easy to emphasize the technical capabilities of IGS, one must not overlook the limitations and disadvantages of this technology. Because commercially available systems are reliable and straightforward, it is easy for surgeons to overly rely on them. It is imperative that surgeons understand the principles of registration and their practical applications to the operating room so that errors in registration can be reduced. Furthermore, such knowledge will also permit surgeons to recognize inaccurate SN before a potentially preventable complication occurs. In the end, IGS is an enabling technology, not a substitute for surgical expertise.[29,49]

An obvious limitation for IGS is that it relies on the imaging dataset. Conventional IGS (i.e., IGS without concomitant II) does not reflect changes in the operative field anatomy due to active surgical intervention. II, as outlined previously, offers a potential solution, because it permits the acquisition of high-quality images, which may be uploaded into the IGS system.

II with CT entails additional radiation exposure for the patient and even for operating room personnel. For this reason, standard precautions must be taken.

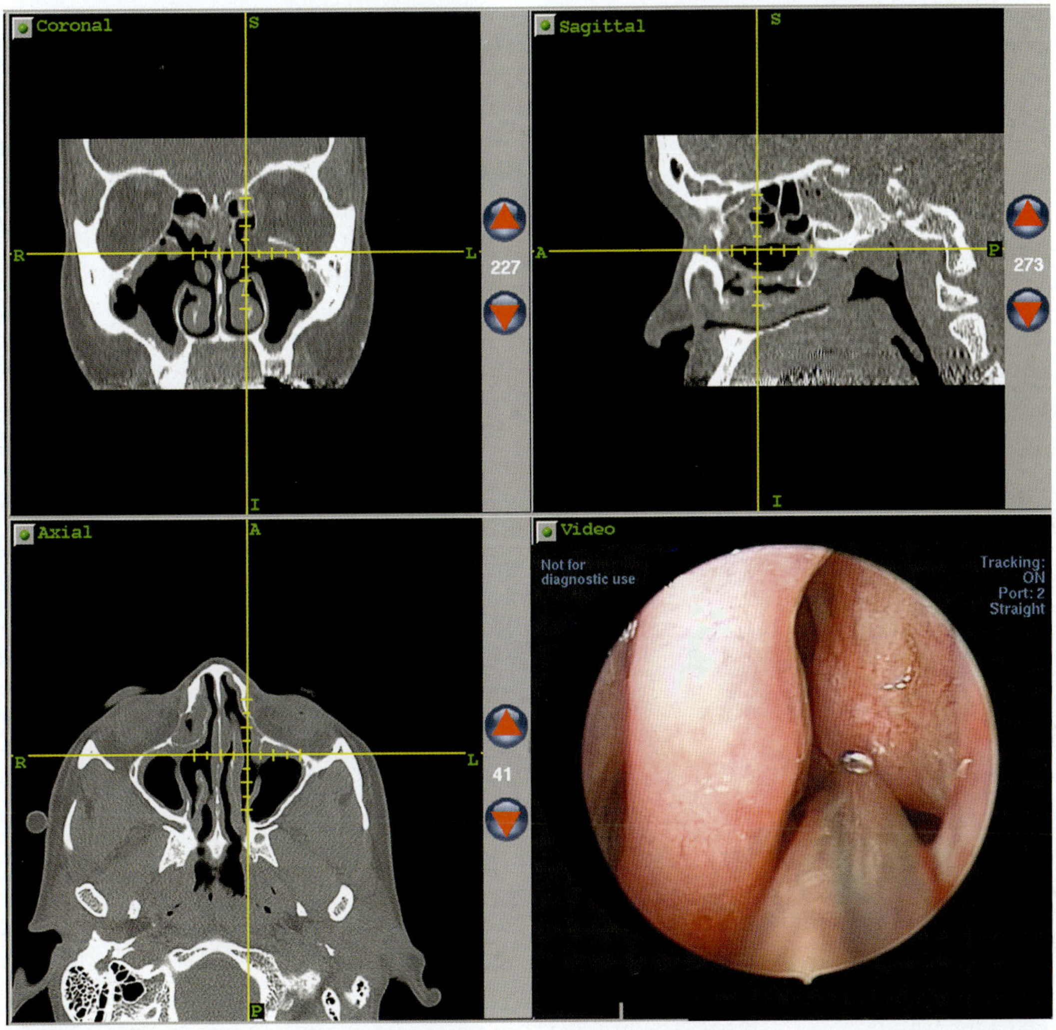

Fig. 23.12 This patient has a dehiscence of the left inferomedial orbital wall with protrusion of fat into the ethmoid cavity. The endoscopic appearance of this dehiscent area looked unremarkable, as seen in the endoscopic picture in the lower right panel of this screen capture, obtained on InstaTrak 3500 Plus (GE Navigation & Visualization, Lawrence, MA). The corresponding orthogonal computed tomography views, however, clearly show the protrusion of orbital contents into the ethmoid cavity.

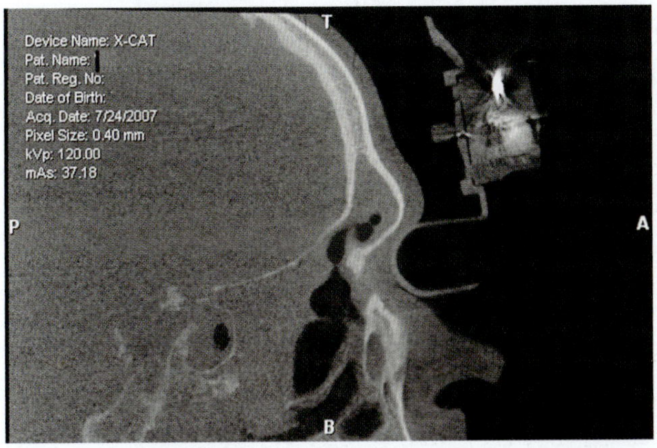

Fig. 23.13 This sagittal computed tomography (CT), obtained intraoperatively on a volume CT scanner (xCAT, Xoran Technologies, Ann Arbor, MI), shows the patent frontal recess after an endoscopic dissection. Intraoperative CT is currently optimized for assessing the extent of bony dissection, although imaging protocol modifications may also allow for the assessment of soft tissue.

Unfortunately, the reported radiation doses in the literature have been reported using inconsistent methodology. The effective dose of radiation from a volume CT scanner has been reported as 0.17 mSv,[50] compared with 2 mSv for a standard-head CT.[51] In a cadaveric study, a radiation dosage from the volume CT scanner was measured as 620 mrad for one scan and 1460 mrad for two scans, compared with a traditional CT cornea exposure of 2950 mrad.[46] Radiation doses to the cornea from CBCTs and fluoroscopic CTs have been reported as 1 mGy[44] and 4.1 mGy,[52] respectively, compared with 24.5 to 29.5 mGy from thin slice, 0.75 to 1.0 axial CTs.[53,54] Of course, II with MRI avoids any exposure to ionizing radiation.

Any new technology entails potential financial costs. Prices for IGS systems for sinus surgery are $100,000 to $250,000 or more, and an intraoperative MRI can cost millions of dollars. An intraoperative volume CT scanner costs approximately $300,000. Other costs include those related to personnel and actual operation of the equipment.

Special Image-Guided Surgery Techniques

Over the past 5 years, specific imaging protocols have been incorporated into IGS. These protocols provide specialized preoperative imaging that can be used for both preoperative planning and intraoperative SN.

Computer Tomography/Magnetic Resonance Imaging Fusion

Under most circumstances, IGS is performed with a single imaging dataset (typically CT scan), but the process of CT/MRI fusion permits the presentation of hybrid CT and MRIs for use by the IGS system. The software for CT/MRI fusion calculates an image-to-image registration (rather than an image-to-patient registration used for SN), which aligns the CT and MRI datasets. After CT/MRI fusion, the surgeon can toggle between CT and MRI, or vary the intensity of the each component of the fused image dataset. Registration for SN is performed to the CT dataset, and then the fused dataset is used for actual SN. Chiu et al. presented an initial report in 2005,[55] and Leong et al. presented a more detailed series in 2006.[56] Indications for CT/MRI fusion include sinonasal tumors, encephaloceles, and mucoceles.[56] In addition, because MRIs provide information about the position of the internal carotid artery (ICA), fused CT/MRIs are helpful for lesions of the sphenoid sinus and adjacent structures (**Fig. 23.14**).

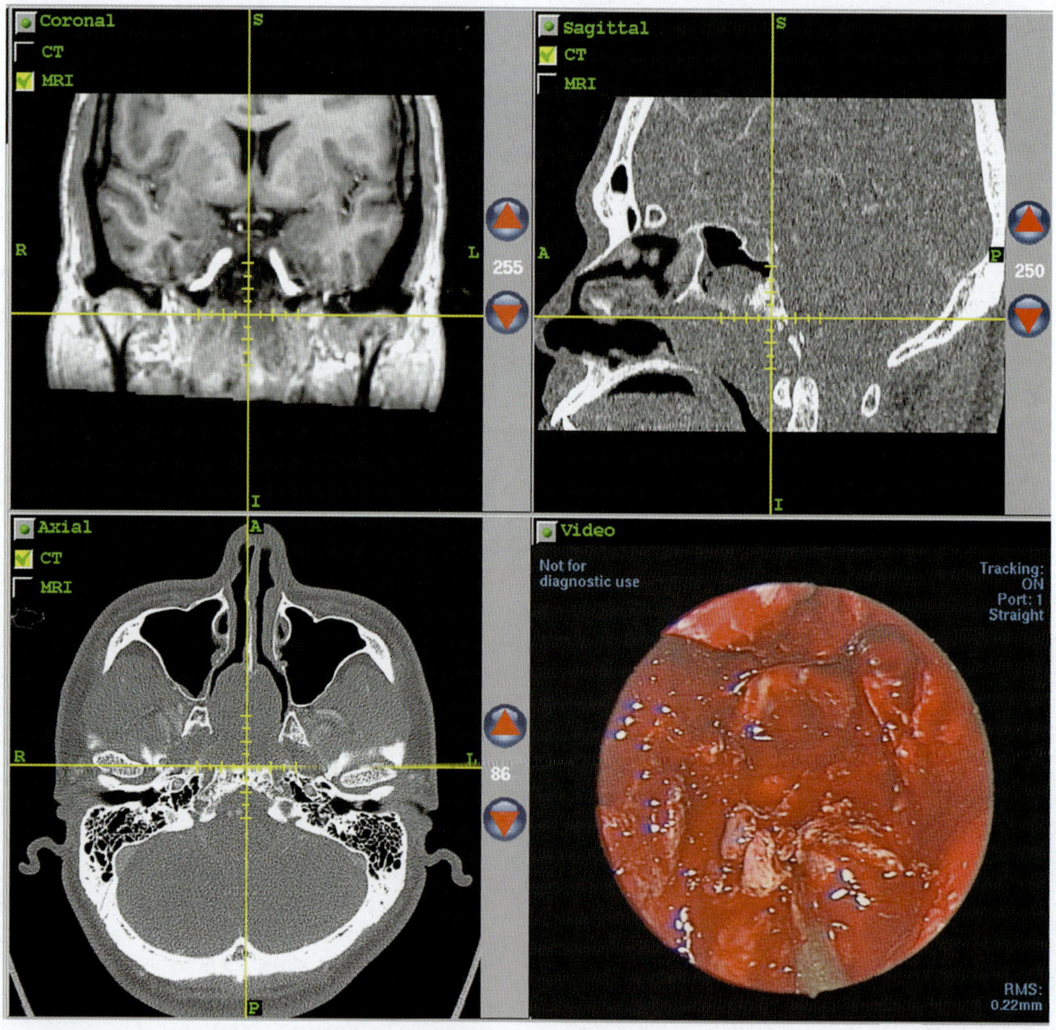

Fig. 23.14 This screen capture, obtained on an InstaTrak 3500 Plus (GE Navigation & Visualization, Lawrence, MA) after a computed tomography/magnetic resonance imaging (CT/MRI) fusion, shows corresponding MRI and CT/MRI fusion images in the upper panels and a CT image in the lower left panel. The endoscopic picture in the lower right panel shows the instrument tip deep in the clivus during the endoscopic resection of a large clival chordoma. Surgical navigation with CT/MRI fusion images was critical for the assessment of the extent of tumor removal as well as the proximity of critical structures (internal carotid artery, cavernous sinus, etc.).

Of course, CT/MRI fusion requires special imaging studies. In general, the MRI is a high-resolution, volumetric T1 acquisition. Standard CT protocols for IGS may be used. Special software packages perform the actual CT/MRI fusion and are compatible with most IGS systems.

Three-Dimensional Computed Tomography Angiography

With the introduction of fast, multidetector CT scanners, 3D CT angiography (3DCTA) has become increasingly popular over the past 10 to 15 years. Such 3DCTA images may be loaded into IGS systems for SN. Leong et al. presented a series of 22 instances of 3DCTA used in preoperative planning, including 18 cases of SN with preoperative 3DCTA.[57] Because 3DCTA can provide critical information about the position of the ICA relative to bony skull base anatomy, indications for IGS with 3DCTA include neoplasm, CSF leak, fibro-osseous lesions, and mucoceles.

The software capabilities of the IGS systems to process 3DCTA data vary greatly. Some systems will support the development of 3D models of the skull base and contrast-filled blood vessels. Even in the absence of such advanced capabilities, the contrast-enhanced ICA may be seen on the standard triplanar CT images.

Conclusion

IGS, a part of the domain of computer-aided surgery, encompasses both computer-enabled CT reviews (for preoperative and intraoperative planning) and intraoperative surgical navigation. Because of the intrinsic limitations of surgical nasal endoscopy and the anatomic complexity of the paranasal sinuses and skull bases, rhinologic surgeons have adopted this technology because it is widely believed to afford more effective and safer surgical interventions. Core principles for all IGS are similar for diverse hardware. Surgeons should understand the concepts of registration, especially as they apply to surgical navigation accuracy. The current consensus statement for indications for IGS emphasizes more complex rhinologic procedures, including revision sinus surgery, frontal sinus surgery, CSF leak repair, and skull base surgery. Intraoperative image acquisition, because it affords a near real-time update of imaging for surgical navigation and intraoperative assessment, has gained considerable interest recently. Intraoperative imaging has great promise, but its ultimate role has yet to be determined. As the technologies of IGS and intraoperative imaging are likely to evolve over the next several years, their importance for rhinologic surgeons and patients is likely to increase.

References

1. International Society for Computer-Aided S. Goals and Missions of ISCAS. www.iscas.net. Accessed April 13, 2008
2. Citardi MJ. Computer-aided frontal sinus surgery. Otolaryngol Clin North Am 2001;34(1):111–122
3. Citardi MJ, Batra PS. Image-guided sinus surgery: current concepts and technology. Otolaryngol Clin North Am 2005;38(3): 439–452, vi.
4. Maurer CR Jr, Rohlfing T, Dean D, et al. Sources of error in image registration for cranial image-guided neurosurgery. In: Geranamo I. Advanced Techniques in Image-Guided Brain and Spine Surgery. New York: Thieme; 2002: 10–36
5. Sibson R. Studies in the robustness of multidimensional scaling: perturbational analysis of classical scaling. JR Stat Soc 1979;41:213–225
6. Maniglia AJ. Fatal and other major complications of endoscopic sinus surgery. Laryngoscope 1991;101(4 Pt 1):349–354
7. West JB, Fitzpatrick JM, Toms SA, Maurer CR Jr, Maciunas RJ. Fiducial point placement and the accuracy of point-based, rigid body registration. Neurosurgery 2001;48(4):810–816, discussion 816–817
8. Snyderman C, Zimmer LA, Kassam A. Sources of registration error with image guidance systems during endoscopic anterior cranial base surgery. Otolaryngol Head Neck Surg 2004;131(3):145–149
9. Knott PD, Batra PS, Butler RS, Citardi MJ. Contour and paired-point registration in a model for image-guided surgery. Laryngoscope 2006;116(10):1877–1881
10. Helm PA, Eckel TS. Accuracy of registration methods in frameless stereotaxis. Comput Aided Surg 1998;3(2):51–56
11. Knott PD, Maurer CR, Gallivan R, Roh HJ, Citardi MJ. The impact of fiducial distribution on headset-based registration in image-guided sinus surgery. Otolaryngol Head Neck Surg 2004;131(5):666–672
12. Berry J, O'Malley BW Jr, Humphries S, Staecker H. Making image guidance work: understanding control of accuracy. Ann Otol Rhinol Laryngol 2003;112(8):689–692
13. Labadie RF, Davis BM, Fitzpatrick JM. Image-guided surgery: what is the accuracy? Curr Opin Otolaryngol Head Neck Surg 2005;13(1):27–31
14. Watanabe E, Watanabe T, Manaka S, Mayanagi Y, Takakura K. Three-dimensional digitizer (neuronavigator): new equipment for computed tomography-guided stereotaxic surgery. Surg Neurol 1987;27(6):543–547
15. Watanabe E, Mayanagi Y, Kosugi Y, Manaka S, Takakura K. Open surgery assisted by the neuronavigator, a stereotactic, articulated, sensitive arm. Neurosurgery 1991;28(6):792–799, discussion 799–800
16. Zinreich SJ, Tebo SA, Long DM, et al. Frameless stereotaxic integration of CT imaging data: accuracy and initial applications. Radiology 1993;188(3):735–742
17. Metson R, Cosenza M, Gliklich RE, Montgomery WW. The role of image-guidance systems for head and neck surgery. Arch Otolaryngol Head Neck Surg 1999;125(10):1100–1104
18. Cartellieri M, Kremser J, Vorbeck F. Comparison of different 3D navigation systems by a clinical "user". Eur Arch Otorhinolaryngol 2001;258(1):38–41
19. Fried MP, Moharir VM, Shin J, Taylor-Becker M, Morrison P. Comparison of endoscopic sinus surgery with and without image guidance. Am J Rhinol 2002;16(4):193–197
20. Raabe A, Krishnan R, Wolff R, Hermann E, Zimmermann M, Seifert V. Laser surface scanning for patient registration in intracranial image-guided surgery. Neurosurgery 2002;50(4):797–801, discussion 802–803
21. American Academy of Otolaryngology-Head and Neck Surgery Policy on Intra-Operative Use of Computer-Aided Surgery.

http://www.entnet.org/Practice/policyIntraOperativeSurgery.cfm. Accessed June 11, 2011
22. Orlandi RR, Petersen E. Image guidance: A survey of attitudes and use. Am J Rhinol 2006;20(4):406–411
23. Smith TL, Stewart MG, Orlandi RR, Setzen M, Lanza DC. Indications for image-guided sinus surgery: the current evidence. Am J Rhinol 2007;21(1):80–83
24. Smith GCS, Pell JP. Parachute use to prevent death and major trauma related to gravitational challenge: systematic review of randomized clinical trials. BMJ 2003;327:20–27
25. Anon JB, Lipman SP, Oppenheim D, Halt RA. Computer-assisted endoscopic sinus surgery. Laryngoscope 1994;104(7): 901–905
26. Fried MP, Kleefield J, Gopal H, Reardon E, Ho BT, Kuhn FA. Image-guided endoscopic surgery: results of accuracy and performance in a multicenter clinical study using an electromagnetic tracking system. Laryngoscope 1997;107(5):594–601
27. Fried MP, Kleefield J, Taylor R. New armless image-guidance system for endoscopic sinus surgery. Otolaryngol Head Neck Surg 1998;119(5):528–532
28. Anon JB. Computer-aided endoscopic sinus surgery. Laryngoscope 1998;108(7):949–961
29. Olson G, Citardi MJ. Image-guided functional endoscopic sinus surgery. Otolaryngol Head Neck Surg 2000;123(3):188–194
30. Metson R, Gliklich RE, Cosenza M. A comparison of image guidance systems for sinus surgery. Laryngoscope 1998;108(8 Pt 1):1164–1170
31. Metson RB, Cosenza MJ, Cunningham MJ, Randolph GW. Physician experience with an optical image guidance system for sinus surgery. Laryngoscope 2000;110(6):972–976
32. Neumann AM Jr, Pasquale-Niebles K, Bhuta T, Sillers MJ. Image-guided transnasal endoscopic surgery of the paranasal sinuses and anterior skull base. Am J Rhinol 1999;13(6):449–454
33. Metson R. Image-guided sinus surgery: lessons learned from the first 1000 cases. Otolaryngol Head Neck Surg 2003; 128(1):8–13
34. Tabaee A, Kacker A, Kassenoff TL, Anand V. Outcome of computer-assisted sinus surgery: a 5-year study. Am J Rhinol 2003;17(5): 291–297
35. Melroy CT, Dubin MG, Hardy SM, Senior BA. Analysis of methods to assess frontal sinus extent in osteoplastic flap surgery: transillumination versus 6-ft Caldwell versus image guidance. Am J Rhinol 2006;20(1):77–83
36. Innis W, Byrne P, Tufano RP. Image-guided osteoplastic frontal sinusotomy. Am J Rhinol 2005;19(5):430–434
37. Sindwani R, Metson R. Impact of image guidance on complications during osteoplastic frontal sinus surgery. Otolaryngol Head Neck Surg 2004;131(3):150–155
38. Tabaee A, Kassenoff TL, Kacker A, Anand VK. The efficacy of computer assisted surgery in the endoscopic management of cerebrospinal fluid rhinorrhea. Otolaryngol Head Neck Surg 2005;133(6):936–943
39. Jagannathan J, Prevedello DM, Ayer VS, Dumont AS, Jane JA Jr, Laws ER. Computer-assisted frameless stereotaxy in transsphenoidal surgery at a single institution: review of 176 cases. Neurosurg Focus 2006;20(2):E9
40. Strauss G, Koulechov K, Röttger S, et al. Evaluation of a navigation system for ENT with surgical efficiency criteria. Laryngoscope 2006;116(4):564–572
41. Fried MP, Hsu L, Topulos GP, Jolesz FA. Image-guided surgery in a new magnetic resonance suite: preclinical considerations. Laryngoscope 1996;106(4):411–417
42. Fried MP, Topulos G, Hsu L, et al. Endoscopic sinus surgery with magnetic resonance imaging guidance: initial patient experience. Otolaryngol Head Neck Surg 1998;119(4):374–380
43. Anand VK, Schwartz TH, Hiltzik DH, Kacker A. Endoscopic transphenoidal pituitary surgery with real-time intraoperative magnetic resonance imaging. Am J Rhinol 2006;20(4): 401–405
44. Rafferty MA, Siewerdsen JH, Chan Y, et al. Investigation of C-arm cone-beam CT-guided surgery of the frontal recess. Laryngoscope 2005;115(12):2138–2143
45. Brown SM, Sadoughi B, Cuellar H, von Jako R, Fried MP. Feasibility of near real-time image-guided sinus surgery using intraoperative fluoroscopic computed axial tomography. Otolaryngol Head Neck Surg 2007;136(2):268–273
46. Das S, Maeso PA, Figueroa RE, et al. The use of portable intraoperative computed tomography scanning for real-time image guidance: a pilot cadaver study. Am J Rhinol 2008;22(2): 166–169
47. Jackman AH, Palmer JN, Chiu AG, Kennedy DW. Use of intraoperative CT scanning in endoscopic sinus surgery: a preliminary report. Am J Rhinol 2008;22(2):170–174
48. Batra PS, Kanowitz SJ, Citardi MJ. Clinical utility of intraoperative volume computed tomography scanner for endoscopic sinonasal and skull base procedures. Am J Rhinol 2008;22(5): 511–515
49. Knott PD, Batra PS, Citardi MJ. Computer aided surgery: concepts and applications in rhinology. Otolaryngol Clin North Am 2006;39(3):503–522, ix
50. MiniCAT. Effective patient radiation dose. http://www.xorantech.com/contentHTML/miniCAT_effective_dose.php. Accessed May 4, 2008.
51. Federal Drug Adminstration. What are the radiation risks from CT? http://www.fda.gov/cdrh/ct/risks.html. Accessed May 4, 2008
52. Manarey CR, Anand VK. Radiation dosimetry of the FluoroCAT scan for real-time endoscopic sinus surgery. Otolaryngol Head Neck Surg 2006;135(3):409–412
53. Zammit-Maempel I, Chadwick CL, Willis SP. Radiation dose to the lens of eye and thyroid gland in paranasal sinus multislice CT. Br J Radiol 2003;76(906):418–420
54. Bassim MK, Ebert CS, Sit RC, Senior BA. Radiation dose to the eyes and parotids during CT of the sinuses. Otolaryngol Head Neck Surg 2005;133(4):531–533
55. Chiu AG, Palmer JN, Cohen N. Use of image-guided computed tomography-magnetic resonance fusion for complex endoscopic sinus and skull base surgery. Laryngoscope 2005;115(4): 753–755
56. Leong JLBP, Batra PS, Citardi MJ. CT-MR image fusion for the management of skull base lesions. Otolaryngol Head Neck Surg 2006;134(5):868–876
57. Leong JL, Batra PS, Citardi MJ. Three-dimensional computed tomography angiography of the internal carotid artery for preoperative evaluation of sinonasal lesions and intraoperative surgical navigation. Laryngoscope 2005;115(9):1618–1623

24 Instrumentation in Sinus Surgery

Troy D. Woodard and James A. Stankiewicz

Throughout the past few decades there has been a dramatic shift in the surgical management of medically refractory chronic rhinosinusitis. Open techniques and stripping diseased mucosa from the sinuses have given way to the more minimally invasive mucosal preserving endoscopic techniques.[1]

Upon its initial implementation, endoscopic sinus surgery primarily focused on opening the blocked sinus ostia and restoring proper ventilation and drainage.[2] However, improvements with surgical instrumentation have led to better visualization, more efficient dissections with mucosal preservation, an expansion in the scope of endoscopic sinus surgery, and improved surgical outcomes. This chapter provides a brief overview of the basic instrumentation used in endoscopic sinus surgery.

Endoscopes

Visualization of the nasal cavity and paranasal sinuses is essential to the successful completion of endoscopic sinus surgery. Although flexible fiberoptic scopes provide a broad visual field, they must be used with both hands, and lack in visual quality compared with rigid scopes. These qualities make flexible scopes inadequate for surgical dissections or procedures. As a result, the rigid endoscope is the premier instrument of visualizing the surgical field. The rigid endoscope not only provides superior lighting and visualization, but also can be held with one hand, allowing for one-handed or two-handed techniques using other surgical instrumentation for procedures.

Surprisingly to many, use of the endoscope has been around for at least a century. In 1879, Maximilian Nitze, an urologist, developed the cystoscope.[1,3,4] This design was used as the basis for the nasal endoscope. In 1901, Hirschman used this scope to view into the maxillary sinus from an enlarged tooth socket.[3,5] He is described as being the first physician to use the endoscope to view the nasal cavity and paranasal sinuses. Over the next few decades, several other versions of the endoscope were designed and used to view the maxillary sinus via the inferior meatus.[3] Like the prior scopes, however, the low illumination of these scopes limited their widespread use.

In the late 1950s, Harold Hopkins, a professor of optical physics at the University of Reading, who had already invented the zoom lens for cameras, developed the rod lens system.[5,6] This invention was patented in 1960 and used glass rods instead of small lenses within the optical shaft. This change resulted in improved resolution, contrast, brightness, and allowed for a smaller diameter.[1,5,6] Soon thereafter, he partnered with Karl Storz. Together, they developed the new generation of endoscopes incorporating the rod lens system coupled with fiberoptic light transmission, another area that he had developed. Unlike its predecessor, this system incorporated glass cables, which transmitted light from a portable light source through a fiberoptic bundle to the endoscope. This resulted in an increase in illumination and optical efficiency up to ninefold.[5,6] In contrast to prior endoscopes, this source is considered to be "cold light," emitting less heat from the tip.

The Hopkins rod system is the primary system used today for endoscopic examinations and surgery. The endoscopes for intranasal use range in size from 2.7 to 4 mm in diameter. The smaller scopes are easier to use in the younger pediatric patient population, whereas the larger scopes are commonly used in the teenaged and adult population.

Although the shape of the optical shaft of the scopes is straight, the field of view varies depending on the specific prism within the scope. The most commonly used endoscopes are the 0-, the 30-, the 45-, and the 70-degree (**Fig. 24.1**). Depending on the surgeon's preference, surgery can be performed with direct visualization through the eyepiece, or a video camera can also be connected to the endoscope and the image displayed on a monitor within the operating room. Although monitors are not essential for endoscopic sinus surgery, they allow the surgeon to operate in the upright position, thus avoiding undue strain on the neck and back (**Fig. 24.2**).

The 0-degree endoscope is primarily used when operating in the ethmoid and sphenoid sinuses. These structures lie in a straight line within the nasal cavity and are therefore within the straight field of view of the 0-degree telescope. This straight axis of the telescope allows for easy orientation and manipulation within the nasal cavity. However, it is difficult to see around certain structures and into angled cavities. As a result, the development of angled endoscopes has become vital in obtaining a comprehensive exam and working in difficult to visualize areas.

The 30-degree telescope is generally used when identifying the natural maxillary os and working within the maxillary and frontal sinuses. Once the maxillary sinus ostium is identified and opened, this scope also allows excellent visualization of the antrum of the maxillary sinus. Depending on how anterior one wants to look, another angled scope (45- or 70-degree) may be used. Of the latter two, the 45-degree scope is generally easier to use because it has a wider angle of view.

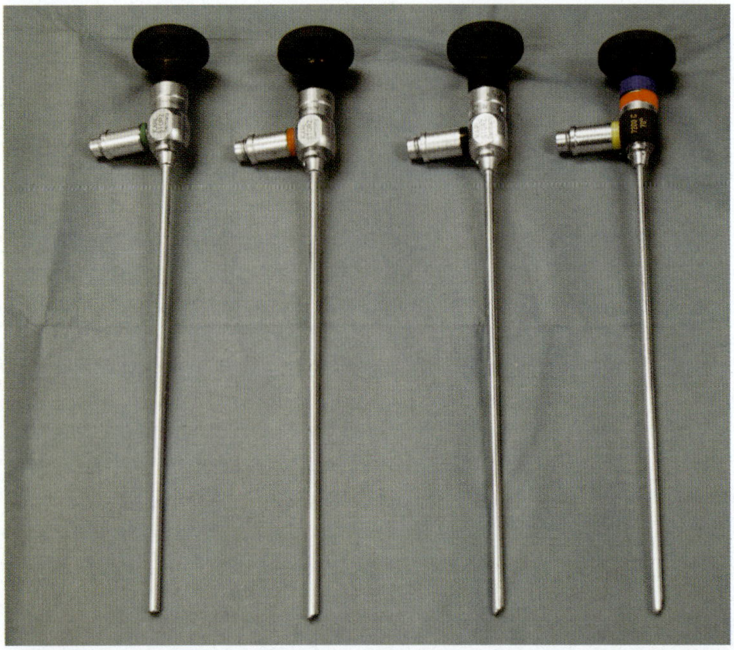

A

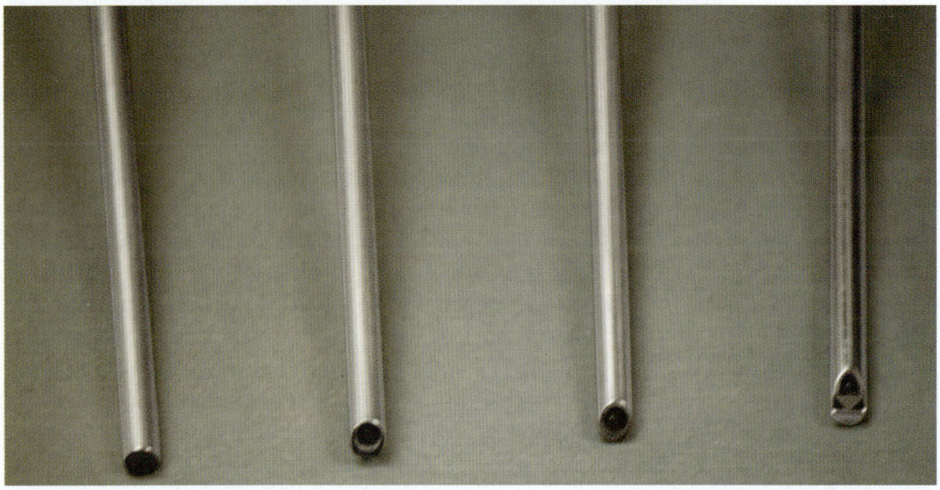

B

Fig. 24.1 (A) Hopkins rod telescopes (4 mm) are used during endoscopic sinus surgery. Pictured from left to right are the 0-, 30-, 45-, and 70-degree angled telescopes. **(B)** An up-close view of the angled tips of the telescopes.

The anterior superior location of the frontal sinuses prohibits the use of a 0-degree telescope unless bone is removed from the lacrimal frontal arch. Angled telescopes must be used to have proper visualization and illumination of the frontal recess. These telescopes are used with curved instrumentation during frontal sinus surgery. Although the 45- and, especially, the 70-degree scope are more difficult to maneuver, they can be very valuable when working at the skull base and in other hard to visualize areas.

Newer rigid scopes with integrated rotatable lenses have recently become available. Although light transmission through these new scopes is reduced compared to standard rigid endoscopes, the scopes offer the advantage of a multidirectional visualization through a single scope.

The gathering of blood on the telescope's lens often impairs visualization during surgery. Consequently, some surgeons prefer to use protective sheaths, which are attached to irrigation systems that clean the lens of the endoscope. Although the sheaths contribute to the size of the diameter of the telescope, they also enable the surgeon to be able to clean the scope without having to withdraw it from the nasal cavity. Despite using these irrigation systems, lens fogging can still occur. Consequently, an antifogging agent is helpful to ensure good visualization.

Traditional Instrumentation

Before the development of powered instrumentation, manual instruments were used to open the diseased sinuses. These handheld instruments include forceps, punches, probes, elevators, and curettes. Use of these diverse instruments has allowed endoscopic sinus surgeons

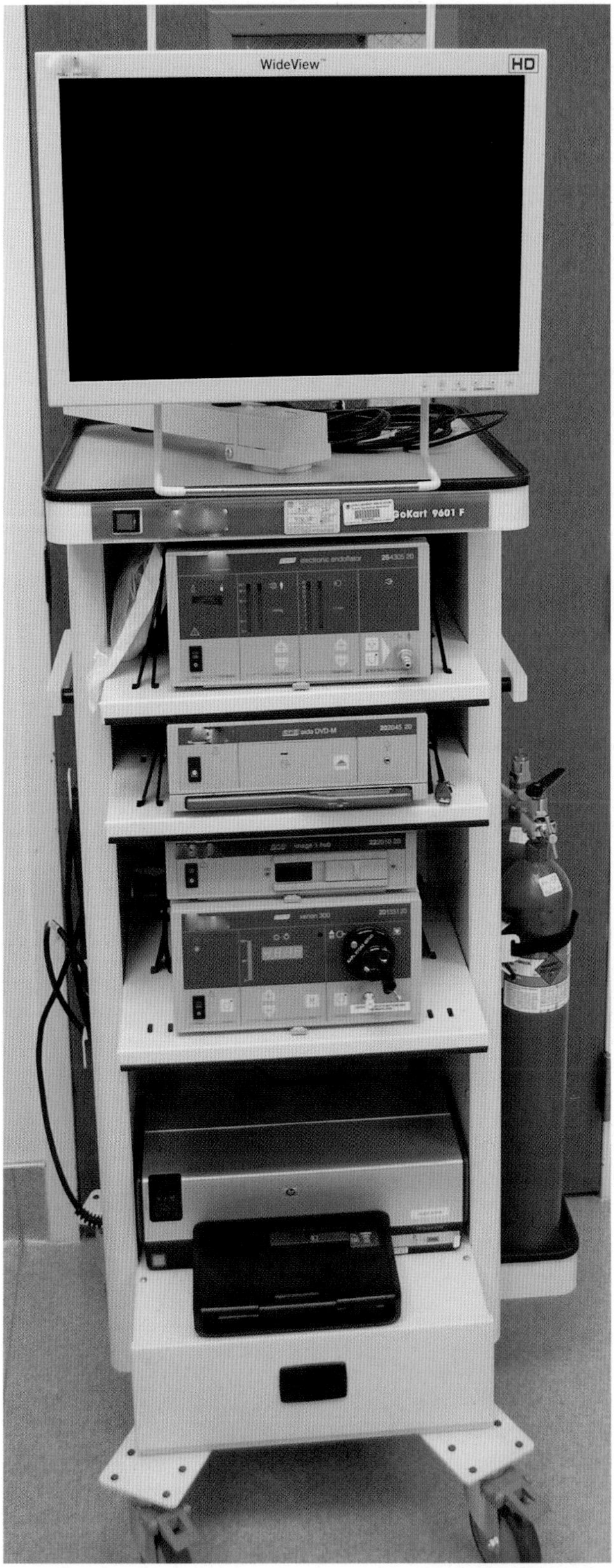

Fig. 24.2 Video monitors allow surgeons to operate in an upright and more comfortable position. This setup includes a high definition video monitor, camera, video recording device, light source, and printer.

to accomplish feats that were once reserved for open techniques.

The most commonly used instruments are the forceps and punches (**Figs. 24.3 and 24.4**). These are commonly used to grasp and bite through tissue and bone. Careful attention must be given when using noncutting, grasping forceps because they have a tendency to tear and strip the sinus mucosa. As a result, noncutting forceps are generally used to grasp loose fragments of tissue or bone. Through-cutting mechanisms have been incorporated into many forceps, which enable these forceps to cut tissue and bone sharply, resulting in a more precise cut and a better preservation of mucosa. The shape and design of forceps and punches have been modified over time to incorporate varying sizes and degrees of rotation, which allow better access to several areas within the nasal cavity. Back-biting, side-biting, and down-biting forceps with through-cutting features are just a few examples of modifications on these instruments.

The unique position of the frontal sinus/recess requires modified instrumentation when operating. Giraffe forceps have been specifically designed to remove loose tissue along the skull base and frontal recess. They have angled shafts in the 55- and 90-degree positions and also have 2- and 3-mm cupped jaws that open in the horizontal and vertical positions (front-to-back and side-to-side positions). Likewise, a variety of frontal sinus punches have been designed to integrate through-cutting jaws, circular shapes, and various opening directions to remove bony partitions (**Fig. 24.5**). The use of through-cutting instrumentation in the frontal recess is particularly important because mucosal preservation is paramount to avoiding postoperative frontal stenosis.

Other commonly used instruments include probes, elevators, knives, and curettes (**Fig. 24.6**). Probes are available in various sizes, shapes, and curvatures. They are commonly used to palpate behind bony partitions before removal. They are also used to aid in the location of the various sinonasal ostia, can be used to tease out bony fragments, and reposition nasal mucosa. Commonly used elevators are the Freer and Cottle elevators. The Freer elevator has two rounded ends, one sharp and one dull, that are shaped for blunt dissection and tissue manipulation. In contrast, the Cottle elevator has one sharpened spade-like end and one dull flat end. The sharp end is often used to initiate the dissection underneath the mucoperichondrium of the nasal septum. Once the proper subperichondrial plane has been found, less traumatic dissection can continue with the blunt end.

Curettes are also used to help break residual ethmoid cells and gain access to the frontal recess. When using the curettes along the skull base, these instruments must be used in a posterior-to-anterior direction. Extra care must be used to avoid upward movements, which may result in an inadvertent iatrogenic violation of the skull base. Like the other manual instruments, curettes come in various shapes, sizes, and curvatures, which aid in accessing various spaces within the sinonasal cavity.

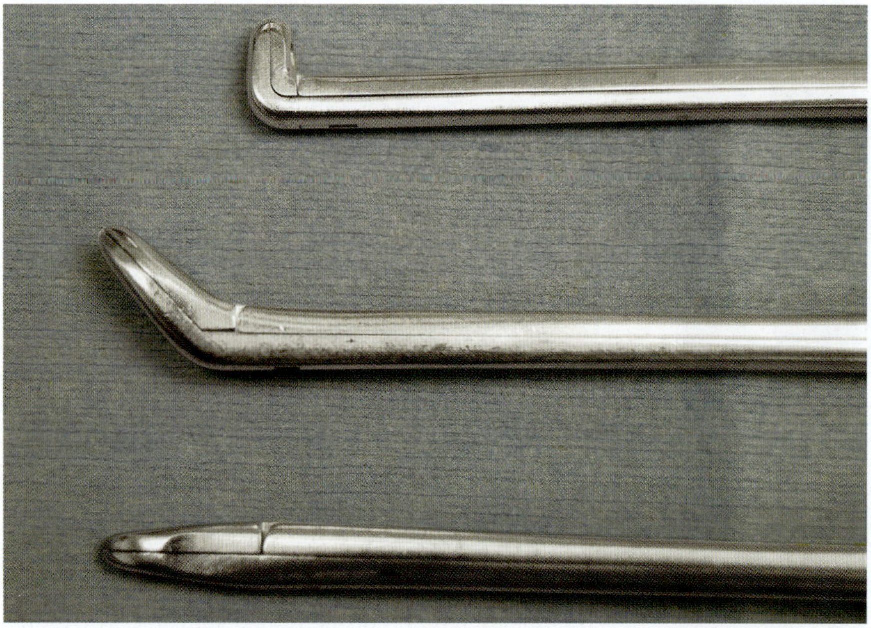

Fig. 24.3 Various forceps used during endoscopic sinus surgery to manipulate or remove loose bony and tissue fragments. Pictured from top to bottom are the 90-, 45-, and 0-degree Blakesley ethmoid forceps.

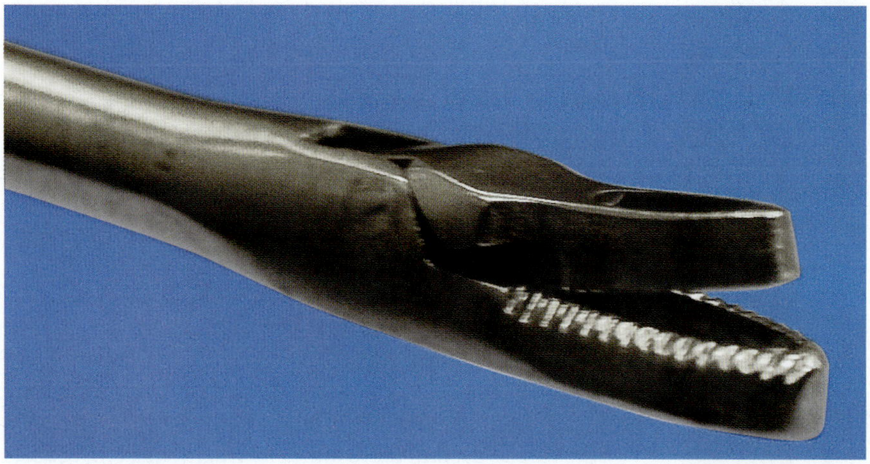

Fig. 24.4 A medium straight punch. Note the through-cutting tip that allows this instrument to cut through bone and cartilage without tearing or stripping the surrounding mucosa.

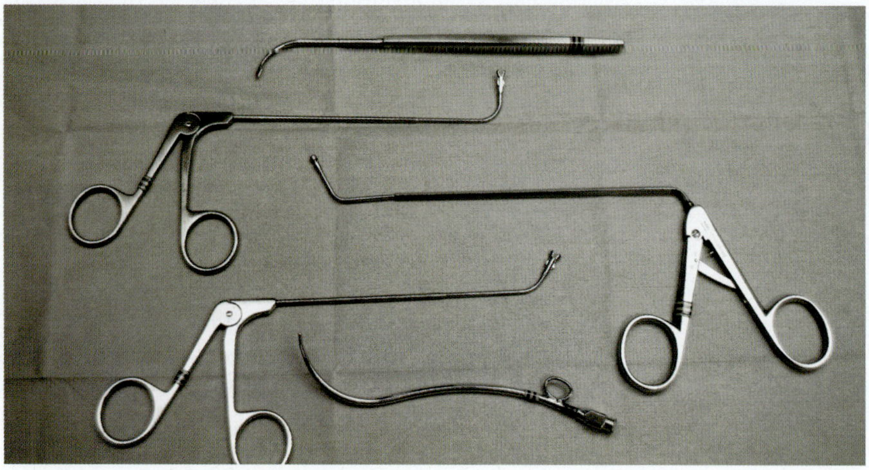

Fig. 24.5 Various instruments used to dissect the skull base and frontal sinus. Pictured from top to bottom are the frontal curette, the 90-degree giraffe forceps, the 45-degree mushroom punch, the 45-degree giraffe forceps, and the Van Alyea frontal sinus cannula.

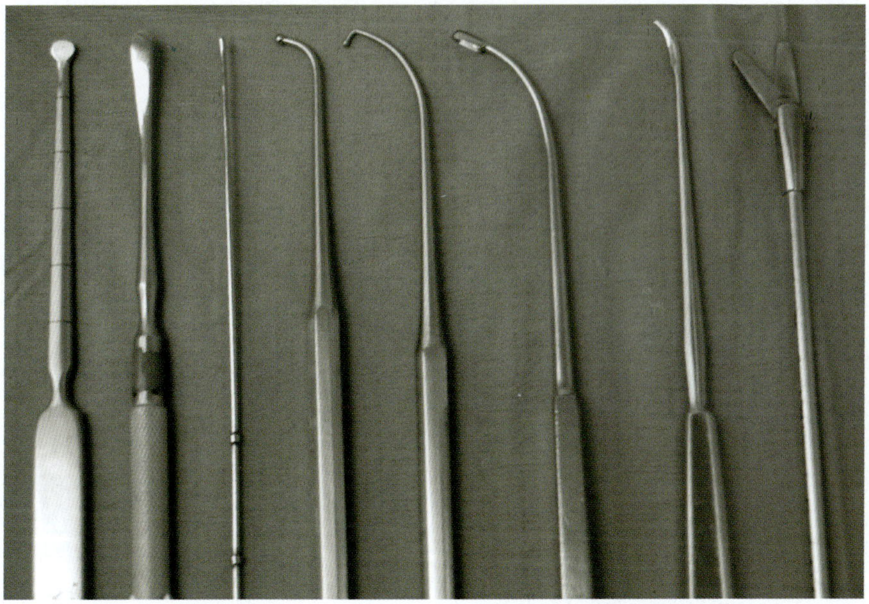

Fig. 24.6 Various instruments used during endoscopic sinus surgery. Pictured from left to right are the Cottle and Freer elevators, the beaded probe, the ball-tip probes, the curette, the sickle knife, and endoscopic scissors.

Powered Instrumentation

The development of power instrumentation has yielded dramatic enhancements to endoscopic surgical techniques. Interestingly, powered dissectors were initially used in the 1970s by orthopedic surgeons during arthroscopic procedures. This method became very popular and resulted in widespread use among orthopedic surgeons.[1] This design was modified and applied to sinus surgery in the 1990s. In 1993, Setliff and Parsons became the first surgeons to report using the powered shavers in the nasal cavity.[7]

Improvements in the microdebrider have allowed the instrument to become one of the most commonly used instruments in endoscopic sinus surgery. Current microdebriders contain a rotating blade that is housed within a sheath that has a small opening at its tip. The shaft is hollow and allows for continuous suction. As soft tissue is suctioned into the tip of the shaft, the oscillating blade cuts the tissue. The suction also removes blood and other debris. Most systems use disposable blades, which allows for a fresh blade to be used on every case. The fresh blade results in more precise cutting and preserves more nasal mucosa.

As with most other instruments, several different companies make these instruments and have slight variations in the design. The blades generally are available in a straight (0-degree) design as well as a curved orientation (40-, 60-, 90-, and 120-degree) (**Fig. 24.7**). Although the straight blades are used to dissect the ethmoidal and sphenoidal regions, the curved blades allow for better dissection of the frontal recess and maxillary sinuses.

The benefits of using the powered microdebrider lie in its ability to provide a more efficient dissection of soft tissue and bone. Its coupled cutting and suction capabilities allow the surgeon to continue operating without stopping to suction the blood. Although the advantages of using powered microdebriders are significant, there are notable risks associated with its use. In inexperienced hands, the microdebrider can become a dangerous weapon. Unlike other manual instruments, it is difficult to use the microdebrider as a probe to palpate bony edges. In addition, the close proximity of the sinuses to the orbit, optic nerve, carotid artery, and anterior cranial fossa make a sound knowledge of the sinonasal anatomy a strict requirement prior to its use. If close attention is not paid, the fast moving blade can cause tremendous damage within a few seconds.

Clogging of the shaft also poses a problem for some microdebriders. This is often caused by large pieces of tissue blocking the suction tubing. As a result, many systems have irrigation systems that have been incorporated into their units to help flush the collected debris through the suction tubing.

Similar to the microdebrider, the endoscopic sinus drill was designed after instruments used in orthopedic arthroscopic surgery. Several endoscopic procedures including the modified Lothrop procedure, choanal atresia repair dacryocystorhinostomy, and various skull base procedures require the removal of dense bone. Otologic drills have been used in the past. However, difficulty with visualization, short unprotected burrs, and the lack of an integrated suction led to a decrease in their usage in rhinologic procedures.

Endoscopic drill burrs come in a variety of sizes and shapes, including straight and curved bits (**Fig. 24.8**). Depending on the manner of drilling, beveled sheaths that cover one side of the drill bit may or may not be used. Beveled sheaths may help prevent circumferential damage to the surrounding tissue that increases the risk of scarring

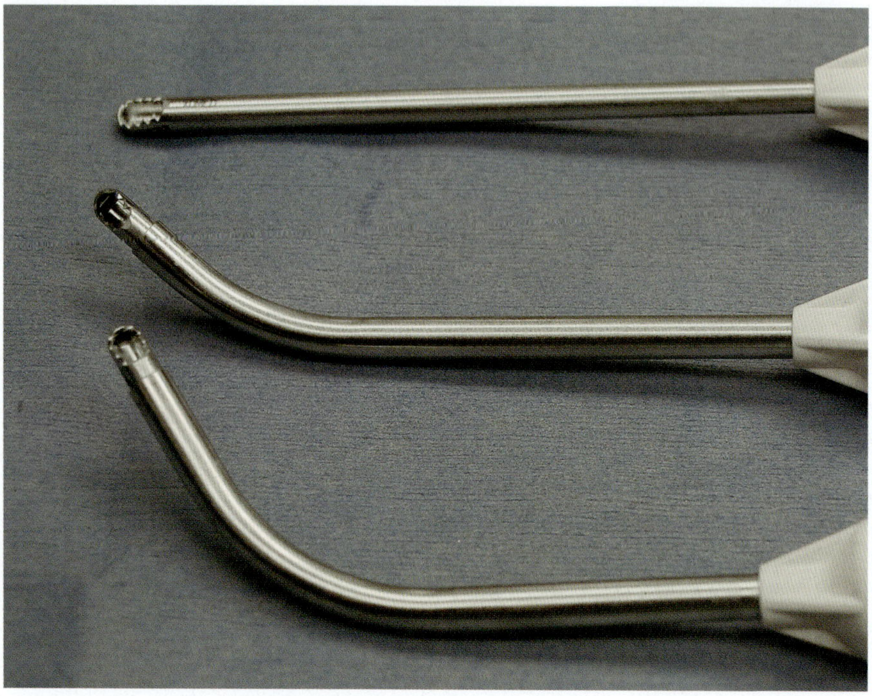

Fig. 24.7 Microdebrider blades with various angles. Pictured from top to bottom are the 0-, 40-, and 60-degree blades.

and stenosis. The drill speed varies but tends to be more precise at increased rotational speeds. One disadvantage of current rhinologic drills is that the revolutions per minute (RPM) are limited to less than 15,000 RPM. This makes thick bone problematic for removal. In this circumstance, a specifically designed skull base drill with enhanced RPMs should be considered.

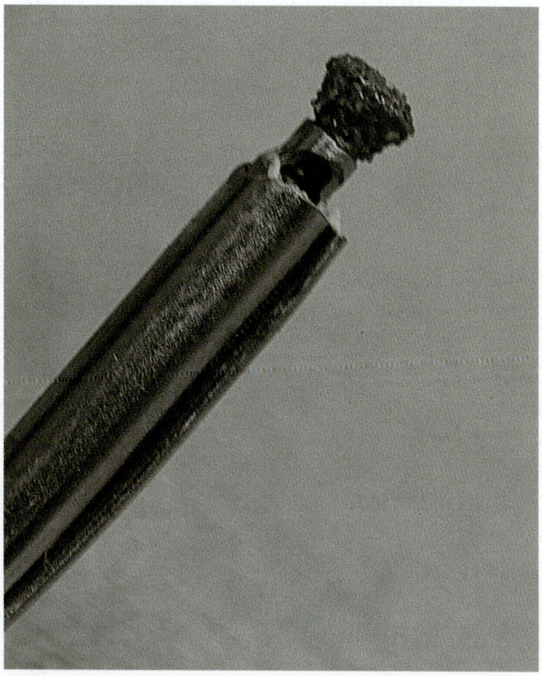

Fig. 24.8 Angled suction-irrigation diamond burr used to drill the skull base.

Stents

Although newly developed devices have improved the surgical management of rhinosinusitis, restenosis following endoscopic sinus surgery is not uncommon. Reported rates of this complication vary within the literature but has been reported to occur in up to 34% of patients.[8–10] In addition, Tran et al. demonstrated in a retrospective review of 77 patients who had an endoscopic-modified Lothrop procedure that the area of the neo-ostium decreased by 33% in the first postoperative year.[9]

Although there are several reasons why stenosis occurs, one major cause is the inappropriate use of the surgical instrumentation. Circumferentially damaging the sinonasal mucosa leads to scar or synechiae formation as well as osteoneogenesis. This results in occlusion of the sinus openings and eventually leads to recurrence of sinusitis. Although all of the sinus ostia have the ability to scar and stenose, the narrow outflow tract and surrounding anatomy associated with the frontal sinus make it particularly susceptible. Other factors that predispose patients to developing stenosis are denuded and remnant osteitic bone, and severe mucosal and polypoid disease.[10] Because of the propensity for the ostia to close, many surgeons believe in making large openings into the sinuses. Stenosis of the frontal sinus has been shown to be more likely when the diameter of the neo-ostium is less than 4 to 5 mm.[10–12] As a result, some surgeons use stents to try to help prevent cicatricial stenosis.

Stents comprised of various substances, including gold, rubber, Dacron, and Silastic, have been described in the literature.[13–16] They are available in a variety of sizes and

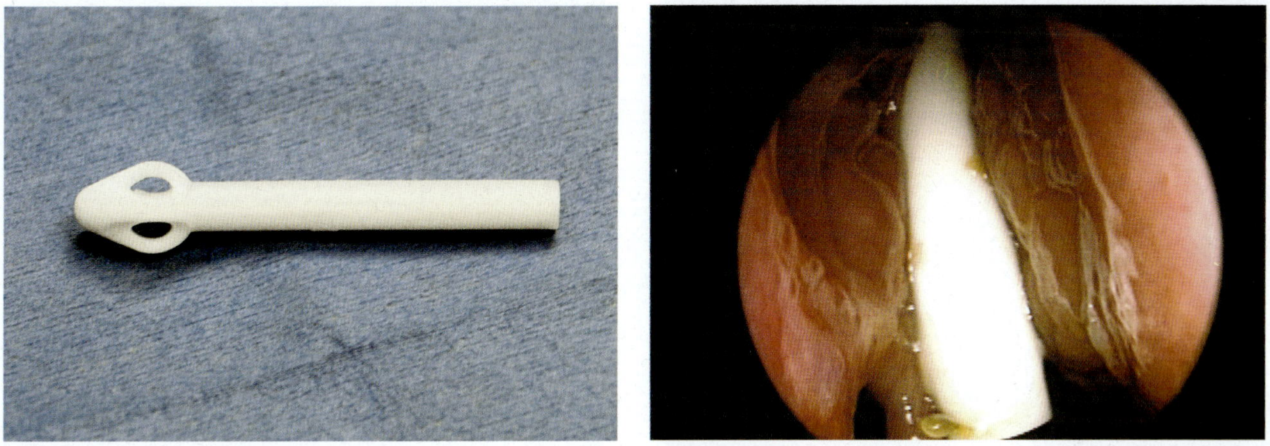

Fig. 24.9 (A) Sinus stent. Note that the stent is dilated at one end to prevent extrusion of the stent from the sinus. (B) Sinus stent placed within the right frontal sinus.

shapes. Although some stents are not self-retaining and require intranasal suturing, other stents have flanges or are dilated at one end, which helps prevent extrusion from the sinus (**Fig. 24.9**). In addition to helping avoid stenosis, some stents can be used as a drain or as an irrigation port for the sinus. Recently, there has been an evolution of the drug-eluting sinus stent.[17] These stents have a reservoir that can be infused with an antibiotic and/or a steroid solution and implanted into the frontal or ethmoid cavities during sinus surgery. The antimicrobial and/or anti-inflammatory solution slowly diffuses out of the stent and bathes the adjacent sinus mucosa, which may help reduce scar formation and help maintain sinus patency. Prefabricated steroid-coated middle meatal stents have also recently become commercially available. These bioabsorbable stents serve dual purposes of slow-release regional steroid delivery and stenting of the ethmoid sinus and middle meatus.[18]

Whether to use stents is a point of considerable debate. Some surgeons believe that stents act as foreign bodies that incite an inflammatory response that may lead to further granulation formation and scarring; others firmly believe in the ability of stents to successfully preserve the outflow tract with minimal inflammation.[10,13,19] Among the stent users, the duration of stent placement varies from weeks to months. Weber et al. found favorable results when stenting for prolonged periods of 6 months or more.[20]

Balloon Dilation

Sinus balloon catheterization is a relatively new technique, first introduced in 2005, that has since gained increasing popularity. It is used to dilate the natural ostia of the frontal, maxillary, or sphenoid sinuses, restoring normal drainage and ventilation with less trauma. No balloon is currently available for ethmoid sinus dilation. Balloon technology can be used as a stand-alone procedure that is amenable to being performed in the operating room suite or under local anesthesia in the office setting. Balloons can also be used in conjunction with more traditional means of sinus dissection in so called "hybrid" procedures.

This procedure uses a balloon catheter technique that is similar to that used in cardiac angioplasty. There are two main approaches for the passage of the balloons: transnasal for maxillary, sphenoid, and frontal sinuses; and transantral for maxillary access only.

Transnasal

The equipment setup for transnasal balloon dilation consists of various introducer guides (which come in a variety of angles for different sinuses), a guide wire, a balloon catheter, an inflation/pump device, a manometer, and a sinus lavage catheter. Depending on the sinus targeted, angled endoscopes may be needed to properly visualize the ostium of the sinus.

First, the guide wire is endoscopically passed transnasally into the outflow region of the targeted sinus and is carefully advanced through the obstructed ostium and into the sinus. In the first-generation device, this was performed under fluoroscopic guidance. An illuminated wire has since replaced the original guide wire, allowing for a confirmation of successful wire placement by direct inspection of sinus illumination, thus obviating the need for a fluoroscopy. Once confirmation of successful wire placement has been made (**Fig. 24.10**), an uninflated balloon catheter is threaded over the guide wire and into the sinus. Once positioning of the balloon across the ostium has been confirmed, the balloon is inflated with saline (**Fig. 24.11**). The balloon is then deflated and the complex is removed, leaving a dilated ostium (**Fig. 24.12**). The dilated opening can then be evaluated to see if the opening is adequate. If not, the ostium can be redilated or a larger sized balloon catheter can be used to redilate the ostium. After dilation, the sinus can be lavaged and aspirated.

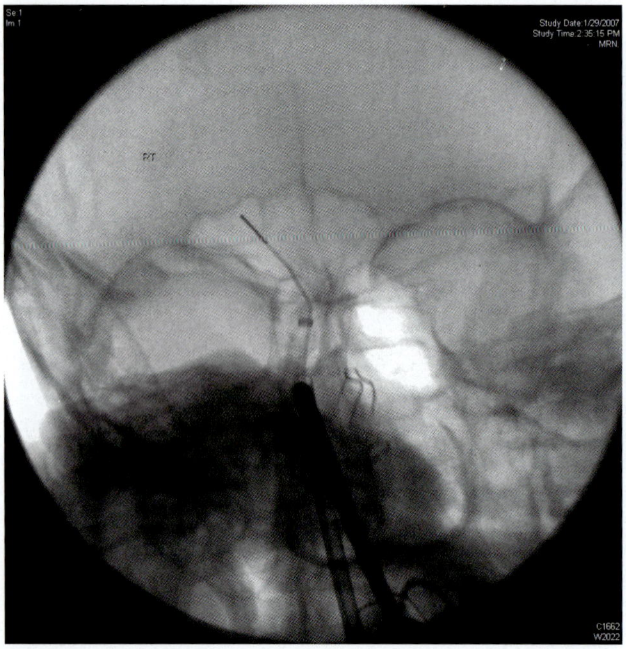

Fig. 24.10 A guide wire passed into the right frontal sinus under fluoroscopic guidance.

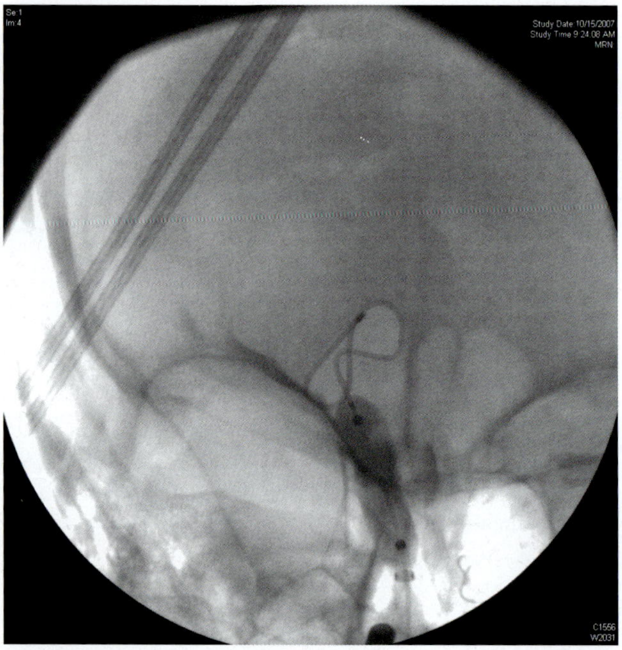

Fig. 24.11 Balloon catheter is threaded over the guide wire and into the frontal sinus. The balloon is inflated once the position across the ostium is confirmed.

Newer balloons designed for hybrid procedures are also now available. These balloons are sheathed over malleable metal probes, designed much like those probes used in traditional endoscopic sinus surgery. After initial sinus dissection, the probe is placed into the target sinus (frontal, sphenoid, or maxillary) under direct endoscopic visualization. The integrated balloon can then be advanced along the probe by a built-in fingertip slider into the ostium for dilation.

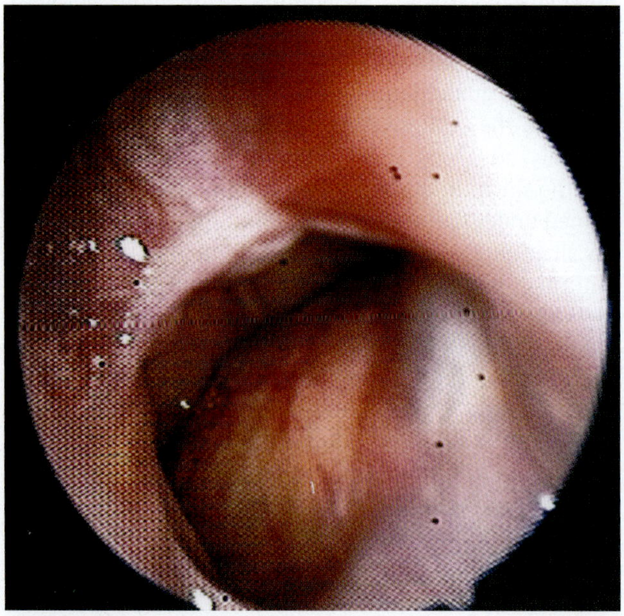

Fig. 24.12 Dilated frontal recess 1 month after balloon catheter sinuplasty.

Transantral

The transantral approach to the maxillary sinus involves sublabial puncture and placement of a trocar across the canine fossa into the maxillary antrum. With specially designed endoscopes, the balloon catheter can be passed through the trocar, across the antrum, and into the maxillary sinus ostium under direct visualization. Balloon inflation and deflation proceeds in a manner similar to the transnasal approach. After withdrawal of the balloon and trocar, the small sublabial puncture site can be left without the need for closure.

Outcomes

Compared with traditional endoscopic sinus surgery, balloon dilation is less invasive and results in less bleeding.[21] It has been associated with less mucosal trauma or stripping that may be found with conventional endoscopic sinus surgery, and under certain circumstances can be performed under local anesthesia.[21] These characteristics make balloon sinuplasty an attractive option in treating select patients whose overall medical status is too poor to subject them to the risks associated with conventional endoscopic sinus surgery.

Several studies demonstrate that balloon dilation is a safe and feasible method of enlarging obstructed sinus ostia in select patients with chronic rhinosinusitis.[21–23] In a multicenter, nonrandomized trial involving 115 patients, the efficacy, safety, and initial outcomes at 24 weeks postoperatively were measured.[22] At 24 weeks postprocedure, 80.5% (247/307) of the previously dilated ostia were patent, 1.6% (5/307) were not patent, and the patency of 17.9% of the ostia could not be determined. This trial also reported a significant improvement in patients' Sino-Nasal Outcome Test (SNOT)-20 scores and demonstrated no serious adverse events associated with sinus balloon catheterization. Conclusions from this trial were that balloon sinus catheterization is a safe and effective tool in dilating the sinus ostia for a durable time period.[22]

More recently, several trials have demonstrated long-term efficacy of balloon dilation. Weiss et al. reported significant improvement in baseline SNOT-20 and Lund-MacKay CT scores 2 years after surgery in patients that underwent balloon-only and hybrid surgeries.[24] Additionally, transantral balloon dilation of the ethmoid infundibulum was substantiated when Stankiewicz et al. reported significant reduction in SNOT-20 scores 1 year posttransantral dilation of the ethmoid infindibulum.[25]

Despite the definite advantages, balloon sinus catheterization is not a panacea and must be used in the proper settings. Patients with extensive previous surgery, sinonasal polyposis, sinonasal osteogenesis, significant ethmoid disease, history of facial trauma, and sinonasal tumors are not appropriate candidates for balloon dilation.[22] One pitfall of balloon dilation lies in the inability of the device to resect inflamed/diseased tissue and bone. Therefore, dilation of sinus ostia and restoration of the natural drainage pathways of the sinus may not be sufficient to eradicate the disease. Because of its versatile nature, sinus balloon catheterization has the potential to have a broad and favorable impact within the field of rhinology. More data regarding long-term outcomes of balloon dilation are necessary to understand the ideal candidates for this technology.

Conclusion

A sound understanding of the sinonasal anatomy and basic instrumentation is a requirement for performing successful endoscopic sinus surgery. With the advent of innovative instrumentation, the realm of endoscopic sinus surgery has broadened tremendously. Improvements in the instrumentation have been vital in providing increased visualization of the paranasal sinuses and allowing a more precise dissection. Although these instruments have led to improved surgical outcomes, they must be managed properly to avoid any inadvertent iatrogenic injuries.

References

1. Kennedy DW. Technical innovations and the evolution of endoscopic sinus surgery. Ann Otol Rhinol Laryngol Suppl 2006;196:3–12
2. Anand VK. Epidemiology and economic impact of rhinosinusitis. Ann Otol Rhinol Laryngol Suppl 2004;193:3–5
3. Jacobs JB. 100 years of frontal sinus surgery. Laryngoscope 1997;107(11 Pt 2):1–36
4. Nogueira JF Jr, Hermann DR, Américo Rdos R, Barauna Filho IS, Stamm AE, Pignatari SS. A brief history of otorhinolaryngolgy: otology, laryngology and rhinology. Braz J Otorhinolaryngol 2007;73(5):693–703
5. Jennings CR. Harold Hopkins. Arch Otolaryngol Head Neck Surg 1998;124(9):1042
6. Linder TE, Simmen D, Stool SE. Revolutionary inventions in the 20th century. The history of endoscopy. Arch Otolaryngol Head Neck Surg 1997;123(11):1161–1163
7. Setliff R, Parsons D. The "Hummer": new instrumentation for functional endoscopic sinus surgery. Am J Rhinol 1994;8:275–278
8. Friedman M, Bliznikas D, Vidyasagar R, Joseph NJ, Landsberg R. Long-term results after endoscopic sinus surgery involving frontal recess dissection. Laryngoscope 2006;116(4):573–579
9. Tran KN, Beule AG, Singal D, Wormald PJ. Frontal ostium restenosis after the endoscopic modified Lothrop procedure. Laryngoscope 2007;117(8):1457–1462
10. Rains BM III. Frontal sinus stenting. Otolaryngol Clin North Am 2001;34(1):101–110
11. Hosemann W, Kühnel T, Held P, Wagner W, Felderhoff A. Endonasal frontal sinusotomy in surgical management of chronic sinusitis: a critical evaluation. Am J Rhinol 1997;11(1):1–9
12. Orlandi RR, Kennedy DW. Revision endoscopic frontal sinus surgery. Otolaryngol Clin North Am 2001;34(1):77–90
13. Freeman SB, Blom ED. Frontal sinus stents. Laryngoscope 2000; 110(7):1179–1182
14. Amble FR, Kern EB, Neel B III, Facer GW, McDonald TJ, Czaja JM. Nasofrontal duct reconstruction with silicone rubber sheeting for inflammatory frontal sinus disease: analysis of 164 cases. Laryngoscope 1996;106(7):809–815
15. Barton RT. Dacron prosthesis in frontal sinus surgery. Laryngoscope 1972;82(10):1799–1805
16. Ijaduola TG. Use of a Foley catheter for short-term drainage in frontal sinus surgery. J Laryngol Otol 1989;103(4):375–378
17. Melroy CT, Kuhn FA. Safety of ethmoid sinus drug-eluting catheter insertion. Ann Otol Rhinol Laryngol 2009;118(10):708–713
18. Murr AH, Smith TL, Hwang PH, Bhattacharyya N, Lanier BJ, Stambaugh JW, Mugglin AS. Safety and efficacy of a novel bioabsorbable, steroid-eluting sinus stent. Int Forum Allergy Rhinol 2011;1:23–32
19. Schlosser R, Gross K. Postoperative management of endoscopic sinus surgery. Curr Opin Otolaryngol Head Neck Surg 2002;10:36–39
20. Weber R, Mai R, Hosemann W, Draf W, Toffel P. The success of 6-month stenting in endonasal frontal sinus surgery. Ear Nose Throat J 2000;79(12):930–932, 934, 937–938 passim
21. Brown CL, Bolger WE. Safety and feasibility of balloon catheter dilation of paranasal sinus ostia: a preliminary investigation. Ann Otol Rhinol Laryngol 2006;115(4):293–299, discussion 300–301
22. Bolger WE, Brown CL, Church CA, et al. Safety and outcomes of balloon catheter sinusotomy: a multicenter 24-week analysis in 115 patients. Otolaryngol Head Neck Surg 2007;137(1):10–20
23. Vaughan WC. Review of balloon sinuplasty. Curr Opin Otolaryngol Head Neck Surg 2008;16(1):2–9
24. Weiss RL, Church CA, Kuhn FA, Levine HL, Sillers MJ, Vaughan WC. Long-term outcome analysis of balloon catheter sinusotomy: two-year follow-up. Otolaryngol Head Neck Surg 2008;139(3, Suppl 3)S38–S46
25. Stankiewicz J, Truitt T, Atkins JJ Jr. One-year results: Transantral balloon dilation of the ethmoid infundibulum. Ear Nose Throat J 2010;89(2):72–77

25 Functional Endoscopic Sinus Surgery: Concepts, Surgical Indications, and Techniques

David W. Kennedy and Vijay R. Ramakrishnan

Since the initial introduction of the concepts of functional endoscopic sinus surgery (FESS) in 1985, there has been some significant improvement in our understanding of the most important factors involved in the pathogenesis of chronic rhinosinusitis. Naumann had originally described the ostiomeatal complex (OMC) nearly 20 years prior to the introduction of the concept of FESS.[1] However, as a result of the area being poorly seen on the plain film imaging available in that era, as well as the very limited use of nasal endoscopes at the time, little attention was paid in clinical practice to the concepts espoused by Naumann, Proctor, and others regarding the importance of the OMC. As endoscopes became more widely used in the clinic setting, and with Zinreich's subsequent development of appropriate computed tomography (CT) parameters that could provide imaging of the detailed anatomy and localized pathology, the clinical importance of the area became significantly more evident.[2]

In fact, following the introduction of endoscopic sinus surgery, many otorhinolaryngologists started to think of the OMC as the underlying cause of chronic rhinosinusitis (CRS), rather than its involvement being an important final common pathway in the pathogenesis of chronic inflammation. Additionally, with the wide anatomic variations of the region now easily visualized, the importance of these variations in the pathogenesis became overemphasized. Indeed, with the strong focus that developed on the OMC, resolution of CRS began to be thought of by some as just a "plumbing problem," and the concept began to predominate that restoration of drainage should resolve the majority of patients with sinusitis, even in the absence of medical therapy or surgical attention to the associated chronic inflammation. Over the subsequent years, it has become very evident that CRS is a complicated multifactorial inflammatory process, and that although anatomy and obstruction may play a contributory role, it is rarely the underlying cause of the chronic disease.

The Influence of Pathogenesis on Surgical Management

Broadly, the factors that predispose to sinusitis can be divided into environmental, general host, and local host factors (**Table 25.1**), and careful assessment and management of the predominant predisposing factors is key to the successful treatment of this disorder in any one patient. Environmental factors include pollution, viruses, bacteria, fungi, and classical allergens, all of which appear to be capable of enhancing the chronic inflammatory response in susceptible individuals. Indeed, it appears that the superimposition of bacteria and fungi may enhance the immunologic response in many patients, regardless of the presence of other predisposing factors.

General host factors include immunodeficiency, either congenital or acquired, primary ciliary abnormalities, cystic fibrosis, and other currently less well-defined genetic predispositions to rhinosinusitis, as well as the presence of atopy. Local factors include the presence of regional persistent inflammation such as inflammation in the underlying bone, the presence of bacterial biofilms, and the influence of anatomic abnormalities and obstructing masses. Although surgery may play some part in the management CRS regardless of underlying cause, the degree to which surgery is effective, and the appropriate physician and patient expectations, are clearly influenced by the underlying pathogenesis, and in some instances, the underlying pathogenesis may be a contraindication to surgery. For instance, surgical correction of an anatomic abnormality such as a concha bullosa in the absence of significant persistent inflammation, in a patient with significant allergies and ongoing environmental exposure, may open up additional virgin mucosa to the same environmental factors that caused the original disease. As such, this can potentially lead to more diffuse chronic inflammation in the long

Table 25.1 Known Etiologic Contributors to Chronic Rhinosinusitis

Environmental Factors	General Host Factors	Local Host Factors
Pollution	Immune deficiency	Persistent localized inflammation
Allergens	Ciliary dyskinesia	Osteitis
Viruses	Cystic fibrosis	Biofilms
Bacteria	Atopy	Anatomic abnormalities
Fungi	Mucosal hyperreactivity	Obstructing masses
Smoking	Stress	Granulomatous disorders

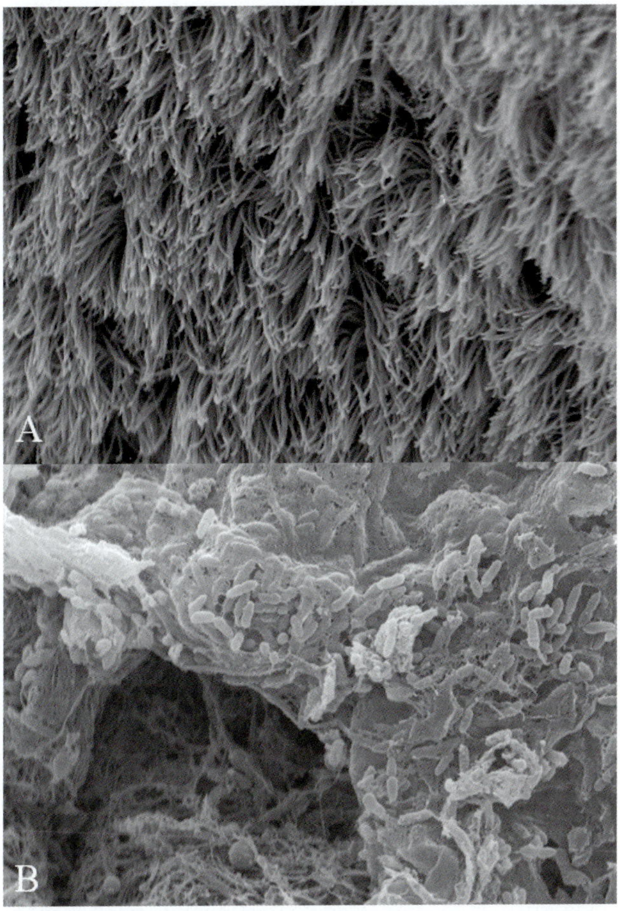

Fig. 25.1 High-power scanning electron micrograph of **(A)** normal ciliated epithelial lining versus **(B)** presence of bacterial biofilm. (Courtesy of Noam Cohen, MD, PhD.)

run. The greatest role of surgery is when local factors predominate in the inflammatory process. One such example is when chronic bacterial and fungal contamination are exacerbating the inflammation (**Fig. 25.1**). Such an inflammatory reaction may then induce additional mucociliary impairment, with the subsequent mucociliary stasis further potentiating the inflammatory cascade.

In recent years there has also been improved and increasing understanding of the potential role of the underlying bone and CRS. Our initial interest in the role of the underlying bone developed because a postoperative endoscopic evaluation demonstrated localized persistence of disease, even when the regional mucosa was removed. Subsequently, we and others have been able to identify the early involvement of bone in the disease process. Human studies demonstrated dramatic remodeling of bone in CRS, and by studying the process in an animal model of chronic sinusitis, the spread of inflammation through the Haversian canals of the bone can be seen, even to a significant distance from the site of primary infection.[3] Such changes are characteristic of chronic osteomyelitis (**Fig. 25.2**). Although there is, to date, no evidence of organisms within the bone, it is our impression that the Haversian canal fibrosis associated with these chronic osteomyelitic findings results in decreased bone viability and localized persistence of inflammation. Medical therapy alone may be unable to resolve such inflammatory processes, and surgical treatment is indicated when medical therapy fails. Removing the inflamed bone and reestablishing drainage in areas of obstruction then allows the residual inflammation to be treated medically with

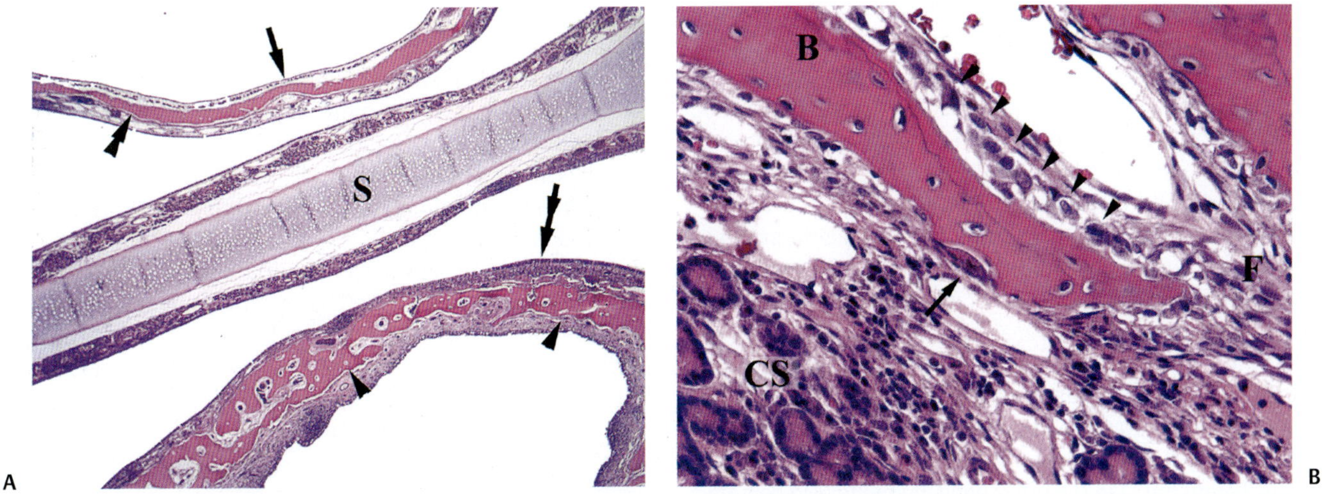

Fig. 25.2 Experimentally induced sinusitis in a rabbit model demonstrates osteitis with inflammation spreading through the bone to the opposite side of the nose. **(A)** On the right side (*double arrow*) of the nasal septum (*S*) with experimentally induced chronic sinusitis there are lymphocytes and plasma cells in the mucous membranes and hyperplastic changes. On the opposite side (*single arrow*), the epithelium appears normal. The bone on the infected side (lower right, *arrowheads*) shows osteitis and the uninfected side (upper left, *double arrowhead*) appears normal. **(B)** A higher power view of the opposite un-inoculated side demonstrates chronic sinusitis (*CS*) and inflammatory bone changes (*B*). There is fibrosis (*F*) and osteoblastic rimming (*arrowheads*), as well as a well-formed Howship's lacuna (*arrow*).

subsequent drainage of the distal sinuses, a reduction in microbial contamination, and secondary improvement in the residual inflammatory process.

Surgical Indications

The most common reasons for surgical intervention are CRS that does not respond to medical intervention and symptomatic polypoid disease, which is not adequately managed on medical therapy alone. However, many other medical problems may require surgical intervention including complicated acute sinusitis, allergic fungal sinusitis, and mucoceles. Indeed, the indications for this type of surgery have extended well beyond inflammatory causes to include intranasal, sinus, and skull base tumor removal; closure of skull base defects; orbital decompression; dacryocystorhinostomy; and resection of medially placed intraorbital lesions.

In inflammatory disease, the functional endoscopic approach is of most benefit when extensive sinus disease results from a limited cause. Thus, frontal sinus obstruction resulting in an extensive frontal sinus mucocele with a posterior table erosion is an ideal case for endoscopic intervention. Such an approach maintains the bony framework of the frontal recess and allows wide marsupialization with minimal morbidity. Indeed, in the presence of posterior table erosion, sinus obliteration is not a good alternative because of the difficulty of completely removing the lining mucosa from the exposed dura.

The more minor the disease, the more difficult the decision regarding surgical intervention. Recurrent acute sinusitis, in the absence of significant persistent disease between episodes, is probably more due to mucosal hyperreactivity or immunodeficiency than to persistent inflammation, and in this situation is usually not a good indication for surgical correction. The relationship between anatomic variations and recurrent disease is also controversial, but it is reasonable to consider surgery when such obstructing anatomic variations correspond to the area of recurrent symptomatology. Similarly, classical headaches are generally a poor indication for surgical intervention. The cause of such headaches is significantly more likely to be vascular in origin in the absence of significant associated disease. Even in the presence of significant disease, it is important to remember that whereas severe pain may occur in acute sinusitis, severe pain is not usually associated with chronic rhinosinusitis. Additionally, several publications have demonstrated radiographic evidence of mucosal thickening of between 30 and 50% in patients undergoing CT for indications other than sinus complaint.[4] On the other hand, it should also be noted that the normal sinus mucosa appears to be more sensitive to pain from ostial obstruction than chronically thickened mucosa, so that pain due to obstruction and barosinusitis in a patient with minimal disease will be greater than in a patient with significant polypoid changes.

Although there are several absolute indications for surgical intervention, there are no absolute indications for using an endoscopic approach rather than an alternative intranasal technique or external operation. The closest situation to an absolute indication is the presence of a mucocele with a posterior table or orbital involvement mentioned previously, because the marsupialization is usually best achieved with minimal trauma under endoscopic visualization (**Fig. 25.3**).

In general, patients with persistent environmental exposures after surgery, uncontrolled allergies, and continuing chemical exposures or who smoke are not good candidates for elective surgical intervention. In the authors' experience, cigarette smokers have such bad outcomes from FESS, both in terms of short-term granulation tissue and scar formation and in terms of revision surgery in the long term, that we consider smoking as a relative contraindication to elective endoscopic sinus surgery.[5] However, a shorter term follow-up by Kountakis et al. and Smith et al. have demonstrated no decrement in symptom improvement in smokers, apparently again demonstrating that patient symptoms in the early and midterm do not correlate well with endoscopic findings and disease resolution.[6,7]

Concurrent septoplasty will be required during FESS when the 0-degree telescope cannot be introduced to the anterior superior attachment of the middle turbinate. Failure to perform a septoplasty in this situation will compromise frontal recess access. Septoplasty in other situations, such as for impacted septal spurs, is usually more elective, although when contributing to nasal obstruction is typically performed in conjunction with sinus procedures.

Preoperative Medical Therapy

Surgery is usually reserved for patients who have failed appropriate, and frequently prolonged, medical therapy. Such therapy typically includes a long-term trial of topical nasal steroids, two or more courses of antibiotics and, frequently, topical nasal irrigations. The antibiotics should be based on endoscopically directed cultures wherever possible. Where allergies are suspected, an allergy evaluation should be performed, and if significant allergies are identified, it is usually better to initiate allergy desensitization prior to surgery. If there is no contraindication, a short course of oral steroids may also be helpful in controlling preexistent disease. Exceptions to these rules of prolonged medical therapy would be patients with a complication of CRS, such as an expansile mucocele.

Once the decision is made to perform surgery, the key is to use medical therapy to reduce intraoperative bleeding and thus improve visualization and thereby the ability to perform a complete surgical procedure. Patients with a significant degree of infection present may require an additional course of antibiotics immediately prior to surgical intervention. When there is reactive nasal mucosa, marked

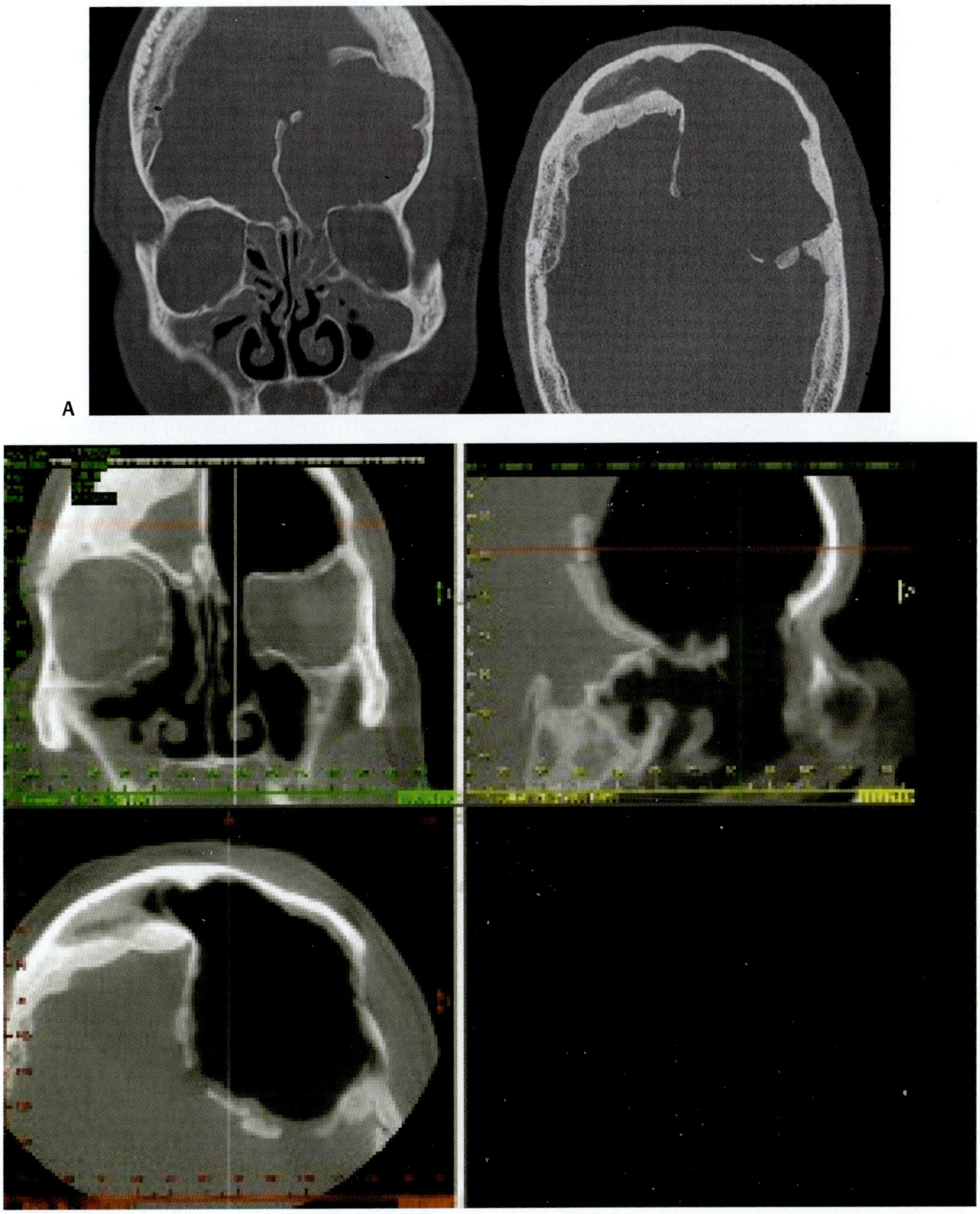

Fig. 25.3 (A,B) Pre- and postoperative computed tomography scans of a patient with a massive frontal mucocele with bony erosion and intracranial involvement who underwent endoscopic sinus surgery.

polyposis, or the patient has significant asthma, additional preoperative oral steroids are indicated. It has been demonstrated that the use of prednisone preoperatively for nasal polyps reduces intraoperative bleeding and improves the surgical field.[8] Depending on the extent of the disease, prednisone at a dosage of 20 to 40 mg per day may be started 4 to 8 days preoperatively, and is typically sufficient to stabilize the mucosa. Additionally, immediately prior to surgery, spraying the patient's nose with oxymetazoline both vasoconstricts the nose and reduces the absorption of cocaine or adrenaline when the latter is used intraoperatively.

Presurgical Evaluation

Because the degree of mucosal inflammation and the presence of mucosal hyperreactivity are important predictors of blood loss during surgery, it is helpful to perform a repeat nasal endoscopy in the weeks prior to the surgery. The presence of reactive nasal mucosa is identified by the tendency to develop marked congestion, sneezing, and hypersecretion during diagnostic endoscopy, despite topical decongestion and anesthesia. In this situation, if the mucosa is not stabilized preoperatively, bleeding will be increased

Table 25.2 Checklist for Preoperative Computed Tomography Evaluation

Anatomic Site	Key Points in Review
Skull base	Slope, height, shape, erosions, relative areas of thickening and thinning
Medial orbital wall	Integrity, shape, infundibular size, and uncinate position
Ethmoid vessels	Position of anterior and posterior ethmoid vessels relative to skull base
Posterior ethmoid	Vertical height, presence of sphenoethmoidal (Onodi) cell
Maxillary sinus	Infraorbital ethmoid (Haller) cells, accessory ostia, medial protrusion
Sphenoid sinus	Relative sizes, intersinus septum position, carotid arteries, optic nerves
Frontal recess and frontal sinus	Frontal sinus pneumatization, frontal recess size, agger nasi and supraorbital ethmoid pneumatization, frontal sinus drainage pathway

and may be intermittently profuse in response to intraoperative mucosal stimulation, even when the site of intranasal stimulation is at a distance from the immediate site of surgery. Prior to the surgery, the nasal anatomy is also reevaluated and any significant deviations from normal are noted. An endoscopic evaluation of the anatomy is particularly important in patients who have had prior surgical intervention. In particular, a prior partial resection of the middle turbinate, if not recognized preoperatively, can be particularly misleading at the time of surgical intervention, and might potentially lead to an inadvertent intracranial entry. An endoscopically directed culture taken preoperatively may aid in directing therapy either during surgery or in the early postoperative period. It is also important to note whether or not the 0-degree 4-mm telescope can be introduced within the nose to the anterior attachment of the middle turbinate bilaterally. As noted previously, if the 0-degree telescope cannot be introduced to this area, septoplasty will be required at the time of surgical intervention.

It is essential that the patient's CT scans be re-reviewed prior to the surgical intervention. This is typically best done shortly before the surgery. Standardized methodology should be used for the review of the films to ensure that no significant anatomic variations are missed (**Table 25.2**). First and foremost in terms of surgical safety, the skull base anatomy deserves particular attention. This evaluation should include an assessment of the vertical height as well as the slope of the skull base medially. The vertical distance between the roof of the maxillary sinus posteromedially and the roof of the ethmoid sinus determines the working room available within the posterior ethmoid for access to the sphenoid sinus. Failure to recognize a narrow vertical height in this area may result in inadvertent intracranial entry (**Fig. 25.4**). In general, the roof is significantly thicker laterally than medially. Any areas of hyperostosis should also be identified because, in these areas, the skull base can probably be approached with relative impunity. If there is an area of mucosal thickening or opacity adjacent to a skull base defect, a magnetic resonance (MR) scan should be performed prior to surgery, so as to determine whether or not a meningoencephalocele may be present.

The medial orbital wall is evaluated for areas of erosion and for any irregularities (**Fig. 25.5**). The relative position of the uncinate process to the orbital wall and the presence of any infundibular atelectasis are noted so that inadvertent orbital entry will not occur during the initial infundibulotomy incision. The anterior ethmoidal artery usually can be identified by a medial indentation ("nipple") pointing medially from the medial orbital wall. This may be seen either at the level of the skull base or some distance below it (**Fig. 25.6**). The posterior ethmoidal artery is typically within the skull base and is significantly more difficult to recognize.

Maxillary sinus pneumatization is evaluated with respect to the presence of any infraorbital ethmoid cells and the medial wall is evaluated for the presence of any accessory ostia that might have been missed during

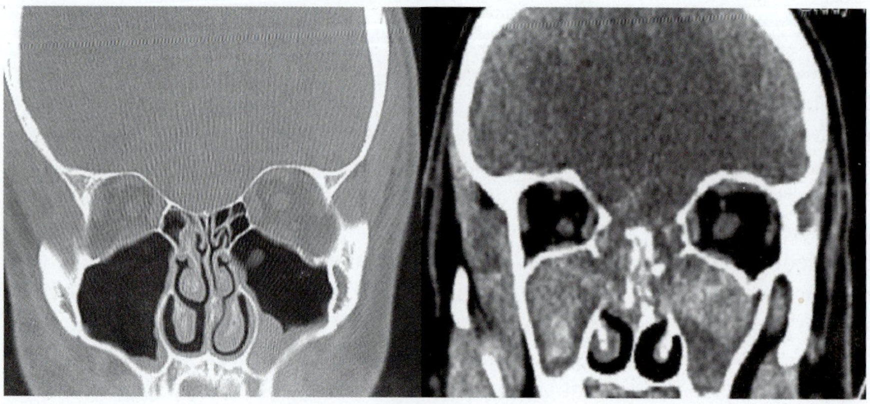

Fig. 25.4 (A,B) Pre- and postoperative computed tomography scans of a major complication as a result of an unrecognized low ethmoid skull base. The patient was referred following surgical intervention. The postoperative scan demonstrates bilateral skull base penetration and severe cerebral edema indicative of intracranial injury. The patient subsequently died from the intracranial injury.

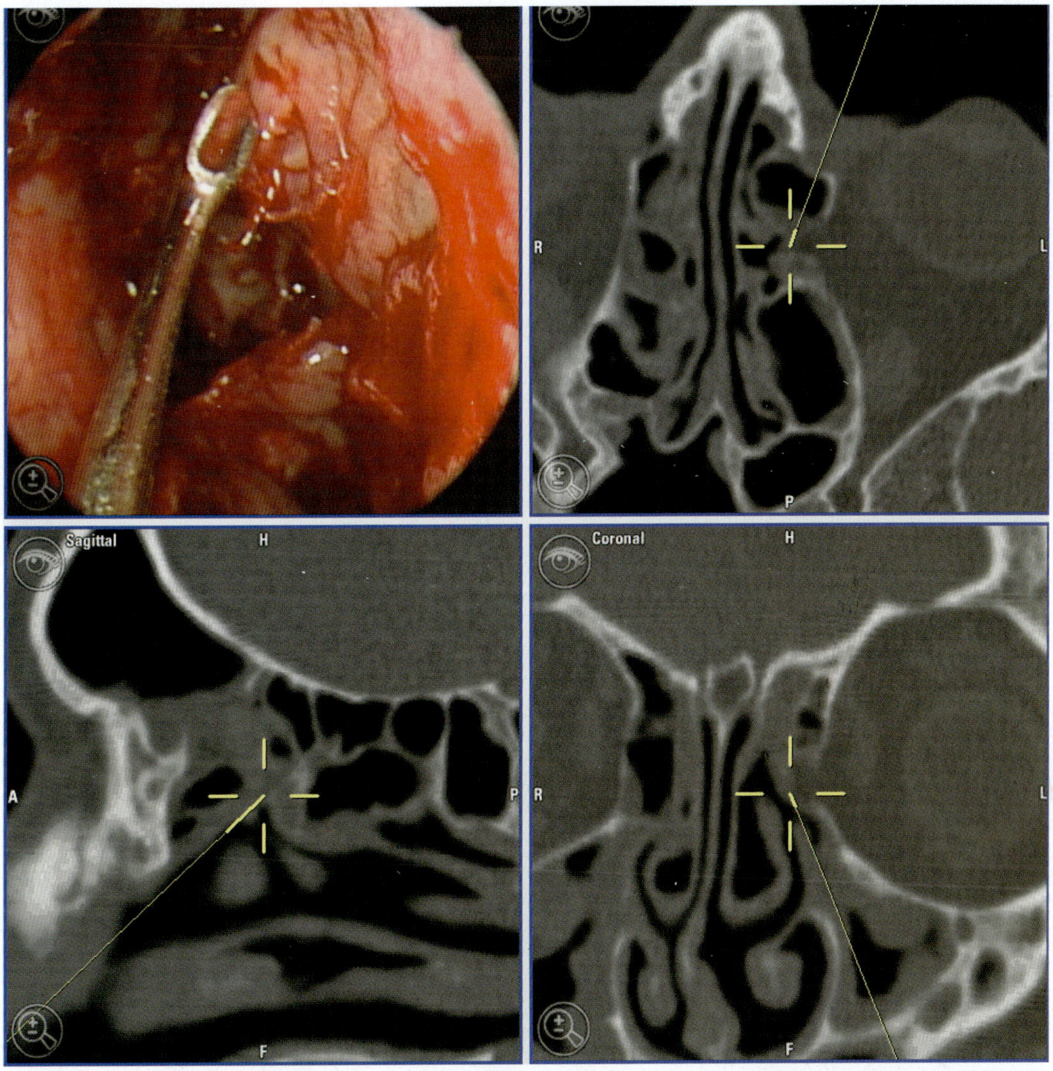

Fig. 25.5 Intraoperative image guidance in a patient with a left medial orbital wall dehiscence and a protuberance of fat into the ethmoid cavity (curette). The protuberance was noted on the preoperative scan. Had this not been so identified, removal of fat with the microdebrider might well have resulted.

nasal endoscopy. The presence of a retracted posterior fontanelle in conjunction with an atelectatic infundibulum suggests that gaining entry into the maxillary sinus will be challenging. However, an uncinate process may be in close relationship to the medial wall of the orbit even in the absence of maxillary atelectasis (**Fig. 25.7**).

Should surgery be necessary in the region of the sphenoid sinus, this is best evaluated in both the axial and the coronal planes. The axial plane demonstrates the relationship of the intersinus septum to the carotid arteries and the relative size of the two sphenoid sinuses, and the coronal view demonstrates the relationship of any sphenoethmoidal (Onodi) cells and of the optic canal to the sinus.

With the review of the films, the surgeon should develop a three-dimensional (3D) understanding of the sinus anatomy and particularly of the frontal sinus anatomy and the likely location of the frontal sinus drainage pathway. This review is best performed using triplanar films or, even better, by carefully and repeatedly scrolling through the planes of an image-guided system until the careful conceptualization of the 3D anatomy is achieved (**Fig. 25.8**).[9] To ensure that the frontal recess anatomy has been properly conceptualized, Wormald has advocated drawing out the anatomy and the relative positions of the frontal recess drainage pathway and the adjacent cells. This exercise does indeed have merit in helping less experienced surgeons visualize the anatomy that they are likely to encounter endoscopically. In patients who have had prior surgical intervention in particular, it is essential to look for significant areas of neo-osteogenesis. Such bony thickening may occasionally require the use of a drill.

Magnetic Resonance Imaging

Although CT is clearly the primary diagnostic modality for sinus disease, preoperative magnetic resonance

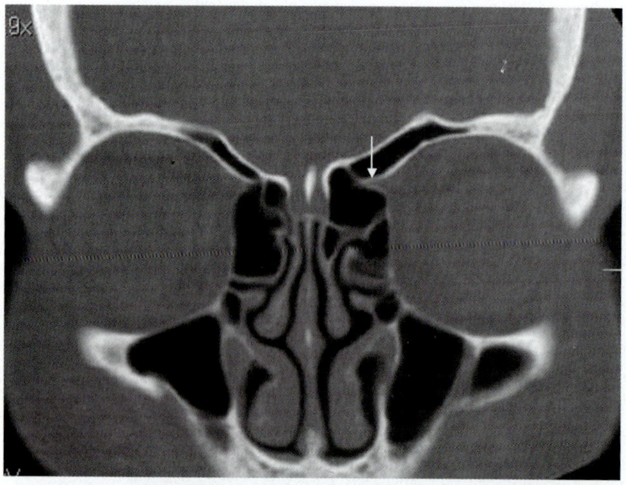

Fig. 25.6 Coronal computed tomography scan identifying the anterior ethmoid artery (*arrow*) at the coronal plane of the posterior globe. The artery is often identified radiographically as a "nipple" protruding medially from the orbit between the superior oblique and medial rectus muscles.

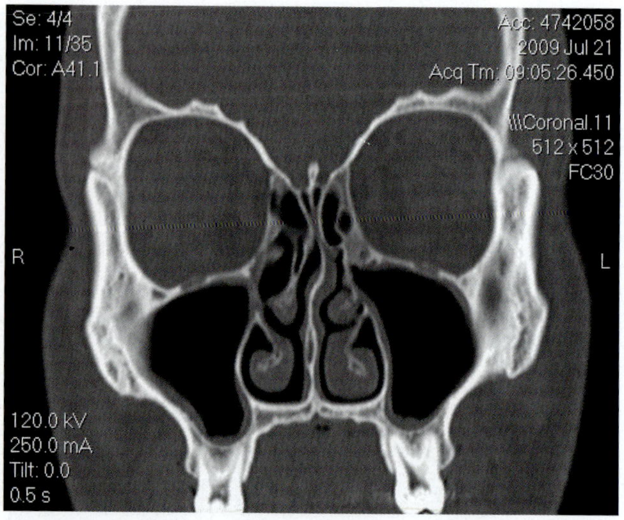

Fig. 25.7 Coronal computed tomography scan of an atelectatic infundibulum. The lateralized uncinate on the right side is immediately adjacent to the medial orbit, making maxillary antrostomy significantly more challenging. In this instance, the associated maxillary sinus is of normal size; however, it is frequently atelectatic.

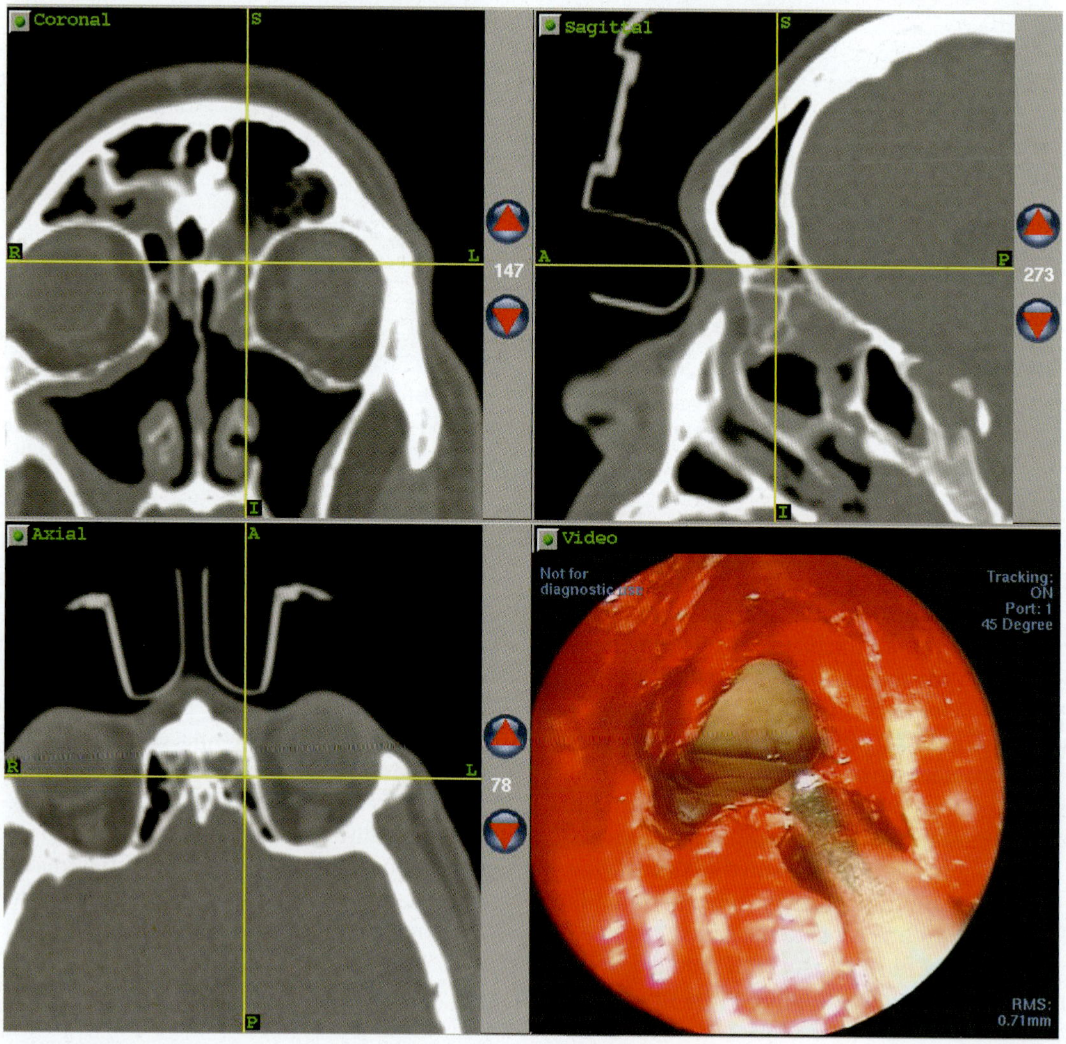

A

Fig. 25.8 Triplanar imaging of the frontal recess is extremely helpful in establishing and conceptualizing the endoscopic anatomy of the drainage pathway prior to surgical intervention. **(A)** In this patient undergoing left revision surgery, the drainage pathway is seen to be quite anterior and medial. *(continued)*

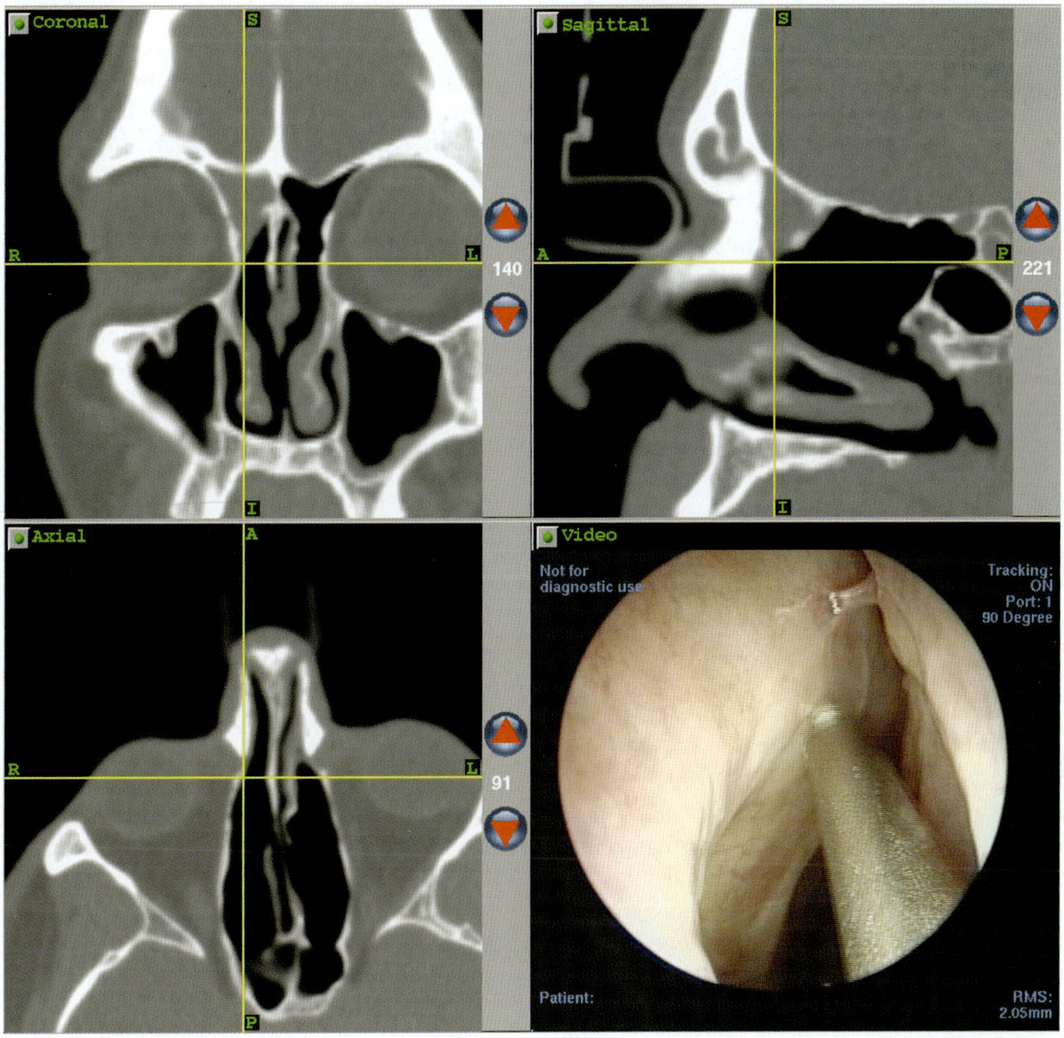

B

Fig. 25.8 *(continued)* **(B)** Triplanar image of a patient undergoing right revision surgery demonstrates a right frontal sinus obstruction due to middle turbinate lateralization.

imaging (MRI) is adjunctive in certain situations. MRI enables the differentiation of tumors or other soft tissue masses from retained secretions. However, as noted previously, it becomes critical when CT reveals disease adjacent to skull base erosion. In this situation, MRI can discern whether the erosion is caused by sinus disease versus a spontaneous or post-traumatic meningoencephalocele (**Fig. 25.9**). The evaluation of dehiscent areas becomes even more important in the sphenoid sinus, raising the possibility of a carotid artery aneurysm.

Anesthesia

A FESS can be performed satisfactorily under either local anesthesia with sedation or general anesthesia. In the early years of FESS, the surgery was typically performed under local anesthesia with sedation. Advantages were reduced bleeding, the avoidance of intubation, and decreased anesthesia risk. Additionally, should the patient have developed an intraorbital hematoma, the patient's vision could be easily monitored. A patient survey performed by Thaler et al. demonstrated patient satisfaction at least equal to that of patients undergoing the surgery under general anesthesia.[10] However, in recent years, the surgery is more frequently performed under general anesthesia. Several reasons account for this change. First, the mucosal preserving techniques used today, and the fact that we now typically like to remove all of the bony partitions within the area of disease, make the operative time longer than in the early days of FESS. Second, the safety of general anesthesia has improved significantly and the advent of total intravenous anesthesia (TIVA) has been demonstrated to be associated with less blood loss from the prior anesthesia using inhalational agents.[11] Accordingly, therefore, TIVA is the most common anesthesia of choice.

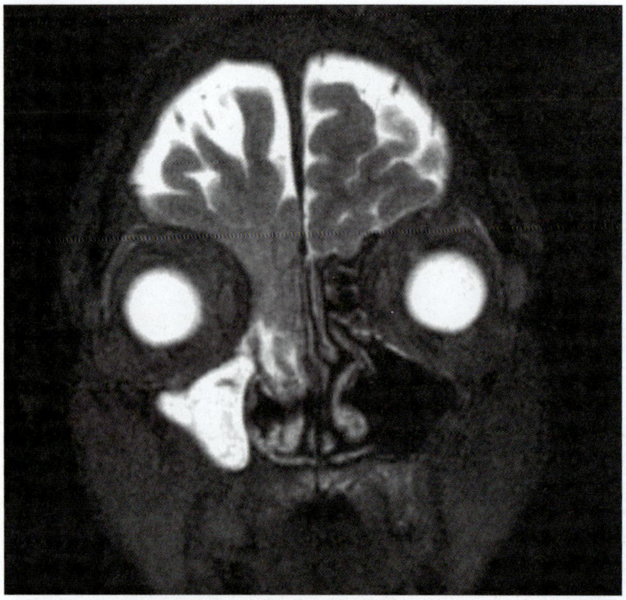

Fig. 25.9 Coronal T2-weighted magnetic resonance image showing a spontaneous massive ethmoid meningoencephalocele with secondary maxillary sinus obstruction.

Intranasal vasoconstriction is essential to endoscopic sinus surgery or other intranasal surgery. This is best initiated by the topical application of oxymetazoline spray prior to anesthesia induction. Oxymetazoline has been demonstrated to decrease subsequent cocaine absorption, and may also decrease adrenaline absorption.[12] Supplemental topical vasoconstriction can then be achieved after the induction of anesthesia either by the application of cocaine powder on nasal applicators, or by the application of 1:1000 topical adrenaline. In either case, the application should be performed slowly, and the patient should be monitored for any change in heart rate or blood pressure. Although the toxic dose of cocaine is quite variable, 2 to 3 mg/kg or 200 mg is considered the safe maximum dosage for topical use.[13]

Surgical Principles

There has been, and still remains, significant controversy regarding the extent of surgery that should be performed for CRS. It is likely that this debate will continue until the pathogenesis of CRS is better understood. In general, the concept of irreversibly diseased mucosa that needs to be removed has been largely abandoned. However, in certain parts of the world, such as France and Belgium, stripping of the ethmoid mucosa is still performed in severe disease in an operation known as nasalization.[14] At the other end of the spectrum, a significant number of people advocate for transition space surgery (MIST) or even balloon sinuplasty.[15,16] Although these procedures have the advantages of causing less mucosal trauma and thereby less scarring, they do not allow for the removal of the inflamed bone and are therefore probably not suitable for treating a well-established disease where there is extensive mucosal and bone involvement, the type of disease typically seen in patients who ordinarily require surgical intervention. However, it is quite possible that, in the long run, the combination of balloon dilatation or a minimal intervention combined with some form of drug-eluting stent or topical therapy may provide a minimally invasive intervention for some patients who truly do not respond to medical therapy and absolutely require surgical intervention. Additionally, early studies suggest that good symptom improvement can be obtained with ostial dilation, particularly in limited disease.[17]

The problems associated with mucosal stripping have been increasingly appreciated. Moriyama and colleagues demonstrated that bone exposure results in extremely delayed healing, and that ciliary density may never return to normal.[18] Additionally, bone exposed during surgery for chronic sinusitis frequently undergoes neo-osteogenesis, may become osteitic and, in some patients, appears to be associated with chronic pain (**Fig. 25.10**). For these reasons, therefore, significant emphasis is usually placed on preserving the mucoperiosteum over the bone whenever possible, and thereby avoiding areas of bone exposure during sinus surgery. Conversely, persistent osteitic bone is frequently a cause for persistent inflammation and scarring, and it is therefore important to ensure that bone that has become osteitic is completely removed whenever possible. For instance, the uncinate process is usually involved early in the disease process, and the residual uncinate process following surgical intervention is one of the most common causes of scarring of the middle turbinate to the lateral nasal wall (**Fig. 25.11**).

In the early days of FESS, the primary goal was to reopen the dependent sinuses, and thus reestablish ventilation and drainage. We now know that in well-established disease, this is usually not sufficient because the involved tissue and bone appears to play a significant part in the inflammatory process. Fortunately, with the advent of through-cutting forceps, microdebriders, and improved hand instrumentation, removal of diseased tissue and bone can now usually be achieved with good mucoperiosteal preservation. However, the surgery tends to take significantly longer and tends to be more meticulous than when FESS was first introduced.

The important question during primary surgical intervention is whether the frontal sinuses should be opened even in the presence of mucosal disease. Performing a frontal sinusotomy creates the potential for significant scarring and, at minimum, requires prolonged postoperative endoscopic follow-up. On the other hand, if disease left in this area does not resolve, it will create bony thickening over time and make subsequent opening of the frontal sinus significantly more difficult. Additionally, opening the frontal sinus provides a clear endoscopic view into the frontal sinus itself and allows any persistent disease to be easily identified. In addition

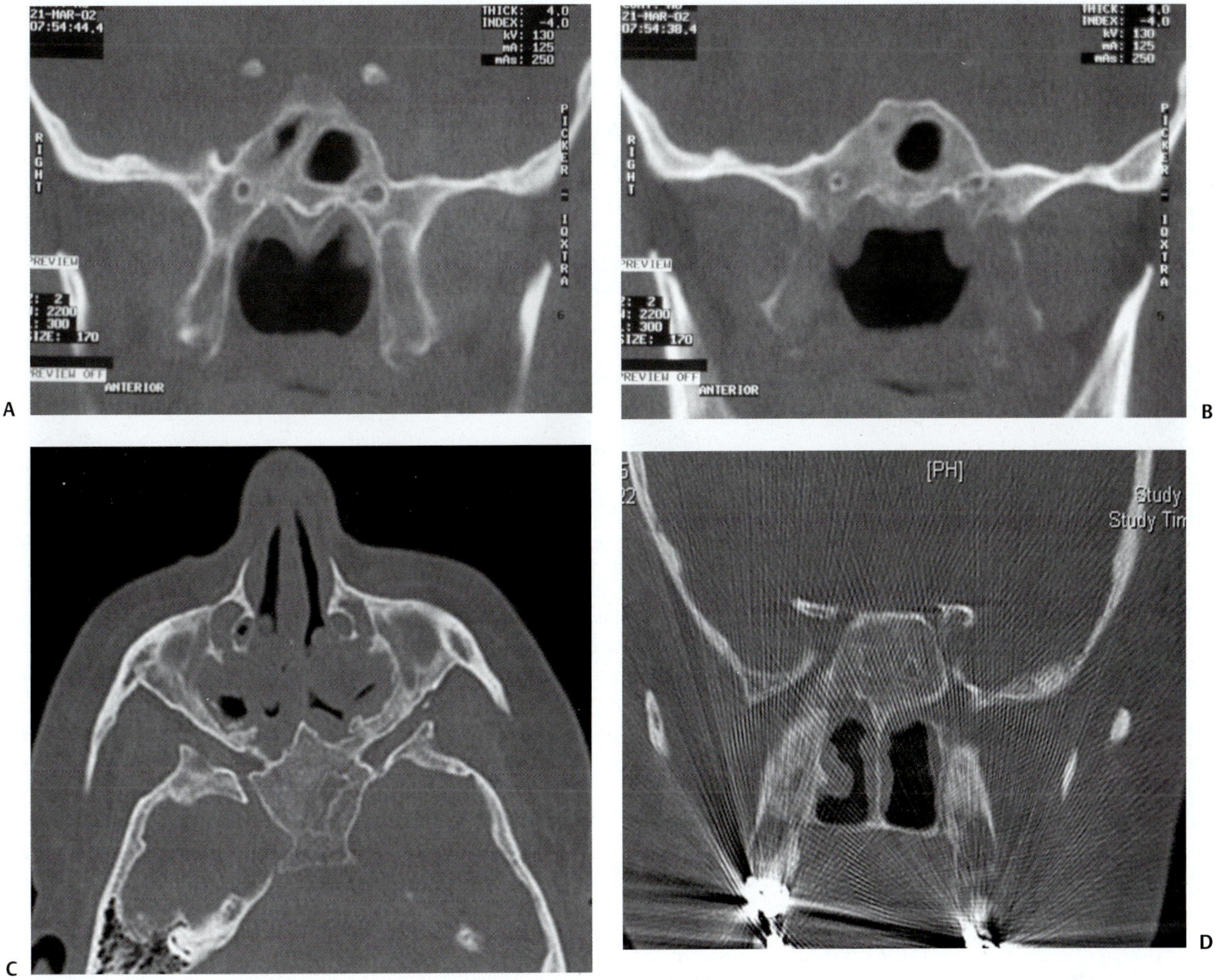

Fig. 25.10 Marked neo-osteogenesis of the sphenoid sinuses. **(A,B)** Coronal computed tomography (CT) scans demonstrate some sphenoid neo-osteogenesis postsurgery. Axial **(C)** and coronal **(D)** CT scans 7 years later demonstrate marked progression of the neo-osteogenesis with entrapped mucosa.

to the extent of the disease, the decision as to whether the frontal sinus should be opened depends to a very significant extent on the skill of the surgeon, the ability of the patient to return for postoperative follow-up, and the frontal sinus instrumentation available (**Fig. 25.12**).

The extent of FESS may vary from a simple uncinectomy to a complete sphenoethmoidectomy, antrostomy, and frontal sinusotomy, but should go one step beyond the extent of disease identified on preoperative imaging or seen at the time of surgical intervention. In general, extended frontal sinus procedures are not performed at the first surgery and are reserved for revision surgical procedures where a simple "uncapping of the egg" is not possible. Overall, the extent of surgery during a revision operation tends to be significantly greater than with a first procedure, and frequently involves opening all of the sinuses and a complete removal of the bony partitions.

Ethmoidectomy

The extent to which an ethmoidectomy should result in the complete removal of the ethmoid bony partitions, and the frequency with which an anterior ethmoidectomy alone results in the resolution of disease still remains a subject of debate. As mentioned previously, the removal of bony partitions within the area of disease should generally be complete and, wherever possible, any exposed bone should be removed. However, there are situations where it is preferable to perform a complete ethmoidectomy, even in the absence of extensive anterior ethmoid disease, particularly if the surgeon is skilled and able to remove the partitions without any bony exposure. Should a complete ethmoidectomy not be performed and residual inflammation persists, the bony partitions will thicken and become more difficult to remove subsequently. Certainly,

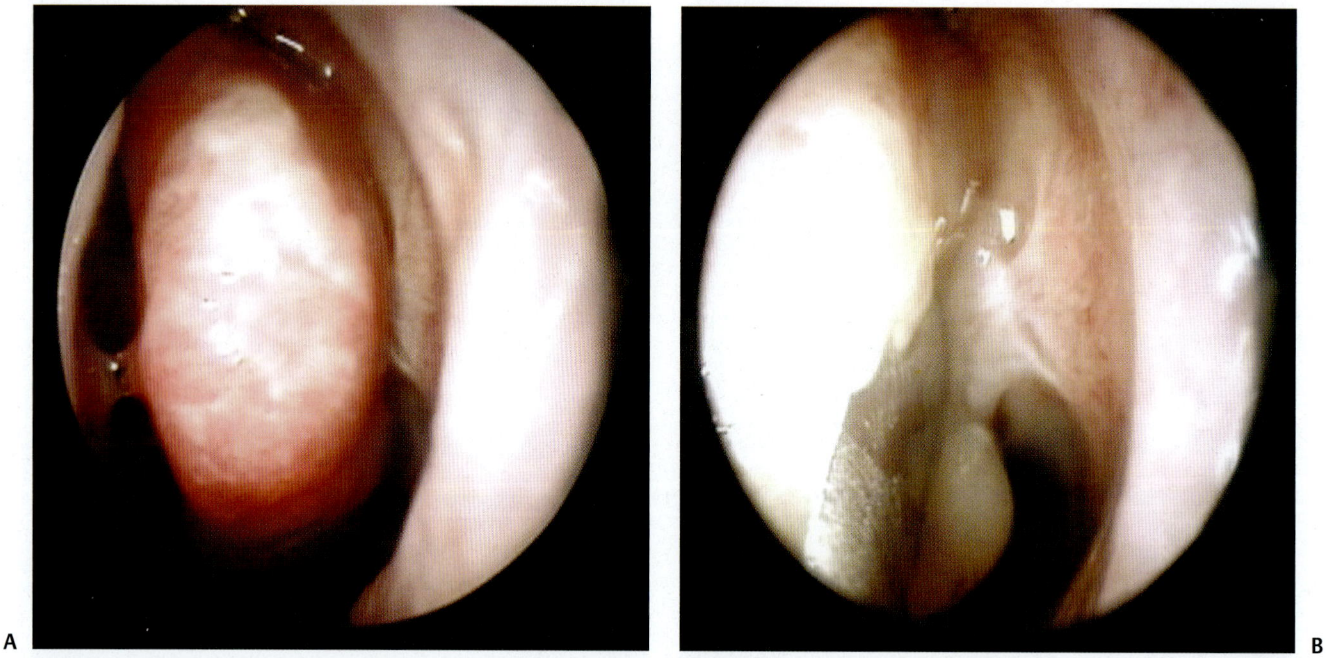

Fig. 25.11 (A) Endoscopic view of the left middle meatus demonstrating the residual uncinate process postsurgery, which frequently leads to middle meatal scarring. **(B)** Medial displacement of the turbinate demonstrates that the turbinate is scarred to the uncinate.

if mucosa is stripped from the basal lamella of the middle turbinate, the basal lamella is better removed and a posterior ethmoidectomy is performed. However, even in the absence of mucosal stripping, we have seen cases where a retained basal lamella is subject to airflow drying and crusting and results in recurrent exacerbations of inflammation. Further experience and long-term studies are really required to identify the best procedure for limited disease and when surgery should be limited to an anterior ethmoid procedure.

Whatever the extent of surgery, the initial steps of the procedure are similar. Following an uncinectomy, the medial orbital wall is identified and provides the first critical landmark for the dissection. The procedure should be performed

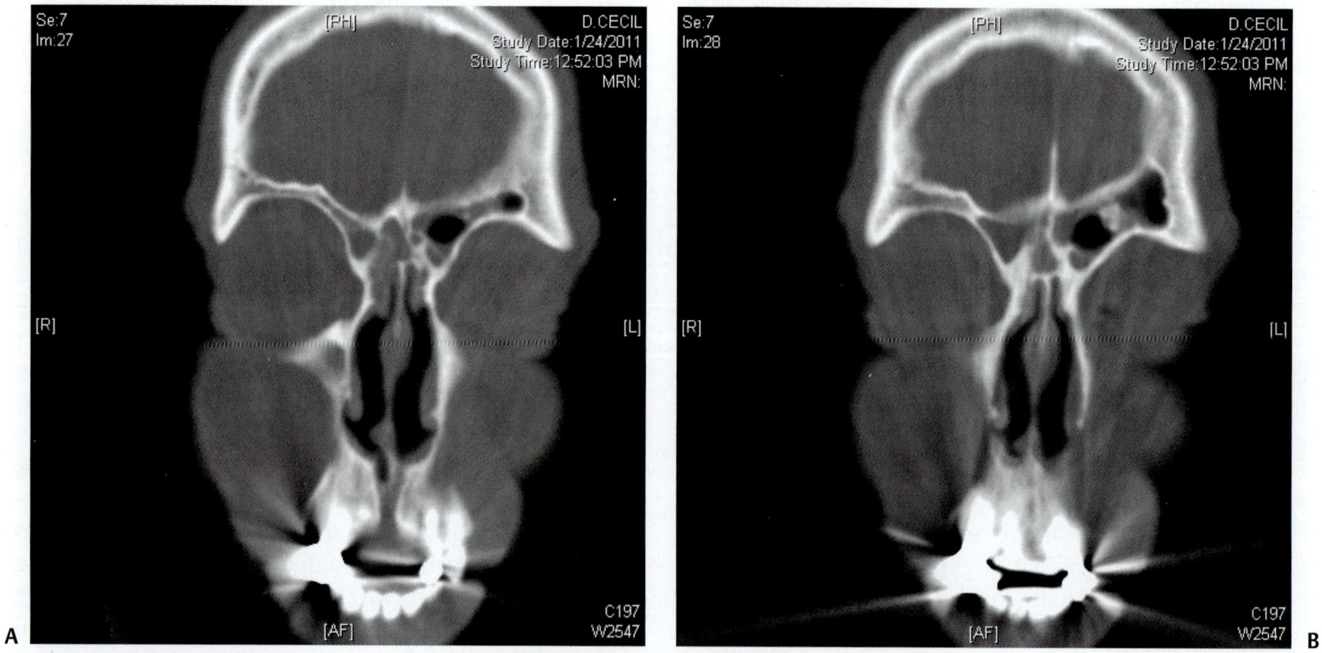

Fig. 25.12 (A) Coronal computed tomography scan demonstrates some bony thickening in the area of the frontal recess bilaterally in this patient with prior surgery. **(B)** A more anterior cut also demonstrates an osteoma arising from a bony partition within the left frontal sinus.

along the medial orbital wall because the skull base laterally is significantly thicker than it is medially where it is both very thin and downsloping into the middle turbinate. Failure to identify the medial orbital wall and to dissect close to it may result in an inadvertent intracranial entry. The procedure is most safely performed with a 0-degree telescope and microdebrider or straight and 45-degree through-cutting forceps. After positive identification is made of the medial orbital wall, the skull base provides the second critical landmark and must be identified carefully. We advocate dissection low in an anterior-to-posterior direction, across the basal lamella to the sphenoid face, and then identification of the skull base in the posterior ethmoid or sphenoid sinus followed by completing the dissection from posterior to anterior (**Fig. 25.13**). This is done by feeling behind the bony partitions with an upbiting forceps as the dissection is performed from posterior to anterior.

Careful attention to bony lamellar remnants, the use of through-cut forceps, as well as the use of a microdebrider

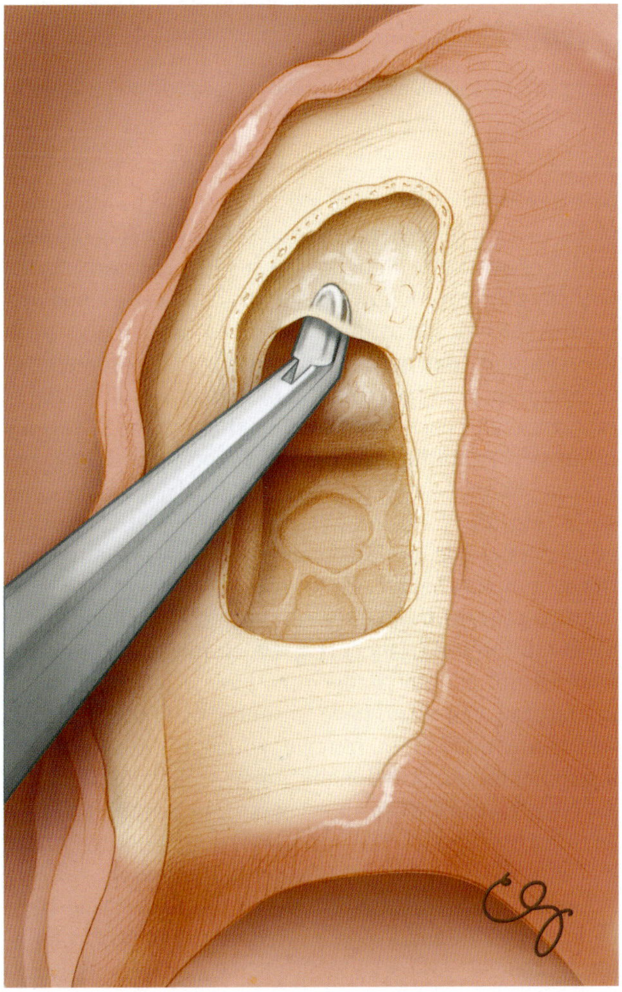

Fig. 25.13 The skull base is identified in the posterior ethmoid sinus, where the bone of the ethmoid roof is frequently thicker and further skeletonized by feeling behind the bony partitions with an upbiting through-cutting forceps and then removing them.

to remove hypertrophic and loose mucosal tags while, at the same time, preserving the mucoperiosteum of the medial orbital wall and skull base helps to achieve the resection of disease and rapid healing (**Fig. 25.14**). Bony partitions within the region of disease are best removed meticulously at the time of initial surgery; residual partitions trap secretions and mucosa, frequently thicken, and become difficult to remove subsequently. As a result of this thickening, on occasion, particularly in revision surgery, a drill may be needed to remove residual osteitic bone. Additionally, if mucosal disease persists, the residual bony partitions may become "layered" in an onionskin fashion against the medial orbital wall or skull base as a result of remodeling from recurrent polyposis.

Some of the more common postoperative findings from an incomplete ethmoidectomy include a retained uncinate process, frequently with scarring of the middle turbinate to the inflamed residual uncinate, and failure to remove the uncinate superiorly (persistent recessus terminalis). Other common problems are residual agger nasi cells and persistent disease along the medial orbital wall (**Fig. 25.15**).

Concepts in Maxillary Antrostomy

The size of a surgically created antrostomy will vary considerably from case to case. However, one aspect is constant: it must communicate with the natural ostium, and ensuring that this has occurred frequently requires a 45- or 70-degree telescope. In considering the most appropriate size for the antrostomy, several theoretical considerations need to be kept in mind. Early on, we demonstrated that experimental exposure of the maxillary sinus to airflow in rabbits results in a dramatic slowing or cessation of mucociliary clearance. Therefore, the maxillary sinus ostium and the maxillary sinus mucosa should ideally remain protected from airflow. It also has been demonstrated that nitric oxide is actively liberated from the sinus mucosa at levels that may reach bacteriostatic concentrations, theoretically creating another advantage for keeping the surgically created ostium small. Conversely, a significant part of the medial wall of the maxillary sinus is composed of the uncinate process, and this bone frequently displays osteitic changes, and when this is not resected and is significantly involved in the disease process, scarring may be seen.

At this point in time, therefore, it appears that when disease is very mild, a minimal opening of the ostium is preferable. However, in the presence of long-standing diffuse chronic sinusitis, especially with evidence of osteitis, or when there is a strong likelihood that significant local care may be required to the maxillary sinus following surgery, a wide middle meatal antrostomy is preferred. The wide middle meatal antrostomy would include the careful and complete removal of the uncinate process both anteriorly and inferiorly. However severe the disease, if

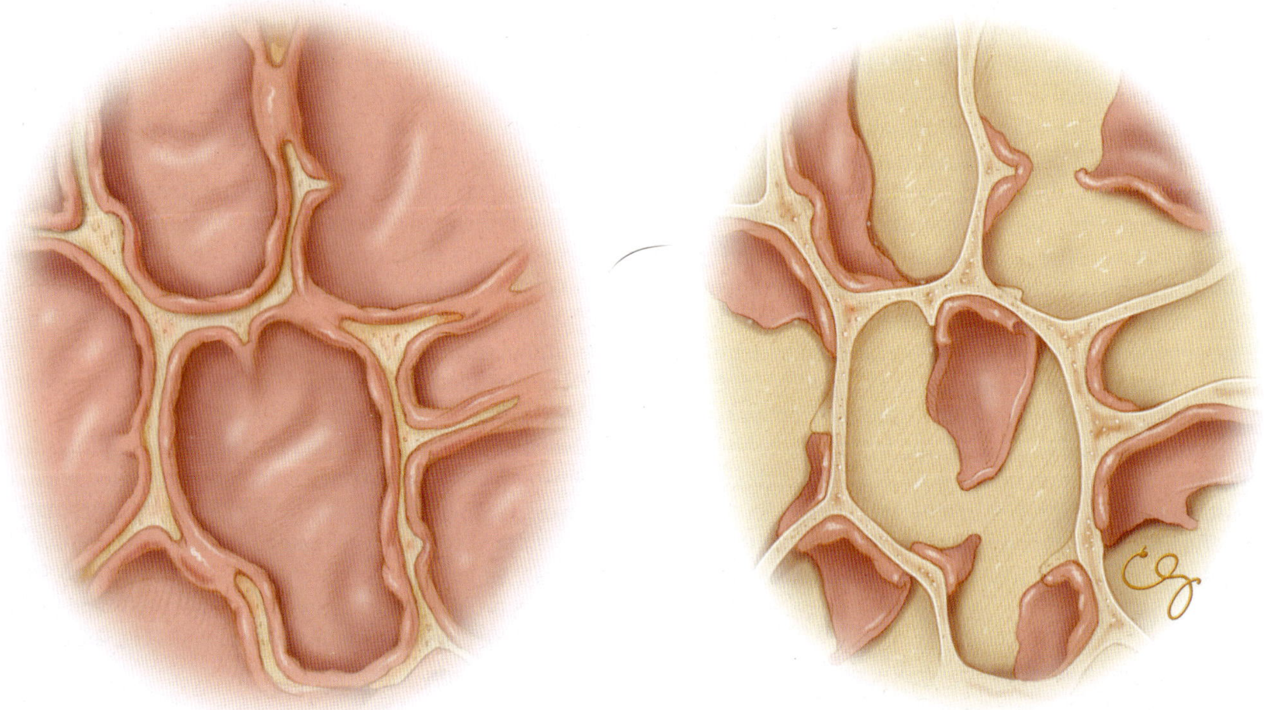

A B

Fig. 25.14 **(A)** Illustration of an ideally performed surgery, in which bony partitions are completely removed with complete preservation of mucosal lining. **(B)** Significant mucosal loss creates the potential for chronic inflammation and neo-osteogenesis.

the maxillary sinus extends medially into the nasal cavity so that the medial wall posterior to the antrostomy is displaced into the nasal air flow, then this medially displaced wall creates an "air scoop" that will dry the mucosa of the posterior maxillary sinus wall and causes mucociliary disturbance within the maxillary sinus, possibly increasing the risk of biofilm formation. In this instance, it is better to extend the antrostomy posteriorly to the pterygoid plate, so as to remove the medial protrusion (**Fig. 25.16**).

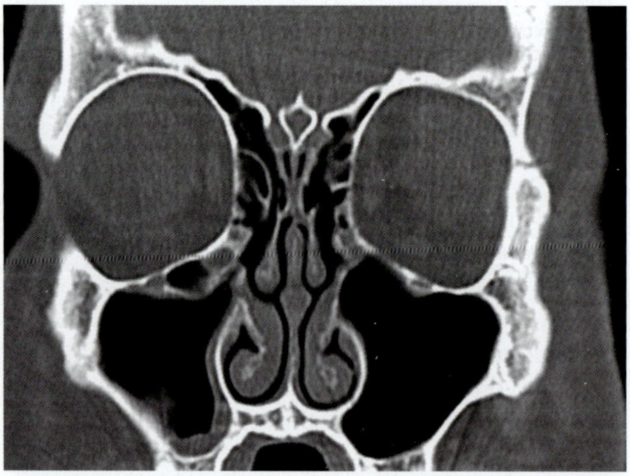

Fig. 25.15 Coronal computed tomography scan of a patient who has undergone incomplete prior sinus surgery. Multiple ethmoid cells are still present along the medial orbital margin bilaterally. Failure to completely identify the medial orbital wall also increases the risk of intracranial entry.

One of the more frequent causes of persistent maxillary sinus disease following surgery is the presence of a middle meatal antrostomy that does not connect with the natural ostium anteriorly, resulting in local pooling of secretion or even recirculation of mucus out of the natural ostium and back into the sinus through the iatrogenic ostium.[19,20] Accordingly, this connection with the natural ostium should be checked with a 45- or 70-degree telescope (**Fig. 25.17**). In some cases, the bone of the uncinate process may become thickened following infection, and the ostium may be difficult to reopen.

Antrostomy is frequently complicated by the presence of an infraorbital (Haller) cell, which makes opening the true natural ostium challenging. Even when opened, an infraorbital cell may have residual osteitic partitions, which are difficult to remove with currently available instrumentation. Occasionally, when such bony partitions are clearly a cause of localized persistent disease, and they are inaccessible from the intranasal route, a limited sublabial approach may be indicated for their removal.

Antrostomy is usually considered the easiest and most basic part of an endoscopic procedure for chronic rhinosinusitis. Indeed, making a middle meatal opening in the maxillary sinus is usually a simple procedure. However, a poorly performed antrostomy is one of the more common causes of failure of an endoscopic procedure for CRS. In addition to difficulties caused by infraorbital cells and bony thickening,

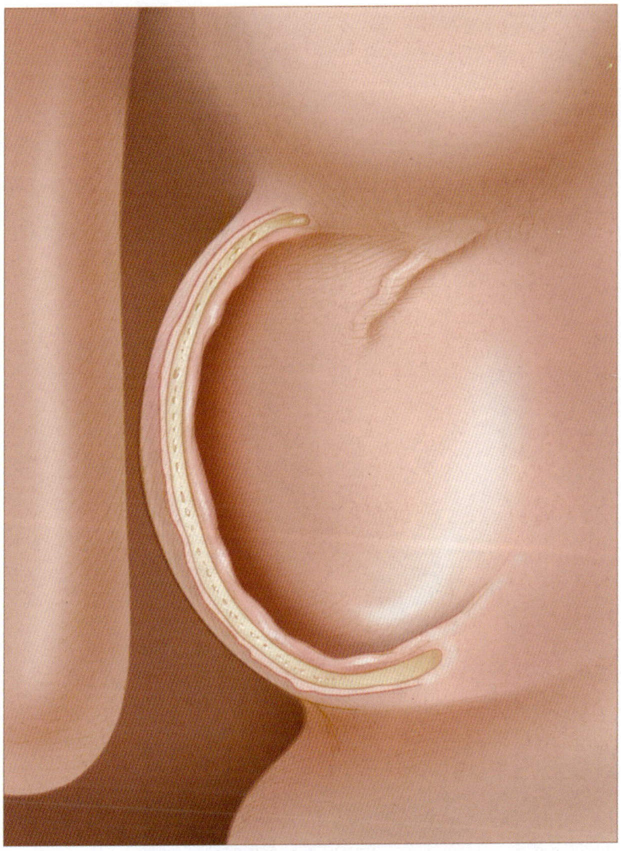

Fig. 25.16 Medial pneumatization of the maxillary sinus may create an "air scoop" phenomenon, where nasal air flow may be directed into the maxillary sinus. In this scenario, the antrostomy is extended posteriorly to the pterygoid plate.

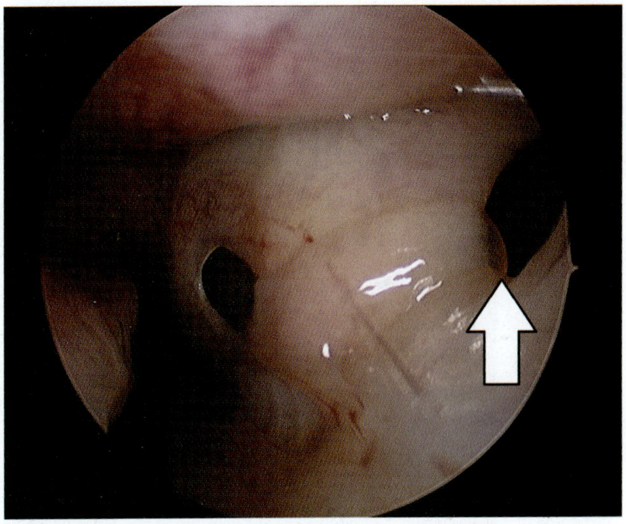

Fig. 25.17 In this previously operated patient with recurrent sinusitis, a nasal endoscopy demonstrates mucus recirculation between the natural ostium *(arrow)* and an accessory or iatrogenic ostium.

there are no easy intranasal landmarks for the extent to which an antrostomy should be brought anteriorly. Using computer-assisted image guidance to identify the nasolacrimal duct can sometimes be helpful in this regard (**Fig. 25.18**).

Sphenoidotomy

Before entering the sphenoid sinus, it is advisable to re-review the radiographic anatomy in both the coronal and axial planes, with particular attention to the presence of any sphenoethmoidal (Onodi) cells and the course of both the carotid arteries and optic nerves. The intersinus septum may be attached to the carotid canal, and it should also be remembered that the carotid artery is "clinically dehiscent" in 23% of sphenoid sinuses and therefore, the potential for serious complication in this region is significant (**Fig. 25.19**).[21]

The approach to the sphenoid will depend, in many cases, on whether the sphenoid disease is isolated or, as in most cases, is accompanied by ethmoid disease. The transethmoidal approach is ideal in a setting where sphenoidotomy is combined with the removal of ethmoid disease or when maximum unilateral sphenoid exposure is required. Following a complete ethmoidectomy, the sphenoid face, skull base, and superior turbinate are identified. The last ethmoid cell is typically identified because of its pyramidal shape with the base facing anteriorly and the apex facing toward the optic nerve superolaterally. In cases where the superior turbinate is difficult to identify from within the ethmoid sinus, a ball-tipped seeker may be helpful in locating the superior meatus medially within the cavity. It can also be helpful to resect the inferomedial portion of the basal lamella of the middle turbinate with a backbiter to further expose both the superior meatus and the superior turbinate (**Fig. 25.20**). Once the appropriate structures are identified, the inferior third of the superior turbinate may be sharply resected and the natural ostium of the sinus is identified medial to it. The ostium is then widened. It is important to create a very wide opening that extends to both the skull base and medial orbital wall if the risk of postoperative stenosis is to be avoided.

The two approaches used for isolated sphenoid sinus disease are the transseptal and the endoscopic transnasal approach. Before the endoscopic era, a transseptal approach to the sphenoid was frequently used because it provided the advantage of keeping the surgeon in the midline of the nasal cavity, as well as allowing excellent bilateral exposure. The endoscopic transnasal approach provides excellent unilateral sphenoid exposure in isolated sphenoid disease and, when combined with a limited posterior septectomy, can provide excellent bilateral exposure. In this situation, the intersinus septum is also removed. The advantage of a transnasal sphenoidotomy is that it avoids disruption to the anatomy of the ethmoid sinuses.

The most common local causes of failure leading to persistent sphenoid disease are inadequate entry and stenosis. The latter may occur as a result of an inadequate sinusotomy, or because of scarring from persistent bony osteitis. In the presence of significant bony thickening on CT, wide bony removal of the anterior wall should be performed if stenosis

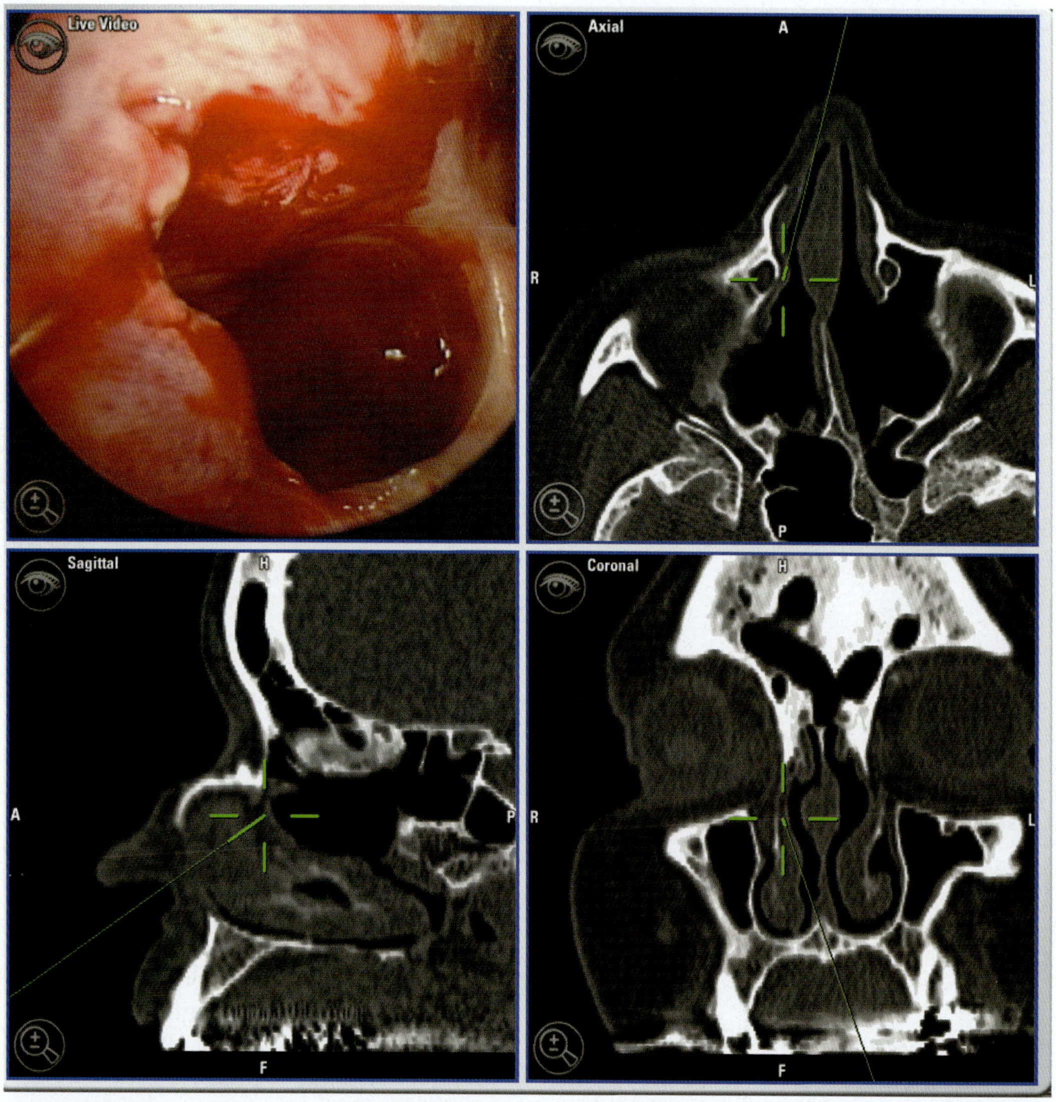

Fig. 25.18 Image-guided screenshot with the probe along the nasolacrimal duct. The maxillary antrostomy may be carried forward to the posterior part of the nasolacrimal duct.

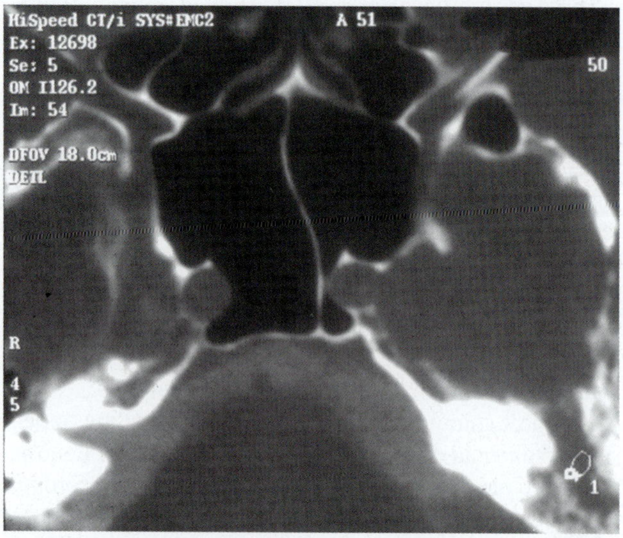

Fig. 25.19 Axial computed tomography scan of the sphenoid sinus. The sphenoid intersinus septum frequently leads to the carotid artery rather than the midline. In this case, dehiscence of the carotid arteries is seen.

is to be avoided. Such surgery frequently requires the use of a drill and, on occasion, a partial posterior septectomy and removal of the intersinus septum (**Fig. 25.21**).

Frontal Sinusotomy

The frontal sinus continues to present the surgeon with the most challenge, both in terms of the surgical procedure and in terms of the potential for persistent and recurrent disease. At a minimum, exploration of the frontal recess commits both the patient and the surgeon to a prolonged period of postoperative care and endoscopic observation. At worst, unnecessary exploration of the frontal sinus or inadvertent stripping of mucosa in this area can result in prolonged morbidity and multiple surgical procedures. Therefore, whether the frontal recess should be explored remains the most difficult decision in FESS. A reasonable potential option is to perform just an ethmoid dissection and then monitor the patient to see if the frontal recess disease resolves. As much as 90% of

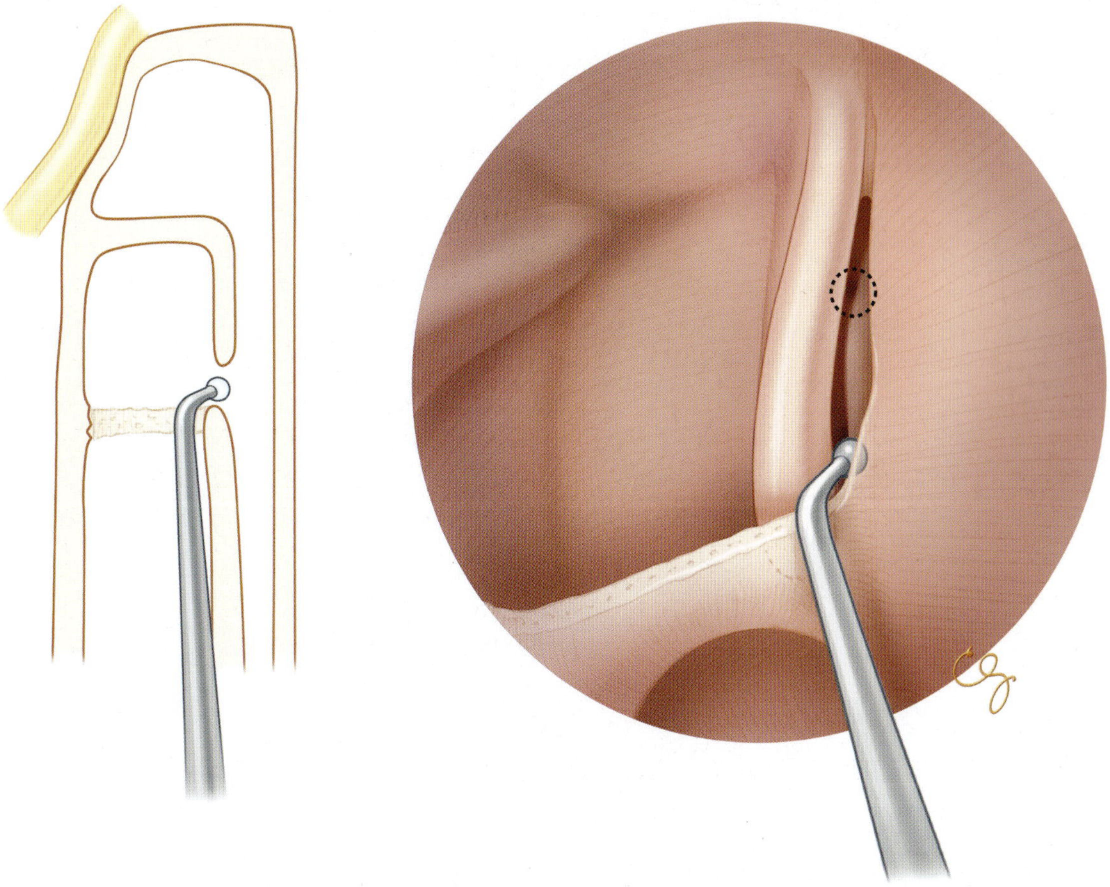

A B

Fig. 25.20 (A,B) Illustrations of the identification of the superior meatus from within the ethmoid sinus with a ball-tipped seeker. The resection of the basal lamella of the middle turbinate reveals the superior turbinate, which forms the medial boundary of the posterior ethmoid sinus. The sphenoid ostium (dotted circle) can be found medial to the superior turbinate in the deepest aspect of the sphenoethmoidal recess.

frontal sinus mucosal thickening may resolve with this minimally invasive approach.[22] As noted previously, the decision should, in part, depend on the surgeon's experience and his or her ability to preserve mucosa, the regional anatomy as seen on CT, and the availability of through-cutting mucosal-sparing instrumentation, as well as the pathology present.

Preoperative evaluation of the frontal sinus and frontal recess anatomy requires a careful evaluation of the coronal and axial CT. A reconstructed sagittal view and the ability to scroll through adjacent cuts, as provided in computer-assisted stereotactic navigation, are also of benefit, particularly in cases of complicated frontal recess

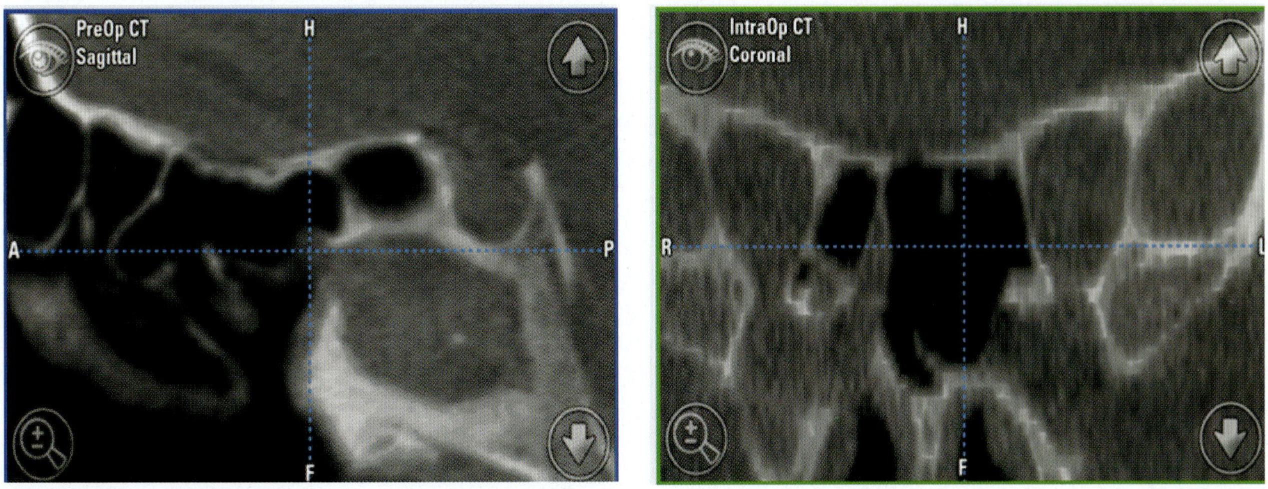

A B

Fig. 25.21 (A) A sagittal computed tomography (CT) scan of a patient with a sphenoid sinus fungal ball and significant neo-osteogenesis. **(B)** Coronal sinus CT scan in the same patient status postbilateral sphenoidotomy with a posterior septectomy.

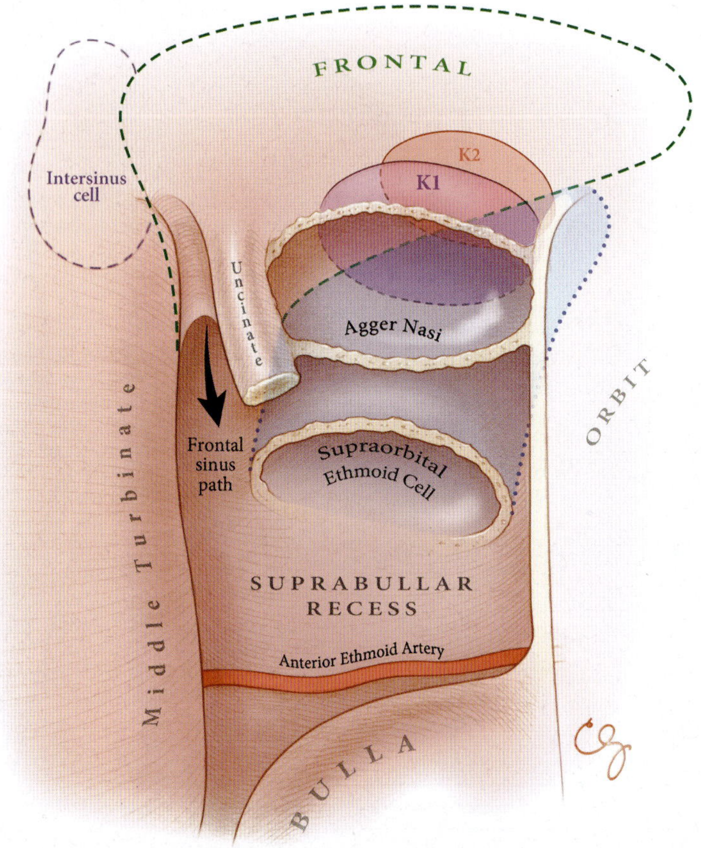

Fig. 25.22 Illustration demonstrating the typical variations in frontal recess pneumatization and the most frequent variation for the frontal sinus drainage pathway. Frequently, more than one supraorbital ethmoid cell may be present. The anterior ethmoidal artery is typically found posterior to the supraorbital ethmoid cells. K1, Kuhn type I cell; K2, Kuhn type II cell.

pneumatization. In evaluating the frontal recess for potential surgical intervention, attention is paid to the frontal sinus drainage pathway and its relative position to the adjacent cells, as well as to the size of the recess in both its anteroposterior and lateral diameters, the presence of neo-osteogenesis, and the extent of the pneumatization of the frontal sinus itself. A hypoplastic frontal sinus appears to be significantly more likely to be associated with frontal recess stenosis than one that is well pneumatized, regardless of the size of the frontal recess. One possible explanation for this phenomenon is that mucociliary clearance from a well pneumatized sinus is greater than from a hypoplastic sinus, and mucociliary flow may aid in maintaining patency.

In our clinical experience, the most common immediate cause of frontal sinus disease is the presence of infundibular disease displacing the uncinate process medially, thereby obstructing a frontal sinus. Indeed, in some cases, the medially displaced uncinate process may undergo fusion to the middle turbinate. The second most common cause of frontal sinus disease appears to be mucosal disease and the expansion of an agger nasi cell, with resultant displacement of the frontal sinus ostium posteriorly.

The initial step in frontal recess dissection involves identification of the appropriate boundaries and the drainage pathway of the frontal recess on CT scan, as well as correlation of this anatomy with the endoscopic view through a 45- or 70-degree telescope (**Fig. 25.22**; **Tables 25.3 and 25.4**). A fine malleable probe can be invaluable in confirming the access to the frontal sinus and, after identifying a pathway, a curette is used to fracture the bone. If the uncinate process inserts on the medial orbit wall, the ethmoid infundibulum will end in a blind pocket called a recessus terminalis. This common anatomic variation (up to 50%) forces the frontal sinus drainage

Table 25.3 Cells and Structures That May Be Encountered in the Frontal Recess

Agger nasi cell
Supraorbital ethmoid cell
Frontal cells (types I–IV)
Interfrontal sinus septal cell
Suprabullar cell
Frontal bullar cell
Uncinate process
Recessus terminalis

Table 25.4 The Anatomic Boundaries of the Frontal Recess

Medial	Skull base attachment of the middle turbinate
Lateral	Lamina papyracea
Superior	Frontal sinus ostium
Anterior	Nasofrontal beak
Posterior	Skull base attachment of the ethmoid bulla
Inferior	Nasal communication

pathway down the medial surface of the uncinate process and thereby directly into the middle meatus. Because of the proximity of the downsloping skull base, dissection of this variant can be tricky, and failure to identify and meticulously dissect this structure is a common cause of failure. Once the wall of an agger nasi cell or recessus terminalis is identified, it can be resected by sliding a 90-degree frontal sinus curette between the skull base and the posterior agger nasi cell wall and fracturing it away from the skull base. Stammberger originally described this gently performed maneuver, and has subsequently very aptly described such maneuvers in his lectures as "uncapping the egg" (**Fig. 25.23**).[23] After fracturing the bone, the loose bony fragments can be teased out with a fine malleable hook and removed with giraffe forceps while preserving the mucosa (**Fig. 25.24**). Mucosal preservation is critically important during frontal recess dissection, and redundant mucosa can be removed with through-cutting forceps or the gentle application of curved powered dissection blades. In general, frontal sinus stents are not used.

Frontal cells originate as anterior ethmoid cells that pneumatize into the frontal recess, creating the potential for compromise of the frontal sinus outflow tract should they overgrow or enlarge, and thus serving as a significant potential cause of persistent disease. Although these cells have been classified depending on the extent to which they pneumatize into the frontal sinus, for a surgeon performing endoscopic sinus surgery, the relationship of the cell to the opening of the frontal sinus outflow tract is typically much more important than the extent of the cell within the frontal sinus. This is best determined by using triplanar reconstructions or, even better, by scrolling through the triplanar cuts on an image-guidance system until the surgeon has developed a true 3D conceptualization of the anatomy and how it will appear endoscopically (**Fig. 25.25**).

Whereas agger nasi cells will pneumatize into the frontal sinus anterior to its drainage pathway, supraorbital ethmoid cells, on the other hand, develop posterior to the frontal sinus and can extend into it from posteriorly, creating an apparent frontal cell as well as narrowing

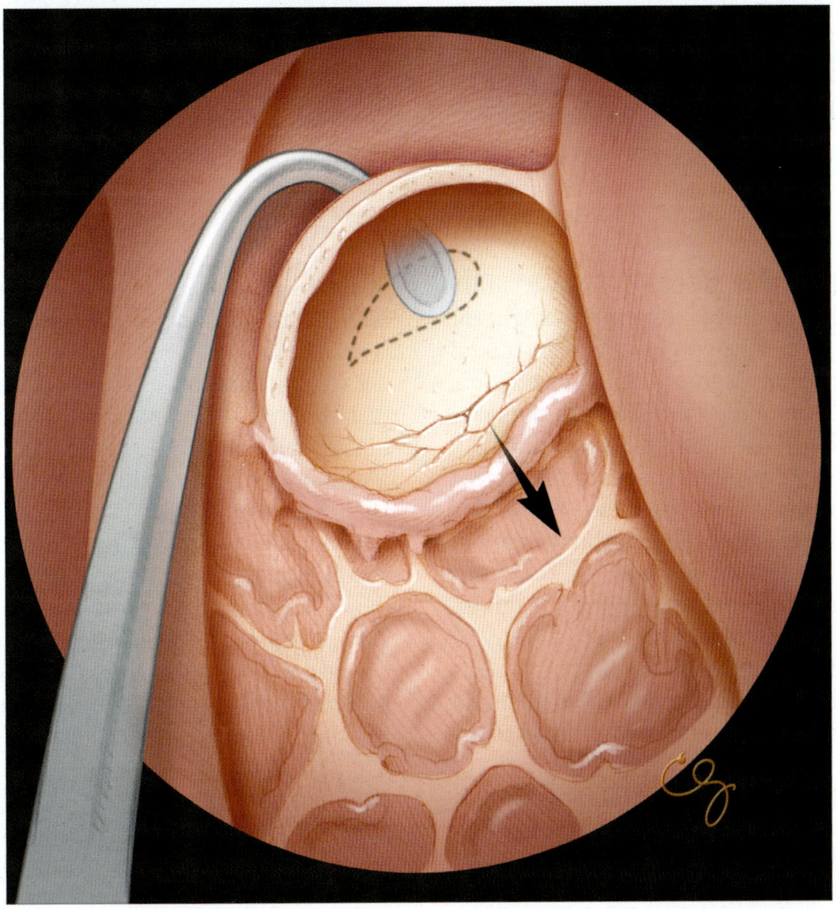

Fig. 25.23 Illustration of using a curette to remove a bony cap (recessus terminalis) from below the frontal recess.

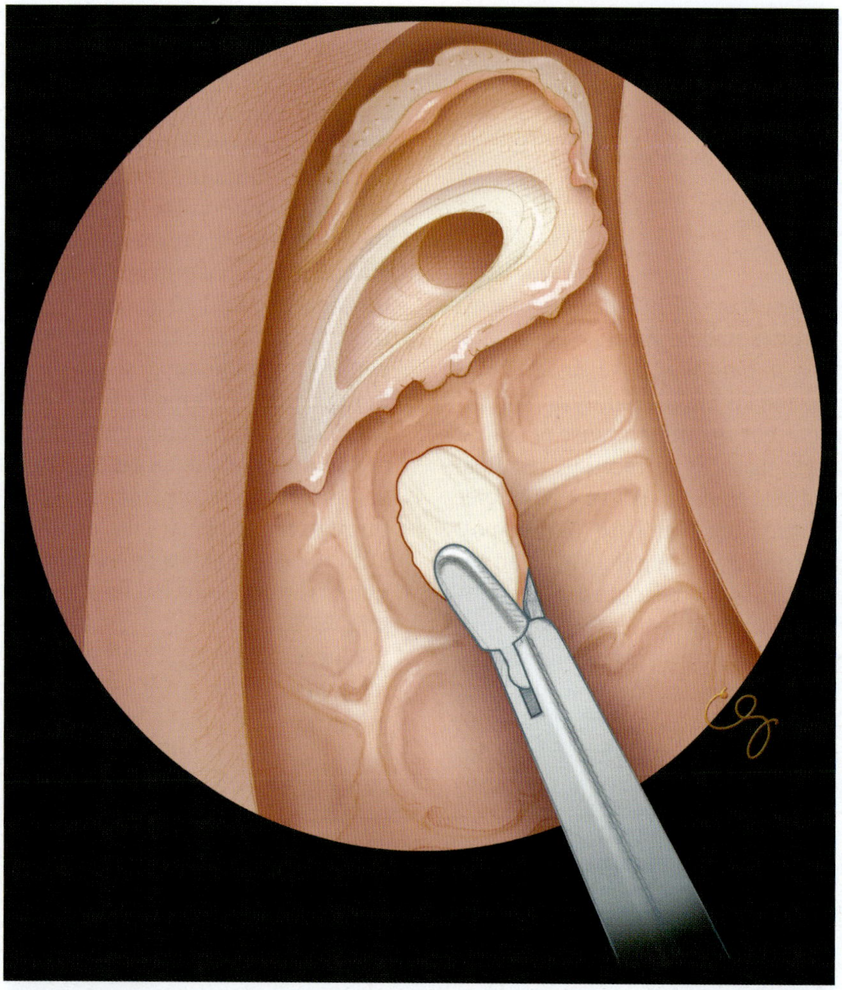

Fig. 25.24 Illustration demonstrating the gentle removal of a small bony partition while, at the same time, preserving the mucosa.

the drainage pathways. Failure to address disease within these cells is also another potential reason for persistent frontal sinus disease. Typically, one or two supraorbital ethmoid cells, with variable degrees of pneumatization, can be identified. Because of their proximity to the frontal sinus, a well pneumatized supraorbital ethmoid cell can easily be confused with an entrance into the frontal sinus ostium. An interfrontal sinus septal cell occurs less frequently than the agger nasi or supraorbital ethmoid cell and develops in the septum between the two frontal sinuses. The cell may pneumatize to different degrees, varying from just the lower septum all the way to the frontal sinus apex or into a pneumatized crista galli. This cell empties into one frontal recess, usually medial and anterior to the internal frontal ostium, and in some situations, into the frontal sinus.

Once the individual cells have been identified, it is important to remove the common walls as far superiorly as possible, preferably to the level of the skull base. Understanding this spatial relationship of supraorbital ethmoid cells or agger nasi cells, as well as the uncinate process to the frontal sinus, orbit, and skull base, is the key to performing a frontal recess dissection. (**Fig. 25.26**).

Extended approaches to the frontal sinus, whether just removing the anterior portion of the middle turbinate and extending the opening to the midline with a drill or punch (Draf IIB) or creating one large inverted U-shaped frontal sinus opening for both frontal sinuses in conjunction with a partial septectomy (Draf III, transseptal frontal sinusotomy or modified Lothrop procedure), have created new options for dealing with frontal sinus disease. However, they should be used sparingly because of the mucosal loss associated with these procedures. Indeed, they are reserved almost exclusively for revision procedures. Additionally, the combination of a Draf III approach with an osteoplastic procedure enables the management of frontal sinus lesions, such as tumors attached laterally within the frontal sinus without the necessity of frontal sinus obliteration (**Fig. 25.26**). This combination of an endoscopic and an external approach means that the big disadvantage of obliteration, the loss

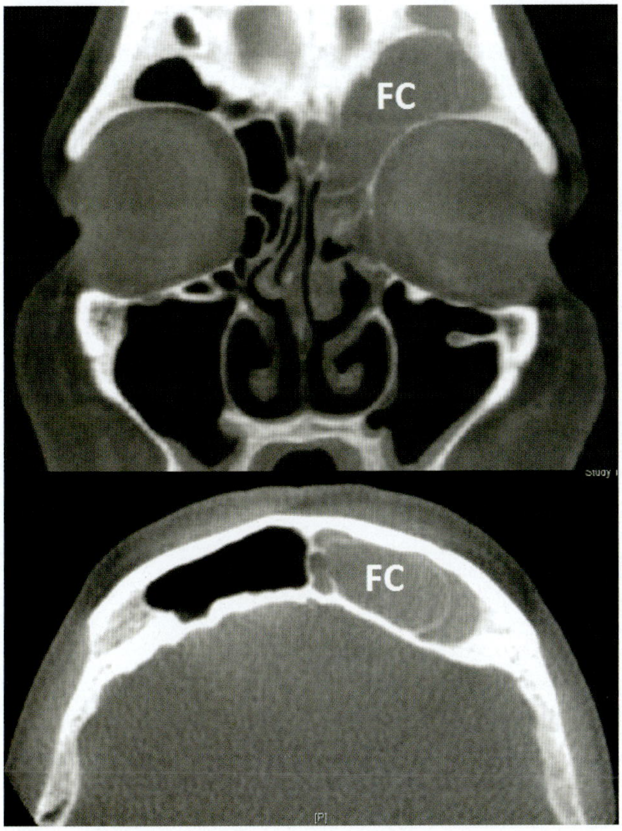

Fig. 25.25 (A,B) A large type 3 frontal cell (*FC*) is seen on the axial and coronal scan. The cell and the true frontal sinus are both associated with disease in this patient, and the frontal sinus drainage pattern is not identified on these routine scans. Three-dimensional conceptualization of the frontal sinus drainage pathway is best achieved by scrolling through triplanar frontal recess images.

of subsequent accurate imaging, is eliminated and the frontal sinus can be directly followed endoscopically with either angled rigid scopes or a flexible endoscope during routine follow-up.

Turbinate Management

At the end of the procedure, after the cavity is carefully rechecked for any residual bone fragments that should be removed, attention is directed to the middle turbinate. Any exposed bone on it should be dissected away and removed. A floppy middle turbinate should be stabilized; frequently, this is done with a controlled scar to the nasal septum (**Fig. 25.27**). At 1 month or more postoperatively, the adhesions between the septum and middle turbinate may be lysed to return the middle turbinate to its normal profile. Another option to stabilize/prevent a lateralized middle turbinate is to suture the turbinate to the septum with an absorbable suture. Routine amputation or resection of the middle turbinate is not recommended because it alters whatever is left of

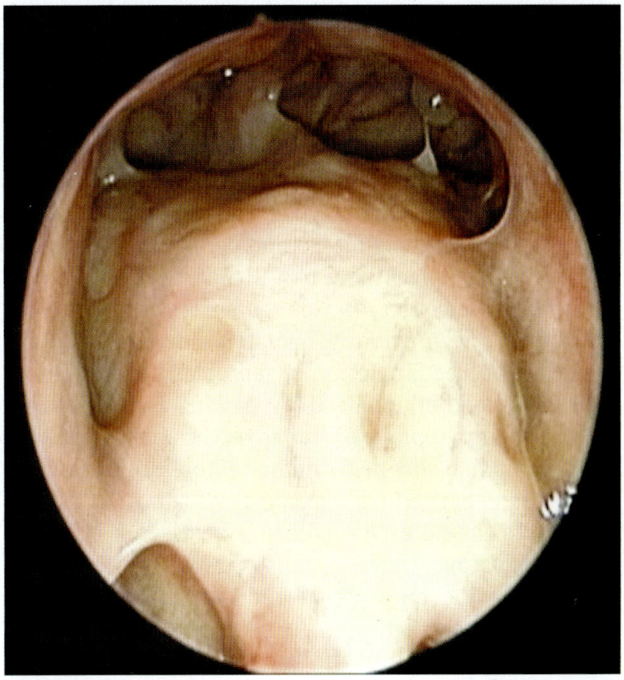

Fig. 25.26 Endoscopic view of the frontal sinus status posttransseptal frontal sinusotomy. Note the inverted U-shape of the frontal sinus around the anterior skull base.

normal physiologic actions of the turbinate and because the stump often still lateralizes and causes iatrogenic frontal sinus disease. However, if the middle turbinate is significantly involved in the disease process, the diseased portions are resected.

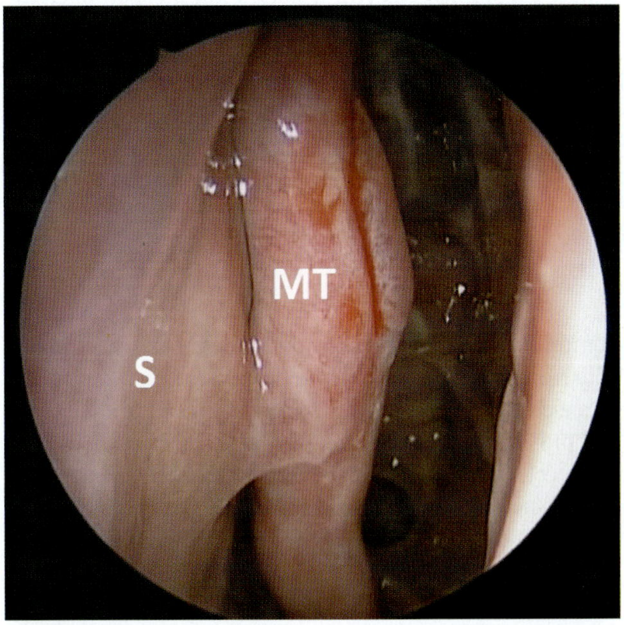

Fig. 25.27 Controlled synechiae formation between the middle turbinate (*MT*) and the septum (*S*) helps prevent lateralization of a destabilized middle turbinate. Persistent edema, which will require continued medical therapy, is seen in the ethmoid cavity of this postoperative patient.

Endoscopic Septoplasty

As noted previously, a concurrent septoplasty is required when a 0-degree telescope cannot be introduced to the anterior attachment of the middle turbinate. In general, such deviations are corrected after the ethmoidectomy has been performed on the wider side and are approached through a hemitransfixion incision performed on the side where the ethmoidectomy has already been performed. Performing the surgery in this sequence and making the incision on the previously operated side decreases the chances that bleeding from the septoplasty will interfere with the second ethmoidectomy, as long as care is taken not to develop a septal perforation on the unoperated side. The authors typically perform the septoplasty endoscopically so as to both provide maximal visualization, as well as to avoid the necessity to change between a headlight and an endoscope. The hemitransfixion incision and initial elevation of the mucoperiochondrial flap is performed with the overhead light.

Once the elevation of the flap has been initiated, the remainder of the septoplasty is performed with a 0-degree endoscope (**Fig. 25.28**). Both the use of the Endoscrub (Medtronic, Jacksonville, FL) and the use of a suction elevator can be extremely helpful in this regard. Once the septal deviation has been corrected, our preference is usually to leave the septal reconstruction, flap quilting, and closure of the hemitransfixion incision until after the second ethmoidectomy has been performed.

When the patient has only an isolated septal spur as a contributory cause of nasal obstruction, it is typically resected after the completion of the sinus procedure. This is best accomplished with a horizontal incision over the apex of the spur and the elevation of mucoperiosteal flaps superiorly and inferiorly, which are limited to the area of resection. Care is taken to keep the opposite mucoperiosteal flap intact and, after the spur is resected, the flaps are simply laid back into place without suturing.

Computer-Assisted Navigation and Intraoperative Imaging

Computer-assisted navigation devices have advanced markedly from the early rigid arm devices that we used nearly 20 years ago. The newer devices are more user friendly and provide reasonable accuracy (generally within 2 mm). However, they are still not a substitute for excellent endoscopic knowledge of the anatomy, and no devices have yet been demonstrated to clearly reduce complications during surgery. On the other hand, they do provide the surgeon with additional information and probably also permit more complete surgery to be performed. The ability to check the anatomy with computer-assisted imaging may have an advantage in any given case, but computer-assisted navigation is particularly important during a transseptal frontal sinusotomy (Draf Type III) procedure, and is almost essential when removing a large fibroosseous tumor that is based in a critical area, or performing extensive bony removal in absence of identifiable landmarks (**Fig. 25.29**). Because computer-assisted surgery is based on computer storage and the manipulation of the preoperative CT, the limitation of this technology is that it does not record any changes in the relative anatomy that occur intraoperatively. However, this shortcoming has recently been overcome by the use of low-dose intraoperative CT. These scanners reduce radiation exposure significantly with a volumetric protocol rather than helical slices, and images taken intraoperatively can be uploaded into the computer-assisted guidance system (**Fig. 25.30**). Future systems will probably combine the advantages of intraoperative CT scanning with image-guided surgery in one machine.

Surgery for Specific Lesions

Complicated Acute Sinusitis

Although endoscopic sinus surgery has been demonstrated to be effective for acute sinusitis, which is either associated with complications or not resolving on appropriate medical therapy, there are special considerations in this situation. The acutely inflamed mucosa tends to be hyperemic and tends to bleed easily, with an increased potential for intraoperative bleeding to obscure vision. Additionally, in chronic sinus disease, if a diseased cell is not opened, the risks of that omission are minor. The same is not true in severe acute sinusitis with threatened or established complications. In the acute situation, leaving a pocket of pus either within the sinuses or immediately adjacent to them could be serious or even life-threatening. Thus, it is more important that the surgeon have a greater skill level in endoscopic surgical techniques if a surgical procedure is undertaken for orbital or intracranial complications of sinusitis.

Mucoceles

Mucoceles are ideally managed through an endoscopic approach. In this situation, there is frequently an extensive disease arising from a limited underlying cause, a situation where endoscopic surgical techniques carry the greatest benefit. This is particularly true where there is erosion of the posterior table of the frontal sinus or of the bony orbit, and mucosa is attached to either the dura or the periosteum (**Fig. 25.31**). In this situation, it is essentially impossible to peel the thin mucosa off the structures, and therefore, marsupialization is by far the best option. However, even in the absence of bony erosion, endoscopic marsupialization of mucoceles results in an excellent resolution of the disease, and the mucosa returns to normal once the underlying inflammation has resolved. However, all osteitic bone in the region of bony closure should be completely

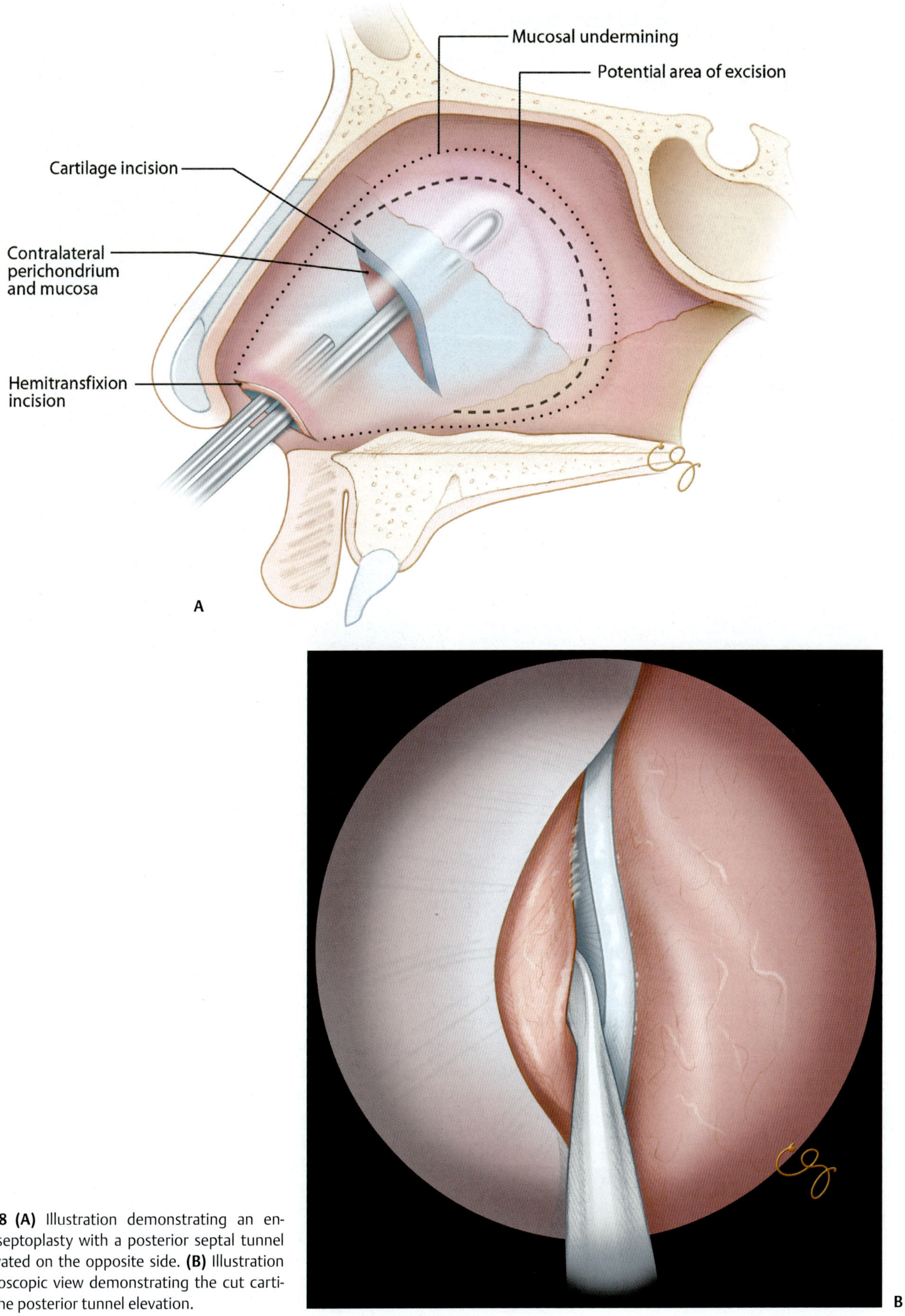

Fig. 25.28 (A) Illustration demonstrating an endoscopic septoplasty with a posterior septal tunnel being elevated on the opposite side. **(B)** Illustration of an endoscopic view demonstrating the cut cartilage and the posterior tunnel elevation.

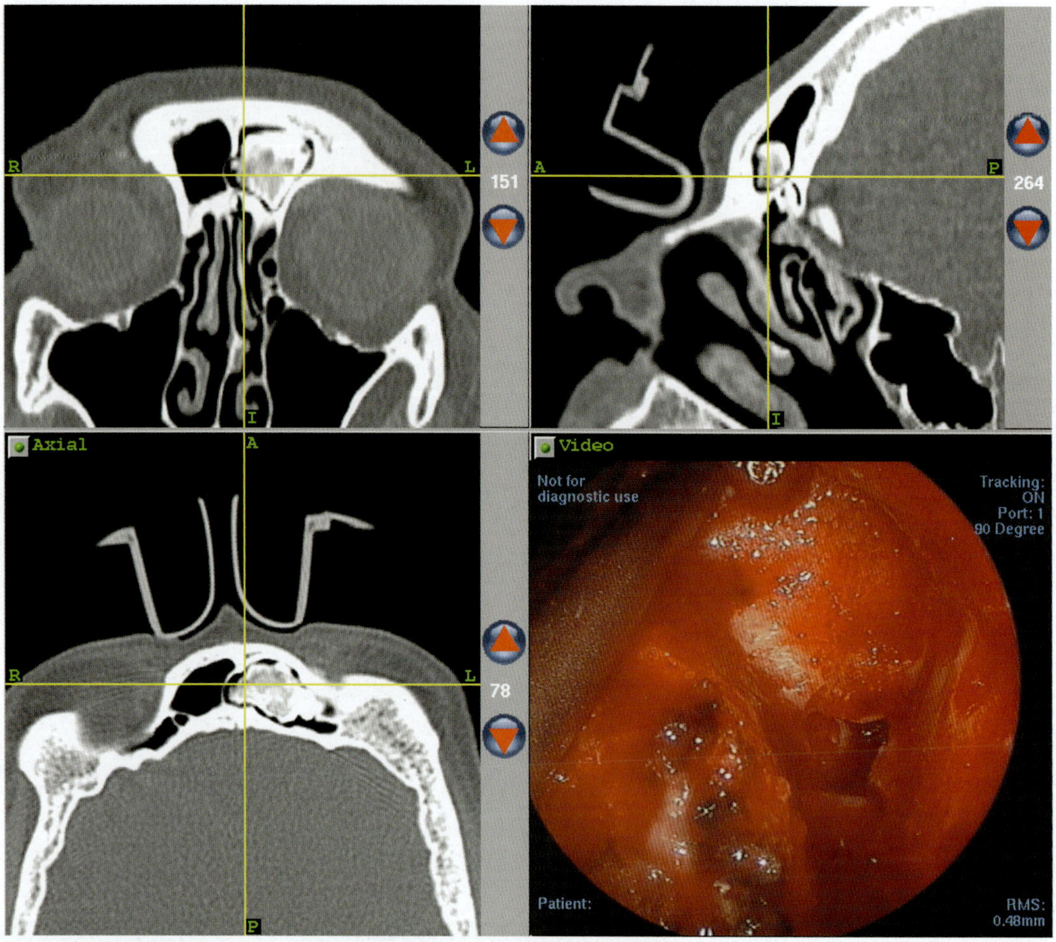

Fig. 25.29 Image guidance is helpful in tumor surgeries where landmarks may be distorted or absent. In this large frontal osteoma, intraoperative image guidance is used to confirm the medial margin of the tumor and to determine the extent to which it has been drilled.

removed if postoperative stenosis is to be avoided. This may frequently involve the use of a drill.

During the preoperative evaluation of the frontal sinus mucocele, the relative position of the bony obstruction to the skull base should be carefully identified, along with the relative position of the anterior ethmoidal neurovascular bundle. At surgery, the skull base is typically identified posteriorly, then is followed anteriorly as it is skeletonized, and the lesion is then identified and opened. Occasionally, particularly in larger lesions, as the mucocele is approached there is clear fluid drainage initially suggesting a cerebrospinal fluid (CSF) leak. However, experience has shown that this just appears to represent marked hypersecretion from the mucosa of the lesion. After the mucocele is opened, the bony margins should be made flush with the surrounding wall, so as to avoid subsequent scarring. In the process, the osteitic bone from this area is also removed.

Fungal Disease

Fungal sinusitis is subdivided into invasive disease and noninvasive disease. Extramucosal manifestations such as fungal balls and allergic fungal sinusitis are included in noninvasive disease. Invasive disease includes both chronic invasive fungal sinusitis and the fulminant invasion that occurs in the immunosuppressed patient. Chronic invasive fungal sinusitis may be subdivided into granulomatous and nongranulomatous manifestations.

Fungal balls occur most frequently in the maxillary sinus, although they are also found less frequently in the sphenoid sinus. Complete removal of the fungal ball results in the resolution of the disease. However, postoperatively, the underlying associated inflammation may need moderately prolonged medical therapy. Sphenoid sinus fungal balls are frequently associated with some bony thickening and osteitis. As with mucoceles, it is very important to ensure that all the thickened bone in the area of drainage is completely removed if stenosis is to be avoided (**Fig. 25.32**).

Removal of fungal balls from the maxillary sinus can usually be performed with a curved suction through a very wide antrostomy. If the mass cannot be satisfactorily removed in this fashion, a canine fossa trocar can be introduced and used as a spoon under endoscopic visualization to scoop the mass toward the antrostomy. Unless a canine

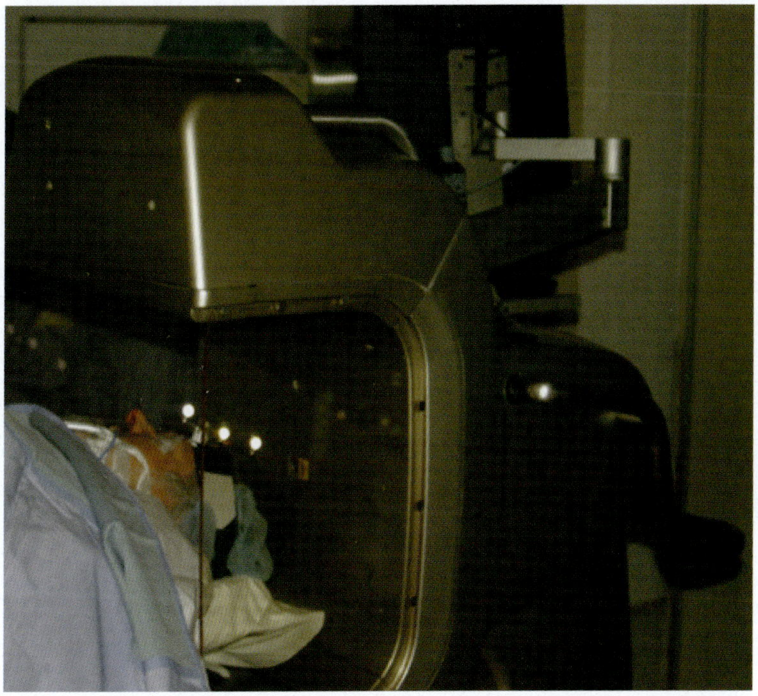

Fig. 25.30 The xCAT intraoperative computed tomography scanner shown here allows for real-time imaging, which can be used for image guidance updates during surgery.

fossa endoscopic visualization is performed, examination with a 70-degree telescope is required to ensure that the mass has been adequately removed from the sinus.

Allergic fungal sinusitis may be associated with a moderate degree of bony remodeling and erosion. This is particularly important from a surgical standpoint because anatomic relationships may be changed dramatically and, in addition, there may be dural exposure or displacement of the optic nerve and the carotid artery when the disease involves the sphenoid or posterior ethmoid sinuses. The aim of surgery in allergic fungal sinusitis is the complete removal of all the inspissated material, as well as the complete removal of the osteitic intersinus partitions and a very wide middle meatal antrostomy. In this situation, a complete sphenoethmoidectomy should essentially always be performed. As in all surgery for inflammatory disease, however, care should be taken to maintain mucoperiosteal coverage of the bone within the cavity. As the degree of inflammation and bleeding in these patients can be significant, preoperative oral steroids are particularly helpful. Postoperatively, the steroid is then slowly tapered and the patient is treated with antibiotics for the associated bacterial inflammation. Therapy with an oral antifungal agent may also reduce the steroid dosage.[24] There is

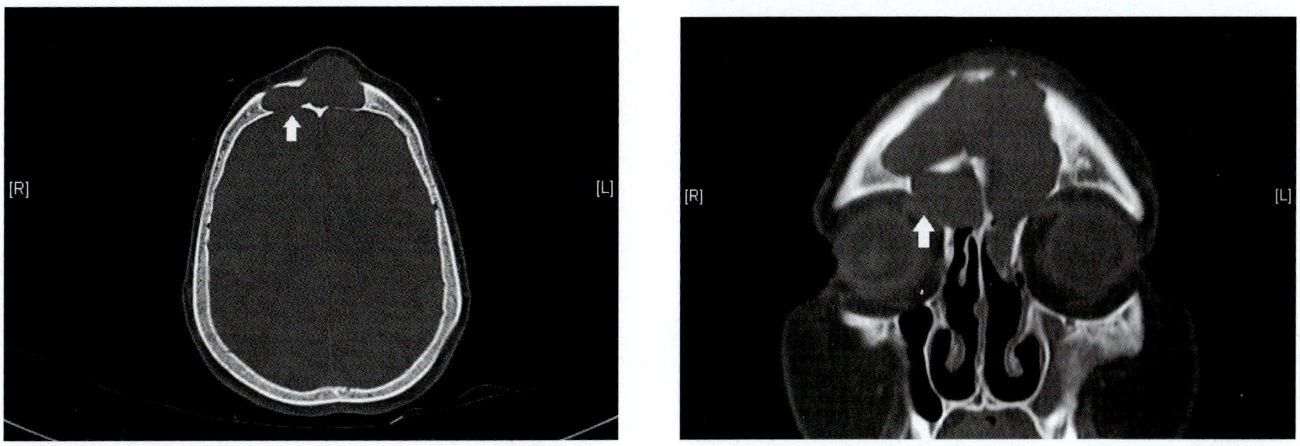

A B

Fig. 25.31 Axial **(A)** and coronal **(B)** computed tomography scan of a patient with large bilateral frontal mucoceles. The mucocele on the left had eroded through the anterior table creating a Pott's puffy tumor and the one on the right has eroded into the orbit and intracranially (*arrows*).

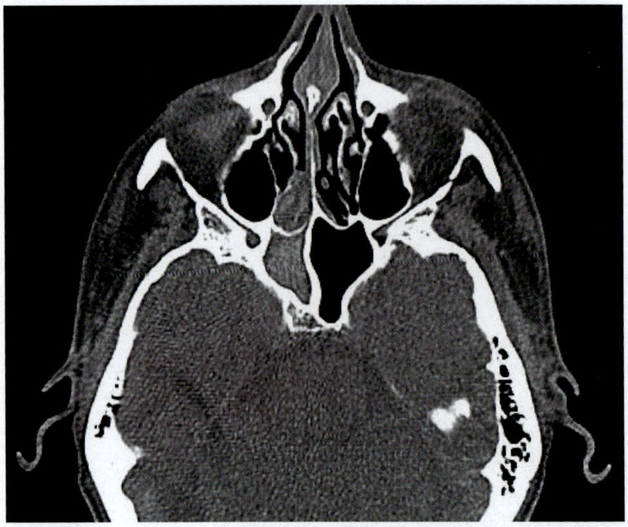

Fig. 25.32 Axial computed tomography scan demonstrating hyperdense material within the sphenoid sinus, which is strongly suspicious of fungal material. In this case, although bony thickening is not appreciated on the scan, the sphenoid sinus needs to be opened widely to avoid recurrent disease.

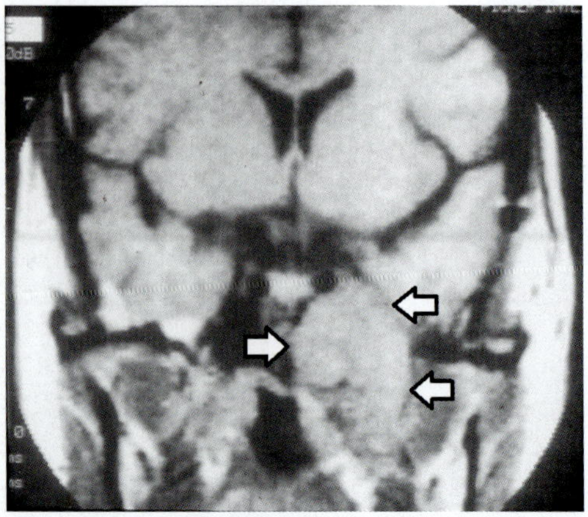

Fig. 25.33 Coronal T1-weighted magnetic resonance image demonstrates a left infratemporal mass extending intracranially and elevating the middle cranial fossa dura (*arrows*). The patient had had three prior surgical resections and has long-standing chronic invasive fungal disease. With endoscopic resections, the patient was followed for over 20 years subsequent to this scan.

evidence that fungal desensitization may be helpful in the long-term management of these patients.[25] Additionally, although the disease does slowly settle down over time, patients may need further boosts of oral steroids in the first year or so after surgical intervention.

Chronic invasive fungal sinusitis typically requires both a "conservative radical" operation and a full course of antifungal therapy. The surgery may be performed through an open approach endoscopically. All involved soft tissue and bone should be removed, but care should be taken to avoid resecting or violating the dura and orbital periosteum. Both structures are relatively good barriers to the fungus, and tears in these structures may allow the fungus to penetrate outside its current boundaries (**Fig. 25.33**).

Nasal endoscopy and biopsy are very helpful in the diagnosis of fulminant fungal sinusitis, and endoscopic techniques have been reported for its resection. However, the classical approach still includes a wide resection of any and all involved areas, as well as the use of systemic antifungal agents and reversal of the underlying cause of immunocompromise.

Tumors, Skull Base Defects, and Other Lesions

Endoscopic transnasal approaches are also effective for lesions such as tumors, skull base defects, orbital decompression, medially placed intraorbital tumors, and dacryocystorhinostomy. The approaches for these pathologies are described in greater detail in other chapters. Yet, a few comments are warranted here. The most important evolutions that allowed the development of these extended surgical approaches are increased familiarity with the anatomy, improved instrumentation, computer-assisted surgical navigation, and the ability to close skull base defects reliably. The latter is particularly important and has continued to evolve. Using primarily free mucosal grafts, we have been able to demonstrate a greater than 90% success rate for skull base defect closure.[26] However, very large defects are more appropriately treated with a vascular pedicled flap, such as the Hadad sphenopalatine flap.[27]

The ability to close large skull base defects, combined with improved understanding of the intracranial endoscopic anatomy, has created the ability to perform true endoscopic oncologic procedures and endoscopically assisted transnasal craniectomies. Contributing improvements have also occurred in instrumentation including the development of the EndoScrub (Medtronic) sheath, which enables the tip of the endoscope to be kept clean and has significantly improved our ability to operate in the presence of bleeding, the development of longer delicate skull base instrumentation, and the introduction of fine slender drills, especially those with simultaneous irrigation and suction.

In all skull base tumors, the key is careful identification of the site or sites of tumor attachment. This requires excellent wide exposure and good hemostasis. In the case of benign tumors, such as an inverted papilloma, the bone is either removed or drilled at the site of the tumor attachment. As with fungal sinusitis, the dura and periorbita usually provide excellent barriers against the spread of the lesion and are generally best left intact. When inverted papilloma involves these structures, the attached tumor is typically bipolarly cauterized. In malignant lesions, in addition to the site of attachment, a margin of normal surrounding tissue must also be resected. In the case of skull base tumors, this will frequently involve a significant portion of the dura and skull base. Close cooperation between a neurosurgeon and an otorhinolaryngologist–head and neck surgeon forming a surgical team is extremely helpful for these lesions. In some situations, postoperative irradiation or proton therapy may be required. Tumors within the frontal sinus may be approached through a Draf III procedure if attached medially, or with a combination of a Draf III procedure and an osteoplastic approach when attached laterally.

Vascular lesions are the most technically demanding tumors for endoscopic resection because any bleeding is the enemy of endoscopic visualization. Endoscopic removal of tumors such as juvenile angiofibroma (JNA) requires excellent interventional angiography and preoperative embolization, in addition to a high level of endoscopic experience. Personal preference is to initially separate the lesion from any blood supply posteriorly in the nasopharynx by the use of a curved bipolar suction forceps administered under direct endoscopic visualization perorally, with the soft palate retracted. The lateral limit of the lesion is approached either transnasally or transseptally after creating a very wide antrostomy, and by removing the posterior wall of the maxillary sinus to provide access to the pterygoid fossa. The primary vascular supply is then clipped and sectioned before further manipulation of the tumor itself is done. The tumor will frequently extend posteriorly in the floor of the sphenoid sinus along the vidian canal, so extensive drilling and removal of the floor of the sphenoid may be required (**Fig. 25.34**).

The variety of procedures currently being performed endoscopically at this point in time is so large and diverse that a discussion of all the endoscopic possibilities is precluded. It is anticipated that the range of procedures where endoscopic intervention can be performed will continue to grow and expand as instrumentation continues to develop and techniques become further refined. Indeed, we anticipate that the possibilities for endoscopic intervention will expand quite dramatically when the mechanical arms of the surgical robot become sufficiently fine that they can be introduced intranasally. Such an advance will create new options for skull base closure and intracranial manipulation and cauterization.

Postoperative Medical Management and Debridement

Medical therapy in the postoperative period includes antibiotic coverage instituted in the operating room prior to the procedure and, when possible in inflammatory cases, adjusted postoperatively based on culture results. In inflammatory disease, long-term antibiotic therapy may be indicated where there is evidence of significant bone inflammation or significant bone exposure. If inflammation increases and pus is seen at any point in the postoperative period, the cavity is recultured, and culture-directed antibiotics are instituted. All inflammatory patients are administered long-term topical steroid sprays to minimize postoperative edema, to reduce the need for oral steroid use, and to decrease the potential for late recurrence. The most common site for disease persistence and recurrence remains the frontal recess. Accordingly, multiple methods have been described to increase topical steroid deposition to this area.

The Moffat head-down position or the Mygind head-hanging in hyperextension are two positions in common use. An alternative approach (the Kennedy position) may allow the patient to maintain the position and hold the spray in the nose for a longer period (**Fig. 25.35**). This relatively comfortable position can be easily maintained for at least 5 minutes. Any oral steroid administration begun in the preoperative setting is slowly tapered based on the endoscopic appearance of the mucosa over days to weeks, but in severe disease the course may need to be prolonged or even slowly reduced to an alternate-day, low-dose maintenance regimen.

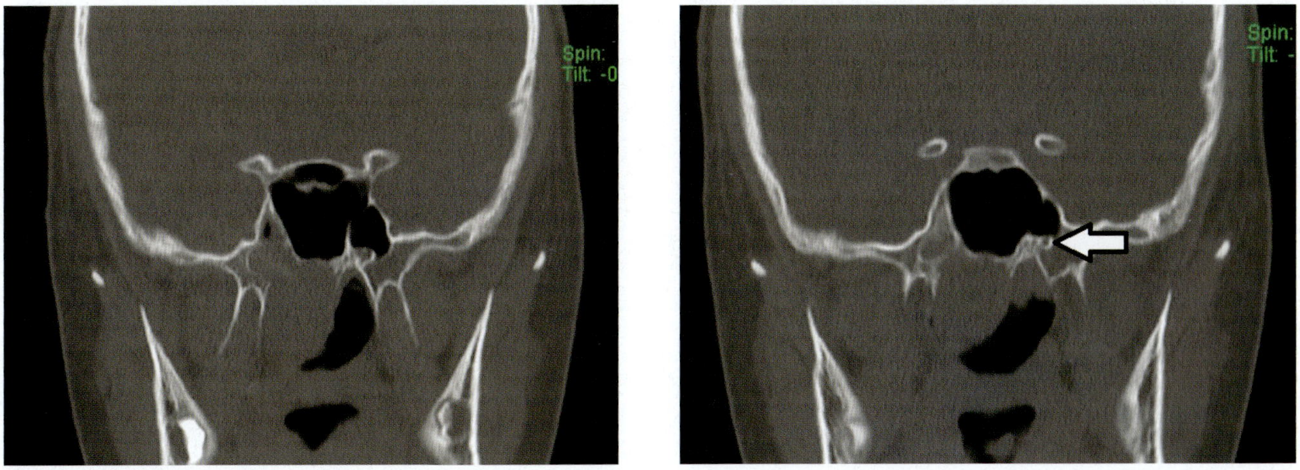

A B

Fig. 25.34 (A,B) Coronal computed tomography scans of a patient with a juvenile nasopharyngeal angiofibroma that has eroded the floor of the sphenoid sinus and extended posteriorly along the right vidian canal. The uninvolved vidian canal on the left side is marked with an arrow. It is important that the involved vidian canal is drilled back toward the carotid artery in these cases.

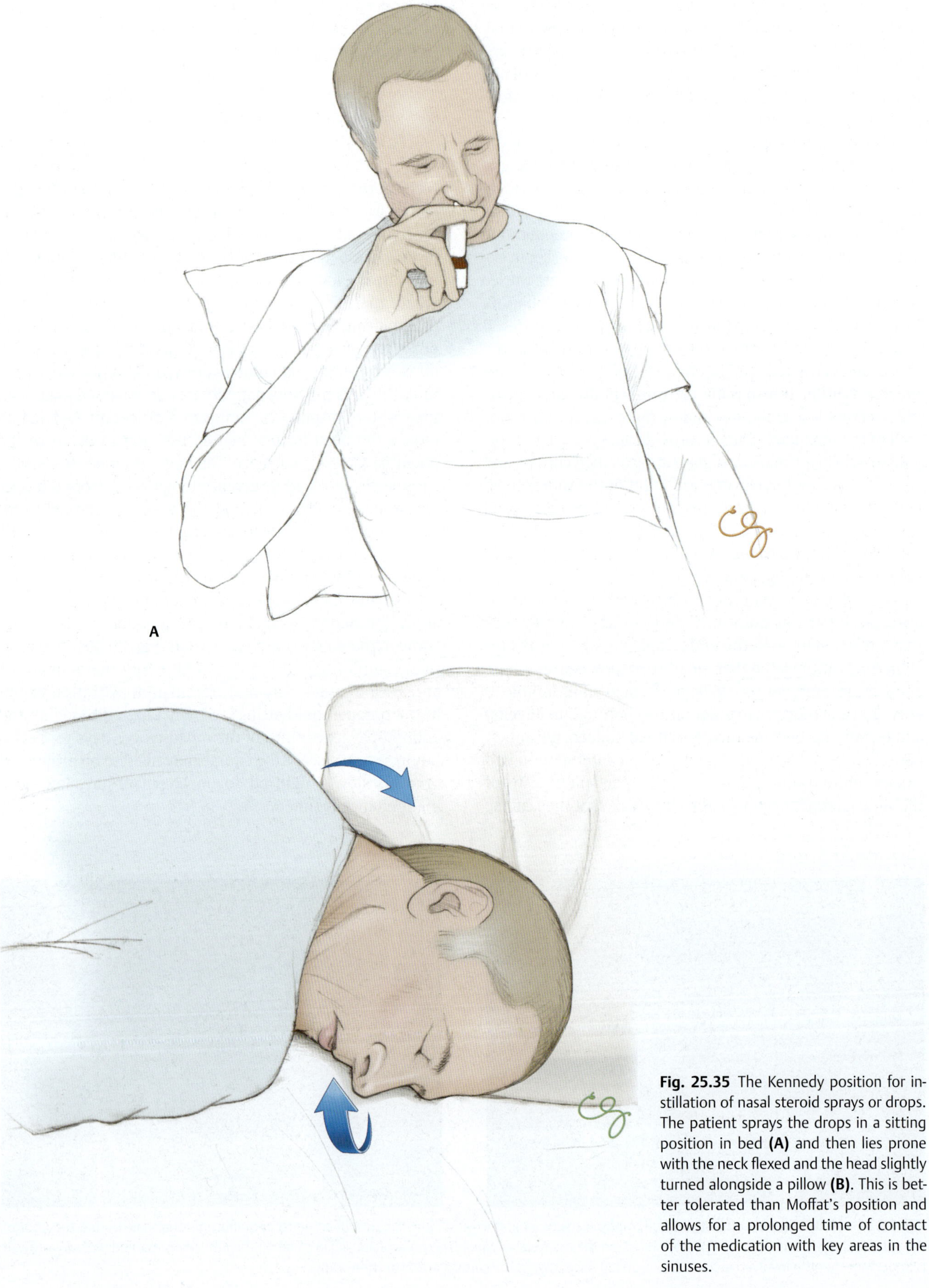

A

B

Fig. 25.35 The Kennedy position for instillation of nasal steroid sprays or drops. The patient sprays the drops in a sitting position in bed **(A)** and then lies prone with the neck flexed and the head slightly turned alongside a pillow **(B)**. This is better tolerated than Moffat's position and allows for a prolonged time of contact of the medication with key areas in the sinuses.

Nasal irrigations may be initiated in the early postoperative period; however, meticulous attention must be paid to cleaning and aseptic technique to prevent the introduction of Gram-negative organisms, and it may be preferable to wait until after the first postoperative week before reintroducing more than just a saline spray.[28] Antibiotics (e.g., mupirocin, gentamicin, tobramycin), antifungals (amphotericin, itraconazole), or steroids (budesonide inhalation suspension) may be added to the saline solution. Additional controlled studies are required, however, to identify the extent to which the addition of medications significantly augments the effects of irrigation alone.

Debridement begins at postoperative day 1, when the Merocel sponges are removed, the cavity is suctioned, and any residual bone fragments are removed. If, as appears likely, the presence of bacteria and mold increases the immunologic response, suctioning the mucus before it becomes heavily contaminated and clearing the mucosal surface during the time between surgery and the time mucociliary clearance response becomes reestablished (typically ~3 to 4 weeks) appears to make sense. This is also one advantage of using a removal sponge as opposed to an absorbable spacer. Debridement is initially performed weekly and subsequently as necessary until the entire cavity is healed, all exposed bone becomes mucosalized, and the mucosa itself has stabilized. The frequency and the amount of debridement is determined primarily by the amount of inflammation present, as greater inflammation increases the tendency for scarring to occur.

In severe disease, debridement can be a labor-intensive process that may require local anesthetic infiltration to make the patient comfortable, in addition to the more frequently used topical analgesia and oral narcotic/analgesic agents. In the office setting, local anesthesia can be achieved using 1% lidocaine with 1:100,000 adrenaline administered with a long, 27-gauge needle attached

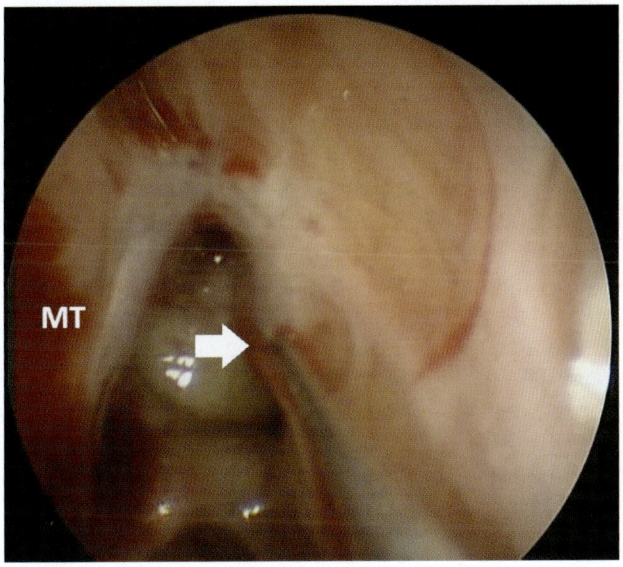

A

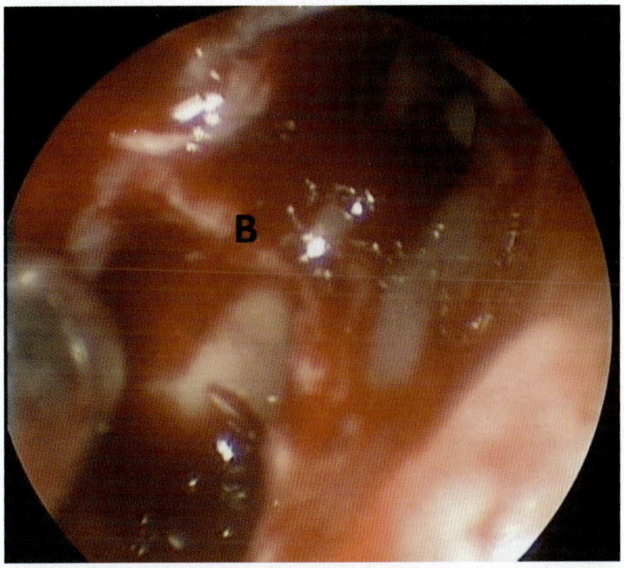

B

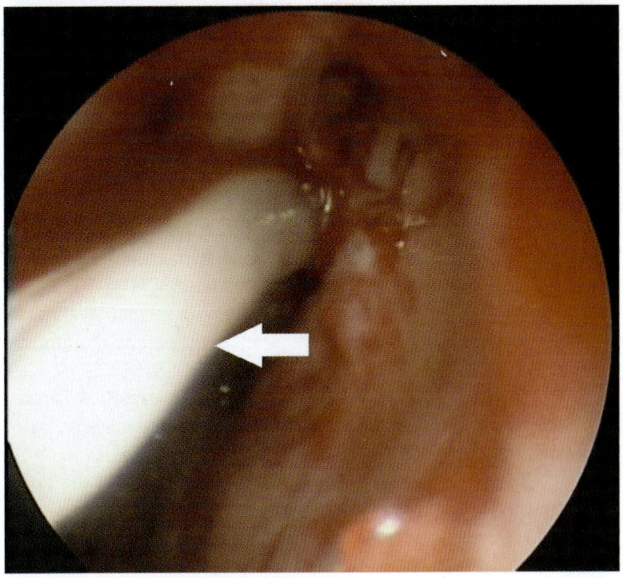

C

Fig. 25.36 Endoscopic views of a postoperative frontal recess debridement. **(A)** The frontal recess is injected with 1% lidocaine with 1:100,000 adrenaline using a bent 2-inch 27-gauge needle (*arrow*). **(B)** Osteitic bone (*B*) is removed with a forward-backward giraffe forceps opening the frontal sinus. **(C)** Thick inspissated mucus (*arrow*) is aspirated from the frontal sinus. These maneuvers are well tolerated by patients in the outpatient clinic setting with appropriate local anesthesia.

to a tuberculin syringe (**Fig. 25.36**). The needle can be bent to allow infiltration directly at the site. More posteriorly, an angled tonsil needle or a spinal needle can be used. Any persistent exposed bone is removed, crusts are cleaned, and blood clots or mucus are suctioned from the cavity. Any cells not removed at surgery and discovered in the postoperative period can be exenterated at this time. Areas of possible stenosis, scarring, or synechiae are lysed and removed with through-cut forceps. The tendency to form scarring slowly decreases as the inflammation decreases with continued medical management.

Asymptomatic persistent inflammation is the rule during the postoperative period and tends to flare up easily and to become diffuse. If not properly managed, this persistent localized asymptomatic disease may eventually lead to a symptomatic diffuse recurrence and the need for revision surgery.[29] Accordingly, it is the appearance of the cavity on nasal endoscopy rather than patient symptoms that determine the intensity and duration of postoperative care and debridement. During this period when the inflammation is settling down, the patient may require multiple courses of oral steroids and culture-directed antibiotics. The occurrence of a viral upper respiratory infection at this point in time may require additional therapy, with either antibiotic coverage or a short course of oral steroids to manage the hyperreactive mucosa. However, over time, the mucosa typically stabilizes and returns toward a more normal function. Symptoms should be monitored closely. Pain and pressure in the postsurgical period are uncommon and should cause further investigation because they are frequently signs of persistent inflammation. On the other hand, postnasal discharge is common, and resolves slowly and sometimes incompletely. Loss of olfaction may be a sensitive indicator of the return of the disease, and is an indication for repeat endoscopic evaluation and possibly additional medical management. In terms of the goal of disease resolution, it is much more effective to intervene earlier in the disease process with debridement, steroids, and antibiotics than to wait until the patient requires another revision surgery for removal of hyperplastic or polypoid disease.

In all situations, the goal is to minimize oral steroid therapy and replace it with a combination of topical and mechanical treatments whenever possible. The use of high-dose topical nasal irrigations (budesonide 0.5 mg) may also be very helpful. In addition to environmental and allergy management, adjunctive therapy with antihistamines, antileukotrienes, and anti-immunoglobulin (Ig)E monoclonal antibody may be considered. Reimaging with a CT scan is not typically required assuming that a nicely patent cavity is achieved. However, repeat CT can be of benefit to evaluate whether any cells were missed in the original surgeries or if frontal stenosis reoccurs.

Conclusion

We have significantly improved our understanding of chronic inflammatory sinus disease, and this has helped to redefine the role of surgery and its adjunctive, but critical, role in the management of chronic inflammatory sinus disease, which is unresponsive to medical management. The surgery itself has become significantly more meticulous and is best based on a clear 3D conceptualization of the anatomy from careful review of multiplanar imaging. The postoperative management is aimed toward resolving the residual asymptomatic disease and avoiding a subsequent revision surgical procedure. However, the surgical techniques have been extended to manage a variety of neoplastic and other lesions of the nose and skull base, and continued refinements in technique and instrumentation will further expand the opportunities for these techniques in the years ahead.

References

1. Naumann H. Pathologische anatomie der chronischen rhinitis und sinusitis. *In:* Proceedings of the Eighth International Congress of Otorhinolaryngology. Amsterdam: Exerpta Medica; 1965: 80
2. Zinreich SJ, Kennedy DW, Rosenbaum AE, Gayler BW, Kumar AJ, Stammberger H. Paranasal sinuses: CT imaging requirements for endoscopic surgery. Radiology 1987;163(3):769–775
3. Kennedy DW, Senior BA, Gannon FH, Montone KT, Hwang P, Lanza DC. Histology and histomorphometry of ethmoid bone in chronic rhinosinusitis. Laryngoscope 1998;108(4 Pt 1) 502–507
4. Havas TE, Motbey JA, Gullane PJ. Prevalence of incidental abnormalities on computed tomographic scans of the paranasal sinuses. Arch Otolaryngol Head Neck Surg 1988;114(8): 856–859
5. Senior BA, Kennedy DW, Tanabodee J, Kroger H, Hassab M, Lanza D. Long-term results of functional endoscopic sinus surgery. Laryngoscope 1998;108(2):151–157
6. Smith TL, Mendolia-Loffredo S, Loehrl TA, Sparapani R, Laud PW, Nattinger AB. Predictive factors and outcomes in endoscopic sinus surgery for chronic rhinosinusitis. Laryngoscope 2005;115(12): 2199–2205
7. Das S, Khichi SS, Perakis H, Woodard T, Kountakis SE. Effects of smoking on quality of life following sinus surgery: 4-year follow-up. Laryngoscope 2009;119(11):2284–2287
8. Sieskiewicz A, Olszewska E, Rogowski M, Grycz E. Preoperative corticosteroid oral therapy and intraoperative bleeding during functional endoscopic sinus surgery in patients with severe nasal polyposis: a preliminary investigation. Ann Otol Rhinol Laryngol 2006;115(7):490–494
9. Kew J, Rees GL, Close D, Sdralis T, Sebben RA, Wormald PJ. Multiplanar reconstructed computed tomography images improves depiction and understanding of the anatomy of the frontal sinus and recess. Am J Rhinol 2002;16(2): 119–123
10. Thaler ER, Gottschalk A, Samaranayake R, Lanza DC, Kennedy DW. Anesthesia in endoscopic sinus surgery. Am J Rhinol 1997;11(6):409–413
11. Ahn HJ, Chung SK, Dhong HJ, et al. Comparison of surgical conditions during propofol or sevoflurane anaesthesia for endoscopic sinus surgery. Br J Anaesth 2008;100(1):50–54

12. Huerter JV, Lydiatt WM, Gupta SK, et al. The effect of intranasal oxymetazoline on serum levels of cocaine after intranasal cocaine application. Am J Rhinol 1991;5(6):235–239
13. Greinwald JH Jr, Holtel MR. Absorption of topical cocaine in rhinologic procedures. Laryngoscope 1996;106(10):1223–1225
14. Jankowski R, Bodino C. Evolution of symptoms associated to nasal polyposis following oral steroid treatment and nasalization of the ethmoid—radical ethmoidectomy is functional surgery for NPS. Rhinology 2003;41(4):211–219
15. Catalano P, Roffman E. Outcome in patients with chronic sinusitis after the minimally invasive sinus technique. Am J Rhinol 2003;17(1):17–22
16. Weiss RL, Church CA, Kuhn FA, Levine HL, Sillers MJ, Vaughan WC. Long-term outcome analysis of balloon catheter sinusotomy: two-year follow-up. Otolaryngol Head Neck Surg 2008;139 (3, Suppl 3)S38–S46
17. Bolger WE, Brown CL, Church CA, et al. Safety and outcomes of balloon catheter sinusotomy: a multicenter 24-week analysis in 115 patients. Otolaryngol Head Neck Surg 2007; 137(1):10–20
18. Moriyama H, Yanagi K, Otori N, Asai K, Fukami M. Healing process of sinus mucosa after endoscopic sinus surgery. Am J Rhinol 1996;10(2):61–66
19. Parsons DS, Stivers FE, Talbot AR. The missed ostium sequence and the surgical approach to revision functional endoscopic sinus surgery. Otolaryngol Clin North Am 1996;29(1):169–183
20. Kane KJ. Recirculation of mucus as a cause of persistent sinusitis. Am J Rhinol 1997;11(5):361–369
21. Kennedy DW, Zinreich SJ, Hassab MJ. The internal carotid artery as it relates to endonasal sphenoethmoidectomy. Am J Rhinol 1990;4(1):7–12
22. Becker SS, Han JK, Nguyen TA, Gross CW. Initial surgical treatment for chronic frontal sinusitis: a pilot study. Ann Otol Rhinol Laryngol. 2007;116(4):286–289.
23. Stammberger H. Endoscopic endonasal surgery—concepts in treatment of recurring rhinosinusitis. Part II. Surgical technique. Otolaryngol Head Neck Surg 1986;94(2):147–156
24. Seiberling K, Wormald PJ. The role of itraconazole in recalcitrant fungal sinusitis. Am J Rhinol Allergy 2009;23(3):303–306
25. Bassichis BA, Marple BF, Mabry RL, Newcomer MT, Schwade ND. Use of immunotherapy in previously treated patients with allergic fungal sinusitis. Otolaryngol Head Neck Surg 2001;125(5):487–490
26. Banks CA, Palmer JN, Chiu AG, O'Malley BW Jr, Woodworth BA, Kennedy DW. Endoscopic closure of CSF rhinorrhea: 193 cases over 21 years. Otolaryngol Head Neck Surg 2009;140(6):826–833
27. Hadad G, Bassagasteguy L, Carrau RL, et al. A novel reconstructive technique after endoscopic expanded endonasal approaches: vascular pedicle nasoseptal flap. Laryngoscope 2006;116(10): 1882–1886
28. Lee JM, Nayak JV, Doghramji LL, Welch KC, Chiu AG. Assessing the risk of irrigation bottle and fluid contamination after endoscopic sinus surgery. Am J Rhinol Allergy 2010;24(3):197–199
29. Senior BA, Kennedy DW, Tanabodee J, Kroger H, Hassab M, Lanza DC. Long-term results of functional endoscopic sinus surgery. Laryngoscope 1998;108(2):151–157

26 Revision Functional Endoscopic Sinus Surgery

Francis T.K. Ling and Stilianos E. Kountakis

Functional endoscopic sinus surgery (FESS) is an important adjunct used in the treatment of chronic rhinosinusitis. It has largely replaced the external approaches for treating chronic rhinosinusitis refractory to medical management. Various instruments were developed over the years that are used to remove anatomic obstruction and to restore function within the drainage pathways of the sinuses.

Long-term success rates of FESS is very high, with over 90% symptomatic improvement.[1,2] Failure does occur, however, with reported rates between 2 and 24% after primary surgery.[2–4] Reasons for failure may be due to several factors including an incorrect diagnosis, a poor surgical technique, an inadequate surgery, postoperative scarring, inadequate postoperative medical therapy, or recurrent disease. A systematic reassessment of the patient to identify the causes of persistent disease is required before revision surgery can be considered. Host and environmental factors contributing to the disease need to be controlled. Repeat nasal endoscopy and radiography is required to identify the possible anatomic and iatrogenic causes while medical management is optimized.

Once it has been determined that the patient is a suitable candidate for revision surgery, the next challenge is to provide safe and complete surgery in a situation where anatomic alterations from previous surgery increase the degree of difficulty and risk of complications.

Preoperative Evaluation

Reassessment of the revision patient is often required, because the etiology of persistent sinus disease is usually multifactorial. A complete history and physical examination is therefore required. It is often helpful to consider the indications for the initial surgery. Was an accurate diagnosis made? Was the patient a good candidate for endoscopic sinus surgery? Preoperative computed tomography (CT) scans of the sinuses prior to the initial procedure may help answer these questions.

Chronic rhinosinusitis is caused by conditions that affect the ostial patency of the sinuses, mucociliary clearance of the nose and sinuses, and quality and quantity of nasal mucus. Common environmental factors include cigarette smoke, chemical irritants, air pollutants, airborne allergens, and mold. These agents hinder normal mucociliary function and incite ongoing mucosal inflammation. It is important that these factors are identified, eliminated, or controlled. Host factors may be systemic or local. Endoscopic sinus surgery, both primary and revision, will not be successful if the underlying systemic disease is not well managed. Often, the cause of ongoing rhinosinusitis in these patients is not anatomic in nature and therefore revision surgery will have limited success without aggressive medical therapy. Conditions such as cystic fibrosis, immunoglobulin deficiency, immunocompromised status, granulomatous disease, autoimmune disease, or genetic diseases such as Kartagener syndrome should therefore be identified.[5] Other systemic factors that can have a negative impact include inflammatory conditions such as reactive airways disease and Samter's triad. Surgery may be beneficial in these patients by removing or reducing the inflammatory load within the nose and sinuses and thus decreasing the systemic inflammatory mediator response.[6] Despite the surgical benefits, a lifetime of ongoing nasal and systemic therapy will be required in these patients and multiple revision surgeries are often expected. Allergy workup may also be beneficial and, if positive, immunotherapy may help reduce chronic sinonasal inflammation.

The surgeon must keep in mind that nonrhinologic conditions such as migraine headaches or neuropathic pain may mimic symptoms of chronic rhinosinusitis. Careful history and corroboration with physical exam, diagnostic endoscopy, and radiography is important to determine whether ongoing symptoms are due to rhinologic versus nonrhinologic causes. Bringing a patient back for revision surgery for nonrhinologic causes only places the patient at unnecessary risk for iatrogenic complications. Consultation with a neurologist may be beneficial in such cases of suspected migraine or neuropathic pain syndromes.

Nasal Endoscopy

Diagnostic nasal endoscopy is an important component in the evaluation of persistent chronic rhinosinusitis. It determines the degree of mucosal inflammation and identifies the presence of recurrent polyps or ongoing purulence. Nasal endoscopy can identify contributing anatomic factors to persistent disease such as a septal deviation, concha bullosa, missed Haller cell, retained uncinate process, or undissected ethmoidal cells. With angled endoscopes, iatrogenic factors can be seen, such as a lateralized middle turbinate, scarring of the frontal recess, or a recirculation phenomenon from a missed ostium of the maxillary sinus (**Fig. 26.1**).

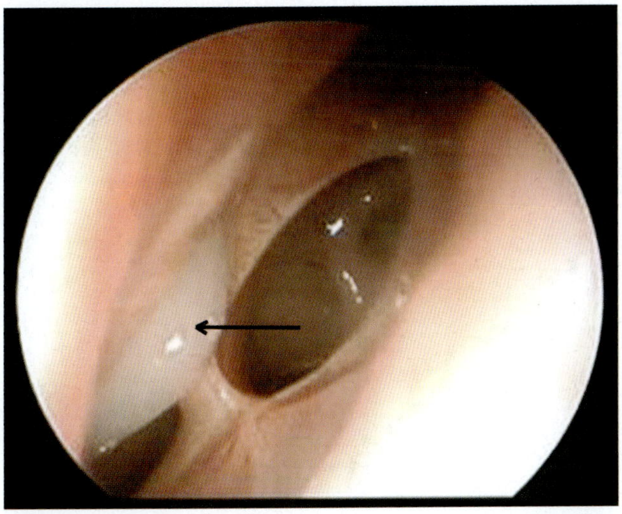

Fig. 26.1 Recirculation phenomenon (*arrow*) from a missed ostium of the maxillary sinus.

Radiology

Whenever possible, the original CT scan is compared with the postoperative scan with the goal of identifying new or residual disease from the initial surgery, as well as postoperative changes such as osteoneogenesis or scarring. Coronal, axial, and sagittal views are especially important in revision surgery to obtain a complete appreciation of the paranasal sinus anatomy for preoperative planning. Magnetic resonance imaging (MRI) may occasionally be indicated when soft tissue detail is required, as in the case of sinonasal tumors or where intracranial or intraorbital extension of disease is suspected.

The authors advocate the routine use of a systematic checklist for the evaluation of the CT scan. The skull base and lamina papyracea must be scrutinized for any breach from previous surgery. The relative position of the ethmoidal vessels to the skull base is determined. Identification of Onodi cells in the posterior ethmoid cells is determined to avoid inadvertent injury to the optic nerve. Maxillary sinus ostia are evaluated for patency with respect to retained Haller cells or retained uncinate processes. The sphenoid sinus is scrutinized for any bony dehiscence of the carotid artery or optic nerve. The frontal recess is examined for the presence of persistent agger nasi cells, undissected frontal cells, supraorbital ethmoid cells, or postoperative scarring.

Computer image guidance systems may assist in the confirmation of anatomic landmarks. Although it should not replace the surgeon's knowledge of sinus anatomy, it may also orient the surgeon during revision sinus surgery where the normal anatomic landmarks may no longer be present. Computer guidance may increase the surgeon's confidence while dealing with disease that abuts the skull base, orbit, optic nerve, or carotid artery. With this technology, high-risk areas such as the frontal recess and skull base can be more confidently accessed to attain the most complete surgery possible.

Causes of Postsurgical Recurrent Sinusitis

Primary sinus surgery failure may be caused by incomplete surgery, technical error, aggressive disease, recurrent nasal polyposis, or excessive resection of sinonasal structures and mucosa.

Lazar et al.[7] reported on 63 patients who underwent revision sinus surgery and found that 43% had significant adhesions, most commonly located between the lateral nasal wall and the middle turbinate with obstruction of the ostiomeatal complex. Twenty-two percent had recurrent polyps in the ethmoid or frontal recess. Chu et al. found that in 153 revision cases, the anterior ethmoid sinus was the sinus most commonly involved by persistent mucosal disease.[8] Partial middle turbinectomy with postoperative scarring in the middle meatus was the most common finding associated with mucosal disease. Chambers[9] also noted that the most common cause of failure was residual ethmoid air cells in addition to scarring in the middle meatus area. Moses et al.[3] found that the most frequent intraoperative findings in patients undergoing revision sinus surgery were adhesions, maxillary ostial stenosis, recurrent polyposis, residual concha bullosa, and incomplete removal of agger nasi cells. In 52 revision cases evaluated by Ramadan, the most common cause of failure was residual air cells and adhesions in the ethmoid area (30.7%), followed by maxillary sinus ostium stenosis (27%), frontal sinus ostium stenosis (25%), and maxillary sinus recirculation (15%).[10] Parsons et al. described "missed ostium sequence" as the most important cause of failure of primary FESS. Failure to identify the maxillary ostium resulted from incomplete resection of the uncinate process, resulting in maxillary sinus recirculation.[11] Musy and Kountakis[12] found that the most common anatomic factor associated with primary surgery failure was lateralization of the middle turbinate (78%) (**Fig. 26.2**) followed by incomplete anterior ethmoidectomy (64%), scarred frontal

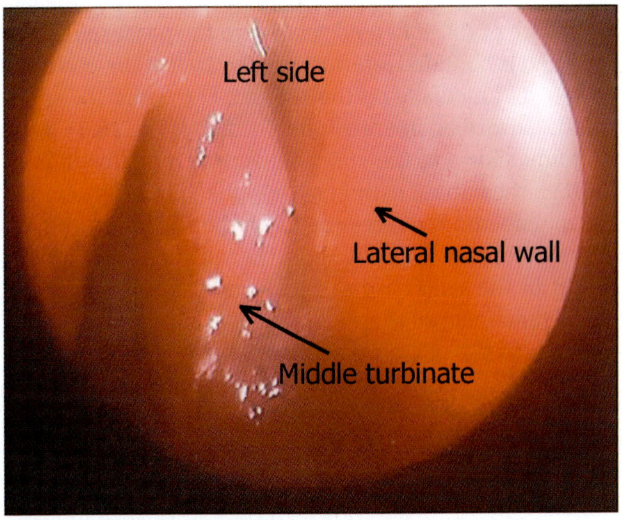

Fig. 26.2 Lateralized middle turbinate.

recess (50%), incomplete posterior ethmoidectomy (41%), and middle meatal antrostomy stenosis (39%). Retained agger nasi cells and a retained uncinate process were identified in 49 and 37% of patients, respectively, whereas recurrent polyposis was seen in 37% percent of patients.

General Concepts in Revision Sinus Surgery

In revision sinus surgery, key anatomic landmarks may be altered or missing, thereby increasing the potential risk of complications such as orbital injury, cerebrospinal fluid (CSF) leak, and excessive bleeding. One of the most commonly used landmarks, the middle turbinate, may have been removed or altered. Barriers such as the skull base and the lamina papyracea may be missing from previous surgery. It is therefore essential that constant landmarks are found and that dissection proceeds from known to unknown territory.

May et al. described consistent anatomic landmarks that may be useful for the revision sinus surgeon.[13] These include the arch formed by the junction of the frontal process of the maxilla and the root of the middle turbinate, the anterosuperior attachment of the middle turbinate, the roof and posterior wall of the maxillary sinus, the lamina papyracea, the nasal septum, and the arch of the posterior choana. The frontal process of the maxillary bone forms the lateral nasal wall. Its fusion with the anterosuperior attachment of the middle turbinate serves as the anterior boundary of the ethmoid complex. The anterosuperior attachment of the middle turbinate inserts at the junction between the medial and lateral lamellae of the cribriform plate. Dissection should be performed lateral to this landmark to avoid injury to the cribriform plate.

The roof of the maxillary sinus approximates the level of the sphenoid ostium and serves as a landmark for a safe height for posterior dissection through the ethmoid sinuses to the sphenoid sinuses (**Fig. 26.3**). The posterior wall of the maxillary sinus is at the approximate depth of the anterior face of the sphenoid relative to the nasal spine. The sphenoid is bounded inferiorly by the arch of the posterior choana and medially by the septum. Entry into the sphenoid is performed inferiorly and medially (**Fig. 26.4**). If the anatomy allows it, the sphenoid is preferentially entered through the natural ostium of the sphenoid sinus found in the sphenoethmoid recess between the superior turbinate and the septum (**Fig. 26.5**). In the sphenoid, the lowest height of the skull base can be identified, and dissection of the remainder of the skull base is facilitated when performed from a posterior to anterior direction. Owing to fewer and larger air cells in the posterior ethmoid labyrinth, identification of the skull base and posterior lamina papyracea is more readily accomplished in the posterior ethmoid sinus. Again, remnant partitions can be removed from a posterior to anterior dissection, thus skeletonizing the skull base and medial orbital wall.

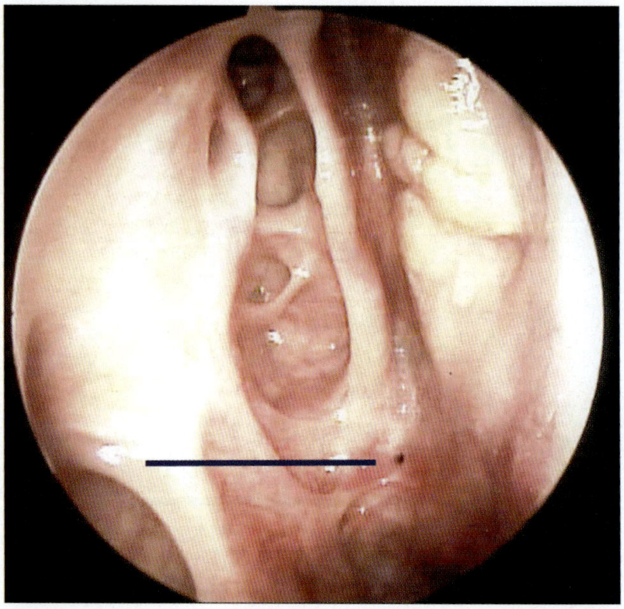

Fig. 26.3 The natural ostium of the sphenoid sinus is found approximately at the level of the roof of the maxillary sinus. *Horizontal bar* indicates the horizontal plane at the level of the orbital floor.

It is known that chronic rhinosinusitis results in an acquired mucosal ciliary dyskinesia.[14] However, because acquired ciliary dyskinesias are potentially reversible with the resolution of inflammatory disease, the principle of mucosal preservation should be upheld whenever possible during revision sinus surgery. Preservation of mucosa also avoids exposing the underlying bone, which when denuded, can result in osteoneogenesis and osteitis. Even without being denuded, the underlying bone in chronic rhinosinusitis demonstrates marked acceleration in bone physiology with histologic changes comparable to osteomyelitis.[15] It is therefore preferable to use techniques that preserve the sinus mucosa and limit the exposure of bone. This is best

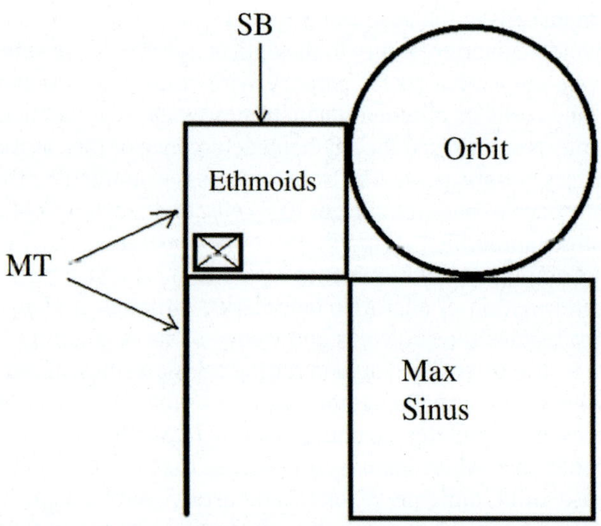

Fig. 26.4 The figure shows safe entry into the sphenoid when performing a transethmoidal sphenoidotomy. *SB*, skull base; *MT*, middle turbinate; *X*, denotes safer entry point.

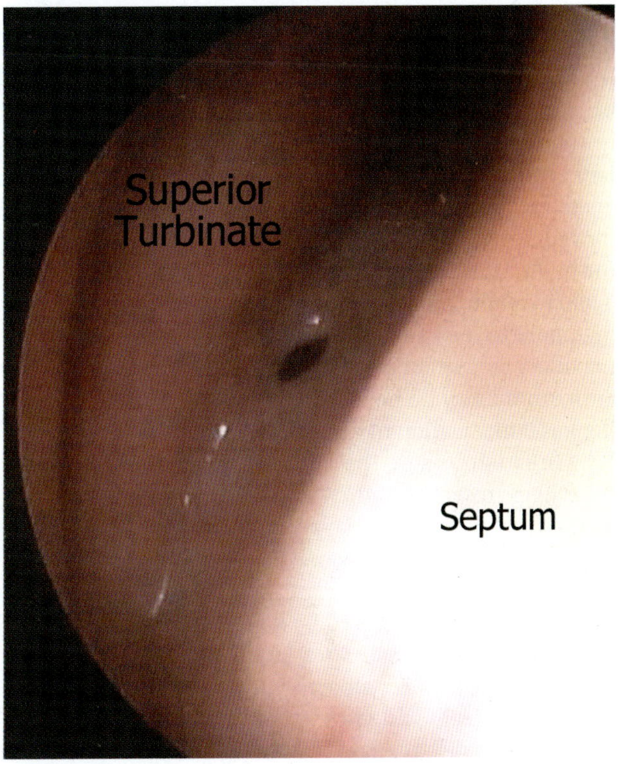

Fig. 26.5 The natural ostium of the sphenoid is found in the spheno-ethmoid recess between the superior turbinate and the septum.

accomplished by the use of through-cutting instruments and judicious use of powered microdebriders.

Revision Surgery of the Maxillary Sinus

Locating the maxillary sinus and defining its limits is an important initial step in establishing surgical orientation within the paranasal sinuses. The maxillary sinus is often the easiest sinus to identify in revision sinus surgery as visualized through the prior antrostomy. It must first be determined whether the surgical antrostomy is in continuity with the natural ostium of the maxillary sinus. Once continuity has been confirmed or established, the maxillary antrostomy can be enlarged posteriorly as needed. Locating the maxillary sinus roof and posterior wall will establish important landmarks for the dissection of other paranasal sinuses. Other landmarks that can then be identified relative to the maxillary sinus include the anterosuperior attachment of the middle turbinate to the lateral nasal wall, the posterolateral attachment of the middle turbinate to the lateral nasal wall at the sphenopalatine foramen, nasal choanae, nasal floor, and eustachian tube orifice.

Persistent disease within the maxillary sinus can be caused by iatrogenic, infectious, and systemic factors. Iatrogenic causes commonly include an unresected uncinate process, stenosis of the middle meatal antrostomy, recirculation of mucus between the natural and surgical

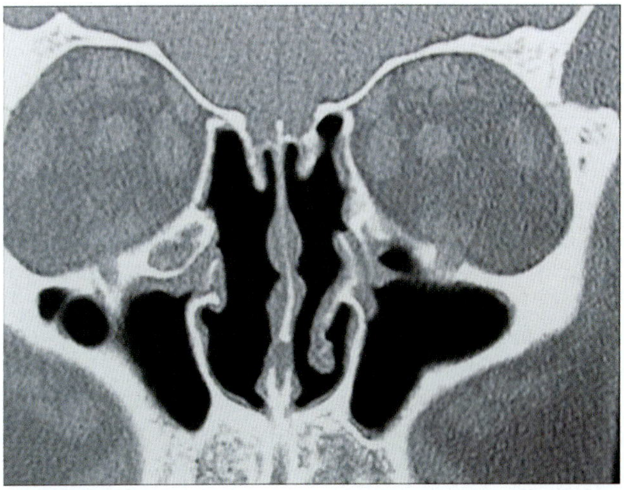

Fig. 26.6 Residual uncinate process and diseased infraorbital ethmoid (Haller) cells causing maxillary sinus disease.

ostia (**Fig. 26.1**), residual infraorbital ethmoid (Haller) cells (**Fig. 26.6**), and entrapment of airflow following the exposure of a medially pneumatized maxillary sinus.

An unresected or partially resected uncinate process can contribute to scarring and stenosis of the middle meatal antrostomy. The resulting persistence of inflammation at the maxillary ostium can impede drainage of the ostiomeatal complex (**Fig. 26.7**). When visualized with a 0-degree endoscope, the unresected anterosuperior portion of the uncinate process can hide the natural ostium. Failure to identify the natural ostium may result in a discontinuity between it and the surgical antrostomy, resulting in the so-called “recirculation phenomenon” (**Fig. 26.1**). In this situation, mucociliary flow leaves the natural ostium and

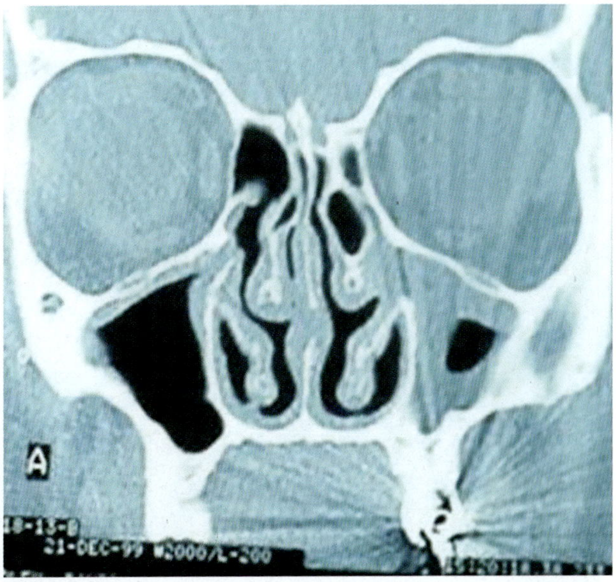

Fig. 26.7 Coronal sinus computed tomography scan showing an unresected right uncinate process with persistent maxillary sinus disease. The left middle turbinate was an interlamellar cell and is scarred laterally.

reenters the surgical antrostomy. Removal of the remnant uncinate process is performed by using a maxillary seeker probe to locate the posterior edge of the uncinate and subsequently medializing it. Removal of this segment is completed using microdebrider, back-biter, or through-cutting instruments. Ideally, complete removal of the anterosuperior uncinate up to the level of the anterior attachment of the middle turbinate to the lateral nasal wall should be done. Next, the posteroinferior segment of the uncinate process is resected similarly. After a complete uncinectomy, the maxillary ostium can then be visualized with a 30- or 45-degree endoscope. If discontinuity between the natural ostium and the surgical antrostomy is identified, the intervening bridge of tissue should be removed to connect the two ostia and thereby eliminate recirculation. Care is taken not to enlarge an antrostomy too far inferiorly to avoid resecting the attachment of the inferior turbinate and entering the inferior meatus. This may cause the problem of mucus entering the inferior meatus, leading to stasis beneath the inferior turbinate or even recirculation circumferentially around the inferior turbinate.

Unresected or residual Haller cells can cause persistent inflammation within the middle meatus by encroaching on the maxillary sinus ostium or by entrapment of mucosal disease within the Haller cell itself. Entry of these cells can be performed with a maxillary seeker or J curette. Ballottement of the eye and an examination of the medial orbital wall verifies that entry into the periorbita has not occurred. Complete removal of the cell and any associated osteitic bony partitions is performed with through-cutting forceps or a microdebrider under visualization with an angled endoscope.

If the medial wall of the maxillary sinus has marked medial pneumatization, the maxillary sinus may encroach on the nasal cavity. Following antrostomy, entrapment of airflow may occur within the medial maxillary sinus, leading to mucosal drying and to secondary impairment of mucociliary clearance. Such a problem can be avoided in the original surgery by limiting the size of the maxillary antrostomy. In revision surgery, if such a problem is encountered, the medial wall of the maxillary sinus is removed using through-cutting instruments so that it is near flush with the posterior wall of the sinus. Care is taken to avoid extending the dissection too far posteriorly and risking injury to the sphenopalatine artery. In cases where the maxillary sinus membrane is chronically thickened, a large antrostomy may be beneficial for the instillation of ongoing nasal medication treatment.

In situations where the middle and superior turbinates have been resected and extensive scarring has occurred in the area of the maxillary sinus, the appearance of an "empty cavity" may offer challenges to safe entry into the maxillary sinus. In such a case, the obstructed maxillary sinus cavity can be entered by using the cephalad surface of the inferior turbinate as a landmark. The frontal process of the maxilla is palpated with a curved suction, and the maxillary sinus is entered just posterior to the maxillary line and just cephalad to the inferior turbinate, orienting the instrument in a lateral and inferior direction (**Fig. 26.8**). Entering more superiorly may result in injury to the orbit, whereas a more anterior entry may injure the nasolacrimal duct, and a more posterior entry may cause injury to the sphenopalatine artery branches.

Infectious causes of persistent maxillary sinus disease may be due to infection draining into the maxillary sinus from the frontal and ethmoid sinuses. Treatment will involve addressing the disease within the affected sinuses in addition to correcting any defects in the maxillary sinus.

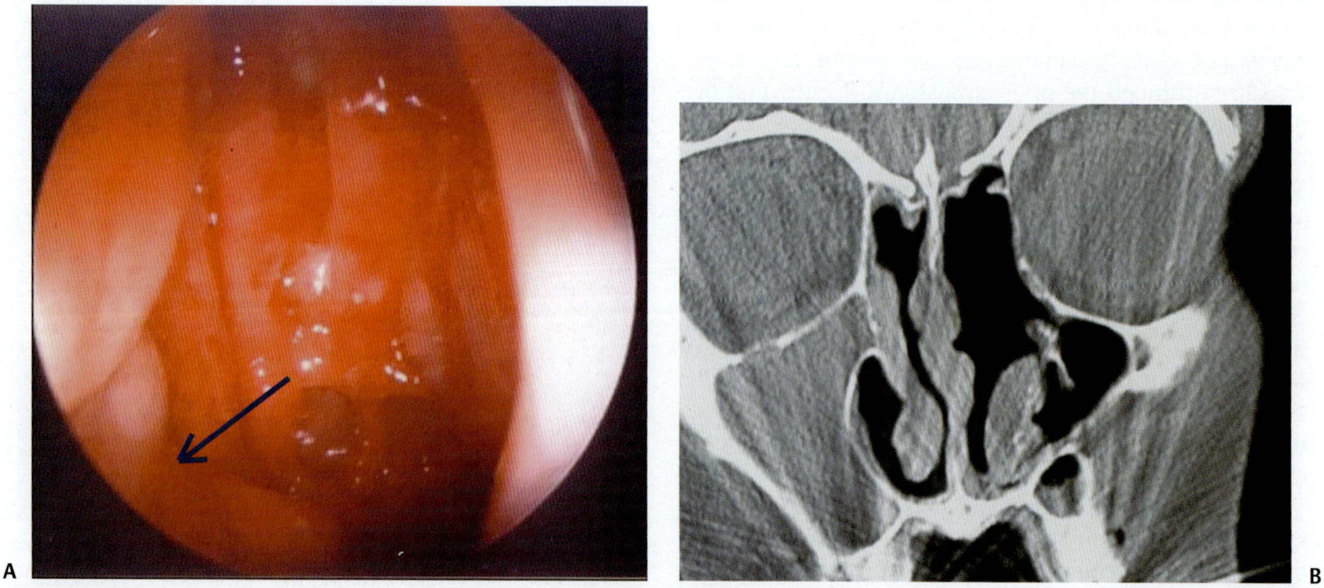

Fig. 26.8 **(A)** Endoscopic picture showing safe entry (*arrow*) into the maxillary sinus cavity. Note the complete absence of the right middle turbinate. **(B)** Coronal computed tomography scan showing maxillary opacification and an absence of the right middle turbinate.

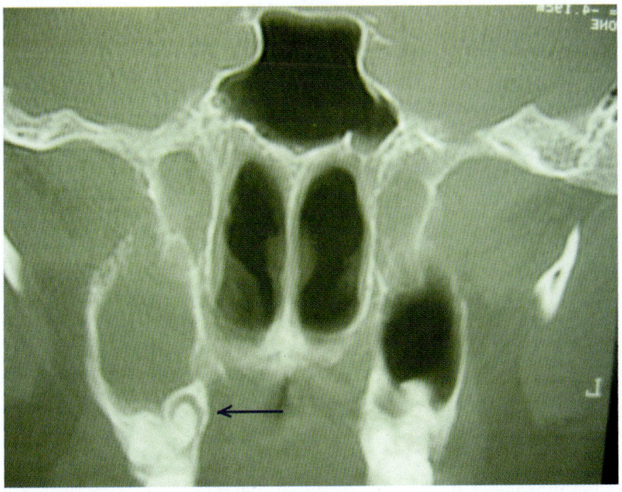

Fig. 26.9 Right maxillary disease associated with dental abscess. Note the lucency surrounding the tooth root (*arrow*).

One must also ensure removal of any retained foreign body such as dental filling material, bone chips, or inspissated concretions of a fungal ball. It is also important to ensure that the patient does not have an associated dental abscess, which may be the nidus of ongoing infection within the maxillary sinus (**Fig. 26.9**).

Finally, in cases where mucociliary transport is presumed to be permanently impaired, a "mega-antrostomy" can be created if there is repeated failure of functional endoscopic surgery. Indications include cystic fibrosis, ciliary dyskinesia, or previous Caldwell-Luc surgery. The mega-antrostomy encompasses most of the medial wall of the maxillary sinus to facilitate nasal irrigation and sinus hygiene. The posterior half of the inferior turbinate is first resected, and the medial wall of the maxillary sinus is then resected to extend the antrostomy to the floor of the nasal cavity. Preservation of the anterior half of the inferior turbinate avoids the risk of empty nose syndrome and preserves lacrimal duct drainage. The mucosa of the maxillary antrum is preserved. Excellent results have been reported using this strategy for "salvage" maxillary sinus surgery.[16,17]

Revision Surgery of the Ethmoid Sinus

The main goal of revision surgery within the ethmoid sinus is to create an open cavity lined by healthy, intact mucosa. Limits of the dissection are the lamina papyracea and skull base. As much osteitic bone is resected as reasonably necessary, and mucosal stripping is avoided. Failure of primary surgery within the ethmoid sinuses is usually due to residual ethmoid cells along the skull base and medial orbital wall, which contribute to persistent inflammation and obstruction. Therefore, a complete ethmoidectomy is required to allow for the drainage of these areas as well as to allow access for saline irrigation and topical medications.

Two important landmarks to identify are the lamina papyracea and the skull base. The preoperative CT scan must be scrutinized for any breach of these barriers from prior surgery. One must be wary of encephaloceles, a dehiscent optic nerve within the posterior ethmoids, and defects in the lamina papyracea and lateral lamella of the cribriform plate.

It is suggested that a 0-degree endoscope be used until the medial orbital wall and skull base have been identified to avoid disorientation. The plane of the lamina papyracea can be identified after completion of the maxillary antrostomy. By locating the roof of the maxillary sinus, one can palpate the floor of the orbit with a maxillary seeker probe and localize the ridge at the junction of the lamina (**Fig. 26.10**). The medial orbital wall is then skeletonized by removing residual ethmoid cells. Using a maxillary seeker probe, palpation behind a cell wall is done to gently feel the lamina and to gauge the lateral limit of the dissection. Once the lateral limit is safely identified, the cell wall is removed with a microdebrider or a through-cutting instrument. A technique that is used to protect the orbit is to gently ballotte the eye and look for transmitted pulsations, which may reveal any dehiscence. Rarely, very thick osteitic bone may cause obstruction and can be removed selectively with a diamond burr.

The basal lamella of the middle turbinate is an important landmark for distinguishing the anterior ethmoid sinus from the posterior ethmoid. After traversing the basal lamella, the surgeon will encounter the posterior ethmoid cavity, which usually contains much larger cells than the anterior ethmoid. The residual ethmoid cells can be cleared systematically, keeping in mind the boundaries of the posterior ethmoid: medially, the

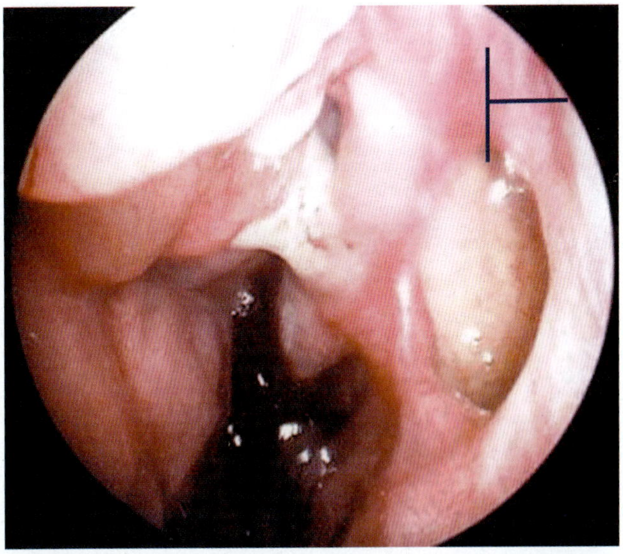

Fig. 26.10 Endoscopic picture of the left nasal cavity in a patient with chronic rhinosinusitis and recurrent nasal polyps. The sagittal plane (*vertical line*), indicating the location of the lamina papyracea, is at the junction of the medial maxillary wall and the orbital floor (*horizontal line*).

superior turbinate; laterally, the orbital wall; and superiorly, the skull base.

Although the bone of the skull base in the posterior ethmoids is usually thicker, it can be very thin close to the location of the posterior ethmoidal artery, which causes a natural weakness of the skull base. Once the skull base is identified, it is cleared of cells by dissecting posterior to anterior and staying adjacent to the medial orbital wall. Palpation behind each bony partition with a seeker probe or tip of a through-cutting instrument is performed to determine the superior limit of the dissection. Removal with a through-cutting instrument or microdebrider can then be performed.

An area of particular danger along the skull base in the ethmoid roof is the lateral lamella of the cribriform plate, which is the thinnest area of the skull base. While dissecting, instruments should be guided away from this area to avoid inadvertent intracranial entry and CSF leak. Care must be taken if using a microdebrider because the suction may inadvertently pull tissue into the teeth of the shaver if a dehiscence is present. Anteriorly, care must be taken not to injure the anterior ethmoidal artery, which may be hanging freely from the ethmoid roof. Injury and retraction of this artery into the orbit may lead to an orbital hematoma.

Revision Surgery of the Sphenoid Sinus

The sphenoid sinus defines the lowest point of the skull base and serves as a posterior landmark for the medial orbital wall. Cephalad to the arch of the choana, the sinus is not located more medially than the septum. The sphenoid sinus is approximately at the level of the roof of the maxillary sinus. In a revision case, the sphenoid sinus may serve as a critical landmark to identify the skull base and the medial orbital wall safely.

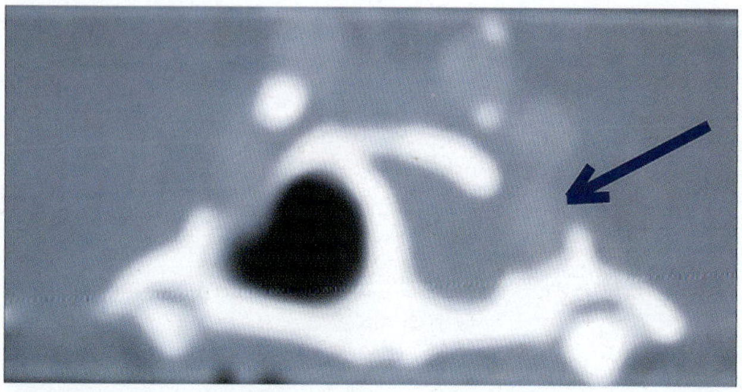

Fig. 26.11 Coronal computed tomography scan at the level of the sphenoid sinuses with a left opacified sphenoid sinus and dehiscent left carotid artery (*arrow*).

Persistent sphenoid sinus disease is caused by a failure to open the sinus in the original surgery, a subsequent stenosis from inadequate postoperative debridement, scarring of the superior turbinate to the face of the sphenoid, or a recurrence of polyps within the sphenoethmoidal recess.[18] The course of the optic nerve and carotid artery is reviewed on the preoperative CT scan. Carotid artery dehiscence can occur in up to 23% of sphenoid sinuses (**Fig. 26.11**). The presence of an Onodi cell should be determined to prevent optic nerve injury (**Fig. 26.12**).

Use of a 0-degree endoscope is preferable to prevent superior migration during dissection. The two endoscopic approaches to the sphenoid sinus are the transethmoidal and transnasal approaches. The transethmoidal approach to the sphenoid sinus follows a total ethmoidectomy. The key step to this approach is the identification of the

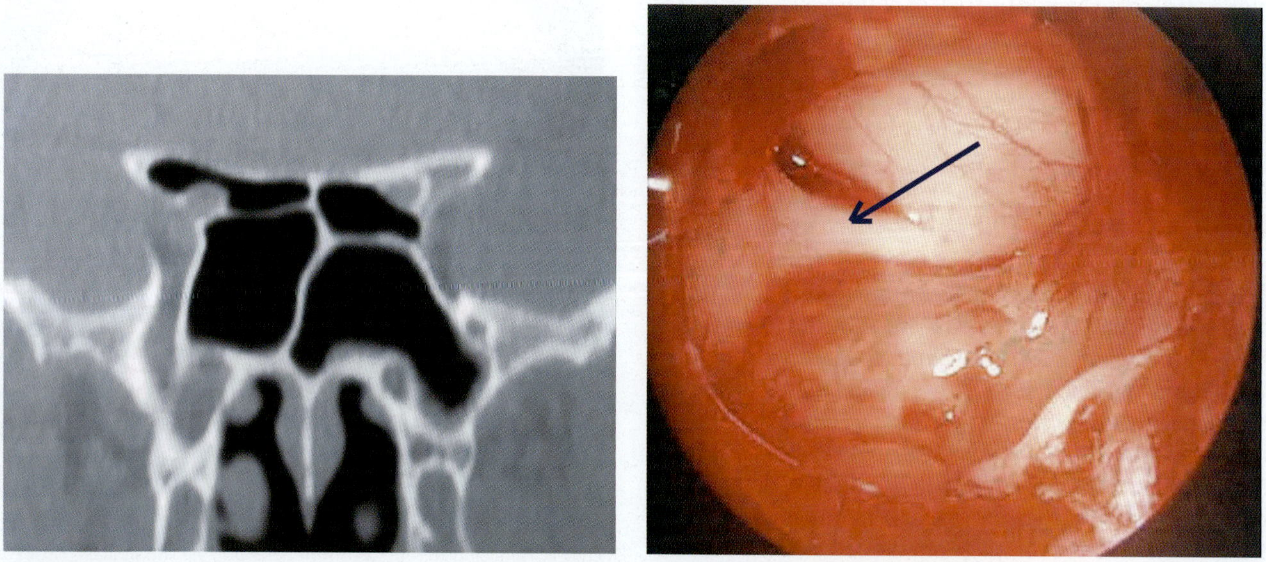

A B

Fig. 26.12 (A) Coronal computed tomography scan showing bilateral sphenoethmoid (Onodi) cells. The optic canal is seen along the floor of the right Onodi cell. **(B)** Endoscopic picture showing the optic nerve bordering the left Onodi cell (*solid arrow*).

superior turbinate, which subsequently leads to the identification of the natural sphenoid sinus ostium. During revision sinus surgery, the anatomy within the ethmoid sinus may be distorted and it may be preferable to identify the key landmarks within the sphenoid sinus first. In such a situation, the transnasal approach medial to the middle turbinate is often helpful. Progressive dilation of the sphenoethmoidal recess is done by packing pledgets soaked with a vasoconstrictive agent just medial to the middle turbinate and lateral to the posterior nasal septum. Next, identification of the superior turbinate followed by resection of its inferior one-third is performed if needed. The natural ostium is located medial to the inferior one-third of the superior turbinate, lateral to the nasal septum, and ~12 mm superior to the posterior nasal choana (**Fig. 26.5**). Entry into the sinus through the natural ostium is preferable; however, in cases where the ostium is heavily scarred or not identifiable, entry into the sinus in a medial inferior location is safe using the roof of the maxillary sinus and the posterior nasal septum as reference points (**Fig. 26.4**).

Once the sinus is entered with a J curette or a Frazier suction, the ostium is enlarged using a mushroom punch, or a Hajek-Koffler sphenoid punch, or Kerrison rongeurs. Diamond burr drills may be necessary in cases of thick osteitic bone. Palpation behind the bone is done before resection to gauge the location of the lateral and superior sinus walls. Ideally, the anterior face of the sinus should be taken down to where it is almost flush with the medial orbital wall and skull base. Inferiorly, one must be aware of the posterior septal branch of the sphenopalatine artery, which courses along the inferior face of the sphenoid, ~1 to 1.5 cm below the sphenoid ostium. Bleeding from this branch can be controlled with a suction cautery if it occurs. Preservation of the inferior region of sphenoid mucosa will avoid bleeding from this branch and will also prevent circumferential stenosis of the sphenoidotomy.

Revision Surgery of the Frontal Sinus

Revision endoscopic frontal sinus surgery remains one of the greatest challenges facing the endoscopic surgeon. Primary complaints of headaches, although more common with frontal sinusitis, are poor predictors of surgically amenable sinus disease. Evaluation for migraines and other causes of headaches by a qualified neurologist should be pursued with a very low threshold for patients with this symptom. Similarly, evaluation for allergic, rheumatologic, psychiatric, and other causes of the patient's symptomatology should always be considered.

If the patient's disease is attributable to chronic frontal sinus pathology, then a thorough analysis for the failure of previous frontal sinus surgery should be performed. Broadly, causes for frontal sinus disease in the setting of previous frontal sinus surgery can represent lack of optimal medical management, persistent disease due to incomplete surgery, iatrogenic disease, and recurrent disease following a successful procedure.

If appropriate medical therapy has been optimized and is unsuccessful in mitigating the patient's disease, then a careful evaluation should be made whether surgery can be effective at treating the patient's disease. The best likelihood of success with a repeat operation is in the setting of persistent disease due to a previous incomplete or inadequate surgery.

Whereas patients with persistent anatomic obstruction often have excellent outcomes with revision surgical techniques, patients with iatrogenic causes of chronic frontal rhinosinusitis are often the most difficult patients to cure. Furthermore, iatrogenic scarring and osteoneogenesis can unfortunately convert a patient with previously mild-to-moderate symptoms into one having a crippling disease. As a result, iatrogenic frontal sinus disease is best avoided by using sound and meticulous techniques when performing primary frontal sinus operations.

Revision frontal sinus surgery poses new anatomic challenges for the sinus surgeon. Evidence of a residual superior uncinate or remaining anterior ethmoid/frontal cells may reveal evidence for previous inadequate surgery. Given the likelihood of distorted anatomy, the sinus surgeon should have a clear three-dimensional understanding of the anatomy of the patient's individual frontal recess prior to commencing with surgery. The skull base and the lamina should be carefully evaluated for any potential dehiscence that may be the result of prior surgery, and intraoperatively, suspicious areas should be considered dehiscent unless bone is palpated or confirmed with accurate image guidance. In revision frontal sinus cases, the surgeon should look for the following common causes of pathology: a partially amputated middle turbinate or lateralization of the entire middle turbinate (due to a complete resection of the basal lamella) causing obstruction of frontal sinus outflow, scarring of the superior uncinate to the middle turbinate medial to the frontal sinus outflow tract, scarring, circumferential stenosis, and/or osteoneogenesis in the frontal ostium area, a remnant ethmoid bulla cap mistakenly considered the frontal recess, agger nasi or frontal cells left undissected (**Fig. 26.13**), and/or recurrence of polyposis in the frontal outflow system.[19]

Surgery for frontal sinus disease should follow an organized progression from least aggressive to most aggressive. The choice of the proper procedure should not only be based on careful review of preoperative CT films, but also on the pathophysiology behind the recurrent or persistent frontal sinus disease. There are multiple procedures from which to choose from; however, endoscopic procedures should be at the forefront of the thought process when considering frontal sinus surgery. The classification of the types of frontal surgery was described by Draf, and the different surgical techniques are described in Chapters 27 and 28 of this book. Endoscopic approaches to the frontal sinus are usually favored; however, there are

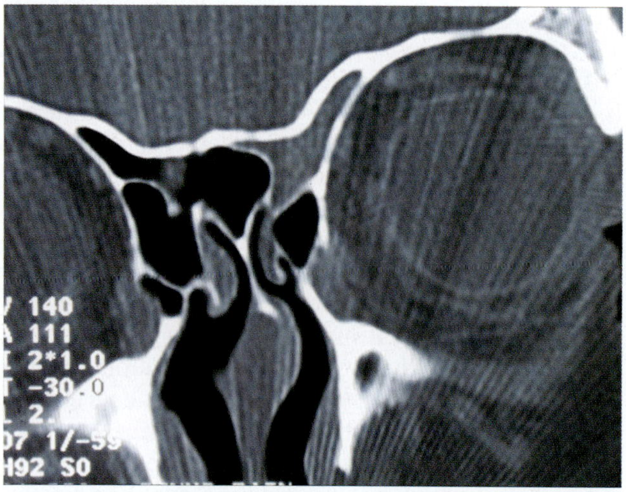

Fig. 26.13 Coronal sinus computed tomography scan showing a left agger nasi cell contributing to obstruction of frontal sinus drainage.

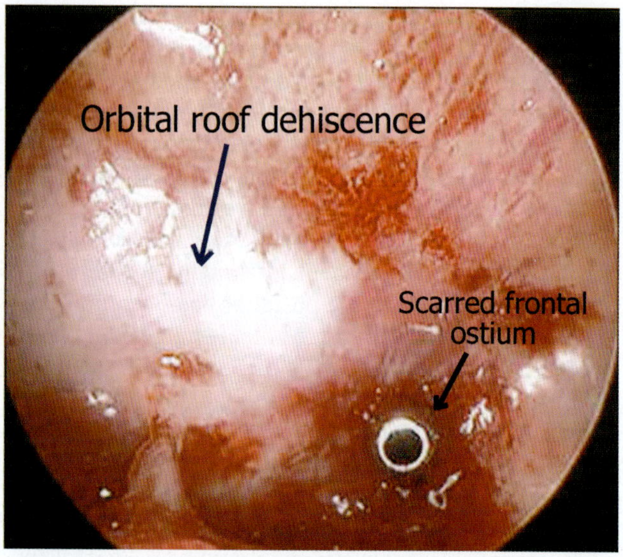

Fig. 26.14 Endoscopic picture illustrates the above and below technique. An endoscope is used through the mini-trephine ("above") to show instrumentation of scarred frontal recess using a curved suction from "below."

some circumstances where the simple trephine along with an endoscopic approach or "the above and below technique" can facilitate the surgery and obviate the need for a more aggressive approach to the frontal sinus. Indications for this procedure are ever expanding because it is minimally invasive and cosmetically appealing yet also allows the surgeon to reach areas that are not available via endonasal techniques. Among the indications for the procedure, the most common remain lateral or cephalad frontal sinus lesions, type II or IV frontal cells that cannot be addressed endoscopically, tumors or inflammatory lesions involving the frontal sinus, frontal sinus trauma, and distorted anatomy of the frontal recess. **Figure 26.14** illustrates the technique by using an endoscope through the mini-trephine ("above") to show instrumentation of scarred frontal recess using a curved suction from "below."

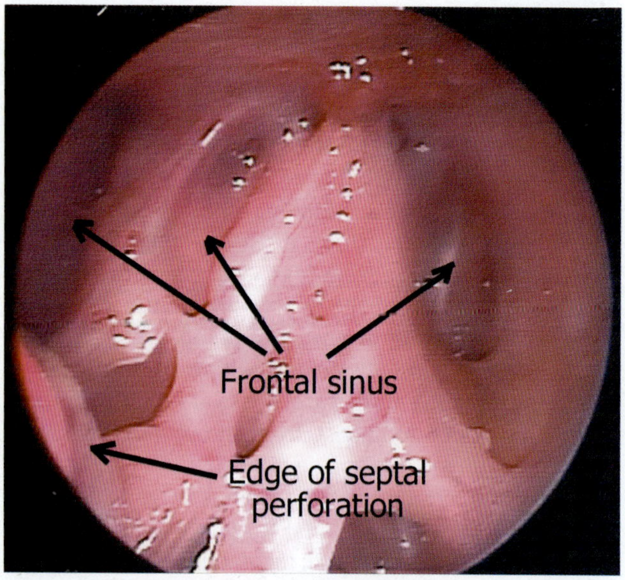

Fig. 26.15 Endoscopic view of the frontal recess and sinus area after the endoscopic modified Lothrop procedure.

The endoscopic modified Lothrop procedure or a Draf type III endonasal median drainage procedure can be used as an alternative to frontal sinus obliteration via an osteoplastic flap procedure. The procedure has the surgical objective of creating a large nasofrontal communication (**Fig. 26.15**) by using a totally intranasal approach and avoiding an external incision while preserving the frontal sinus mucosa.[20] The indications for the procedure are varied and include failed endoscopic sinus surgery techniques, significant osteoneogenesis in the frontal recess and frontal ostium, frontal recess adhesions, disease processes that have resulted in the loss of the posterior wall or floor of the frontal sinus, failed previous osteoplastic flap with obliteration with mucocele formation, and tumor removal from the frontal sinus.[21] Frontal sinus obliterations are now infrequently used with the advent of improved frontal sinus instruments and technology.

Complications and Success Rates of Revision Surgery

The risk of complications is thought to be higher in revision surgery than in primary surgery. Absence of anatomic landmarks, increased bleeding, osteoneogenesis, and extensive adhesions all contribute to this increased risk. Major complication rates have been reported to be 0.3% to more than 1.3%, and have included violation of the lamina papyracea and CSF leaks.[3]

The success rate for revision cases tends to be lower than that of primary cases and is in the range of 50 to 90.9%.[3,12] Poor prognostic factors are the extent of mucosal disease, underlying medical disease such as asthma, the presence of polyps, prior ethmoidal surgery, and the degree of osteoneogenesis.[22,23] With proper medical management, however, symptomatic relief that revision surgery can provide is similar to that following a primary surgery.[24]

Postoperative Care and Medical Management for Revision Sinus Surgery

Postoperative care in revision surgery is similar to that of primary surgery. It is most important that the patient understands the benefits of postoperative endoscopic debridements and that he or she adheres to ongoing medical therapies. Failure to do so will only lead to a recurrence or persistence of the disease. Postoperative debridements in the office to remove crusts, blood clots, or inflamed tissue should be done when possible to help reduce inflammation or local infection, which contribute to scarring. If needed, synechiae formation between the middle turbinate and lateral nasal wall can be taken down using a freer elevator or through-cutting instruments in the office. Ideally, debridements should start 1 week postoperatively, with subsequent endoscopic evaluations and debridements of the nasal cavity done based on the response of the patient to medical therapy.

Medical therapy includes the use of antibiotics, topical steroids, leukotriene antagonists, or oral steroids. Nasal saline irrigations are an important adjunct to medical therapy and should be done at least twice daily during the first few months following surgery. Hypertonic saline nasal irrigations have been found to improve the quality of life in patients with chronic rhinosinusitis.[25,26] Concentrations of saline should not reach 7% because such a concentration has been shown to be ciliostatic.[27] A short burst of high-dose oral steroids may be required in cases of refractory inflammation and polyps. The limitations of oral steroids are based on their potential short- and long-term adverse side effects. Topical steroid sprays are usually the mainstay of medical therapy. To limit the adverse effects of oral steroids and to increase the delivery of steroids within the nasal cavity, nasal steroid irrigations have been used. Budesonide mixed in with saline irrigation has been used with reported success.[28] Persistent purulent infections are treated with oral antibiotics, whereas the option of nebulized or nasal spray antibiotics can be considered in patients with low-grade local nasal infections. Finally, leukotriene antagonists or lipo-oxygenase inhibitors can be considered in patients with concomitant asthma and refractory sinonasal symptoms. Long-term follow-up should be individualized for each patient according to the pathophysiology of his or her sinus disease.

Conclusion

Patients who require revision sinus surgery are a challenge from both a technical and a medical management perspective. The revision surgeon should first undertake a thorough reevaluation of the patient's disease, followed by efforts to optimize medical therapy. Next, a thorough investigation into the causes of previous surgical failure should ensue. The choice of procedure should be dictated by the anatomy and CT findings, as well as by the underlying pathology. Surgery should be as conservative as possible to reduce the chance of further scarring and osteoneogenesis. The dependence on image guidance should be cautioned, and safe endoscopic sinus surgery should be based on the surgeon's experience and knowledge of key anatomic landmarks. In cases of disorientation or uncertainty, it is always wise to stop the surgery rather than risk serious and irreversible damage. Completeness of surgery is secondary to patient safety and one should be mindful that one can always bring the patient at a later day to complete the surgery if excessive bleeding, poor visualization, or uncertainty is present. Aggressive postoperative debridements and individualized medical therapy are key to the successful treatment of refractory sinonasal disease in this difficult subset of patients.

References

1. Ling FT, Kountakis SE. Important clinical symptoms in patients undergoing functional endoscopic sinus surgery for chronic rhinosinusitis. Laryngoscope 2007;117(6):1090–1093
2. Senior BA, Kennedy DW, Tanabodee J, Kroger H, Hassab M, Lanza D. Long-term results of functional endoscopic sinus surgery. Laryngoscope 1998;108(2):151–157
3. Moses RL, Cornetta A, Atkins JP Jr, Roth M, Rosen MR, Keane WM. Revision endoscopic sinus surgery: the Thomas Jefferson University experience. Ear Nose Throat J 1998;77(3):190, 193–195, 199–202
4. Jiang RS, Hsu CY. Revision functional endoscopic sinus surgery. Ann Otol Rhinol Laryngol 2002;111(2):155–159
5. Cullen MMBW. Revision endoscopic sinus surgery for recurrent rhinosinusitis. In: Kennedy DW, Bolger WE, Zinreich SJ, ed. Diseases of the Sinuses - Diagnosis and Management. Hamilton - London: BC Decker Inc.; 2001:245–253
6. Senior BA, Kennedy DW, Tanabodee J, Kroger H, Hassab M, Lanza DC. Long-term impact of functional endoscopic sinus surgery on asthma. Otolaryngol Head Neck Surg 1999;121(1):66–68
7. Lazar RH, Younis RT, Long TE, Gross CW. Revision functional endonasal sinus surgery. Ear Nose Throat J 1992;71(3):131–133
8. Chu CT, Lebowitz RA, Jacobs JB. An analysis of sites of disease in revision endoscopic sinus surgery. Am J Rhinol 1997;11(4): 287–291

9. Chambers DW, Davis WE, Cook PR, Nishioka GJ, Rudman DT. Long-term outcome analysis of functional endoscopic sinus surgery: correlation of symptoms with endoscopic examination findings and potential prognostic variables. Laryngoscope 1997;107(4): 504–510
10. Ramadan HH. Surgical causes of failure in endoscopic sinus surgery. Laryngoscope 1999;109(1):27–29
11. Parsons DS, Stivers FE, Talbot AR. The missed ostium sequence and the surgical approach to revision functional endoscopic sinus surgery. Otolaryngol Clin North Am 1996;29(1):169–183
12. Musy PY, Kountakis SE. Anatomic findings in patients undergoing revision endoscopic sinus surgery. Am J Otolaryngol 2004; 25(6):418–422
13. May M, Schaitkin B, Kay SL. Revision endoscopic sinus surgery: six friendly surgical landmarks. Laryngoscope 1994;104(6 Pt 1): 766–767
14. Al-Rawi MM, Edelstein DR, Erlandson RA. Changes in nasal epithelium in patients with severe chronic sinusitis: a clinicopathologic and electron microscopic study. Laryngoscope 1998;108(12): 1816–1823
15. Kennedy DW, Senior BA, Gannon FH, Montone KT, Hwang P, Lanza DC. Histology and histomorphometry of ethmoid bone in chronic rhinosinusitis. Laryngoscope 1998;108(4 Pt 1): 502–507
16. Cho DY, Hwang PH. Results of endoscopic maxillary mega-antrostomy in recalcitrant maxillary sinusitis. Am J Rhinol 2008; 22(6):658–662
17. Woodworth BA, Parker RO, Schlosser RJ. Modified endoscopic medial maxillectomy for chronic maxillary sinusitis. Am J Rhinol 2006;20(3):317–319
18. Cohen NA, Kennedy DW. Revision endoscopic sinus surgery. Otolaryngol Clin North Am 2006;39(3):417–435, vii.
19. Friedman M. Frontal sinus surgery 2004: Update of clinical anatomy and surgical techniques. Oper Tech Otolaryngol—Head Neck Surg 2004;15:23–31
20. Farhat FT, Figueroa RE, Kountakis SE. Anatomic measurements for the endoscopic modified Lothrop procedure. Am J Rhinol 2005;19(3):293–296
21. Wormald PJ. Salvage frontal sinus surgery: the endoscopic modified Lothrop procedure. Laryngoscope 2003;113(2):276–283
22. Wynn R, Har-El G. Recurrence rates after endoscopic sinus surgery for massive sinus polyposis. Laryngoscope 2004;114(5): 811–813
23. King JM, Caldarelli DD, Pigato JB. A review of revision functional endoscopic sinus surgery. Laryngoscope 1994;104(4):404–408
24. Bhattacharyya N. Clinical outcomes after revision endoscopic sinus surgery. Arch Otolaryngol Head Neck Surg 2004;130(8):975–978
25. Rabago D, Zgierska A, Mundt M, Barrett B, Bobula J, Maberry R. Efficacy of daily hypertonic saline nasal irrigation among patients with sinusitis: a randomized controlled trial. J Fam Pract 2002;51(12):1049–1055
26. Rabago D, Pasic T, Zgierska A, Mundt M, Barrett B, Maberry R. The efficacy of hypertonic saline nasal irrigation for chronic sinonasal symptoms. Otolaryngol Head Neck Surg 2005;133(1):3–8
27. Boek WM, Keleş N, Graamans K, Huizing EH. Physiologic and hypertonic saline solutions impair ciliary activity in vitro. Laryngoscope 1999;109(3):396–399
28. Lavigne F, Cameron L, Renzi PM, et al. Intrasinus administration of topical budesonide to allergic patients with chronic rhinosinusitis following surgery. Laryngoscope 2002;112(5):858–864

27 Endoscopic Frontal Sinusotomy

Yvonne Chan, Christopher T. Melroy, and Frederick A. Kuhn

The frontal sinus is the most challenging of the four paranasal sinuses to treat endoscopically because frontal sinus surgery often has a higher failure rate than surgery on other sinuses, encompasses multiple surgical approaches, and represents more anatomically difficult dissections. Surgery for frontal sinus disease can induce complications related to the skull base, the anterior ethmoid artery, and the periorbital tissue. Failure is often a result of multiple factors, principal among which is incomplete surgery. Other factors include excessive mucosa removal, edema, infection, scar tissue formation, and osteoneogenesis.

Surgical management of frontal sinus disease has evolved from external obliterative procedures to endoscopic mucosal preserving ones.[1,2] Classically, the treatment of chronic frontal sinusitis has been directed at the sinus itself. As frontal sinus anatomy has been studied and understood over the past 20 years,[3] it has become clear that the underlying problem in chronic frontal sinusitis is not the sinus, but rather its drainage pathway, the frontal recess. Consequently, redirecting our efforts from destructive frontal sinus procedures to function-restoring frontal recess procedures has yielded far better long-term results.

The complex and intricate anatomy of the inverted funnel-like frontal recess and its anterosuperior location can limit endoscopic frontal recess dissection and visualization. This area is predisposed to incomplete dissection and stenosis because of surgeons' unfamiliarity with the difficult anatomy, the 70-degree telescope, and the frontal sinus instruments. When performing frontal sinus surgery, it is important to tailor the procedure to the individual patient and the extent of the disease. The general tenet is to employ the least invasive procedure that will accomplish the task of restoring frontal sinus function. Most cases can be managed endoscopically; however, if the disease cannot be resolved, then additional, more aggressive procedures can be added in a stepwise fashion using an integrated approach to frontal sinus surgery (**Table 27.1**).[4] The different frontal sinus surgical techniques that have been collected into an integrated approach to frontal sinus surgery will be discussed individually, some in other chapters. This chapter focuses on intranasal endoscopic techniques without the use of intranasal drills.

Table 27.1 The Integrated Approach to Frontal Sinus Surgery

- Endoscopic frontal sinusotomy (instruments and balloon dilation)
- Endoscopic frontal sinus rescue procedure
- Endoscopic extended frontal sinus rescue procedure
- Above and below technique (frontal sinus trephination and transnasal endoscopic)
- Endoscopic modified Lothrop with punches (Draf III)
- Above and below technique (Osteoplastic flap and endoscopic approach)
- Frontal sinus obliteration
- Frontal sinus unobliteration

Source: Data from Kuhn FA. An integrated approach to frontal sinus surgery. Otolaryngol Clin North Am 2006;39(3):437–461.

Patient Selection/Indications

Indications for Endoscopic Frontal Sinusotomy (Draf Type I, IIa, and IIb)

Endoscopic frontal sinusotomy encompasses the Draf I, IIa, and IIb variants, depending on the extent of dissection required.[2] Endoscopic frontal sinusotomy can be functionally defined as the intranasal endoscopic removal of the frontal recess structures necessary to restore physiologic mucus clearance. This may include removal of all frontal recess cells[5] (i.e., agger nasi cells, types I through IV frontal cells), the common wall between the frontal sinus and a supraorbital ethmoid cell, suprabullar cells, the frontal bulla, and/or the interfrontal sinus septal cells. This technique may also involve removing the medial and lateral frontal sinus floor, which in most cases is simply the roof of the frontal recess cells.

The most common indication for endoscopic frontal sinusotomy is chronic frontal sinusitis not controlled with maximal medical management. Common etiologies of chronic frontal sinusitis include (1) mechanical obstruction; (2) eosinophilic inflammatory chronic sinusitis (including allergic fungal sinusitis); (3) nasal polyposis; and (4) frontal sinus mucoceles. Endoscopic frontal sinusotomy may also be indicated in patients with severe acute frontal sinusitis refractory to medical management, and those with intracranial or orbital complications. Other indications include benign and malignant neoplasms involving the frontal sinus, as well as frontal sinus anterior table fractures that extend into the frontal recess.

Indications for Frontal Sinus Rescue Procedure

The frontal sinus rescue procedure was designed to address recurrent frontal sinusitis in patients whose middle turbinate has been "trimmed" or partially amputated, resulting in a lateralized remnant that is scarred to the medial orbital wall. This produces a bony stenosis of the frontal recess. This anatomic configuration is very difficult to address with a standard frontal sinusotomy as it creates a circumferential opening that is prone to stenosis.

Indications for Extended Frontal Sinus Rescue Procedure

This procedure was designed for patients who have an intact middle turbinate and a narrowed or collapsed frontal recess, which does not function. The frontal recess may be so narrow that a mild amount of edema obstructs it and prevents physiologic drainage. If this is the case, the standard endoscopic approach will have no chance of success in the nonfunctional frontal recess. Consequently, something else must be done to divert frontal mucous clearance around the frontal recess.

Indications for Endoscopic Modified Lothrop with Punches (Draf III)

The Draf III with punches is intended for difficult revision surgery where endoscopic frontal sinusotomy has failed multiple times. This procedure also may be performed primarily in patients with benign or malignant neoplasms involving the frontal sinus for intraoperative or postoperative access into the sinus.

Diagnostic Workup

The surgical management of acute or chronic frontal sinusitis should be tailored to the individual patient's needs according to the underlying pathology. Thus, a detailed history and physical examination is of utmost importance. The history should document common sinonasal symptoms, episodes of recurrent sinusitis, previous antibiotic and/or systemic corticosteroid therapy, previous surgical management, and the presence of other systemic diseases such as asthma and autoimmune diseases. Physical examination, including anterior rhinoscopy and a nasal endoscopy using the 0-, 30-, and, 70-degree telescopes, should be performed to assess for normal/abnormal anatomy, evidence of previous surgery, and presence of pathology (i.e., nasal polyps, polypoid edema, purulent drainage, scar tissue, and tumors). Thin axial computed tomography (CT) imaging of the paranasal sinuses with coronal and sagittal reconstructions are always required in the diagnostic workup of frontal sinusitis. CT enables an assessment of the extent of disease and can identify anatomic contributors to frontal recess obstruction. The sagittal views are crucial for diagnostic and surgical planning purposes because they allow direct visualization of the frontal sinus drainage pathway. In reviewing the CT scans, the location of the ethmoid bulla lamella, the anterior ethmoid artery, agger nasi cells, supraorbital ethmoid cells, and frontal cells should be noted because these structures need to be identified in the course of any frontal recess dissection.

Surgical Anatomy

The frontal recess, the frontal sinus drainage pathway, is an inverted funnel-shaped space that connects the frontal sinus to the anterior ethmoid region. Although the concept of the frontal recess re-emerged with the development of endoscopic sinus surgery, the three-dimensional frontal recess was first mentioned by Killian in 1896.[6] The embryologic development of the frontal recess was described by Schaeffer[7] and Kaspar,[8] and the surgical anatomy as well as clinical significance was illustrated by Van Alyea.[9] Being mindful of the frontal sinus ciliary beat pattern described by Messerklinger,[10] frontal recess mucosal preservation is key to successful frontal recess surgery. Messerklinger demonstrated that frontal sinus cilia sweep the mucus up the interfrontal sinus septum, across the frontal sinus roof laterally, and medially along the frontal sinus floor to the ostium (**Fig. 27.1**). 40 to 60% of the mucus is cleared out of the frontal sinus along the lateral aspect of the frontal recess, either along the medial orbital wall or over the medial aspect of the agger nasi cell. The remainder of the mucus recirculates up the interfrontal sinus septum, potentially carrying debris or microbes from the frontal recess up into the frontal sinus.

Surgical Technique

Endoscopic Frontal Sinusotomy (Draf Type I and IIa)

Over the last two decades, endoscopic frontal sinusotomy gradually has been accepted as the procedure of choice for the surgical management of chronic frontal sinusitis.[11–13] Improved surgeon experience, the development of specialized frontal sinus instruments, and image-guided surgery have allowed endoscopic frontal sinusotomy to supplant external approaches.[14–16] The advantages include preservation of the lateral bony frontal recess wall (otherwise removed in the Lynch procedure), decreased morbidity, shorter hospital stay, reduced convalescent period, lack of external scar, and restoration of normal sinus function.

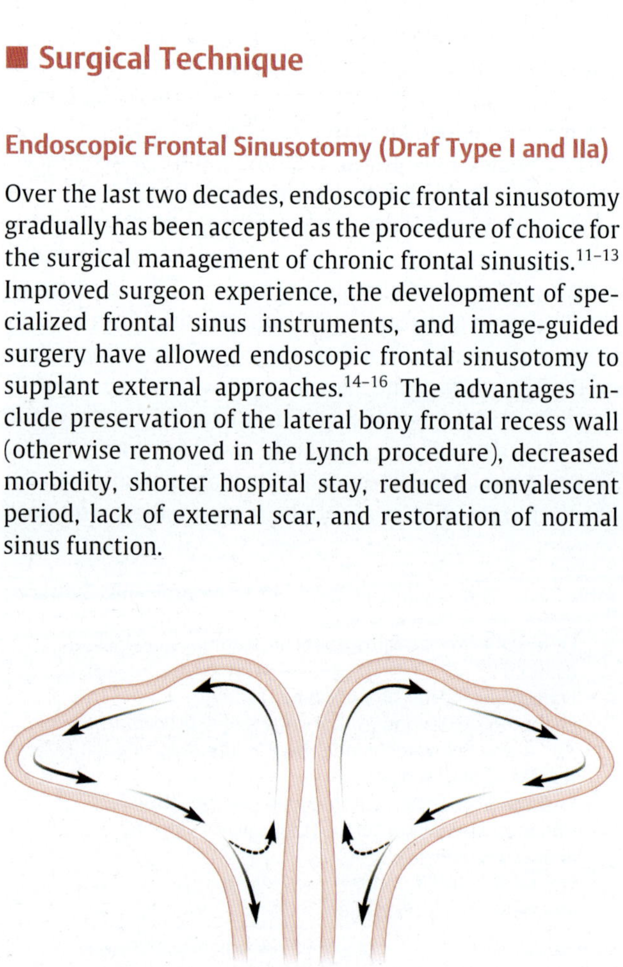

Fig. 27.1 Frontal sinus mucociliary flow pattern.

Preservation of mucous membrane in the frontal sinus drainage pathway is the key to a successful functional outcome. The ideal method of dealing with the frontal sinus drainage pathway is to carry out delicate dissection with the appropriate instrumentation while causing minimal damage to the mucosa. The development of frontal sinus instruments such as angled through-cutting punches, curettes, giraffe cup forceps, and seekers have enabled surgery in the narrow confines of the frontal recess (**Fig. 27.2**). Familiarization

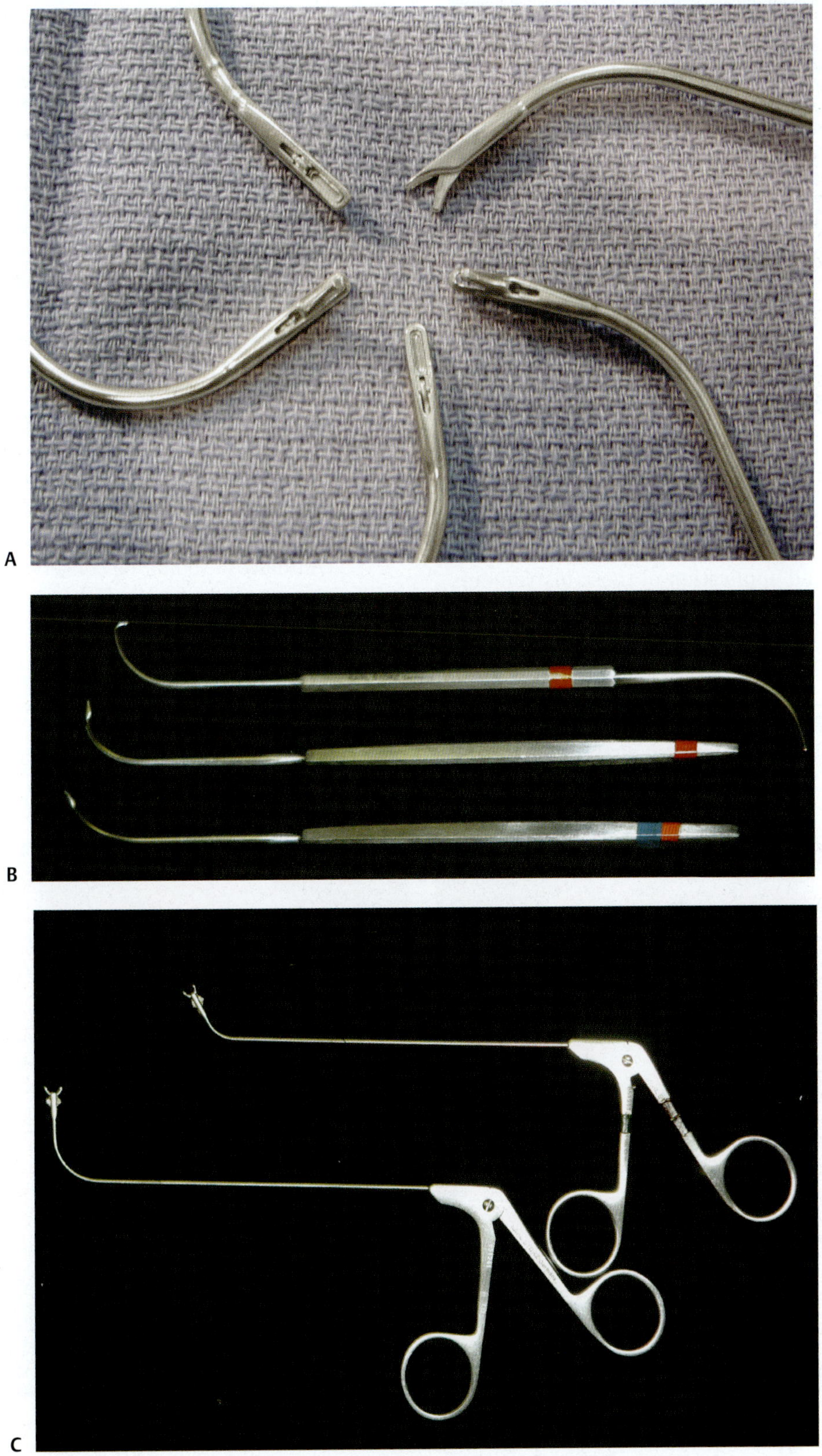

Fig. 27.2 (A) New style frontal sinus punches. **(B)** Frontal sinus curettes and seeker. **(C)** Frontal recess giraffe forceps.

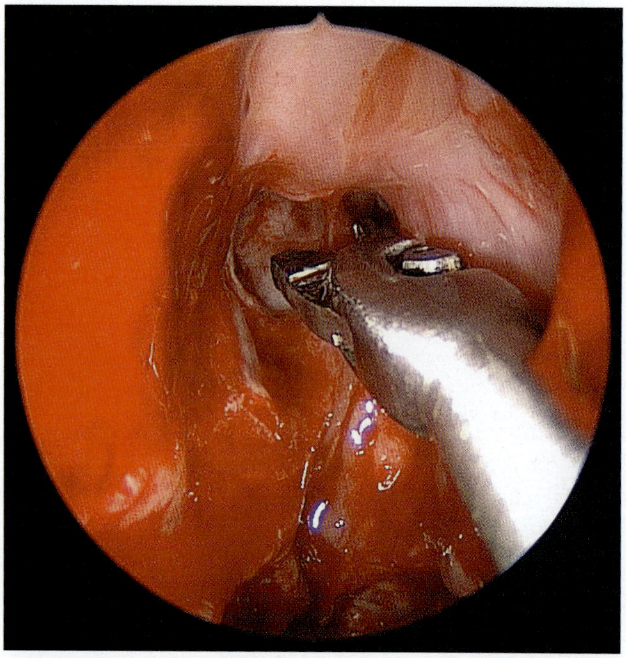

Fig. 27.3 Intraoperative photo demonstrating the use of a 90-degree side-to-side frontal sinus punch removing a partition between the frontal sinus ostium and an interfrontal sinus septal cell.

with the function and application of these instruments will prove invaluable to successful surgical outcomes. Five surgical principles in the approach to the frontal recess should be noted:

1. An ethmoidectomy based on extent of disease should be performed first to allow room for the dissection of the frontal recess from posterior-to-anterior along the skull base.
2. Frontal recess dissection should be approached in a posterior-to-anterior and a medial-to-lateral direction to avoid penetration of the thinnest bony skull base areas surrounding the frontal recess. These include the posterior table of the frontal recess and the lateral lamella of the cribriform plate.
3. The medial and posterior walls of the agger nasi cell are not part of the skull base; therefore, they are the two walls which can and should be removed.
4. Frontal recess cells may be resected with angled frontal sinus punches (**Fig. 27.3**) or fractured from a posterior-to-anterior direction with frontal recess curettes under visualization with a 30- or 70-degree telescope. The fragments can then be gently removed with giraffe forceps (**Fig. 27.4**) or by using short bursts of an angled tissue debrider.
5. The array of frontal sinus seekers may be used to retrieve small bony fragments obstructing the ostium or to divide flaps of mucosa to drape them flat along the bony surfaces. This process should be repeated until the frontal sinus ostium is clear. All mucosa should be conserved, especially in the vicinity of the frontal ostium.

The dissected frontal ostium may be stented or left alone depending on the resultant diameter of the internal frontal ostium and how well the mucosa is aligned. Because Neel and Lake demonstrated that semirigid stents induced

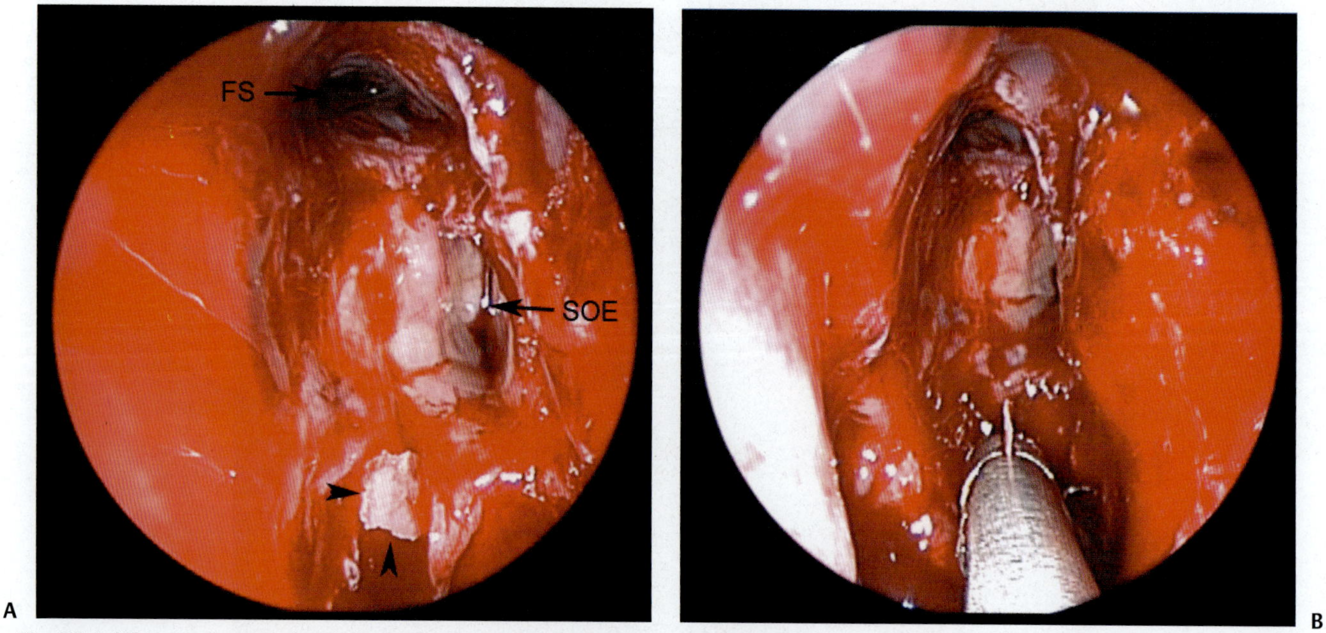

Fig. 27.4 (A) Intraoperative photo of a small bony fragment (*arrows*) in the left frontal recess. *FS*, frontal sinus; *SOE*, supraorbital ethmoid cell. **(B)** Intraoperative photo of the bony fragment being removed with a pair of 90-degree side-to-side biting giraffe forceps.

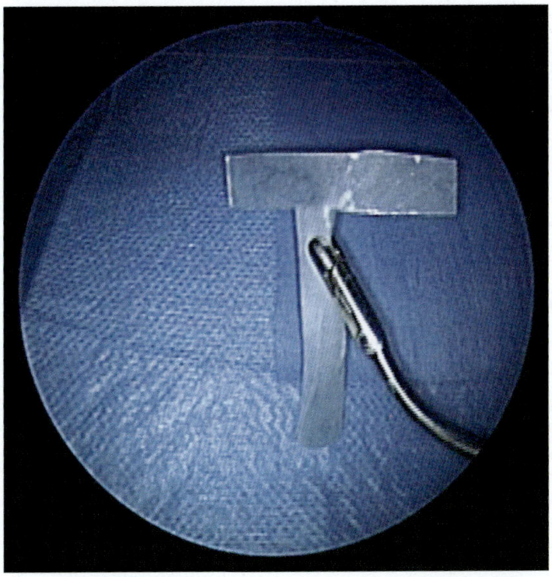

Fig. 27.5 Frontal sinus stent fashioned from a piece of 0.01-inch thick soft silastic sheeting.

circumferential scarring and osteoneogenesis in animal studies of frontal sinus healing, we advocate, as they did, the use of soft flexible silastic stents, as described in previous articles (**Fig. 27.5**).[4]

The following case example illustrates some of the commonly encountered anatomic causes of frontal sinusitis in revision sinus surgery, namely undissected cells in the frontal recess. The patient in **Fig. 27.6** has had a previous ethmoidectomy and an attempted frontal sinusotomy; however, there is a retained agger nasi cell cap that can be seen impinging on the lateral surface of the middle turbinate. It is this area that was retaining the infected secretions. An undissected type I frontal cell was also identified above the agger nasi cell (**Fig. 27.6**). The endoscopic view in the figure demonstrates the agger nasi cell with the InstaTrak suction behind it. The sagittal view illustrates the type I frontal cell encroaching on the posterior frontal sinus table. Each of these cells needs to be removed to ensure an adequate egress of mucus from the frontal sinus.

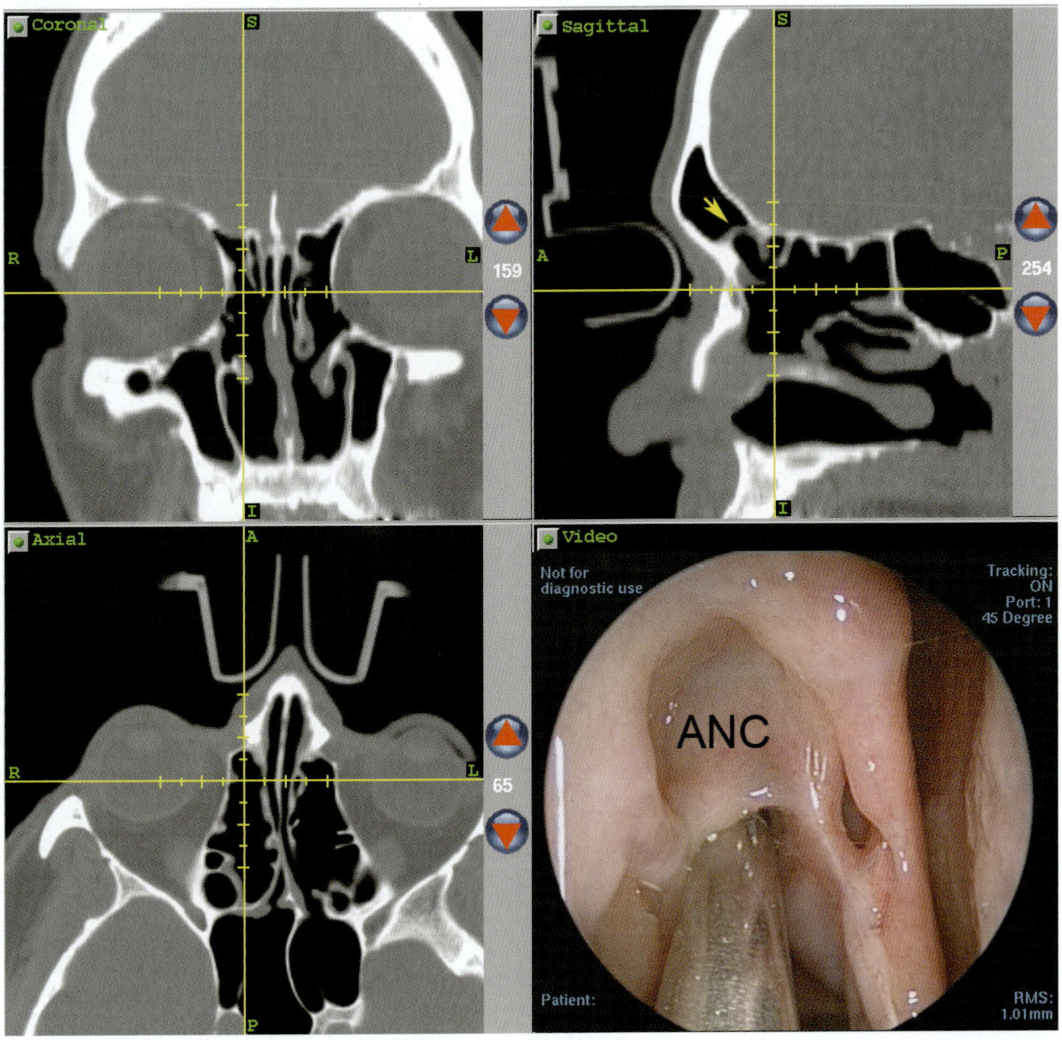

Fig. 27.6 Intraoperative view of the agger nasi cell (*ANC*) cap with a suction tip behind it. The sagittal computed tomography image demonstrates a type I frontal cell (*arrow*) impinging on the posterior frontal sinus table.

Endoscopic Frontal Sinusotomy with Balloon Dilating Catheters

Because the frontal recess still represents a challenge for many surgeons, the development of novel devices allowing for less invasive dissection has improved access to the frontal sinus. One useful adjunct to frontal sinus instruments in our armamentarium is the balloon dilation catheter. Since the introduction of this device in 2005, several studies have been conducted demonstrating its safety and efficacy.[17,18] This technology is an adaptation of cardiac dilation devices to open sinus drainage pathways. The underlying principle is to pass a balloon catheter over a guidewire through a sinus ostium and dilate the surrounding tissue. This is illustrated in **Fig. 27.7**. A range of sinus guides with varying angles (0, 30, 70, and 110 degrees) was designed to guide the wire through specific sinus ostia (**Fig. 27.8A**). The balloon catheters are also available in different sizes tailored to the dimensions of different sinus ostia (**Fig. 27.8B**). The advent of the balloon device allows the sinus surgeon to use this as the sole tool in certain select patients, especially those with isolated or unilateral diseases. Other patients, however, may require a mixture of endoscopic dissection, specifically ethmoidectomy, along with ostial dilation of the other sinuses. This type of procedure is referred to as a "hybrid" case.

Several studies examining the accessibility, efficacy, safety, and patency rates of frontal recess endoscopic dilation have been conducted. A multicenter prospective trial demonstrated high patient tolerability of the device with no serious adverse effects.[18] Patient symptom responses on the Sino-Nasal Outcome Test (SNOT-20) showed a significant improvement over baseline values. This study also reported an endoscopic frontal sinus patency rate of 82% at 6 months.[18] The 1-year endoscopic patency in this same cohort of patients is 85%.[19] When the functionally patent frontal sinuses—that is, those whose ostia cannot be visualized but who have frontal sinuses completely clear on a CT scan (Lund/McKay score 0)—are added to the endoscopically patent sinuses, the 1-year frontal sinus patency was 91.9%. After revision of two additional frontal sinuses, the patency was 94.6%.[19] Rehl and Vaughan reviewed 136 frontal recesses that underwent a balloon dilation with 91% accessibility rate and 99% patency rate of the 95 frontal recesses examined with endoscopy at 6 months.[20]

The frontal recess endoscopic dilation is performed using a 70- or 90-degree sinus guide along with a 5-mm balloon catheter. The sinus guide is placed into the middle

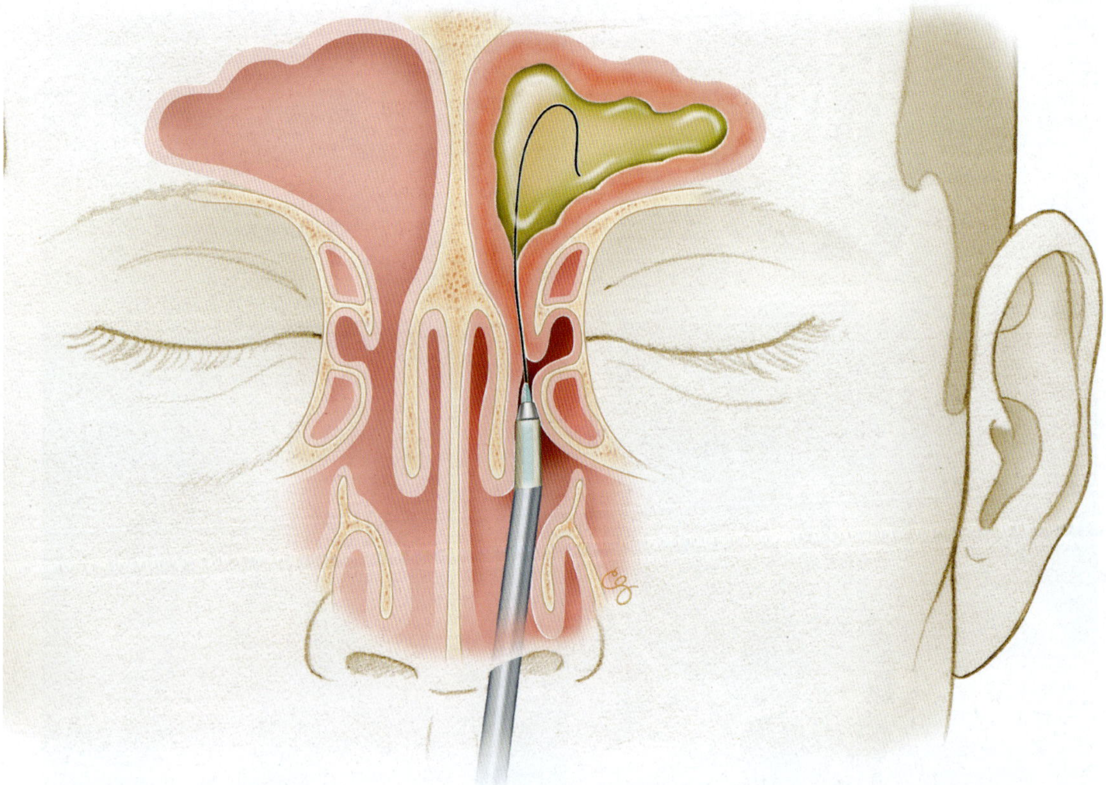

A

Fig. 27.7 Illustration of frontal balloon catheter dilation. **(A)** A guidewire is first passed through the frontal sinus ostium into the frontal sinus via an introducer sheath.

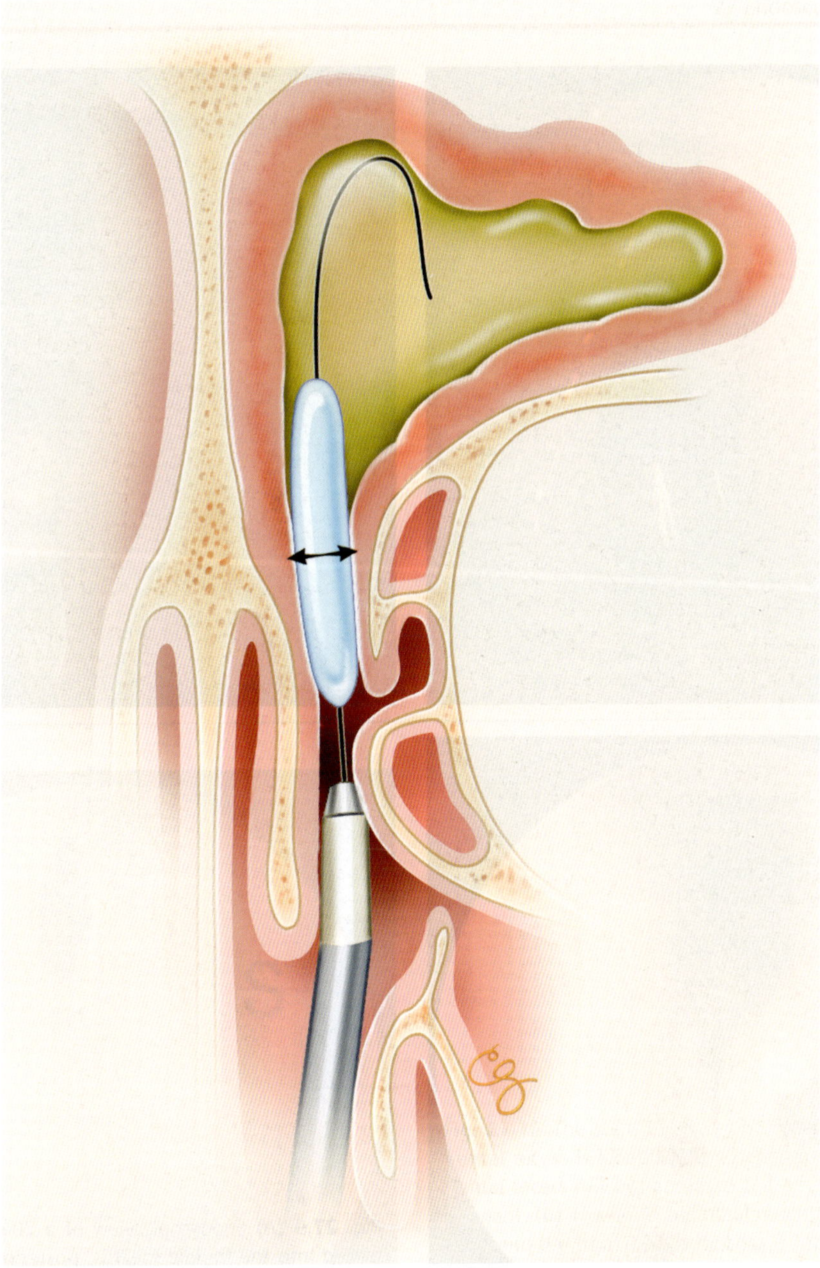

B

Fig. 27.7 (B) The balloon is then advanced over the guidewire and insufflated with saline to dilate the ostium and surrounding structures.

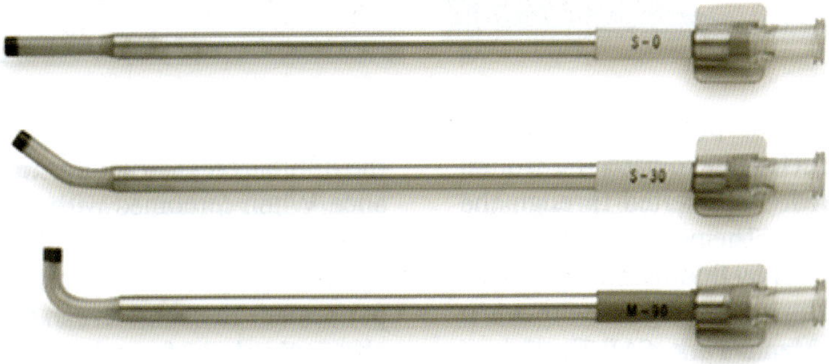

A

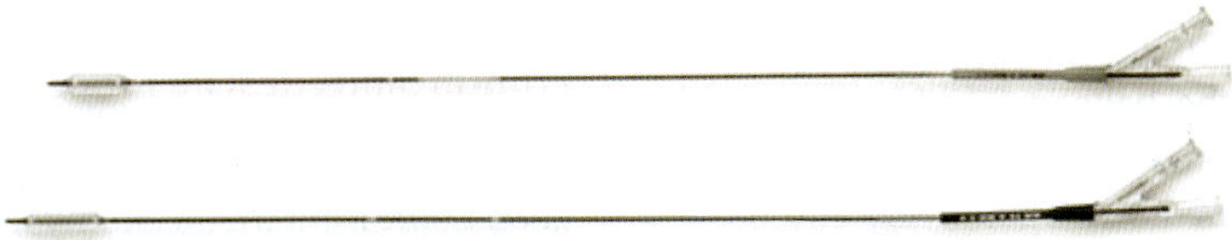

B

Fig. 27.8 (A) A range of sinus guides with varying angles. **(B)** Balloon catheters of different dimensions.

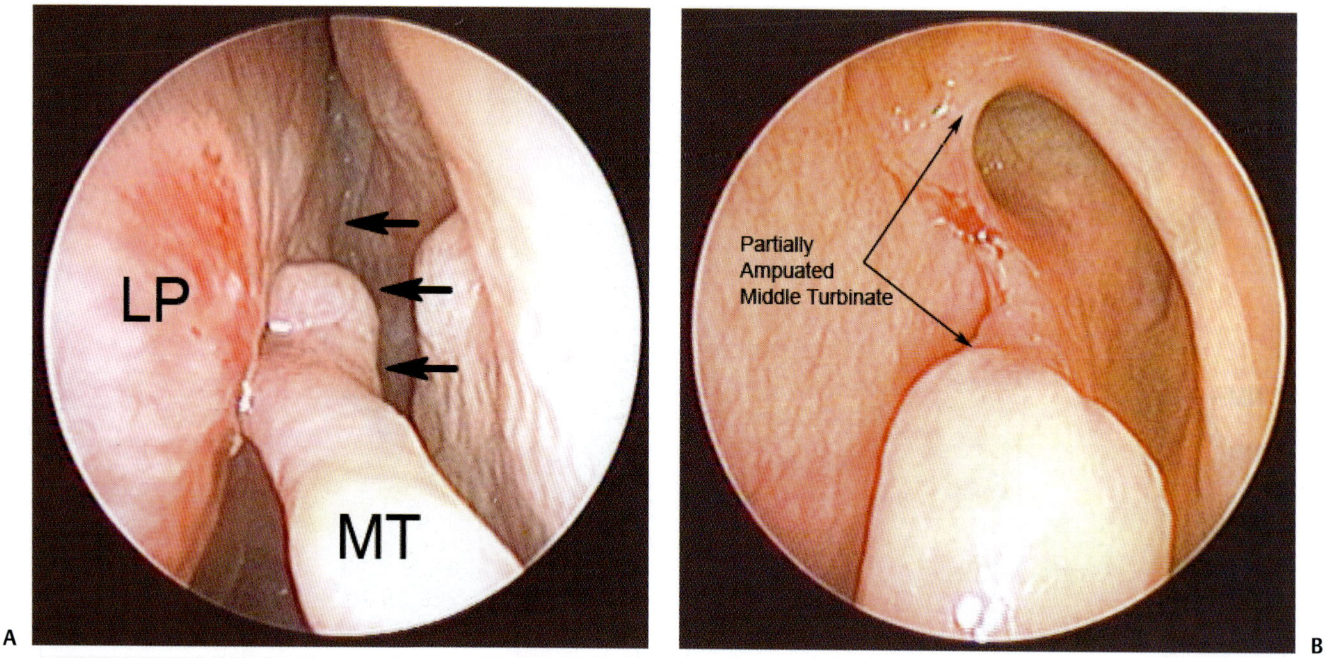

Fig. 27.11 (A) Endoscopic view demonstrating a collapsed right middle turbinate (*arrows*), which is obstructing the frontal sinus drainage pathway. *LP*, lamina papyracea; *MT*, middle turbinate. **(B)** Endoscopic view of a healed left extended frontal sinus rescue frontal ostium demonstrating a partially amputated middle turbinate.

narrow to heal properly or to allow normal mucus clearance if a standard endoscopic frontal sinusotomy is performed. The extended frontal sinus rescue (exFSR) procedure involves cutting a channel into the middle turbinate from its attachment at the agger nasi region obliquely up to its skull base attachment (**Fig. 27.11B**).[4] After the channel is established, an FSR procedure is performed as described previously. Once the new frontal ostium is formed, the middle turbinate frequently attaches itself to the lateral nasal wall below the frontal ostium, diverting frontal mucus clearance directly into the nasal cavity and not the middle meatus.

Endoscopic Modified Lothrop with Punches (Draf III)

Draf first described the endoscopic intranasal modification of the Lothrop procedure in 1991.[7] The Draf III refers to a procedure that uses a drill to create a common drainage pathway for both frontal sinuses by removing the upper nasal septum, the interfrontal sinus septum, the agger nasi regions, and the floor of each frontal sinus. This is commonly referred to as the "drill out" procedure. Several studies advocate the Draf III as a successful alternative to the more morbid osteoplastic flap with or without obliteration. They claim sustained frontal ostium patency and improved symptomatology.[22,23] The one drawback of the procedure is the use of a high-speed drill within the narrow confines of the frontal recess. The removal of the bony structures by drilling can lead to circumferential injury to the frontal recess mucosa with possible subsequent osteoneogenesis and scar tissue formation. In 2001, Lanza introduced a transseptal approach with drill to avoid the problem of circumferential injury and scarring.[24] More recently, Dubin and Kuhn described a Draf III procedure with punches to address this concern. This procedure preserves the important lateral frontal recess mucous membrane commonly injured with a drill (**Fig. 27.12**).[25]

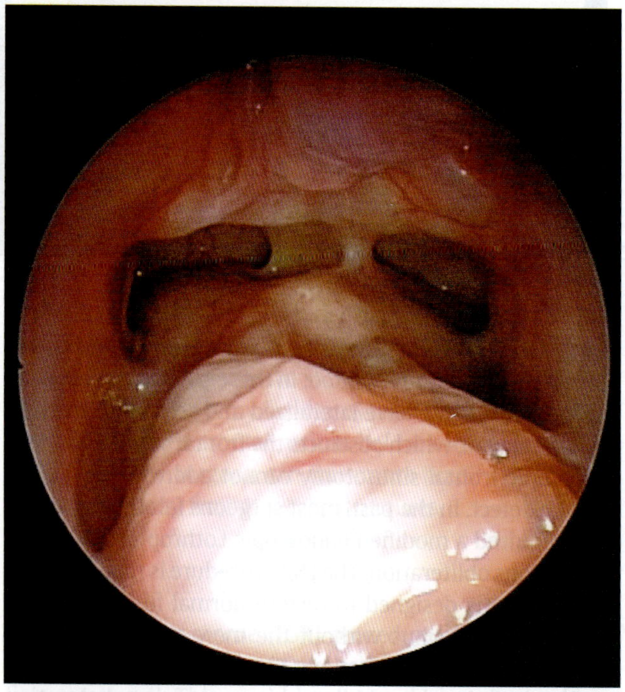

Fig. 27.12 Endoscopic view of a healed modified Lothrop procedure with punches. Lateral frontal recess mucous membrane is intact.

A standard endoscopic frontal sinusotomy is performed using a 70-degree telescope, through-cutting punches, and image guidance. The position of the nasal septum and the anterior ends of the middle turbinates immediately inferior to the frontal sinus floor are identified using image guidance. An inferiorly based mucoperiosteal flap on the septum is then delineated using a sickle knife and raised using a Cottle elevator. The septum and the anterior agger nasi region are removed up to the frontal sinus floor. The creation of the common cavity is achieved by resection of bone between the two frontal sinus ostia using punches instead of a drill. The resection of the frontal sinus floor is accomplished using a combination of 45- and 90-degree frontal sinus front-to-back and side-to-side punches, the frontal sinus mushroom punch, the Hosemann frontal sinus punch, and the frontal sinus Kerrison. Thick bony fragments that cannot be punched through directly may be grasped and rocked loose using the punches as graspers or by using an osteotome. Other instruments that may be helpful are the frontal sinus 45- and 90-degree curettes, curved osteotomes, frontal sinus seekers, and giraffe forceps.

Complications

Due to its proximity to vital structures, dissection of the frontal sinus drainage pathway may lead to specific intraoperative and postoperative complications. Possible complications include hemorrhage, cerebrospinal fluid leak, anterior ethmoid artery laceration, orbital injury, disease recurrence, and frontal sinus ostial stenosis.

Postoperative Care

Regular endoscopic surveillance and debridement in the postoperative period is important. Removal of fibrin clots and crusts, separation of synechiae, and suctioning secretions during postoperative visits are helpful in clearing the mucosal surface for better healing. Patients are asked to irrigate the sinonasal cavities with normal buffered saline solution (8 oz/nostril) three times per day for 3 to 5 weeks. Systemic antibiotics are prescribed only as directed by intraoperative or postoperative cultures. Oral corticosteroids are indicated in patients with allergic fungal sinusitis, eosinophilic inflammatory rhinosinusitis, and nasal polyps.

Outcomes

The frontal recess has been the most challenging region of the paranasal sinuses in which to achieve good surgical results. The anatomy is difficult to understand and visibility is often limited, leading to higher disease recurrence rates. Short-term frontal sinusotomy outcomes have been reported in several studies in the literature. Friedman et al. reported a short-term (12.2 months) frontal sinus patency rate of 90% after endoscopic frontal sinus surgery.[26] Other more recent studies demonstrated short-term (10 to 30 months) patency rates ranging between 82 and 86%.[27,28] An 80% endoscopic frontal sinus patency rate, achieved after a Draf II procedure, was reported by Weber et al. after a follow-up of 12 to 16 months.[29] Unfortunately, there is a paucity of literature on long-term frontal sinus ostial patency after endoscopic frontal sinus surgery. Friedman's original cohort of patients at 4 years follow-up was reported to have 67.6% patency (71.1% with revision).[30] Of the senior authors' patients operated over 18 months from July 1, 1999, to December 31, 2000, 161 were followed for an average of 45.9 months. They were found to have a long-term frontal ostium patency rate of 87% after only one procedure; however, a rate of 94% was achieved with revision surgery.[31] These findings by Chan et al. clearly demonstrate that an endoscopic frontal sinusotomy provides excellent durable results over the long term.

Conclusion

The frontal sinus is the most challenging of the four paranasal sinuses in terms of obtaining good and long-lasting endoscopic surgical results. The complex anatomy and its anterosuperior location render endoscopic dissection and visualization more difficult, hence an increased failure rate. This chapter has summarized an integrated approach to endoscopic frontal sinusotomy, ranging from less to more invasive. This approach includes dissection of the frontal recess with instruments and balloon catheters, the FSR procedure, the exFSR procedure, and the modified intranasal endoscopic Lothrop procedure with punches, each of which has its own unique application as discussed. These techniques are essential to each surgeon's armamentarium of frontal sinus surgical techniques. Greater than 90% of all frontal sinusitis should be manageable with these procedures.

References

1. Lothrop HA. Frontal sinus suppuration. Ann Surg 1914;59(6): 937–957
2. Draf W. Endonasal microendoscopic frontal sinus surgery: the Fulda concept. Oper Tech Otolaryngol—Head Neck Surg 1991;2:234–240
3. Kuhn FA. Operative techniques in chronic frontal sinusitis: the endoscopic frontal recess approach. Oper Tech Otolaryngol—Head Neck Surg 1996;7:222–229
4. Kuhn FA. An integrated approach to frontal sinus surgery. Otolaryngol Clin North Am 2006;39(3):437–461, viii
5. Kuhn FA. Surgery of the frontal sinus. In: Kennedy DW, Bolger WE, Zinreich SJ, ed. Diseases of the Sinuses: Diagnosis and Management. London: B.C. Decker Inc; 2001: 281–301
6. Killian G. Zur anatomie der Nase menschlicher Embryonen. Arch Laryngol Rhinol 1896;4:1–45

7. Schaeffer JP. The genesis, development and adult anatomy of the nasofrontal region in man. Am J Anat 1916;20:125–145
8. Kasper KA. Nasofrontal connections: a study based on one hundred consecutive dissections. Arch Otolaryngol 1936;23: 322–343
9. Van Alyea OE. Frontal sinus drainage. Ann Otol Rhinol Laryngol 1946;55:267–277
10. Messerklinger W. On the drainage of the normal frontal sinus of man. Acta Otolaryngol 1967;63(2):176–181
11. Kennedy DW, Josephson JS, Zinreich SJ, Mattox DE, Goldsmith MM. Endoscopic sinus surgery for mucoceles: a viable alternative. Laryngoscope 1989;99(9):885–895
12. Har-El G, Lucente FE. Endoscopic intranasal frontal sinusotomy. Laryngoscope 1995;105(4 Pt 1):440–443
13. Metson R. Endoscopic treatment of frontal sinusitis. Laryngoscope 1992;102(6):712–716
14. Kuhn FA, Javer AR. Primary endoscopic management of the frontal sinus. Otolaryngol Clin North Am 2001;34(1):59–75
15. Fried MP, Kleefield J, Gopal H, Reardon E, Ho BT, Kuhn FA. Image-guided endoscopic surgery: results of accuracy and performance in a multicenter clinical study using an electromagnetic tracking system. Laryngoscope 1997;107(5):594–601
16. Olson G, Citardi MJ. Image-guided functional endoscopic sinus surgery. Otolaryngol Head Neck Surg 2000;123(3):188–194
17. Brown CL, Bolger WE. Safety and feasibility of balloon catheter dilation of paranasal sinus ostia: a preliminary investigation. Ann Otol Rhinol Laryngol 2006;115(4):293–299, discussion 300–301
18. Bolger WE, Brown CL, Church CA, et al. Safety and outcomes of balloon catheter sinusotomy: a multicenter 24-week analysis in 115 patients. Otolaryngol Head Neck Surg 2007;137(1): 10–20
19. Kuhn FA, Church CA, Goldberg AN, et al. Balloon catheter sinusotomy: one-year follow-up—outcomes and role in functional endoscopic sinus surgery. Otolaryngol Head Neck Surg 2008;139 (3, Suppl 3)S27–S37
20. Rehl RM, Vaughan WC. Initial use of balloon dilation in the frontal recess. Presented at the Triological Society Annual Meeting. San Diego, CA; 2007
21. Citardi MJ, Javer AR, Kuhn FA. Revision endoscopic frontal sinusotomy with mucoperiosteal flap advancement: the frontal sinus rescue procedure. Otolaryngol Clin North Am 2001;34(1):123–132
22. Gross CW, Harrison SE. The modified Lothrop procedure: indications, results, and complications. Otolaryngol Clin North Am 2001;34(1):133–137
23. Wormald PJ. Salvage frontal sinus surgery: the endoscopic modified Lothrop procedure. Laryngoscope 2003;113(2):276–283
24. Lanza DC, McLaughlin RB Jr, Hwang PH. The five year experience with endoscopic trans-septal frontal sinusotomy. Otolaryngol Clin North Am 2001;34(1):139–152
25. Dubin MG, Kuhn FA. Endoscopic modified Lothrop (Draf III) with frontal sinus punches. Laryngoscope 2005;115(9):1702–1703
26. Friedman M, Landsberg R, Schults RA, Tanyeri H, Caldarelli DD. Frontal sinus surgery: endoscopic technique and preliminary results. Am J Rhinol 2000;14(6):393–403
27. Chandra RK, Palmer JN, Tangsujarittham T, Kennedy DW. Factors associated with failure of frontal sinusotomy in the early follow-up period. Otolaryngol Head Neck Surg 2004;131(4):514–518
28. Chiu AG, Vaughan WC. Revision endoscopic frontal sinus surgery with surgical navigation. Otolaryngol Head Neck Surg 2004;130(3):312–318
29. Weber R, Draf W, Kratzsch B, Hosemann W, Schaefer SD. Modern concepts of frontal sinus surgery. Laryngoscope 2001;111(1): 137–146
30. Friedman M, Bliznikas D, Vidyasagar R, Joseph NJ, Landsberg R. Long-term results after endoscopic sinus surgery involving frontal recess dissection. Laryngoscope 2006;116(4):573–579
31. Chan Y, Melroy CT, Kuhn CA, Daniel WT, Dempsey SI, Kuhn FA. Long term frontal sinus patency after endoscopic frontal sinusotomy. Presented at the Combined Otolaryngological Spring Meeting. Orlando, FL; 2008

28 Advanced Frontal Surgery Techniques

Karen A. Bednarski and Brent A. Senior

Chronic and recurrent disease of the frontal sinus presents many challenges given the complex anatomy and difficult access for adequate treatment. Early procedures, both extra- and intranasal, were fraught with complications secondary to poor visualization and radical resection of bony support and mucosal surfaces. These early procedures were associated with a high rate of stenosis. In the 1960s, the osteoplastic obliteration was introduced and failure rates dropped precipitously. For some this has remained the gold standard, with a quoted success rate of up to 90% for the treatment of recurrent frontal sinusitis. However, there are significant morbidities that may be associated with frontal obliteration, including chronic pain, hypesthesia, and delayed mucocele development. Furthermore, surgical failures may persist despite frontal obliteration, and when this occurs, diagnosis and treatment can be fraught with challenges.[1]

With the advent of endoscopic techniques, intranasal approaches once again came to the forefront, as endoscopic frontal sinusotomy became the treatment of choice for frontal sinus surgery. Combined external and endoscopic procedures were also introduced to augment the exposure and access that were possible through solely endoscopic approaches. The main advantages that endoscopic-based techniques have over obliteration are shorter postoperative hospitalization, less pain and hypesthesia, preservation or reestablishment of a functional frontal sinus, and ease of follow-up (including endoscopic examination as well as radiographic imaging). There is, however, no single approach that is universally applicable, and therefore, the choice of technique must be based on the individual disease process, the patient's anatomy, and the patient's tolerance for future procedures, postoperative care, and follow-up.[2]

In this chapter, endoscopic procedures including Draf IIb, modified Lothrop (Draf III), and transseptal frontal sinusotomy are discussed, as well as the combined above-and-below approach. All of these techniques should be considered only after maximal medical therapy and more standard endoscopic approaches have failed for chronic inflammatory disease. These advanced approaches may be indicated as the first-line treatment for tumors such as osteomas or inverted papillomas, mucoceles, or in the setting of previous trauma. Finally, in the setting of previous obliteration or cranialization, these advanced procedures can re-create functional frontal sinus outflow. All of the techniques have three common goals: (1) to create a functional frontal sinus; (2) to eradicate the underlying disease process; and (3) to relieve the patient's symptoms. We consider intraoperative image guidance a tremendous aid for performing advanced frontal sinus surgery.

Draf IIb

As initially described by Draf in 1991, "extended drainage" consists of the removal of the frontal sinus floor between: (1) the lamina papyracea and the middle turbinate (type IIa); and (2) the lamina papyracea and the nasal septum (type IIb).[3] The Draf IIa procedure has been previously discussed in Chapter 27; therefore, our discussion focuses on the Draf IIb procedure.

Patient Selection/Indications

The indications for all advanced approaches to the frontal sinus are summarized in **Table 28.1**. As described by Draf, the decision to create a more aggressive nasofrontal connection may in fact be made intraoperatively when the frontal sinus ostium created in the Draf IIa procedure is smaller than 5 × 7 mm.[3,4]

Surgical Anatomy

Frontal sinus surgery is challenging, owing to the complexity of the drainage pathway from the frontal ostium through the frontal recess. The frontal recess is a potential space occupied by various types of ethmoid cells, and in most cases, chronic

Table 28.1 Indications for Advanced Frontal Sinus Techniques

Recalcitrant chronic frontal sinusitis • Failing maximal medical therapy • Failing previous, more conservative surgical management
Mucocele or mucopyocele
Osseous lesions: osteoma, ossifying fibroma, fibrous dysplasia
Inverted papilloma
Failed frontal sinus obliteration
Trauma
Revision frontal sinusotomy with extensive scarring and previous resection of middle turbinate
Consider in patients with frontal sinusitis and significant comorbidities: primary ciliary dyskinesia, cystic fibrosis, aspirin-exacerbated respiratory disease

frontal sinusitis can be managed adequately by the targeted removal of the ethmoid cells around which the frontal drains. The middle turbinate attaches posterolaterally at the crista ethmoidalis, and as it courses superiorly and medially, it attaches to the skull base at the lateral aspect of the cribriform plate. In addition, the olfactory fibers are closely associated with the middle turbinate mucosa at the level of the skull base. When partially resected, the middle turbinate may tend to scar laterally and obstruct the outflow from the frontal sinus. When the middle turbinate remnant has scarred in this manner, a traditional endoscopic frontal sinusotomy is often much more difficult. In the Draf IIb procedure, the anteriormost portion of the middle turbinate, which inserts on the floor of the frontal sinus, is resected to allow enlargement of the frontal ostium medially toward the septum.

With regard to the frontal sinus itself, it should also be remembered that the ciliary beat pattern creates a circular mucus flow pattern superiorly along the interfrontal sinus septum, laterally across the roof, and inferomedially across the frontal sinus floor to the frontal ostium. Therefore, the mucosa at the lateral aspect of the frontal ostium should be respected and managed delicately.[5]

Surgical Techniques

Common to all procedures, the patient is under general anesthesia, and standard length 0-, 30-, 45-, and 70-degree, 4-mm endoscopes fitted with scope irrigation are used to afford the best visualization. The patient is positioned in the "beach chair" position and the head rests in a gel or foam donut. The right arm is tucked by the patient's side, and it may be necessary to tilt the patient toward the surgeon, especially in a patient with large body habitus. Greater palatine blocks are performed to aid in hemostasis by injecting 1.5 mm of 1% lidocaine with 1:100,000 epinephrine transorally into each greater palatine canal (at a height of 2.5 cm above the hard palate mucosa). The patient is then registered with stereotactic computer guidance software and the patient is draped. The surgeon sits to the patient's right when not precluded by body habitus. Under endoscopic guidance, neuro-patties soaked with oxymetazoline hydrochloride are placed in each nasal cavity for decongestion, and then additional lidocaine is injected into the superior lateral nasal wall anterior to the uncinate, posteriorly at the junction of the horizontal portion of the basal lamella and the lateral nasal wall, and in the septum if indicated. The surgeon then proceeds with standard endoscopic sinus surgery addressing the concurrent sinus disease, when present, before addressing the frontal recess. A total ethmoidectomy should be performed with care taken to remove all septations at the lamina papyracea and the skull base.

Using the middle turbinate or the middle turbinate remnant and the anterior ethmoid artery as landmarks and with the assistance of image guidance, the frontal recess is identified and widened with frontal sinus punches and Kerrison-type instruments, as described in the previous chapter. If drainage remains inadequate, the remnant of the middle turbinate is resected in small pieces from anterior to posterior, ending at the middle turbinate's attachment to the skull base. The first olfactory fiber should be identified at this time emanating from the skull base and medial to the origin of the middle turbinate. This marks the posterior extent of the dissection. A burr is placed into the frontal infundibulum, and the floor of the frontal sinus is removed in an anterosuperior direction to the septum, again remaining anterior to the first olfactory fiber.[4] At the completion of the procedure, the floor of the frontal sinus has been removed unilaterally (**Fig. 28.1**).

Instrumentation: Drills Versus Punches

When creating the neo-frontal ostium, the surgeon is confronted with the challenge of removing bone, which can be quite thick, in an atraumatic manner to avoid mucosal disruption and secondary scarring. Proper instrumentation, therefore, plays a vital role in surgical outcomes. In 2004, Hosemann et al. created an experimental model using cadaver specimens to evaluate drill models including the straight burr, a modified dental drill with a right angle, and frontal sinus burrs with a curved shaft. The amount of mucosal destruction, exposed bone, and the size of the neo-ostium were calculated following a microscopic dissection. All drills had some shortcomings. Although the straight drill was restricted in an anterior dissection, the right angle drill was limited in the superior and lateral directions, but spared more mucosa. The drill with the curved shaft had technical problems and was not fully evaluated.[6] Also in 2004, Chandra et al. described the use

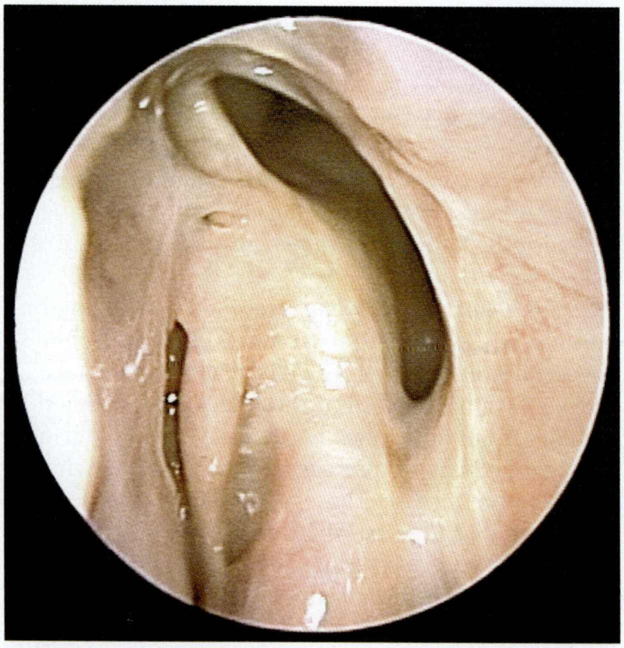

Fig. 28.1 Endoscopic view at the completion of Draf IIb on the left. The limits of dissection are the lamina papyracea laterally and the nasal septum medially.

of a 70-degree drill to remove bone at the floor of the frontal sinus with a 4-mm diamond burr. This angle allowed for instrumentation within the frontal sinus while maintaining visualization with a 45- or 70-degree telescope. The 4-mm diamond burr resisted skipping and created less mucosal trauma than a cutting burr.[7] Since 2004, there have been no published comparisons between drills; however, advances have been made with thinner self-irrigating drills that maximize visualization and limit thermal injury to the mucosa. In the authors' experience, a drill with a 70-degree curved shaft and a round burr affords the best visualization, although the anterior aspect of the burr may still not be visible during dissection.

To minimize the mucosal trauma associated with drilling, Dubin and Kuhn described the use of frontal sinus punches for extended frontal sinus instrumentation (Draf III, discussed further later). The authors recognize that in cases of significantly thickened bone, this technique may not be feasible, but should in fact be considered to spare mucosa and avoid circumferential damage.[8] At our institution, we advocate atraumatic dissection whenever possible and rely on the drill only in the setting of significantly thickened and osteitic bone when punches are not adequate.

Complications

Potential complications for all advanced frontal sinus procedures are similar to those encountered in any endoscopic sinus surgery, and result from the close association of the paranasal sinuses with the orbit and the anterior cranial fossa. Intraoperative complications, including cerebrospinal fluid (CSF) leak, intraorbital penetration, hemorrhage, and damage to the lacrimal sac, can all occur. Postoperative complications include epistaxis, diplopia, blindness, and epiphora. Recurrence of the underlying pathology and stenosis of the nasofrontal communication will be discussed further in the outcomes section.

Postoperative Care

Postoperative care is similar for all procedures. When possible, patients are placed on culture-directed antibiotic therapy during the healing process. Broad-spectrum antibiotics are used when cultures to direct therapy are lacking. An oral steroid taper is used to modulate the inflammatory response and to decrease the risk of postoperative scarring. Most patients return 1 week following the procedure and then every 1 to 2 weeks for gentle debridement. Fibrinous debris is carefully cleared to prevent postoperative scarring until healing is complete. Saline irrigation is instituted 1 week postoperatively to aid in gentle debridement and twice daily intranasal topical steroids are also initiated at that time in the head-down position. Treatment of concomitant medical problems, especially allergies, is of vital importance for successful surgical outcomes.

Outcomes

The largest series reported to date evaluated both the symptomatic improvement and the endoscopic appearance of the frontal ostium following Draf IIb procedure. Follow-up was a minimum of 1 year and revealed 51% of patients to be asymptomatic and another 32.6% to have significant improvement in their symptoms. In addition, an endoscopic examination revealed that 91.5% of patients had no or minimal inflammatory changes at the ostium.[4,9] On the other hand, Kikawada et al. compared the outcomes of unilateral (Draf IIb) versus bilateral (Draf III) approaches in patients with obstructive frontal sinusitis secondary to scarring. The overall patency rate following the IIb procedure was 42% at 1 year postoperatively, and when compared with the results of the bilateral procedure (88% patency at 1 year), this group concluded that the Draf III procedure was the more reliable method for treating refractory frontal sinusitis caused by scarring of the anterior ethmoid sinus.[10]

Endoscopic Modified Lothrop Procedure (Draf III)

In 1914, Lothrop described a combined transnasal and external procedure, which created a single, common frontal sinus outflow tract by removing the frontal sinus floor from orbit to orbit.[11] Due to bilateral removal of the lamina, papyracea as orbital contents prolapsed into the nose obstructing the outflow tract, and the procedure was largely abandoned. This was later modified to spare the lamina, and with the advent of endoscopic techniques, it regained favor in the 1990s.[12] In 1991, Draf described a median drainage approach, the Draf III, using the same underlying principle.[3] Thus, both names are used to describe the creation of a common median drainage pathway for both frontal sinuses, from lamina to lamina. The extent of this resection is compared with that of the IIb procedure in **Fig. 28.2**.

Patient Selection/Indications

Patients undergoing the endoscopic modified Lothrop procedure (EMLP) are a highly select population. Of 371 frontal sinus procedures performed during a 3-year period in a tertiary referral practice, only 18 were EMLPs.[13] Indications, listed in **Table 28.1**, are held in context with anatomic factors. This procedure holds the advantage of bilateral exposure, which can increase lateral reach into the frontal sinus, especially when instruments are directed from one naris to the contralateral frontal sinus. In addition, because this procedure creates median drainage, it can be optimal for mucoceles and tumors associated with the midline. Posterior table dehiscence is not a contraindication, and mucoceles, which have eroded the posterior table, can be successfully treated without complication.[14]

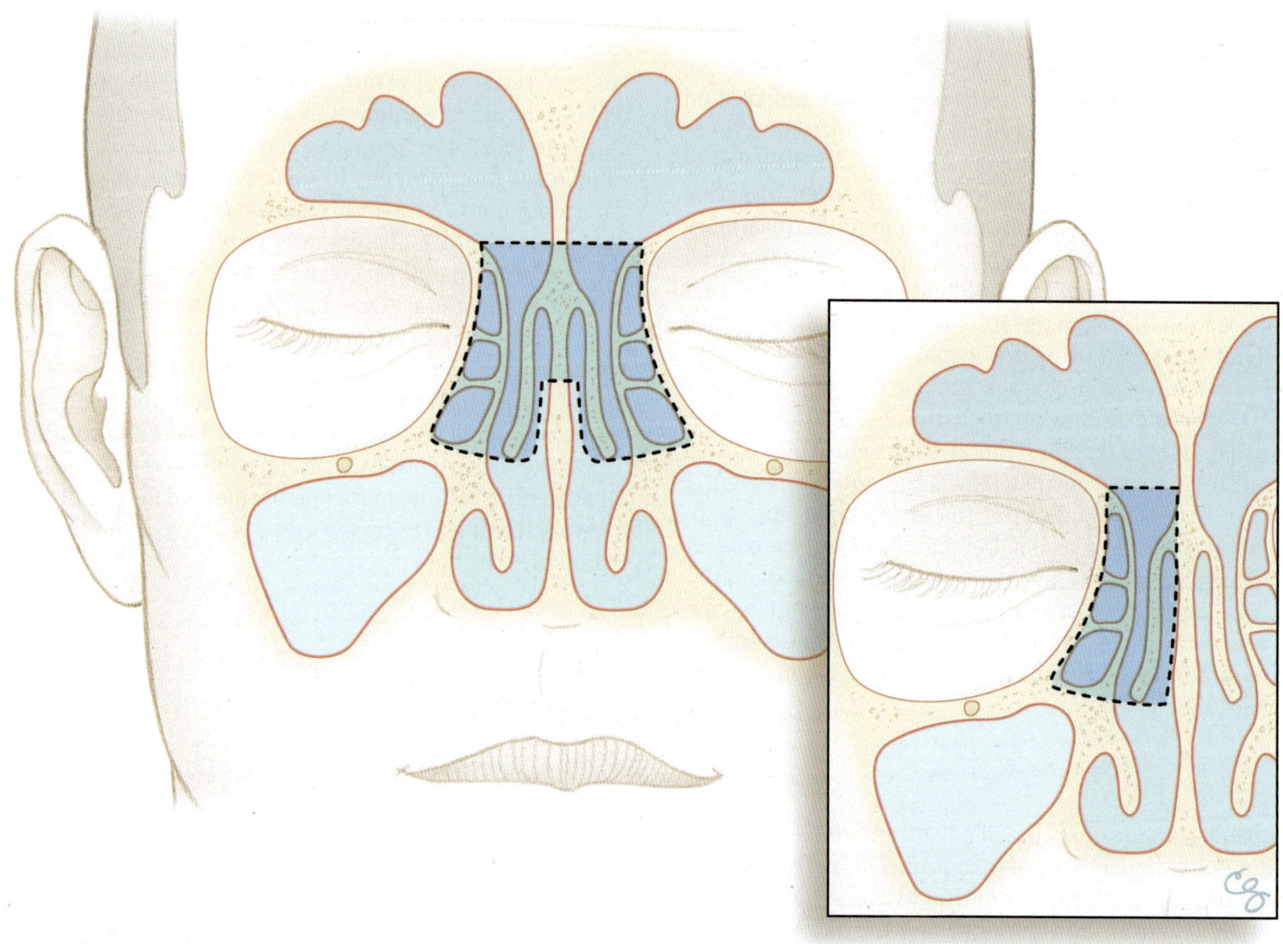

Fig. 28.2 Illustration showing comparison of Draf IIb and Draf III (endoscopic modified Lothrop procedure [EMLP]) procedures. The inset picture on the right depicts the area of resection (shaded) in the Draf IIb, involving the superior anterior ethmoid cells, the anterior aspect of the middle turbinate, and the floor of the frontal sinus from the lamina papyracea to the nasal septum. The Draf III (left) incorporates a similar resection (shaded) performed bilaterally and also includes resection of the superior nasal septum.

The EMLP is also a viable alternative for selected patients who have failed previous frontal sinus obliteration with an osteoplastic flap. Failure in these cases is most commonly associated with incomplete removal of mucous membrane and most often occurs in the frontal recess, which can be addressed with the EMLP. An advantage of endoscopic revision over a repeat osteoplastic flap is that endoscopic EMLP affords a wide intranasal view of the frontal sinusotomy and frontal sinus, thereby allowing improved postoperative monitoring. Patients must be appropriately selected, however, and limitations are the same regardless of the indication.[15,16]

The main limiting factor to safely perform the EMLP is a narrow anteroposterior depth of the frontal sinus. This can manifest through a deeply set nasion, hypoplastic or poorly pneumatized frontal sinuses, and/or a thick nasal beak. A frontal sinus floor with a depth of less than 1.5 cm is considered a relative, but not absolute, contraindication to safely performing the procedure.[17] Careful review of triplanar reconstructions of thin-section CT scans of the frontal sinus can aid in predicting surgical amenability to the EMLP.[18]

Surgical Anatomy

As mentioned previously, the anatomy of the frontal sinus, and most importantly the frontal sinus floor, is critical when selecting patients for candidacy for the EMLP. The total anteroposterior dimension at the floor of the frontal sinus should be at least 1.5 cm (**Fig. 28.3**). This includes the anteroposterior thickness of the nasal beak (which should not exceed 1 cm) and the distance from the beak to the anterior skull base.[17,19] As the anteroposterior dimension narrows, it becomes increasingly difficult to manipulate instruments within the frontal sinus. As a result, there is an increased risk of skull base injury and CSF leak. In addition, the "accessible dimension" represents the working

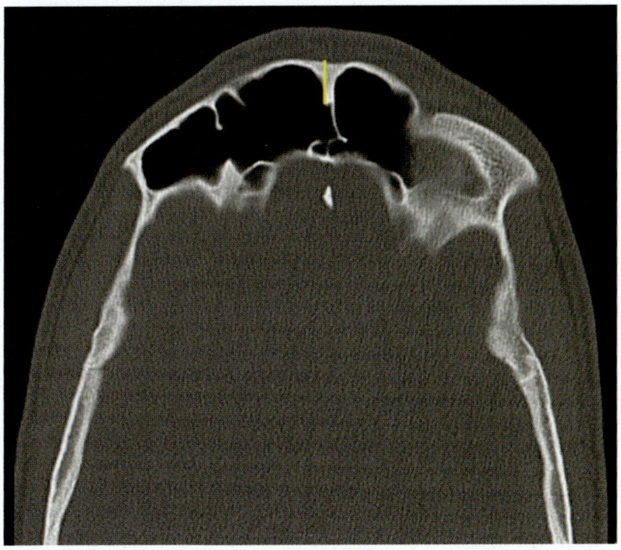

Fig. 28.3 Axial computed tomography image demonstrating a favorable anteroposterior diameter of the frontal sinus, including the component of the nasal beak (*yellow*).

space available to maneuver instruments within the frontal ostium and remove the frontal sinus floor. This space should be at least 5 mm, and is defined by two parallel lines, the first tangential to the skull base and the second, parallel to the first, and tangential to the posterior margin of the nasal beak (**Fig. 28.4**).[20]

Surgical Technique

The initial approach to the frontal sinus is commenced on the side where naso-frontal communication is the most straightforward. Concomitant sinus disease should be addressed and a complete ethmoidectomy should be performed bilaterally. When Becker and Gross initially described the procedure, a wire was used to cannulate the frontal sinus, which marked the posterior extent of the dissection.[21,22] Following a total ethmoidectomy, the middle turbinate remnant is resected from anterior to posterior as described in the Draf IIb procedure with identification of the first olfactory fibers. When identified on both sides, these first olfactory fibers help delineate what Draf describes as the "frontal T," which ensures adequate exposure in the anteroposterior direction. The long limb of the T is represented by the perpendicular plate of the ethmoid (with the first olfactory fibers lying laterally), and the short limb is the posterior margin of the frontal sinus floor resection.[4]

Following the anterior resection of the middle turbinate, dissection continues anterosuperiorly toward the septum (**Fig. 28.5**). The crista galli lies medial to the frontal recess and thus the direction of drilling should be in the anterosuperior direction as opposed to the medial. A superior septectomy is performed to facilitate the binarial placement of instruments and to enhance visualization of the ipsilateral and contralateral frontal infundibula. An endoscopic shaver is used to remove mucosa over the perpendicular plate of the ethmoid, or alternatively, a sickle knife is used to create a mucosal flap. When resecting the septum, the center of the defect should be inferior to the floor of the frontal sinus and should be ~2 cm in diameter. The posterior aspect of the septal defect should be level with the anterior end of the resected middle turbinate stump.[14]

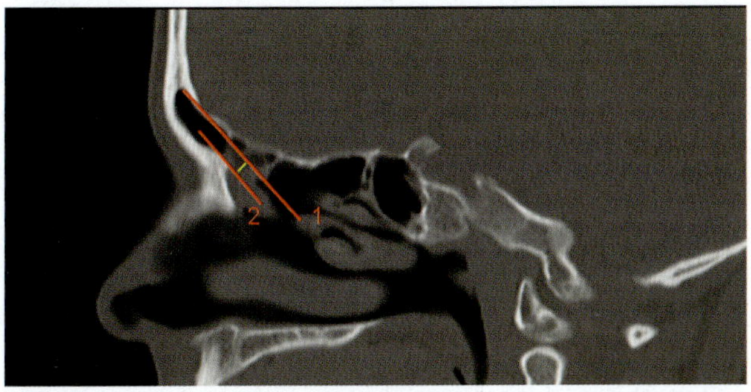

Fig. 28.4 Computed tomography image in the parasagittal plane representing the "accessible dimension" as described by Farhat and colleagues. This space (*yellow line*), bound by line 1 (tangential to the skull base) and line 2 (tangential to the posterior aspect of the nasal beak), should be greater than 5 mm to ensure adequate instrumentation of the frontal sinus.

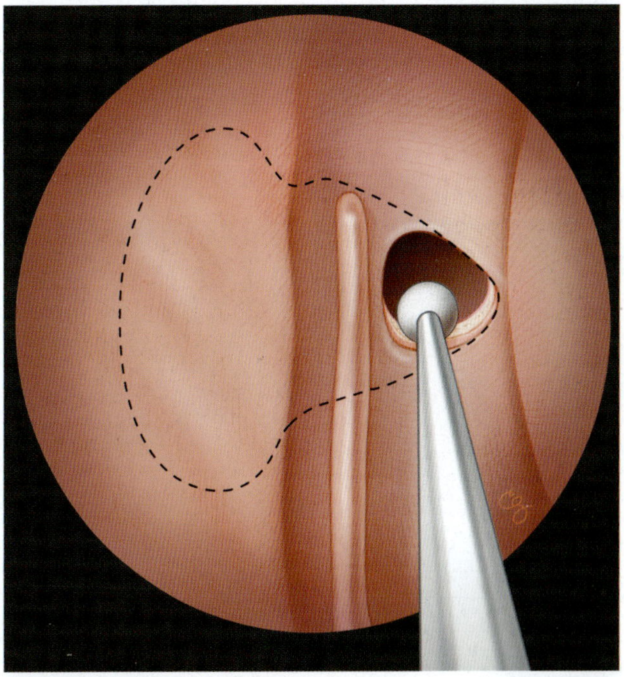

Fig. 28.5 Illustration of dissection during endoscopic modified Lothrop procedure. The drill is depicted within the accessible frontal sinus on the left and the middle turbinate remnant has been removed. Dissection continues anterior-superiorly, as shown by the broken line, followed by a superior septectomy.

At this point of the procedure, after the level of the skull base has been established and the superior portion of the septum has been resected, the floor of the frontal sinus can be safely removed. A drill or a frontal sinus punch is used to remove bone from the floor beginning from the frontal ostium and working medially toward the midline. The bone removal can also be extended anteriorly toward the anterior face of the frontal sinus, known as the nasofrontal "beak."[8,19,21,22] After the completion of bone removal of the frontal sinus floor, the intersinus septum is drilled or removed with through-cutting instruments up to the roof of the frontal sinus. Completion of the dissection results in a common median drainage pathway with exposure from lamina to lamina, which should be at least 20 × 15 mm (**Fig. 28.6**).[14] During dissection, the utmost care must be taken to avoid circumferential mucosal injury; therefore, the lateral and posterior mucosal margins should remain undisturbed.

Complications

CSF leak is the most frequent major complication during EMLP. This occurs in 1.2 to 7.8% of procedures, which is greater than in standard endoscopic sinus surgery.[13,14,23] When identified and repaired intraoperatively, there have been no reports of sequelae. Other complications include frontal stenosis secondary to adhesions (7.8%) and postoperative anosmia (15%).[13,14] With an increased risk of violating the cranial vault, other rare complications may occur, including tension pneumocephalus as reported by Schlosser et al. in 2002.[24] Injury to the anterior ethmoid artery has not been reported, but Samaha et al. reported four cases of postoperative epistaxis in their series of 100 patients, one which ultimately required ligation of the sphenopalatine artery.[25]

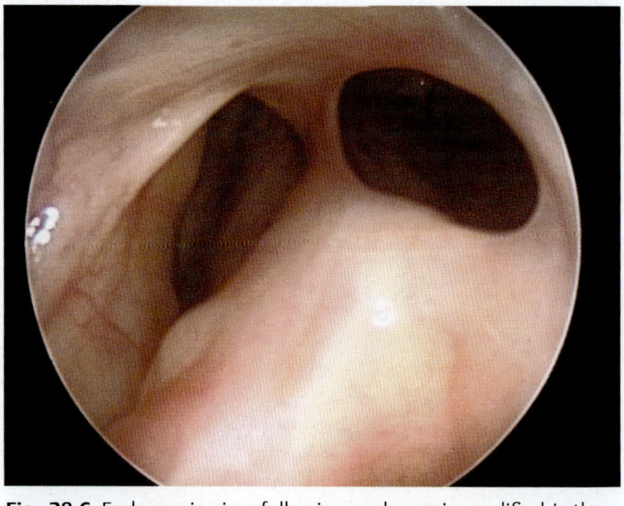

Fig. 28.6 Endoscopic view following endoscopic modified Lothrop procedure. The left and right frontal sinuses connect to a common median drainage pathway.

Postoperative Care

General postoperative care is as described previously. Most authors do not advocate packing. Draf, however, promotes the use of packing postoperatively, specifically rubber finger stalls (Rhinotamp, Vostra, Aachen, Germany), to minimize crusting and to promote wound healing. These are commercially available latex or latex-free finger cots filled with sponges, which are left in place for 7 days postoperatively.[4,26,27] Silastic (pliable silicone) sheeting can also be cut to form a customized stent that can be left in for several days to months after surgery. Silastic sheeting 0.04-inch thick can be cut into a U-shape and placed over the septum to help maintain patency postoperatively.

When closely examining the time course of wound healing following EMLP, Tran et al. reported two important findings related to postoperative care. First, there was a significant difference in frontal ostium size 3 months postoperatively in those patients most likely to require revision surgery. This indicated that patients most at risk of stenosing can be identified early and treated with aggressive medical management. Second, restenosis is a process that continues for at least the first year postoperatively, and therefore, patients should be closely followed for this time frame at a minimum.[28]

Outcomes

Initial outcomes of the EMLP were encouraging. Becker et al. reported that all 14 patients in their series had patent frontal ostia and only two (14%) had persistent symptoms 9 months postoperatively.[22] However, with increased length of follow-up, the patency rate decreased. In Wormald's series of 83 patients undergoing EMLP with a mean follow-up of 21.9 months, there was a frontal sinus patency rate of 93%. Interestingly, stenosis of the frontal ostium occurred in all patients within the first year of the procedure. Seventy-five percent of patients were asymptomatic during this follow-up period.[14] In the most recent review, Shirazi et al. included data from 97 patients undergoing EMLP over a 7-year period with a mean follow-up of 1.5 years. Twenty-three percent required revision surgery due to recalcitrant frontal sinusitis. Even in the setting of recurrent disease, postoperative surveys showed at least some degree of symptomatic improvement in 98% of patients.[23]

One of the difficulties in comparing outcomes is the definition of frontal sinus stenosis. Some authors classify results as patent versus stenosed, whereas others use a grading system. Tran et al. have recently tried to establish what constitutes an adequately sized frontal ostium following EMLP. In their study, they defined abnormal restenosis as being a reduction in size of more than 60% of the original. Based on a scatterplot analysis of postoperative frontal ostium cross-sectional areas, 41% of those with more than 60% decrease in frontal ostium size required revision surgery. Only one patient who did not have this decrease in frontal sinus ostium size required revision surgery, for severe fungal recurrence. The total revision rate was 13%, and eosinophilic chronic rhinosinusitis was the only statistically significant predictive factor for revision surgery.[28]

Outcomes of EMLP may vary depending on the indication of the procedure, but this is not well addressed by the literature. Many reports in the literature have a mixed population, but most focus on recalcitrant chronic rhinosinusitis as the main indication. Looking specifically at EMLP salvage following failed frontal sinus obliteration, Stankiewicz and Wachter reported a revision rate of 50% in the first year, but symptomatic improvement was noted in more than 90% of patients.[16] A systematic review of outcomes of EMLP by Anderson and Sindwani in 2009 offers perhaps the most comprehensive overview of the cumulative published experience thus far in EMLP. There were 612 patients that met inclusion criteria and were followed for a mean period of 28.5 months. The major complication rate was <1%, and minor complication rate was 4%. Frontal sinus patency or partial stenosis was achieved in 95.9%, but 14% failed their first EMLP, requiring either revision EMLP or obliteration. Symptomatic improvement was achieved in 82.2% of cases, with 16% reporting no significant change and 1.2% reporting worsening of symptoms.[29]

Unfortunately, the creation of a functional and patent frontal sinus does not always correlate with an improvement in the patient's symptoms. As a rule, patients undergoing EMLP have recalcitrant disease, and the majority has had multiple previous procedures. Thus, patients may have persistent symptoms from underlying pathology that cannot be completely eradicated surgically, such as allergic fungal sinusitis, aspirin-exacerbated respiratory disease, or atopy.

Endoscopic Transseptal Frontal Sinusotomy

Patient Selection/Indications

Similar to the EMLP and Draf III, the endoscopic transseptal frontal sinusotomy (TSFS) results in common median drainage, but exploits the relationship of the nasal septum and the midline floor of the frontal sinus where the bone is the thinnest. One advantage this technique holds over the EMLP is that it can be performed when the frontal sinus cannot be cannulated from below. A significant disadvantage is that the frontal sinus is entered "blind," and not through the natural outflow tract of the frontal sinus. Secure transseptal entry to the frontal sinus may be facilitated by intraoperative computer navigation. Similar to the EMLP, the main contraindication is a narrow anteroposterior dimension of the frontal sinus. Lanza recommended refraining from performing the procedure if the anteroposterior depth of the frontal sinus floor are less than 1.2 cm, citing an increased risk of skull base injury and CSF leak.[30]

Surgical Anatomy

The TSFS uses the relationship of the frontal sinus floor to the septum. The midline position of the floor of the frontal sinus is located posterior-superior to the septal bony-cartilaginous junction. This location can also be approximated adjacent to the most anterior remnant of the middle turbinate and the agger nasi. The frontal recess consistently lies posteriorly to this area.[30,31]

The nasofrontal beak and anterior table of the frontal sinus are part of the bony support of the nose. If the bone is removed too aggressively, the radix may lose support and secondary cosmetic deformity may ensue. Anatomic variants of the superior nasal septum and nasal floor should be observed carefully because they may affect surgical access positively or negatively. For example, 9% of patients have a septum that splits as it creates part of the midline floor of the frontal sinus. As a result of the septal bifurcation, the bony floor is quite thin and anatomically favorable for a successful procedure.[30] Another anatomic variant, the interfrontal septal cell or frontal wishbone, may complicate the transseptal approach. It is present in 77% of the population.[32] Interfrontal septal cells usually drain to one side (right 54%, left 45%), but rarely may drain bilaterally (0.8%).

Surgical Technique

A hemitransfixion incision is made under endoscopic guidance with an ophthalmic crescent knife (Alcon Laboratories, Ft. Worth, TX). A mucoperichondrial flap is elevated and the quadrangular cartilage is disarticulated at the bony-cartilaginous junction with subsequent mobilization of the anterior septum off of the maxillary spine. Any obstructing cartilage may be removed at this time. A high septal perforation is then created, and the superior portion of the septum is removed using microdebrider and through-cutting instruments. The floor of the frontal sinus is then entered using an endoscopic drill or curette depending on the thickness of the floor. The opening is then widened anteriorly and laterally, and may be extended to the frontal ostium/recess. It is recommended to place two fingers on the nasion while drilling to avoid overaggressive anterior bone resection. In addition, the inferior portion of the intersinus septum is removed to create the neo-ostium. At the completion of the procedure, the hemitransifixion incision is closed using 5–0 chromic and the septal flaps are reapproximated with a "whip-stitch" using 4–0 plain gut on a Keith needle. Packing and nasal splints are not routinely used.[30,31,33] **Figure 28.7** depicts the common central drainage pathway that is obtained.

Postoperative Care

Similar to other procedures, debridement, saline, and topical and oral steroids with culture-directed antibiotics are indicated with close monitoring until the patient has fully healed.

Complications

As with other advanced frontal sinus procedures, TSFS carries the potential for being complicated by CSF leak. In Lanza's series, two CSF leaks (6.9%) occurred during widening of the frontal sinus (not during entrance into the floor). One occurred secondary to surgical trauma from drilling in a frontal sinus with a narrow anteroposterior, whereas the second occurred during debridement of scarred mucosa in the setting of a dehiscent posterior table. Both were repaired intraoperatively with no secondary sequelae. The risk of dural violation can be mitigated by minimizing the use of the drill when the frontal sinus has a narrow anteroposterior diameter, and by using curettes whenever possible in lieu of the drill.

Unique to the TSFS, unintended anterior inferior septal perforation and chronic crusting can occur. Previous septoplasty is a risk factor. In addition, overly aggressive bony removal in the anterior dimension can cause cosmetic deformity due to depression of the radix. Other minor sequelae include transient postoperative frontal headaches and early synechiae formation.[30,31,33]

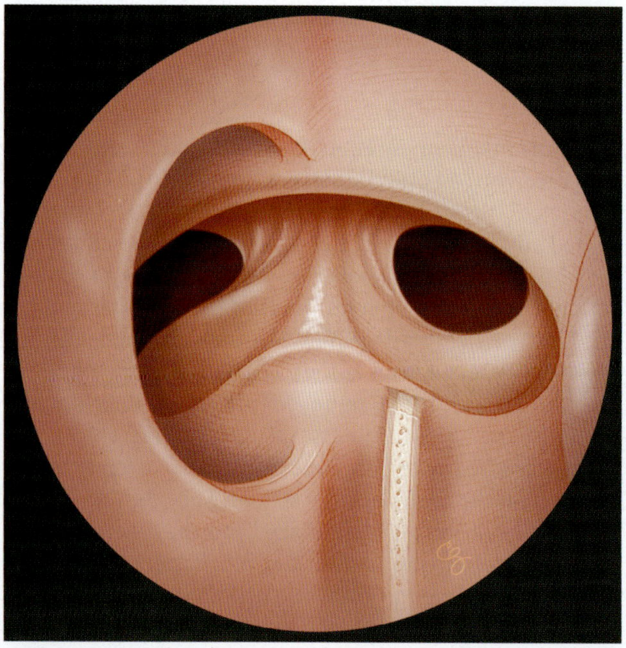

Fig. 28.7 Illustration of common median drainage pathway following an endoscopic modified Lothrop procedure/Draf III/transseptal frontal sinusotomy.

Outcomes

Lanza et al. reported on long-term follow-up on 24 of the 29 patients who had undergone TSFS in their series for frontal sinus stenosis and mucocele. At a mean follow-up of 45 months, 16.6% had required revision surgery. Of those patients not receiving revision surgery, 75% reported a 50% improvement in their symptoms and 58% reported an 80% improvement in their symptoms. All patients with symptomatic improvements also reported less frequent use of systemic antibiotics and steroids.[30,31]

Combined Above-and-Below Approach (Trephine + Endoscopic)

Patient Selection/Indications

There are situations where visualization from above is required, but it is desirable and/or possible to avoid an osteoplastic flap. Combining endoscopic frontal sinusotomy with frontal trephination offers superb visualization and access for all regions of the frontal sinus. The combined above-and-below approach may be indicated where larger supraorbital ethmoid and type III or type IV frontal sinus cells have obstructed the frontal outflow tract. Complete removal of these cells may not be possible via an endonasal transethmoidal approach. Even with the wide exposure of the Draf III, the superolateral extent of these cells may not be visible or reachable with standard instrumentation. In addition, the above-and-below technique may be indicated for frontal lesions confined to the superiormost or lateralmost extent of the frontal sinus. This approach may also be useful to reestablish patency of a stenotic frontal sinusotomy when no visible pathway from below can be appreciated.

The advantages of the combined above-and-below approach, when compared with those already discussed, are numerous. This technique is safe in patients whose frontal sinus floor is narrow in the anteroposterior dimension, where use of powered instrumentation carries a risk for CSF leak. This procedure is technically more straightforward than other advanced frontal techniques and uses skills familiar to most otorhinolaryngologists; it therefore may be considered a safer choice for the occasional frontal sinus surgeon. In addition, the superior access allows for irrigation postoperatively, and less postoperative debridement is necessary than with the aforementioned procedures.[34] These advantages should be considered when determining the appropriate approach for a given patient.

Surgical Anatomy

The supratrochlear and surpraorbital neurovascular bundles exit the skull in the orbit and supraorbital foramen, respectively. Both nerves are branches of the trigeminal nerve and provide general sensory afferent innervation to the forehead. The supratrochlear nerve lies more medially and courses superiorly on the undersurface of the corrugator.

The floor of the frontal sinus generally sits at the level of the supraorbital rim. Pneumatization patterns vary greatly, and thus, variants such as supraorbital ethmoid and frontal cells should be carefully identified on preoperative imaging. Optimum placement of the trephination may be affected by frontal sinus pathology such as mucocele or previous trauma (**Fig. 28.8**).

Surgical Techniques

The frontal sinus is initially approached and, if possible, opened from below in the standard fashion discussed in Chapter 27. The standard trephine incision is placed in the medial brow, medial to the supratrochlear neurovascular bundle. The incision should be made parallel to the hair follicles and dissection should be carried down through the periosteum to expose the anterior table. A diamond drill is then used to remove the frontal bone and care should be taken not to damage the mucosa by inadvertently entering into the sinus. Once adequately exposed, the frontal sinus is entered using a scalpel. In general, the size of the trephination should be limited to ~5 mm.[35,36] However, in selected cases, a Kerrison rongeur can be used to enlarge the trephination more inferiorly in the floor of the frontal sinus, allowing for simultaneous instrumentation and visualization with the endoscope without significant risk for cosmetic deformity. Care must be taken, however, not to enter directly into the frontal recess.

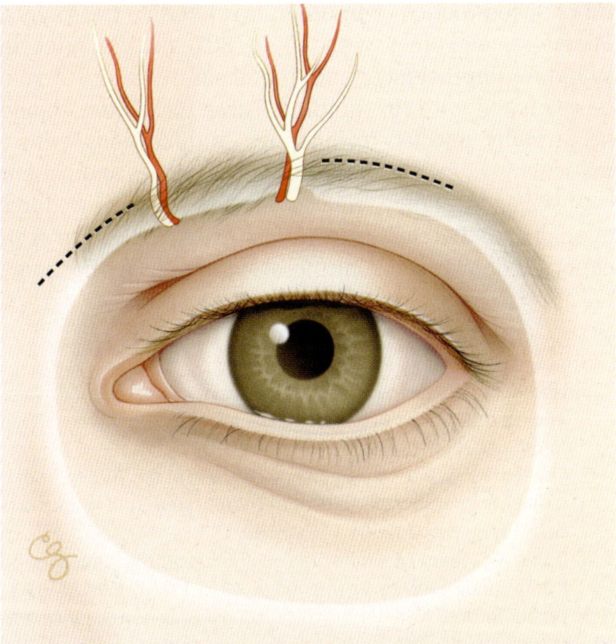

Fig. 28.8 Illustration of possible incisions for left-sided trephination. Standard incision lies medial to the neurovascular bundle; however, the incision is guided by frontal sinus anatomy.

In Batra's report in 2005, it was noted that the trephination may be placed in various locations to be of greatest assistance with respect to the underlying frontal pathology. The classic incision, as described previously, through the anterior table of the frontal sinus affords a view of the frontal recess from above and the entire frontal sinus when an endoscope is placed through the trephine. The frontal sinus may also be instrumented through this trephination with the 30-degree endoscope held back at the entrance, creating a panoramic view. In addition, the trephine may be placed lateral to the supraorbital neurovascular bundle for the management of a far-lateral disease process.[35] Computer navigation can be helpful in selecting a safe point of entry into the frontal sinus in close proximity to the targeted frontal pathology.[37]

There may be times when the frontal sinus outflow tract is stenotic and it is not possible to safely open it from below. At our institution, we have used the above-and-below approach successfully in these patients by performing a trephination and instilling dilute methylene blue into the frontal sinus from above while viewing from below to identify the frontal sinus outflow tract (**Fig. 28.9**). In addition to aiding in a safe dissection, it also allows for the irrigation of purulence and mucus from the affected sinus.

Complications

Complications specific to the above-and-below approach include hypesthesia of the forehead secondary to damage to the supratrochlear or supraorbital nerves; wound breakdown with subsequent sino-cutaneous fistula; loss of hair at the incision; and keloid or hypertrophic scar formation. Cosmetic deformity at the trephination can be minimized by limiting the size of the trephine to ~5 mm; this allows for adequate manipulation without the risk of soft tissue prolapsing into the defect. Anterior table trephination should also be avoided in the setting of acute frontal sinusitis, as the incision may lead to bacterial seeding of the frontal bone leading to frontal osteomyelitis (Pott's puffy tumor).[35]

Postoperative Care

Close follow-up continues to be important following the above-and-below approach, and postoperative debridement remains important for maintenance of a patent frontal outflow tract.[38] However, there is relatively less postoperative debridement required with the above-and-below approach than with the EMLP or Draf procedures. In addition, postoperative irrigation can be instilled through

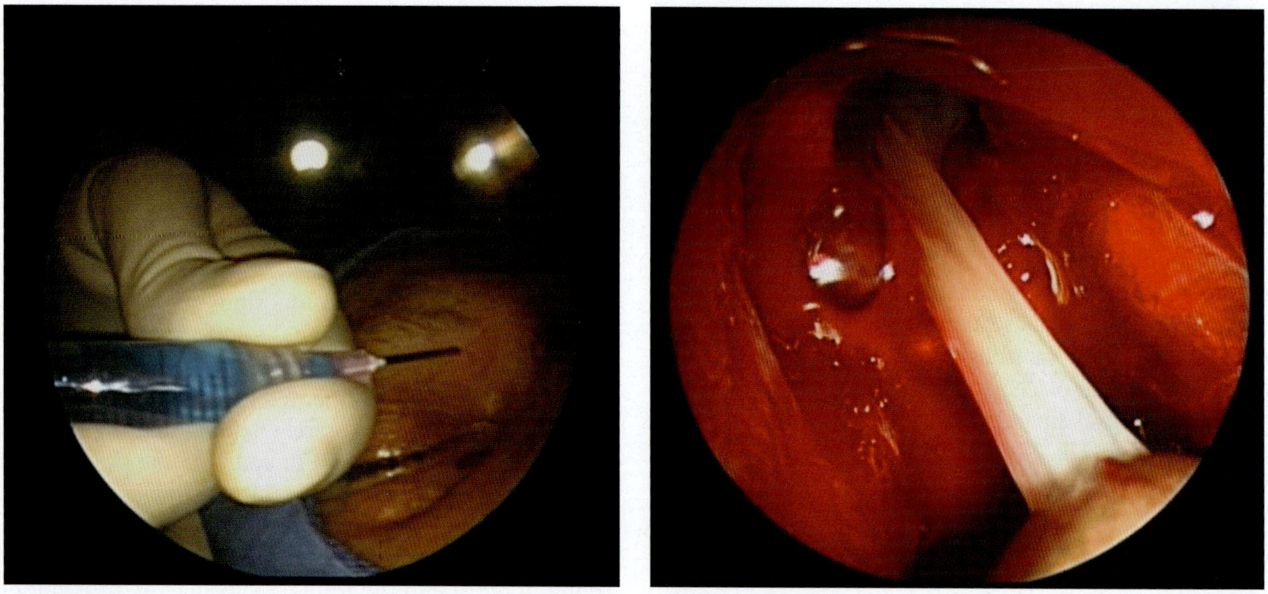

A B

Fig. 28.9 (A) Dilute methylene blue is instilled under stereotactic guidance into a dehiscence in the anterior table. **(B)** During instillation of the methylene blue, the frontal recess is visualized from below to trace the origin of the blue irrigant to the frontal ostium.

a red rubber or angio-catheter placed through the trephination and secured to the skin at the time of surgery. This can aid in flushing the sinus of purulence as well as fibrin clots to help avoid postoperative scarring.

Outcomes

When compared with the EMLP and Draf procedures, the outcomes are similar with the above-and-below approach. Benoit and Duncavage reported on a retrospective review of 40 patients who underwent combined an above-and-below approach with a mean follow-up of 12 months. In this series, 78% of patients had subjective improvement in their symptoms and 79% had a patent outflow tract, results that are similar to the EMLP.[36] In 2005, Batra et al. reported a similar patency rate of 86% of the frontal outflow tract at a mean follow-up of 16.2 months.[35]

Conclusion

All of the procedures discussed previously are intermediate procedures to avoid an osteoplastic flap with or without obliteration, or to be used in patients with a tumor or other process that necessitates increased exposure. The procedures are safe in experienced hands, although they do carry an increased risk of CSF leak. Patients undergoing these procedures for chronic rhinosinusitis have, by definition, been refractory to other, less invasive treatments. Therefore, outcomes with 70 to 80% success rates in symptom improvement and frontal sinus patency should be evaluated with this in mind. These techniques should be carefully selected to minimize complications, with a meticulous review of preoperative CT images and patient counseling. As noted, indications for these procedures overlap and, therefore, patient factors and physician skill/expertise do play a significant role in approach selection.

References

1. Hardy JM, Montgomery WW. Osteoplastic frontal sinusotomy: an analysis of 250 operations. Ann Otol Rhinol Laryngol 1976;85 (4 Pt 1):523–532
2. McLaughlin RB Jr. History of surgical approaches to the frontal sinus. Otolaryngol Clin North Am 2001;34(1):49–58
3. Draf W. Endonasal micro-endoscopic frontal sinus surgery: the Fulda concept. Oper Tech Otolaryngol—Head Neck Surg 1991;2:234–240
4. Draf W. Endonasal frontal sinus drainage type I–III according to Draf. In: The Frontal Sinus. Berlin: Springer-Verlag; 2005: 219 -232
5. Kuhn FA. An integrated approach to frontal sinus surgery. Otolaryngol Clin North Am 2006;39(3):437–461, viii
6. Hosemann W, Herzog D, Beule AG, Kaftan H. Experimental evaluation of drills for extended frontal sinusotomy. Otolaryngol Head Neck Surg 2004;131(3):187–191
7. Chandra RK, Schlosser R, Kennedy DW. Use of the 70-degree diamond burr in the management of complicated frontal sinus disease. Laryngoscope 2004;114(2):188–192
8. Dubin MG, Kuhn FA. Endoscopic modified Lothrop (Draf III) with frontal sinus punches. Laryngoscope 2005;115(9):1702–1703
9. Weber R, Draf W, Keerl R, Schick B, Saha A. Endonasal microendoscopic pansinusoperation in chronic sinusitis. II. Results and complications. Am J Otolaryngol 1997;18(4):247–253
10. Kikawada T, Fujigaki M, Kikura M, Matsumoto M, Kikawada K. Extended endoscopic frontal sinus surgery to interrupted

nasofrontal communication caused by scarring of the anterior ethmoid: long-term results. Arch Otolaryngol Head Neck Surg 1999;125(1):92–96

11. Lothrop HA. Frontal sinus suppuration. Ann Surg 1914;59(6): 937 -957
12. Gross WE, Gross CW, Becker D, Moore D, Phillips D. Modified transnasal endoscopic Lothrop procedure as an alternative to frontal sinus obliteration. Otolaryngol Head Neck Surg 1995;113(4):427–434
13. Schulze SL, Loehrl TA, Smith TL. Outcomes of the modified endoscopic Lothrop procedure. Am J Rhinol 2002;16(5):269–273
14. Wormald PJ. Salvage frontal sinus surgery: the endoscopic modified Lothrop procedure. Laryngoscope 2003;113(2):276–283
15. Wynn R, Vaughan WC. Treatment of failed frontal sinus obliteration. Oper Tech Otolaryngol 2006;17:13–18
16. Stankiewicz JA, Wachter B. The endoscopic modified Lothrop procedure for salvage of chronic frontal sinusitis after osteoplastic flap failure. Otolaryngol Head Neck Surg 2003;129(6):678–683
17. Gross CW, Harrison SE. The modified Lothrop procedure: indications, results, and complications. Otolaryngol Clin North Am 2001;34(1):133–137
18. Burkart CM, Zimmer LA. Endoscopic modified Lothrop procedure: a radiographic anatomic study. Laryngoscope 2011;121(2): 442–445
19. Kountakis S. The Frontal Sinus. Berlin: Springer-Verlag; 2005: 233–241
20. Farhat FT, Figueroa RE, Kountakis SE. Anatomic measurements for the endoscopic modified Lothrop procedure. Am J Rhinol 2005;19(3):293–296
21. Gross WE, Gross CW, Becker D, Moore D, Phillips D. Modified transnasal endoscopic Lothrop procedure as an alternative to frontal sinus obliteration. Otolaryngol Head Neck Surg 1995;113(4):427–434
22. Becker DG, Moore D, Lindsey WH, Gross WE, Gross CW. Modified transnasal endoscopic Lothrop procedure: further considerations. Laryngoscope 1995;105(11):1161–1166
23. Shirazi MA, Silver AL, Stankiewicz JA. Surgical outcomes following the endoscopic modified Lothrop procedure. Laryngoscope 2007;117(5):765–769
24. Schlosser RJ, Zachmann G, Harrison S, Gross CW. The endoscopic modified Lothrop: long-term follow-up on 44 patients. Am J Rhinol 2002;16(2):103–108
25. Samaha M, Cosenza MJ, Metson R. Endoscopic frontal sinus drillout in 100 patients. Arch Otolaryngol Head Neck Surg 2003;129(8):854–858
26. Vostra. Rhinotamp. http://www.vostra.de/index.php/nasal-tamponades.html. Accessed March 15, 2008
27. Weber R, Keerl R, Hochapfel F, Draf W, Toffel PH. Packing in endonasal surgery. Am J Otolaryngol 2001;22(5):306–320
28. Tran KN, Beule AG, Singal D, Wormald PJ. Frontal ostium restenosis after the endoscopic modified Lothrop procedure. Laryngoscope 2007;117(8):1457–1462
29. Anderson P, Sindwani R. Safety and efficacy of the endoscopic modified Lothrop procedure: a systematic review and meta-analysis. Laryngoscope 2009;119(9):1828–1833
30. Lanza DC, McLaughlin RB Jr, Hwang PH. The five year experience with endoscopic trans-septal frontal sinusotomy. Otolaryngol Clin North Am 2001;34(1):139–152
31. Batra PS, Lanza D. The Frontal Sinus. Berlin: Springer-Verlag; 2005:252–259
32. Goldsztein H, Pletcher SD, Reh DD, Metson R. The frontal wishbone: anatomic and clinical implications. Am J Rhinol 2007;21(6):725–728
33. McLaughlin RB, Hwang PH, Lanza DC. Endoscopic trans-septal frontal sinusotomy: the rationale and results of an alternative technique. Am J Rhinol 1999;13(4):279–287
34. Benoit CM, Duncavage JA. Combined external and endoscopic frontal sinusotomy with stent placement: a retrospective review. Laryngoscope 2001;111(7):1246–1249
35. Batra PS, Citardi MJ, Lanza DC. Combined endoscopic trephination and endoscopic frontal sinusotomy for management of complex frontal sinus pathology. Am J Rhinol 2005;19(5): 435–441
36. Wigand ME, Steiner W, Jaumann MP. Endonasal sinus surgery with endoscopical control: from radical operation to rehabilitation of the mucosa. Endoscopy 1978;10(4): 255–260
37. Zacharek MA, Fong KJ, Hwang PH. Image-guided frontal trephination: a minimally invasive approach for hard-to-reach frontal sinus disease. Otolaryngol Head Neck Surg 2006;135(4): 518–522
38. Benoit CM, Duncavage JA. Combined external and endoscopic frontal sinusotomy with stent placement: a retrospective review. Laryngoscope 2001;111(7):1246–1249

29 Complications of Endoscopic Sinus Surgery: Prevention and Management

Ralph B. Metson and Michael P. Platt

Since the introduction of endoscopic sinus surgery in the 1980s, numerous innovations in operative techniques and technology have advanced the efficacy and safety of this procedure. Nevertheless, sinus surgery, which requires deft manipulation of tissues within a relatively confined space, continues to be associated with complications of both minor and major consequence.

The reported incidence of complications associated with endoscopic sinus surgery ranges from 0.3 to 22.4% (median 7.0%).[1–4] The majority of these complications cause minimal patient morbidity and require nominal treatment. Major complications, such as cerebrospinal fluid (CSF) leak or orbital hemorrhage, are seen in less than 1% of patients.[1,4] Most major complications occur in the presence of excessive bleeding, which leads to reduced intraoperative visualization and loss of anatomic landmarks. In such cases, the surgeon may become disoriented and may extend instrumentation beyond the confines of the paranasal sinuses.

Proper knowledge of sinonasal anatomy, meticulous surgical technique, and adequate intraoperative hemostasis are the keys to the performance of safe and effective sinus surgery. The avoidance of complications associated with such surgery begins with proper preoperative evaluation of the surgical patient.

■ Preoperative Considerations

An appropriate patient history can reduce the incidence of complications related to sinus surgery. Such a history should include screening for risk factors associated with bleeding, including the use of antiplatelet medication (e.g., aspirin and clopidogrel), a history of excessive bleeding with prior surgery, and family history of bleeding disorders. Preoperative medical treatment with antibiotics or corticosteroids for patients with severe mucosal inflammation or polyposis may decrease intraoperative blood loss and may allow for better visualization.

Review of pertinent radiologic imaging studies can alert the sinus surgeon to potential surgical pitfalls, such as a defect in the lamina papyracea (**Fig. 29.1**), low-lying cribriform plate (Keros type 3),[5] or dehiscence of a carotid canal. This review is especially important in revision surgery, where protective bone in these regions may have been removed. Preoperative recognition of anatomic variants, such as a hypoplastic maxillary sinus, sphenoethmoidal (Onodi) cell (**Fig. 29.2**), or undeveloped frontal sinus may avert intraoperative complications.

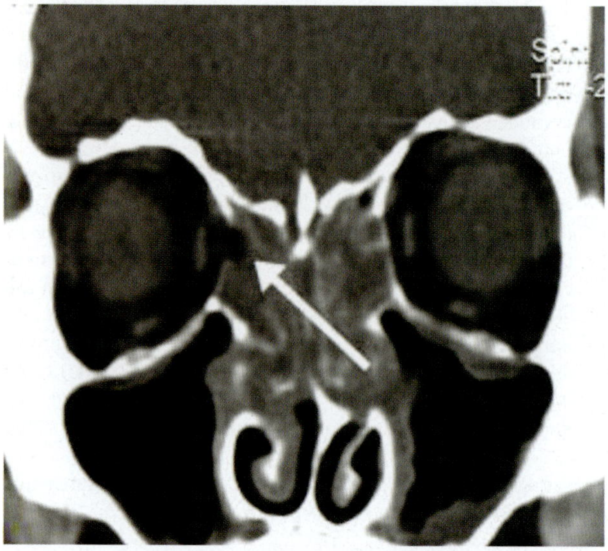

Fig. 29.1 A defect in the right lamina papyracea with herniation of orbital fat (*arrow*) into the ethmoid sinus is evident on this preoperative computed tomography scan. Identification of this finding prior to surgery can help prevent injury to the orbital contents during an ethmoidectomy.

Although image-guidance technology has not been definitively shown to decrease complications related to sinus surgery,[6] its use has become widely accepted for advanced sinonasal procedures. Image-guidance systems provide the surgeon with immediate anatomic localization during challenging surgeries and should be considered for those cases where anatomic landmarks have become obscured from prior surgery or extensive disease.

Obtaining an informed consent, with discussion of the potential risks, complications, and alternatives to surgery, is important in today's healthcare environment. Such a discussion enhances patient understanding of the surgical process and serves to provide proper legal documentation when poor outcomes occur.

■ Intraoperative Complications

Intranasal Complications

Diffuse Hemorrhage

Diffuse bleeding, which arises from small caliber vessels, typically occurs in the setting of extensive mucosal inflammation or large nasal polyps. Adequate hemostasis begins

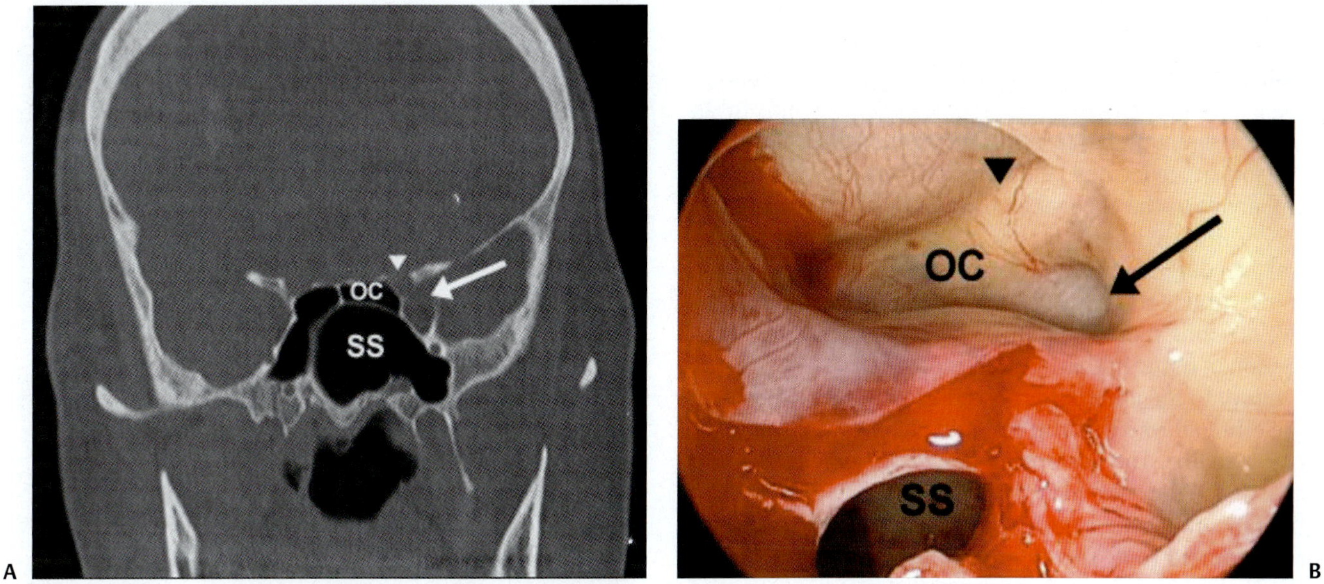

Fig. 29.2 (A) Preoperative computed tomography scan demonstrates the presence of an Onodi cell (*OC*) located above the left sphenoid sinus (*SS*). The optic nerve (*arrowhead*) and carotid artery (*arrow*), which run along the lateral wall of this cell, are at increased risk for injury during a posterior ethmoidectomy. **(B)** Intraoperative view of the Onodi cell at the time of a sphenoethmoidectomy.

with the proper preparation of the sinonasal tissues, including the use of topical decongestants (e.g., oxymetazoline 0.5% or cocaine 4%) and a submucosal injection of vasoconstrictive agents (e.g., 1% lidocaine with 1:100,000 epinephrine) prior to surgery. Communication with the anesthesia team to maintain systolic pressures of 80 to 100 mm Hg, when appropriate, can also help to minimize intraoperative bleeding.[7]

Intraoperative mucosal bleeding can usually be managed with intermittent nasal packs soaked in a topical decongestant medication, such as oxymetazoline 0.5% or epinephrine 1:50,000. Microdebrider instrumentation can also be helpful in such cases because of its ability to simultaneously suction blood from the surgical field and remove tissue. When bleeding cannot be sufficiently controlled to see anatomic landmarks, surgery should be halted to prevent inadvertent injury to surrounding structures. In such circumstances, a staged second procedure to remove residual disease when bleeding is no longer an issue is a safe and prudent choice.

Arterial Injury

Intraoperative arterial bleeding typically occurs at specific sites within the paranasal sinuses when larger blood vessels are disrupted. Resection of the middle turbinate near its posterior insertion site along the lateral nasal wall can result in pulsatile bleeding from the sphenopalatine artery or one of its branches. This complication may be prevented by preservation of the posterior third of the middle turbinate. Overly aggressive enlargement of the maxillary ostium in a posterior direction can also result in bleeding from the region of the sphenopalatine foramen. When such bleeding does occur, it can often be controlled by the use of either monopolar or bipolar cautery. If bleeding is brisk, suction cautery may be helpful; however, excessive cauterization in the region can cause delayed healing and postoperative discomfort from crust formation and osteitis. A more definitive control of arterial bleeding may be achieved through an endoscopic placement of a clip on the sphenopalatine artery where it exits from the pterygopalatine fossa (**Fig. 29.3**).

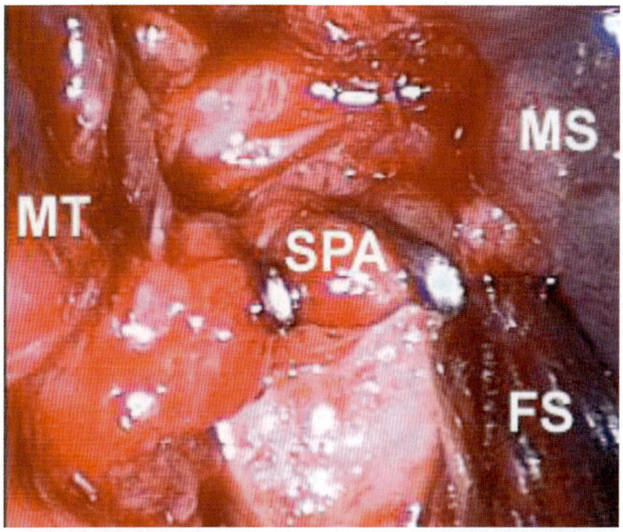

Fig. 29.3 Endoscopic image of two clips placed on the left sphenopalatine artery (*SPA*) for control of severe epistaxis following endoscopic sinus surgery. The SPA is located between the posterior wall of the maxillary sinus (*MS*) and the horizontal insertion of the middle turbinate (*MT*). FS, Frazier suction tip.

Pulsatile bleeding from the posterior septal branch of the sphenopalatine artery can occur along the anterior wall of the sphenoid sinus. Injury to this vessel is typically seen during enlargement of the sphenoid ostium in an inferior direction because the vessel runs transversely in the soft tissue located below the natural sphenoid ostium and above to the choanal arch. Monopolar or bipolar cautery, with or without suction, is usually sufficient to control bleeding at this site. Prophylactic cauterization and transection of this vessel to avoid troublesome intraoperative bleeding should be considered when an extensive dissection of tissue in this location is planned.

Injury to the anterior or posterior ethmoid artery along the ethmoid roof can also result in significant intraoperative bleeding. The posterior ethmoid artery runs ~5 mm anterior to the sphenoethmoid angle, which is formed by the junction of the anterior sphenoid wall and the posterior ethmoid roof. The anterior ethmoid artery traverses the skull base ~12 mm anterior to the posterior ethmoid artery. Injury to these vessels can occur when there is bony dehiscence of their canals or when they are mistaken for an ethmoid septation and disrupted. In the extensively pneumatized ethmoid labyrinth, the anterior ethmoid artery (and, rarely, the posterior ethmoid artery) may lie below the level of the skull base, traversing the ethmoid along a mesentery. In such cases, the artery may be particularly susceptible to injury, but this anatomic variant can be anticipated by a careful preoperative review of the computed tomography (CT) images.

Because blood flow through the ethmoid arteries occurs from a lateral to a medial direction (via ophthalmic artery), their disruption must be meticulously managed to avoid retraction of the arterial stump into the orbit. Such an occurrence could lead to a complicated intraorbital hemorrhage (see later). If electrocautery is used to control bleeding from these vessels, bipolar cautery is preferred, so as to avoid transmitting the electrical current to the skull base and orbit. Ligation of the anterior ethmoid artery through an external approach is well described, although recent reports suggest that endoscopic ligation may be an alternative that avoids the need for a facial incision.[8]

Intraorbital Complications

Orbital Fat Exposure

Injury to the thin bone that forms the medial orbital wall may occur during uncinectomy near the start of sinus surgery. An incision of the uncinate process that is directed too far lateral or posterior can enter the orbit through the lamina papyracea. This injury is more likely in the setting of a hypoplastic or atelectatic maxillary sinus (**Fig. 29.4**). Similarly, aggressive lateral dissection during ethmoidectomy can result in lamina papyracea disruption. The inadvertent penetration or removal of the lamina with exposure of the periorbita usually does not have adverse consequences if it is recognized promptly and the periorbita has not been violated. Routine palpation of the globe is critical when operating in this region. Even a small defect in the lamina papyracea can be seen as movement along the medial orbital wall when the globe is gently compressed during surgery.

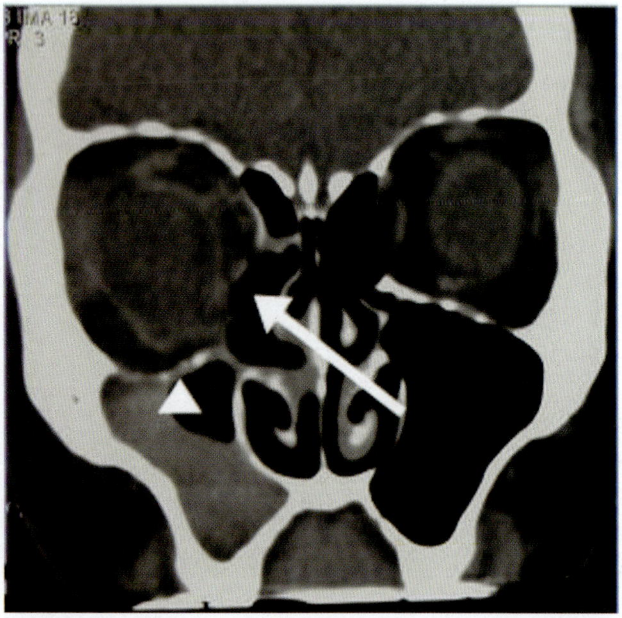

Fig. 29.4 Postoperative computed tomography scan of a patient who suffered orbital injury during sinus surgery. Passage of a motorized instrument through the lamina papyracea resulted in transection of the medial rectus muscle (*arrow*). Preoperative recognition of the atelectatic right maxillary sinus with an unusually low right orbital floor (*arrowhead*) might have prevented the injury.

If the periorbita has been violated and orbital fat is seen, manipulation of exposed fat within the ethmoid sinus should be avoided to prevent further injury. No repair of this defect is needed. So long as protruding fat does not obscure visualization, surgery may be continued as planned. Serial examinations of the eye should be performed during the remainder of surgery to ensure that intraorbital hemorrhage has not developed.

Nasal packing is usually avoided in such cases. Placement of packing over the orbital defect at the conclusion of surgery can create a one-way valve and trap air or blood within the orbital tissues should the patient strain, cough, or vomit. In such cases, periorbital edema, ecchymosis, subcutaneous emphysema, or proptosis may result. Prompt removal of any packing usually eliminates the ball-valve effect and halts progression of symptoms, but continued close monitoring of the eye, including vision testing, is needed to ensure clinical stability.

Intraorbital Hematoma

An intraorbital hematoma (also known as retro-orbital or retrobulbar hemorrhage) is a potentially devastating complication of endoscopic sinus surgery,[9] but one that can have a favorable outcome if recognized promptly and

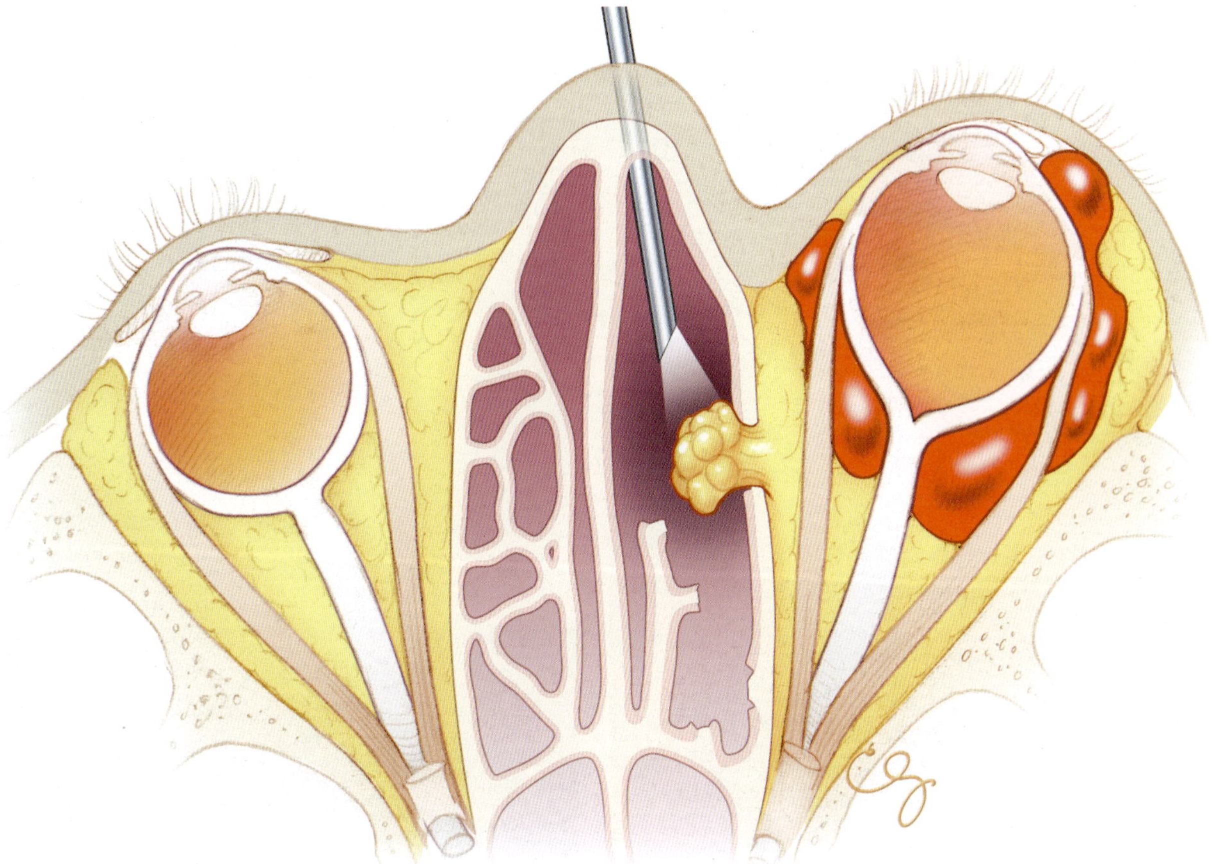

Fig. 29.5 Intraorbital hemorrhage may result from injury to the lamina papyracea and orbital vessels. Accumulation of blood within the orbit increases pressure on the retina and optic nerve, which may result in irreversible ischemic injury. Herniation of orbital fat into the ethmoid cavity alerts the surgeon to violation of the lamina papyracea and underlying periorbita.

treated appropriately. Bleeding into the orbit from injury to vessels within the orbit, or retraction of a bleeding anterior or posterior ethmoid artery, can cause increased intraorbital pressure with retinal ischemia (**Fig. 29.5**). The retina can tolerate 30 to 90 minutes of ischemia before irreversible damage ensues. Signs and symptoms of intraorbital hemorrhage include a tense globe, increased intraocular pressure, loss of pupillary reflex, eye pain, limitation of eye mobility, and decreased vision.

Medical management of a slowly expanding orbital hematoma without visual loss includes removal of nasal packing and eye massage. Administration of systemic steroids (dexamethasone 0.2 mg/kg intravenous [IV]), mannitol (1 to 2 g/kg IV), and acetazolamide (10 to 15 mg/kg IV) can reduce edema and aqueous humor production. The importance of immediate ophthalmic consultation with serial examination of visual acuity and intraocular pressures cannot be overstated.

For rapidly expanding hematomas identified during or at the conclusion of sinus surgery, emergent treatment is warranted to prevent or reverse loss of vision. A lateral canthotomy and cantholysis to increase orbital volume and thereby reduce intraorbital pressure should be performed without delay. It is a simple and effective procedure that can be done in the operating room, recovery room, or at the bedside. Local anesthetic may be used to infiltrate the lateral canthus, but is usually not necessary. To perform lateral canthotomy, a hemostat is advanced to the bone of the lateral orbital rim with one tine anterior and the other tine posterior to the skin of the lateral canthus, and closed for 15 to 30 seconds to compress the tissues in preparation for their incision. Once the clamp is removed, a dissecting scissor is used to incise the full thickness of the skin and underlying canthal tendon (**Fig. 29.6A**).

To further increase the orbital volume, a lateral cantholysis may also be performed by making a second incision across the lateralmost aspect of the lower lid in an inferior direction. The goal of cantholysis is to completely transect the inferior half of the lateral canthal tendon, thereby completely mobilizing the lateral lower lid. The orbital contents can then decompress forward unimpeded by the orbital septum or canthal tendon (**Fig. 29.6B**). These incisions heal well by secondary intention, usually without the need for secondary repair (**Fig. 29.6C,D**).

If these measures do not lead to clinical improvement, medial orbital decompression may be necessary. This

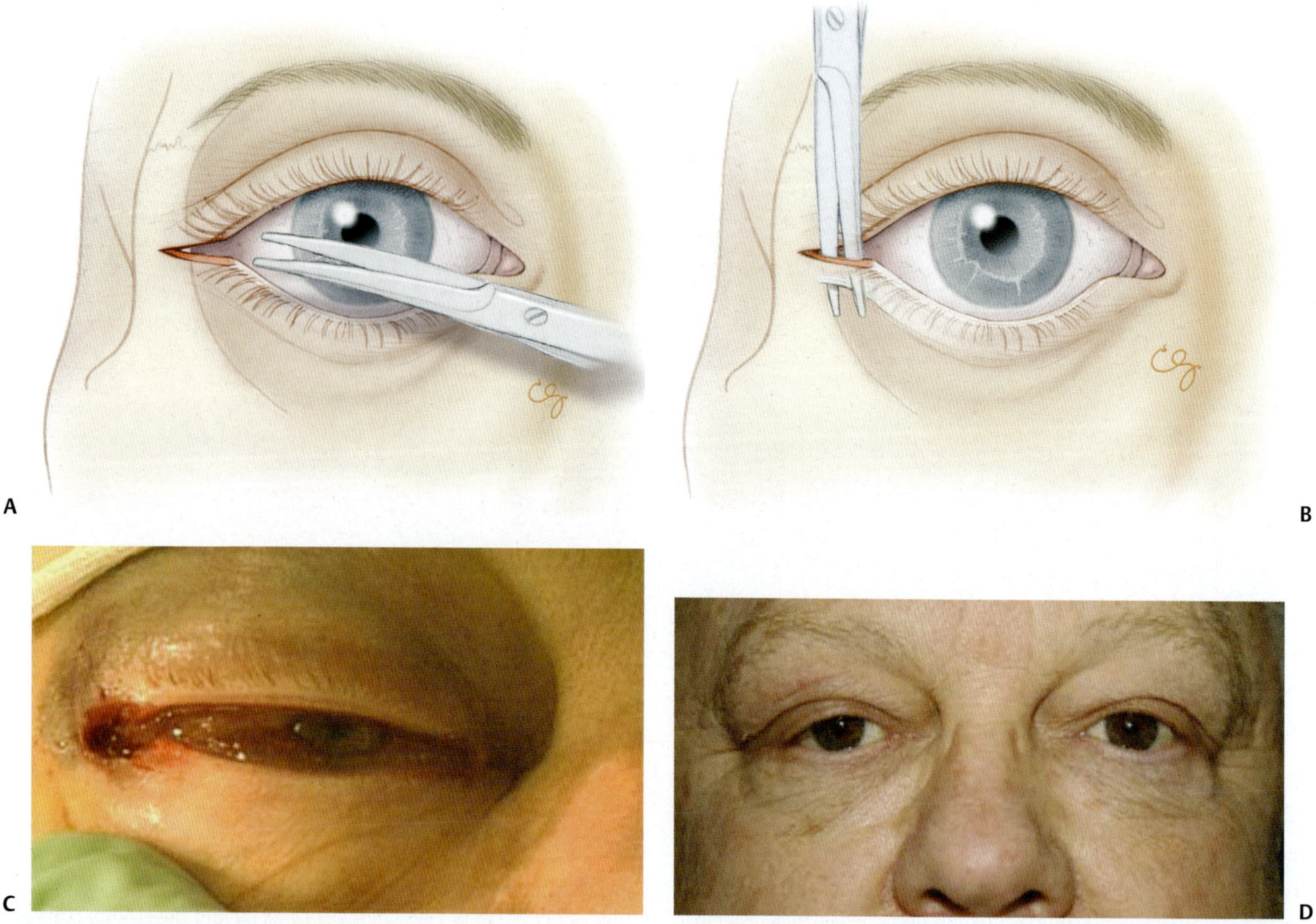

Fig. 29.6 (A) When an intraorbital hematoma occurs, a lateral canthotomy is performed by advancing a dissecting scissor to the bone of the lateral orbital rim and incising the full thickness of skin and underlying canthal tendon. **(B)** Additional reduction in intraorbital pressure can be achieved with an inferior cantholysis performed by directing the scissors inferiorly to release and transect the inferior half of the canthal tendon within the lower eyelid. **(C)** Right eye of a patient who underwent a lateral canthotomy with cantholysis for an intraorbital hematoma that developed following sinus surgery. Diagnosis was made by signs of conjunctival edema and hemorrhage, a tense globe with proptosis, and a visual loss with no light perception. **(D)** The lateral canthotomy and cantholysis healed well by secondary intention without the need for additional repair. This patient regained full visual acuity (20/20) and ocular function.

procedure can be performed effectively through either an endoscopic or external approach with removal of the lamina papyracea. Exploration of the orbit for ligation of a specific bleeding vessel can result in further injury and is not generally recommended.

Extraocular Muscle Injury

If violation of the lamina papyracea is not recognized at the time of surgery and dissection continues through the periorbita, damage to the underlying extraocular muscles can occur with resultant diplopia (**Fig. 29.4**). The medial rectus is most susceptible to such injury because of its proximity to the lateral boundary of the ethmoid sinus, particularly in the posterior ethmoid sinus; however, injury to the inferior rectus and the superior oblique muscles has also been described.[10] The incorporation of microdebrider devices in sinus surgery, with their rapid suctioning and cutting of soft tissue, has been associated with greater risks of injury to the extraocular muscles.[11] Injuries may range from muscle contusion to complete transection. If an extraocular muscle injury is recognized at the time of surgery, intraoperative consultation with an ophthalmologist can help to determine the extent of injury and the need for immediate orbital exploration with muscle repair. Although strabismus surgery may be performed to treat diplopia from rectus muscle injury, it is not always successful in restoring the full range of motion of the globe.

Optic Nerve Injury

Prevention of optic nerve injury during endoscopic surgery is critical given the severity of its associated morbidity and the lack of treatment options. If the surgeon is not aware that the lamina papyracea has been violated, inadvertent instrumentation within the orbital apex can result in optic nerve injury with a partial loss of vision or blindness. Similar injury can occur during manipulation within the superolateral sphenoid sinus if the optic canal is dehiscent. Sphenoidotomy should therefore be performed by careful enlargement of the natural sphenoid ostium, located at the anteromedial aspect of the sphenoid, so that bone removal begins as far away from the optic nerve as possible.

An unrecognized Onodi (sphenoethmoid) cell can place patients at risk for optic nerve injury during a posterior ethmoidectomy. This anatomic variation can be identified on the preoperative CT scan. If an Onodi cell is present, care should be taken during surgery to limit dissection in this region (**Fig. 29.2**).

If injury to the optic nerve is suspected during surgery, high-dose systemic corticosteroids should be administered, ophthalmologic consultation should be obtained, and the patient awakened in a timely fashion to assess visual acuity. A postoperative CT scan is necessary to evaluate the location and extent of this injury.

Intracranial Complications

Cerebrospinal Fluid Leak

CSF leaks and intracranial injuries occur when there has been violation of the skull base during endoscopic sinus surgery. These complications typically arise in the setting of excessive intraoperative bleeding, which can obscure intranasal landmarks and lead to surgical disorientation. Image guidance technology can help to confirm the location of the skull base in this scenario, but should not be solely relied on for identification of such a critical structure. When sinus surgery becomes technically difficult and anatomic landmarks are obscured, it is better to leave the disease along the skull base and terminate the procedure rather than risk injury to this region.

The incidence of CSF leak from inadvertent penetration of the skull base and underlying dura is ~0.5% of surgical cases.[11] The bone of the skull base is thinnest and most susceptible to injury at the junction of the anterior ethmoid artery and the middle turbinate along the anterior ethmoid roof[12]; however, injury may occur anywhere along the skull base, including the posterior ethmoid roof, cribriform plate, posterior wall of the frontal sinus, and roof of the sphenoid sinus.

Intraoperatively, a CSF leak often appears as a stream of darker fluid coursing through red blood. If only minimal bleeding is present, alternating streams of clear CSF and red blood are seen. When confronted with an intraoperative CSF leak, it is best for the surgeon step back and collect his or her thoughts. When recognized at the time of surgery and managed correctly, such complications have a greater than 90% likelihood of success with good clinical outcomes.[13,14]

For most intraoperative CSF leaks, repair with a single layer consisting of a free intranasal mucosal graft harvested from the septum or turbinate is all that is necessary to seal the defect. Occasionally, larger defects require an additional structural layer, such as septal bone or cartilage placed on the intracranial side of the defect. The mucosal graft is stabilized and protected with a generous layer of absorbable packing material such as Surgicel (Johnson & Johnson, Piscataway, NJ) or Gelfoam (Pfizer, New York, NY). An additional layer of nonabsorbable packing, such as strip gauze or Merocel (Medtronic, Jacksonville, FL) may be placed to further secure the repair. The nonabsorbable packing is removed after 1 week, whereas the absorbable packing is left in place and allowed to dissolve.

Once the patient is awake and out of the operating room, a CT scan should be obtained to assess for pneumocephalus or intracranial injury. Oral antistaphylococcal antibiotics are recommended during the perioperative period. Intravenous antibiotics with a CSF penetration may be administered instead, although their use is controversial, because they may mask signs of impending meningitis. A CT scan is performed 3 to 6 months after surgery for the surveillance of the repair.

Carotid Artery Injury

Injury to the internal carotid artery is one of the most catastrophic complications that can occur during endoscopic sinus surgery. Although this complication occurs in less than 0.1% of cases,[4] its consequences can be devastating, leading to an intracranial injury with stroke. The internal carotid artery courses along the lateral wall of the sphenoid sinus just inferior to the opticocarotid recess. Injury to the carotid may occur when the sphenoid sinus is entered too far laterally or when surgical dissection is performed along the lateral sphenoid wall and the carotid canal is penetrated. This complication can be avoided by entering the sphenoid sinus medially through the natural sphenoid ostium and enlarging this opening in an inferior and medial direction away from the laterally positioned carotid artery. Instrumentation within the lateral sphenoid sinus is not usually necessary during routine sinus surgery and, when performed, should be approached with extreme caution. The intersphenoid septum can insert onto the bony canal overlying the carotid artery, and arterial injury has been reported with the removal of this partition.

When injury to the carotid artery does occur, profuse bleeding will rapidly fill the nasal cavity. The surgeon must gain control of bleeding by packing the sphenoid sinus. Aggressive fluid resuscitation should be begun immediately, and hemodynamic control must be achieved to maintain cerebral perfusion. A blood sample should also be typed and cross-matched for the transfusion of blood products. Once stabilized, a patient may be considered for further intervention. Definitive treatment is performed by the interventional radiologist, who uses angiography to identify the site and extent of vascular injury. Treatment may include the use of detachable coils to seal a hole in the vessel wall, or balloons to occlude the carotid artery. A balloon occlusion test to verify adequate cross-perfusion may be performed by the interventional neuroradiologist prior to permanent occlusion of the internal carotid artery. If internal carotid artery occlusion is not a viable option due to cerebral ischemia, cross-cranial vascular bypass may be needed to prevent brain ischemia and stroke.

Postoperative Complications

Intranasal Complications

Epistaxis

Epistaxis following sinus surgery occurs in 2% of patients.[1] It is typically seen immediately following surgery from inadequate hemostasis or 5 to 7 days after surgery when intranasal scabs dislodge. The most common sites of postoperative bleeding include the turbinates and septum, when turbinate reduction or septoplasty has been performed as an adjunct to sinus surgery. Routine placement of packing material or absorbable hemostatic agents within the sinonasal cavities at the conclusion of surgery may help decrease the incidence of postoperative bleeding; however, such materials may contribute to the delayed restoration of normal sinus drainage and increased patient discomfort. If excessive bleeding is not present at the conclusion of surgery, studies have suggested that nasal packing need not be placed at the conclusion of routine endoscopic sinus surgery.[15,16]

Mild cases of postoperative epistaxis can often be managed with topical decongestant sprays. Patients who present to the emergency department with active bleeding require more aggressive intervention. Vital signs should be monitored and hypertension, if present, should be controlled. A blood sample may be drawn to determine hemoglobin level and to obtain a clot for the blood bank if necessary. Intravenous access allows for volume replacement and the administration of blood replacement products.

Epistaxis treatment protocols use a stepwise treatment approach based on the severity and site of bleeding. In general, one should first attempt to identify the site of bleeding with an endoscope. If possible, the bleeding vessel is cauterized with silver nitrate under direct visualization. Otherwise, the placement of absorbable or nonabsorbable nasal packing is necessary. A variety of tamponade balloons are available for this purpose and usually leads to successful control of postoperative epistaxis. For bleeding that is not controlled with conservative measures, operative exploration with electrocauterization or vessel ligation may be performed. Bleeding from the sphenopalatine, anterior ethmoid, or posterior ethmoid arteries can be controlled through either an open or endoscopic approach, as described previously. For persistent postoperative epistaxis, embolization of the bleeding vessel by a skilled interventional radiologist is comparable to surgical ligation and should be considered as a treatment alternative.

Sinusitis

Postoperative sinusitis is one of the most common complications of endoscopic sinus surgery, occurring in up to 16% of patients.[17] Raw mucosal surfaces, intranasal bacterial colonization, and decreased mucociliary clearance of nasal secretions contribute to sinus infection during the healing period. Prophylactic use of antistaphylococcal antibiotics, frequent nasal saline irrigations, and postoperative sinus debridement can reduce the incidence of such sinusitis by reducing bacterial growth in stagnant nasal secretions. If sinusitis develops in the postoperative period, endoscopically directed cultures are helpful in identifying the pathogens involved and selecting the appropriate antibiotic regimen.

Olfactory Dysfunction

During the postoperative healing period, alteration in olfaction is commonly observed for 1 to 2 weeks following surgery as a result of edema and secretions within the sinonasal cavities. If abnormal olfaction persists after the healing of the sinus cavities is complete, a nasal endoscopy and a sinus CT scan can be helpful to look for anatomic obstruction of the olfactory cleft or persistent sinus disease. If symptoms do not respond to topical or oral corticosteroids, formal olfactory testing may be considered.[18]

With the high incidence of preoperative smell dysfunction in patients undergoing sinus surgery, it is often difficult to determine whether postoperative changes in olfaction are secondary to the surgical procedure or to preexisting conditions. Nonetheless, care should be taken to avoid mucosal trauma along the olfactory cleft or cribriform plate during surgery. Postoperative adhesions spanning the middle turbinate and septum can prevent odor molecules from reaching their receptors within the superior nasal cavity.

Synechiae

Small, asymptomatic adhesions are often noted as incidental findings at the time of nasal endoscopy following sinus surgery. Dense adhesions and synechiae, however, can be a source of postoperative anosmia, recurrent sinusitis, and mucocele formation (**Fig. 29.7**). In a series of patients undergoing revision sinus surgery, adhesions were found to be present in 56% of cases and were felt to be a contributing factor for failure in up to 31% of patients.[19]

If the middle turbinate mucosa is traumatized during surgery, an adhesion may form between the middle turbinate and the lateral nasal wall, resulting in obstruction of sinus drainage pathways. Adhesion between the medial surface of the middle turbinate and septum can result in postoperative anosmia. Postoperative nasal airway

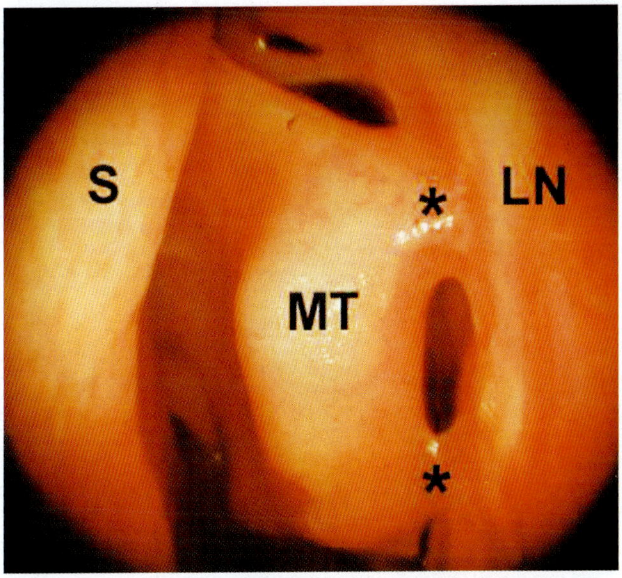

Fig. 29.7 Endoscopic view of synechial bands between the left middle turbinate (*MT*) and lateral nasal wall (*LN*) that formed after endoscopic sinus surgery. These adhesions can obstruct the natural drainage pathways and can lead to suboptimal surgical outcomes. *S*, septum.

obstruction may occur when a dense adhesion forms between the inferior turbinate and septum.

A spacer or packing material placed at the time of surgery may decrease the incidence of adhesion formation and turbinate lateralization. If adhesions are noted at the time of office endoscopy during the first postoperative week, they can usually be divided with minimal patient discomfort. Once healing is completed, however, resection of synechiae in the office setting is more difficult, and lysis of symptomatic adhesions may require the use of either local or general anesthesia.

Myospherulosis is an infrequent postoperative complication of sinus surgery caused by foreign body reaction to petrolatum or lanolin found in some antibiotic ointments used to coat packing material placed in the nose at the completion of sinus surgery.[20] This reaction results in the formation of profuse granulation tissue and dense adhesions, leading to an increased incidence of postoperative sinusitis and revision sinus surgery. Myospherulosis is diagnosed by the presence of multinucleated giant cells and granulomatous inflammation surrounding lipid vacuoles seen by the pathologist on a histologic evaluation of surgical specimens. This complication may be avoided by the use of water-soluble antibiotic gels, instead of petrolatum-containing ointments, in patients undergoing sinonasal surgery.

Orbital Complications

Corneal Abrasion

During endoscopic sinus surgery, the orbits need to be draped within the surgical field to serve as external anatomic landmarks and to allow for monitoring of the globes. This draping method, however, makes the surfaces of the eyes susceptible to injury from inadvertent contact with the surgeon's hands or instruments. Corneal abrasion presents with eye pain and foreign body sensation during the immediate postoperative period. Diagnosis is made by the ophthalmologist with the aid of supravital fluorescence staining and slit-lamp examination. When corneal abrasion does occur, conservative medical management with topical antibiotic ointment and patching of the eye usually results in resolution of the symptoms within 48 hours.

During surgery, the use of ophthalmic ointment and taping of the eyelids can help protect the cornea. For prolonged sinus procedures, a scleral shell or a large contact lens can be placed in the eye at the start of surgery to provide additional corneal protection.

Diplopia

Double vision following endoscopic sinus surgery is indicative of asymmetric eye movement caused by injury to an extraocular muscle or its motor nerve. Violation of the lamina papyracea and periorbita with the passage of an instrument into the orbital cavity can result in rectus muscle injury. The medial rectus is the muscle most commonly injured during sinus surgery because of its close proximity to the ethmoid sinus. Complete rectus muscle transection has been associated with microdebrider use.[11] When postoperative diplopia is reported by the patient, an evaluation should include an ophthalmic consultation to document visual acuity and globe status, and CT scan to localize the site and extent of injury.

Spontaneous resolution of diplopia can be seen when the etiology is intraorbital inflammation or superficial muscle injury. The use of an eye patch or an eyeglass prism may improve mild diplopia, but is not a good long-term treatment option. For more extensive muscle injury, strabismus surgery is needed to correct persistent double vision. With severe injury or the complete transection of a rectus muscle, diplopia may remain despite surgical repair.[21,22]

Epiphora

Injury to the nasolacrimal duct can occur during the performance of maxillary sinus antrostomy. This complication is most commonly seen when the back-biting forceps or microdebrider is used to enlarge the maxillary ostium too far in an anterior direction, resulting in a transection of the duct (**Fig. 29.8**). Nasolacrimal obstruction presents with persistent tearing (epiphora) or lacrimal sac infection (dacryocystitis).[23] The nasolacrimal duct, which is located ~10 mm anterior to the natural maxillary ostium, is protected by the thick bone of the frontal process of the maxilla, which should not be violated. Injury to the lacrimal drainage system can be prevented by avoiding removal

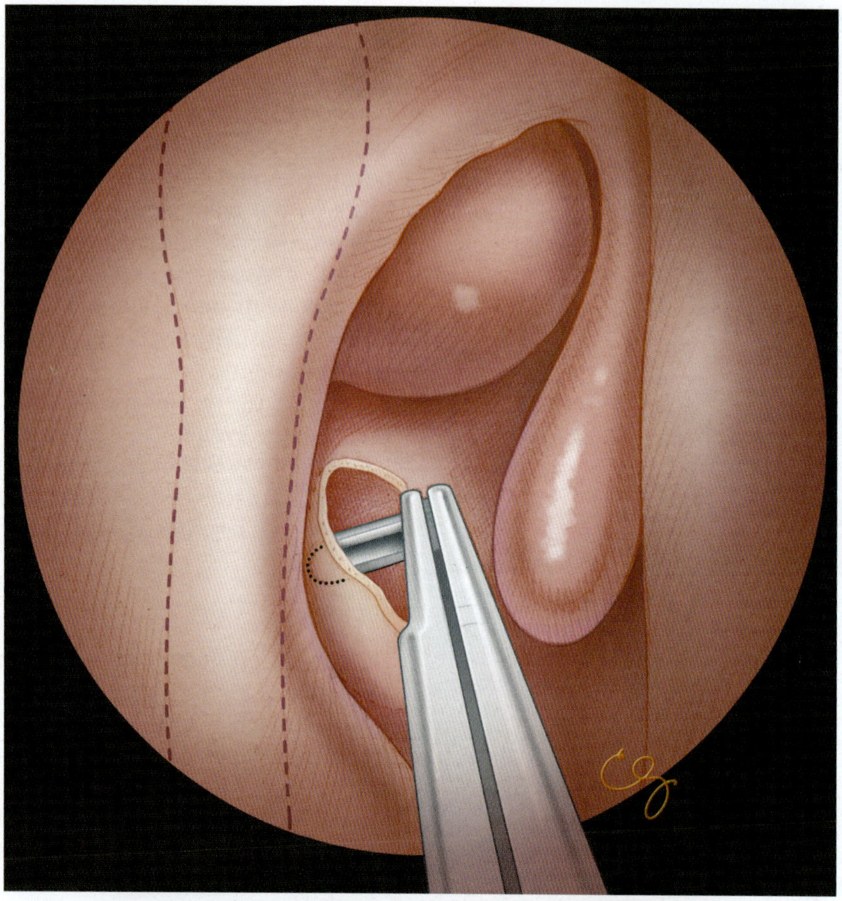

A

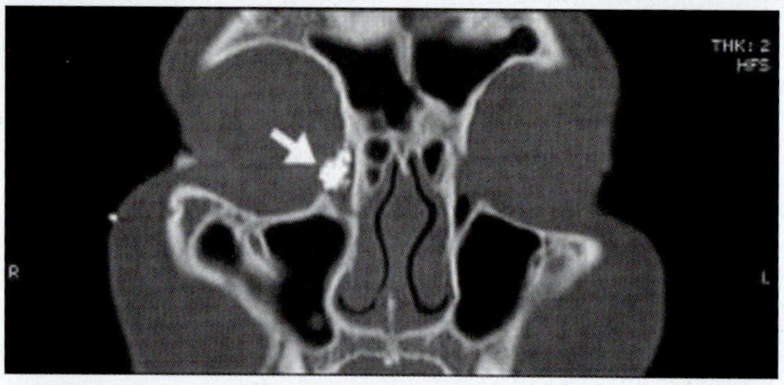

B

Fig. 29.8 (A) When using a back-biting instrument to enlarge the natural maxillary ostium, injury to the nasolacrimal duct can occur if dissection proceeds too far anteriorly through the thick bone of the frontal process of the maxilla. **(B)** Computed tomography dacryocystogram following sinus surgery shows the retention of contrast material in the right lacrimal sac (*arrow*) indicative of injury to the nasolacrimal duct.

of the bone anterior to the maxillary line when enlarging the ostium.

Postoperative epiphora is treated with probing, irrigation, or intubation of the lacrimal system. If epiphora persists despite conservative measures or is accompanied by recurrent dacryocystitis, endoscopic dacryocystorhinostomy (DCR) is recommended to reestablish lacrimal drainage.[24–26]

Orbital Infection

Postoperative orbital infection secondary to extension of sinusitis can occur from either the direct spread of bacteria through bony dehiscence in the lamina papyracea or through retrograde thrombophlebitis from valveless veins that drain both the sinuses and the orbits. Patients who develop signs of periorbital cellulitis, including eye pain, periorbital edema, and erythema, should be treated with broad-spectrum oral or intravenous antibiotics. Removal of any intranasal packing and close monitoring for an extension of the infection into the orbital compartment are also recommended. Worsening symptoms with restricted eye mobility and vision changes require CT imaging to rule out an orbital cellulitis, abscess, or cavernous sinus thrombosis.

Intracranial Complications

Cerebrospinal Fluid Leak

Patients who report persistent, unilateral, and watery rhinorrhea following sinus surgery may have a CSF leak. Nasal endoscopy can be useful to look for pulsatile tissue or clear fluid drainage suggestive of a skull base defect. In most cases, however, clear nasal drainage is evident when the patient leans forward. A CT scan is needed to evaluate the integrity of the skull base, looking for the presence of a bony defect or pneumocephalus (**Fig. 29.9**).

If there is question of whether the drainage is CSF or mucus, which can be difficult to differentiate in the early postoperative period, a sample of nasal fluid should be collected for beta-2 transferrin assay. This test is highly specific for CSF fluid, although false negatives and positives have been reported, particularly when the sample size is small. Use of prophylactic oral antibiotics in patients with CSF leaks is controversial, as they may mask impending meningitis or may select for resistant organisms. While awaiting definitive treatment, patients must be counseled regarding the signs and symptoms of meningitis and instructed to seek immediate medical care should any clinical changes develop. Although conservative measures, including lumbar drainage catheter and bed rest, have been described for the treatment of CSF leaks, when such leaks occur following sinus surgery, early surgical repair is recommended to decrease the risk of meningitis.

Parenchymal Brain Injury

Parenchymal brain injury and intracranial bleeding during endoscopic sinus surgery may occur if an instrument is passed through an unrecognized skull base defect. Mental status change or neurologic deficits in the immediate postoperative period are suggestive of such neurologic injury. In these cases, an immediate CT scan or magnetic resonance imaging (MRI) and neurosurgical consultation are needed to determine the site and extent of brain tissue injury. If intracranial bleeding is identified, control through an open or endovascular approach may be necessary.

Central Nervous System Infection

Although rare, infectious intracranial complications, including meningitis, intracranial abscess, and cavernous sinus thrombosis, have been reported following endoscopic sinus surgery. Meningitis is usually the result of an unidentified CSF leak, where there is direct bacterial spread from the sinonasal cavity through a skull base defect. When a patient develops severe headache, high fever, photophobia, and nuchal rigidity after sinus surgery, emergent evaluation with CT scan, lumbar puncture, and neurologic consultation is indicated. Intravenous antibiotics are the mainstay of treatment for meningitis.

Intracranial abscesses can develop in the epidural, subdural, or intraparenchymal spaces, necessitating neurosurgical drainage. Cavernous sinus thrombosis occurs from venous extension of sinus or orbital infection, and presents with signs of proptosis, chemosis, and ophthalmoplegia. The diagnosis is confirmed by MRI/magnetic resonance venography. Intravenous antibiotics and anticoagulation should be administered under the care of infectious disease and neurology consultants.

A B

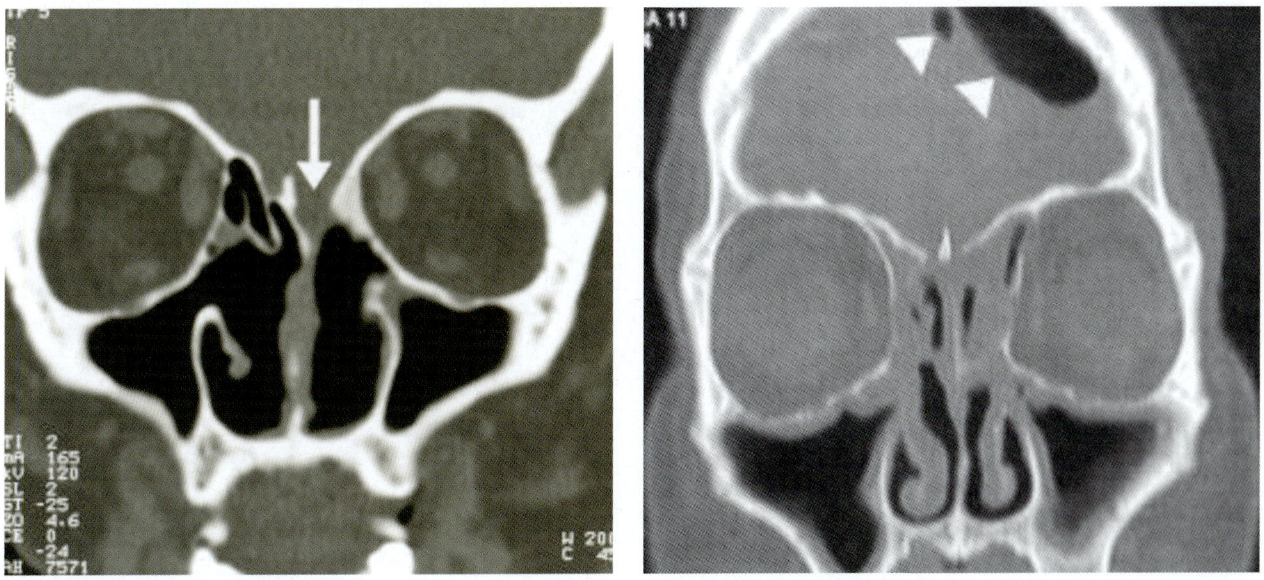

Fig. 29.9 **(A)** Computed tomography (CT) scan of a patient with a cerebrospinal fluid (CSF) leak following sinus surgery reveals a defect in the cribriform plate (*arrow*). **(B)** CT scan of a patient with mental status changes following endoscopic sinus surgery demonstrates pneumocephalus (*arrowheads*). A skull base defect was identified in the anterior ethmoid roof. Endoscopic repair resulted in resolution of the CSF leak, resorption of the intracranial air, and return of normal neurologic function.

Conclusion

Complications of both minor and major consequence are associated with the performance of endoscopic sinus surgery. Their avoidance depends on preoperative awareness of potential surgical pitfalls, proper knowledge of sinonasal anatomy, meticulous surgical technique, and adequate intraoperative hemostasis. When complications do occur, prompt recognition and appropriate management usually result in good patient outcomes.

References

1. Dalziel K, Stein K, Round A, Garside R, Royle P. Endoscopic sinus surgery for the excision of nasal polyps: A systematic review of safety and effectiveness. Am J Rhinol 2006;20(5):506–519
2. Stankiewicz JA. Complications in endoscopic intranasal ethmoidectomy: an update. Laryngoscope 1989;99(7 Pt 1): 686–690
3. Kennedy DW, Shaman P, Han W, Selman H, Deems DA, Lanza DC. Complications of ethmoidectomy: a survey of fellows of the American Academy of Otolaryngology-Head and Neck Surgery. Otolaryngol Head Neck Surg 1994;111(5):589–599
4. May M, Levine HL, Mester SJ, Schaitkin B. Complications of endoscopic sinus surgery: analysis of 2108 patients—incidence and prevention. Laryngoscope 1994;104(9):1080–1083
5. Stankiewicz JA, Chow JM. The low skull base: an invitation to disaster. Am J Rhinol 2004;18(1):35–40
6. Smith TL, Stewart MG, Orlandi RR, Setzen M, Lanza DC. Indications for image-guided sinus surgery: the current evidence. Am J Rhinol 2007;21(1):80–83
7. Blackwell KE, Ross DA, Kapur P, Calcaterra TC. Propofol for maintenance of general anesthesia: a technique to limit blood loss during endoscopic sinus surgery. Am J Otolaryngol 1993;14(4):262–266
8. Pletcher SD, Metson R. Endoscopic ligation of the anterior ethmoid artery. Laryngoscope 2007;117(2):378–381
9. Stankiewicz JA. Blindness and intranasal endoscopic ethmoidectomy: prevention and management. Otolaryngol Head Neck Surg 1989;101(3):320–329
10. Thacker NM, Velez FG, Demer JL, Wang MB, Rosenbaum AL. Extraocular muscle damage associated with endoscopic sinus surgery: an ophthalmology perspective. Am J Rhinol 2005;19 (4):400 -405
11. Bhatti MT, Giannoni CM, Raynor E, Monshizadeh R, Levine LM. Ocular motility complications after endoscopic sinus surgery with powered cutting instruments. Otolaryngol Head Neck Surg 2001;125(5):501–509
12. Kainz J, Stammberger H. The roof of the anterior ethmoid: a place of least resistance in the skull base. Am J Rhinol 1989;3:191–199
13. Hegazy HM, Carrau RL, Snyderman CH, Kassam A, Zweig J. Transnasal endoscopic repair of cerebrospinal fluid rhinorrhea: a meta-analysis. Laryngoscope 2000;110(7):1166–1172
14. Banks CA, Palmer JN, Chiu AG, O'Malley BW Jr, Woodworth BA, Kennedy DW. Endoscopic closure of CSF rhinorrhea: 193 cases over 21 years. Otolaryngol Head Neck Surg 2009;140(6):826–833
15. Orlandi RR, Lanza DC. Is nasal packing necessary following endoscopic sinus surgery? Laryngoscope 2004;114(9):1541–1544
16. Mo JH, Han DH, Shin HW, Cha W, Chang MY, Jin HR. No packing versus packing after endoscopic sinus surgery: pursuit of patients' comfort after surgery. Am J Rhinol 2008;22(5):525–528
17. Venkatachalam VVP, Bhat A. Comparative evaluation of endoscopic and conventional surgical techniques in the management of nasal polyposis. JK Pract 1998;5:295–299
18. Jafek BW, Murrow B, Johnson EW. Olfaction and endoscopic sinus surgery. Ear Nose Throat J 1994;73(8):548–552
19. Ramadan HH. Surgical causes of failure in endoscopic sinus surgery. Laryngoscope 1999;109(1):27–29
20. Sindwani R, Cohen JT, Pilch BZ, Metson RB. Myospherulosis following sinus surgery: pathological curiosity or important clinical entity? Laryngoscope 2003;113(7):1123–1127
21. Penne RB, Flanagan JC, Stefanyszyn MA, Nowinski T. Ocular motility disorders secondary to sinus surgery. Ophthal Plast Reconstr Surg 1993;9(1):53–61
22. Dawson EL, Boyle NJ, Lee JP. Full-tendon nasal transposition of the vertical rectus muscles: a retrospective review. Strabismus 2007;15(3):133–136
23. Serdahl CL, Berris CE, Chole RA. Nasolacrimal duct obstruction after endoscopic sinus surgery. Arch Ophthalmol 1990;108(3):391–392
24. Metson R. Endoscopic surgery for lacrimal obstruction. Otolaryngol Head Neck Surg 1991;104(4):473–479
25. Tsirbas A, Davis G, Wormald PJ. Mechanical endonasal dacryocystorhinostomy versus external dacryocystorhinostomy. Ophthal Plast Reconstr Surg 2004;20(1):50–56
26. Leong SC, Macewen CJ, White PS. A systematic review of outcomes after dacryocystorhinostomy in adults. Am J Rhinol Allergy 2010;24(1):81–90

30 Congenital Sinonasal Disorders

Man-Kit Leung, Paul R. Krakovitz, and Peter J. Koltai

A variety of congenital sinonasal disorders can afflict the newborn child. These anomalies may be due to maldevelopment of structures intrinsic to the nose and nasal cavity or to maldevelopment of paranasal structures extrinsic to the nose but involving the nose. Moreover, these anomalies may occur in isolation or in association with craniofacial syndromes. This chapter reviews several congenital sinonasal disorders and their management.

Disorders of the Nose and Nasal Cavity

A broad range of nasal maldevelopments can occur with a structure as complex as the nose. These include partial and complete failure of nasal development or, on the opposite extreme, duplications. The degree and location of nasal dysgenesis leads to a variety of both cosmetic and nasal obstructive abnormalities.

Arhinia, Polyrrhinia, and Proboscis Lateralis

Complete congenital nasal agenesis, or arhinia, is extremely rare (**Fig. 30.1**). It is considered an anomaly in the spectrum of holoprosencephaly, a disorder caused by the failure of the prosencephalon to divide into the double lobes of the cerebral hemispheres. This results in a single-lobed brain structure with severe skull and facial defects. Little is known about the pathogenesis of arhinia and most cases appear to occur sporadically. Because of the rarity of this disease, established management protocols do not exist. In general, congenital absence of the nose is compatible with life and can be treated with supportive measures, such as a McGovern nipple or an oral airway, followed by delayed reconstruction.[1] When airway distress is present, a tracheotomy should be considered.

Polyrrhinia, or double nose, is another extremely rare disorder. It can be associated with pseudohypertelorism,

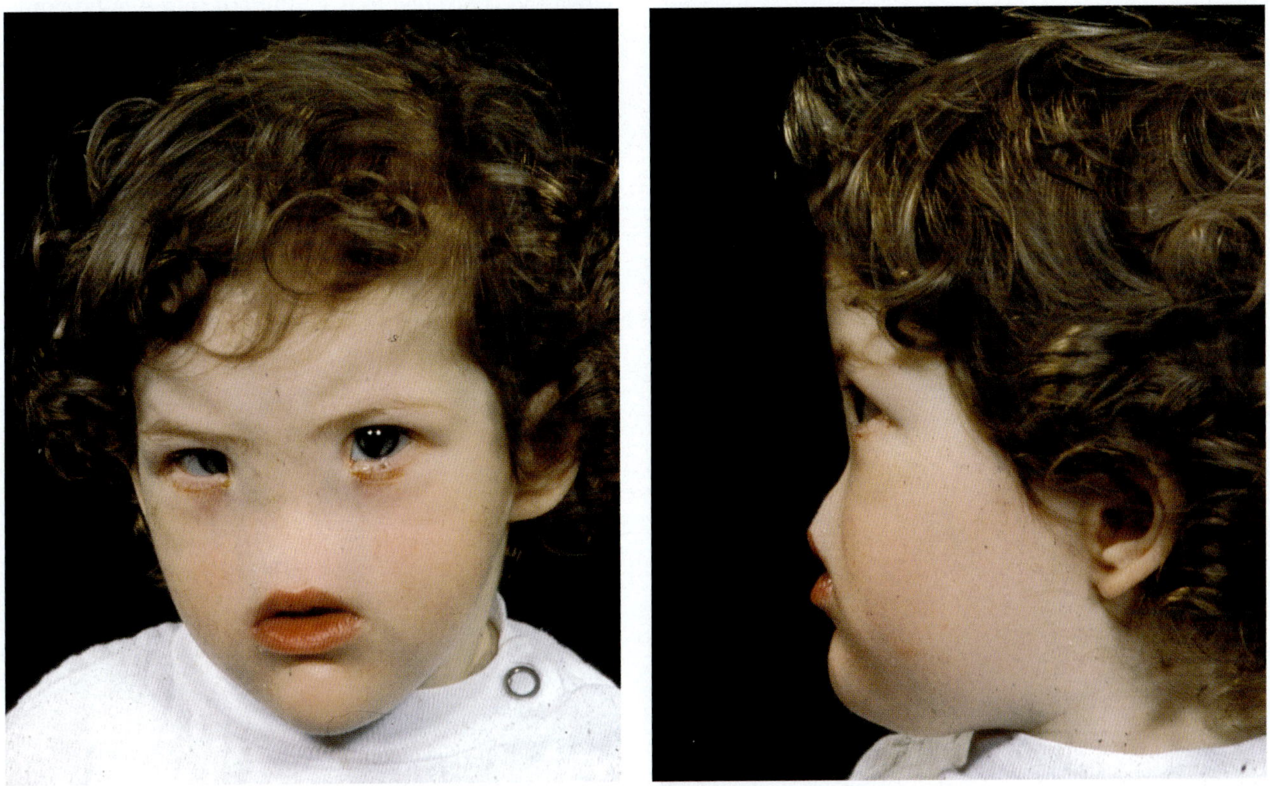

A B

Fig. 30.1 (A,B) Frontal and lateral views of a child with arhinia.

but it can also be an isolated anomaly. Patients usually present with bilateral choanal atresia. Treatment includes an initial repair of choanal atresia followed by correction of the external nasal duplication deformity.[2]

Proboscis lateralis typically presents as a tubular sleeve of skin originating from the region of the medial canthus of the orbit. It is characterized by a central tract lined with squamous and ciliated respiratory epithelium.[3] Proboscis lateralis is associated with ipsilateral sinonasal hypoplasia or aplasia. Diagnostic imaging includes computed tomography (CT) and/or magnetic resonance imaging (MRI) to delineate the extent of the malformation. Treatment involves the excision of the proboscis and reconstruction of the ipsilateral nose and nasal cavity. Occasionally, soft tissue and skin from the proboscis can be used in the reconstruction of the nose and should be considered prior to a complete excision. Nasal stents and postoperative serial dilations are usually necessary.

Congenital Nasal Tip Deviation

Asymmetrical nasal tip deformity is an occasional problem found in newborns. These neonates typically present with a flattening of the nasal tip to one side with the septum deviated in the same direction (**Fig. 30.2**). The bony dorsum is invariably straight. This type of deformity may be the result of acute traumatic birth injury or, more likely, prolonged intrauterine positional pressure.

Although some reports have advocated immediate surgical reduction by straightening and relocating the septum, in the authors' experience these deformities tend to straighten over time without intervention and without late sequelae. Treatment for these infants is to reassure the parents that the nose will straighten out in time. In general, even severe nasal tip deformities have not been found to cause airway obstruction in the nasally obligate neonate.[4]

Nasal Hemangiomas

Hemangiomas are benign vascular tumors that commonly occur in the head and neck and appear during the first several weeks of life. Nasal hemangiomas may present as an asymptomatic external or internal nasal mass (**Fig. 30.3**). Whereas external nasal hemangiomas can be found anywhere along the entire length of the nose, intranasal hemangiomas typically occur on the turbinates or septum. Aesthetic deformity is the norm. Intranasal hemangiomas can cause varying degrees of nasal obstruction, whereas large paranasal hemangiomas can be associated with visual obstruction. Because hemangiomas can have superficial cutaneous and/or deep soft tissue components, an MRI may be useful in delineating the full extent of these lesions. The classic natural history of hemangiomas is characterized by a rapid proliferation phase during the first year of life, followed by a quiescence and an involution phase that can last until 9 years of age.

Consensus over the best treatment of nasal hemangiomas continues to evolve. Given the natural course of these lesions to spontaneously regress, some recommend serial observation for lesions that do not obstruct the airway, impair feeding, or bleed from ulceration. Oral steroids can be used during the proliferative phase; however, rebound growth is a concern as are the well recognized side effects of systemic corticosteroids. Recent studies have demonstrated a growing role for oral propranolol, a nonselective beta-blocker that has been shown to accelerate involution of infantile hemangiomas. In a randomized, double-blind, placebo-controlled trial, a 6-month course of propranolol was found to reduce hemangioma color, volume, and elevation.[5] For nonsegmental, localized nasal tip lesions, intralesional steroid (Kenalog 40 mg/mL) injection is an excellent treatment option, although there are theoretical concerns of upper or lower lateral cartilage degeneration. Pulse dyed laser therapy can be used to address the cutaneous components but will not affect the subcutaneous parts of the lesion. Historically, surgical excision was reserved for lesions that obstruct the airway, impair vision, or cause

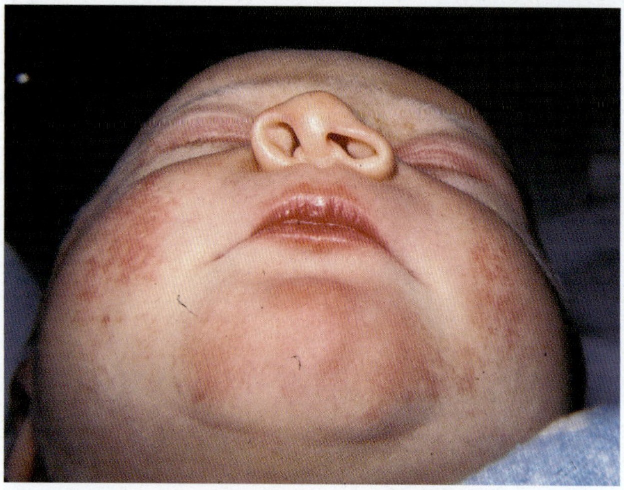

Fig. 30.2 Newborn with congenital septal deviation.

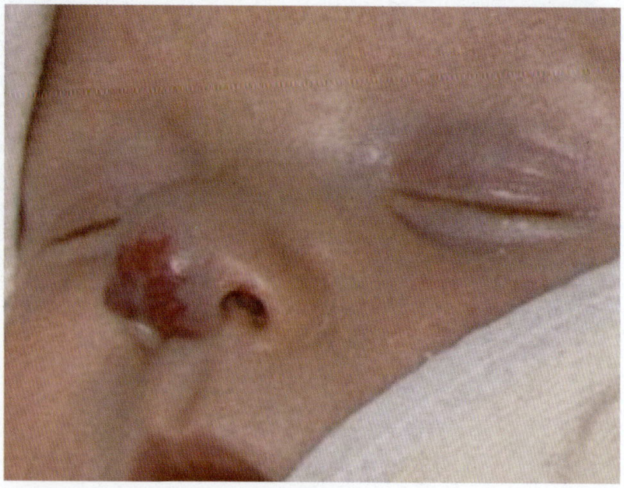

Fig. 30.3 Newborn with nasal tip hemangioma.

severe cosmetic deformities. However, there is a growing body of literature supporting early surgical resection after a trial of observation, arguing that nasal hemangiomas can distort the growing nasal architecture, can cause undue psychological disturbance in childhood development, and can be excised with aesthetic results that may be superior to their natural course.[6,7] Using each of these treatment modalities allows for case-specific therapy depending on the characteristics of the lesion.

Pyriform Aperture Stenosis

Pyriform aperture stenosis (PAS) was first recognized as a distinct clinical entity in 1989 and is characterized by bony narrowing of the premaxillary pyriform aperture with resultant anterior nasal obstruction. The pyriform aperture is the narrowest part of the newborn nasal airway, and even small changes in the diameter can affect nasal resistance. Newborns can present with varying degrees of airway compromise with symptoms similar to choanal atresia. PAS may occur in isolation or in association with other congenital abnormalities, such as holoprosencephaly, submucous cleft palate, an absence of anterior pituitary gland, or hypoplastic maxillary sinuses.[8]

On physical exam, an anterior rhinoscopy reveals narrowed nasal passageways with difficulty passing a 2.5-mm endoscope. A single central maxillary incisor has been associated with PAS. CT scans are diagnostic, revealing extreme narrowing at the level of the pyriform aperture and bony compression of the nasal soft tissues (**Fig. 30.4**). A pyriform aperture with a width of <11 mm on an axial CT at the level of the inferior meatus for a term infant has been considered diagnostic for PAS.[9]

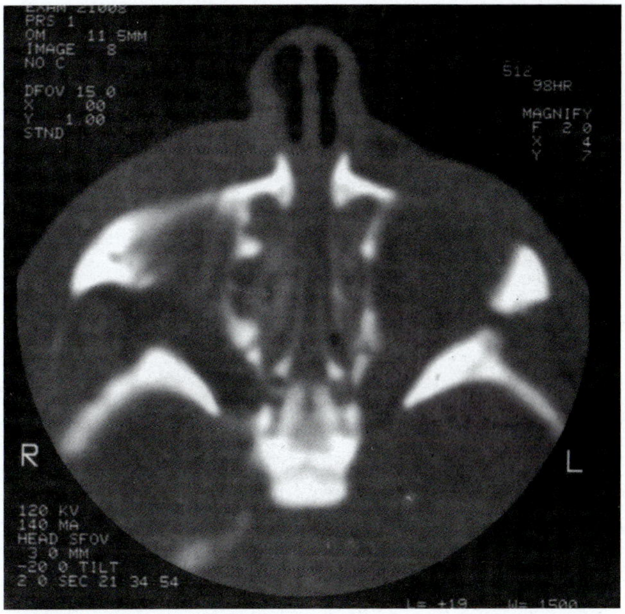

Fig. 30.4 Axial computed tomography image showing extreme narrowing at the level of the pyriform aperture indicative of pyriform aperture stenosis.

Mild cases of PAS may be handled with conservative management, including topical steroid drops, careful suctioning, and humidification. More severe cases may require a more aggressive management with an oral airway, gavage feedings, and surgical correction. When surgical intervention is warranted, the premaxillary soft tissues are elevated via a sublabial incision, thus exposing the caudal septum and pyriform aperture (**Fig. 30.5**). The pyriform aperture is enlarged with an otologic diamond drill

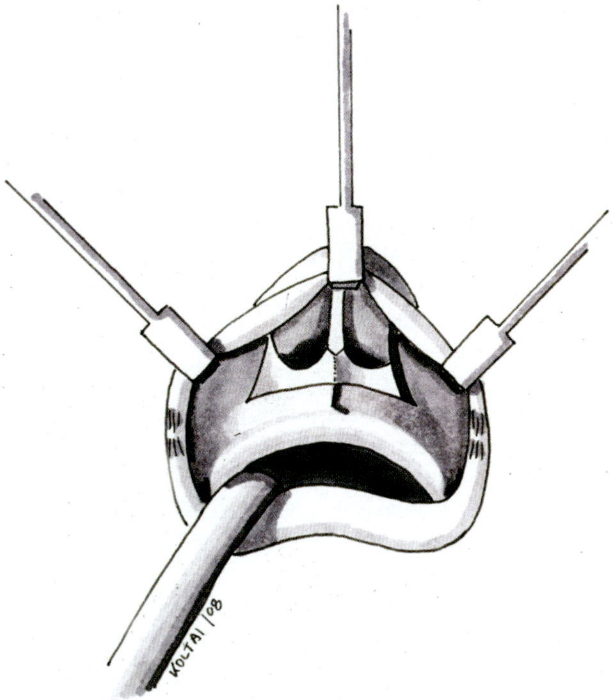

A

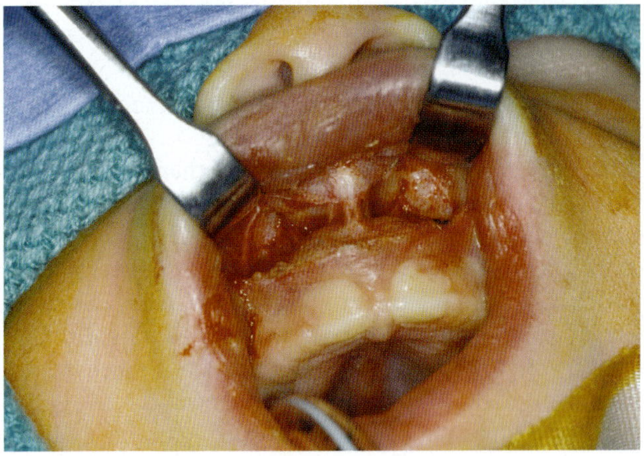

B

Fig. 30.5 **(A)** Illustration of the sublabial approach to repair a nasal pyriform aperture stenosis. **(B)** Intraoperative view of the sublabial approach to repair of a nasal pyriform aperture stenosis.

laterally to the maxillary sinus and sagittally to the inferior turbinate. Care must be taken to avoid injury to the nasolacrimal system and to tooth buds, which may abut the nasal floor. Postoperatively, the nasal airway is stented with a 3.5-mm endotracheal tube for 1 week. We prefer to keep the infant on oral antibiotics while the stents are in place. When the stents are removed, we use topical steroid/antibiotic drops to facilitate mucosal healing.

Choanal Atresia

Choanal atresia (CA) is characterized by a narrowing of the posterior opening of the nasal cavity into the nasopharynx (**Fig. 30.6A,B**). The condition occurs in 1:5000 to 1:8000 live births and affects females twice as often as males. Unilateral CA accounts for 65 to 75% of all cases. Bilateral CA is frequently associated with other anomalies; the most common associated syndrome is CHARGE (*c*oloboma and cranial nerve palsies, *h*eart defects, *a*tresia of the choanae, *r*etardation of growth and development, *g*enitourinary anomalies, *e*ar malformations, and hearing loss). Polydactyly, nasal, auricular and palatal deformities, Crouzon syndrome, craniosynostosis, microencephaly, meningocele, facial asymmetry, cleft palate, and hypertelorism are also often seen in patients with CA. In utero exposure to methimazole has been associated with increased rates of CA.[10]

CA is believed to be caused by persistence of the buccopharyngeal membranes or by failure of the oronasal membranes to rupture. The four parts of the anatomic deformity include a narrow nasal cavity, medialization of the lateral pterygoid plate, widening of the vomer into a diamond shape, and a thinning of the atresia plate inferomedially. Historically, cases of CA have been classified as 90% bony and 10% membranous, but recent reviews using CT studies suggest that 30% are pure bony, whereas 70% are mixed bony-membranous.[11] In the authors' experience, we have never seen a purely membranous choanal atresia.

The presentation of bilateral CA is characterized by respiratory distress at birth and cyclic cyanosis that is relieved with crying and is exacerbated with feeding. In contrast, a unilateral CA may not present until later in life as complaints of unilateral rhinorrhea and nasal obstruction. Exam findings include the inability to pass a small catheter into the nasopharynx and a lack of condensation on a mirror placed at the nares. The diagnosis is made with nasal endoscopy and is further classified with the use of a noncontrast CT (**Fig. 30.6C,D**). On CT imaging, CA is diagnosed if the posterior choanal orifice measures less than 0.34 cm unilaterally or if the posterior vomer measures greater than 0.55 cm.[12]

Unilateral atresia generally is managed with elective surgery after the first postnatal year. In contrast, bilateral atresia will cause significant respiratory distress in a newborn and must be addressed in the perinatal period. Immediate management of a bilateral CA involves training the infant to breathe through the mouth with an indwelling oral appliance such as a McGovern nipple or an oral airway. In an emergency, the infant can be stimulated to cry or be intubated. Although a bilateral CA should be corrected in the perinatal period, it cannot be overemphasized that a full multisystem evaluation must be completed prior to surgical correction. Tracheotomy can be considered if definitive surgery must be delayed because of associated anomalies.

Surgery for CA can be approached through transnasal, transseptal, or transpalatal routes. Regardless of the approach, the key to a successful repair is creating an adequate three-dimensional opening by removing the widened posterior vomer and thinning the lateral pterygoid plate. With the transnasal approach, a nasal endoscopy is performed and a perforation is made in the atretic plate at the junction of the nasal floor and septum using a no. 10 curved urethral sound. Subsequently, the posterior vomer is resected and the lateral nasal wall and pterygoid plates are thinned under direct visualization with a drill. Mucosal flaps should be preserved wherever possible. When a direct nasal endoscopy with resection is difficult, we prefer a sublabial transseptal approach using endoscopy. This allows for direct submucosal access to the vomer and the atresia plate. The vomer is resected en bloc via a common cavity provided by lateralization of the anterior septum. Moreover, by initially performing the bony resection, the mucosa in the posterior nose is preserved and one can create mucosal flaps that cover the neo-choanae in a practical and consistent fashion. Historically, once the choanae were opened appropriately, stents made from polyethylene endotracheal tubes were placed for 1 to 8 weeks. Recent literature, however, has challenged the necessity for stents, citing high rates of long-term nasal patency without stenting.[13,14]

The transpalatal approach is often used by surgeons comfortable with palatal surgery in the newborn or in revisions of transnasal failures. There is controversy with this approach due to concerns about orthodontic growth and development. Although the reported incidence of malocclusion has been reported to be as high as 50% in young patients undergoing transpalatal repair, we question the validity of these findings. With this approach, the mucosa is elevated off the hard palate back to its posterior edge and pedicled on the greater palatine artery. The atresia plate and a substantial portion of the posterior vomer are obliterated with an otologic drill. A passage between the nose and the nasopharynx is thus established.

Both the transnasal and transpalatal approaches result in a functional nasal airway in ~50 to 80% of children. Postsurgical topical medications, such as mitomycin C, have shown promise in preventing restenosis. In addition, the authors will occasionally inject steroids (Kenalog 40 mg/mL) to the borders of the neo-choanae.

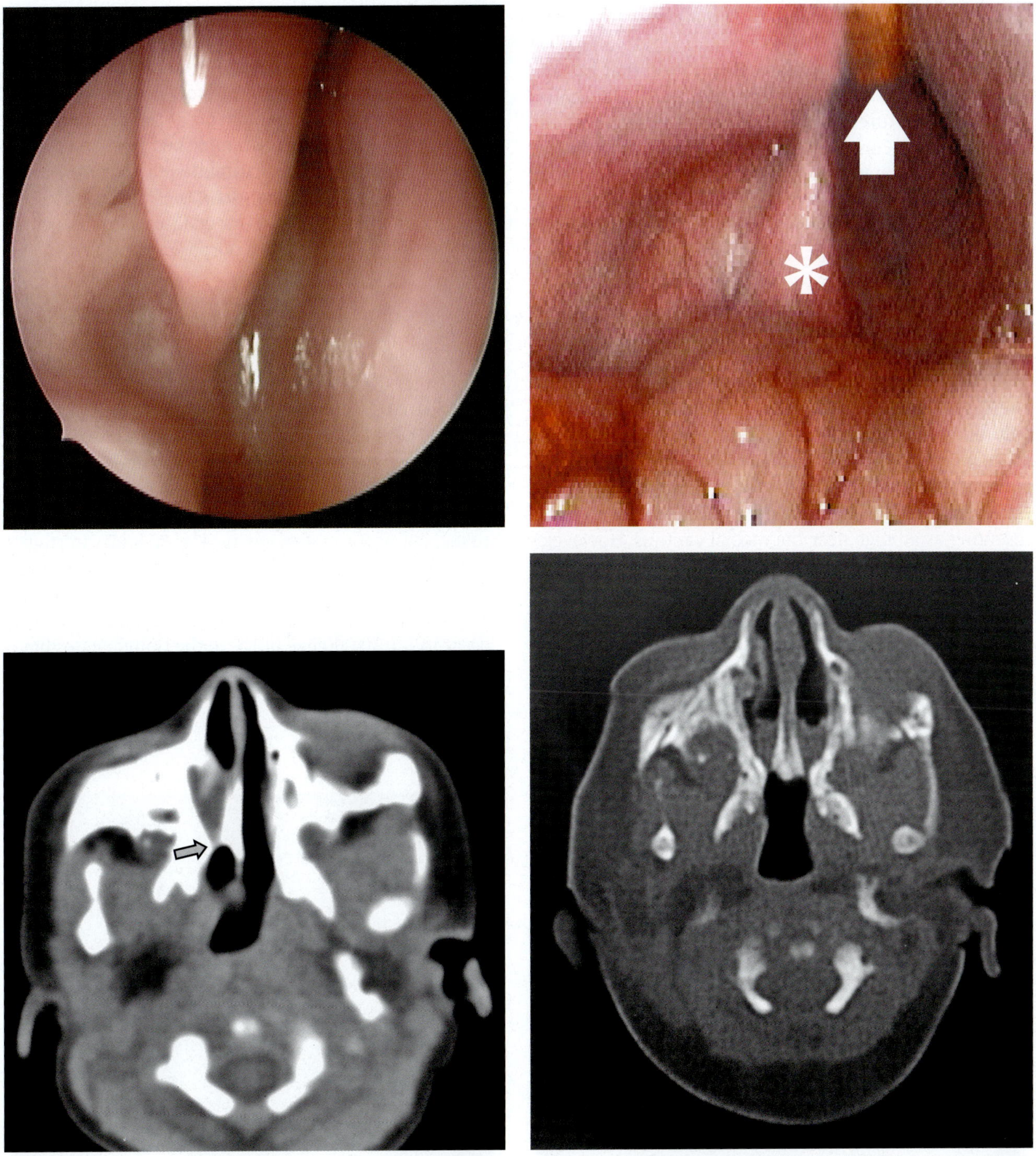

A B C D

Fig. 30.6 **(A)** Endoscopic view of a right-sided choanal atresia. **(B)** Transoral mirror view of a unilateral, right-sided choanal atresia. A red rubber catheter has been passed through the patent left choana (*arrow*) lateral to the nasal septum (*asterisk*). **(C)** Axial computed tomography (CT) image depicting a unilateral right-sided choanal atresia (*arrow*). **(D)** Axial CT image depicting a bilateral choanal atresia.

Nonetheless, restenosis requiring serial dilatation is common. In the authors' experience, attention to adequate resection of the offending vomer, mucosal preservation, and short-term stenting when necessary, followed by diligent postoperative wound care, are keys to a high success rate. We prefer bringing the children back to the operating room after 1 week to remove the stents. The operative site is endoscopically debrided, mitomycin (0.4 mg/mL) is applied, and Kenalog (40 mg/mL) is injected. This process is repeated 2 weeks later. It should be emphasized that this is not for dilatation but for wound care, similar to what is provided in the outpatient setting for patients who have had endoscopic sinus surgery.

Disorders of Paranasal Structures

The nose is situated in an anatomic location that has an important relationship to the eye and brain. Maldevelopment of structures around the nose can manifest as nasal disorders. Common disorders of paranasal structures that can manifest as nasal anomalies include lacrimal cysts and congenital midline nasal masses, which include nasal gliomas, encephaloceles, and nasal dermoids.

Lacrimal Cysts

Lacrimal cysts form when there is both proximal and distal obstruction of the lacrimal drainage system. Accumulation of mucus results in cyst formation. Lacrimal cysts are generally unilateral but can be bilateral and have a strong female preponderance. Patients typically present with epiphora and varying degrees of nasal obstruction. These cysts commonly develop near the medial canthal tendon, presenting as a bulge near the medial canthus. However, intranasal lacrimal cysts can form, often originating beneath the inferior turbinate at the valve of Hasner. Endoscopically, their appearance is similar to a large polyp originating underneath the inferior turbinate (**Fig. 30.7**). When these cysts are large, their origin may not be apparent; consequently, it is important to differentiate them from encephaloceles with appropriate imaging. The obstruction of the lacrimal drainage system resolves spontaneously in 85% of infants by ~9 months. Indications for surgery include infection, respiratory distress, feeding difficulties, or failure to spontaneously regress. Surgical repair, when necessary, is accomplished by marsupializing the cyst into the nose, concurrently relieving the obstruction and restoring lacrimal drainage.[15] The authors have found a small caliber (2.9 mm) endoscopic microdebrider or sickle knife useful for this purpose.

Congenital Midline Nasal Masses: Nasal Gliomas, Encephaloceles, and Nasal Dermoids

Congenital midline nasal masses are rare anomalies that include nasal gliomas, encephaloceles, and nasal dermoids. These lesions are differentiated by their tissues of origin. Whereas gliomas are composed of unencapsulated glial cells within a connective tissue matrix, encephaloceles are herniations of meninges, with or without brain tissue, out of the cranial cavity (**Fig. 30.8A,B**). In contrast, dermoids are lesions derived from entrapped ectoderm and mesoderm and contain skin, hair follicles, sebaceous glands, and sweat glands. Congenital midline nasal masses occur in ~1:30,000 live births in the United States but are more common among Asians, occurring in ~1:6000 live births.

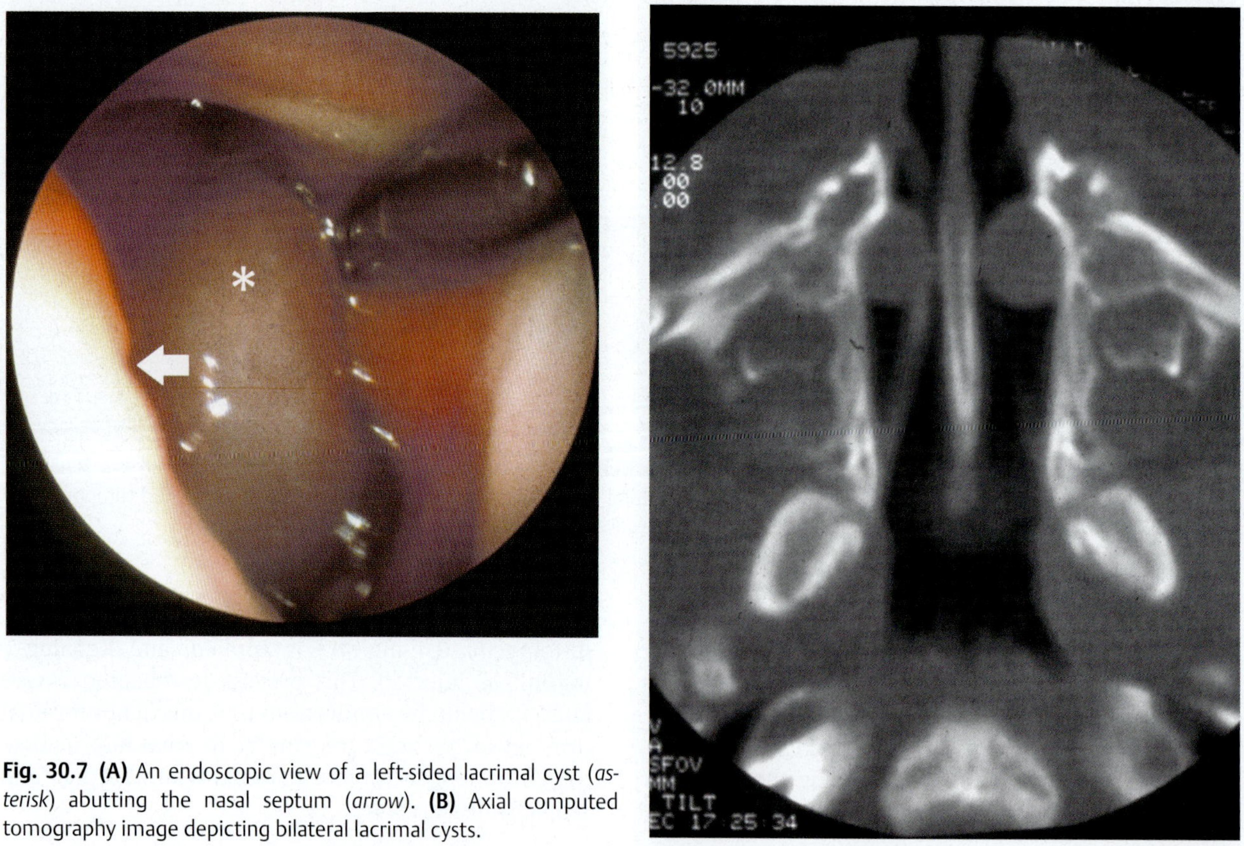

A

B

Fig. 30.7 (A) An endoscopic view of a left-sided lacrimal cyst (*asterisk*) abutting the nasal septum (*arrow*). **(B)** Axial computed tomography image depicting bilateral lacrimal cysts.

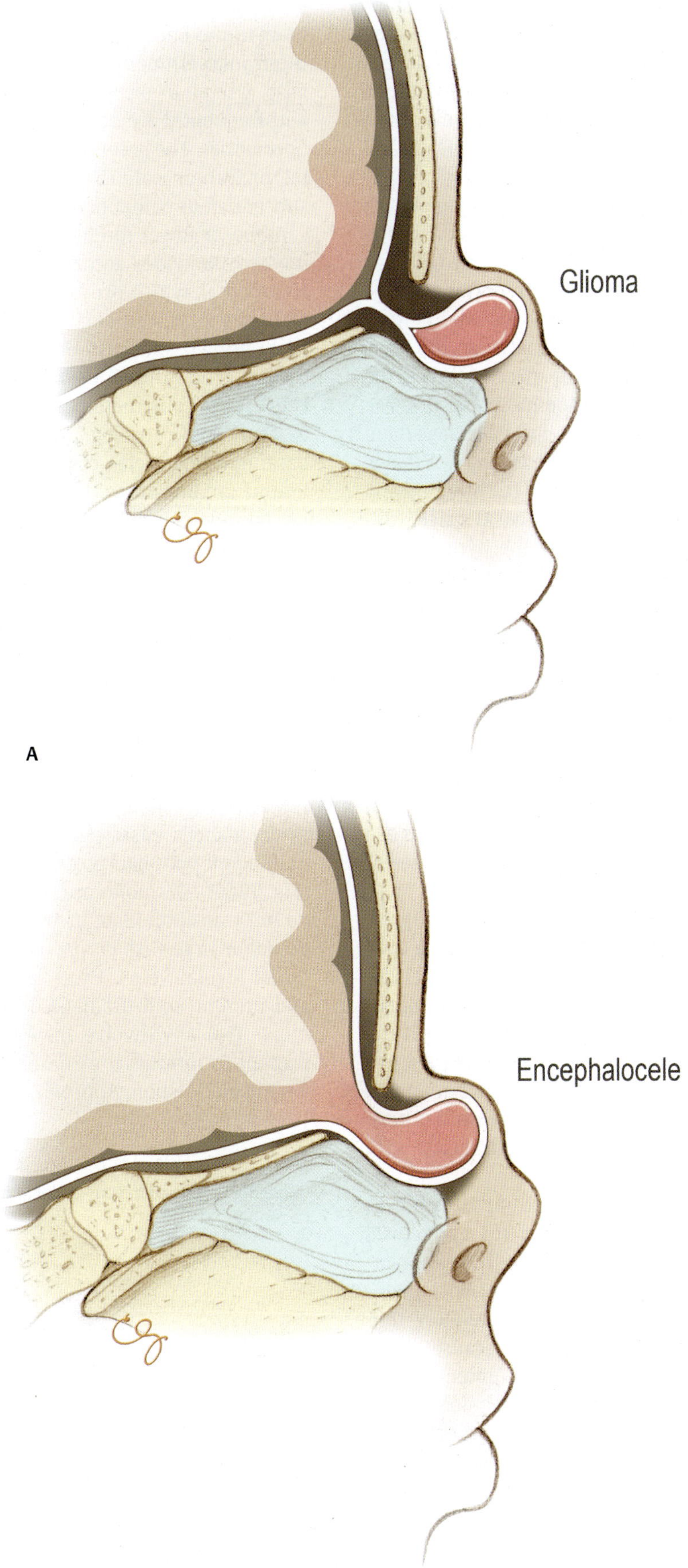

Fig. 30.8 (A) Intranasal glioma with a stalk connection to the dura. **(B)** Encephalocele with herniation of the meninges and brain tissue.

An understanding of these masses requires understanding the embryology of the anterior skull base. Neural tube closure occurs during the 4th week of gestation. Closure begins in the midportion before progressing both anteriorly and posteriorly. The anterior neuropore forms at the optic recess of the sphenoid sinus. The frontal, nasal, and ethmoid structures form proximal to the anterior neuropore. Neural crest cells migrate through this region rich with ectoderm and mesoderm, which form skin, cartilage, and bone. Once in position, the mesenchyme organizes into skeletal structures, forming important spaces that are normally closed by birth. These include the fonticulus nasofrontalis, which is the gap between the frontal and nasal bones, and the prenasal space, which is the area between the nasal bones and the nasal capsule. The nasal capsule is the precursor of the nasal cartilages and septum and is continuous with the ethmoid bone. Finally, the foramen cecum is the region between the ethmoid and frontal bones and connects with the prenasal space. Failure of these spaces to close allows for the herniation of glial tissue and intracranial contents, forming gliomas and encephaloceles. Similarly, ingrowth and entrapment of ectodermal and mesodermal elements through these spaces can lead to dermoid formation.[16]

Gliomas, encephaloceles, and dermoids usually present as midline external or internal nasal masses that are apparent at birth. However, occasionally, the presentation may be subtle, with some children presenting with widened noses, hypertelorism, or nasal obstructions that may not be clinically evident until they are older. These lesions can vary in size and location, and large lesions can cause respiratory distress.

Nasal gliomas may present as extranasal (60%), intranasal (30%), or combined (10%) lesions. If intranasal, they may resemble a unilateral large polyp, which is neither compressible nor pulsatile. They are reddish, firm masses that do not transilluminate or increase in size with the Valsalva maneuver or crying. Gliomas also do not enlarge with the Furstenberg test (a compression of bilateral internal jugular veins). Although 15% of gliomas retain a fibrous attachment to the dura, gliomas do not communicate with the cerebrospinal fluid (CSF).

Like gliomas, encephaloceles can also masquerade as nasal polyposis. In contrast, encephaloceles are bluish, soft, compressible masses that are pulsatile. They are typically attached to the superior nasal septum. Encephaloceles expand with crying and with the Furstenberg test. These lesions should not be manipulated because of the risk of neurologic changes, seizures, and potential meningitis. Biopsy is not advised, because encephaloceles can contain brain tissue that lies in continuity with the CSF. As a general rule, midline nasal masses should not be manipulated or biopsied until a thorough workup, including imaging, is completed.

Encephaloceles can be classified by their content or by their location. Whereas meningoceles contain only meninges, meningoencephaloceles contain meninges and brain tissue. Encephaloceles can occur in the occipital area, the frontal ethmoidal region, or along the anterior skull base. Occipital encephaloceles are most common (75%) and frequently are associated with other congenital abnormalities. The second most common location is sincipital, or frontonasal (15%). These encephaloceles can have subcutaneous components over the nose, glabella, medial canthus, or lower forehead. Sincipital encephaloceles are further subdivided according to location into three types: nasofrontal, which protrude between the nasal and frontal bones; nasoethmoidal, which protrude from the lateral nasal bridge; and naso-orbital, which protrude near the medial orbit. The sincipital encephaloceles occasionally cause nasal obstruction but more typically present as aesthetic and neurologic challenges. Finally, intranasal or basal encephaloceles comprise 10% of the lesions. These lesions can present with nasal obstruction at birth or may not become clinically evident until the child is old enough to complain of unilateral nasal obstruction. Basal encephaloceles can be transethmoidal, sphenoethmoidal, transsphenoidal, or spheno-orbital herniations (**Table 30.1**).

Nasal dermoids are the most common of the congenital midline nasal masses and constitute ~10% of all facial dermoids. Most lesions are present at birth and are diagnosed during childhood. Inheritance is generally sporadic, although rare hereditary forms have been reported. Nasal dermoids can present as a cyst, sinus, or fistula anywhere along the midline nose, from the columella to the glabella. Classically, these lesions can present as a midline pit with hair protrusion, which is pathognomonic (**Fig. 30.9A**). Dermoids are slow-growing, firm masses that do not transilluminate or pulsate. Like gliomas, they also do not enlarge with crying or with compression of the internal jugular veins. These lesions may become infected and present with drainage or an abscess. Although dermoids typically involve the external nose, they can also present as intranasal or nasopharyngeal masses, causing airway obstruction. Approximately 30% of nasal dermoids

Table 30.1 Classification of Encephaloceles by Content and Location

1. Contents:
    a. Meninges (Meningocele)
    b. Meninges + brain tissue (Meningoencephalocele)
2. Location:
    a. Occipital
    b. Sincipital
        i. Nasofrontal
        ii. Nasoethmoidal
        iii. Naso-orbital
    c. Basal
        i. Transethmoidal
        ii. Sphenoethmoidal
        iii. Transsphenoidal
        iv. Spheno-orbital

communicate with the dura, and there is no correlation between an external presentation and an intracranial extension. Consequently, nasal dermoids should not be manipulated or biopsied until imaging has been obtained to rule out intracranial communication (**Table 30.2**).

Regardless of the diagnosis, both CT and MRI are crucial for the evaluation of any congenital midline nasal mass. CT details the bony anatomy that serves as a roadmap for surgical excision and can identify skull base defects. An enlarged foramen cecum or bifid crista galli found on CT should raise suspicion, but is not diagnostic, for intracranial involvement (**Fig. 30.9B,C**). On the other hand, an absent foramen cecum or normal crista galli on CT makes intracranial extension unlikely.[17] MRI can characterize the soft tissue component, delineate boundaries, and determine if an intracranial extension is present (**Fig. 30.9D**). Normally, the crista galli in infants is unossified and does not contain marrow fat. Any high-intensity

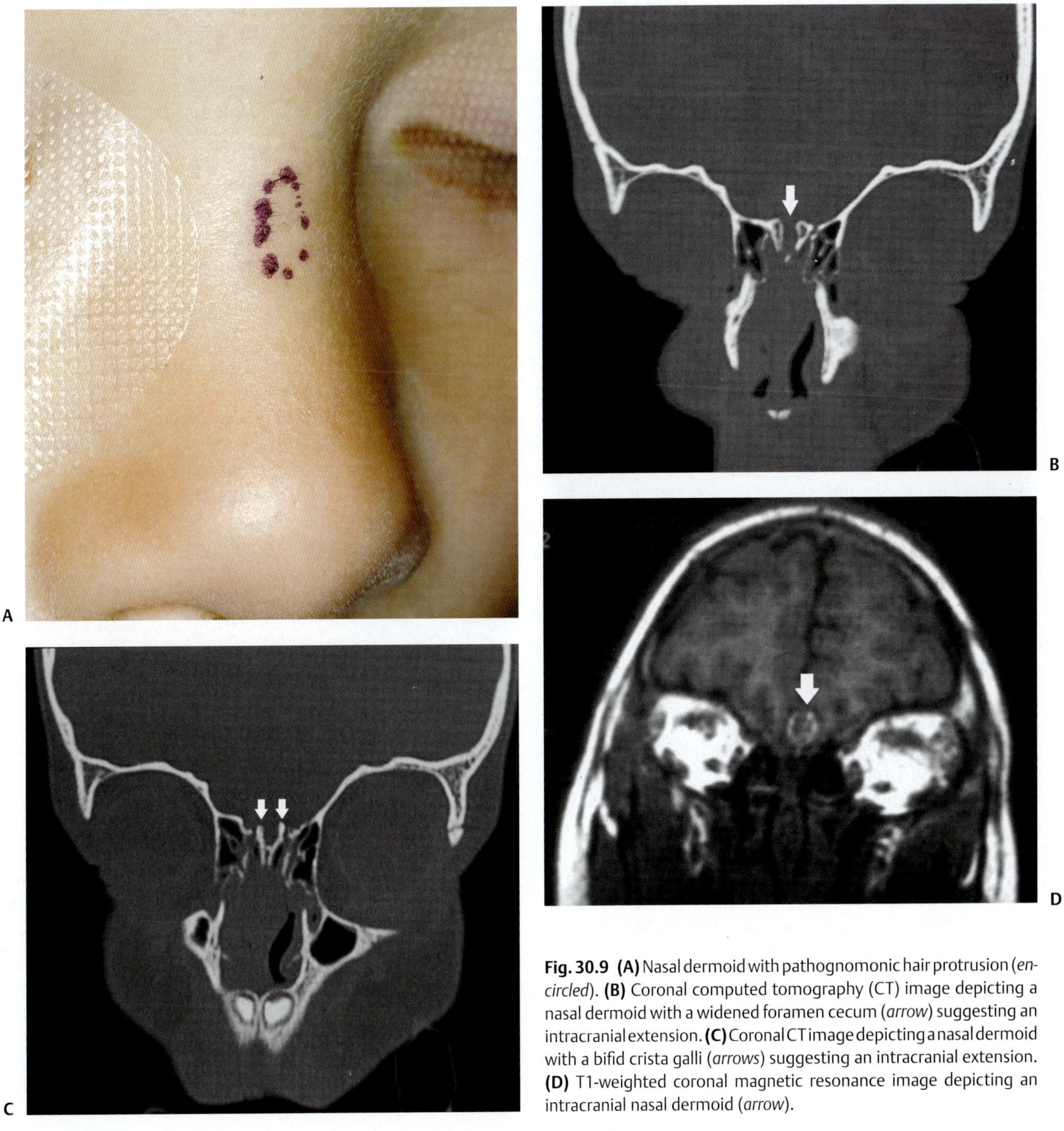

Fig. 30.9 **(A)** Nasal dermoid with pathognomonic hair protrusion (*encircled*). **(B)** Coronal computed tomography (CT) image depicting a nasal dermoid with a widened foramen cecum (*arrow*) suggesting an intracranial extension. **(C)** Coronal CT image depicting a nasal dermoid with a bifid crista galli (*arrows*) suggesting an intracranial extension. **(D)** T1-weighted coronal magnetic resonance image depicting an intracranial nasal dermoid (*arrow*).

Table 30.2 Distinguishing Features of Congenital Midline Nasal Masses

	Gliomas	Encephaloceles	Dermoids
Contents	Glial cells	Meninges ± brain tissue	Ectodermal/mesodermal derivates (i.e., skin, hair, sweat glands)
Characteristics	Reddish, firm, nonpulsatile	Bluish, soft, pulsatile	Nonpulsatile cyst, sinus, or fistula
Furstenberg test	Negative	Positive	Negative
Intracranial extension	~15%	100%	~30%

signal on T1-weighted images in the vicinity of the crista galli in a newborn should suggest the possibility of an intracranial dermoid.[18]

Surgical excision is the mainstay of treatment for congenital midline nasal masses and often requires a two-teamed approach involving neurosurgeons and otorhinolaryngologists–head and neck surgeons. Although the rare lesion causing airway obstruction should be resected early in life to aid in airway management, in general, the surgical management of both intracranial and extracranial dermoids can be safely delayed until the infant is over 1 year of age. Indications for intervention include recurrent infections, rapid expansion, or facial deformity.

The surgical approach depends on the location and extent of the mass. Pollock and colleagues reviewed the surgical treatment of the nasal dermoid cyst and recommended four criteria for a surgical approach. First, the approach should provide exposure to all midline masses and should readily permit medial and lateral osteotomies, if required. Second, the surgical exposure should favor the rapid repair of cribriform defects, should they be present, and would permit the control of CSF rhinorrhea if it develops. Third, the surgical approach should allow reconstruction of the nasal dorsum, if it is required. Fourth, the approach should offer the probability of acceptable scar formation.[19] To these criteria we suggest the addition of ease of intracranial access with minimal brain retraction.

For lesions with extranasal components, external incisions are often necessary. Traditional incisions include the vertical midline rhinotomy, the lateral rhinotomy, and, more recently, the external rhinoplasty. These incisions can be used in conjunction with a bicoronal incision for a combined extracranial and intracranial approach. When appropriate, the external rhinoplasty with or without a vertical rhinotomy incision can provide excellent exposure through cosmetic incision lines (**Fig. 30.10A,B**).[20] If the lesion tracts deep to the nasal bones, nasal osteotomies may be required and subsequently reconstructed with wire and/or plate fixation. Alternatively, the nasal bones may be removed en bloc via the bicoronal exposure to give wider access to the subosseous portion of the dermoid. A frozen section analysis of the tract at the skull base, which shows only fibrous tissue without an epithelial tract, indicates that the residual tract can be ligated at the skull base without entering the cranial cavity.

Intranasal lesions can be managed with the transnasal endoscopic approach and facilitated by intraoperative image guidance systems. Although there have been many reports documenting successful endoscopic excisions of anterior skull base lesions and repairs of skull base defects in the pediatric population, current technical limitations still favor traditional craniotomy approaches for lesions with intracranial extensions or large skull base defects.[21,22]

A formal anterior bifrontal craniotomy has been the standard approach used to address intracranial components of congenital midline nasal masses. With this approach, a bicoronal incision is made and subpericranial flaps are elevated. A frontal bone flap is created in the skull to allow access into the cranium. Because the frontal bar is left intact, retraction of the frontal lobes of the brain is necessary to visualize the anterior skull base. For lesions tracking to the inferior aspect of the nose, the frontal craniotomy can be combined with a craniofacial approach from below. Because of brain edema and olfactory filament injury associated with a brain retraction, however, alternatives to the bifrontal craniotomy have been developed.

The subcranial approach was initially described for the management of craniofacial trauma, but its role was later extended for the management of skull base tumors.[23] Recent reports have advocated the use of this approach for the management of midline nasal masses in the pediatric population.[24] After en bloc removal of the nasal bones, a limited inferior midline bifrontal craniotomy is performed with superior osteotomies made across the frontal bones, lateral osteotomies made vertically through the supraorbital rims and lateral nasal bones, and inferior osteotomies at the nasofrontal suture (**Fig. 30.10C–E**). Posteriorly, the bone flap is separated carefully from the nasal septum and the crista galli. This approach provides excellent exposure of the floor of the anterior cranial fossa and eliminates the need for brain retraction. Advantages of this approach include lower risks of anosmia, CSF leaks, and brain edema. Moreover, a recent study showed a minimal effect on long-term facial skeleton growth with this approach.[25]

Craniofacial Malformations

The classic craniofacial syndromes that are associated with sinonasal anomalies and neonatal nasal obstruction are Apert, Crouzon, Pfeiffer, and Treacher-Collins. The hallmark of these craniofacial syndromes is midfacial hypoplasia, which results in a very shallow nasopharynx and often a small nose that can compromise nasal respiration. Nonetheless, most affected patients have adequate nasal airways and can be treated by the optimization of nasal hygiene.[16]

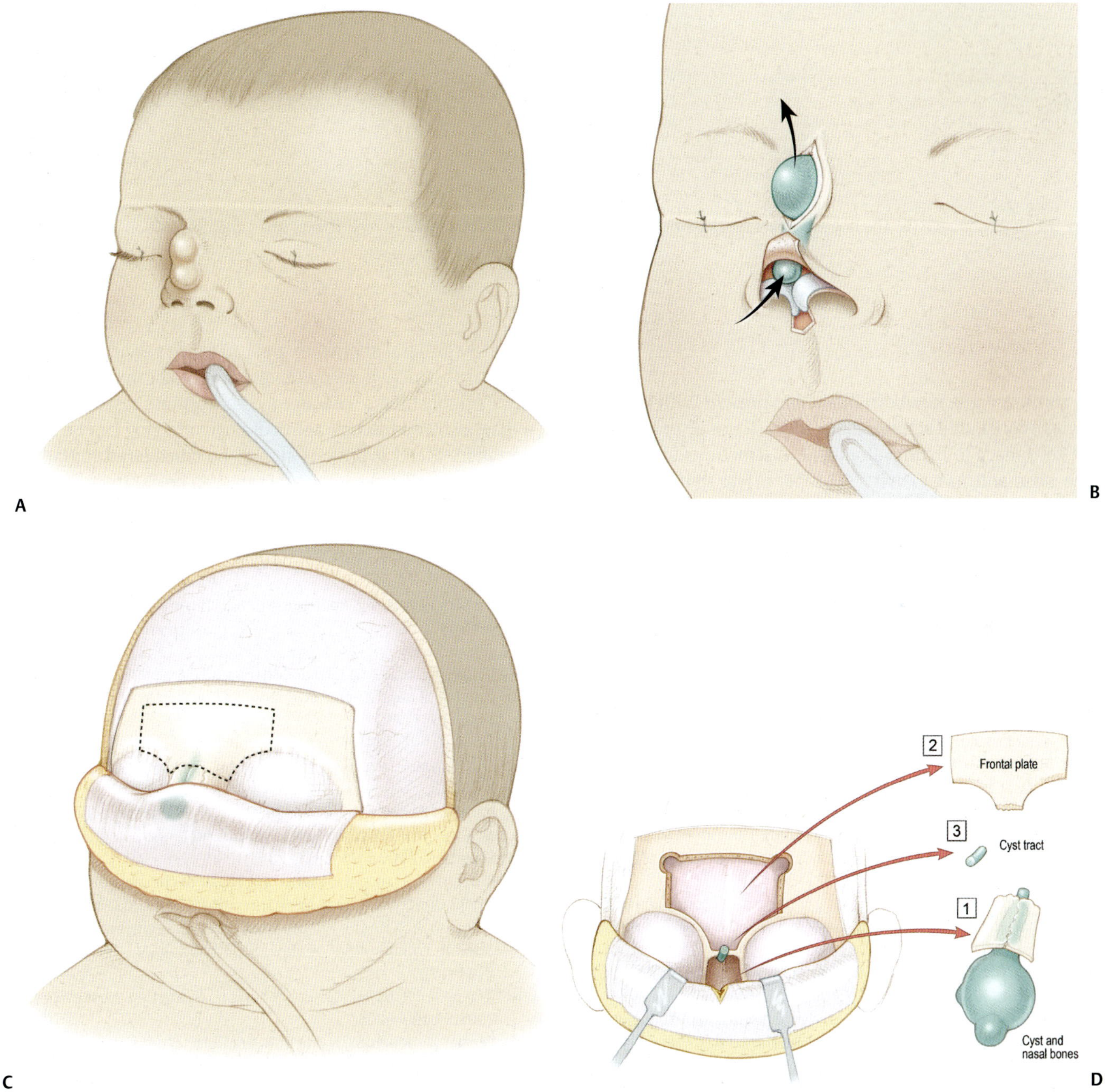

Fig. 30.10 (A) Preoperative depiction of a child with a nasal dermoid. **(B)** Removal of a nasal dermoid via an external rhinoplasty and vertical rhinotomy incisions. **(C)** Removal of a nasal dermoid via a subcranial approach. Subpericranial flaps have been elevated and osteotomy lines are marked. **(D)** Intraoperative depiction of a nasal dermoid cyst and the tract removed along with nasal bones and the frontal plate. *(continued)*

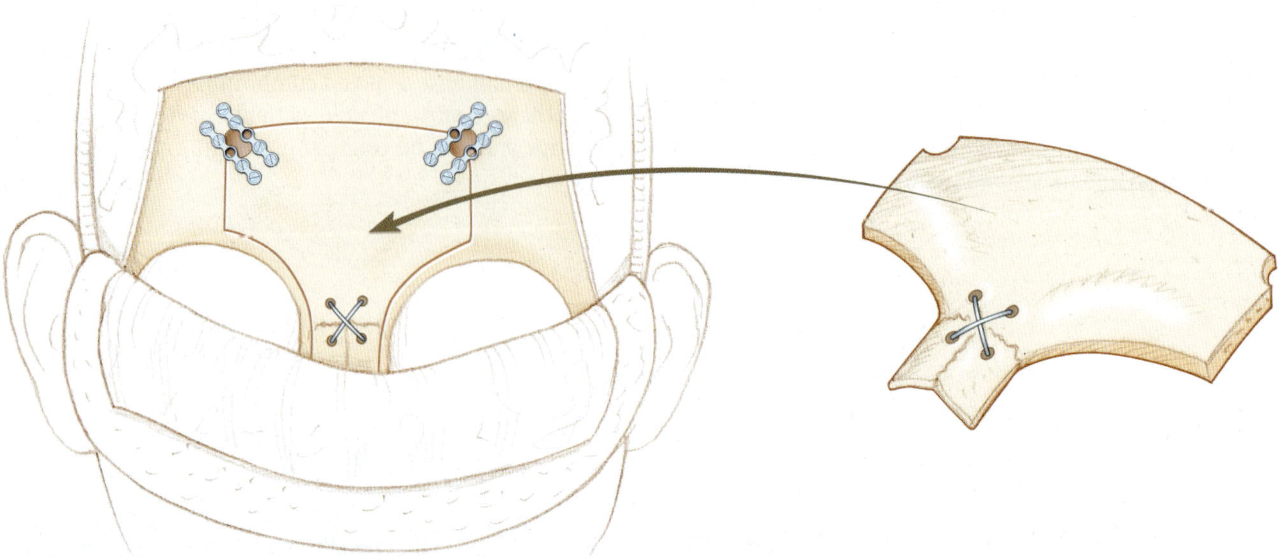

E

Fig. 30.10 *(continued)* **(E)** The bone flaps are repaired and replaced with titanium plates, wires, and screws to its original position.

Conclusion

In summary, the newborn infant can present with a multitude of congenital sinonasal disorders. These disorders may be secondary to maldevelopment of structures intrinsic to the nose and nasal cavity or to paranasal structures that manifest as nasal anomalies and can cause varying degrees of nasal obstructive, cosmetic, and neurologic impairments. After establishing a safe airway, appropriate tests such as a diagnostic endoscopy and radiologic imaging can be undertaken. Medical options should be considered initially. When appropriate, surgical therapy can be curative.

References

1. Olsen ØE, Gjelland K, Reigstad H, Rosendahl K. Congenital absence of the nose: a case report and literature review. Pediatr Radiol 2001;31(4):225–232
2. Brown K, Rodriguez K, Brown OE. Congenital malformations of the nose. In: Cummings CW, Flint PW, Harker LE, et al., eds. Cummings Otolaryngology–Head and Neck Surgery. 4th ed. Philadelphia: Elsevier Mosby; 2005: 4099–4109
3. Thorne MC, Ruiz RE, Carvalho J, Lesperance MM. Proboscis lateralis: case report and review. Arch Otolaryngol Head Neck Surg 2007;133(10):1051–1053
4. Koltai PJ. Maxillofacial injuries in children. In: Smith JD, Bumsted RM, eds. Pediatric Facial Plastic and Reconstructive Surgery. New York: Raven Press, Ltd.; 1993: 283–316
5. Hogeling M, Adams S, Wargon O. A randomized controlled trial of propranolol for infantile hemangiomas. Pediatrics 2011;128(2): e259–266
6. McCarthy JG, Borud LJ, Schreiber JS. Hemangiomas of the nasal tip. Plast Reconstr Surg 2002;109(1):31–40
7. Hochman M, Mascareno A. Management of nasal hemangiomas. Arch Facial Plast Surg 2005;7(5):295–300
8. Shikowitz MJ. Congenital nasal pyriform aperture stenosis: diagnosis and treatment. Int J Pediatr Otorhinolaryngol 2003;67(6): 635–639
9. Belden CJ, Mancuso AA, Schmalfuss IM. CT features of congenital nasal piriform aperture stenosis: initial experience. Radiology 1999;213(2):495–501
10. Barbero P, Valdez R, Rodríguez H, et al. Choanal atresia associated with maternal hyperthyroidism treated with methimazole: a case-control study. Am J Med Genet A 2008;146A(18):2390–2395
11. Keller JL, Kacker A. Choanal atresia, CHARGE association, and congenital nasal stenosis. Otolaryngol Clin North Am 2000;33(6): 1343–1351, viii
12. Slovis TL, Renfro B, Watts FB, Kuhns LR, Belenky W, Spoylar J. Choanal atresia: precise CT evaluation. Radiology 1985;155(2): 345–348
13. Van Den Abbeele T, François M, Narcy P. Transnasal endoscopic treatment of choanal atresia without prolonged stenting. Arch Otolaryngol Head Neck Surg 2002;128(8):936–940
14. Schoem SR. Transnasal endoscopic repair of choanal atresia: why stent? Otolaryngol Head Neck Surg 2004;131(4):362–366
15. Mansour AM, Cheng KP, Mumma JV, et al. Congenital dacryocele. A collaborative review. Ophthalmology 1991;98(11): 1744–1751
16. Krakovitz PR, Koltai PJ. Neonatal nasal obstruction. NeoReviews. 2007;8:e199–e205
17. Pensler JM, Bauer BS, Naidich TP. Craniofacial dermoids. Plast Reconstr Surg 1988;82(6):953–958
18. Szeremeta W, Parikh TD, Widelitz JS. Congenital nasal malformations. Otolaryngol Clin North Am 2007;40(1):97–112, vi–vii
19. Pollock RA. Surgical approaches to the nasal dermoid cyst. Ann Plast Surg 1983;10(6):498–501

20. Koltai PJ, Hoehn J, Bailey CM. The external rhinoplasty approach for rhinologic surgery in children. Arch Otolaryngol Head Neck Surg 1992;118(4):401–405
21. Woodworth BA, Schlosser RJ, Faust RA, Bolger WE. Evolutions in the management of congenital intranasal skull base defects. Arch Otolaryngol Head Neck Surg 2004;130(11):1283–1288
22. Kanowitz SJ, Bernstein JM. Pediatric meningoencephaloceles and nasal obstruction: a case for endoscopic repair. Int J Pediatr Otorhinolaryngol 2006;70(12):2087–2092
23. Raveh J, Vuillemin T. The surgical one-stage management of combined cranio-maxillo-facial and frontobasal fractures. Advantages of the subcranial approach in 374 cases. J Craniomaxillofac Surg 1988;16(4):160–172
24. Goyal P, Kellman RM, Tatum SA III. Transglabellar subcranial approach for the management of nasal masses with intracranial extension in pediatric patients. Arch Facial Plast Surg 2007;9(5):314–317
25. Shlomi B, Chaushu S, Gil Z, Chaushu G, Fliss DM. Effects of the subcranial approach on facial growth and development. Otolaryngol Head Neck Surg 2007;136(1):27–32

31 Benign Sinonasal Tumors

Kristin Seiberling and Peter-John Wormald

There is a multiplicity of benign tumors that arise within the sinonasal cavity. Although by histologic definition they are classified as benign neoplasms, local expansion and growth into surrounding critical structures may make these tumors aggressive in behavior. The proximity of vital structures (i.e., orbit, brain, skull base) to the nasal cavity necessitates prompt treatment in most cases. In small tumors, minimal if any symptoms may be present initially. As the tumor enlarges, symptoms of nasal obstruction, epistaxis, rhinorrhea, headache, and facial pain or pressure may occur. Given the nonspecific early symptoms, it is not uncommon for patients to be initially misdiagnosed with recurrent sinusitis or allergies. As the tumor continues to grow, more concerning symptoms may develop. Diplopia or proptosis may result from compression of the orbit or from direct involvement of the optic or oculomotor nerves at the orbital apex or the cavernous sinus. Facial numbness may develop as pressure is put on the trigeminal nerve. The presence of epiphora may indicate obstruction of the nasolacrimal duct situated in the anteromedial aspect of the maxilla. Hearing loss may be the first sign of a nasopharyngeal mass with obstruction of the eustachian tube. Thus, early diagnosis and treatment is essential to prevent the development of these later symptoms and complications.

Benign sinonasal tumors may be classified by histologic type: epithelial, mesenchymal, neural, vascular, and fibro-osseous lesions (**Table 31.1**). Endoscopic evaluation and radiographic analysis may help narrow the differential diagnosis and, in a few select cases, confirm the diagnosis. However, ultimately, histologic analysis of the tissue is needed for confirmation in the majority of tumors.

Treatment of benign sinonasal neoplasms depends on tumor histology, location, and the extent of disease, as well as the physical status of the patient. Historically, even benign tumors were removed with open approaches to ensure adequate exposure and removal. These open approaches included, but were not limited to, lateral rhinotomy, midface degloving, and medial maxillectomy. However, over the last decade with the advancement of endoscopic technique and introduction of image guidance surgery, endoscopic endonasal removal has become the procedure of choice in most teaching institutions. Proponents of endoscopic surgery cite several advantages, including less morbidity, shorter hospital stays, decreased blood loss, and lack of an external incision as compared with the traditional open techniques. In addition, endoscopes allow for better visualization and magnification of the tumor. Endoscopes improve definition and may narrow the resection field, avoiding unnecessary resection of healthy mucosa and anatomic structures. The endoscopic technique is, without doubt, advantageous as compared with the external approaches for the treatment of large juvenile angiofibroma as it avoids violation of the facial skeleton and osteotomies. Osteotomies and nonabsorbable osteosynthetic plates used in open approaches have the potential to negatively influence the development of facial skeleton growth in children.[1] Endonasal removal may be used alone or in combination with external approaches in cases with extension beyond the reach of the endoscope. This chapter focuses on patient selection, surgical anatomy, and the technique for the more common benign tumors of the sinonasal cavity: inverted papilloma (IP) and juvenile nasopharyngeal angiofibroma (JNA). The principles of surgical resection in these tumor types are broadly applicable to other types of benign sinonasal tumors.

Table 31.1 Benign Sinonasal Neoplasms

Benign Sinonasal Neoplasms
Epithelial
Keratotic papilloma
Schneiderian papilloma
Fungiform
Inverted
Cylindrical
Mesenchymal
Osteoma
Chondroma
Fibroma
Juvenile nasopharyngeal angiofibroma
Neural
Schwannoma
Neurofibroma
Meningioma
Fibro-osseous
Fibrous dysplasia
Ossifying fibroma
Giant cell tumor
Giant cell granuloma
Aneurysmal bone cyst
Vascular
Hemangioma
Hemangiopericytoma
Pyogenic granuloma

Inverted Papilloma

IP represents one of the most common benign sinonasal tumors with an incidence of 0.2 to 0.6% per 100,000 people per year. IP accounts for 0.4 to 4.7% of all nasal tumors.[2] Known by several names (inverting papilloma, inverted papilloma, schneiderian papilloma, soft papilloma), all show the characteristic inverted epithelium into the underlying connective tissue on pathology. Inverting papillomas affect men more than women (3:1) and may present at any age, although peak incidence is between the fifth and sixth decades of life. Most cases are unilateral with no side predilection; bilateral IPs have been reported in 4.9% of cases.[3] The exact etiology of IPs remains uncertain. IPs appear to occur in isolation (with normal sinuses) or in association with chronic sinusitis. There is some debate whether chronic inflammation induces a monoclonal cell expansion resulting in the formation of an IP. Although under debate, a link to human papilloma virus (HPV) has also been reported in the literature. Kashima demonstrated an increased risk of malignant transformation with those that harbor HPV types 6, 11, or 16, and a higher likelihood of recurrence.[4] IPs are histologically benign, but aggressive in nature due to local destruction, bony remodeling and erosion, intracranial extension, propensity for recurrence, and associated malignancy. The incidence of malignant transformation into squamous cell carcinoma has been reported between 5 and 15%.[5] Whether IPs represent a true premalignant lesion is still under debate. To date there are no documented histologic, radiographic, or pathologic findings predictive of malignant transformation. Wormald suggests that malignancy tends to be associated with bilateral IPs, severe hyperkeratosis, a mitotic index of more than two mitoses per high-power field, the absence of inflammatory of polyps and neutrophils, and the presence of plasma cells.[6] However, when Suh and associates looked at atypical features in benign IP, they failed to find a correlation with malignant transformation or recurrence.[7] The number of recurrences fails to show a relation to malignancy.

Clinical Presentation

The most common initial symptom is that of unilateral nasal obstruction. Other associated symptoms include rhinorrhea, postnasal drainage, headache/facial pain, and epistaxis. Larger tumors may extend into the sinuses causing obstruction and infection, or may compress the orbit leading to diplopia, proptosis, and even blindness. Physical examination usually reveals a unilateral polypoid mass off the lateral nasal wall filling the nasal cavity. Grossly, IP tends to have an irregular friable appearance and often bleeds with manipulation. However, they can also be hidden amongst inflammatory polyp disease and identified only with a high index of suspicion, or on pathology. The tumor may grow in size to involve the maxillary and ethmoid sinuses and, less commonly, into the frontal and sphenoid sinuses. Primary lesions of the sphenoid and frontal sinus have been reported; however, these are infrequent in nature. Eighty percent of all lesions occupy both the sinuses and the nasal cavity, with either the maxillary and/or ethmoid sinus involved in 50 to 80%.[8] Tumors found exclusively within the sinus without extension into the nasal cavity are rare, with a reported incidence of 5%.[9]

Diagnostic Workup

The workup for IP includes a comprehensive physical examination with nasal endoscopy, radiographic studies, and ultimately, tissue biopsy. Imaging should be obtained prior to performing a biopsy to rule out an intracranial mass extending into the nasal cavity or a vascular lesion. Radiology is imperative in the workup and diagnosis of the disease and to assess the resectability of the tumor. Computed tomography (CT) and magnetic resonance imaging (MRI) are complementary and both are needed to plan the appropriate surgical approach. CT is used to define the extent of the disease and to identify areas of bony erosion. Up to 75% of patients with IPs have evidence of various degrees of bone destruction, which may appear as cortical thinning, remodeling, erosion, or sclerotic changes. Areas of bony thickening may represent the site of attachment of the tumor. CT scans used alone frequently overestimate the extent of disease due to the lack of differentiation of tumors from adjacent inflammatory mucosa or retained secretions. CT alone has a sensitivity of 69% and a specificity of 20%.[10] T2-weighted images and contrast-enhanced T1-weighted MRIs are used in conjunction to further evaluate the surrounding soft tissue and to define the extent of orbital or intracranial involvement. MRI allows for excellent delineation of the tumor from the surrounding soft tissues, inflammation, and retained secretions. Tumors will be of intermediate intensity on T2-weighted images, whereas the inflammatory component will be of high signal intensity (**Fig. 31.1**). Additionally, the tumor will have intermediate intensity on T1 images with intravenous gadolinium enhancement; retained secretions will not enhance but will be rimmed by a bright signal from the inflamed mucosa.

Patient Selection

Several staging systems have been developed to aid the classification of disease extent and to help guide management options. Although no single staging system is universally adopted, their use should be encouraged to optimize patient care and to facilitate further research. In 2000, Krouse proposed a four-stage system for IPs based on the degree of invasion of the tumor into the paranasal sinuses and the associated malignancy (**Table 31.2**). Using this staging system, he advocated the endoscopic removal of T1, T2, and certain T3 tumors.[3] Until recent years, the endoscopic removal of lesions up to a T3 lesion was recommended, but now, T4 lesions are routinely resected endoscopically. A review published by Weissler looked at three treatment options for IPs: transnasal polypectomy, external (Caldwell-Luc, external ethmoidectomy), and open (lateral rhinotomy, midface degloving).[11] The recurrence rate was found to be inversely related to the extent of the procedure—71% for intranasal procedures, 56% for external, and 29% for open. However, with improved endoscopic techniques, resection of all structures traditionally resected by an open approach

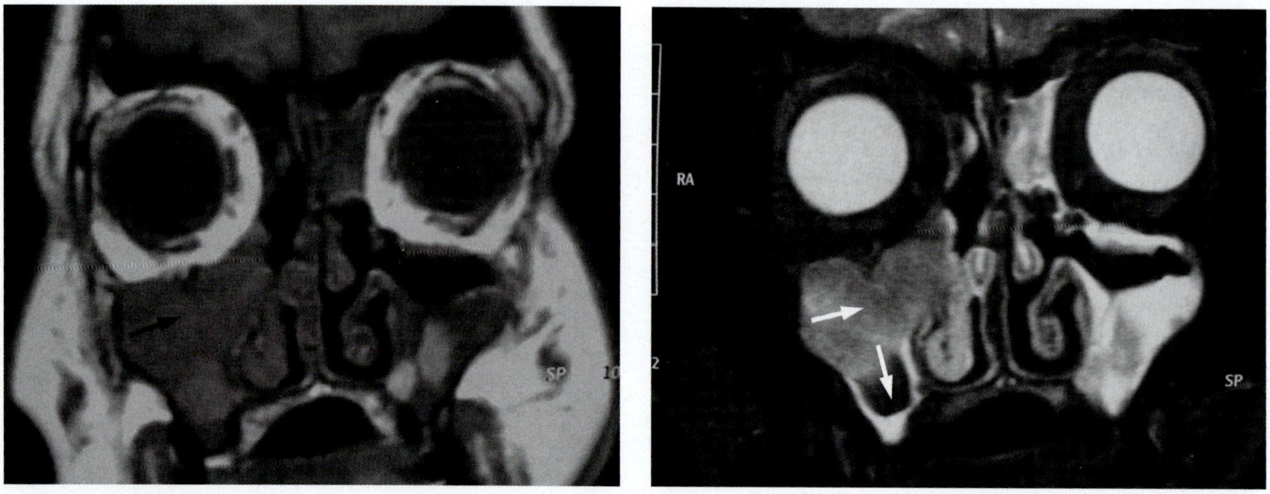

A B

Fig. 31.1 **(A)** Coronal T1-weighted magnetic resonance image (MRI) demonstrating a tumor (*black arrows*) with intermediate intensity in the right maxillary sinus. **(B)** Coronal T2-weighted MRI demonstrating a tumor with intermediate intensity and surrounding secretions with high signal intensity (*white arrows*).

can be performed resulting in lower recurrence rates than that seen by the open approaches. Krouse published a 30-year review on 1426 patients in which the recurrence rates of IPs using different surgical approaches for removal were analyzed. He categorized the surgical approaches into four groups: nonendoscopic intranasal, conservative (Caldwell-Luc, transnasal, and transantral procedures short of an en bloc resection), aggressive (en bloc resection of tumor by means of midface degloving, lateral rhinotomy, or Weber-Ferguson incision), and endoscopic (including all endoscopic approaches). The recurrence rates for these groups were 67.3%, 44.0%, 18.0%, and 11.8%, respectively.[3] In a more recent comprehensive literature review, Busquets looked at a total of 49 articles published between 1992 and 2004 combined with data from the authors' own institution.[12] In total, the cohort included 1060 patients: 714 patients treated endoscopically and 346 patients treated nonendoscopically. The overall recurrence rate was 15% with a weighted average follow-up time of 44 months (3.7 years). The recurrence rate was significantly lower at 12% ($p = 0.001$) for the endoscopic subgroup compared with 20% for the nonendoscopic subgroup. The incidence of carcinoma was 5% (**Table 31.3**).

Table 31.2 IP Staging System Developed by Krouse

Stage	Description
T1	Tumors limited to the nasal cavity
T2	Tumors limited to the ethmoid sinus and/or medial and superior portions of maxillary sinus
T3	Tumors involving lateral, inferior, anterior, or posterior walls of maxillary sinus, sphenoid sinus, or frontal sinus
T4	Tumors extending outside sinonasal cavities (i.e., orbital or intracranial extension) or tumors associated with malignancy

Source: Data from Krouse JH. Endoscopic treatment of inverted papilloma: safety and efficacy. Am J Otolaryngol 2001;22:87–99.

Endoscopic Removal of IP: Surgical Technique

The extent of surgery should be tailored to the size and location of the tumor. The surgeon must meticulously remove all of the tumor with a cuff of normal mucosa and drill the bone underlying the attachment site of the tumor. In most cases, the tumor needs to be judiciously debulked with the microdebrider until the exact site and extent of its origin is identified. Tissue traps are placed in the suction line to collect all debrided tissue for histology. In most cases, the site of origin can be identified on the CT scan as there tends to be new bone formation in this area (**Fig. 31.2**).[13] This bone should be drilled down with a diamond burr to remove microscopic mucosal remnants, which if left, may result in tumor recurrence. Early recurrence often occurs at the bony buttress (the junction of maxillary antrostomy and lamina papyracea)[14] and at the site of the original tumor due to incomplete local resection.[15]

IP of the Maxillary Sinus

The use of an angled endoscope will allow the surgeon to precisely evaluate the majority of the maxillary sinus mucosa. Depending on the extent and location of the tumor, an endoscopic removal may be supplemented with targeted additional approaches. For example, a canine fossa trephination may aid in dissection when the tumor involves the medial wall, floor, or posterior walls of the maxillary sinus. Tumors involving some of these areas, especially more anteriorly in the maxillary sinus, cannot be accessed through a maxillary antrostomy irrespective of how large the antrostomy is made. A canine fossa trephine is created to allow for placement of the dissecting instrument while the endoscope is placed into the maxillary antrostomy. Using this technique, the entire maxillary sinus except for a small area of the anterior wall can be accessed and visualized. The instruments may also be reversed to allow for

Table 31.3 Endoscopic Resection of Sinonasal Inverted Papilloma: A Meta-Analysis

Authors	Year of Publication	Endoscopic Cases	Endoscopic Recurrence (%)	External Cases	External Recurrence (%)	Total Cases	Total Recurrence (%)	Carcinomas (%)	Mean Follow-up (Months)
Waitz et al.[34]	1992	35	6 (17)	16	3 (19)	51	9 (18)	1 (2)	46
Stankiewicz et al.[35]	1994	15	5 (33)	0		15	5 (33)	1 (7)	36
McCary et al.[36]	1994	4	0 (0)	20	4 (20)	24	4 (17)	0 (0)	30
Buchwald et al.[37]	1995	5	0 (0)	0		5	0 (0)	0 (0)	24
Kamel[38]	1995	12	0 (0)	0		12	0 (0)	0 (0)	35
Raveh et al.[39]	1996	9	2 (22)	39	14 (36)	48	16 (33)	4 (8)	26
Sham et al.[15]	1998	22	6 (27)	0		22	6 (27)	1 (4)	53
Chee et al.[40]	1999	18	1 (5)	0		18	1 (5)	0 (0)	33
Tufano et al.[16]	1999	33	5 (15)	0		33	5 (15)	0 (0)	20
Bertrand et al.[41]	2000	84	15 (18)	0		84	15 (18)	3 (3)	42
Sukenik et al.[10]	2000	19	4 (21)	0		19	4 (21)	0 (0)	36
Klimek et al.[42]	2000	33	6 (18)	22	4 (18)	55	10 (18)	3 (5)	36
Lund[43]	2000	13	1 (8)	24	5 (21)	37	6 (16)	0 (0)	45
Krouse[3]	2001	7	1 (14)	5	0 (0)	12	1 (8)	0 (0)	40
Schlosser et al.[14]	2001	20	4 (20)	1	0 (0)	21	4 (19)	1 (5)	42
Han et al.[44]	2001	15	2 (13)	12	1 (8)	27	3 (11)	3 (11)	54
Thorp et al.[45]	2001	2	0 (0)	41	11(27)	43	11 (26)	5 (12)	32
Keles et al.[46]	2001	13	3 (23)	0		13	3 (23)	1 (7)	27
Kuhn et al.[47]	2001	28	2 (7)	0		28	2 (7)	2 (7)	22
Baruah et al.[48]	2003	6	1 (17)	0		6	1 (17)	0 (0)	21
Sadeghi et al.[49]	2003	5	0 (0)	6	0 (0)	11	0 (0)	0 (0)	66
Wormald et al.[6]	2003	17	1 (6)	0		17	1 (6)	1 (6)	39
Pasquini et al.[50]	2003	1	0 (0)	0		1	0 (0)	1 (100)	53
Kaza et al.[51]	2003	51	7 (14)	0		51	7 (14)	4 (8)	30
Kraft et al.[52]	2003	26	2 (8)	8	3 (37)	34	5 (15)	4 (12)	62
Lawson et al.[53]	2003	41	5 (12)	119	18 (15)	160	23 (14)	11 (7)	62
Llorente et al.[54]	2003	26	2 (8)	0		26	2 (8)	0 (0)	60
Lee et al.[55]	2004	43	4 (9)	0		43	4 (9)	1 (2)	25
Tomenzoli et al.[56]	2004	47	0 (0)	0		47	0 (0)	0 (0)	55
Pasquini et al.[57]	2004	36	1 (3)	32	6 (19)	68	7 (10)	8 (12)	74
Authors' series[12]	2006	28	3 (11)	1	0 (0)	29	3 (10)	0 (0)	22
Total		714	89 (12)	346	69 (20)	1,060	158 (15)	55 (5)	44

Source: Adapted with permission from Busquets JM, Hwang PH. Endoscopic resection of sinonasal inverted papilloma: a meta-analysis. Otolaryngol Head Neck Surg 2006;134:476–482.

additional views. Care must be taken not to use this technique for tumors that originate from the anterior face of the maxillary sinus because placement of the trephine through the tumor may result in an incomplete removal.

If the tumor originates from the anterior wall or has a large area of origin within the maxillary sinus, an endoscopic medial maxillectomy is recommended for complete tumor removal. Prior to the start of surgery, neuropatties soaked in cocaine or adrenaline should be placed within the nasal cavity. The lateral nasal wall, septum, and greater palatine canal are injected with 2% lidocaine and 1:80,000 adrenaline. After allowing adequate time for vasoconstriction, the procedure begins with an uncinectomy and exposure of the maxillary sinus ostium. The maxillary antrum is enlarged posteriorly until the posterior wall of the sinus is encountered and the medial wall of the orbit is visualized. Next, the inferior turbinate is medialized and crushed with Tilley packing forceps just distal to the point where the anterior

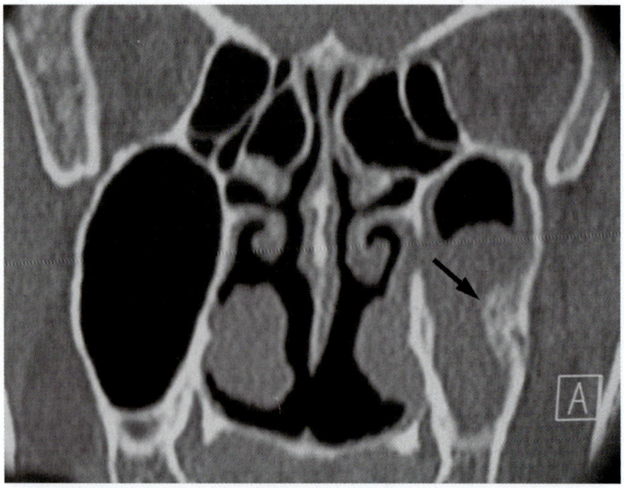

Fig. 31.2 New bone formation in the lateral wall of the left maxillary sinus (*black arrow*). This signifies the site of origin of the tumor and must be drilled down after the removal of the tumor.

end meets the lateral nasal wall. Turbinectomy scissors are used to cut the turbinate up to the point where it reaches the lateral nasal wall (**Fig. 31.3**). Mucosal cuts are made with a scalpel from a point just below the orbit through the cut turbinate to the floor of the nose. This cut is continued posteriorly, turning vertically at the posterior region of the inferior turbinate to reach the posterior end of the maxillary antrostomy. A sharp osteotome is used to cut the bone after the mucosal incisions have been made (**Fig. 31.4A**). After the bone cuts have been made, the medial maxillary wall should be mobile and tethered only by the nasolacrimal duct anteriorly. This duct is visualized and transected with a scalpel. The specimen may be removed in its entirety, allowing for excellent visualization into the maxillary sinus (**Fig. 31.4B**). Care must be taken at the end of the case to open the end of the nasolacrimal duct widely to prevent postoperative scarring and epiphora. This may be done using a dacryocystorhinostomy spear knife (**Fig. 31.5**).

If more exposure is needed to visualize the anterior face of the maxillary sinus, two other techniques may be of benefit. First, the anteromedial wall and frontal process of the maxilla can be drilled down (**Fig. 31.6**). Furthermore, this may be combined with the transseptal route, which changes the angle that instruments are passed into the sinus and improves access to the anterior wall. To create a transseptal passageway for the instruments, a hemitransfixion incision is made and a small piece of septal cartilage opposite the anterior maxillary sinus is removed. A horizontal incision is made in the opposite septal flap, making sure that this incision does not overlap

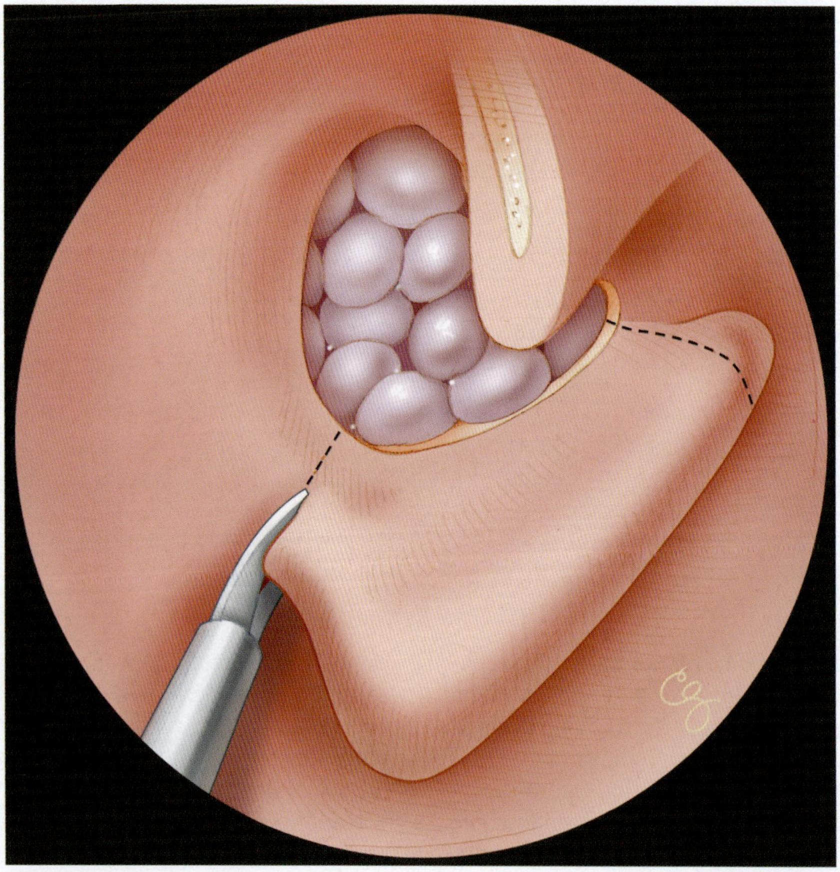

Fig. 31.3 The inferior turbinate has been medialized and scissors are used to cut the inferior turbinate along the crushed portion of the turbinate as flush as possible to the lateral nasal wall.

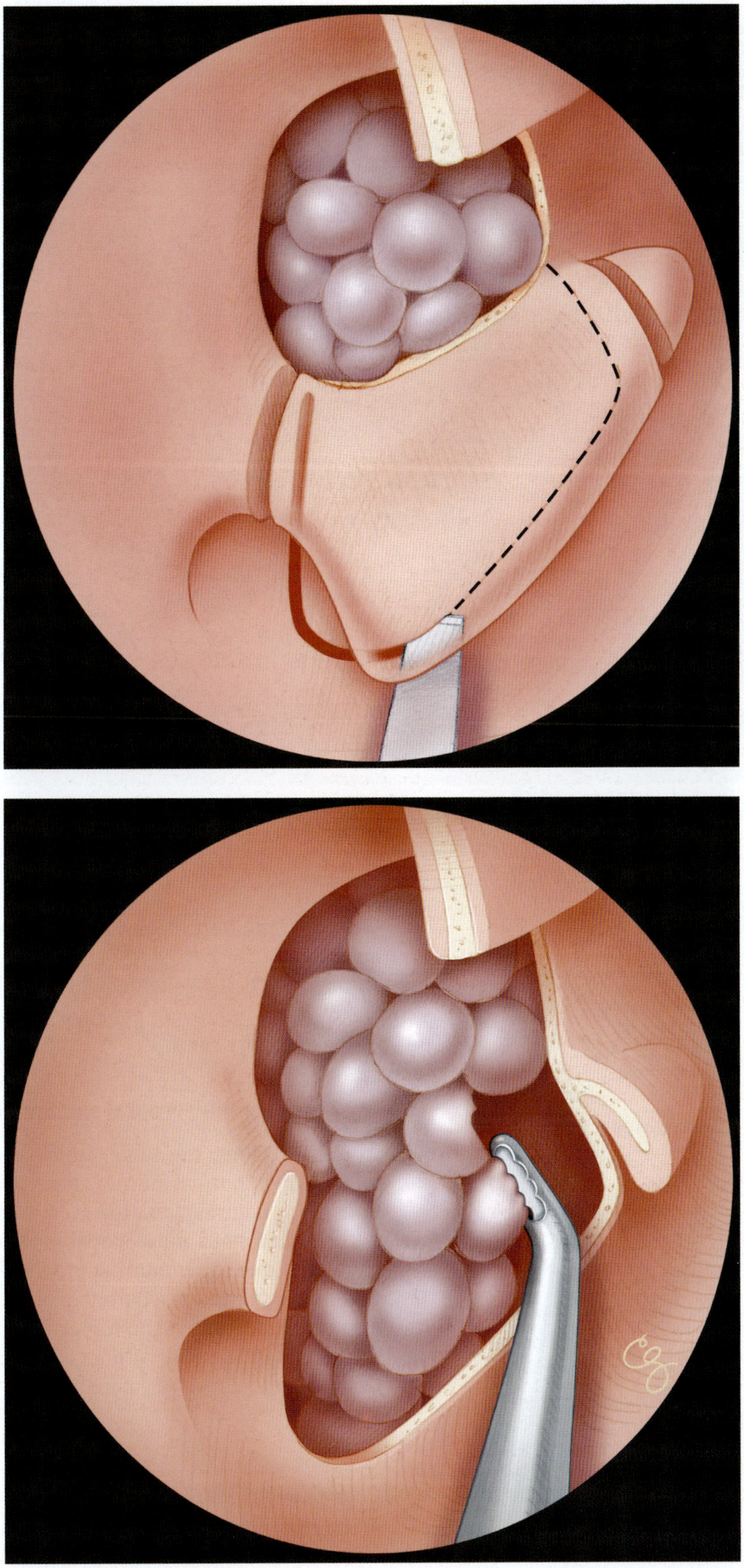

A

B

Fig. 31.4 (A) Bone cuts are made with an osteotome along the mucosal incision lines along the floor of the nose to the posterior wall of the maxillary sinus. **(B)** The medial wall of the maxillary sinus has been removed to allow for visualization of the tumor within the maxillary sinus. Non-attached portions of tumor may be debulked with a microdebrider.

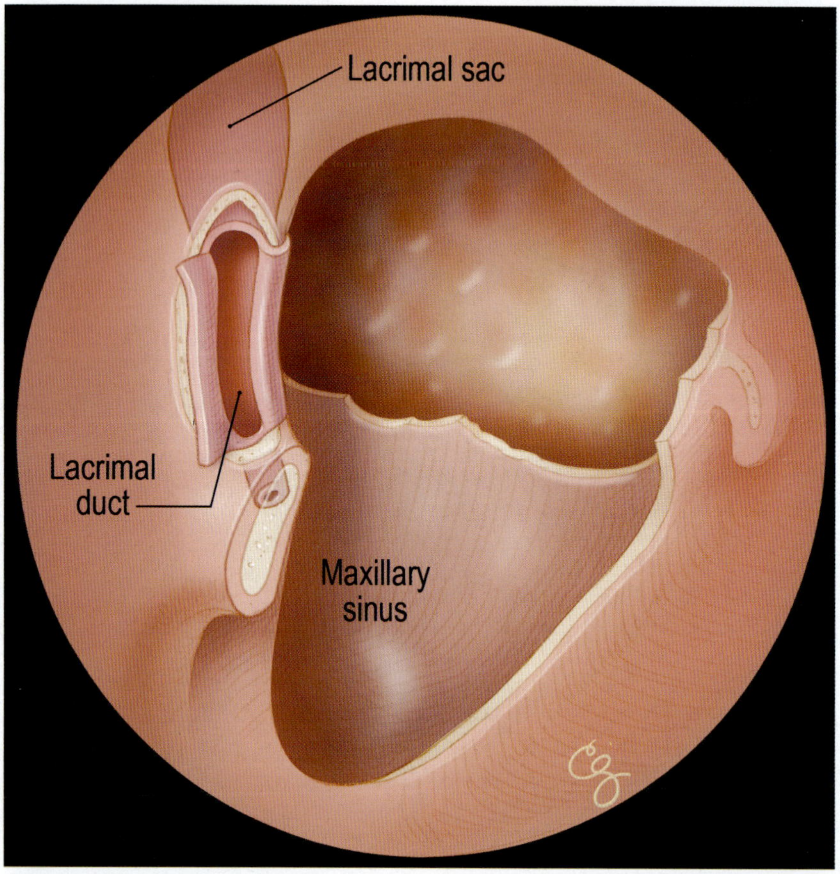

Fig. 31.5 The lacrimal sac has been widely opened with a spear knife. The mucosal edges of the sac have been opened and positioned against the lateral nasal wall.

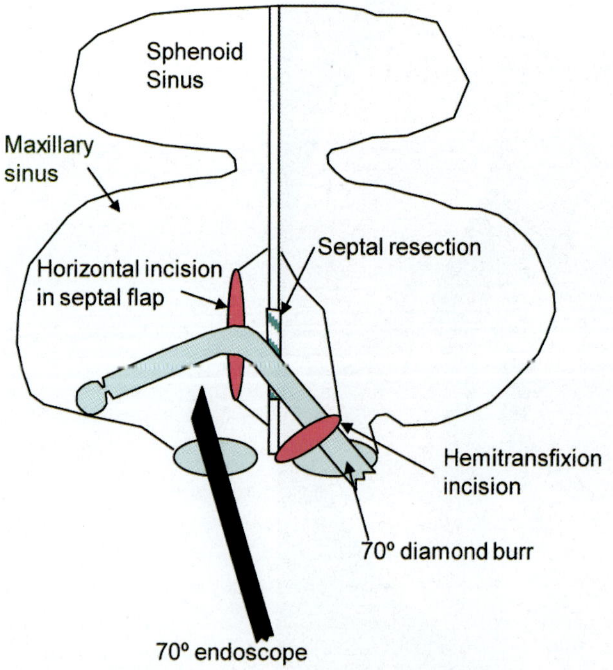

Fig. 31.6 Using a septal window approach, a 70-degree diamond burr can be placed through the window and onto the frontal process of the maxilla. The frontal process may be drilled down to gain further exposure of the tumor.

with the hemitransfixion incision. The instruments may subsequently be passed from the hemitransfixion incision through the cartilage window to the opposite side of the nasal cavity, improving the angle and thereby the access to the maxillary sinus.

IP of the Ethmoid, Frontal and Sphenoid Sinus

In these regions, the same principle of tumor removal with a cuff of normal mucosa and diamond drilling of the underlying bone applies. However, access may be difficult in the frontal sinus and all patients who have extension of the tumor into the frontal ostium undergo an endoscopic modified Lothrop procedure to allow for a complete and clear identification of the tumor and precise removal of the tumor attachment with a cuff of normal mucosa and drilling of the underlying bone.[14,16]

Complications

Complications are similar to those encountered with any endoscopic sinus surgery. Potential complications include a cerebrospinal fluid (CSF) leak, orbital injury (blindness, hematoma, and diplopia), epiphora, prolonged crusting, infection, synechia/scarring, and bleeding.

Postoperative Care

Frequent follow-up of these patients is critical to detect early recurrence. In the immediate postoperative period, the patient should come to the office regularly for a nasal endoscopy with debridement of crusts and suctioning of old blood and mucus from the sinuses. Antibiotics are generally given for the first week after surgery. The patient should be instructed to judiciously use saline rinses until the mucosal surfaces have healed. Nasal steroid sprays may help reduce inflammation and improve postoperative healing in some cases. In patients in whom the entire maxillary mucosa has been removed and the underlying bone has been drilled, the cavity may fill with granulation tissue during the first 6 months. If there is concern about recurrence, this can be regularly biopsied, but the granulations tend to gradually settle down with a partial obliteration of the maxillary sinus. When this occurs, repeat MRI scanning may be necessary at 1 to 2 years. However, routine postoperative imaging is seldom necessary unless there is a question of incomplete removal or the patient continues to be symptomatic.

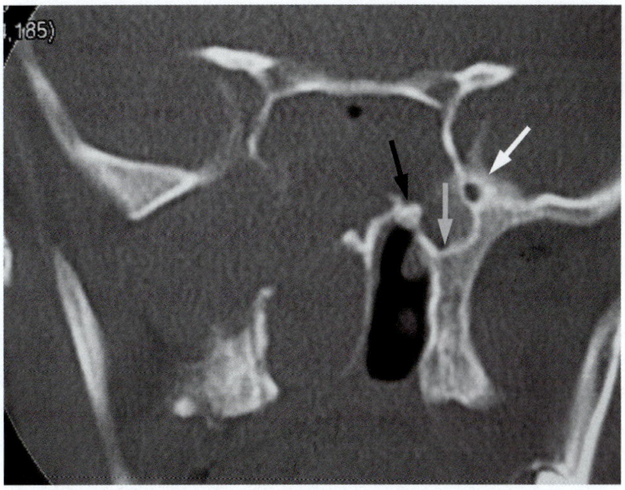

Fig. 31.7 A coronal computed tomography scan of a juvenile nasopharyngeal angiofibroma originating from the trifurcation of the palatine bone, the horizontal ala of the vomer, and the root of the pterygoid process. The tumor has eroded the pterygoid process and expanded the vidian canal on the right. The left side demonstrates the normal position of the foramen rotundum (*white arrow*), vidian canal (*black arrow*), and pterygoid plate (*gray arrow*).

Juvenile Nasopharyngeal Angiofibroma

Juvenile nasopharyngeal angiofibroma (JNA) is a highly aggressive locally invasive vascular neoplasm found almost exclusively in prepubescent and pubescent boys. It accounts for 0.05% of all head and neck tumors[17] and is the most common benign tumor involving the pterygopalatine and infratemporal fossa. Although histologically benign, it is locally invasive and, if left untreated, has the potential to erode through the skull base.[18] The embryology of JNA is unclear, but it appears to originate from the superior margin of the sphenopalatine foramen formed by the trifurcation of the palatine bone, the horizontal ala of the vomer, and the root of the pterygoid process (**Fig. 31.7**). The neoplastic growth of the tumor can occur through several pathways. The tumor may grow in the submucosal plane of the nasopharyngeal roof, reaching the posterior choana and septum. It may erode through the anterior face of the sphenoid sinus or go laterally into the pterygomaxillary fissure, causing the pathognomonic bowing of the posterior wall of the maxillary sinus. If not caught early, the tumor may grow into the infratemporal fossa, orbit, and middle cranial fossa. Most studies report a 10 to 20% incidence of intracranial extension.[19–21]

Clinical Presentation

Patients typically present with nasal obstruction (80%), epistaxis (45 to 60%), headache (25%), and facial swelling (10 to 18%). Other symptoms may include unilateral rhinorrhea, anosmia, hyposmia, hyponasal speech, proptosis, hearing loss, facial asymmetry, and nasal dorsum deformities. On physical exam, a smooth firm purple-reddish mass is typically seen filling the nasopharynx and nasal cavity.

Diagnostic Workup

The diagnosis of JNA relies heavily on radiographic signs. The location and radiographic appearance of the tumor are generally diagnostic. Biopsy is rarely needed to confirm the diagnosis and is not recommended due to the highly vascular nature of the tumor. If a biopsy is needed to confirm the diagnosis in cases that are atypical, the biopsy should not be performed in the office but in the operating room with adequate equipment available to control bleeding. The radiographic signs thought to be classic for JNA are listed in **Table 31.4**. The anterior bowing of the posterior wall of the antrum is pathognomonic for JNA. Both CT and MRI are complementary, as described in the previous section, and used in the diagnosis and staging of JNA.

Table 31.4 Radiographic Signs of Juvenile Nasopharyngeal Angiofibroma

Radiographic signs
Nasopharyngeal mass
Anterior bowing of the posterior wall of the maxillary sinus*
Erosion of the sphenoid sinus
Expansion of the pterygomaxillary fissure
Erosion of the hard palate
Erosion of the maxillary sinus
Displacement of the nasal septum
Widening of the sphenopalatine foramen

* Hollman-Miller sign: pathognomonic for juvenile nasopharyngeal angiofibroma.

In reviewing the scans, careful attention must be paid to the degree of involvement of the pterygopalatine fossa and surrounding structures. The pterygopalatine fossa may act as a conduit, allowing the tumor to pass from one area to the next (i.e., infratemporal fossa, nasal cavity, orbit). Tumors that expand within the pterygopalatine fossa may extend into the inferior orbital fissure, infiltrate around the infraorbital nerve, and grow posteriorly toward the foramen rotundum and vidian canal. Furthermore, the degree of involvement of the vidian canal must be assessed preoperatively on imaging studies. Tumors may expand this canal, erode the floor of the sphenoid sinus, and extend posteriorly along the vidian canal until it abuts the carotid artery (**Fig. 31.8**). Angiography confirms the vascularization of this tumor and is used both in the diagnosis and treatment. The main arterial supply comes from the ipsilateral internal maxillary artery. In addition, some tumors may be supplied by the contralateral external carotid artery and may receive contributions from branches of one or both internal carotid arteries.[22] The characteristic blush seen on the angiography confirms the diagnosis and also allows for embolization of the tumor preoperatively. Embolization should be performed 24 hours or less preoperatively to help minimize intraoperative blood loss, a major source of morbidity. In addition, if major hemorrhage occurs during surgery, an incomplete tumor removal due to inadequate visualization may occur. Antonelli et al. reported a 60% average reduction in intraoperative blood loss when preoperative embolization was performed.[23] Although some authors do not recommend preoperative embolization, there has been a decrease in recurrence rates with the use of preoperative embolization.[24] This is thought to result from a higher percentage of cases having complete tumor removal due to improved visualization with less intraoperative bleeding.[25,26]

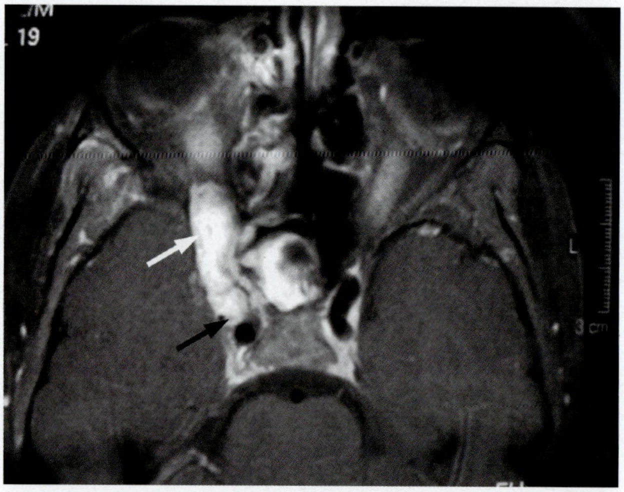

Fig. 31.8 An axial T1-weighted magnetic resonance image demonstrating the tumor infiltrating the orbital apex (*white arrow*) and extending up to the carotid canal (*black arrow*).

Table 31.5 Staging System for Juvenile Nasopharyngeal Angiofibroma

Stage	Description
I	Tumor limited to the nasopharynx and nasal cavity; bone destruction is negligible or limited to the sphenopalatine foramen
II	Tumor invading the PF or maxillary, ethmoidal, and sphenoid sinuses; with bone destruction
IIIa	Tumor invading the ITF or orbital region without intracranial involvement
IIIb	Tumor invading the ITF or orbital region with extradural intracranial involvement (parasellar)
IVa	Tumor with intradural intracranial involvement without infiltration of cavernous sinus, pituitary fossa, or optic chiasma
IVb	Tumor with infiltration of cavernous sinus, pituitary fossa, or optic chiasma

Source: Data from Andrews JC, Fisch U, Valavanis A, Aeppli U, Makek MS. The surgical management of extensive nasopharyngeal angiofibromas with the infratemporal fossa approach. Laryngoscope 1989;99:429–437.
Abbreviations: PF, pterygopalatine fossa; ITF, infratemporal fossa.

Patient Selection

Multiple staging systems have been developed to classify tumors according to location and extent of spread. Two staging systems that must be recognized are those of Andrews and Radkowski, both of which may be used to aid surgical decision making in the treatment of JNA. The staging system developed by Andrews is depicted in **Table 31.5**.[27]

Treatment Options

The preferred management for JNA is a complete surgical removal. Various medical treatments have been used, all with variable results. Hormonal regulation was thought to decrease tumor volume; however, its current use has been limited due to side effects and inconsistent tumor response. Low dose external beam radiation has been shown to decrease tumor size over a period of 12 to 36 months. Cummings reported a series of 42 patients with JNA, stage IIIb or greater, treated with primary radiotherapy. In this paper, tumor control was obtained in 80% of the patients who received 3000 to 3500 cGy. A second course of radiotherapy achieved tumor control in 94% of patients. However, radiotherapy is not a cure, nor is it a benign treatment regimen. Radiation-induced malignancies have been reported in the literature over a decade after treatment.[28] It is recommended that the use of radiation be limited to those patients unable to undergo surgery; as an aid to preoperatively reduce tumor bulk when vital structures are involved; and to help in the management of inoperable recurrence.

There are numerous approaches for surgical removal; the choice depends on the extent and location of the tumor as well as the skills of the surgical team. Acceptable approaches include transpalatine, transzygomatic, transmandibular, transhyoid, transantral, medial maxillectomy,

Le Fort 1, and infratemporal.[22,29] Endoscopic removal has been shown to be successful and is widely accepted for smaller tumors but more recently has been recommended for large tumors without intracranial extension.[26,30,31] As endoscopic instrumentation and surgical technique improve, the boundaries of minimally invasive paranasal surgery continue to expand.

Surgical Anatomy

Pterygopalatine Fossa

The pterygopalatine fossa is a fat-filled space between the posterior wall of the maxillary sinus and the pterygoid process of the sphenoid bone (**Fig. 31.9**). The space is shaped like an inverted, quadrangular pyramid with the base directed superiorly and the apex inferiorly. It communicates via six foramen and canals with the middle cranial fossa, orbit, nasal cavity, oral cavity, and the infratemporal fossa. For this reason, the pterygopalatine fossa represents a major pathway for the spread of the tumor. The medial wall of the pterygopalatine fossa is formed by the palatine bone, sphenopalatine foramen (access to the nasal cavity), and sphenopalatine artery (SPA); the roof is formed by the infraorbital fissure and foramen rotundum; the floor is formed by the greater palatine canal; and the lateral wall is formed by the pterygomaxillary fissure. As described previously, the pterygopalatine fossa is intimately associated with the inferior orbital fissure. It is through this fissure that tumors may extend from the pterygopalatine fossa and infratemporal fossa up toward the orbital apex and posteriorly toward the cavernous sinus and carotid artery. The pterygopalatine fossa contains the distal branches of the maxillary artery (sphenopalatine and greater palatine artery). The vidian nerve can be seen transversing the posterior aspect of the fossa before moving laterally to join the pterygopalatine ganglion. The maxillary nerve courses from the foramen rotundum from medial to lateral across the roof of the fossa just below the orbital apex. The maxillary nerve may be followed posteromedial to the foramen rotundum. The foramen rotundum links the pterygopalatine fossa with the Gasserian ganglion and carries the maxillary nerve (V2). The vidian canal is slightly inferior and medial to the foramen rotundum and carries the vidian nerve and a small branch of the inferior mesenteric artery. Three foramina—rotundum, vidian canal, and the palatovaginal canal—all enter through the

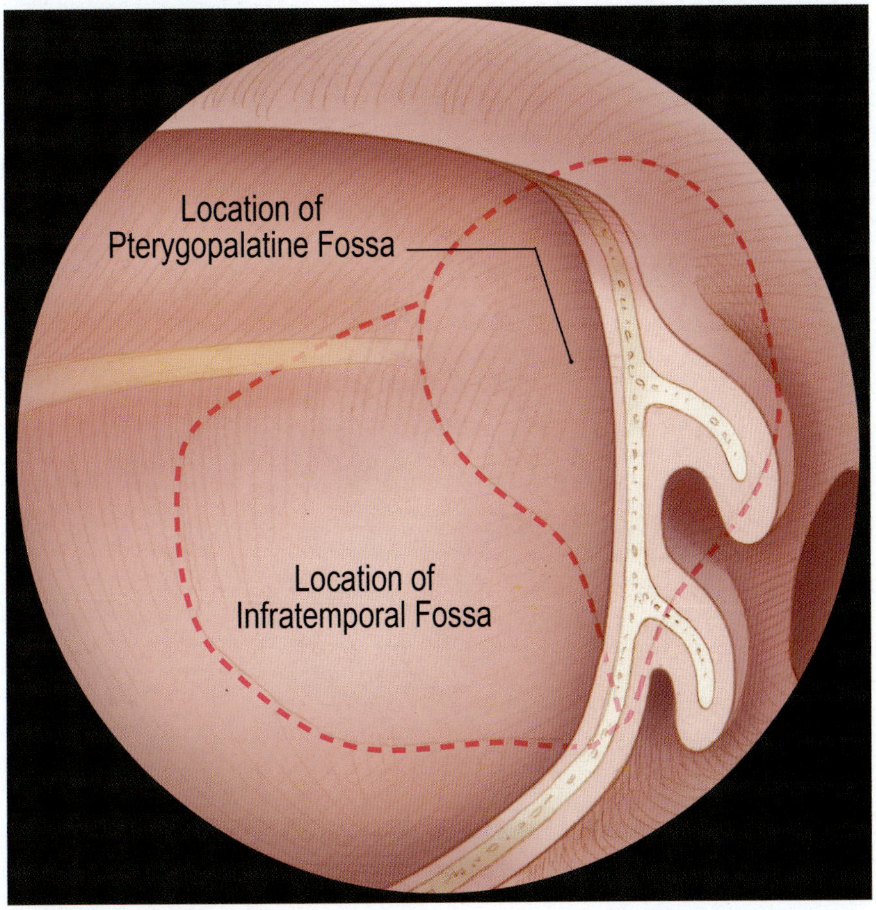

Fig. 31.9 The medial wall of the maxillary sinus has been removed, allowing exposure of the posterior wall. The dotted lines represent the pterygopalatine fossa (medial) and infratemporal fossa (lateral).

posterior wall of the pterygopalatine fossa (**Fig. 31.10**). When dissecting in this area, it must be kept in mind that the first structures encountered are the blood vessels followed by the deeper neural structures.

Infratemporal Fossa

The infratemporal fossa is the space deep to the zygomatic arch. The roof is formed by the greater wing of the sphenoid and temporal bone. The lateral wall is formed by the ramus of the mandible. The medial wall is formed by the lateral pterygoid plate and the pterygomaxillary fissure, which communicates directly with the pterygopalatine fossa (**Fig. 31.9**). The anterior wall is formed by the posterior maxilla and the inferior orbital fissure. To expose the contents of the infratemporal fossa, the bone of the posterior and lateral wall of the maxillary sinus must be removed. The contents of the infratemporal fossa include: pterygoid muscles, the maxillary artery and its branches, the pterygoid venous plexus, and branches of the mandibular division of the trigeminal nerve. Within the infratemporal fossa, the fat and blood vessels are located anteromedial to the neural structures. The fat must be removed first to expose the vessels and muscles. The maxillary artery can be seen entering the infratemporal fossa between the two heads of the lateral pterygoid muscle (LPM) (**Fig. 31.11**). The temporalis muscle and the deep portion of the masseter muscle occupy the lateral part of the fossa. Deep to the masseter muscle lies the ramus of the mandible.

Surgical Technique

Prior to undertaking any surgical approach, preoperative embolization should be performed to reduce the vascularity of the tumor and to improve visualization during surgical removal. Both carotid systems should be visualized during an angiography and contributions should be selectively embolized whether on the ipsilateral or contralateral side. Due to the highly vascular nature of these tumors, the surgeon must be prepared to deal with intraoperative hemorrhage if it occurs. In addition, any surgeon

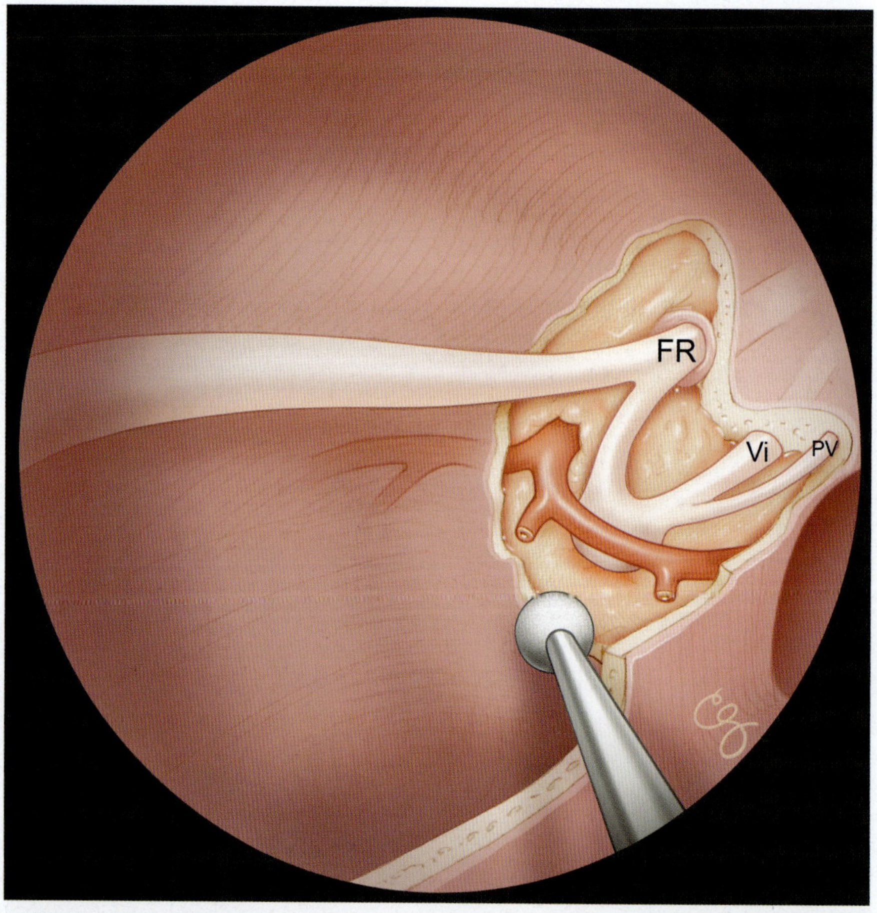

Fig. 31.10 The pterygopalatine fossa is a fat-filled space that is occupied by the maxillary nerve, vidian nerve, and branches of the internal maxillary artery. The three foramina—foramen rotundum (*FR*), vidian canal (*Vi*) and palatovaginal canal (*PV*)—can be seen entering the pterygopalatine fossa from the posterior wall.

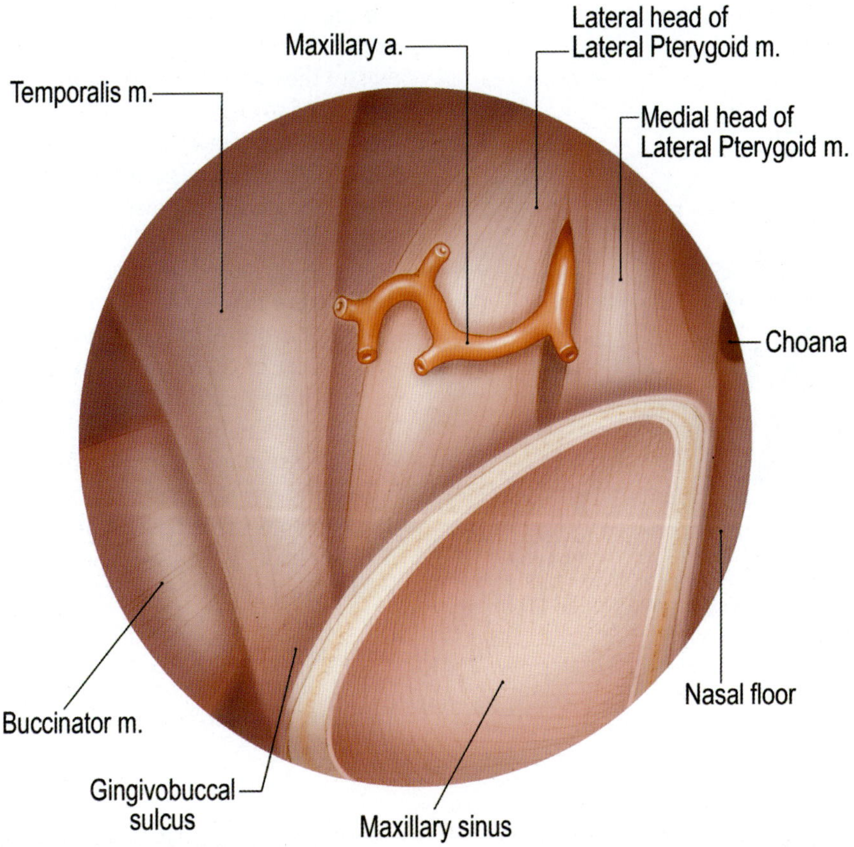

Fig. 31.11 The maxillary artery can be seen entering the infratemporal fossa between the medial and lateral pterygoid muscle.

attempting an endoscopic removal should be prepared to convert to an open approach if the circumstance necessitates greater exposure. A meticulous review of imaging studies must be performed prior to surgery to ensure endoscopic resectability. Special attention must be paid to tumor involvement of the inferior orbital fissure and vidian canal. [32] Failure to fully evaluate the vidian canal for tumor extension may result in incomplete tumor removal and recurrence. Computer-aided navigation should be set up and used throughout the case to help confirm the position of vital anatomic structures.

At the beginning of the case, the pterygopalatine fossa can be infiltrated with local anesthetic transorally by way of the greater palatine foramen. The injection of a vasoconstrictor into the pterygopalatine fossa at the start of the case may reduce intraoperative blood loss and may aid in visualization during the tumor resection. Surgical access to the pterygopalatine fossa is achieved by performing an uncinectomy, a large maxillary antrostomy with removal of the posterior fontanelle, and a sphenoethmoidectomy. This exposes the posterior wall of the maxillary sinus and sphenopalatine foramen. In most cases, except small tumors occupying the nasal cavity alone, a two-surgeon approach is advocated.[33] Having two surgeons allows one surgeon to place a high-volume suction in the surgical field if significant bleeding occurs or allows traction to be placed on the tumor, facilitating dissection around the tumor (**Fig. 31.12**). If there is a bulky endonasal component of the tumor that hinders the dissection, it may be separated from the deeper portion of the tumor and removed transorally. This is done with a Coblation wand to minimize bleeding from the cut edge of the tumor. An endoscopic medial maxillectomy is typically required in cases in which there is significant extension into the infratemporal fossa. Once this has been performed, the posterior wall of the maxillary sinus is removed starting at the sphenopalatine foramen using angled through-biting Blakesley forceps and Hajek Koeffler or Kerrison punches. With the wall removed, the contents of the pterygopalatine fossa and infratemporal fossa are exposed (**Fig. 31.13**). If needed, a canine fossa puncture can be performed to allow the second surgeon to place instruments through this additional access port to aid in tumor dissection or visualization if necessary.

The bone of the posterior wall is further removed up to the vertical process of the palatine bone medially and to the infraorbital nerve laterally. The infraorbital nerve is then followed posteriorly above the tumor and dissected

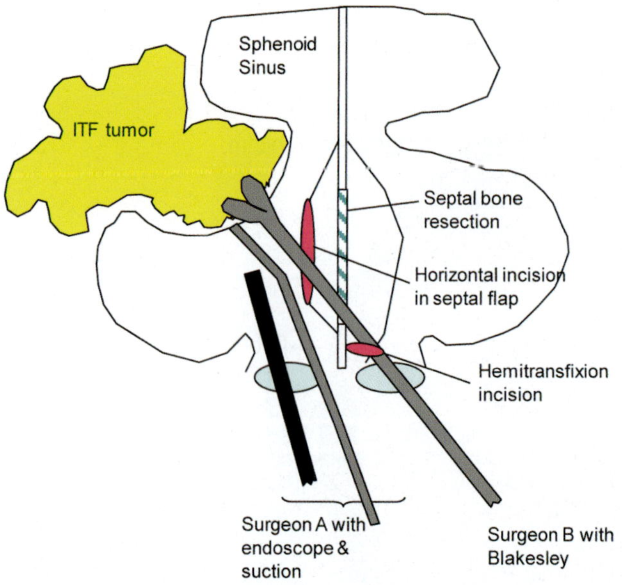

Fig. 31.12 Two-surgeon approach using a septal window to remove tumors in the infratemporal fossa.

off the upper aspect of the tumor, thereby preserving the nerve. If the tumor infiltrates around the nerve and traverses the inferior orbital fissure, the nerve may need to be sacrificed to ensure a complete tumor removal. The tumor at this point is put under traction by the second surgeon, which allows for dissection on the surface of the tumor. As the posterolateral aspect of the tumor is approached, the maxillary artery will be seen to enter and tether the tumor. This should be clipped with vascular clips and cautery before being cut. This allows further mobilization of the tumor out of the infratemporal fossa. As the posterior aspect of the tumor is approached, the vidian canal is identified and fully drilled out to ensure that no tumor remnants remain in the canal. Neglect of the vidian canal is the most common reason for recurrence of the tumor after surgery. This dissection can often be bloody with large venous lakes opened in the trabeculae of the bone. This bleeding is controlled with Gelfoam powder mixed with saline to form a paste and injected with a syringe and through a 14-gauge intravenous cannula onto the bleeding bone.

The region is packed with a neuropattie and once the bleeding is controlled, further drilling is done until the

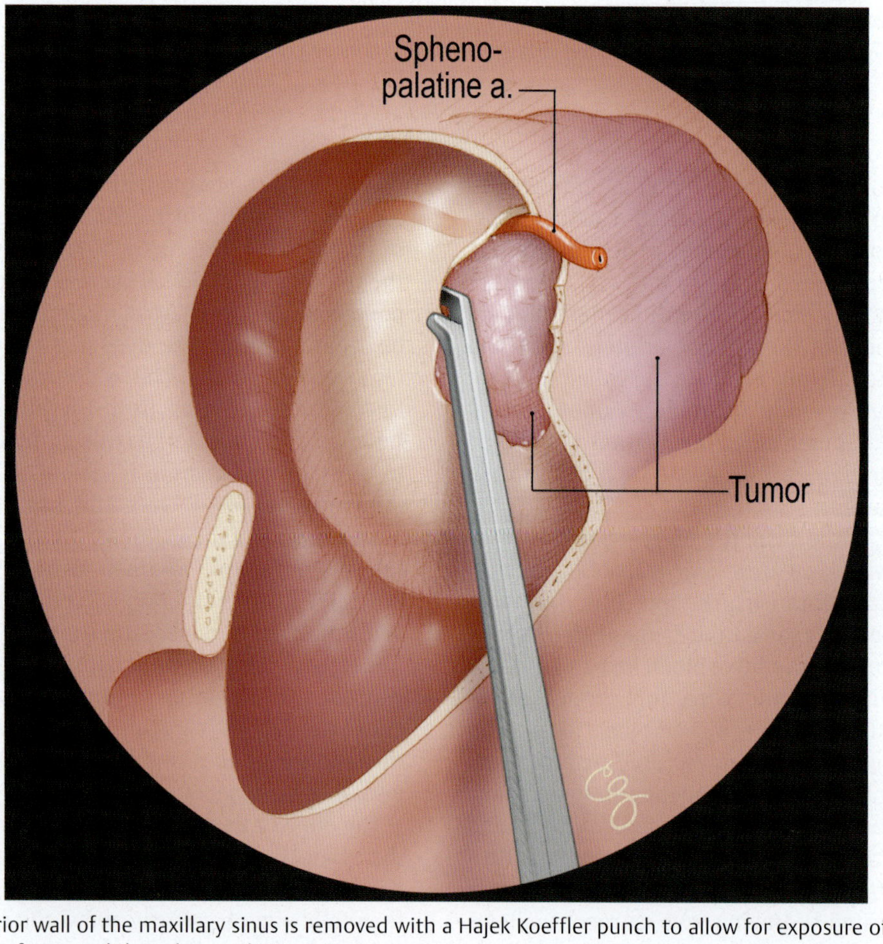

Fig. 31.13 The posterior wall of the maxillary sinus is removed with a Hajek Koeffler punch to allow for exposure of the pterygopalatine fossa, tumor within the fossa, and the sphenopalatine artery.

vidian canal has been fully explored and all tumors have been removed. Endoscopic resection of tumors with extensive involvement of the infratemporal fossa and intracranial extension should be done with a neurosurgeon, and it may be better to approach these lesions through an open infratemporal approach to facilitate the control of the vascular supply from the internal carotid artery. In all patients in whom an endoscopic medial maxillectomy has been performed, the lacrimal sac is opened at the end of surgery. Once exposure of the sac is complete, a vertical incision is made into the sac and the anterior and posterior walls splayed to ensure that no obstruction of tear drainage will occur postoperatively (**Fig. 31.5**).

Complications

The most important complication is hemorrhage, which if failed to be controlled, can result in significant patient morbidity. Hemorrhage from the maxillary artery can usually be controlled but a hemorrhage from either an internal carotid feeding branch or from the carotid itself can result in stroke or even death of the patient. Tumors that involve the cavernous sinus may also result in cranial nerve injury in addition to the risk posed to the carotid artery. In addition, the possible injury or sacrificing of the infraorbital nerve may result in cheek numbness. If the lacrimal sac is not formally opened after an endoscopic medial maxillectomy, an epiphora from stenosis of the nasolacrimal duct may result.

Postoperative Care

Postoperatively patients are put on broad-spectrum antibiotics for 5 to 7 days. Patients should be advised to avoid straining, heavy lifting, nose blowing, and strenuous exercise in the immediate postoperative period. Aggressive saline irrigations may be started from the day after surgery and are performed four to six times a day. Routine office endoscopy with the removal of crusts and debris in the early postoperative period is crucial for proper healing. Because of the high rate of recurrence of these tumors, postoperative surveillance with imaging and endoscopy is essential. Tumors may recur early in the recovery period (3 to 4 months). A postoperative contrast enhanced MRI scan at 6 months is advocated.[32]

Conclusion

Endoscopic surgery is currently advocated for the treatment of most benign tumors of the nasal cavity and paranasal sinuses. The use of image guidance systems and dedicated surgical instruments and tools has allowed the boundaries of endoscopic sinus surgery to expand immensely. Advanced endoscopic resections should be limited to experienced surgeons who have a strong foundation in the complex anatomy of the sinonasal cavity and surrounding regions. When compared with traditional external approaches, endoscopic surgery is characterized by less morbidity, shorter recovery time, and reduced complications. It is expected that with continued advancement in endoscopic techniques, the limits to their use will decrease.

References

1. Imola MJ, Hamlar DD, Shao W, Chowdhury K, Tatum S. Resorbable plate fixation in pediatric craniofacial surgery: long-term outcome. Arch Facial Plast Surg 2001;3(2):79–90
2. Buchwald C, Nielsen LH, Nielsen PL, Ahlgren P, Tos M. Inverted papilloma: a follow-up study including primarily unacknowledged cases. Am J Otolaryngol 1989;10(4):273–281
3. Krouse JH. Endoscopic treatment of inverted papilloma: safety and efficacy. Am J Otolaryngol 2001;22(2):87–99
4. Kashima HK, Kessis T, Hruban RH, Wu TC, Zinreich SJ, Shah KV. Human papillomavirus in sinonasal papillomas and squamous cell carcinoma. Laryngoscope 1992;102(9):973–976
5. Lesperance MM, Esclamado RM. Squamous cell carcinoma arising in inverted papilloma. Laryngoscope 1995;105(2):178–183
6. Wormald PJ, Ooi E, van Hasselt CA, Nair S. Endoscopic removal of sinonasal inverted papilloma including endoscopic medial maxillectomy. Laryngoscope 2003;113(5):867–873
7. Suh KW, Facer GW, Devine KD, Weiland LH, Zujko RD. Inverting papilloma of the nose and paranasal sinuses. Laryngoscope 1977; 87(1):35–46
8. Clarke SR, Amedee RG. Schneiderian papilloma. J La State Med Soc 1997;149(9):310–315
9. Phillips PP, Gustafson RO, Facer GW. The clinical behavior of inverting papilloma of the nose and paranasal sinuses: report of 112 cases and review of the literature. Laryngoscope 1990;100(5):463–469
10. Sukenik MA, Casiano R. Endoscopic medial maxillectomy for inverted papillomas of the paranasal sinuses: value of the intraoperative endoscopic examination. Laryngoscope 2000;110(1):39–42
11. Weissler MC, Montgomery WW, Turner PA, Montgomery SK, Joseph MP. Inverted papilloma. Ann Otol Rhinol Laryngol 1986; 95(3 Pt 1):215–221
12. Busquets JM, Hwang PH. Endoscopic resection of sinonasal inverted papilloma: a meta-analysis. Otolaryngol Head Neck Surg 2006;134(3):476–482
13. Chiu AG, Jackman AH, Antunes MB, Feldman MD, Palmer JN. Radiographic and histologic analysis of the bone underlying inverted papillomas. Laryngoscope 2006;116(9):1617–1620
14. Schlosser RJ, Mason JC, Gross CW. Aggressive endoscopic resection of inverted papilloma: an update. Otolaryngol Head Neck Surg 2001;125(1):49–53
15. Sham CL, Woo JK, van Hasselt CA. Endoscopic resection of inverted papilloma of the nose and paranasal sinuses. J Laryngol Otol 1998;112(8):758–764
16. Tufano RP, Thaler ER, Lanza DC, Goldberg AN, Kennedy DW. Endoscopic management of sinonasal inverted papilloma. Am J Rhinol 1999;13(6):423–426
17. Gullane PJ, Davidson J, O'Dwyer T, Forte V. Juvenile angiofibroma: a review of the literature and a case series report. Laryngoscope 1992;102(8):928–933

18. Granato L. Juvenile nasopharyngeal angiofibroma. In: Otolaryngology Textbook. Sao Paulo: Roca; 2002: 701–710
19. Jafek BW, Krekorian EA, Kirsch WM, Wood RP. Juvenile nasopharyngeal angiofibroma: management of intracranial extension. Head Neck Surg 1979;2(2):119–128
20. Standefer J, Holt GR, Brown WE Jr, Gates GA. Combined intracranial and extracranial excision of nasopharyngeal angiofibroma. Laryngoscope 1983;93(6):772–779
21. Krekorian EA, Kato RH. Surgical management of nasopharyngeal angiofibroma with intracranial extension. Laryngoscope 1977;87(2):154–164
22. Mann WJ, Jecker P, Amedee RG. Juvenile angiofibromas: changing surgical concept over the last 20 years. Laryngoscope 2004; 114(2):291–293
23. Antonelli AR, Cappiello J, Di Lorenzo D, Donajo CA, Nicolai P, Orlandini A. Diagnosis, staging, and treatment of juvenile nasopharyngeal angiofibroma (JNA). Laryngoscope 1987;97(11): 1319 –1325
24. Lloyd G, Howard D, Phelps P, Cheesman A. Juvenile angiofibroma: the lessons of 20 years of modern imaging. J Laryngol Otol 1999;113(2):127–134
25. Siniluoto TM, Luotonen JP, Tikkakoski TA, Leinonen AS, Jokinen KE. Value of pre-operative embolization in surgery for nasopharyngeal angiofibroma. J Laryngol Otol 1993;107(6):514–521
26. Pryor SG, Moore EJ, Kasperbauer JL. Endoscopic versus traditional approaches for excision of juvenile nasopharyngeal angiofibroma. Laryngoscope 2005;115(7):1201–1207
27. Andrews JC, Fisch U, Valavanis A, Aeppli U, Makek MS. The surgical management of extensive nasopharyngeal angiofibromas with the infratemporal fossa approach. Laryngoscope 1989;99(4):429–437
28. Cummings BJ, Blend R, Keane T, et al. Primary radiation therapy for juvenile nasopharyngeal angiofibroma. Laryngoscope 1984;94(12 Pt 1):1599–1605
29. Neel HB III. Nasopharyngeal carcinoma. Clinical presentation, diagnosis, treatment, and prognosis. Otolaryngol Clin North Am 1985;18(3):479–490
30. Roger G, Tran Ba Huy P, Froehlich P, et al. Exclusively endoscopic removal of juvenile nasopharyngeal angiofibroma: trends and limits. Arch Otolaryngol Head Neck Surg 2002;128(8):928–935
31. Andrade NA, Pinto JA, Nóbrega MdeO, Aguiar JE, Aguiar TF, Vinhaes ES. Exclusively endoscopic surgery for juvenile nasopharyngeal angiofibroma. Otolaryngol Head Neck Surg 2007;137(3):492–496
32. Douglas R, Wormald PJ. Endoscopic surgery for juvenile nasopharyngeal angiofibroma: where are the limits? Curr Opin Otolaryngol Head Neck Surg 2006;14(1):1–5
33. Robinson S, Patel N, Wormald PJ. Endoscopic management of benign tumors extending into the infratemporal fossa: a two-surgeon transnasal approach. Laryngoscope 2005;115(10): 1818 –1822
34. Waitz G, Wigand ME. Results of endoscopic sinus surgery for the treatment of inverted papillomas. Laryngoscope 1992;102(8):917–922
35. Stankiewicz JA, Girgis SJ. Endoscopic surgical treatment of nasal and paranasal sinus inverted papilloma. Otolaryngol Head Neck Surg 1993;109(6):988–995
36. McCary WS, Gross CW, Reibel JF, Cantrell RW. Preliminary report: endoscopic versus external surgery in the management of inverting papilloma. Laryngoscope 1994;104(4):415–419
37. Buchwald C, Franzmann MB, Tos M. Sinonasal papillomas: a report of 82 cases in Copenhagen County, including a longitudinal epidemiological and clinical study. Laryngoscope 1995;105(1): 72–79
38. Kamel RH. Transnasal endoscopic medial maxillectomy in inverted papilloma. Laryngoscope 1995;105(8 Pt 1):847–853
39. Raveh E, Feinmesser R, Shpitzer T, Yaniv E, Segal K. Inverted papilloma of the nose and paranasal sinuses: a study of 56 cases and review of the literature. Isr J Med Sci 1996;32(12):1163–1167
40. Chee LW, Sethi DS. The endoscopic management of sinonasal inverted papillomas. Clin Otolaryngol Allied Sci 1999;24(1):61–66
41. Bertrand B, Eloy P, Jorissen M, et al. Surgery of inverted papillomas under endoscopic control. Acta Otorhinolaryngol Belg 2000;54(2):139–150
42. Klimek T, Atai E, Schubert M, Glanz H. Inverted papilloma of the nasal cavity and paranasal sinuses: clinical data, surgical strategy and recurrence rates. Acta Otolaryngol 2000;120(2):267–272
43. Lund VJ. Optimum management of inverted papilloma. J Laryngol Otol 2000;114(3):194–197
44. Han JK, Smith TL, Loehrl T, Toohill RJ, Smith MM. An evolution in the management of sinonasal inverting papilloma. Laryngoscope 2001;111(8):1395–1400
45. Thorp MA, Oyarzabal-Amigo MF, du Plessis JH, Sellars SL. Inverted papilloma: a review of 53 cases. Laryngoscope 2001;111(8): 1401–1405
46. Keleş N, Değber K. Endonasal endoscopic surgical treatment of paranasal sinus inverted papilloma—first experiences. Rhinology 2001;39(3):156–159
47. Kühn UM, Mann WJ, Amedee RG. Endonasal approach for nasal and paranasal sinus tumor removal. ORL J Otorhinolaryngol Relat Spec 2001;63(6):366–371
48. Baruah P, Deka RC. Endoscopic management of inverted papillomas of the nose and paranasal sinuses. Ear Nose Throat J 2003;82(4):317–320
49. Sadeghi N, Al-Dhahri S, Manoukian JJ. Transnasal endoscopic medial maxillectomy for inverting papilloma. Laryngoscope 2003;113(4):749–753
50. Pasquini E, Sciarretta V, Compadretti GC, Cantaroni C. A case report of inverted papilloma associated with esthesioneuroblastoma treated by endoscopic sinus surgery. Am J Otolaryngol 2003;24(3):181–182
51. Kaza S, Capasso R, Casiano RR. Endoscopic resection of inverted papilloma: University of Miami experience. Am J Rhinol 2003;17(4):185–190
52. Kraft M, Simmen D, Kaufmann T, Holzmann D. Long-term results of endonasal sinus surgery in sinonasal papillomas. Laryngoscope 2003;113(9):1541–1547
53. Lawson W, Kaufman MR, Biller HF. Treatment outcomes in the management of inverted papilloma: an analysis of 160 cases. Laryngoscope 2003;113(9):1548–1556
54. Llorente JL, Deleyiannis F, Rodrigo JP, et al. Minimally invasive treatment of the nasal inverted papilloma. Am J Rhinol 2003;17(6):335–341
55. Lee TJ, Huang SF, Huang CC. Tailored endoscopic surgery for the treatment of sinonasal inverted papilloma. Head Neck 2004; 26(2):145–153
56. Tomenzoli D, Castelnuovo P, Pagella F, et al. Different endoscopic surgical strategies in the management of inverted papilloma of the sinonasal tract: experience with 47 patients. Laryngoscope 2004;114(2):193–200
57. Pasquini E, Sciarretta V, Frank G, et al. Endoscopic treatment of benign tumors of the nose and paranasal sinuses. Otolaryngol Head Neck Surg 2004;131(3):180–186

32 Malignant Sinonasal Tumors

Valerie J. Lund

Malignant tumors in the nose and paranasal sinuses pose many problems due to their rarity, late presentation, and proximity to important structures such as the orbit and skull base. They also represent the area of greatest histologic diversity in the body with every type of tumor occurring, each with differing natural histories. This makes it difficult for any individual to accrue large numbers of patients for statistical analysis and optimum management can only really be offered in tertiary referral centers where expert imaging and histopathology underpin the medical and surgical oncology. Malignant sinonasal tumors affect less than 1 in 100,000 individuals per year in most countries. They can occur at any age though the majority present in the sixth and seventh decades with some (e.g., malignant melanoma) more often affecting the elderly. When occupational factors are excluded, the male to female ratio is ~2:1.

Unlike tumors elsewhere in the head and neck, smoking and alcohol have little role in the development of malignant sinonasal tumors. Certain occupations, however, notably those with exposure to hardwood dust, are a recognized factor in the etiology of ethmoidal adenocarcinoma as was first described in 1968.[1] Only those jobs such as lathing and sanding that create dust particles greater than 5 μm diameter seem susceptible, increasing the relative risk as compared with the normal population 70-fold, although it is not yet known which component of the dust is responsible. The duration of exposure and interval between exposure and development of the tumor was initially reported as over 20 years in both respects. However, it is clear that there are several individuals who develop the tumor with much shorter exposure and lag time.

The nose and sinuses are included in conventional classification systems (e.g., TNM; see **Table 32.1**),[2] but these are of less prognostic value than elsewhere in the head and neck due to the wide range of pathologies, relatively large primary size, initially low metastatic spread, and long natural histories. Attempts to classify according to extent (e.g., Kadish) staging for olfactory neuroblastoma remain relatively crude, though a study by Cantu et al. found this approach was more successful than the American Joint Committee on Cancer (AJCC) or Union for International Cancer Control (UICC) systems for the ethmoids.[3,4] Histologic classification based on the degree of differentiation may be of some help in predicting prognosis (e.g., in adenocarcinoma).

Histology and Patient Selection

Although squamous cell carcinoma remains the most common, it is interesting to consider why such a diversity of different types of tumors is found in the nose and sinuses (**Table 32.2**). Consequently, an expert pathologist is often needed. The distinction between benign and malignant is also less clear in this area where a malignant tumor may overwhelm a patient with local intracranial spread before manifesting metastatic spread, whereas very large benign tumors may also lead to the demise of their host. As tumors often present late, it can often be difficult to say exactly where they arose.

Squamous Cell Carcinoma

Most squamous cell carcinomas probably arise in the maxillary sinus (**Fig. 32.1**) and are generally treated with combined surgery and chemoradiation; although, in poorly differentiated or undifferentiated sinonasal carcinomas, chemoradiation alone may be curative. Occasionally, this tumor affects the nasal septum or columella, which is associated with a particularly poor prognosis partly due to the possibility of bilateral metastatic spread to the cervical nodes.

Adenocarcinoma

Adenocarcinomas usually arise in the middle meatus and spread into the ethmoid from which they may spread forward into the glabella or backward into the sphenoethmoidal recess and nasopharynx (**Fig. 32.2**). The association with the woodworking trade is well known, but the tumor can occur without this exposure. It is relatively radioresistant, but combined therapy is usually offered. A craniofacial resection is often used but endoscopic surgery may be possible in selected cases.[5–7] Surgical debulking combined with topical 5-fluoro-uracil has been used by some.[8]

Adenoid Cystic Carcinoma

Adenoid cystic carcinoma has a propensity for direct and embolic dissemination along perineural lymphatics and by blood-borne metastases, which makes curative excision difficult, especially since the natural history of late

Table 32.1 TNM Classification of Sinonasal Tumors

Primary Tumor (T)	
Maxillary Sinus	
TX	Primary tumor cannot be assessed
TO	No evidence of primary tumor
Tis	Carcinoma in situ
T1	Tumor limited to the maxillary sinus mucosa with no erosion or destruction of bone
T2	Tumor causing bone erosion or destruction including extension into the hard palate and/or middle nasal meatus, except extension to posterior wall of maxillary sinus and pterygoid plates
T3	Tumor invades any of the following: bone of the posterior wall of maxillary sinus, subcutaneous tissues, floor or medial wall of orbit, pterygoid fossa, ethmoid sinuses
T4a	Moderately advanced local disease
	Tumor invades anterior orbital contents, skin of cheek, pterygoid plates, infratemporal fossa, cribriform plate, sphenoid, or frontal sinuses
T4b	Very advanced local disease
	Tumor invades any of the following: orbital apex, dura, brain, middle cranial fossa, cranial nerves other than maxillary division of trigeminal nerve V_2, nasopharynx, or clivus
Nasal Cavity and Ethmoid Sinus	
TX	Primary tumor cannot be assessed
TO	No evidence of primary tumor
Tis	Carcinoma in situ
T1	Tumor restricted to any one subsite, with or without bony invasion
T2	Tumor invading two subsites in a single region within the nasoethmoidal complex, with or without bony invasion
T3	Tumor extends to invade the medial wall or floor of the orbit, maxillary sinus, palate, or cribriform plate
T4a	Moderately advanced local disease
	Tumor invades any of the following: anterior orbital contents, skin of the nose or cheek, minimal extension to anterior cranial fossa, pterygoid plates, sphenoid, or frontal sinuses
T4b	Very advanced local disease
	Tumor invades any of the following: orbital apex, dura, brain, middle cranial fossa, cranial nerves other than V_2, nasopharynx, or clivus
Regional Lymph Nodes (N)	
NX	Regional lymph nodes cannot be assessed
NO	No regional lymph node metastasis
N1	Metastasis in a single ipsilateral lymph node, 3 cm or less in greatest dimension
N2	Metastasis in a single ipsilateral lymph node, more than 3 cm but not more than 6 cm in greatest dimension, or in multiple ipsilateral lymph nodes, none more than 6 cm in greatest dimension, or in bilateral or contralateral lymph nodes, none more than 6 cm in greatest dimension
N2a	Metastasis in a single ipsilateral lymph node, more than 3 cm but not more than 6 cm in greatest dimension
N2b	Metastasis in multiple ipsilateral lymph nodes, none more than 6 cm in greatest dimension
N2c	Metastasis in bilateral or contralateral lymph nodes, none more than 6 cm in greatest dimension
N3	Metastasis in a lymph node, more than 6 cm in greatest dimension
Distant Metastasis (M)	
MO	No distant metastasis
M1	Distant metastasis

Source: Data from Edge S, Byrd D, Compton C, Fritz A, Greene F, Trotti A, eds. American Joint Committee on Cancer Staging Manual. 7th ed. New York: Springer; 2010: 69–78.

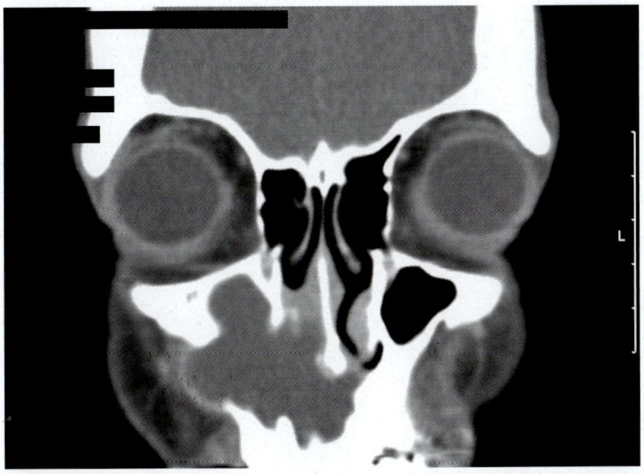

Fig. 32.1 Coronal computed tomography scan showing squamous cell carcinoma arising within maxillary antrum and eroding through bony walls.

Table 32.2 Histology of Malignant Sinonasal Neoplasia

Epithelial Epidermoid	• Squamous cell carcinoma (spindle cell, verrucous, transitional)
Epithelial Nonepidermoid	• Adenoid cystic carcinoma • Adenocarcinoma • Mucoepidermoid carcinoma • Acinic cell carcinoma
Neurectodermal	• Malignant melanoma • Olfactory neuroblastoma • Neuroendocrine carcinoma • Primitive peripheral neuroectodermal tumor and Ewing sarcoma • Sinonasal undifferentiated carcinoma
Odontogenic tumors	• Ameloblastoma
Vascular	• Angiosarcoma • Kaposi sarcoma • Hemangiopericytoma
Muscular	• Leiomyosarcoma • Rhabdomyosarcoma
Cartilaginous	• Chondrosarcoma (+ mesenchymal)
Osseous	• Osteosarcoma
Lymphoreticular	• Burkitt lymphoma • Non-Hodgkin lymphoma • Extramedullary plasmacytoma • T and natural kill cell lymphoma • Histiocytic/dendritic cell malignancies
Mesenchymal	• Fibrosarcoma • Liposarcoma • Malignant fibrous histiocytoma • Alveolar soft-part sarcoma
Metastases	

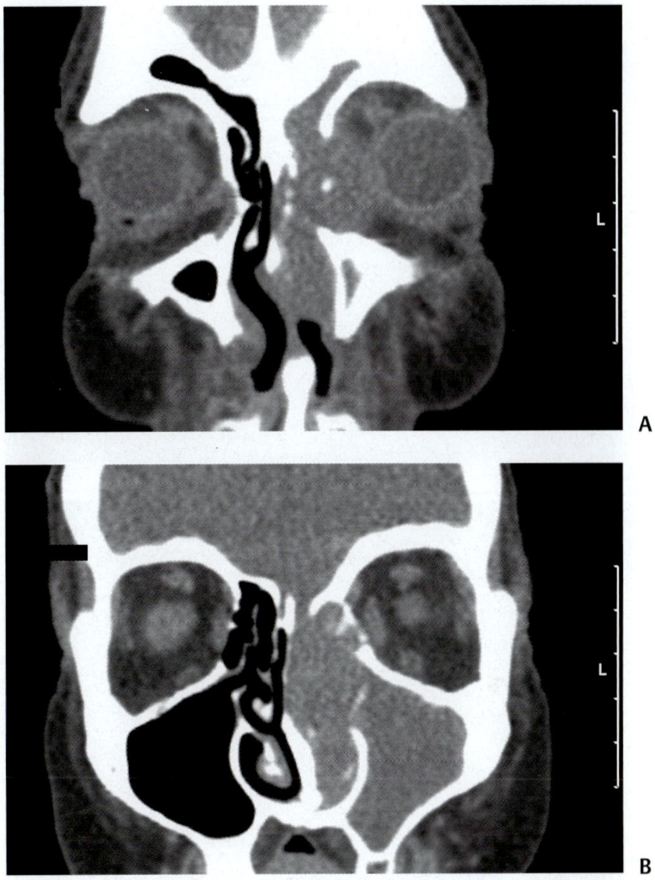

Fig. 32.2 Coronal computed tomography scans showing **(A)** adenocarcinoma eroding anterior lamina papyracea, and **(B)** anterior skull base.

recurrence can be long.[9] Thus, although 5-year survival figures may be encouraging, by 20 years, less than 5% may be alive.[5] Treatment is again combined surgery and radiotherapy, although radiotherapy only delays recurrence rather than increasing cure.

Olfactory Neuroblastoma

Olfactory neuroblastoma, or esthesioneuroblastoma, classically arises from olfactory epithelium in the upper nasal cavity and therefore spreads intracranially at an early stage to involve the olfactory bulb and tracts (**Figs. 32.3 and 32.4**). It is more common than once thought due to improved diagnostic techniques. The age range was from 12 to 70 years (mean 46 years) in a cohort of 42 patients.[10] Cervical metastases have been described in up to 23%.[11] The craniofacial resection was specifically designed to deal with this tumor because it allows for a complete resection of the olfactory apparatus.[12] Outcome analysis showed a higher rate of recurrence when craniofacial resection was not combined with radiotherapy, so this should always be offered.[10] Adjuvant chemotherapy is also being offered in many protocols.[13] Endoscopic resection is increasingly being used for

A

B

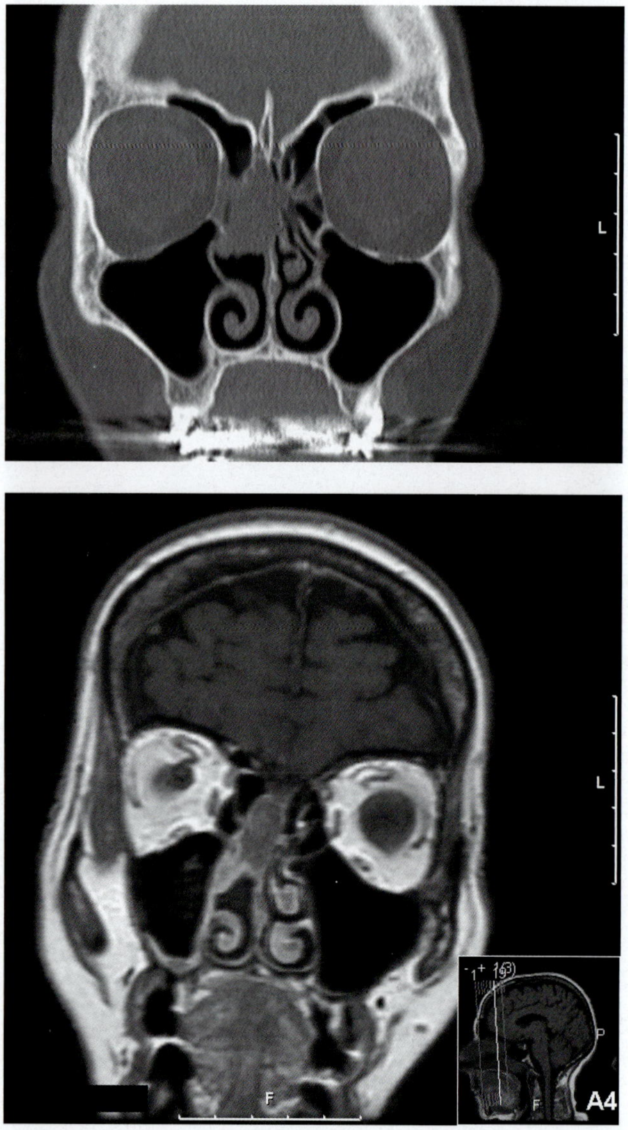

Fig. 32.3 (A) Coronal computed tomography scan showing olfactory neuroblastoma arising in superior nasal cavity. **(B)** Coronal magnetic resonance image (T1 with gadolinium).

this tumor, particularly when it arises from the middle and superior turbinates[6,14] and should be combined with radiotherapy. Long-term follow-up is important because late recurrence has been observed up to 14 years after the initial treatment, sometimes at some distance from the original lesion.[10]

Malignant Melanoma

Malignant melanoma is a rare mucosal neoplasm originating from neural crest tissue and often affects the elderly. Typically, it arises in the nose on the septum or inferior turbinate and can be associated with satellite lesions and areas of an amelanotic tumor (**Fig. 32.5**). It is a capricious and unpredictable disease in which some patients are

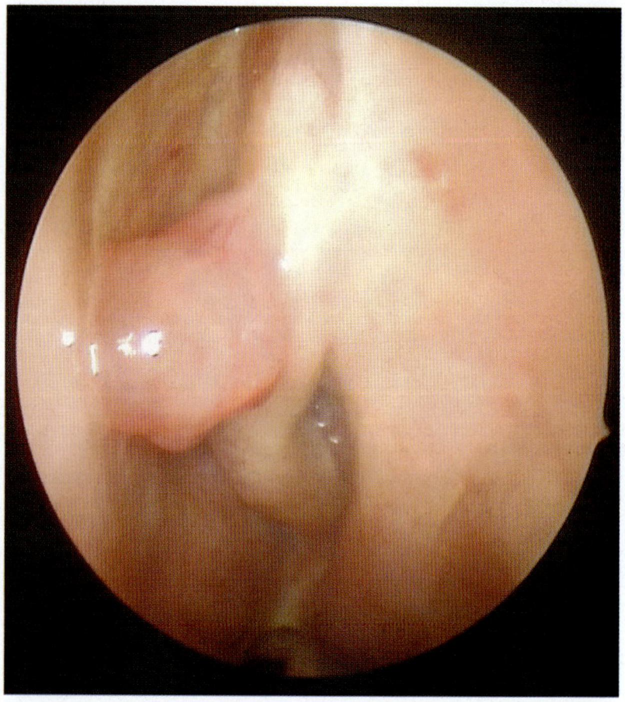

Fig. 32.4 Endoscopic view of an olfactory neuroblastoma arising from the medial surface of the superior turbinate.

rapidly overwhelmed in a few months, whereas others survive for years with residual disease.[15] Thus, endoscopic surgery is as effective as more radical procedures and a craniofacial is contraindicated. The role of radiotherapy is debated but may confer a small advantage.

Chondrosarcoma

Chondrosarcoma arises in the nasal cavity, often from the septum and spreading into the skull base and palate (**Fig. 32.6**).[16] It may be multifocal and can be quite indolent with frequent "recurrences" over many years.[5] Although often well differentiated, the term chondroma should not be used because these tumors ultimately produce major problems due to cranial nerve involvement as the disease inexorably spreads across the skull base. Any age can be affected and it is generally more aggressive in younger patients, especially the mesenchymal variety. Craniofacial resection usually offers the best oncologic approach, particularly as these tumors are not radiosensitive, although endoscopic resection is sometimes possible.

Lymphomas

Lymphomas comprise ~6% of malignant sinonasal tumors and less than 1% of lymphomas occur in this area. Extranodal lymphomas, such as sinonasal B cell and T and natural killer (T/NK) cell lymphomas, present particular problems. B cell tumors present as an infiltrating indurated mass often affecting the external nose and soft tissues,

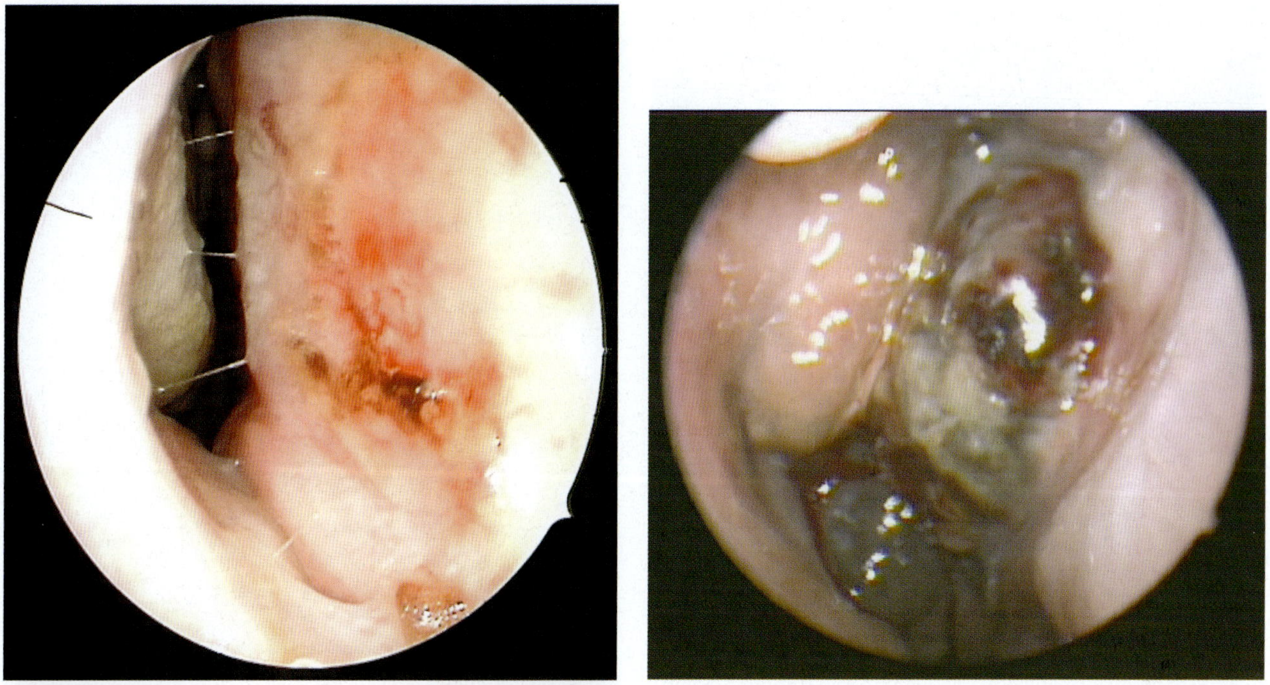

A B

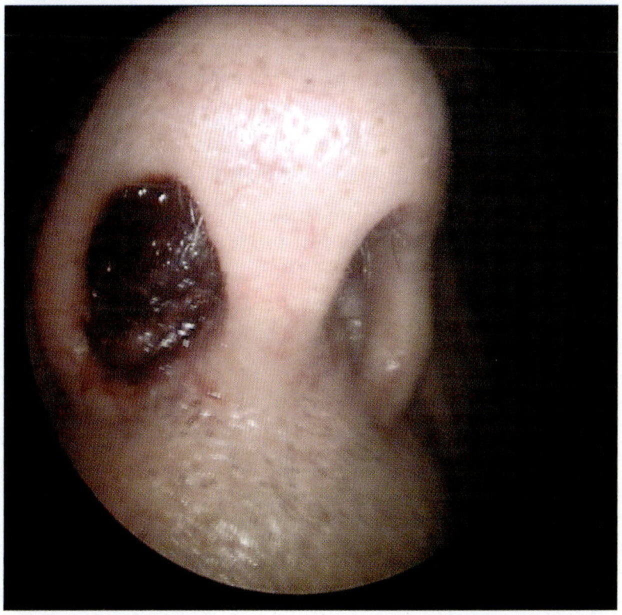

C

Fig. 32.5 Endoscopic views of malignant melanoma **(A)** with associated melanosis on nasal septum, **(B)** melanotic mass arising from septum with necrosis and bleeding, and **(C)** completely filling nasal cavity.

whereas T/NK cell tumors produce aggressive destructive lesions of the midface, previously referred to as lethal midline granulomas and many other terms, and are associated with Epstein-Barr exposure.[17] Suspecting the diagnosis and taking representative tissue is very important as they are often associated with significant inflammation and necrosis. Once diagnosed, a full staging is undertaken and treatment is by established chemoradiotherapy regimens dependent on the extent of spread.[18]

Ultimately, patient selection will depend on: (1) histology, type and extent; and (2) patient factors such as comorbidities, psychological factors, and social factors. In most centers, these will be the subject of a multidisciplinary team discussion.

Diagnostic Workup

Clinical Presentation

The presenting features of a sinonasal tumor are often subtle and easily confused with inflammation or allergy. The warning features are that they start unilaterally and spontaneously. Tumors arising in the nasal cavity will

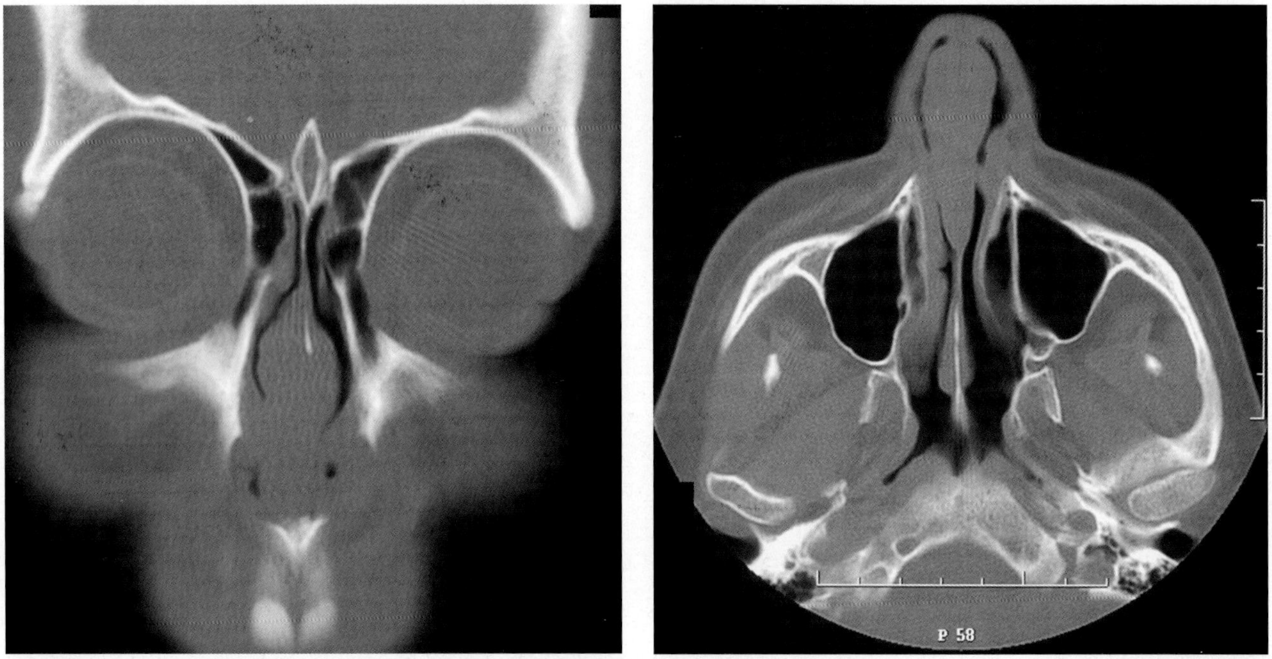

A B

Fig. 32.6 (A) Coronal computed tomography scan showing chondrosarcoma arising from the septum. **(B)** Axial view.

present earlier than those in the sinuses, which have to break out of the bony confines into the nose itself, the orbit, or the intracranial cavity. As these initial symptoms are often ignored by the patient and clinicians, the tumor often involves several sites at presentation, and therefore, it can be difficult to determine the original point of origin. Conversely, sometimes apparently extensive tumors can have a limited origin from the lateral wall of the nose.

Depending on the series, squamous cell carcinoma of the maxilla probably remains the most common tumor in this area even if it is difficult to estimate the percentage of the whole group due to changing referral patterns. Ethmoidal tumors (e.g., adenocarcinomas) spread into the nasal cavity but also involve the orbit, skull base, and contralateral side reasonably quickly, as well as involving the glabella anteriorly and the sphenoethmoidal recess and the nasopharynx posteriorly. Tumors arising on the lateral wall of the nose will involve the nasal cavity, ethmoid, and maxilla at an early stage. From this point, disease may spread into the sphenoid and/or frontal sinus, whereas primary tumors of these sinuses are extremely rare for reasons that are unclear. Those arising on the septum may affect the soft tissue of the external nose or may spread posterosuperiorly to affect the sphenoid and optic chiasm.

Thus, the most common symptoms are unilateral nasal obstruction, discharge that may be blood-stained, and a reduction in the sense of smell. As the tumor erodes through the lamina papyracea, the eye is displaced anteriorly, which may produce double vision if it happens relatively quickly. Rapid displacement may result in exposure of the cornea, keratosis, and ulceration. Epiphora will occur with obstruction of the nasolacrimal apparatus. The tumor may penetrate the periosteum, infiltrating muscles and increasing diplopia and proptosis, and affecting vision. From the orbital apex, the tumor can spread posteriorly either intra- or extraperiosteally to affect the cavernous sinus with its respective cranial nerves, the internal carotid artery, and then can reach the middle cranial fossa. If the sphenoid is involved (e.g., chondrosarcoma), one or both orbital apices can be affected, as can the optic chiasm, resulting in devastating bilateral visual loss. Orbital symptoms occur in over 50% of patients with malignant sinonasal tumors, more often with ethmoidal tumors (62%) than nasal (42%) and in 60 to 80% of maxillary sinus malignancies. Ianetti et al. have identified three stages of orbital invasion: (1) erosion or destruction of the medial orbital wall; (2) extraconal invasion of periorbital fat; and (3) invasion of the medial rectus muscle, optic nerve, ocular bulb, or eyelid skin.[19]

The skull base, in contrast, is a symptomatically silent area with cerebrospinal fluid (CSF) leaks and meningitis extremely rare, pain unusual, and any personality changes associated with extensive frontal lobe infiltration usually too subtle to be noticed. Pain and paraesthesia may occur with involvement of the infraorbital nerve, the pterygoid region, and the infratemporal fossa, which may also produce trismus. Tumor can also spread directly into the soft tissues of the face, producing a mass in the cheek that may ulcerate or extend into the gum, again producing a mass, the loosening of teeth, and/or an oroantral fistula.

It is relatively uncommon for a sinonasal malignancy to present with lymphatic or hematogenous metastases; though this more frequently occurs in the terminal stages, especially when local disease is uncontrolled. An incidence of cervical lymphadenopathy of <10% is cited, most often with squamous cell carcinoma of the maxilla, and is associated with a poor prognosis.[20] In addition, sinonasal undifferentiated carcinoma (SNUC), olfactory neuroblastoma, and lymphoma may all present with neck nodes. The submandibular, jugulodigastric, prefacial, and postfacial nodes are most commonly involved with tumors from the septum and, in particular, the columellar region, which sometimes spread bilaterally. This is invariably associated with a poor prognosis.

Not only can adenoid cystic carcinoma spread along perineural lymphatics to present at some distance from the original tumor, but it can also produce secondary deposits in the lung, although these may be quite indolent in their behavior and may occur in the presence of local control. Thus, although systemic problems are rare, particularly at presentation, complaints of an unresolving nonproductive cough, bone pain, or significant fatigue should prompt further investigation.

Imaging

The availability of fine detail and rapidly performed computed tomography (CT) in the coronal, axial, and sagittal plane combined with magnetic resonance imaging (MRI) provide an accurate depiction of tumor extent and sometimes an indication of the tumor type (**Table 32.3**).[21] Earlier studies suggest that a combination of these modalities produced an accuracy of 98% in predicting the extent of the tumor, although the assessment of spread through the orbital periosteum and dura still requires macro- and microscopic confirmation. MRI alone is not sufficient because early erosion of the cribriform plate is still best shown on coronal CT.

Table 32.3 Protocol for Investigation of Sinonasal Malignancy

Preoperative
1. Endoscopic examination under anesthesia
2. Imaging
CT: fine detail coronal, axial ± sagittal; contrast enhancement if skull base affected
MRI: coronal, axial, and sagittal T1 sequences; pre- and post-gandolinium-DTPA; axial T2-weighted sequences
± CXR/ CT chest*
± CT abdomen*
Postoperative Follow-up Protocol
1. Endoscopic examination under anesthesia
2. Imaging
MRI: coronal, axial, and sagittal T1 sequences; pre- and post-gadolinium T1 sequences; axial T2-weighted sequences
Every 4 months for first two years, then 6 month thereafter depending on histology

Source: Data from Lloyd GAS, Lund VJ, Howard DJ, et al. Optimum imaging for sinonasal malignancy. J Laryngol Otol 2000;114:557–562.
Abbreviations: CXR, chest x-ray; CT, computed tomography; DTPA, diethylenetriaminepentaacetic acid
*Dependent on histology.

The extent to which imaging beyond the nose and sinuses is undertaken will depend to some extent on the histology and the patient's symptoms. For most malignant tumors, it is not routinely undertaken, but poorly differentiated tumors such as SNUCs, neuroendocrine carcinomas, and lymphomas require more extensive staging using CT, MRI, or positron emission tomography (PET)-CT.[22] Similarly, adenoid cystic carcinomas, which have a propensity to spread to the lung, require a chest X-ray and/or chest CT.

For those tumors associated with higher rates of cervical metastases, such as olfactory neuroblastomas and SNUCs, an ultrasound of the neck combined with a fine-needle aspiration biopsy (FNAB) are recommended. This offers more accurate staging and an important baseline for subsequent follow-up.[23]

Biopsy

Although this can sometimes be performed under no or local anesthesia in the outpatient setting, it is generally more appropriate to perform a biopsy under endoscopic control and general anesthesia because this is most likely to produce representative tissue without the transgression of normal tissue planes in a controlled setting.

Additional Tests

In patients where bone metastases are suspected, a formal radionucleotide bone scan should be undertaken. Hematologic investigations, including bone marrow aspirate, may be appropriate in cases of chloroma (leukemic deposits), lymphoma, and individuals where bone and liver secondaries are suspected.

Surgical Anatomy

A late presentation and a close proximity of the orbit, skull base, pterygoid, and infratemporal regions mean that tumors have often spread into these adjacent areas at presentation (**Fig. 32.1**). Both the lamina papyracea and the skull base are composed of thin bone, with natural dehiscences where neurovascular structures cross. Although the roof of the ethmoids is largely composed of hard frontal bone, the lateral lamella of the cribriform niche is thin and divides the ethmoids from the anterior cranial fossa. Fortunately, the dura and orbital periosteum are comparatively strong and resist tumor spread for some time. However, tumors invading the medial orbit may run subperiosteally to the apex and thence into the middle cranial fossa. The superior and inferior orbital fissures also offer routes of tumor exit and entry. The inferior fissure communicates with the pterygopalatine fossa medially and the infratemporal fossa laterally, whereas the superior fissure leads to the cavernous sinus.

The cribriform niche varies considerably in length (15.5 to 25.8 mm) and in depth (0 to 15.5 mm),[24] and the dura is closely applied in this area, requiring sharp dissection during a craniofacial resection. An emissary vein to the sagittal sinus and the olfactory fibers themselves provide routes for the tumor to spread. The sphenoid jugum and optic chiasm lie behind the cribriform plate (mean 21 mm).[24]

The optic nerve and internal carotid artery run in the lateral wall of the sphenoid and may be exposed by natural anatomic variation or bone erosion. The bone overlying these structures has been estimated to be clinically dehiscent in up to 20% of cases. This is particularly the case in the presence of a sphenoethmoidal (Onodi) cell, which pneumatizes laterally and superiorly to the sphenoid. Septations, including an asymmetric intersinus septum, can attach to bone overlying the carotid. The cavernous sinus lies laterally, and the foramen rotundum (V2) and pterygoid canal may impinge on the sinus cavity, especially if well pneumatized.

Tumors in the maxillary sinus may spread through natural areas of weakness into the nose via the ostium and fontanelles, into the mouth via the premolar and molar teeth roots, and into the eye and cheek via the infraorbital canal and foramen. Posteriorly, the bone is strong but once the tumor reaches the pterygomaxillary fissure, pterygopalatine fossa, and the infratemporal fossa, the excellent blood supply of these areas facilitates tumor dissemination and the prognosis is much reduced.

The nasal septum consists of the quadrilateral cartilage, the vomer, and perpendicular plate of the ethmoid. Anteriorly, it is contiguous with the medial crura of the lower lateral cartilages. Tumors in this area can escape superiorly into the external nasal structures and inferiorly into the upper lip and gingivobuccal sulcus.

Fortunately, the lymphatic drainage from the sinuses is relatively poor, going to the retropharyngeal and jugulodigastric nodes, but squamous cell carcinomas affecting the nasal vestibule, anterior septum, and/or columella can spread bilaterally to level I nodes in the submandibular region.

Surgical Techniques

Principles

1. To completely resect the tumor
2. To reconstruct and rehabilitate the patient
3. If complete resection is not possible, to genuinely palliate

Although most sinonasal tumors are managed by surgery, often in combination with chemoradiation, some such as lymphomas or sinonasal undifferentiated carcinomas are treated by chemoradiation alone. Sometimes this modality alone is used for palliation due to the extent of the tumor at presentation (**Fig. 32.7**).

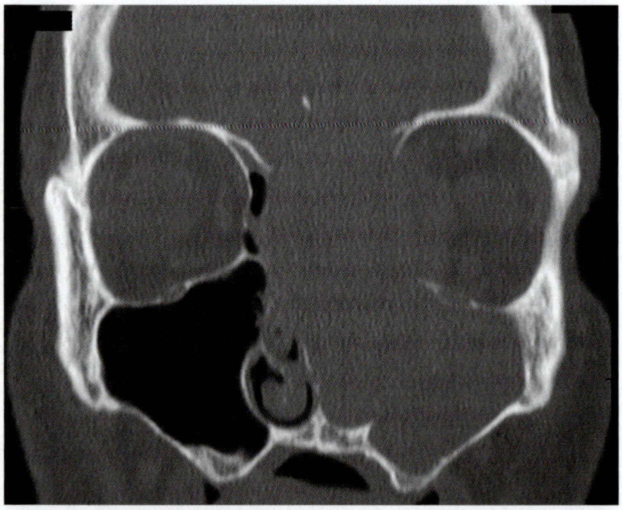

A

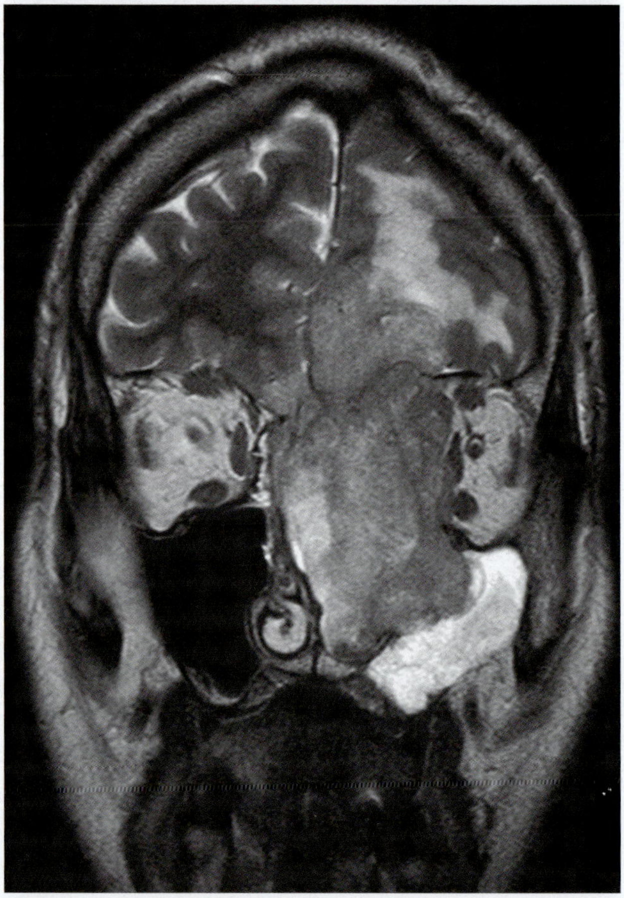

B

Fig. 32.7 (A) Coronal computed tomography scan of extensive sinonasal undifferentiated carcinoma. **(B)** Coronal magnetic resonance image (T1 with gadolinium).

Anesthesia

All the following procedures are performed under general anesthesia in the reversed Trendelenburg position with 15 to 20 degrees of head elevation. Vasoconstriction of the nasal mucosa is effected by instilling 2 to 4 mL of Moffat's solution (10% cocaine, 2 mL; 1:1000 adrenaline, 2 mL; and

0.9% sodium bicarbonate, 1 mL) in the anesthetic room with the patient in the head down position for ~10 minutes. Any incision line(s) is infiltrated with 2% Xylocaine and adrenaline 1:80,000, and during the procedure, ribbon gauzes soaked in 1:1,000 adrenaline are applied to the surgical field.

In the case of a craniofacial resection, the patients are started on phenytoin 200 mg/day for 48 hours before surgery as a prophylaxis against seizure activity. During the surgery, manipulation of the blood pressure and pCO_2 are generally sufficient to reduce brain mass without using systemic diuretics.[25]

A broad-spectrum antibiotic (e.g., amoxicillin/clavulanate) or cephalosporin and metronidazole is generally administered with induction and continued while any packing is in place.

Craniofacial Resection

This approach, in its many variations, offered for the first time the possibility of oncologic resection of tumors affecting the anterior skull base and has thus become the "gold standard" for tumors affecting this area.[26] However, it can only be regarded as palliative in the presence of extensive frontal lobe, middle cranial fossa, bilateral orbital, or optic chiasm involvement or in the presence of systemic metastases. It has been of particular value for cases of adenocarcinoma and olfactory neuroblastoma, which have a predilection for this area, but it is not useful for certain histologies such as mucosal malignant melanoma where the extent of surgery does not influence the outcome and in those where surgery is not appropriate such as for sinonasal undifferentiated carcinoma, lymphoma, and plasmacytoma.

Incision

Following bilateral temporal tarsorrhaphies, an extended lateral rhinotomy is made on the side of maximal tumor involvement. Alternatively, a coronal flap combined with a midfacial degloving or an endoscopic approach has been advocated, among other options.[27–29]

Technique

The soft tissues of the face are mobilized by subperiosteal elevation to expose the nasal bones, the frontal processes of the maxilla, and the frontal bone up to the hairline.[5] The incision may be carried on into the vestibule, although, if possible, this attachment is preserved to reduce alar lift. A self-retaining retractor is then placed superiorly. If a coronal scalp incision is used, the forehead is elevated in the subperiosteal plane, whereas the middle third of the face is elevated via a midfacial degloving approach.

The orbital periosteum is dissected from the lamina to expose the lacrimal fossa and the medial orbital wall, and the nasolacrimal duct may be cut obliquely without significant sequelae. The trochlea is sharply detached from the superomedial socket, and the anterior and posterior ethmoidal arteries are divided after bipolar coagulation, allowing lateral retraction of the orbital contents. At this point, if the tumor is adherent to the orbital periosteum, this area should be resected for frozen section assessment.

The size and shape of the frontal craniotomy also varies from surgeon to surgeon, but it is not necessary to have a large "neurosurgical" approach. A shield-shaped craniotomy ~$3 \times 3 \times 3.5$ cm is generally all that is required, placed above the level of the supraorbital rim to include the frontal sinus. This can be done with any high-speed drill, including an otologic drill, using either a small rosehead or fissure burr until the dura is just visible. Miniplates are then drilled and attached. The bone flap is then removed using straight and curved osteotomes and stored for subsequent reconstruction.

The frontal sinus, which has been opened by this maneuver, is cleared of its mucosa and the posterior wall is removed together with a wide dissection of the dura. It is important that this is carried far laterally to allow the dura to fall back as the brain shrinks with the anesthesia. Using an operating microscope helps with the sharp dissection of the dural prolongations and olfactory fibers as they traverse the cribriform plate. The dissection continues at least as far as the jugum of the sphenoid. If a tumor is encountered, this will necessitate resection of the adjacent dura. Thus, the extent of the dural resection will depend on the extent of the tumor; but, in cases of olfactory neuroblastoma, the olfactory bulb and tracts are routinely removed in continuity as it is known that there can be microscopic involvement of these structures. The ethmoidal arteries can be coagulated with the bipolar diathermy as they cross the plate, but care must be exercised as the optic nerve is approached.

Cuts are then made using a burr or osteotome through the bone surrounding the cribriform plate into the ethmoids and the sphenoid below, and are joined with those through the lamina papyracea and the perpendicular plate of the ethmoid. The most posterior osteotomy crosses the planum sphenoidale to include the anterior face of the sphenoid, and the nasal septum is separated by quadrilateral cuts. The specimen, thus mobilized, can be removed, any bleeding is dealt with, and the cavity is inspected for further resection. An operating microscope or endoscope facilitates the complete clearance of any residual ethmoidal cells and the removal of sphenoid and maxillary mucosa, if required. A large middle meatal antrostomy is usually performed to reduce the risk of subsequent infection.

Small dural defects can be repaired primarily, but more often, a formal repair is required. This can be done with a fascia lata or a pericranial flap held in place with fibrin glue to which a split skin graft taken from the thigh is applied inferiorly. A layer of Gelfoam soaked with dexamethasone, framycetin sulfate, and gramicidin (Sofradex) is applied to the skin graft, and the cavity is packed with 5-cm ribbon gauze soaked in Whitehead's varnish (compound iodoform paint: iodoform, benzoin prepared storax, tolu balsam, and solvent ether).[30] A wide variety of other repair techniques have been described.

The frontal bone flap is repositioned using the miniplates, the periosteum, and subcutaneous layer closed with absorbable sutures, and the skin is closed with clips or fine skin sutures. A pressure dressing is applied to both the head and the donor sites.

Complications

Although several serious complications have been described, they have been relatively few using the extended lateral rhinotomy and fascia lata/skin graft repair (**Table 32.4**).[5] It is unavoidable that patients lose their sense of smell, which has a significant impact on quality of life.

Postoperative Care

Patients are kept in a neutral position of ~15 degrees for the first 2 or 3 days and then gently elevated, and usually getting out of bed on the 5th day. Neurologic observations continue for at least 24 hours. Fluid intake is initially restricted to match the inevitable diuresis experienced in the first 24 to 36 hours. The urinary catheter is removed on the second or third day and facial sutures after 5 to 7 days. All patients experience some degree of cerebrospinal rhinorrhea initially, so broad-spectrum antibiotics are continued until the nasal packing is removed at 10 to 12 days. We perform the packing removal under a general anesthetic. The anticonvulsant is continued for 6 weeks following the operation, and patients must douche the nose with saline or alkaline solution long-term (**Fig. 32.8**).

Lateral Rhinotomy

This is a quick procedure that gives excellent access to the nasal cavity through which a medial maxillectomy, a frontoethmosphenoidectomy, and/or a resection of the septum can be undertaken. It can be extended both superiorly for a craniofacial to encompass the skull base or inferiorly for a formal maxillectomy, if required. It is particularly suitable for malignant melanomas or any malignancy confined to the nose and adjacent sinuses and in the elderly where a facial scar may be of less concern.

Table 32.4 Complications of Surgery for Sinonasal Tumors

	Craniofacial Resection	Lateral Rhinotomy	Midfacial Degloving	Maxillectomy	ESS
Early					
Convulsions	+				
Hemorrhage	+	+	+	+	+
Air embolism	+				
Infection	+	+	+	+	+
Intermediate/Late					
CVA	+				
Confusion	+				
Pulmonary embolism	+				
CSF leak/meningitis	+	+	+	+ (if eye removed)	+
Aerocele (pneumoencephalocele)	+				
Frontal abscess/ encephalitis	+				
Bone necrosis/fistula	+		+ (oro-antral)		
Epilepsy	+				
Epiphora	+	+	+	+	
Diplopia	+	+	+	+	
Serous otitis media	+		+	+	
Sinusitis/mucocele	+	+		+	
Paraesthesia	+	+	+	+	
Pituitary deficiency	+				
Cosmetic	+	+	+	+	

Abbreviations: CVA, cerebrovascular accident; CSF, cerebrospinal fluid; ESS, endoscopic sinus surgery.

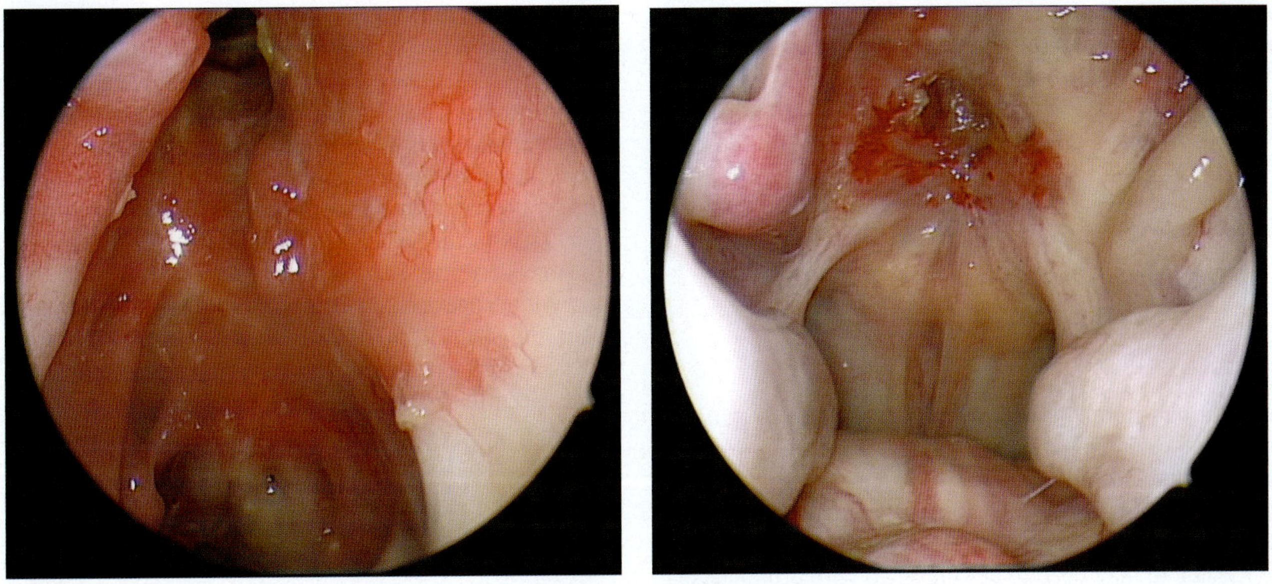

A B

Fig. 32.8 Endoscopic views of a craniofacial cavity 15 years postoperative: **(A)** superior cavity with access to the frontal region and **(B)** inferior cavity with view onto the face of the sphenoid with small granulations and into the nasopharynx.

Incision

After a temporary tarsorrhaphy, the incision runs from the level of the medial canthus, midway between the canthus and nasal bridge in the nasomaxillary groove, and curving round the lower ala into the nasal cavity. If possible, the incision should stop before the ala to avoid postoperative alar lift.

Technique

The orbital periosteum can be dissected from the lamina, and the nasolacrimal duct can be mobilized. The duct can be cut obliquely adjacent to the sac with little risk of stenosis, although sometimes a stent may be inserted or the sac opened as a formal rhinostomy. The ethmoidal arteries can be ligated or bipolar diathermized, taking care posteriorly where one may be close to the optic nerve. An en bloc or piecemeal removal of the lateral nasal wall can be undertaken, including the pyriform aperture, the nasal bones, the frontal process of the maxilla and anterior maxillary wall, the medial orbital floor and rim, ethmoids, lamina papyracea, and lacrimal fossa, dependent on the extent of the tumor. Then, the sphenoid sinus can be opened and, if the incision is extended superiorly, the frontal can be accessed. Orbital periosteum can be resected if required and grafted with skin or fascia. The cavity may be packed, and the incision is closed with absorbable subcutaneous and skin sutures.

Midfacial Degloving

The degloving approach can be used alone or in combination with a coronal scalp incision for a craniofacial resection or with an endoscope or even microscope to improve visualization. It offers excellent access to the middle third of the face and can be used for selected malignant tumors that affect the nasal cavity, maxilla, ethmoids, sphenoid, pterygopalatine, and infratemporal fossae. A bilateral maxillectomy can be performed via this approach if required.[31] It is particularly suitable for chondrosarcomas and other malignant tumors that have not reached the anterior skull base. However, access is restricted if it is necessary to reach the posterior wall of the sphenoid, the skull base, and coronoid process of the mandible.

Incision

After temporary tarsorrhaphies, a bilateral sublabial incision is made down to bone from maxillary tuberosity to tuberosity. Routine rhinoplasty intercartilaginous incisions are made, extending into a transfixion incision along the dorsal and caudal borders of the cartilaginous septum, separating it from the medial crura of the lower lateral cartilages. The circumferential incisions are joined across the floor of the nose just anterior to the pyriform aperture.

Technique

The soft tissues of the midface are elevated subperiosteally as far as the infraorbital nerve on each side to display the pyriform aperture. The soft tissues over the nasal bridge are elevated as far as the root of the nose and laterally so that the middle third of the face is completely elevated and can be lifted superiorly over the nasal skeleton. Thereafter, the nasal cavities and maxillary sinuses can be opened using drills, osteotomes, and upcutting bone forceps, and the maxillary and sphenopalatine arteries are ligated. Further resection of the ethmoids, sphenoid, nasopharynx, and structures posterior and lateral to the maxillae can be undertaken as indicated by the extent of the tumor. The incisions must be sutured carefully using absorbable suture material to avoid distortion, fistulas, and stenoses. The bridge of the nose may be taped or a rhinoplasty dressing applied for a few days.

Complications

Complications are generally rare; see **Table 32.4**.[31]

Maxillectomy

A traditional total maxillectomy via a Weber-Fergusson or Weber-Dieffenbach incision may still be employed but has been replaced by midfacial degloving, particularly in younger patients. It is used for malignant tumors of the maxilla involving the inferior, superior, anterior, or posterior wall and may need to be combined with orbital clearance or exenteration. Extension into the skull base will require an additional craniofacial approach. An impression of the upper alveolus should be taken preoperatively by a prosthetic orthodontist for future reconstruction.

Incision

After temporary tarsorrhaphy, the classic Weber-Fergusson incision extends 1 cm lateral to the lateral canthus and medially ~3 mm below the lower eyelash. If the incision is too close to the lashes, an ectropion results. If it is too low, an edema may occur. At the medial canthus, the incision curves inferiorly into the nasomaxillary groove down to the alar margin. It then continues medially to the midline where it turns at a right angle, dividing the upper lip. The incision then extends around the upper alveolus in the gingivobuccal sulcus as far as the maxillary tuberosity. Medially, the incision passes onto the hard palate between the central incisors as far as the junction of the hard and soft palate, where it crosses laterally toward the posterior aspect of the maxillary tuberosity. The incision on the palate should lie ~3 mm lateral to the midline so that a mucoperiosteal flap can be formed to cover the raw bony edge.

Technique

The entire soft tissues of the cheek are raised subperiosteally off the anterior maxilla from the pyriform aperture to the zygomatic arch, including the buccinator. If tumor extends through the anterior wall, a layer of soft tissues should be left on the tumor. The orbicularis oculi is left intact around the eye, but the orbital periosteum is incised at the bony rim so that the orbital contents can be dissected off the orbital floor. The infraorbital neurovascular bundle is cut at the infraorbital foramen.

Osteotomies are made through the zygoma, beneath the infraorbital rim if the eye is being preserved, across the frontal process of the maxilla, into the pyriform fossa, and inferiorly through the central upper alveolus using a drill, saw, or osteotomes. The lateral nasal wall is divided below the superior turbinate. The hard palate is divided from front to back, just lateral to the septum, and the maxillary tuberosity is separated from the pterygoid plates with a curved osteotome. Any remaining soft tissue attachments are divided with curved Mayo scissors and, once the bone is removed, bleeding from the maxillary artery can be controlled with ligatures.

A wide range of reconstructions are available from a split-skin graft held in place on the cavity walls with quilting incisions, biological glues, a Whitehead's varnish pack,[30] and a temporary gutta percha prosthesis to a free flap such as a rectus abdominis, a latissimus dorsi, or osteocutaneous flaps (e.g., radial or fibular with or without osseointegration).[32] Regardless of the method used, the patient should be able to eat and speak in the immediate postoperative period. Closure of the flap can then be effected with absorbable subcutaneous and skin sutures, taking particular care to align the vermillion border.

Malposition of the globe results in diplopia and poor cosmesis (**Table 32.4**). Small defects in the floor can be left, but larger ones need repair using a fascia lata sling secured to the edges of the bony margins or some form of rigid reconstruction.

The artificial prosthesis will need refashioning, and a permanent prosthesis/denture is made once the cavity has healed, and is ideally held in place using an osseointegration system.

Extension posteriorly into the pterygoid region has a serious effect on prognosis. Limited areas of pterygoid muscle can be removed, but a partial mandibulectomy may be required. Further clearance of the pterygopalatine and infratemporal fossae can be undertaken, bearing in mind the close relationship of the internal carotid artery. Involvement of facial skin can be repaired using a local pedicled or free microvascular flap.

Endoscopic Resection

Shortly after its inception, endoscopic sinus surgery was extended to CSF repair and orbital decompression, then to benign tumors, and more recently to selected malignancies. When resecting tumors, it can be used alone or in combination with a craniotomy, but the principle of complete excision must be observed and the options must be discussed with the patient, who should understand that a craniofacial may still be required if there is significant dural invasion and/or infiltration of the superior sagittal sinus.

Technique

Although resection of the tumor is necessarily often piecemeal, surgical resection adheres to basic oncologic principles with focused resection with wide margins at all points of tumor attachment. A wide field clearance of adjacent

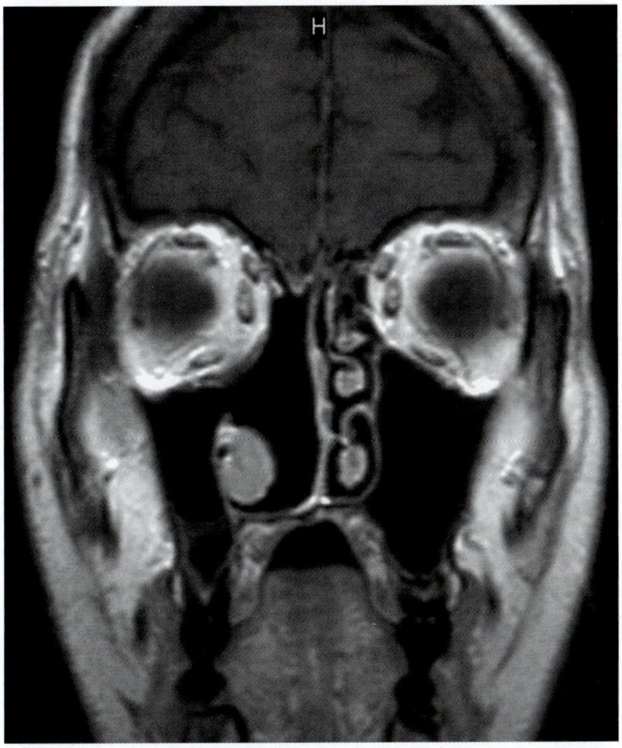

Fig. 32.9 A coronal magnetic resonance image (T1 with gadolinium) of a postoperative cavity after an endoscopic resection of an adenocarcinoma at 8 years follow-up.

mucosa, bone, and periorbita/dura is still undertaken with the intention of curative resection (**Fig. 32.9**).[33] Bone and dural defects can be repaired using combinations of fascia, pinna cartilage, contralateral nasal mucosa, and pedicled flaps, dependent on the size of the defect, and orbital periosteum can be resected and repaired with contralateral mucosa or a split skin graft held with fibrin glue, a gelatin sponge, and some form of packing (e.g., a Whitehead's varnish pack).[6,33,34] Resection is determined by the extent of the tumor, but in practice, a complete frontoethmosphenoidectomy is generally undertaken (on one or both sides depending on the tumor), combined with the removal of the lateral nasal wall (from a middle meatal antrostomy to a medial maxillectomy) and/or septal resection. The frontal sinus should be widely opened in most cases (Draf III) to provide adequate exposure for future inspection, as should the sphenoid. Image guidance is often employed and two surgeons using a four-handed technique can be extremely helpful.

The advent of neuroendoscopic techniques is pushing the boundaries of what can be resected via an endonasal approach, although careful patient selection remains paramount to maximizing cure and minimizing morbidity.[33]

Complications

Although the complications are theoretically the same as for a craniofacial, thus far, the reported problems have been few. However, significant hemorrhage poses a serious risk if the internal carotid artery is opened, and surgeons must be prepared to deal with this should it occur. As the extent of skull base resections increased, there were also problems with reconstruction, leading to CSF leaks and meningitis. The use of vascular pedicled flaps (e.g., the Hadad-Bassagasteguy nasoseptal flap) has improved this situation significantly (**Table 32.4**).[35]

Total Rhinectomy

Extensive tumors in the nasal cavity will sometimes involve the external nose, resulting in the need to completely excise the nose (e.g., squamous cell carcinoma of the columella, vestibule, and septum; malignant mucosal melanoma).

Incision

A circumferential cut down to the bone is made around the pyriform aperture, while bearing in mind that the tumor can escape submucosally into the upper lip and premaxilla, therefore, a wide margin is recommended.

Technique

The entire cuff of the nasal mucosa can be removed together with septum, lateral wall, and floor as dictated by the tumor. Skin grafts may be applied to exposed bone, but this will mucosalize with time. A Whitehead's varnish pack is placed in the cavity for a few days. The superstructure of the nose can be replaced with an artificial prosthesis secured by osseointegration or by a variety of pedicled or free microvascular flaps. Reconstruction will be helped if some nasal bone can be preserved. A palatal prosthesis or a modification of an existing denture may be required if the premaxilla has been resected.

Management of the Orbit

Involvement of the orbit is an important predictor of survival and, in the past, if tumor had reached the orbital periosteum, the patient was advised to have the eye removed. However, it appears that a more conservative strategy can be adopted without adversely affecting outcome.[5,36,37] Thus, if the tumor has eroded through lamina and onto orbital periosteum but has not penetrated into the orbital fat, the periosteum can be widely resected and repaired with split skin or fascia. Frozen section is invaluable in making this assessment. In cases where the tumor has spread through the periosteum and a cure is otherwise impossible, the eye should be sacrificed but, in most cases, the eyelids can be spared because there is no lymphatic drainage anteriorly and preseptal spread is rare. This is an orbital clearance as opposed to orbital exenteration where the lids are sacrificed.

When preserving the lids, cuts are made leaving the lash margin on the specimen, and the skin and subcutaneous tissues are dissected off the tarsal plates. A circumferential incision is made around the socket, down to bone, and the canthal ligaments divided. The periosteum is then elevated

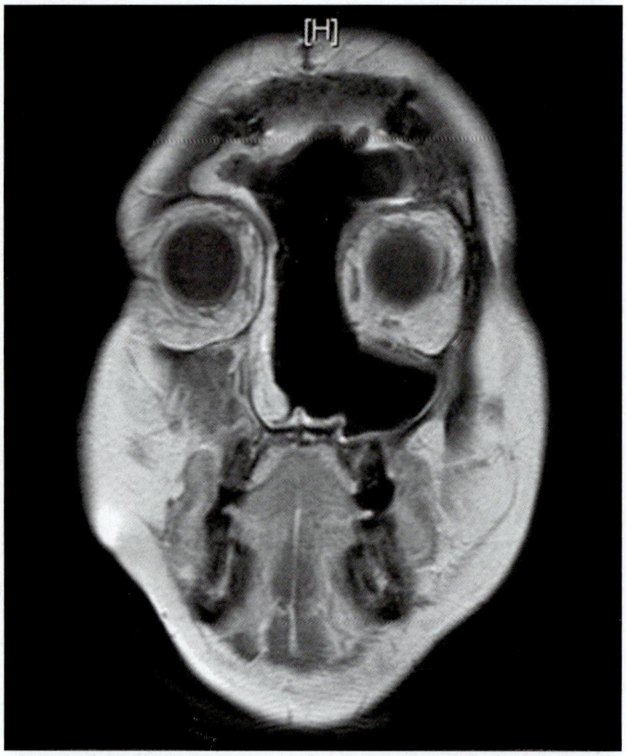

Fig. 32.10 Coronal magnetic resonance image (T1 with gadolinium) of postoperative cavity after craniofacial resection of an olfactory neuroblastoma at 10 years follow-up.

using a Freer and ribbon gauze soaked in 1:1000 adrenaline, taking care not to extend out through the fissures. Once the orbital contents are mobilized, the apex is divided with curved Mayo scissors. The anesthesiologist should be warned that patients often develop a marked bradycardia as the optic nerve is cut. Significant bleeding is encountered from the ophthalmic artery, although this quickly vasoconstricts. It is advisable to put a stay suture through the optic neurovascular bundle not only for hemostasis but also to close the CSF space around the nerve. The lids are closed without tension using dissolvable sutures. However, they will sometimes break down, especially after radiotherapy or if they are intentionally sacrificed in an exenteration, and the socket may be filled with a free microvascular flap or a temporalis muscle flap to which a split skin graft can be applied. Osseointegrated implants may be placed in the orbital rim at the time of the resection or any time thereafter, but integration can take up to a year, especially if radiotherapy is given. An orbital prosthesis held with adhesives or on a spectacle frame can be fitted once the lids have sunk back to form a skin-lined socket while integration takes place.

Postoperative Care

In the absence of complications, patients generally make a rapid recovery from all of these procedures. Many have a pack inserted (e.g., Whitehead's varnish),[30] which is removed under sedation or even under a general anesthetic some days later. Thereafter, patients are asked to douche the nose with saline or an alkaline solution to reduce crusting. Careful long-term follow-up is required because malignant sinonasal tumors can recur many years later and can affect areas that are difficult to visualize in the clinic. Dependent on the pathology, patients undergo regular MRI and endoscopic examinations (**Table 32.3**; **Fig. 32.10**), and can be salvaged if recurrence is detected sufficiently early.

Outcomes

Although lateral rhinotomy, midfacial degloving, and maxillectomy still have a role for selected malignancies, craniofacial resection has substantially improved the outcome for those tumors affecting the anterior skull base, doubling survival in many cases.[26] In a cohort of 308 patients undergoing a craniofacial resection, of whom 259 had malignant tumors, actuarial disease-free survival was 59% at 5 years, dropping to 40% at 10 years, and 33% at 15 years (**Table 32.5**).[5] Prior to craniofacial the 5-year survival figure for olfactory neuroblastoma was 35%, whereas it is now 77%.[10] However, these studies also show

Table 32.5 Craniofacial Resection: Actuarial Survival for Whole Group and Individual Histologies

Histology	5 year (%)	10 year (%)	15 year (%)	No. of patients
Overall	65	47	41	308
Benign	92	82	76	49
Malignant	59	40	33	259
Adenocarcinoma	58	40	33	62
Olfactory neuroblastoma	74	50	40	56
Squamous cell carcinoma	53	35	35	34
Chondrosarcoma	94	56	37	24
Adenoid cystic carcinoma	61	31	31	19

Source: Data from Howard DJ, Lund VJ, Wei WI. Craniofacial resection for sinonasal neoplasia – a twenty-five year experience. Head Neck 2006;28:867–873.

that late recurrence occurs with many of these tumors, so 5-year actuarial survival does not predict a cure.

In the nasal cavity, and the maxillary and ethmoid sinuses, prognosis is determined by involvement of the brain, the type of histology, and involvement of the orbit.[5,26,38–42] Even when orbital clearance is undertaken, tumor at the orbital apex significantly reduces survival and is worse with certain types of tumor (e.g., squamous cell carcinoma).[43] However, survival is not affected when invasion is limited to the orbital periosteum, which is resected with orbital preservation.[5]

For some tumors, irrespective of treatment, overall survival may be poor. In a cohort of 58 patients with a malignant mucosal melanoma, 5-year actuarial survival was 28%, falling to 20% at 10 years.[15]

Recurrence most often occurs locally and can be treated with further surgery, including craniofacial or endoscopic resection, on numerous occasions with the intention to cure or palliate because morbidity is generally low.

So far, the number and follow-up of patients undergoing endoscopic resection is relatively small, making it difficult to compare the technique with conventional approaches. Also, these patients will generally have a more limited disease, so one would anticipate similar if not better results, which appears to be the case in emerging series.[6,7,14,29,34] A review of all the available literature shows at least comparable results to conventional open techniques, and there are obviously advantages in terms of lower morbidity, shorter hospital stay, and the ability to start chemoradiation shortly after surgery.[33] However, the principle of oncologic resection must be observed wherever possible, and the full menu of surgical (and medical) approaches should be available if required.

Conclusion

Malignant sinonasal tumors are rare, are histologically diverse, and present late. They require radical treatment, usually a combination of surgery, radiotherapy, and, in some cases, chemotherapy, and must be followed up for at least 20 years due to the possibility of late recurrence. This is optimally provided in centers with a particular interest in these problems because expertise in imaging and histology as well as the therapeutic options is required. The proximity of the eye and the skull base presents particular problems in management. A range of surgical options are available, of which the craniofacial resection has provided a dramatic improvement in outcome. However, a significant and increasing number of cases are now being dealt with endoscopically, which, with careful patient selection, can achieve the same surgical clearance with reduced morbidity. Careful long-term follow-up with multicenter collaboration will provide comparative data in the future.

References

1. Acheson ED, Cowdell RH, Hadfield EH, Macbeth RG. Nasal cancer in woodworkers in the furniture industry. BMJ 1968;2(5605):587–596
2. Edge S, Byrd D, Compton C, Fritz A, Greene F, Trotti A, eds. American Joint Committee on Cancer Staging Manual. 7th ed. New York: Springer; 2010.
3. Kadish S, Goodman M, Wang CC. Olfactory neuroblastoma. A clinical analysis of 17 cases. Cancer 1976;37(3):1571–1576
4. Cantù G, Solero CL, Miceli R, et al. Which classification for ethmoid malignant tumors involving the anterior skull base? Head Neck 2005;27(3):224–231
5. Howard DJ, Lund VJ, Wei WI. Craniofacial resection for tumors of the nasal cavity and paranasal sinuses: a 25-year experience. Head Neck 2006;28(10):867–873
6. Lund VJ, Howard DJ, Wei WI. Endoscopic resection of malignant tumors of the nose and sinuses. Am J Rhinol 2007;21(1):89–94
7. Goffart Y, Jorissen M, Daele J, et al. Minimally invasive endoscopic management of malignant sinonasal tumours. Acta Otorhinolaryngol Belg 2000;54(2):221–232
8. Knegt PP, de Jong PC, van Andel JG, de Boer MF, Eykenboom W, van der Schans E. Carcinoma of the paranasal sinuses. Results of a prospective pilot study. Cancer 1985;56(1):57–62
9. Howard DJ, Lund VJ. Reflections on the management of adenoid cystic carcinoma of the nasal cavity and paranasal sinuses. Otolaryngol Head Neck Surg 1985;93(3):338–341
10. Lund VJ, Howard D, Wei W, Spittle M. Olfactory neuroblastoma: past, present, and future? Laryngoscope 2003;113(3):502–507
11. Rinaldo A, Ferlito A, Shaha AR, Wei WI, Lund VJ. Esthesioneuroblastoma and cervical lymph node metastases: clinical and therapeutic implications. Acta Otolaryngol 2002;122(2):215–221
12. Dulguerov P, Allal AS, Calcaterra TC. Esthesioneuroblastoma: a meta-analysis and review. Lancet Oncol 2001;2(11):683–690
13. Kim DW, Jo YH, Kim JH, et al. Neoadjuvant etoposide, ifosfamide, and cisplatin for the treatment of olfactory neuroblastoma. Cancer 2004;101(10):2257–2260
14. Casiano RR, Numa WA, Falquez AM. Endoscopic resection of esthesioneuroblastoma. Am J Rhinol 2001;15(4):271–279
15. Lund VJ, Howard DJ, Harding L, Wei WI. Management options and survival in malignant melanoma of the sinonasal mucosa. Laryngoscope 1999;109(2 Pt 1):208–211
16. Rassekh CH, Nuss DW, Kapadia SB, Curtin HD, Weissman JL, Janecka IP. Chondrosarcoma of the nasal septum: skull base imaging and clinicopathologic correlation. Otolaryngol Head Neck Surg 1996;115(1):29–37
17. Harabuchi Y, Yamanaka N, Kataura A, et al. Epstein-Barr virus in nasal T-cell lymphomas in patients with lethal midline granuloma. Lancet 1990;335(8682):128–130
18. Logsdon MD, Ha CS, Kavadi VS, Cabanillas F, Hess MA, Cox JD. Lymphoma of the nasal cavity and paranasal sinuses: improved outcome and altered prognostic factors with combined modality therapy. Cancer 1997;80(3):477–488
19. Iannetti G, Valentini V, Rinna C, Ventucci E, Marianetti TM. Ethmoido-orbital tumors: our experience. J Craniofac Surg 2005;16(6):1085–1091
20. Cantù G, Bimbi G, Miceli R, et al. Lymph node metastases in malignant tumors of the paranasal sinuses: prognostic value and treatment. Arch Otolaryngol Head Neck Surg 2008;134(2):170–177
21. Lloyd GAS, Lund VJ, Howard DJ, Savy L. Optimum imaging for sinonasal malignancy. J Laryngol Otol 2000;114(7):557–562

22. Koshy M, Paulino AC, Howell R, Schuster D, Halkar R, Davis LW. F-18 FDG PET-CT fusion in radiotherapy treatment planning for head and neck cancer. Head Neck 2005;27(6):494–502
23. Collins BT, Cramer HM, Hearn SA. Fine needle aspiration cytology of metastatic olfactory neuroblastoma. Acta Cytol 1997;41(3):802–810
24. Lang J. Clinical Anatomy of the Nose, Nasal Cavity and Paranasal Sinuses. New York: Thieme; 1989
25. Lund VJ, Howard DJ, Wei WI, Cheesman AD. Craniofacial resection for tumors of the nasal cavity and paranasal sinuses—a 17-year experience. Head Neck 1998;20(2):97–105
26. Ganly I, Patel SG, Singh B, et al. Craniofacial resection for malignant paranasal sinus tumors: Report of an International Collaborative Study. Head Neck 2005;27(7):575–584
27. Shah JP, Kraus DH, Bilsky MH, Gutin PH, Harrison LH, Strong EW. Craniofacial resection for malignant tumors involving the anterior skull base. Arch Otolaryngol Head Neck Surg 1997;123(12): 1312–1317
28. Raveh J, Laedrach K, Speiser M, et al. The subcranial approach for fronto-orbital and anteroposterior skull-base tumors. Arch Otolaryngol Head Neck Surg 1993;119(4):385–393
29. Thaler ER, Kotapka M, Lanza DC, Kennedy DW. Endoscopically assisted anterior cranial skull base resection of sinonasal tumors. Am J Rhinol 1999;13(4):303–310
30. Lim M, Lew-Gor S, Sandhu G, Howard D, Lund VJ. Whitehead's varnish nasal pack. J Laryngol Otol 2007;121(6):592–594
31. Howard DJ, Lund VJ. The role of midfacial degloving in modern rhinological practice. J Laryngol Otol 1999;113(10):885–887
32. Cordeiro PG, Santamaria E. A classification system and algorithm for reconstruction of maxillectomy and midfacial defects. Plast Reconstr Surg 2000;105(7):2331–2346, discussion 2347–2348
33. Lund VJ, Stammberger H, Nicolai P, et al; European Rhinologic Society Advisory Board on Endoscopic Techniques in the Management of Nose, Paranasal Sinus and Skull Base Tumours. European position paper on endoscopic management of tumours of the nose, paranasal sinuses and skull base. Rhinol Suppl 2010;(22):1–143
34. Carrau R, Kassam A, Snyderman C, Duvvuri U, Mintz A, Gardner P. Endoscopic transnasal anterior skull base resection for the treatment of sinonasal malignancies. Oper Tech Otolaryngol—Head Neck Surg 2006;17:102–110
35. Hadad G, Bassagasteguy L, Carrau RL, et al. A novel reconstructive technique after endoscopic expanded endonasal approaches: vascular pedicle nasoseptal flap. Laryngoscope 2006;116(10):1882–1886
36. Imola MJ, Schramm VL Jr. Orbital preservation in surgical management of sinonasal malignancy. Laryngoscope 2002;112 (8 Pt 1):1357–1365
37. Suárez C, Ferlito A, Lund VJ, et al. Management of the orbit in malignant sinonasal tumors. Head Neck 2008;30(2):242–250
38. Cantù G, Solero CL, Mariani L, et al. Anterior craniofacial resection for malignant ethmoid tumors—a series of 91 patients. Head Neck 1999;21(3):185–191
39. Dulguerov P, Jacobsen MS, Allal AS, Lehmann W, Calcaterra T. Nasal and paranasal sinus carcinoma: are we making progress? A series of 220 patients and a systematic review. Cancer 2001;92(12):3012–3029
40. Bhattacharyya N. Cancer of the nasal cavity: survival and factors influencing prognosis. Arch Otolaryngol Head Neck Surg 2002;128(9):1079–1083
41. Carrillo JF, Güemes A, Ramírez-Ortega MC, Oñate-Ocaña LF. Prognostic factors in maxillary sinus and nasal cavity carcinoma. Eur J Surg Oncol 2005;31(10):1206–1212
42. Diaz EM Jr, Johnigan RH III, Pero C, et al. Olfactory neuroblastoma: the 22-year experience at one comprehensive cancer center. Head Neck 2005;27(2):138–149
43. Suarez C, Llorente JL, Fernandez De Leon R, Maseda E, Lopez A. Prognostic factors in sinonasal tumors involving the anterior skull base. Head Neck 2004;26(2):136–144

33 Endoscopic Applications in Orbital Surgery

Todd T. Kingdom and Vikram D. Durairaj

Applying endoscopic techniques to orbital pathology is a logical extension of the rhinologist's armamentarium given the close proximity of the orbit to the sinuses. Continued advances in endoscopic surgical instrumentation and growing clinical experience have helped expand the rhinologist's role in managing select conditions of the orbit and the related structures. Perhaps even more important than the many technological advancements is the working relationship between the rhinologist and our ophthalmology colleagues. The patient clearly benefits from a team approach in this area. This chapter discusses the relevant orbital anatomy as it relates to the endoscopic surgeon and reviews the current applications of these techniques to the orbit.

Orbital Anatomy

The understanding of orbital disease requires a thorough and clear understanding of anatomic relationships. Endoscopic orbital and lacrimal surgery demands an accurate intraoperative identification of orbital anatomy.

Osteology of the Orbit

The bony orbit is a pyramidal shaped space that is ~4 cm deep with a volume of 30 mL. The width of the orbit is greatest 1 cm posterior to the entrance of the orbit and this location corresponds to the equator of the globe. The orbit is composed of seven bones that, with the exception of fissures and foramina, form a closed compartment that is open anteriorly. The medial walls of the two orbits are parallel to each other, and the lateral walls are 45 degrees to the medial wall and 90 degrees to each other (**Tables 33.1 and 33.2**). The orbits are lined by periosteum (often referred to as periorbita), which is loosely adherent to bone except at the arcus marginalis (orbital margin representing the fusion of the orbital septum and periorbita), sutures, fissures, foramina, and lacrimal sac (**Fig. 33.1**).

Table 33.1 Typical Dimensions of the Adult Orbit

Volume	30 mL
Entrance height	35 mm
Entrance width	40 mm
Medial wall length	45 mm
Orbital segment length of optic nerve	25–30 mm

Orbital Rim

The orbital rim protects the eye from injury. It is thickened and forms a spiral, with the two ends originating at the anterior and posterior aspect of the lacrimal sac fossa at the inferior medial aspect of the orbit. The superior rim is formed by the frontal bone, and the medial third contains a notch that transmits the supraorbital neurovascular bundle in two-thirds of all orbits (one-third of orbits have a closed foramen just above the rim). The lateral rim is composed of the zygomatic process of the frontal bone and the frontal process of the zygoma meeting at the frontozygomatic suture. The lateral orbital tubercle (Whitnall's tubercle) is located 11 mm inferior to the frontozygomatic suture and 3 mm posterior to the orbital rim. It serves as the attachment site for the posterior crus of the lateral canthal tendon, the inferior suspensory ligament (Lockwood's ligament), the lateral rectus muscle check ligaments, and the lateral horn of the levator aponeurosis. Proper realignment of these structures at the lateral orbital tubercle is necessary during eyelid and orbit procedures to achieve normal aesthetic and functional reconstruction. The inferior rim is formed by the zygomatic bone laterally and the maxillary bone medially, and meeting at the zygomaticomaxillary suture. The infraorbital foramen, which transmits the infraorbital artery and nerve, is located 4 to 10 mm inferior to the central portion of the rim. The inferior orbital rim curves in a superior and medial direction to form the anterior lacrimal crest (the frontal process of the lacrimal bone). The superior rim curves in an inferior and medial direction to form the posterior lacrimal crest and the entrance into the lacrimal canal.

Table 33.2 Bony Composition of Orbital Walls

Roof of the orbit	Frontal bone Lesser wing of the sphenoid
Lateral wall of the orbit	Zygomatic bone Greater wing of the sphenoid
Medial wall of the orbit	Ethmoid bone Lacrimal bone Maxillary bone Sphenoid bone
Floor of the orbit	Maxillary bone Palatine bone Zygomatic bone

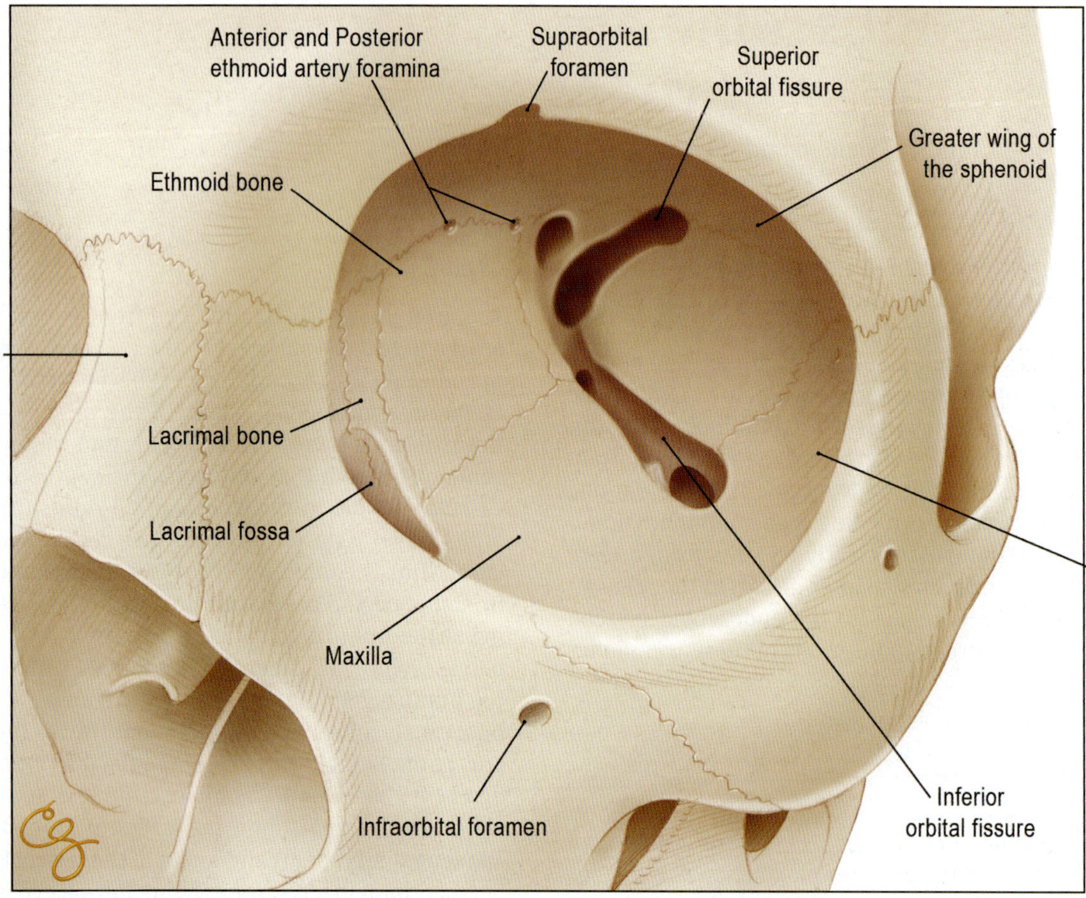

Fig. 33.1 Orbital bones, foramina, and fissures (frontal view).

The rim is discontinuous at the lacrimal sac fossa. The supratrochlear and infratrochlear nerves and dorsal nasal artery emerge from the superior aspect of the medial rim. The cartilaginous trochlea of the superior oblique tendon is also located just inside the medial rim.

Orbital Roof

The orbital roof is triangular shaped and composed mainly of the orbital plate of the frontal bone and, to a lesser contribution, from the lesser wing of the sphenoid. The orbital roof is thinnest just behind the orbital rim and is ~3 mm thick at its posterior aspect. The lacrimal gland fossa is contained anterolaterally, and the trochlear fossa is contained anteromedially 4 mm from the orbital margin.

Lateral Orbital Wall

The lateral orbit wall is formed from two bones: the zygomatic bone and greater wing of the sphenoid. It is the strongest and thickest of the orbital walls. The lateral orbital tubercle is a small elevation of the zygomatic bone and is the site for several important attachments (see orbital rim section).

Orbital Floor

The floor of the orbit is the roof of the maxillary sinus and is composed of three bones: the maxillary, the palatine, and the orbital plate of the zygomatic. The orbital floor slopes downward 20 degrees from posterior to anterior. The infraorbital nerve travels along the floor and descends anteriorly into a canal. It exits in the maxillary bone 4 to 10 mm inferior to the orbital margin. It transmits the infraorbital nerve, which is a branch of V_2 (the maxillary division of cranial nerve V).

Medial Orbital Wall

Four bones form the medial wall of the orbit: the frontal process of the maxillary, the lacrimal, the orbital plate of the ethmoidal, and the lesser wing of the sphenoid. The medial wall, appropriately termed the lamina papyracea ("paper-like sheet"), is the thinnest of the orbital walls. The ethmoidal bone makes up the largest portion of the medial wall. The inferior anterior aspect of the medial wall contains the lacrimal fossa, which is formed by the frontal process of the maxillary and the lacrimal bone. The nasolacrimal canal is continuous with the inferior medial wall of the orbit and descends inferiorly from the lacrimal fossa into the inferior meatus of the nose.

Orbital Foramina and Fissures

Foramina

The optic foramen passes through the lesser wing of the sphenoid and contains the optic nerve, the ophthalmic artery, and sympathetic fibers from the carotid plexus. It extends from the orbital apex to the middle cranial fossa. The supraorbital foramen or notch transmits the supraorbital nerve, artery, vein, and is located at the medial third of the superior margin of the orbital rim. The anterior ethmoidal foramen transmits the anterior ethmoidal vessel and nerve and is located at the frontoethmoidal suture 24 mm posterior to the orbital rim. The posterior ethmoidal foramen transmits the posterior ethmoidal vessels and nerve, and is located 12 mm posterior to the anterior ethmoidal foramen at the junction of the medial wall and the orbital roof. The zygomaticotemporal and zygomaticofacial foramina are located in the lateral wall of the orbit and transmit branches of the zygomatic nerve and artery.

Fissures

The superior orbital fissure is formed by the greater and lesser wing of the sphenoid. It is 22 mm in length and lies below and lateral to the optic foramen. The superior orbital fissure is divided into superior and inferior parts by the origination of the lateral rectus. The superior part transmits frontal and lacrimal branches of the cranial nerve V_1 and cranial nerve IV. The inferior part transmits the superior and inferior divisions of cranial nerve III, the nasociliary branch of cranial nerve V_1, cranial nerve VI, the superior ophthalmic vein, and the sympathetic nerve plexus. The inferior orbital fissure is between the lateral wall and floor of the orbit and lies below the superior orbital floor. It transmits branches of cranial nerve V_2 and the inferior ophthalmic vein.

Extraocular Muscles

All extraocular muscles, with the exception of the inferior oblique, originate at the orbital apex. The four rectus muscles originate from the annulus of Zinn, a tendinous ring that encircles the inferior portion of the superior orbital fissure and optic foramen. The medial, inferior, lateral, and superior recti insert on the anterior portion of the globe. The medial rectus inserts closest to the limbus (5.5 mm), and the superior rectus inserts farthest from the limbus (7.7 mm). The superior oblique travels 40 mm from the orbital apex to the trochlea and makes a 54-degree turn to insert on the globe. The inferior oblique arises from a shallow depression in the orbital plate of the maxillary bone just below the lacrimal fossa and passes posteriorly, laterally, and superiorly to insert on the globe.

Cranial nerve III innervates the medial, superior, and inferior rectus along with the inferior oblique muscle. Cranial nerve IV innervates the superior oblique muscle, and cranial nerve VI innervates the lateral rectus muscle. The vascular supply of the extraocular muscles is provided by the inferior and superior muscular branches of the ophthalmic artery, lacrimal artery, and infraorbital artery. Each rectus muscle is supplied by two vascular branches except for the lateral rectus, which is supplied by one.

Orbital Vasculature

The arterial supply of the orbit arises from the internal carotid artery via the ophthalmic artery, which anastomoses with branches of the superficial facial artery arising from the external carotid artery. The ophthalmic artery enters the orbit via the optic canal, inferior and lateral to the optic nerve. In 80 to 85% of orbits, the ophthalmic artery crosses over to the medial orbit over the optic nerve. In the remaining 15 to 20%, the artery courses under the nerve. The branches of the ophthalmic artery include the central retinal; the lateral and medial posterior ciliary; the lacrimal, muscular, supraorbital, anterior, and posterior ethmoidal; and the supratrochlear, nasofrontal, and dorsonasal arteries. The lacrimal artery anastomoses with the external carotid system via the transverse facial and superficial temporal arteries. Medially, the dorsonasal vessels provide anastomosis with the external carotid system via the angular vessels. The maxillary artery contributes arterial supply to the orbit through its infraorbital branch.

The venous drainage of the orbit occurs through the superior and inferior ophthalmic veins. The inferior ophthalmic vein originates from a small plexus of vessels in the inferior orbit; a branch exits through the inferior orbital fissure to join the pterygoid plexus before the vessel terminates at the superior ophthalmic vein before entering the cavernous sinus. The superior ophthalmic vein originates at the superior medial orbit and crosses at mid orbit just below the superior rectus muscle. The lacrimal vein joins at this point and the superior ophthalmic vein exits through the superior orbital fissure into the cavernous sinus.

Orbital Nerves

Five of the 12 cranial nerves innervate the orbit. The optic nerve, which contains 1 million nerve fibers, extends from the brain into the orbit and is covered by meninges and is surrounded with cerebrospinal fluid. Its trajectory can be divided into four anatomic segments: intraocular, intraorbital, intracanalicular, and intracranial. The intraocular portion measures 1 mm in length and 3 mm in diameter. As the optic nerve exits the globe, the diameter doubles in size due to the acquisition of myelin. The intraorbital portion of the optic nerve is ~25 mm and has a sinusoidal course toward the orbital apex, allowing for globe movement without stretching of the nerve. The intracanalicular segment begins as the optic nerve exits the orbital apex and enters the optic canal. The optic canal is 5 to 10 mm long and 5 to 7 mm wide, and the bony wall is thinnest medially where the nerve is separated from the sphenoid and ethmoid sinuses. In the canal, the dura of the optic nerve and the periosteum of the bone are fused. The optic nerve exits the canal, and the intracranial portion measures 12 mm to 18 mm on its way to join the optic chiasm. Often, the lateral aspect of the optic nerve is immediately adjacent to the cavernous sinus.

The oculomotor nerve (cranial nerve III) enters the orbit as superior and inferior divisions. The superior division innervates the superior rectus and the levator aponeurosis. The inferior branch innervates the medial rectus, inferior rectus, and inferior oblique. The branch of the inferior division of cranial nerve III that travels along the lateral rectus and innervates the inferior oblique also contains parasympathetic fibers to the ciliary ganglion that is responsible for pupillary contraction. The trochlear nerve (cranial nerve IV) is the longest intracranial nerve and enters the orbit outside of the annulus of Zinn to eventually innervate the superior oblique. The abducens nerve (cranial nerve VI) enters the orbit through the annulus of Zinn and superior orbital fissure to innervate the lateral rectus muscle.

The ophthalmic and maxillary branches of the trigeminal nerve (cranial nerve V) provide sensory innervation to the orbit. The three branches of the ophthalmic division (V_1) are the lacrimal, frontal, and nasociliary nerves, which enter the orbit through the superior orbital fissure. The lacrimal nerve supplies the lacrimal gland, conjunctiva, and lateral upper eyelid. The frontal nerve divides into the supraorbital and supratrochlear nerve, and supplies the forehead, frontoparietal scalp, and medial upper eyelid. The nasociliary nerve gives rise to the anterior and posterior ethmoidal nerves, long ciliary nerve to the globe, and sensory root to the ciliary ganglion. The maxillary division of the trigeminal nerve (V_2) emerges from the cranial cavity through foramen rotundum and enters the orbit through the inferior orbital fissure. It enters the infraorbital sulcus as the infraorbital nerve and gives off three branches: the anterior superior alveolar, zygomaticofacial, and zygomaticotemporal. The infraorbital nerve then exits the orbit via the infraorbital foramen to supply sensory innervation to the lateral forehead, skin and conjunctiva of the lower eyelid, skin and septum of the nose, and skin and mucosa of the upper lip.

Sympathetic innervation to the orbit arises from the superior cervical ganglion, providing pupillary dilation, constriction of eyelid smooth muscle, vasoconstriction, and hidrosis. The sympathetic nerves travel along the internal carotid artery in its course through the cavernous sinus. The deep petrosal nerve carries postganglionic sympathetic nerve fibers from the carotid plexus via the pterygoid (vidian) canal to the pterygopalatine ganglion. Sympathetic fibers pass through the pterygopalatine ganglion without synapsing while en route to distal targets of innervation.

Parasympathetic innervation to the orbit arises from the Edinger-Westphal (cranial nerve III) nucleus, facial (cranial nerve VII) nucleus, and parasympathetic ganglia, providing pupillary constriction, lacrimal gland innervation, and vasodilation. Preganglionic parasympathetic fibers enter the orbit along the inferior division of the oculomotor nerve, synapsing at the ciliary ganglion (located between the lateral rectus muscle and optic nerve 15 mm posterior to the globe). Parasympathetic innervation to the lacrimal gland originates from the lacrimal nucleus of the facial nerve. Preganglionic parasympathetic nerve fibers are transmitted by the greater superficial petrosal nerve through the pterygoid (vidian) canal, where it meets the deep petrosal nerve to form the vidian nerve. The preganglionic parasympathetic nerves synapse at the pterygopalatine ganglion, beyond which postganglionic parasympathetic nerve fibers are distributed to the lacrimal gland.

Lacrimal Anatomy

Secretory System

The lacrimal gland is located in the lacrimal gland fossa in the orbital portion of the frontal bone and is responsible for reflex tearing. The gland is divided by the lateral horn of the levator aponeurosis into the palpebral lobe and the main orbital lobe. The smaller palpebral lobe is often visible in the superior conjunctival fornix. Eight to 12 lacrimal gland ductules empty into the superior lateral conjunctival fornix. The accessory lacrimal glands, the glands of Krause and Wolfring, are located in the eyelid and are responsible for basal tear secretion.

Excretory System

The lacrimal papillae are located on the posterior edge of the upper and lower eyelids ~6.0 mm from the medial canthus. Each opening is ~0.3 mm in diameter and leads to the lacrimal canaliculi. The lacrimal canaliculi have a 2 mm vertical component and an 8 mm horizontal length on the way to the lacrimal sac. In 90% of subjects, the canaliculi join to form a single common canaliculus before entering the lacrimal sac. At the medial end of the common canaliculus, the valve of Rosenmuller prevents tear reflux. The lacrimal sac is located in the lacrimal fossa and measures 12 mm in height with 5 mm superior to the medial canthal tendon. The lacrimal sac continues inferiorly to the nasolacrimal duct, which extends 10 to 12 mm within the bony nasolacrimal canal. The nasolacrimal canal continues 2 to 5 mm and drains into the inferior meatus of the nose beneath the inferior turbinate, where the valve of Hasner is present (**Fig. 33.2A,B**).

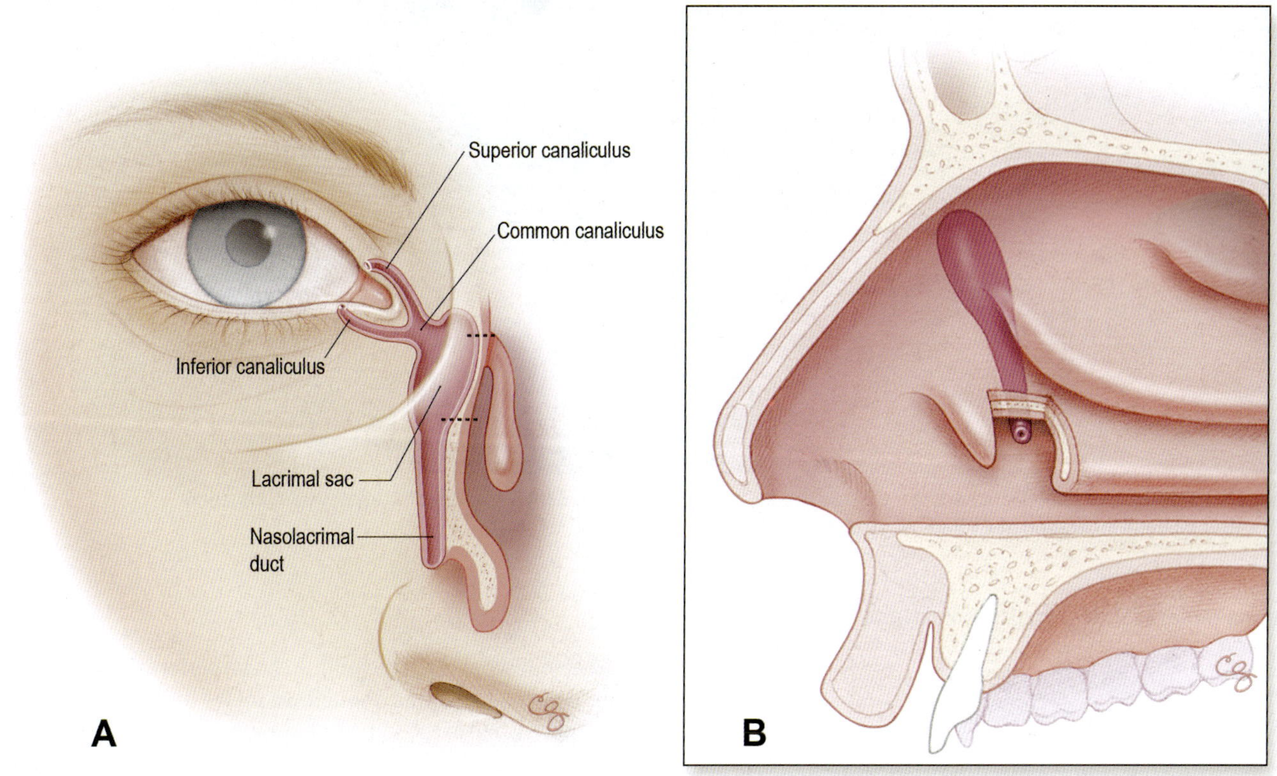

Fig. 33.2 (A) Normal adult lacrimal system. **(B)** View of the lateral nasal wall showing the position of the lacrimal sac and duct relative to the middle and inferior turbinates.

Endoscopic Dacryocystorhinostomy

Introduction and Background

Historically, the majority of surgery for nasolacrimal duct obstruction (NLDO) has been performed through external techniques with excellent outcomes. Intranasal techniques for dacryocystorhinostomy (DCR) were introduced in the early 1900s, and the modern endonasal endoscopic technique was first described in 1989 by McDonogh and Meiring.[1] Acceptance of transnasal approaches had been guarded, however, due to inconsistent success rates. Poor visualization, limited understanding of the intranasal anatomy, and suboptimal surgical instrumentation had been identified as the main reasons for the inferior outcomes compared with external techniques. Continued advances in videoscopic visualization, development of new rhinologic instrumentation, and a growing clinical experience have addressed many of these issues. There is now a growing body of literature validating the endoscopic approach to DCR with reported success rates comparable to the traditional external techniques.[2–5] The advantages of endoscopic DCR include the absence of skin incision and scar, the preservation of the pump mechanism of the orbicularis oculi muscle, less disruption of the medial canthal anatomy, decreased operating time, decreased intraoperative bleeding, and the ability to concurrently address nasal cavity or paranasal sinus abnormalities.[6,7]

Indications and Evaluation

Acquired tearing results from either hypersecretion of tears (lacrimation) or impairment of drainage (epiphora). Acquired nasolacrimal duct obstruction presents with epiphora and/or infection. Epiphora can be unilateral or bilateral and can be constant or intermittent. It can be associated with midfacial trauma, sinus disease or surgery, systemic inflammatory disease, and previous episodes of inflammation of the lacrimal sac. Nasolacrimal duct obstruction can be confirmed by several lacrimal diagnostic tests including the dye disappearance test, lacrimal drainage system irrigation and probing, scintigraphy, and contrast dacryocystography. Persistence of dye or an asymmetric clearance after the instillation of 2% fluorescein solution in the conjunctival cul-de-sac after 5 minutes indicates decreased outflow (**Fig. 33.3**). Irrigation of the lacrimal system with a blunt-tipped 23-gauge irrigating cannula with reflux through the opposite punctum indicates either partial or complete nasolacrimal duct obstruction (**Fig. 33.4**). Scintigraphy using gamma ray–emitting radionucleotides can be used to evaluate physiologic flow, and a contrast dacryocystography can radiologically define lacrimal sac anatomy. The definitive

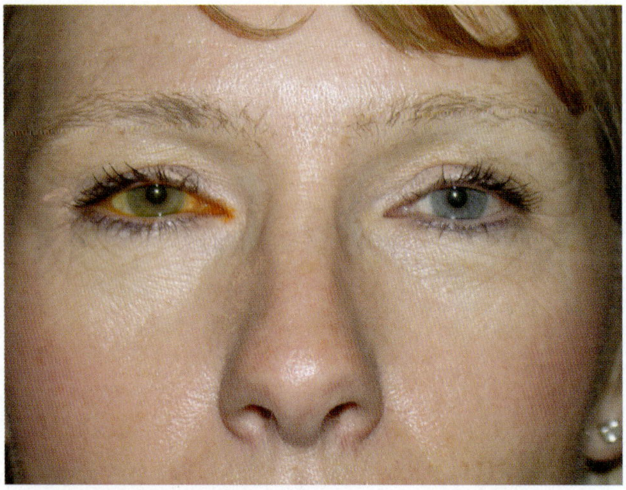

Fig. 33.3 Positive dye disappearance test—retained dye on the right side after bilateral instillation of 2% fluorescein dye.

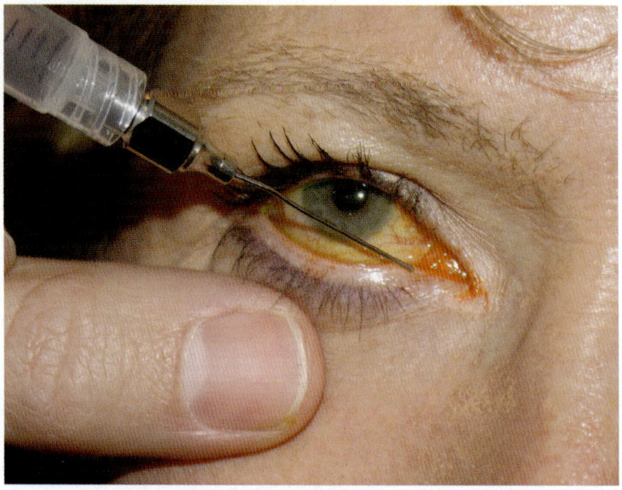

Fig. 33.4 Diagnostic lacrimal system irrigation.

management of acquired nasolacrimal duct obstruction is DCR.

Anatomic Considerations

Tears are primarily secreted by both the lacrimal gland and the accessory lacrimal gland, and collect at the medial eyelid commissure where they drain into the canaliculi through the superior and inferior puncta. In 90% of patients, the superior and inferior canaliculi combine into one common canaliculus and enter into the lateral aspect of the lacrimal sac. The lacrimal sac rests in an oval-shaped fossa measuring ~15 × 10 mm. The thick bone from the frontal process of the maxilla forms the anterior lacrimal crest, whereas the thin lacrimal bone forms the posterior crest. The suture line formed by these two bones corresponds to the maxillary line, an important landmark seen endoscopically (**Fig. 33.5**).

The intranasal anatomic landmarks important to successful endoscopic DCR have historically been poorly understood, but in recent years, have been well studied and documented. In 2000, Wormald et al. published a detailed characterization of the intranasal location of the lacrimal sac.[8] Using computed tomography (CT) dacryocystograms and sinus CT scans, they demonstrated that the mean height of the lacrimal sac is 8.8 mm above the middle turbinate insertion and 5.3 mm above the common canaliculus. These findings confirmed that the location of the sac is higher relative to the middle turbinate insertion and the common canaliculus than previously described. Based on this more detailed appreciation of the anatomic relationships, subsequent modifications of the endoscopic surgical technique were developed, especially related to bone removal. Because the extent of bone removal correlates with both the extent of sac exposure and, ultimately, the outcome, a more thorough removal superior to the frontal process of the maxilla is mandatory.

Surgical Technique

The endoscopic DCR technique can be performed under local or general anesthesia, though we prefer the latter. The setup is approached in the same fashion as routine endoscopic sinus surgery. Topical decongestion with oxymetazoline is applied in the preoperative holding area followed by intranasal placement of pledgets soaked in 1:1000 parts epinephrine in the operating room. Under endoscopic visualization the maxillary line, the uncinate process, and the superior attachment of the middle turbinate are identified as important landmarks and infiltrated with 1% lidocaine with epinephrine.

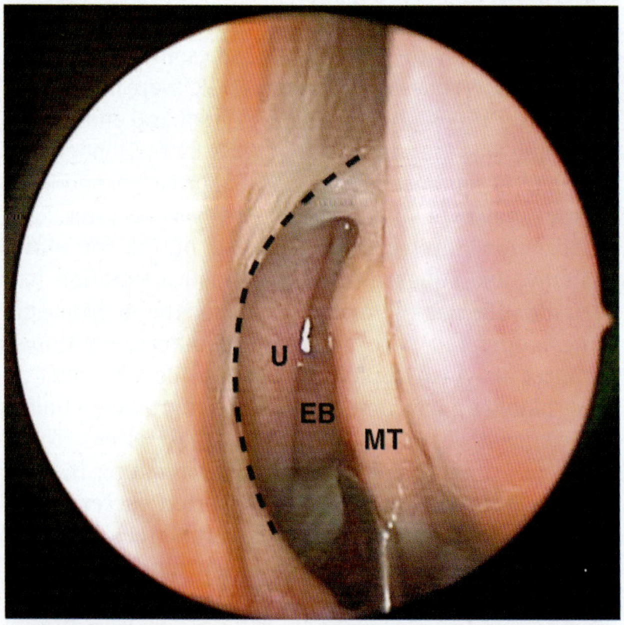

Fig. 33.5 Endoscopic view of the maxillary line. Note the relationship between the maxillary line (*dashed line*), uncinate (*U*), ethmoid bulla (*EB*), and middle turbinate (*MT*).

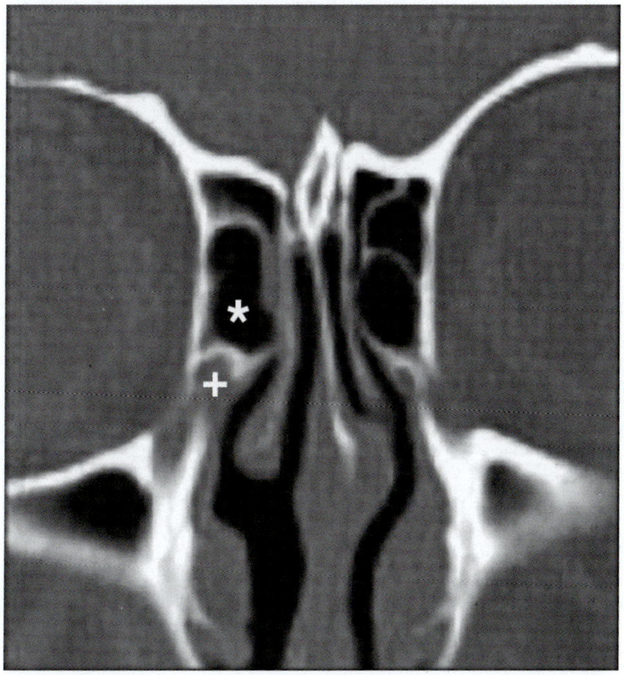

Fig. 33.6 Coronal computed tomography scan showing the relationship between the agger nasi cell (*asterisk*) and the lacrimal sac (*plus sign*).

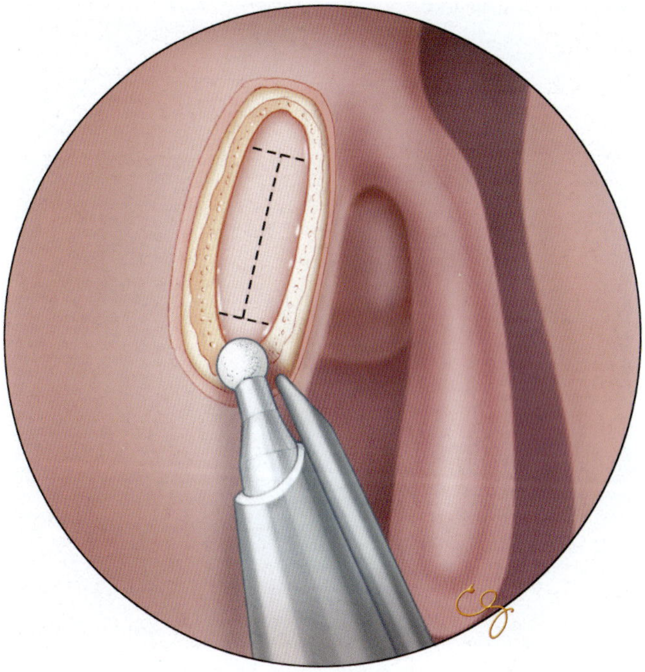

Fig. 33.7 Removal of the frontal process of the maxilla to expose the lacrimal sac using a high-speed burr.

The maxillary line corresponds to the suture line between the frontal process of the maxilla and the lacrimal bone, which runs vertically through the lacrimal fossa. This serves as a consistent endoscopic landmark for the lacrimal sac.

A mucosal flap is typically fashioned using a sickle knife on the lateral nasal wall over the location of the lacrimal fossa. The incision is started ~5 to 6 mm above the insertion of the middle turbinate and carried anteriorly for ~5 mm. A vertical mucosal cut is created inferiorly to about the midway point between the middle turbinate insertion and the inferior turbinate, then taken posteriorly to the uncinate process. A suction elevator is used to elevate the mucosa from the underlying bone along the maxillary line posteriorly to the thin lacrimal bone. The raised mucosal flap is then debulked or trimmed using either a small microdebrider blade or fine cutting forceps. The thin lacrimal bone is easily dissected free of the posterior aspect of the lacrimal sac with the suction elevator or curette. The superior origin of the uncinate process may be encountered in this region and will often be removed with the lacrimal bone. In some patients, a well pneumatized agger nasi will border the lacrimal sac superiorly and posteriorly (**Fig. 33.6**). When present, the agger nasi cell should be dissected thoroughly to optimize lacrimal sac exposure. The thick bone of the frontal process of the maxilla is initially removed using a small Kerrison rongeur to begin the exposure of the inferior portion of the lacrimal sac. As the dissection proceeds, the bone becomes thick and access is limited, thus necessitating the use of a drill to remove bone. Use of a high-speed burr is ideal for efficient and controlled removal of the remainder of the bone overlying the sac (**Fig. 33.7**). An angled (20-degree, 2.5-mm) diamond burr attached to a powered microdebrider set at 12,000 rpm (Medtronic, Inc., Jacksonville, FL) is used to continue the dissection superiorly above the middle turbinate insertion to ensure complete sac exposure (**Fig. 33.8**). The design of the diamond burr minimizes skipping as well as injury to the medial wall of the lacrimal sac; however, the surgeon must be careful to avoid soft tissue injury (**Fig. 33.9**).

After the medial wall of the lacrimal sac has been exposed, a lacrimal probe is passed from the canaliculi to tent the medial wall of the sac and to confirm adequate bony removal. While tented by the lacrimal probe, the medial sac wall is incised and superior and inferior releasing incisions are created. Microscopic scissors or a small aperture microdebrider blade can be used to carefully open the medial wall of the lacrimal sac. The lacrimal probe should be readily visualized in the lumen of the sac

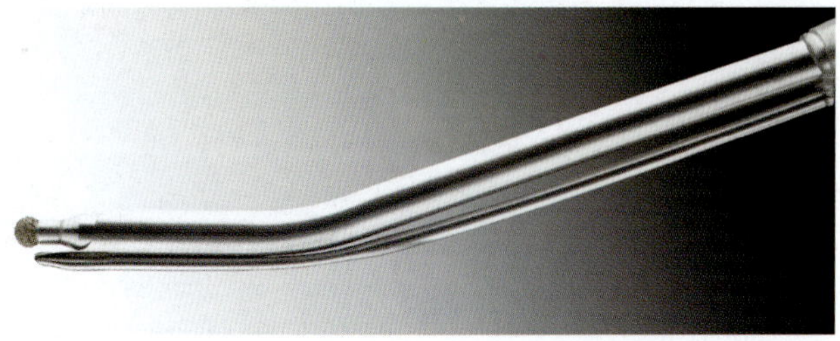

Fig. 33.8 High-speed diamond burr used for bone removal during dacryocystorhinostomy (Medtronic, Inc., Jacksonville, Florida).

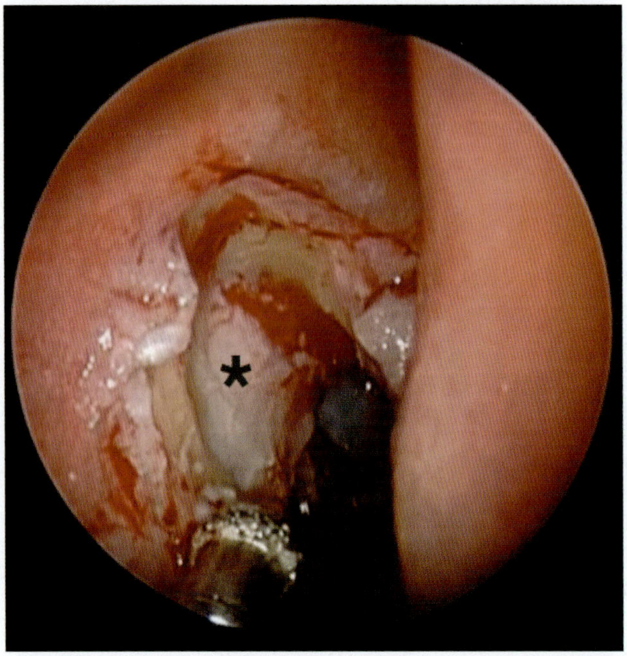

Fig. 33.9 Intraoperative view during a right dacryocystorhinostomy. The medial wall of the lacrimal sac (*asterisk*) has been exposed after removal of the bone with the burr.

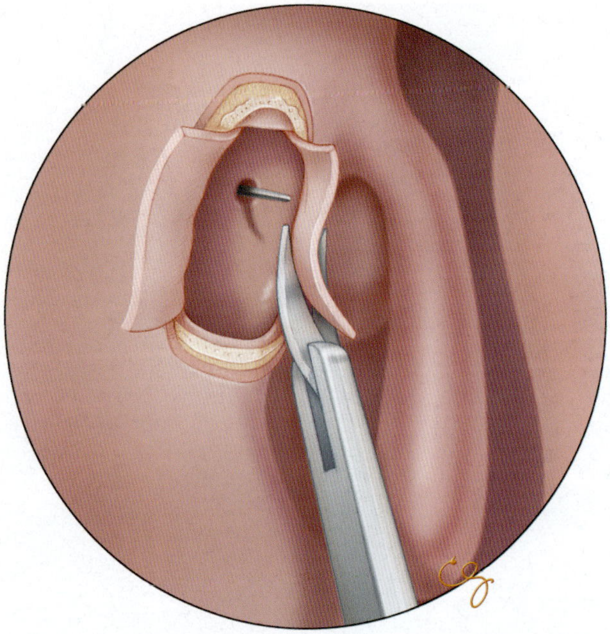

Fig. 33.10 The lacrimal sac is opened and the incised edges are removed using microscissor, small cutting forceps, or an angled microdebrider blade. The lacrimal probe is seen passing through the common internal punctum.

once the sac is opened. The goal is to achieve wide exposure of the common internal punctum with a minimum of several millimeters of sac exposure above this opening (**Fig. 33.10**). Microscopic scissors, cutting forceps, or angled narrow microdebrider blades are used to remove the redundant tissue along the incised sac edges (**Fig. 33.11**). This step is in contrast to the mucosal-sparing technique described by Wormald, but we believe this may actually reduce the opportunity for postoperative stenosis due to mucosal web formation. Ultimately, the exposure should range from 10 to 20 mm in the vertical dimension and 10 to 15 mm in width. Silicone lacrimal intubation stents are typically placed and tied intranasally (**Fig. 33.12**). Nasal packing is not routinely used.

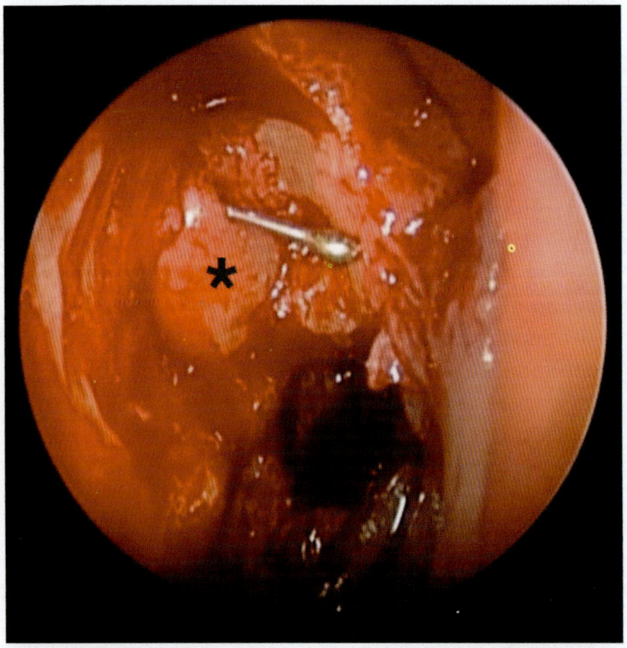

Fig. 33.11 The medial wall of the lacrimal sac (*asterisk*) has been removed and wide exposure of the common internal punctum achieved. Note the lacrimal probe passing through the common internal punctum.

Outcomes

The important role of endoscopic DCR in the treatment of NLDO has been established, with published success rates comparable to the external DCR techniques. Generally speaking, a variety of endoscopic surgical techniques and modifications have been reported with success rates ranging from 80% to greater than 95%.[3,4,9–11] Despite these many described modifications, a direct comparison between endoscopic techniques is lacking in the literature. An improved instrument design coupled with an improved understanding of the relevant anatomy paved the way for a more refined application of powered instrumentation in DCR. The use of drills or burrs during endoscopic DCR was described in the mid-1990s, but it was the recent work of Wormald et al. that helped establish the current efficacy of powered instrumentation.

Tsirbas et al. compared 31 powered endoscopic DCRs to 24 external procedures.[2] The reported success rates were statistically equivalent for the two techniques (93.5% vs.

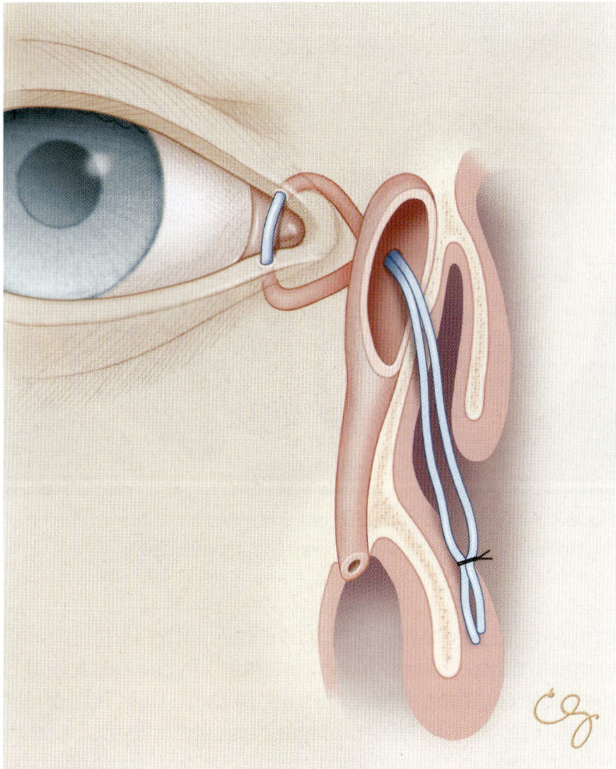

Fig. 33.12 Silicone lacrimal intubation stents are typically placed at the conclusion of the procedure.

95.8%). The technique used by these authors emphasized the importance of complete bone removal as well as mucosal flap preservation. The results from this group are excellent and may very well be a function of these technical considerations. However, the importance of using the mucosal flap technique remains unclear because success rates appear to be reasonable with a variety of approaches. In our approach, we elect to trim or debulk the mucosal flap raised early in the procedure, and to eliminate the redundant lacrimal sac edges at the conclusion of the procedure. In 2007, we published our initial experience using this technical modification.[5] Twenty patients underwent 27 procedures with a mean follow-up of 16 months. A subjective resolution of epiphora and an objective assessment of anatomic patency were recorded. A subjective improvement in epiphora was noted in 100% of procedures with a complete resolution noted in 93% (25 out of 27). Anatomic patency was noted in 100% of our procedures. These data, combined with previously reported outcomes by other authors, suggest preservation of mucosal flaps is not essential for successful patient outcomes.[4,9,11] The mucosal sparing technique has been shown to produce a large and stable ostium with excellent functional outcomes.[12] The technique we advocate does rely on healing by secondary intention and may be associated with a greater risk of granulation tissue formation and mucosal contraction. We did not find this to be an issue in our series, however, as evidenced by comparable outcomes. Meticulous surgical techniques minimizing the degree of exposed bone during the removal of the frontal process of the maxilla will mitigate these risks.

Successful endoscopic DCRs appear to be dependent on three key factors: (1) a thorough understanding of the endoscopic anatomy and location of the lacrimal sac; (2) complete removal of the frontal process of the maxilla to expose the medial wall of the lacrimal sac; and (3) careful incision of the lacrimal sac to achieve adequate exposure of the common internal punctum. Powered endoscopic DCRs, with or without mucosal flap preservation, appear to satisfy these criteria and produce excellent results comparable to widely accepted outcomes following external techniques. All clinicians must remember that tearing is often multifactorial, and even patients with patent ostia may have epiphora from increased lacrimation from an exposure keratopathy or decreased drainage from poor lacrimal pump function. Recently, Mansour et al. demonstrated a persistently abnormal tear drainage function by scintigraphy in patients after DCR with anatomically patent ostia as compared with controls.[13] It is likely, therefore, that even a procedure that achieves 100% anatomic patency may still result in a small minority of patients with continued epiphora.

The role of silicone intubation following endoscopic DCR is debated. The insertion of silicone stents after DCR is generally encouraged both in the ophthalmology and otorhinolaryngology–head and neck surgery literature. However, silicone stents may cause granulation tissue formation, predisposing the patient to infection, adhesions, and possible surgical failure. Unlu et al. reported similar outcomes in patients undergoing endoscopic DCR independent of whether silicone intubation tubes were used.[14] They did, however, note an increased incidence of granulation tissue at the rhinostomy site in their intubation group. Smirnov et al. recently published a prospective randomized study evaluating the clinical value of lacrimal intubation.[15] They found that all of their failures were in the silicone intubation group and concluded that the insertion of silicone tubes does not appear to contribute any benefit. This question requires further study before definitive recommendations can be given.

Summary

Endoscopic DCR has been established as a viable alternative for the management of nasolacrimal duct obstruction. By working closely with colleagues in ophthalmology, the rhinologist should be comfortable at and skilled in providing this service. Although several surgical modifications have been published over the years, the technique of a powered endoscopic DCR appears to provide excellent outcomes with minimal patient morbidity. Proper instrumentation, skill with advanced techniques, and a thorough understanding of the relevant anatomy is essential to optimize outcomes.

Orbital Decompression

Introduction

Ophthalmopathy associated with thyroid dysfunction has been recognized since Graves' description in 1835. Thyroid eye disease (also known as Graves' ophthalmopathy, thyroid-related ophthalmopathy, thyrotoxic exophthalmos, dysthyroid ophthalmopathy, and several other terms) is the most common extrathyroidal manifestation of Graves' disease and is the leading cause of orbital inflammation and proptosis in adults. Thyroid eye disease is considered an autoimmune process. Thyroid-stimulating hormone (TSH) receptor is the likely autoantigen in both the thyroid gland and orbit. Fibroblasts and adipocytes act as effector cells, inducing a complex cytokine-mediated immunologic response marked by tissue inflammation and hypertrophy.

Bartley et al. reviewed the incidence of thyroid eye disease, the chronology of ophthalmopathy, and the clinical features of thyroid eye disease in an incidence cohort.[16] The incidence rate for thyroid eye disease was 16 cases per 100,000 population per year for women and 3 cases per 100,000 for men. The median age at the time of diagnosis was 43 years, and thyroid eye disease affected women 6 times more frequently than men. Ninety percent of patients in the incidence cohort had Graves' hyperthyroidism, 3% had Hashimoto thyroiditis, 1% had primary hypothyroidism, and 6% were euthyroid. Durairaj et al. reported on the clinical features and treatment of thyroid eye disease in the pediatric population and concluded that although thyroid eye disease has similar clinical manifestations in pediatric and adult populations, the disorder is less severe in children than in adults.[17]

Common symptoms of thyroid eye disease include blurred vision, foreign body sensation, photophobia, tearing, double vision, dull pain, and discomfort. Clinical features of thyroid eye disease include eyelid retraction, periorbital soft tissue swelling, lid lag, lagophthalmos, conjunctival injection, exposure keratopathy, restrictive myopathy (strabismus), exophthalmos, and optic neuropathy.[18] Eyelid retraction is the most common sign, occurring in more than 90% of patients (**Fig. 33.13**). Neuroimaging usually reveals fusiform enlargement of the extraocular muscles with tendon sparing. Magnetic resonance imaging (MRI) is more sensitive than CT for showing optic nerve compression at the orbital apex. CT scan is performed before orbital decompression to assess the bony architecture of the orbit (**Fig. 33.14**). Approximately 20% of patients with thyroid eye disease undergo surgery. Surgical rehabilitation is usually staged with orbital decompression first, followed by strabismus surgery, and finally, eyelid surgery. Approximately 5% of patients will experience severe orbital inflammation and congestion resulting in compressive optic neuropathy, requiring urgent treatment.

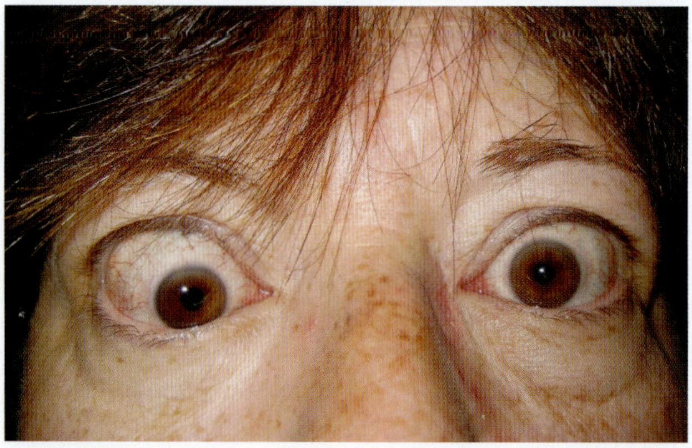

Fig. 33.13 Thyroid eye disease manifested by eyelid retraction, exophthalmos, restrictive myopathy (strabismus), and soft tissue swelling.

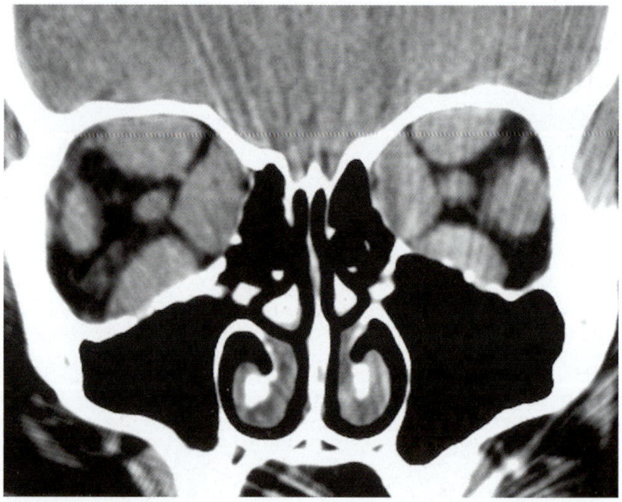

Fig. 33.14 Coronal computed tomography scan of the orbits showing fusiform enlargement of the extraocular muscles.

Nonsurgical Management of Thyroid Eye Disease

Thyroid eye disease is usually self-limited and the majority of patients require only supportive care, including aggressive ocular surface lubrication, cool compresses, and sunglasses to manage light sensitivity and glare. Correction of thyroid dysfunction is important because this may aid in improving orbitopathy. Corticosteroids are the most common immunomodulator prescribed for clinically active thyroid eye disease. They are typically administered orally or intravenously and have an overall favorable response in the majority of patients. Local injections of steroids into the orbit have had mixed results. Other immunomodulators, including cyclosporine, azathioprine, and intravenous immunoglobulin, have also been used in small, retrospective studies. Antioxidant agents such as allopurinol and nicotinamide have also been investigated.[19] The goal of medical therapy is to minimize the severity and shorten the duration of inflammation and associated fibrosis.

Orbital radiation is widely used to treat orbital inflammation and compressive optic neuropathy associated with thyroid eye disease. Typical doses for external beam orbital radiation are 20 Gy over 10 sessions. The role of radiotherapy in the treatment of thyroid-associated orbitopathy has been widely debated. Gorman et al. conducted a prospective, randomized, double-masked, placebo-controlled clinical trial and concluded that, when assessed at 1 year after treatment, radiotherapy had been ineffective in managing patients with mild-to-moderate thyroid eye disease.[20] This study excluded patients with compressive optic neuropathy. Critics of this study state that orbital radiotherapy is effective in patients with active orbitopathy and is indicated for optic neuropathy, steroid-dependent orbital inflammation, and rapidly progressing orbitopathy. A combination of external beam orbital radiation and corticosteroids is the most effective nonmedical treatment for clinically active thyroid eye disease.[21]

Surgical Management of Thyroid Eye Disease

Surgical decompression of the orbit is an accepted and validated treatment of thyroid eye disease. Indications include compressive optic neuropathy, exposure keratopathy, and disfiguring proptosis. Multiple surgical approaches can be used to decompress the orbit by removing bone and fat; however, the superiority of one approach over the others has not clearly been established. Surgical approaches for decompressing the orbit include transcranial, coronal flap, transconjunctival/transcaruncular, transantral, and endonasal. Decompression of the anterior orbit is effective for reducing proptosis. In cases of compressive optic neuropathy, it is important to decompress the posterior aspect of the medial and inferior walls of the orbit.

The degree of recession of the exophthalmos achieved by orbital decompression is directly related to the number of walls surgically decompressed. Depending on the severity of preoperative exophthalmos, patients should be evaluated for a graded surgical approach to orbital decompression, targeting the lateral wall, medial wall, and/or posterior orbital floor along with orbital fat decompression.[22] Surgical decompression of the orbital roof is generally not performed routinely due to the morbidity of the required frontal craniotomy, as well as the potential for resultant transmission of intracranial pulsations to the eye that can be a bothersome side effect. The surgical approaches employed and the extent of orbital decompression pursued are based on the operative goals defined by the surgical team.

Anatomic Considerations

Decompression of the lateral wall can be accomplished with a lid crease incision, subperiosteal dissection plane, and removal of portions of the greater wing of the sphenoid and areas surrounding the inferior orbital fissure using a high-speed diamond burr. Access to the medial wall can be accomplished through endonasal techniques or a transcaruncular approach. Orbital floor decompression is performed via a transconjunctival, inferior fornix approach. Orbital fat decompression is usually performed in the lateral portion and inferomedial quadrant of the orbit after the periorbita has been opened. In our practice, we favor the graded 3-wall (lateral, medial, orbital floor) decompression with preservation of the inferomedial orbital strut in conjunction with orbital fat decompression (**Figs. 33.15 and 33.16**).

Surgical Technique: Endoscopic Medial Decompression

General anesthesia is used for all decompressions in our practice and the order of procedures is not crucial. The operating room setup and patient positioning for endoscopic decompression of the medial orbit is the same as for routine endoscopic sinus surgery. We prefer to use image-guided surgical (IGS) navigation on all our cases to assist with the identification of relevant anatomy. The multiplanar images are carefully reviewed preoperatively on the IGS computer to aid in surgical planning.

The surgical dissection begins with a wide maxillary antrostomy using standard techniques. It is important to widely open the maxillary sinus to completely visualize the floor of the orbit and to prevent ostial obstruction from orbital fat following the decompression. The antrostomy should be widened in the posterior direction, avoiding an anterior dissection that may lead to nasolacrimal duct injury. This wide exposure provides access to the infraorbital nerve canal and the inferomedial orbital strut for extended endoscopic decompression, depending on the surgical plan. A complete sphenoethmoidectomy is then performed using standard technique. The primary goals of this portion of the dissection are (1) fully expose the skull base and its relationship to the medial orbit; (2) widely open the sphenoid sinus exposing the orbital apex and optic canal; and (3) completely skeletonize the lamina papyracea. During the ethmoidectomy, important anatomic variations such as a sphenoethmoidal (Onodi) cell, dehiscent carotid artery, dehiscent optic nerve, low hanging skull base, or exposed ethmoidal artery must be considered (**Fig. 33.17A,B**). The final step during the initial exposure of the orbit may include a frontal recess dissection depending on the extent of pneumatization in this region. In some patients, extensive frontal recess pneumatization can provide easy access to the superomedial bony orbit. It is reasonable to consider maximizing the decompression by removing the select orbital bone in this area. However, the benefit is unclear and the risk of anterior ethmoidal artery injury increases. Preservation of bone in the lateral aspect of the frontal recess may also mitigate the risk of postoperative frontal sinus obstruction from prolapsed fat. Thus, a conservative approach should be considered. Although previous authors have advocated middle

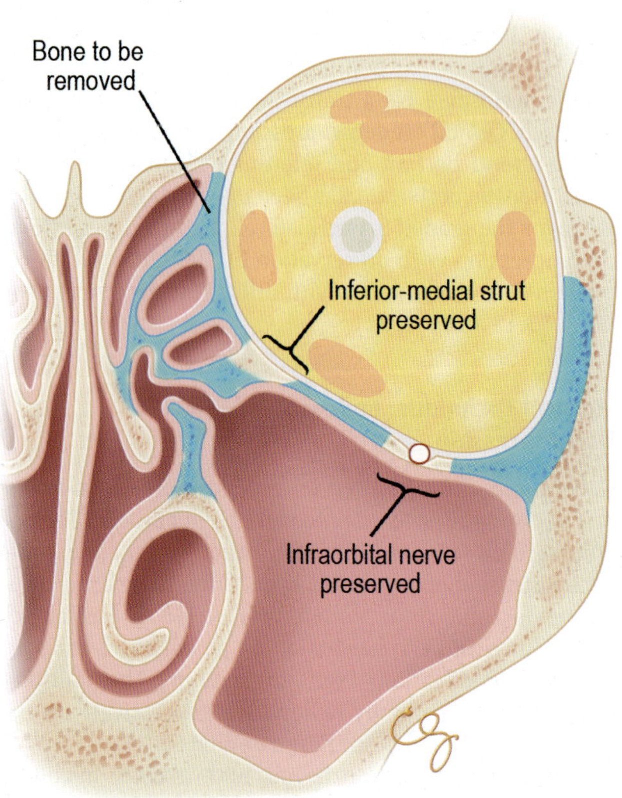

Fig. 33.15 Drawing showing the potential areas of bone removal for medial, inferior, and lateral orbital decompressions. Note the preservation of the inferomedial orbital strut and the infraorbital nerve canal.

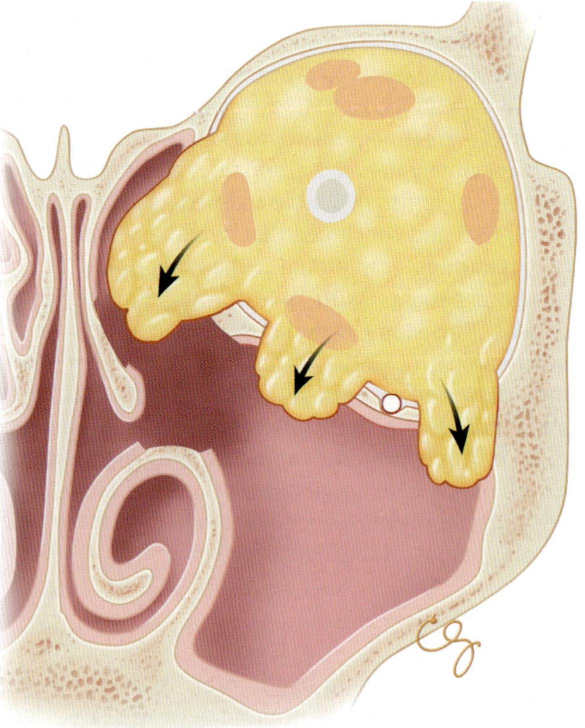

Fig. 33.16 Drawing in the coronal plane showing the release of orbital fat after medial, inferior, and lateral decompressions.

A

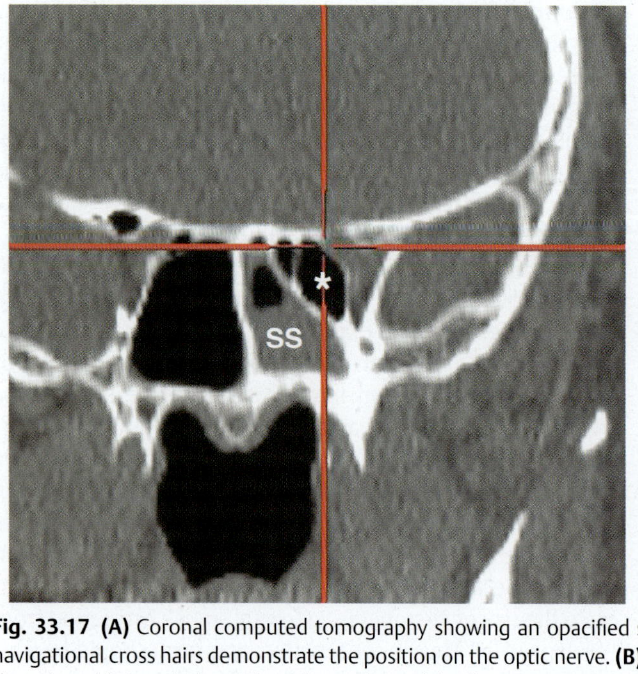

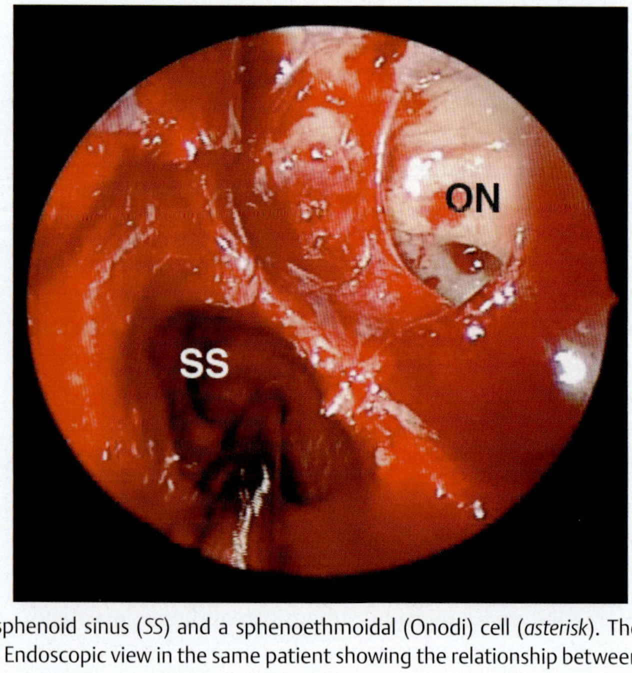

B

Fig. 33.17 **(A)** Coronal computed tomography showing an opacified sphenoid sinus (*SS*) and a sphenoethmoidal (Onodi) cell (*asterisk*). The navigational cross hairs demonstrate the position on the optic nerve. **(B)** Endoscopic view in the same patient showing the relationship between the sphenoid sinus (*SS*) and the sphenoethmoidal cell containing the exposed optic nerve (*ON*).

turbinate removal for aid in the extent of decompression, we elect to preserve this structure and believe there are no adverse consequences in doing so.

Once the medial orbital wall has been completely skeletonized, the thin bone of the lamina papyracea is entered with an elevator, curette, or similar instrument. Entry must be controlled and ideally should not violate the periorbita. Bone is then removed superiorly toward the ethmoid roof and skull base, inferiorly to the inferomedial orbital strut, and anteriorly to the maxillary line (**Fig. 33.18**). The preservation of the inferomedial strut has been advocated as a means to prevent displacement of the globe position and hence reduce the incidence of new or worsened postoperative diplopia. As the dissection moves posteriorly, the thick bone of the optic strut will be encountered. This represents the region of the orbital apex just proximal to the annulus of Zinn. Standard medial orbital decompression will stop 2 to 5 mm anterior to the optic strut. However, in cases of optic nerve compression or when maximum decompression is desired, bone removal may continue through the optic strut to include the optic canal.

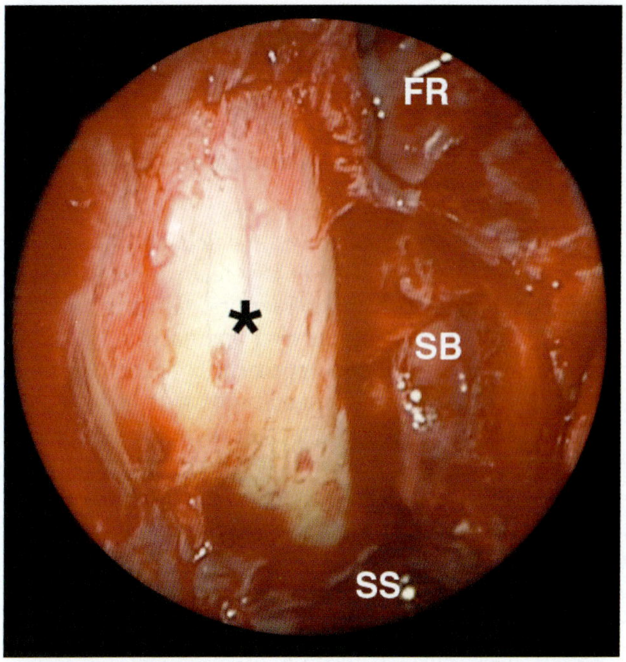

Fig. 33.18 Intraoperative view of the exposed periorbita (*asterisk*) after removal of the right medial orbital wall. Limits of exposure include the frontal recess (*FR*), skull base (*SB*), and sphenoid sinus (*SS*).

With the medial wall bone appropriately removed, the periorbita is opened using a sickle knife. Parallel incisions are performed starting posteriorly and carried anteriorly (**Fig. 33.19**). In the typical setting of a "tight" orbit, there is a brisk prolapse of fat immediately after the periorbita is incised. The surgeon then uses the sickle knife or a blunt ball probe to release the remaining fascial bands between the original incisions until orbital fat fills the ethmoid cavity (**Fig. 33.20**). Gentle ballottement of the orbit may aid in the delivery of the orbital fat into the ethmoid and may help to reveal any residual nonlysed periorbital bands. Several authors have advocated sharply removing the periorbita with forceps, but we find this unnecessary in the vast majority of cases. Although we prefer to completely release all aspects of the exposed periorbita, Metson and

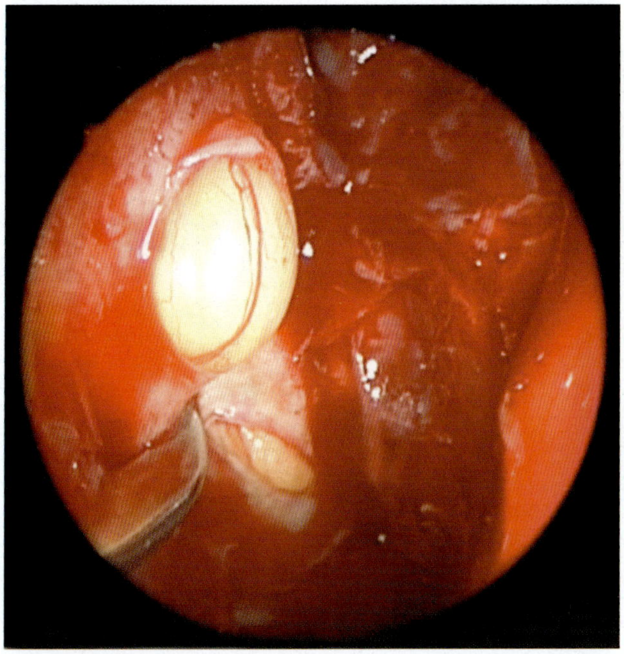

Fig. 33.19 A sickle knife is typically used to incise the periorbita. Parallel incisions are performed from posterior to anterior while working from superior to inferior.

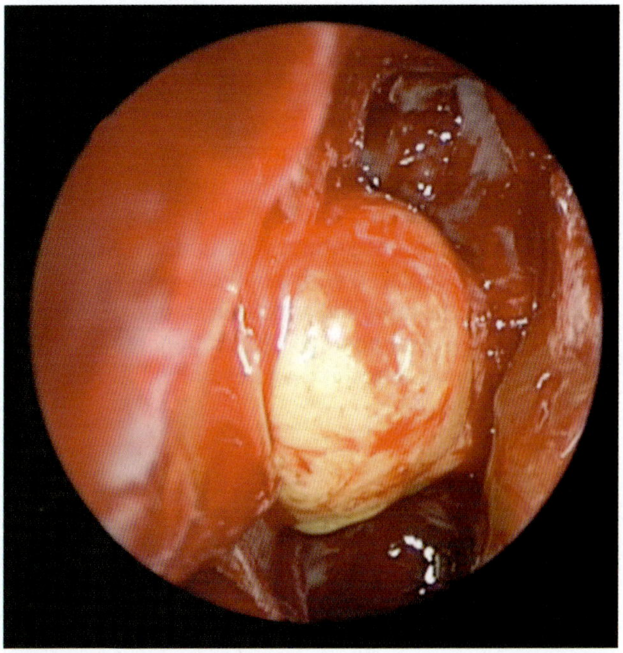

Fig. 33.20 Intraoperative view showing prolapse of fat into the ethmoid cavity once the release of the periorbita is complete.

Samaha described preserving a 10-mm wide sling of periorbita overlying the medial rectus to reduce the risk of postoperative diplopia.[23]

Surgical Technique: Inferior and Lateral Decompression

Surgical decompression of the orbital floor and lateral wall is performed by the ophthalmology team. Removal of the orbital floor medial to the infraorbital nerve is typically handled via the transconjunctival approach in our practice. The authors favor this approach for several reasons: (1) we preserve the inferomedial orbital strut to reduce the risk of diplopia; (2) it is technically easier to remove bone medial to the nerve while preserving the strut with this technique; and (3) the transconjunctival approach is routinely planned for inferior/lateral decompression in all of our cases.

Local infiltrative anesthesia, consisting of 2 mL of 1% lidocaine with 1:100,000 epinephrine (Abbott Laboratories, Chicago, IL) is injected into the lower eyelid and lateral canthus. A lateral canthotomy and inferior cantholysis are performed, followed by a transconjunctival incision from the canthotomy to the caruncle. The swinging eyelid flap is used to widely expose the lateral and inferior wall. A subperiosteal dissection plane is used to elevate the periorbita and expose the bony orbit. Bone from the orbital floor medial and lateral to the inferior orbital neurovascular bundle is carefully removed using Kerrison rongeurs. The bony canal over the inferior orbital neurovascular bundle and the inferomedial orbital strut is left intact. Bone from the lateral wall is decompressed using a high-speed diamond burr. Next, the inferotemporal and inferomedial periorbita are opened with scissors, and blunt dissection is used to prolapse orbital fat. Orbital fat is carefully removed with monopolar cautery. Neurosurgical cottonoids soaked in Neo-Synephrine (Bayer, Morristown, NJ) are used to aid in hemostasis. The transconjunctival incision is closed with one 7–0 Vicryl suture and the lateral canthus is reconstructed with deep 5–0 Vicryl suture and superficial 6–0 fast absorbing gut suture. A temporary suture tarsorrhaphy is then placed with a 5–0 silk suture in a horizontal mattress fashion, and antibiotic/steroid ointment is applied. After several hours of observation, the patient is discharged from the hospital and examined in the clinic the following morning.

Postoperative Care

This procedure, in our hands, is typically performed in the outpatient setting. The patient is seen the next morning by the ophthalmology team and 1 week postoperatively by the rhinology team. Postoperative antibiotics are not typically used and oral steroids are selectively prescribed based on the presence of optic nerve compression. The patient is instructed to start nasal saline irrigations 24 to 72 hours after surgery. Postoperative care follows that used for routine endoscopic surgery except that less vigorous debridements are performed. Mucosal recovery is typically rapid, with eventual remucosalization of all exposed orbital fat (**Fig. 33.21**).

Outcomes

There are several goals of surgical intervention in orbital decompression, including treatment of compressive optic neuropathy, excessive proptosis, and exposure keratopathy. In patients with optic nerve compression, a reversal or the prevention of worsening visual acuity and visual field deficits will be the critical outcome measure. In patients with excessive proptosis and exposure keratopathy, exophthalmometry measurements and ocular surface examination will be the primary outcome measure. Analysis of reported outcomes is difficult because of the wide range of patient indications and the many surgical approaches used. Nonetheless, orbital decompression strikes a delicate balance between achieving maximal reduction of proptosis versus causing new or worsening diplopia. As the indications for surgical intervention continue to shift toward correction of cosmetic deformities, this challenging balance becomes even more relevant.

The transantral (Walsh-Ogura) technique for inferomedial orbital decompression was reported in 1957, and several large series using this technique were subsequently published in 1989 and 1993.[24,25] Reported outcomes with this technique include average decompression of 4.7 mm, worsening visual acuity in 5 to 15% of patients, and postoperative diplopia in as many as 67% of patients. In 1990,

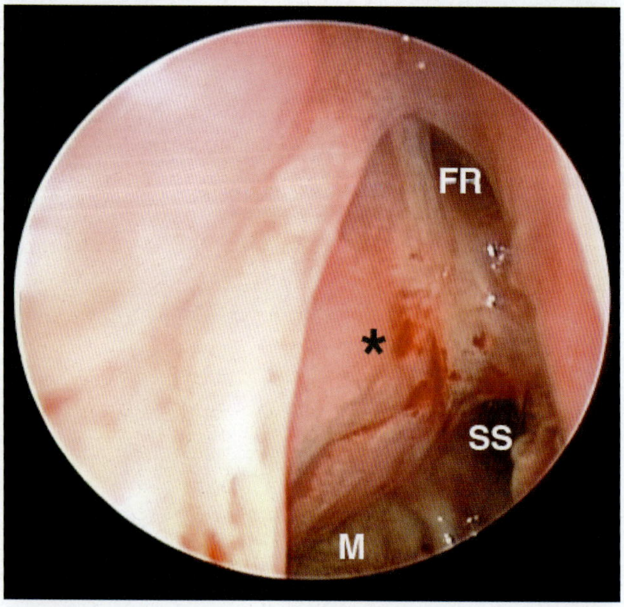

Fig. 33.21 Postoperative view 6 weeks after right endoscopic orbital decompression. *M*, maxillary sinus; *FR*, frontal recess; *SS*, sphenoid sinus; *asterisk*, orbit.

Kennedy et al. introduced the endoscopic transnasal approach for orbital decompression in 8 patients (13 orbits).[26] This technique included the removal of bone from the medial wall extending to and including the orbital floor bone medial to the infraorbital nerve. Thus, the inferomedial strut was removed in all cases. An average decompression of 4.7 mm was reported for the transnasal technique and 5.7 mm when a lateral orbitotomy was added. Two (25%) of their patients reported postoperative diplopia. Using the same technique in 14 patients (22 orbits), Metson et al. reported a reduction of 3.2 mm with endoscopic decompression alone and a reduction of 5.6 mm when a lateral decompression was added.[27]

More recently, the principle of "balanced decompression" has gained favor. The concept behind this technique is the combination of medial and lateral decompression to achieve a symmetric and balanced anatomic result, thus reducing the risk of diplopia. Lateral decompression is not a new concept and was described by both Kennedy and Metson in combination with endoscopic medial decompression. Shepard et al. published their experience with a balanced approach in 1998.[28] Endoscopic medial and external lateral decompressions were performed on 11 patients (18 orbits). Inferior decompression via a transconjunctival approach was also used in 11 of these orbits. However, in all cases, the inferomedial orbital strut was preserved. The reported mean decompression was 4.6 mm and a new onset diplopia was noted in 40% (2 of 5 patients) undergoing decompression for visual deficits. None of the patients undergoing surgery for cosmetic improvement or exposure keratopathy (6 patients) experienced postoperative diplopia. Using a similar technique of balanced decompression with inferomedial orbital strut preservation, Unal et al. reported no new postoperative onsets of diplopia in 11 patients (18 orbits).[29] The incidence of diplopia, however, increased to 57% when they added an inferior wall decompression.

In addition to the well-defined risk of diplopia, postoperative complications after orbital decompression may include cerebrospinal fluid (CSF) leak, visual acuity change, hemorrhage, intranasal scarring with obstruction, and rhinosinusitis. Although surprisingly rare, rhinosinusitis may occur postoperatively due to prolapsed fat obstructing one or more of the sinuses. The technical steps outlined should minimize this complication, and medical management often helps avoid the need for surgery. We have found the frontal sinus to be the most likely site of involvement (**Fig. 33.22A,B**).

Summary

Orbital decompression for Graves' eye disease is an important treatment option in symptomatic patients. A customized surgical approach should be pursued based on clinical indications and patient goals. For patients with purely cosmetic concerns or mild-to-moderate exposure keratopathy, a conservative approach is warranted. In our practice we favor an endoscopic medial decompression combined with a conservative inferolateral decompression via a transconjunctival approach. We preserve

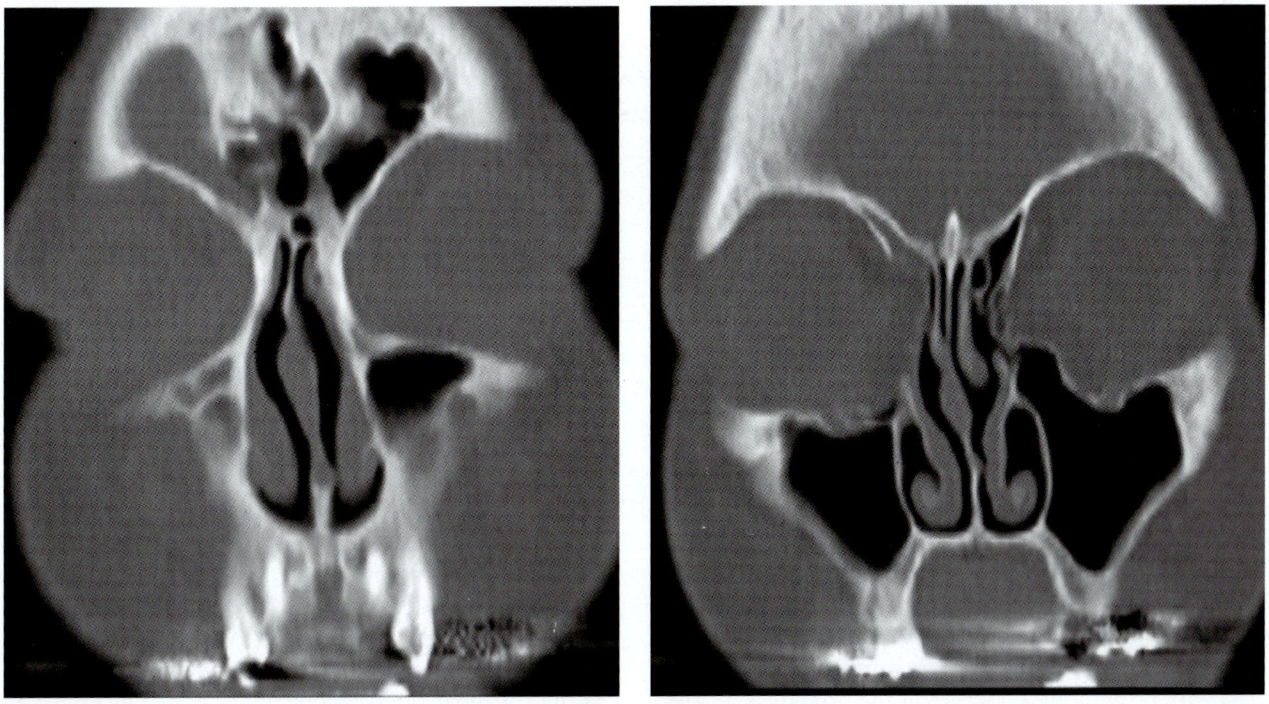

A B

Fig. 33.22 (A,B) Coronal computed tomography views showing right frontal sinus obstruction after orbital decompression due to prolapse of fat across the frontal outflow tract.

the inferomedial strut and limit our posterior dissection in the region of the orbital apex. In our hands, this measured approach has proven very successful in mitigating the risk of diplopia. The approach for patients with severe exophthalmos and/or optic nerve compression with visual deficits is different. In these cases, we pursue a more aggressive lateral decompression, as well as extend our posterior decompression to the optic strut and beyond, as indicated. The inferomedial strut is preserved, except in the most severe cases. The surgical management of the Graves' patient requires a close working relationship between the orbital surgeon and the rhinologist at all levels of planning and care.

Endoscopic Optic Nerve Decompression

Introduction

Refinements in surgical instrumentation and a continued growing surgical experience with advanced rhinologic techniques have made the endoscopic approach to the optic nerve possible. For the experienced rhinologist who is comfortable with endoscopic approaches to the sphenoid, skull base, and orbit, approaching the optic canal is a logical extension of these advanced techniques and concepts. Traumatic optic neuropathy remains the most common indication for which endoscopic optic nerve decompression is considered. Management of these injuries remains controversial due to the lack of evidence-based data to guide decisions. In patients with nontraumatic compressive optic neuropathy (i.e., Graves' optic neuropathy, intracanalicular neoplasms, fibro-osseous lesions) the benefits of surgical decompression appear to be more established. Traditional surgical approaches to the optic nerve include transcranial (craniotomy), extranasal transfacial, transorbital, transantral, and microscopic transnasal. The endoscopic approach affords many potential advantages over these traditional techniques. Decreased morbidity, preservation of olfaction, rapid recovery time, more acceptable cosmetic results, and minimal or no hospitalization requirement are a few of the benefits to this technique.[30]

Indications

Traumatic optic neuropathy (TON) can be categorized as indirect or direct. Direct TON typically results from a penetrating injury and involves the intraorbital portion of the optic nerve. Optic nerve decompression is generally not recommended in such cases. Indirect TON results from blunt trauma to the head and is not an infrequent consequence of head injury. Injury to the optic nerve can occur with or without a fracture of the orbital canal. The pathophysiology of visual loss in the setting of indirect TON is not always clear. Potential causes include intraneural edema, hematoma, shearing injury to the nerve, vascular disruption, compression by displaced bone fragment, and interruption of axonal transport. In cases of hematoma, edema, or disruption of the bony canal with compression, decompression may be indicated. Optic nerve decompression would not be indicated in the presence of nerve transaction.

There is no evidence-based consensus on how to manage TON. Systemic corticosteroids and surgical decompression have been the mainstays of treatment, although neither has been shown to definitively improve outcomes when compared with observation alone. The International Optic Nerve Trauma Study was designed as a randomized, controlled trial looking at outcomes in the management of TON.[31] Due to limited patient numbers, this effort was ultimately reported as a nonrandomized, nonstandardized study with 127 patients. The authors concluded that there was no clear benefit for either corticosteroid therapy or surgical decompression, and management should be based on a case-by-case basis. Subsequent studies, though uncontrolled, have suggested a potential benefit of surgical decompression in patients with TON who fail to respond to a trial of systemic corticosteroids.[31–35] This appears to apply to patients who do not have complete visual loss. The management of TON continues to be both controversial and challenging. In patients with incomplete visual loss that deteriorates or fails to improve while receiving systemic corticosteroids, surgical decompression of the optic nerve appears to be a reasonable consideration.

Anatomic Considerations

The optic nerve is divided into four segments: intraocular, intraorbital, intracanalicular, and intracranial segments. The typical target of endoscopic optic nerve decompression is the intracanalicular segment. The optic canal is formed by the two struts of the lesser wing of the sphenoid and carries both the optic nerve and ophthalmic artery. The optic nerve, in contrast to a peripheral nerve, is a direct continuation of the brain and contains all three meningeal layers: pia, arachnoid, and dura. The dural covering of the optic nerve consists of two layers: (1) the outer layer arising at the orbital apex where the dura splits to form the optic nerve sheath and the periorbita; and (2) the arachnoid, which is attached to the inner portion of the dural sheath. This anatomic relationship has theoretical clinical implications if one elects to incise the nerve sheath. CSF leak is possible if the sheath is incised and must be considered carefully in such cases. Just inferior to the optic canal will sit the carotid canal. The degree of sphenoid sinus/lesser sphenoid wing pneumatization determines the anatomic proximity of these two important structures along the lateral wall of the sphenoid sinus. Preoperative CT in the coronal and axial planes is essential to fully assess these relationships.

In some patients, the optic nerve will course through a posterior ethmoid cell, also known as a sphenoethmoid or Onodi cell (**Fig. 33.17A,B**). This important relationship must be appreciated by the surgeon to ensure proper optic nerve identification and avoidance of injury.

Surgical Technique

Preparation for endoscopic optic nerve decompression should be similar to the approach for standard endoscopic sinus surgery. Careful preoperative review of multiplanar CT imaging is critical to understand the location of the optic canal, carotid artery, and the accessibility of the intracanalicular segment of the nerve. We elect to use IGS navigation in all of our optic nerve decompression cases. The preoperative surgical planning possible by reviewing the multiplanar imaging is invaluable and the intraoperative validation of anatomy is important. The initial step is to perform a complete endoscopic ethmoidectomy and a sphenoidotomy to provide full access to the medial orbital wall and the lateral sphenoid anatomy.

Following exposure of the medial orbit, a small elevator or curette is used to remove the lamina papyracea along the posterior aspect of the orbit. This dissection starts ~10 to 15 mm anterior to the optic strut and will expose the orbital apex. Care should be exercised to avoid penetration of the periorbita because herniation of orbital fat may obstruct the surgical field. As the thin bone of the lamina papyracea is removed, the thick bone of the lesser wing of the sphenoid will be encountered as the optic canal is approached. The initial thick bone represents the optic strut or optic tubercle, and the annulus of Zinn lies deep to this structure. It is at this point that a high-speed drill or burr should be used for efficiently thinning the bone. We prefer to use a self-irrigating straight diamond or 15-degree DCR diamond burr at 12,000 rpm. A variety of burrs are now available with varying lengths, shaft angles, and cutting surfaces. The diamond head is preferable to avoid skipping and to mitigate soft tissue damage. The drill is used only to thin the overlying bone of the canal; exposure of the nerve is to be avoided while using powered instrumentation. These devices now have constant suction and irrigation at the burr tip to optimize visualization and minimize thermal damage to neural structures. Once the bone has been sufficiently thinned, a curette or small elevator is used to remove the remaining fragments to expose the nerve. The dissection should be slow and tedious with precise thinning and subsequent removal of bone until the desired degree of nerve decompression has been accomplished (**Figs. 33.23 and 33.24**).

The general tenet is to remove as much bone as can be done safely in order to maximize decompression. The degree of sphenoid pneumatization will largely dictate what portion of the canal can be accessed (i.e., a 180-degree vs. a 270-degree exposure of the nerve). There are no data to suggest the optimal length of nerve that should be decompressed. In a similar fashion, the role of nerve sheath incision is unclear. Optic nerve sheath incision has been advocated by some authors, but there are no studies to indicate proper patient selection.[30,33,36] In certain cases, such as intrasheath hematoma or neoplasm, nerve sheath incision may be reasonable. CSF leak, nerve fiber injury, and

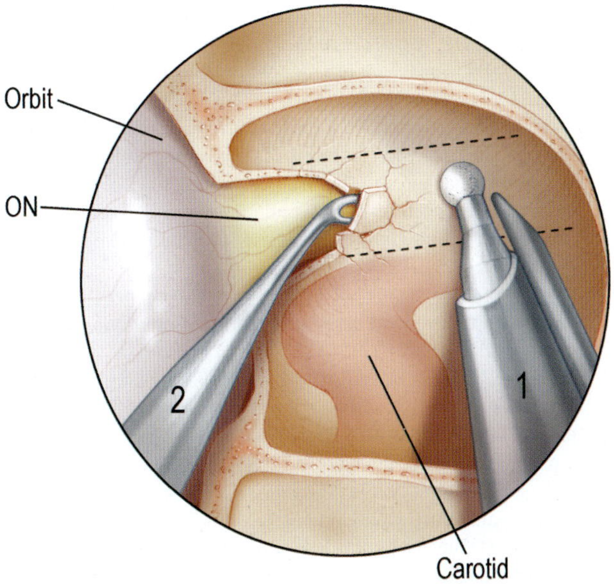

Fig. 33.23 Drawing of a right endoscopic optic nerve decompression. The high-speed burr (*1*) is used to thin the bone overlying the nerve followed by blunt removal using a curette (*2*).

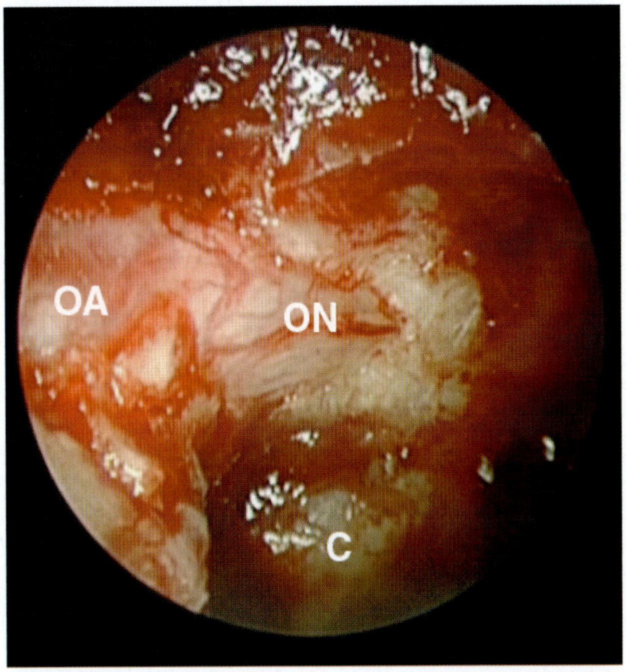

Fig. 33.24 Intraoperative view after right endoscopic optic nerve decompression. OA, orbital apex; C, carotid artery; ON, optic nerve.

hemorrhage are possible adverse consequences of incising the sheath.

Postoperative care mirrors that following standard endoscopic sinus surgery. In select cases, the surgery can be performed as an outpatient procedure with close follow-up by both the rhinology and ophthalmology services. Assessment of visual acuity is performed immediately after the procedure and the following day.

Summary

Safe and efficient decompression of the optic nerve via an endoscopic approach is now possible through refinements in surgical technique, instrumentation, and clinical experience. The endoscopic approach, however, only provides for medial and inferior decompression of the optic nerve. Thus, other techniques are typically required to access the superior or lateral portions of the nerve. The greatest obstacle we face currently is the absence of evidence-based data defining the indications for optic nerve decompression. Endoscopic optic nerve decompression requires significant experience with advanced rhinologic techniques, comfort with and access to advanced instrumentation, and a close working relationship with our ophthalmology colleagues.

Conclusion

Continued advances in endoscopic surgical instrumentation and technique and growing clinical experience have helped expand the rhinologist's role in managing select conditions of the orbit. A close working relationship between the rhinologist and the orbital surgeon is imperative to optimize safety and outcomes. The patient clearly benefits from this team approach. The value of transnasal endoscopic techniques for managing nasolacrimal duct obstruction, orbital decompression, and optic nerve decompression has been established.

References

1. McDonogh M. Endoscopic transnasal dacryocystorhinostomy. Results in 21 patients. S Afr J Surg 1992;30(3):107–110
2. Tsirbas A, Davis G, Wormald PJ. Mechanical endonasal dacryocystorhinostomy versus external dacryocystorhinostomy. Ophthal Plast Reconstr Surg 2004;20(1):50–56
3. Cokkeser Y, Evereklioglu C, Er H. Comparative external versus endoscopic dacryocystorhinostomy: results in 115 patients (130 eyes). Otolaryngol Head Neck Surg 2000;123(4):488–491
4. Ben Simon GJ, Joseph J, Lee S, Schwarcz RM, McCann JD, Goldberg RA. External versus endoscopic dacryocystorhinostomy for acquired nasolacrimal duct obstruction in a tertiary referral center. Ophthalmology 2005;112(8):1463–1468
5. Ramakrishnan VR, Hink EM, Durairaj VD, Kingdom TT. Outcomes after endoscopic dacryocystorhinostomy without mucosal flap preservation. Am J Rhinol 2007;21(6):753–757
6. Nussbaumer M, Schreiber S, Yung MW. Concomitant nasal procedures in endoscopic dacryocystorhinostomy. J Laryngol Otol 2004;118(4):267–269
7. Kamel R, El-Deen HG, El-Deen YS, et al. Manometric measurement of lacrimal sac pressure after endoscopic and external dacryocystorhinostomy. Acta Otolaryngol 2003;123(2):325–329
8. Wormald PJ, Kew J, Van Hasselt A. Intranasal anatomy of the nasolacrimal sac in endoscopic dacryocystorhinostomy. Otolaryngol Head Neck Surg 2000;123(3):307–310
9. Sprekelsen MB, Barberán MT. Endoscopic dacryocystorhinostomy: surgical technique and results. Laryngoscope 1996;106(2 Pt 1):187–189
10. Massegur H, Trias E, Ademà JM. Endoscopic dacryocystorhinostomy: modified technique. Otolaryngol Head Neck Surg 2004;130(1):39–46
11. Yoon SW, Yoon YS, Lee SH. Clinical results of endoscopic dacryocystorhinostomy using a microdebrider. Korean J Ophthalmol 2006;20(1):1–6
12. Mann BS, Wormald PJ. Endoscopic assessment of the dacryocystorhinostomy ostium after endoscopic surgery. Laryngoscope 2006;116(7):1172–1174
13. Mansour K, Blanksma LJ, Vrakking H, Jager PL. Scintigraphic evaluation for tear drainage, after dacryocystorhinostomy, in relation to patient satisfaction. Eye (Lond) 2008;22(3):414–419
14. Unlu HH, Toprak B, Aslan A, Guler C. Comparison of surgical outcomes in primary endoscopic dacryocystorhinostomy with and without silicone intubation. Ann Otol Rhinol Laryngol 2002;111(8):704–709
15. Smirnov G, Tuomilehto H, Teräsvirta M, Nuutinen J, Seppä J. Silicone tubing is not necessary after primary endoscopic dacryocystorhinostomy: a prospective randomized study. Am J Rhinol 2008;22(2):214–217
16. Bartley GB, Fatourechi V, Kadrmas EF, et al. Chronology of Graves' ophthalmopathy in an incidence cohort. Am J Ophthalmol 1996;121(4):426–434
17. Durairaj VD, Bartley GB, Garrity JA. Clinical features and treatment of Graves ophthalmopathy in pediatric patients. Ophthal Plast Reconstr Surg 2006;22(1):7–12
18. Durairaj VD. Clinical perspectives of thyroid eye disease. Am J Med 2006;119(12):1027–1028
19. Bradley EA. Graves ophthalmopathy. Curr Opin Ophthalmol 2001;12(5):347–351
20. Gorman CA, Garrity JA, Fatourechi V, et al. A prospective, randomized, double-blind, placebo-controlled study of orbital radiotherapy for Graves' ophthalmopathy. Ophthalmology 2001;108(9):1523–1534
21. Kazim M. Perspective—Part II: radiotherapy for Graves orbitopathy: the Columbia University experience. Ophthal Plast Reconstr Surg 2002;18(3):173–174
22. Kikkawa DO, Pornpanich K, Cruz RC Jr, Levi L, Granet DB. Graded orbital decompression based on severity of proptosis. Ophthalmology 2002;109(7):1219–1224
23. Metson R, Samaha M. Reduction of diplopia following endoscopic orbital decompression: the orbital sling technique. Laryngoscope 2002;112(10):1753–1757
24. Garrity JA, Fatourechi V, Bergstralh EJ, et al. Results of transantral orbital decompression in 428 patients with severe Graves' ophthalmopathy. Am J Ophthalmol 1993;116(5):533–547
25. Warren JD, Spector JG, Burde R. Long-term follow-up and recent observations on 305 cases of orbital decompression for dysthyroid orbitopathy. Laryngoscope 1989;99(1):35–40
26. Kennedy DW, Goodstein ML, Miller NR, Zinreich SJ. Endoscopic transnasal orbital decompression. Arch Otolaryngol Head Neck Surg 1990;116(3):275–282

27. Metson R, Dallow RL, Shore JW. Endoscopic orbital decompression. Laryngoscope 1994;104(8 Pt 1):950–957
28. Shepard KG, Levin PS, Terris DJ. Balanced orbital decompression for Graves' ophthalmopathy. Laryngoscope 1998;108(11 Pt 1): 1648–1653
29. Unal M, Leri F, Konuk O, Hasanreisoğlu B. Balanced orbital decompression combined with fat removal in Graves ophthalmopathy: do we really need to remove the third wall? Ophthal Plast Reconstr Surg 2003;19(2):112–118
30. Luxenberger W, Stammberger H, Jebeles JA, Walch C. Endoscopic optic nerve decompression: the Graz experience. Laryngoscope 1998;108(6):873–882
31. Levin LA, Beck RW, Joseph MP, Seiff S, Kraker R. The treatment of traumatic optic neuropathy: the International Optic Nerve Trauma Study. Ophthalmology 1999;106(7):1268–1277
32. Thakar A, Mahapatra AK, Tandon DA. Delayed optic nerve decompression for indirect optic nerve injury. Laryngoscope 2003; 113(1):112–119
33. Kountakis SE, Maillard AAJ, El-Harazi SM, Longhini L, Urso RG. Endoscopic optic nerve decompression for traumatic blindness. Otolaryngol Head Neck Surg 2000;123(1 Pt 1):34–37
34. Rajiniganth MG, Gupta AK, Gupta A, Bapuraj JR. Traumatic optic neuropathy: visual outcome following combined therapy protocol. Arch Otolaryngol Head Neck Surg 2003;129(11):1203–1206
35. Li KK, Teknos TN, Lai A, Lauretano AM, Joseph MP. Traumatic optic neuropathy: result in 45 consecutive surgically treated patients. Otolaryngol Head Neck Surg 1999;120(1):5–11
36. Pletcher SD, Sindwani R, Metson R. Endoscopic orbital and optic nerve decompression. Otolaryngol Clin North Am 2006;39(5): 943–958, vi

34 Surgery of the Septum and Turbinates

Parul Goyal and Peter H. Hwang

Septoplasty and turbinate procedures are among the most commonly performed surgical procedures in otolaryngology.[1] This chapter reviews the surgical anatomy, indications, and techniques of commonly performed septal and turbinate procedures.

Surgery of the Septum

The basic principles of septoplasty were described by several authors in the early 20th century and have evolved over time. In recent years, the use of endoscopic techniques has allowed for further refinement of septoplasty surgical techniques. Modern septoplasty techniques allow for definitive correction of septal deviations while minimizing complications.

Patient Selection/Indications

Septal surgery may be indicated for correcting septal deflections that are causing nasal airway obstruction, limiting access during endoscopic sinus surgery, or leading to contact point headaches. Surgery may also be indicated when the nasal septum is to be used as a source for cartilage, bone, or mucosal grafts in patients undergoing endoscopic skull base surgical procedures.

Diagnostic Workup

Patients undergoing septoplasty for nasal obstruction should undergo a thorough nasal examination to define areas of narrowing leading to the obstruction. Anterior rhinoscopy using a nasal speculum allows for adequate visualization of the anteriormost aspect of the nasal septum and nasal cavities. This evaluation should be performed before and after decongestion to evaluate the contribution of vasoactive tissue along the turbinates and nasal septum to nasal airway obstruction. It is difficult to obtain a complete evaluation of patients' nasal airways using anterior rhinoscopy alone. This is because anterior rhinoscopy alone may not provide an adequate assessment of the posterior aspects of the nasal cavity. Additionally, use of a nasal speculum during anterior rhinoscopy can distort the nasal valve. For patients with nasal obstruction, rigid nasal endoscopy is routinely performed in the office because it offers an excellent visualization of the nasal valve, nasal septum, turbinates, and any other sinonasal pathology that may contribute to nasal airway obstruction. This provides the surgeon with a complete assessment of the sites of nasal airway obstruction.

Septoplasty may also be indicated in conjunction with endoscopic sinus surgery when septal deflections limit access to the middle meatus. Preoperative endoscopy will allow the surgeon to determine when septoplasty may be necessary in these situations. Correction of these deflections improves access during the course of surgery, and also helps to improve access for postoperative debridement and surveillance.

Contact point headaches may result from septal deflections and spurs that lead to areas of contact between the septum and turbinates. These areas are best identified at the time of office endoscopy, and the diagnosis can be supported by selectively anesthetizing the contact points using topical anesthetic agents on cotton-tipped applicators. Reproducible reduction in patients' headaches after the application of anesthetic agents may confirm the diagnosis by indicating sites along which contact points are contributing to headaches.

Rhinomanometry and acoustic rhinometry provide objective measures of nasal resistance and cross-sectional area. Because these objective measures do not correlate well with subjective symptoms, these techniques are not used routinely in the preoperative evaluation of patients undergoing septal or turbinate surgery.[2,3]

Surgical Anatomy

The nasal septum has cartilaginous and bony components. A thorough understanding of the structure and function of these components is important. The cartilaginous portion of the septum is formed by the quadrangular cartilage. The bony components are formed by the maxillary crest, the perpendicular plate of the ethmoid bone, the vomer, and the perpendicular plate of the palatine bone. The quadrangular cartilage is fused with the upper lateral cartilages. The area along the junction of the upper lateral cartilages and the nasal septum has been termed the internal nasal valve, which provides significant nasal resistance.[4] A detailed discussion of nasal valve pathology is beyond the focus of this chapter (see instead Chapter 35), but the preoperative evaluation should examine this region carefully because it can often be an overlooked site of significant pathology leading to nasal obstruction.

The anteroinferior aspect of the quadrangular cartilage articulates with the maxillary crest. Posteriorly, the cartilaginous component of the septum articulates with the ethmoid bone and the vomer. At the junction of the

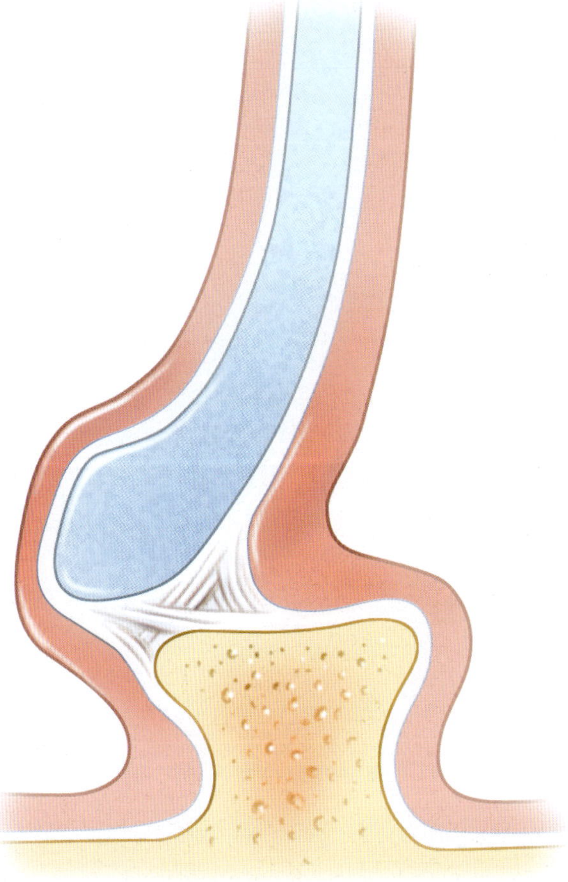

Fig. 34.1 Illustration shows a right-sided septal spur at the junction of the quadrangular cartilage and the maxillary crest. The decussating fibers are shown at the confluence of the perichondrium and periosteum.

cartilaginous and osseous components of the septum, the perichondrium and periosteum are not contiguous. Instead, there are dense decussating fibers at the junction of these components because the perichondrium and periosteum pass around their respective bony or cartilaginous component to the opposite side (**Fig. 34.1**). These fibers must be sharply divided during the course of surgery to maintain a subperichondrial/subperiosteal plane of dissection.

Surgical Technique

Septoplasty has traditionally been performed using a headlight and nasal speculum. In recent years, endoscopic techniques have been used for septal surgery.[5,6] These techniques take advantage of the improved magnification and illumination provided by the endoscope. Whether the procedure is performed with a headlight or an endoscope, the general techniques and principles remain the same. The technique described in this section is an endoscopic one; the same sequence of steps can be used for traditional nonendoscopic septoplasty.

For patients with broad septal deflections, the procedure starts with a hemitransfixion incision at the caudal aspect of the nasal septum. This incision is made using a nasal speculum and an overhead light for illumination. Optimal positioning of the nasal speculum allows the mucosa over the caudal edge of the septum to be placed on stretch, facilitating visualization of the layers of soft tissue as the dissection is carried down to the cartilage. A scalpel is used to incise through the soft tissue layers down to the level of the cartilage. Initial identification of the subperichondrial plane can be difficult because of the tight adherence of the perichondrium to the cartilage. However, it is important to take time to identify the correct dissection plane because this decreases bleeding and preserves maximal flap vascularity and strength.[7]

The initial flap elevation is performed using a Freer elevator, a nasal speculum, and overhead lighting. Once a small pocket has been elevated, the endoscope can be used to continue the dissection. The magnified view available with the endoscope allows the surgeon to confirm that all of the perichondrial layers have been elevated. In the subperichondrial plane, the cartilage has a characteristic bright white appearance (**Fig. 34.2**).

With the endoscopic technique, it is helpful to have a suction elevator and a lens irrigation system to maintain visualization. Our preferred technique is to incise and elevate on the side of the greater septal deviation. As the dissection continues posteriorly, the bony-cartilaginous junction is identified, and elevation continues along the bony septum to the extent necessary to adequately expose the deviated portions of the septum. The initial flap elevation is along the quadrangular cartilage and ethmoid bone, above the level of the decussating fibers (**Fig. 34.3**). Once an adequate ipsilateral dissection has been performed, an incision is made just anterior to the areas of greatest deflection. This incision is most frequently made just anterior to the bony-cartilaginous

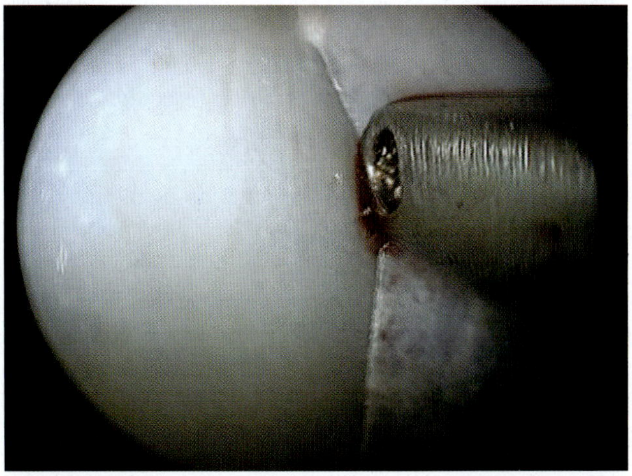

Fig. 34.2 An endoscopic dissection in the subperichondrial plane along the left side of a patient's septum shows the characteristic bright white appearance of the cartilage.

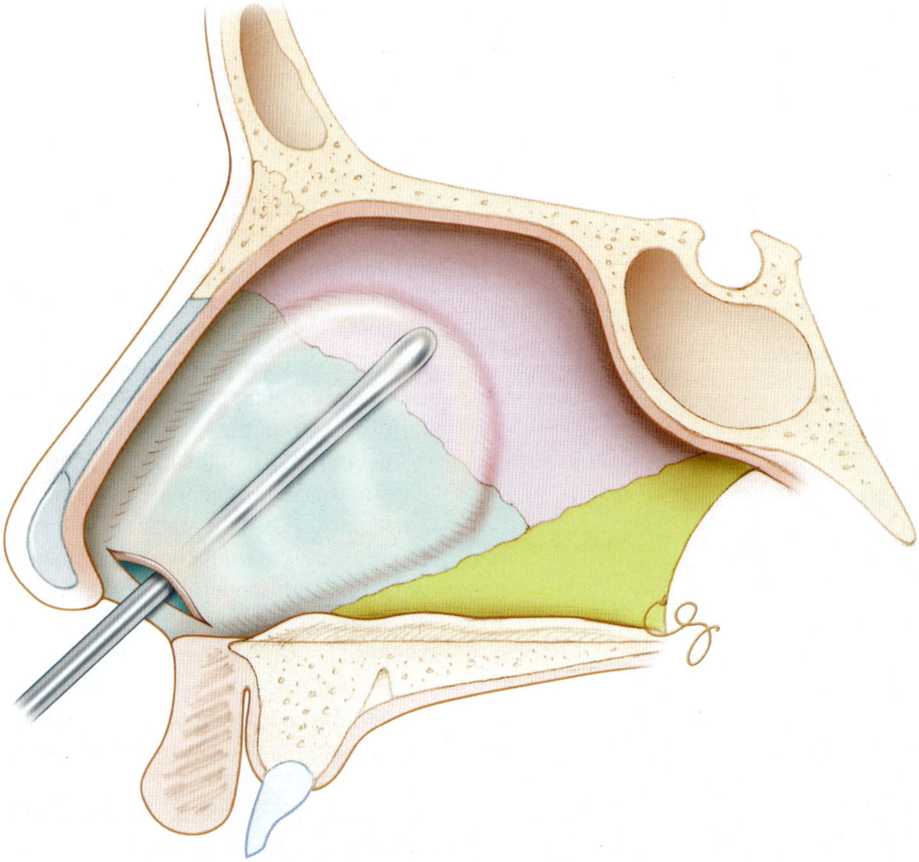

Fig. 34.3 Illustration shows the cartilaginous and bony components of the nasal septum. Components shown include the quadrangular cartilage, maxillary crest, perpendicular portion of the ethmoid bone, and vomer. Initial flap elevation is along the quadrangular cartilage and ethmoid bone, above the decussating fibers.

junction, but may be made more anteriorly if there is a significant cartilaginous deflection (**Fig. 34.4**).

After the incision is made, a contralateral subperichondrial/subperiosteal dissection is performed through the septotomy. The deviated portions of the septum are isolated after flaps have been elevated bilaterally, and these portions can then be removed. Through-cutting instruments are used to make a cut superiorly along the portion of the cartilage and bone that will be resected. Once the superior cut is complete, the cartilage and bone inferior to this cut can be removed using noncutting forceps.

Spurs frequently occur at the junction of the quadrangular cartilage and maxillary crest or vomer (**Fig. 34.5**). Dissection in these areas can be difficult, and flap tears are sometimes unavoidable at these sites. Because the perichondrium of the quadrangular cartilage and the periosteum of the maxillary crest are not contiguous, it is necessary to sharply divide the decussating fibers at the junction of these components of the septum. Typically, it is helpful to remove a strip of cartilage parallel to the maxillary crest. The height of the strip is determined by the deflection point of the cartilaginous portion of the spur. Once the strip of cartilage is removed, the maxillary crest is more easily visible and dissected. A scalpel or very sharp Freer elevator is usually sufficient to cut through the decussating fibers to allow flap elevation from the maxillary crest and vomer down to the level of the nasal floor. In some instances, a more traditional "two-tunnel" technique is helpful to complete the dissection and minimize the risk of large flap perforations. The "two-tunnel" technique involves the dissection of a "superior tunnel" over the cartilaginous septum and an "inferior tunnel" over the maxillary crest at the start of the dissection, extending to the nasal floor. These two tunnels can then be joined along the apex of the spur.

The maxillary crest bone is quite thick and is typically removed using closed Jansen Middleton forceps as a rongeur (**Fig. 34.6**). Alternatively, an osteotome or a drill can be used to address thickened and deviated portions of the crest.

Relatively large portions of the bony septum can be removed without compromising the support of the nasal tip and dorsum. However, when resecting the cartilaginous portions of the nasal septum, it is important to be conservative. Adequate amounts of the dorsal and caudal septum must be preserved to avoid disrupting the support of the tip and dorsum. Scoring, shaving, and suturing are alternatives to cartilage resection for the treatment of

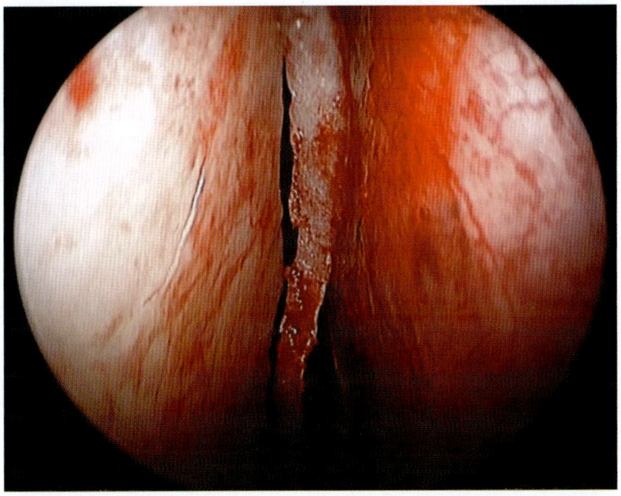

Fig. 34.4 A vertical incision has been made in the cartilage just anterior to the bony-cartilaginous junction. Flaps have been elevated from both sides of the septum posterior to the incision.

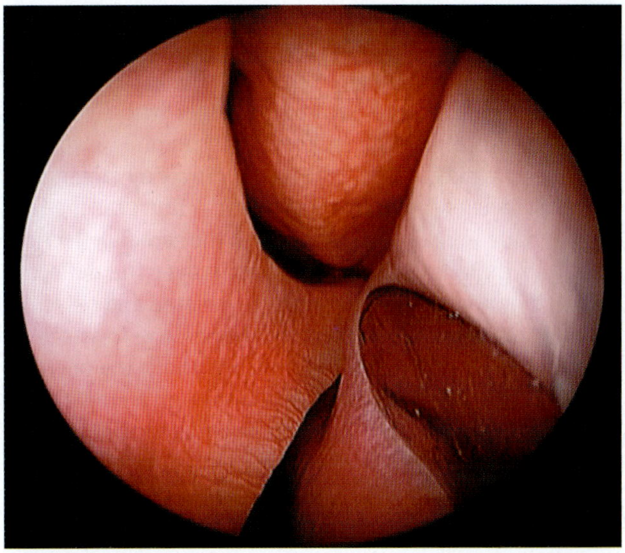

Fig. 34.5 An endoscopic view of the left nasal cavity shows a prominent septal spur at the junction of the quadrangular cartilage with the bony components of the septum. The Freer is along the inferior turbinate, and the middle turbinate is seen just superior to the spur.

cartilaginous deformities. Deflections involving the caudal and dorsal septum are very difficult to address surgically. To reconstitute adequate support for the nasal framework, caudal septal deflections are best approached with reconstructive rhinoplasty techniques such as extracorporeal septoplasty, directed grafting, or suturing.[8,9]

After the deflected portions of the cartilaginous and bony septum have been adequately addressed, the hemitransfixion incision is closed using a fast-absorbing suture. The flaps can be reapproximated using sutures, splints, or packing. We prefer to avoid splints or packing and use a quilting suture to reapproximate the flaps. This maneuver is performed using a 4-0 plain gut quilting suture on a Keith needle. We typically start suturing anteriorly, pass the suture back and forth along the septum as the suture progresses posteriorly, and then return to the initial site of suture placement to tie the suture to itself. Careful placement of sutures in the area of the septal body ensures excellent apposition of the flaps where they may be susceptible to billowing, especially when subsequent access to the middle meatus is required.

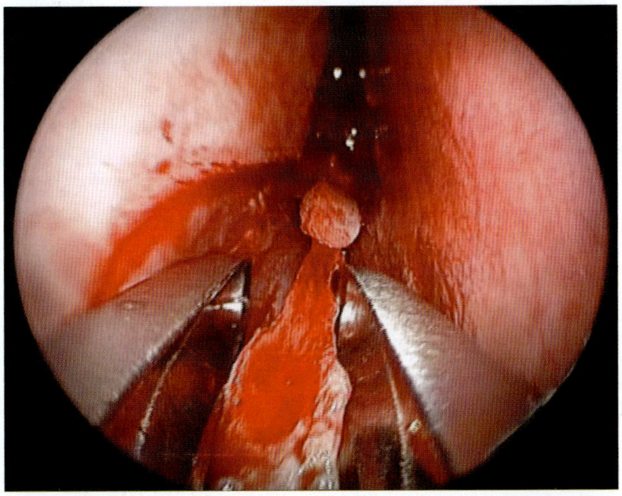

Fig. 34.6 After the decussating fibers have been divided and the maxillary crest has been isolated, closed Jansen Middleton forceps can be used to remove a broad or deviated maxillary crest.

Using endoscopic techniques has several advantages.[5,6] These techniques allow surgeons to visualize certain portions of the dissection more clearly than traditional headlight techniques, especially as the dissection proceeds posteriorly. When a monitor is used, other members of the operative team are able to visualize the procedure. This makes it easier to demonstrate surgical techniques to trainees and allows other operating room staff to remain engaged in the case. When septoplasty is performed in conjunction with endoscopic sinus surgery, endoscopic techniques allow for a more natural transition between the septoplasty and the sinus surgical procedures. It is also easy for the surgeon to determine when an adequate septoplasty has been performed by easily passing the scope into the nasal cavity and visualizing the middle meatus. In revision septoplasty procedures, endoscopic techniques allow for a more limited septoplasty to be performed, avoiding repeat dissection of anterior aspects of the septum.

Limited Septoplasty

Patients with isolated spurs or patients who have undergone a septoplasty previously may have focal deflections for which they are undergoing surgery. In these instances, a more limited dissection may be possible using endoscopic techniques. A limited dissection may be advantageous in both primary and revision septoplasty.[10] In patients undergoing primary septal surgery, a limited septoplasty can minimize the amount of surgical dissection, and thus shorten the postoperative healing period. For patients undergoing revision septal surgery, elevating the mucosal flaps over the quadrangular cartilage may be very difficult because the flaps may be scarred together where cartilage has been resected. Using endoscopic techniques, it may be possible to avoid these scarred areas entirely by moving the mucosal incision posteriorly. A vertical mucosal incision can be made immediately anterior to the septal deflection. Flaps can then be elevated posteriorly over the deflected cartilage or bone, which can then be isolated and resected. When using the more limited techniques, the flaps can be repositioned and generally heal well without the need for packing. Alternatively, a quilting suture or a single mattress suture can be placed to reapproximate the flaps.

For patients with isolated spurs, an incision can be made along the apex of the spur. Subperiosteal flaps can then be elevated above and below the spur, and the spur can then be resected using noncutting forceps. Alternatively, an osteotome can be used to resect the spur along its base.[5] The septal flaps typically approximate very well without the need for suturing.

Complications

Complications of septal surgery include bleeding, septal hematoma or abscess formation, septal perforation, loss of nasal tip support, and cerebrospinal fluid (CSF) leak. Many patients have small amounts of bleeding after surgery, but bleeding significant enough to necessitate significant postoperative intervention is seen in less than 1% of cases.[11] Bleeding between the flaps can result in a septal hematoma, and this in turn can lead to abscess formation and cartilage necrosis. The use of a quilting stitch or splints to reapproximate the septal flaps to the underlying cartilage or bone in the early postoperative period is helpful in preventing hematoma formation. Early recognition and drainage of a septal hematoma can prevent long-term complications. Questionable areas of fullness can be easily aspirated in the office setting to rule out a fluid collection requiring incision and drainage.

Septal perforations are relatively rare complications of septoplasty. The incidence of septal perforation has been reported to be as high as 25% with submucosal resection techniques.[12] Modern septoplasty techniques have been reported to carry a much lower likelihood of perforation, with rates of less than 5% being reported.[12] Perforations most commonly arise when bilateral opposing mucosal tears arise during the course of surgical dissection. Preventing such tears may be the best way to decrease the likelihood of postoperative septal perforations. When such tears are encountered, mucosal rotation flaps can be designed and elevated to cover areas of flap tears. It may also be helpful to place cartilage between the flaps at the site of the tear to decrease the likelihood of a perforation.[13] A preliminary report found that stabilizing such cartilage grafts with fibrin glue may further decrease the likelihood of a long-term perforation.[14]

Excessive loss of septal cartilage, due either to extensive intraoperative resection or to postoperative complications, can lead to a loss of nasal dorsum and tip support. With extensive cartilage loss, a saddle nose deformity may result. To prevent such complications, it is important to be conservative when removing cartilaginous portions of the septum intraoperatively. Postoperatively, techniques that prevent the likelihood of septal hematoma and abscess formation, as discussed previously, will decrease the chance for cartilage necrosis and loss.

Skull base fracture leading to CSF leak is a very rare complication of septal surgery.[15] A CSF leak may result from aggressive manipulation of the attachment of the septum in the region of the skull base. It is important to use cutting instruments when the septum is manipulated along its skull base attachment to avoid disrupting the skull base.

Postoperative Care

Patients generally undergo septoplasty on an outpatient basis and are discharged after a short period of recovery. We do not use packing or splints. Patients are instructed to keep their nose moist through the use of frequent saline nasal sprays and nasal irrigations. Crusting is generally minimal, even in the presence of small mucosal tears along the flap. Patients are seen 1 week postoperatively. If any synechiae are noted between the septum and turbinates, these can be divided using through-cutting forceps. Over the course of the first 3 to 4 weeks, patients should notice improvements in their nasal obstruction as the mucosal edema resolves.

Outcomes

Septal surgery has been shown to be very effective in the surgical treatment of patients with nasal obstructions.[16] Because most patients undergo such surgery for the symptomatic relief of their nasal obstruction, data incorporating symptoms scores provide the most useful information regarding the efficacy of septal surgery. Another reason that symptoms scores provide the most meaningful information is that physician ratings of septal deviation severity and objective measures of airflow have been found to correlate poorly with patients' symptoms.[17]

Septal surgery has been found to lead to significant improvement in disease-specific quality of life. A prospective study of 93 patients undergoing septoplasty found a significant improvement in Nasal Health Survey scores at a mean follow-up of 9 months.[18] Interestingly, there was no significant change in patients' general health status when measured by the Medical Outcome Study Short Form 12-Item Health Survey. In 2004, Stewart et al. published a multi-institutional prospective study that used a validated questionnaire to assess the effectiveness of septal and turbinate surgery for the treatment of nasal obstruction.[17] Using the nasal obstruction symptom evaluation (NOSE) scale, the authors found significant improvement in patients' symptoms after a septoplasty with or without a concurrent inferior turbinate surgery. The authors reported that 94% of patients were pleased with the outcomes of their surgery.

Several authors have reported favorably on the results of endoscopic techniques for the treatment of septal deviation. Hwang et al., in an early series of patients undergoing endoscopic septoplasty,[5] reported improved visualization, the ability to address deviations with less mucosal dissection, and few complications using endoscopic techniques. Dolan[19] and Chung et al.[6] found endoscopic techniques to have comparable rates of efficacy and complications to traditional techniques. These authors reported that using video monitors in conjunction with endoscopes enhanced the ability to teach septal surgical techniques.

Septal Perforation Repair

The surgical techniques of septoplasty can be applied to elective closure of septal perforations. Before considering surgical repair in a patient with a septal perforation, the surgeon should ensure that the perforation is stationary in size through serial exams. A thorough workup of etiologies is necessary, including ruling out past or ongoing cocaine use, granulomatous diseases, or malignancy. Biopsy of the septal perforation may be warranted.

Because of the inherent challenges of achieving complete surgical closure of septal perforation, patients with septal perforation should be offered nonsurgical options for management. Patients with only minor complaints of whistling and crusting may be best served by aggressive nasal hygiene alone, using saline irrigations and sprays. More symptomatic patients may be candidates for the placement of a silicone septal button, although the tendency for prostheses to develop crusting may make septal buttons a poorly tolerated option for many patients.

As in septoplasty, the techniques for repair of small septal perforations are similar whether executed endoscopically or traditionally. A variety of mucosal rotation flaps have been described, and successful endoscopic closures of perforations up to 3 to 4 cm in diameter have been reported using bilateral pedicled mucosal flaps.[20,21] However, more typically for perforations larger than 2 to 3 cm, open rhinoplasty techniques are favored. For large perforations, composite reconstructions involving regional flaps or even free flaps may be considered.[22] Correction of saddle nose deformities may be concurrently performed when using open rhinoplasty techniques for closure of large septal perforations.

Surgery of the Inferior Turbinate

The inferior turbinate is a structure that plays an important role in normal nasal physiology by contributing to the regulation of nasal airflow as well as the warming and humidification of inspired air.[23] When the turbinate is hypertrophic, it can interfere with nasal airflow and can contribute to nasal obstruction. A wide variety of procedures have been described over the years for the management of prominent inferior turbinates.

Patient Selection/Indications

Surgery of the inferior turbinate is most frequently performed for the purpose of improving the nasal patency of patients with nasal obstruction related to inferior turbinate hypertrophy. Patients being evaluated for nasal obstruction should undergo a comprehensive medical history, including an assessment of allergic or other environmental etiologies or triggers. Patients should undergo anterior rhinoscopy and nasal endoscopy to evaluate the patency of the nasal airways. It is important to evaluate these patients before and after decongestion to determine which components (bony or soft tissue) of the inferior turbinates contribute more significantly to an individual's nasal obstruction. As mentioned in the section on septal surgery, the use of diagnostic testing such as rhinomanometry or acoustic rhinometry is generally not useful for clinical decision making. Surgical candidates should first undergo a trial of medical therapy, which may include topical nasal steroids, topical nasal antihistamines, and nasal irrigations.

Inferior turbinate procedures may also be indicated in some patients undergoing maxillary sinus surgery. In some situations, it may be desirable to create a large maxillary antrostomy (or a "mega-antrostomy") extending down to the level of the nasal floor.[24] Indications for a mega-antrostomy include impaired mucociliary clearance requiring gravity-dependent drainage and neoplasms involving the maxillary sinus. In these situations, a partial resection of the posterior aspect of the inferior turbinate may be indicated to create a large maxillary antrostomy. Complete resection of the inferior turbinate should be avoided if at all possible and should be reserved only as needed for tumor extirpation.

Surgical Anatomy

The inferior turbinate is composed of a central bony portion surrounded by layers of soft tissue and mucosa on its medial, lateral, and inferior aspects. The inferior turbinate bone is a distinct bone that attaches to the medial aspects of the maxillary and palatine bones. The pseudostratified ciliated columnar epithelium of the turbinate overlies seromucinous glands and venous sinusoids. The vascular components of the turbinate allow the turbinate to expand, and hypertrophy of the soft tissue components of the turbinate can contribute to nasal obstruction. The soft tissue layer along the medial aspect of inferior turbinate is thicker than the lateral layer.[25] Because the inferior turbinate is thought to play an important role in normal nasal physiology, preservation of the functional components of the turbinate may prevent complications such as nasal dryness, crusting, and atrophic rhinitis.[25]

Surgical Technique

Many different surgical techniques have been described for the treatment of inferior turbinate hypertrophy. Improved understanding of the role of the inferior turbinates in nasal physiology has led surgeons to focus on less invasive procedures that allow for adequate improvement in the nasal airways while maintaining the functional properties of the turbinates. Many turbinate procedures can be performed under local anesthesia in an office setting. The following techniques offer varying levels of tissue preservation, and patients may benefit from a combination of complementary techniques.

Turbinate Lateralization

Lateralizing or outfracturing the turbinate changes the turbinate's position within the nasal cavity. The goal is to change the angle at which the turbinate bone attaches to the maxillary and palatine bones, thus allowing for improved nasal airflow through the central aspect of the nasal cavity. This procedure is generally not sufficient as a stand-alone procedure for the management of significant turbinate hypertrophy, but can be helpful when used in conjunction with other turbinate reduction procedures.

The procedure is performed by using a Boies/Goldman elevator to direct force inferiorly and laterally along the turbinate's attachment site to the lateral nasal wall. The instrument is placed under endoscopic visualization, allowing for an accurate positioning along the turbinate attachment site. It can be helpful to first "infracture" the turbinate to ensure maximal lateralization. This is done by placing the elevator lateral to the turbinate in the inferior meatus to fracture the turbinate medially and superiorly. This avoids greenstick fracturing and promotes complete fracturing at the attachment site, thus leading to more effective lateral displacement when an outfracture is performed.

Soft Tissue Reduction

The soft tissue components of the turbinate can be reduced using different thermal techniques. Monopolar electrocautery, bipolar electrocautery, and radiofrequency tissue ablation have all been used to perform an inferior turbinate reduction. Each of these techniques relies on the creation of an area of submucosal thermal injury, which ultimately heals by fibrosis and scar contracture, leading to reduction in the size of the turbinate.

Monopolar electrocautery is most commonly applied by inserting a needle along the length of the turbinate. Electrocautery is then applied as the needle is slowly withdrawn. Bipolar forceps with needle tips are also available to apply electrocautery to the submucosal tissue of the turbinate.

Radiofrequency tissue reduction techniques have been used extensively to treat soft tissue inferior turbinate hypertrophy. These techniques differ from electrocautery techniques in several ways. The maximal temperature generated within the tissue is significantly lower with radiofrequency techniques than with electrocautery. In addition, the dissipation of the heat is limited, allowing for a more focused reduction of the deeper components of the inferior turbinate tissue.[26] Radiofrequency devices are available from several different companies, with probe designs incorporating both a monopolar and a bipolar delivery of radiofrequency energy. For each device, a probe is inserted into the submucosal tissue to apply energy to the area. Multiple lesions can be created along different aspects of the turbinate to allow for a reduction along the most prominent sites of the turbinate. Care must be taken to limit the amount of energy delivered to protect the surface mucosa from injury.

Soft Tissue Resection

Soft tissue resection of the inferior turbinate allows for precise and targeted removal of the hypertrophic portions of the turbinate. In recent years, this procedure has been made easier with the availability of specialized microdebrider blades designed specifically for submucosal turbinate resections. As with the thermal methods used to treat turbinate hypertrophy, submucosal resection methods aim to reduce the bulk of the submucosal erectile tissue of the turbinate while avoiding injury to the overlying epithelium.

At the start of the procedure, the turbinate is infiltrated with an anesthetic agent containing epinephrine. The infiltration helps to expand the soft tissue of the turbinate, and this makes it easier for the surgeon to perform targeted sculpting of the turbinate. Certain microdebrider devices accept blades designed specifically for inferior turbinate resection. These blades have a sharp dissecting tip that allows for the elevation of a submucosal flap. Typically, the tip is used to make a stab incision along the anteroinferior aspect of the turbinate (**Fig. 34.7**).

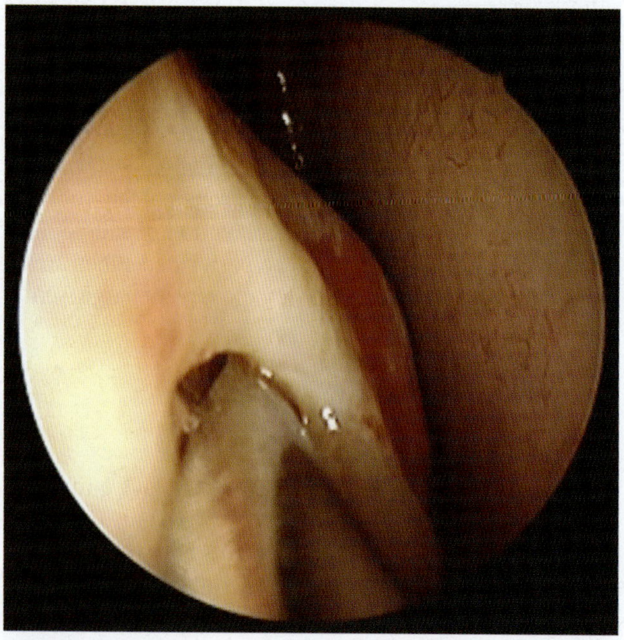

Fig. 34.7 An inferior turbinate microdebrider blade is used to make a stab incision into the anterior aspect of the turbinate.

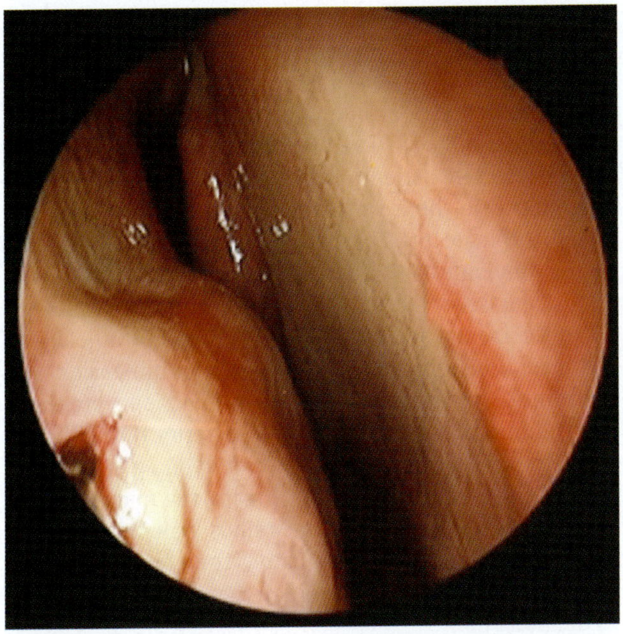

Fig. 34.8 After an adequate submucosal flap has been elevated, the blade is activated to resect the submucosal tissue. In this image, the puckering of the flap is seen at the superior aspect of the inferior turbinate as the blade is used to debride tissue from that area.

With the cutting face of the blade directed toward the turbinate bone, the tip is then used as an elevator to raise a submucosal flap. If the surgeon plans to also resect some of the inferior turbinate bone, it is helpful to stay subperiosteal during the elevation of the flap. The flap elevation is performed primarily along the medial and inferior aspects of the turbinate because these are the areas that contribute most significantly to the prominence of the turbinate.[25] If the specialized blade is not available, the incision can be made using a scalpel, and the flap dissection can be performed using a Cottle or Freer elevator.

When an adequate flap has been elevated, the cutting face of the microdebrider blade is turned toward the submucosal soft tissue and is activated (**Fig. 34.8**). It is important to use the microdebrider in a measured, controlled fashion to allow for adequate tissue resection while minimizing the chance for flap perforation. Attention is focused on the anterior half of the turbinate because this is the portion of the turbinate that contributes most significantly to nasal airflow obstruction. It is especially important to address the tissue along the anterior tip of the inferior turbinate because this portion contributes most significantly to the airway at the nasal valve. Dissection and submucous resection can be successfully extended to the posterior aspect of the turbinate, but this may be associated with higher risks of bleeding related to feeding arterial branches from the sphenopalatine artery. As the blade is manipulated, the surgeon should try to avoid extending the original stab incision. At the completion of the procedure, packing is not typically used. A small incision heals well without any sutures. An immediate intraoperative reduction in the size of the turbinate can be seen at the time of the procedure (**Fig. 34.9**).

Bone Resection

Submucosal resection of the bony component of the turbinate may be indicated if the bony component is a significant contributor to a patient's turbinate hypertrophy. The need for this type of procedure is best determined by careful inspection of the turbinate before and after

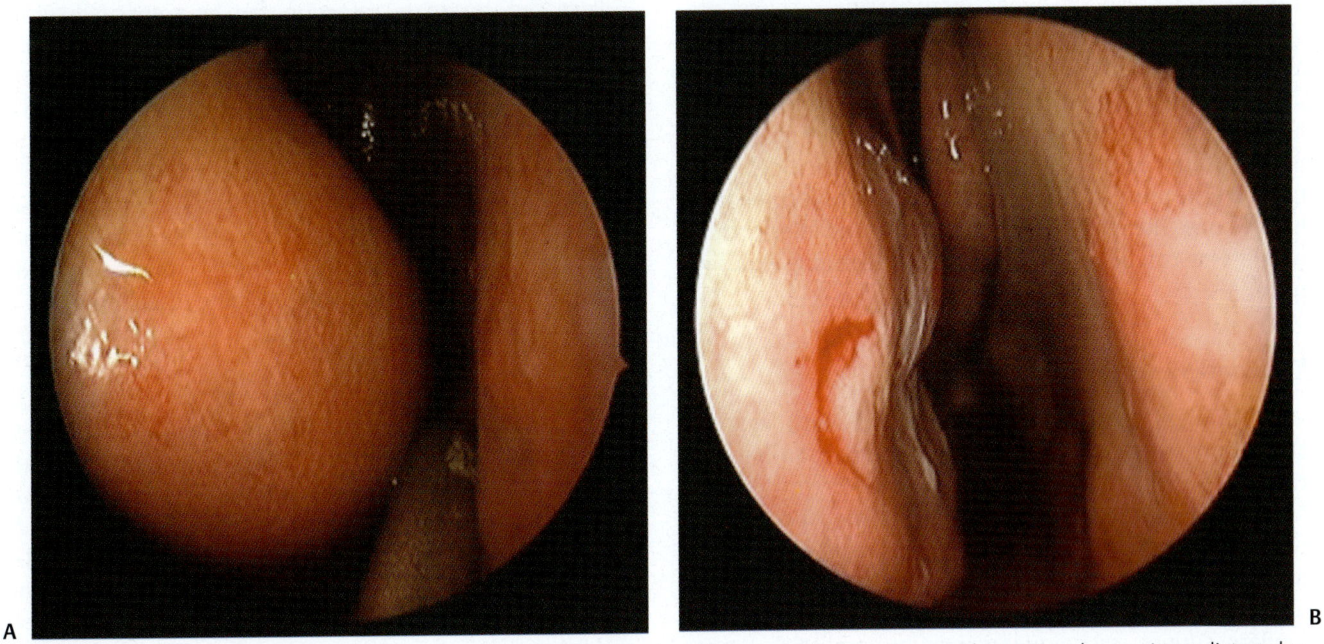

Fig. 34.9 Intraoperative views of an inferior turbinate before **(A)** and after **(B)** a microdebrider submucosal resection show an immediate reduction in the size of the turbinate.

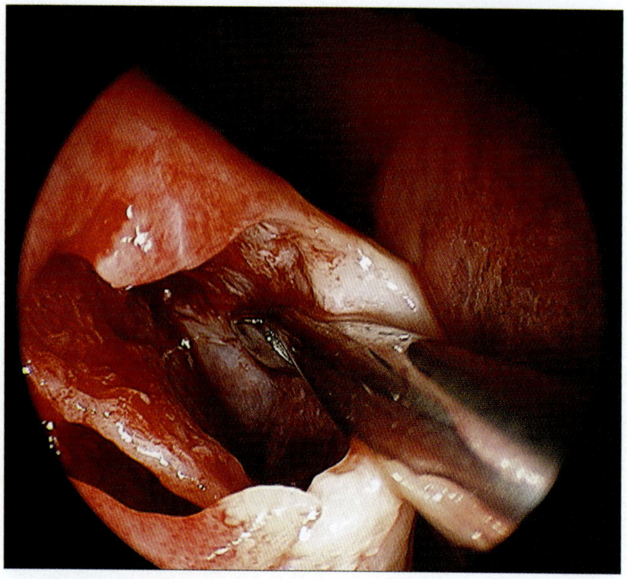

Fig. 34.10 An incision along the anterior aspect of the inferior turbinate allows for adequate exposure for a resection of the turbinate bone. This patient underwent a submucosal resection of the soft tissue component of the turbinate with a microdebrider before a dissection and resection of the bony component.

decongestion. Resection of the bone may be indicated if the office evaluation reveals persistent turbinate hypertrophy after adequate decongestion.

It is possible to perform limited bone resection using the microdebrider technique by directing the cutting face of the microdebrider toward the turbinate bone when it is activated. However, large amounts of bone cannot typically be resected using this technique. More extensive bony resection may require a formal dissection and submucous resection of the bone. This may require a larger incision at the anterior aspect of the turbinate or an incision along the length of the inferior turbinate. A subperiosteal flap can then be elevated, allowing the turbinate bone to be exposed. This bone can then be resected (**Fig. 34.10**). Some authors have also described using a microdebrider to resect the mucosa attached to the lateral aspect the turbinate bone. The remaining flap of medial and inferior mucosal tissue can be rolled to cover any remaining exposed bone.[27]

Turbinate Resection

Full thickness turbinate resection is the most aggressive technique available for the treatment of an inferior turbinate hypertrophy. Turbinate resection procedures range from limited resection of the anterior aspect of the turbinate to extensive total turbinate resections. These procedures are typically performed using heavy scissors to partially or completely resect the turbinate. Although modern surgical techniques generally emphasize tissue conservation, a limited anterior full thickness turbinate resection can be performed without adverse sequelae in most patients. More extensive subtotal or total resections have been hypothesized to predispose one to a paradoxic nasal obstruction or atrophic rhinitis.

Resection of a portion of the inferior turbinate may be indicated in patients undergoing a maxillary mega-antrostomy. In these situations, a part of the midportion of the turbinate may be resected to extend a maxillary antrostomy inferiorly to the floor of the nasal cavity. Endoscopic scissors are placed with the tines positioned along the medial and lateral aspects of the turbinate. The turbinate is bisected in an anteroposterior dimension, and the anterior turbinate is preserved for functional preservation. Additional scissor cuts at the posterior turbinate and along the root attachment of the intervening segment of the turbinate enable its removal using the microdebrider or forceps. The medial maxillary sinus wall below the attachment of the inferior turbinate is thereby exposed, and the middle meatal antrostomy can then be extended down to the nasal floor.[24]

Complications

Complications after inferior turbinate procedures include bleeding, nasal dryness, crusting, scarring, and atrophic rhinitis.[26] The frequency with which these complications have been reported in the literature varies widely based on the techniques used.

Techniques that sacrifice the nasal mucosa have been found to cause a greater disruption of nasal physiology. Comparing the techniques of CO_2 laser ablation, radiofrequency ablation, and partial turbinectomy, Sapci et al. found the greatest increase in mucociliary transport time in patients undergoing laser ablation.[28]

Excessive turbinate resection can be associated with paradoxical complaints of nasal obstruction and atrophic rhinitis. In reviewing a large group of patients with atrophic rhinitis, Moore and Kern found that many had subjective complaints of nasal obstruction despite widely patent nasal airways and normal or low nasal resistance.[29] Atrophic rhinitis is characterized by nasal crusting, nasal obstruction, and a foul odor. Moore and Kern found that 80% of their patients with secondary atrophic rhinitis had a history of partial or complete turbinate resection.[29]

Postoperative Care

Packing is generally not required in patients undergoing inferior turbinate procedures. Patients are asked to keep their nose moist with saline nasal sprays and irrigations to promote the clearance of mucus, clots, and crusts after surgery. Crusting is minimal with contemporary mucosal-preserving techniques. Patients are seen in the office for their first postoperative visit 1 to 2 weeks after the procedure. Any areas of crusting can be gently debrided at that time. Endoscopy allows evaluation to assess for any scars or synechiae. Patients undergoing partial turbinate resection may have more postoperative crusting and may thus need additional debridement.

Outcomes

Good results have been reported with techniques ranging from minimally invasive thermal methods to more invasive total turbinectomy procedures.[30] The results reported in this section focus on the more conservative techniques because these techniques allow for the maximal preservation of functional tissue.

Kizilkaya et al. performed a single-blinded randomized trial comparing the use of radiofrequency reduction and microdebrider submucosal resection in patients with symptomatic inferior turbinate hypertrophy.[31] Each of the 30 subjects in the study underwent a radiofrequency reduction of the inferior turbinate on one side and a microdebrider submucosal resection on the other side. At 6-month follow-up, patients had significant improvement in subjective nasal obstruction scores on both sides. There were no significant differences between the two techniques in symptoms scores or in measures of epithelial function. Although both techniques offered excellent results at 6 months, other studies have shown radiofrequency techniques can be associated with a recurrence of turbinate hypertrophy and nasal obstruction when patients are followed for a year or more. In contrast, microdebrider resection appears to be associated with more enduring results.[32,33] In addition, submucosal cauterization has been reported to lead to more crusting than submucosal resection methods.[34] When comparing unipolar versus bipolar radiofrequency techniques, the degree of improvement appears to be equivalent.[35]

Passali et al. reported on a series of 382 patients treated with a variety of turbinate reduction methods.[36] Patients were randomized to undergo reduction by one of six methods: turbinectomy, laser cautery, electrocautery, cryotherapy, submucosal resection, and submucosal resection with lateralization. The authors found the greatest improvement in symptom scores in patients undergoing a submucosal resection with or without outfracture. Objective measures of nasal patency based on an acoustic rhinometry and an anterior rhinomanometry were initially improved in all groups, but long-term follow-up showed a worsening of these measures in patients treated with electrocautery or cryotherapy. Crusting was seen much less frequently in patients treated with the submucosal resection methods than in those treated with the other methods. In this study, patients treated with a submucosal resection in conjunction with lateral displacement achieved the best results.

Yañez and Mora published the largest series to date reporting long-term results of microdebrider submucosal inferior turbinate resections.[37] The study group consisted of 341 patients who were followed for 10 years. The authors found long-lasting improvements in nasal obstructions, with 91% of patients reporting a complete relief of nasal obstructions. An additional 5% of patients reported a partial relief of nasal obstructions at 10 years. A histologic analysis on 35 patients showed preserved respiratory epithelium that remained retracted onto the turbinate bone due to scar tissue formation within the submucosal region. Complications of the technique included one patient with bleeding requiring cautery under local anesthesia, and minor crusting in 35% of patients that resolved by 2 weeks postoperatively.

Surgery of the Middle Turbinate

Middle turbinate surgery is most often indicated at the time of endoscopic sinus surgery because prominent middle turbinates may impair access to the middle meatus. Patients with a pneumatized middle turbinate, termed a concha bullosa, may undergo a resection of a portion of the turbinate to improve middle meatus access and ventilation. Patients may also have limited middle meatus access in the absence of pneumatized middle turbinates. In these patients, medializing the middle turbinates may be helpful to maintain access during and after endoscopic sinus surgery.

Patient Selection/Indications

Patients undergoing endoscopic sinus surgery are evaluated preoperatively with a nasal endoscopy and a computed tomography (CT) scan. Patients who are candidates for middle turbinate procedures are those in whom access to the middle meatus is limited due to prominent or pneumatized middle turbinates. Often, this determination is best made intraoperatively when the turbinates cannot be maintained in a medial position at the time of the procedure.

Surgical Technique

Concha Bullosa Resection

Although concha bullosa itself is a normal variant, a large concha bullosa may require reduction if it impairs middle meatal access or encroaches on the ostiomeatal complex. In addition, the air cell of the turbinate itself can be a site of inflammatory disease. The lateral aspect of the concha bullosa can be resected in these instances. It is important to avoid excessive manipulation of the medial aspect of the concha bullosa because the medial lamella attaches to the skull base.

A sickle knife is used to enter the pneumatized portion of the middle turbinate. The incision is carried anteriorly in a parasagittal plane. Further anteriorly, the bone can be thick, and a gentle sawing motion with the sickle knife can be helpful in incising this area. Small scissors or through-cutting forceps can then be used to resect the lateral aspect

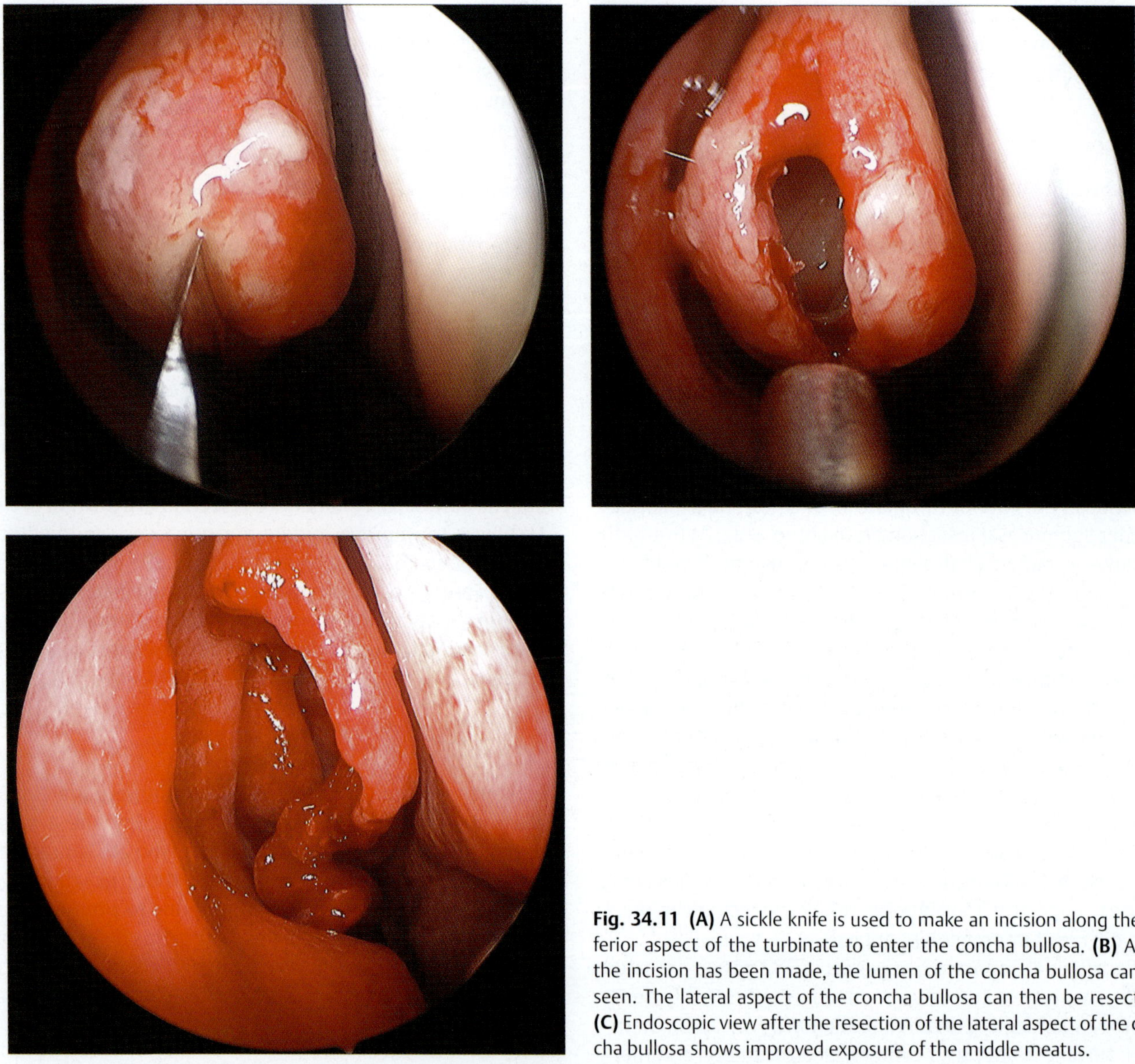

Fig. 34.11 **(A)** A sickle knife is used to make an incision along the inferior aspect of the turbinate to enter the concha bullosa. **(B)** After the incision has been made, the lumen of the concha bullosa can be seen. The lateral aspect of the concha bullosa can then be resected. **(C)** Endoscopic view after the resection of the lateral aspect of the concha bullosa shows improved exposure of the middle meatus.

of the air cell (**Fig. 34.11**). The outflow tract of the concha bullosa is generally located along its posteromedial aspect. This ostium is connected with the resected portion of the turbinate to avoid mucus recirculation.

Middle Turbinate Medialization

Synechiae formation between the middle turbinate and the lateral nasal wall can be associated with persistent obstruction of the paranasal sinus outflow tracts after endoscopic sinus surgery. Several techniques are available for medialization of the middle turbinates after sinus surgery. These techniques include suturing and controlled synechiae formation between the nasal septum and the middle turbinate.

Suturing allows for the temporary medialization of the middle turbinates during the healing process. A 4–0 plain gut suture on a straight needle can be used to place a mattress suture through both turbinates across the nasal septum. In patients who undergo a concurrent septoplasty, the middle turbinates can be incorporated into the quilting stitch. This allows the turbinates to be medialized against the nasal septum temporarily. This allows adequate time for the turbinate and lateral nasal wall mucosa to heal, decreasing the likelihood of synechia formation between the turbinate and the lateral nasal wall.

Creating synechiae between the middle turbinates and the nasal septum can allow for more lasting medialization of the middle turbinates.[38] The mucosa of the medial aspect of the middle turbinate and the adjacent portion of the nasal septum can be abraded using a microdebrider, sinus probe, or scalpel. The turbinate is then juxtaposed against the septum to promote adhesion formation between the raw surfaces, thereby medializing the middle turbinate. It may be helpful to use a suture or to place a middle meatal spacer to maintain medialization of the turbinate long enough for scar tissue to form between the turbinates and the nasal septum.

Complications

If the middle turbinate lateralizes, synechiae can form between the turbinate and lateral nasal wall. This can impair access for endoscopic surveillance, and can impair sinus function. In particular, if middle turbinate resection has been performed, lateralization of the remaining turbinate stump may obstruct the frontal sinus, causing iatrogenic frontal sinusitis. It is important to monitor for such scarring during the postoperative time period. When synechiae are noted, they can be divided using through-cutting forceps in the office. If necessary, a spacer can be placed between the middle turbinate and lateral nasal wall to allow the opposing surfaces to mucosalize and prevent future scarring.

It is important to remember that the superior aspect of the middle turbinate attaches to the skull base. Excessive manipulation of this attachment can cause a fracture and resultant CSF leak.

Conclusion

A thorough preoperative evaluation, meticulous surgical technique, and adequate postoperative care are important factors in optimizing outcomes in patients undergoing septal and turbinate surgery. Modern septoplasty techniques emphasize the preservation of structural support while correcting obstructive deflections. Turbinate procedures focus on mucosal preservation to allow for the maintenance of turbinate function. Surgical advancements have led to an ongoing refinement of techniques for septal and turbinate procedures, allowing for improved outcomes and decreased morbidity.

References

1. Manoukian PD, Wyatt JR, Leopold DA, Bass EB. Recent trends in utilization of procedures in otolaryngology-head and neck surgery. Laryngoscope 1997;107(4):472–477
2. Larsson C, Millqvist E, Bende M. Relationship between subjective nasal stuffiness and nasal patency measured by acoustic rhinometry. Am J Rhinol 2001;15(6):403–405
3. Yaniv E, Hadar T, Shvero J, Raveh E. Objective and subjective nasal airflow. Am J Otolaryngol 1997;18(1):29–32
4. Huang C, Manarey CR, Anand VK. Endoscopic placement of spreader grafts in the nasal valve. Otolaryngol Head Neck Surg 2006;134(6):1001–1005
5. Lanza DC. DF Rosin DF, Kennedy DW. Endoscopic septal spur resection. Am J Rhinol 1993;7:213–216
6. Chung BJ, Batra PS, Citardi MJ, Lanza DC. Endoscopic septoplasty: revisitation of the technique, indications, and outcomes. Am J Rhinol 2007;21(3):307–311
7. Kim DW, Egan KK, O'Grady K, Toriumi DM. Biomechanical strength of human nasal septal lining: comparison of the constituent layers. Laryngoscope 2005;115(8):1451–1453
8. Gubisch W. Extracorporeal septoplasty for the markedly deviated septum. Arch Facial Plast Surg 2005;7(4):218–226
9. Haack J, Papel ID. Caudal septal deviation. Otolaryngol Clin North Am 2009;42(3):427–436
10. Cantrell H. Limited septoplasty for endoscopic sinus surgery. Otolaryngol Head Neck Surg 1997;116(2):274–277
11. Marks S. Nasoseptal surgery. In: Marks S, ed. Nasal and Sinus Surgery. Philadelphia, PA: W.B. Saunders; 2000:193–214
12. Schwab JA, Pirsig W. Complications of septal surgery. Facial Plast Surg 1997;13(1):3–14
13. Kridel RW. Considerations in the etiology, treatment, and repair of septal perforations. Facial Plast Surg Clin North Am 2004;12(4):435–450, vi
14. Lee JY, Lee SH, Kim SC, Koh YW, Lee SW. Usefulness of autologous cartilage and fibrin glue for the prevention of septal perforation during septal surgery: a preliminary report. Laryngoscope 2006;116(6):934–937
15. Onerci TM, Ayhan K, Oğbretmenoğlu O. Two consecutive cases of cerebrospinal fluid rhinorrhea after septoplasty operation. Am J Otolaryngol 2004;25(5):354–356
16. Rowe-Jones J. Nasal surgery: evidence of efficacy. Septal and turbinate surgery. Rhinology 2004;42(4):248–250
17. Stewart MG, Smith TL, Weaver EM, et al. Outcomes after nasal septoplasty: results from the Nasal Obstruction Septoplasty Effectiveness (NOSE) study. Otolaryngol Head Neck Surg 2004;130(3):283–290
18. Siegel NS, Gliklich RE, Taghizadeh F, Chang Y. Outcomes of septoplasty. Otolaryngol Head Neck Surg 2000;122(2):228–232
19. Dolan RW. Endoscopic septoplasty. Facial Plast Surg 2004;20(3):217–221
20. Giacomini PG, Ferraro S, Di Girolamo S, Ottaviani F. Large nasal septal perforation repair by closed endoscopically assisted approach. Ann Plast Surg 2011;66(6):633–636
21. Presutti L, Alicandri Ciufelli M, Marchioni D, Villari D, Marchetti A, Mattioli F. Nasal septal perforations: our surgical technique. Otolaryngol Head Neck Surg 2007;136(3):369–372
22. Watson D, Barkdull G. Surgical management of the septal perforation. Otolaryngol Clin North Am 2009;42(3):483–493
23. Lee KC, Hwang PH, Kingdom TT. Surgical management of inferior turbinate. hypertrophy in the office: three mucosal sparing techniques. Oper Tech Otolaryngol—Head Neck Surg 2001;12(2):107–111
24. Han JK, Smith TL, Loehrl TA, Fong KJ, Hwang PH. Surgical revision of the post-Caldwell-Luc maxillary sinus. Am J Rhinol 2005;19(5):478–482
25. Berger G, Balum-Azim M, Ophir D. The normal inferior turbinate: histomorphometric analysis and clinical implications. Laryngoscope 2003;113(7):1192–1198
26. Cavaliere M, Mottola G, Iemma M. Comparison of the effectiveness and safety of radiofrequency turbinoplasty and traditional surgical technique in treatment of inferior turbinate hypertrophy. Otolaryngol Head Neck Surg 2005;133(6):972–978
27. Bielamowicz S, Hawrych A, Gupta A. Endoscopic inferior turbinate reduction: a new technique. Laryngoscope 1999;109(6):1007–1009
28. Sapçi T, Sahin B, Karavus A, Akbulut UG. Comparison of the effects of radiofrequency tissue ablation, CO2 laser ablation, and partial turbinectomy applications on nasal mucociliary functions. Laryngoscope 2003;113(3):514–519

29. Moore EJ, Kern EB. Atrophic rhinitis: a review of 242 cases. Am J Rhinol 2001;15(6):355–361
30. Talmon Y, Samet A, Gilbey P. Total inferior turbinectomy: operative results and technique. Ann Otol Rhinol Laryngol 2000;109(12 Pt 1):1117–1119
31. Kizilkaya Z, Ceylan K, Emir H, et al. Comparison of radiofrequency tissue volume reduction and submucosal resection with microdebrider in inferior turbinate hypertrophy. Otolaryngol Head Neck Surg 2008;138(2):176–181
32. Lee JY, Lee JD. Comparative study on the long-term effectiveness between coblation- and microdebrider-assisted partial turbinoplasty. Laryngoscope 2006;116(5):729–734
33. Liu CM, Tan CD, Lee FP, Lin KN, Huang HM. Microdebrider-assisted versus radiofrequency-assisted inferior turbinoplasty. Laryngoscope 2009;119(2):414–418
34. Joniau S, Wong I, Rajapaksa S, Carney SA, Wormald PJ. Long-term comparison between submucosal cauterization and powered reduction of the inferior turbinates. Laryngoscope 2006;116(9):1612–1616
35. Cavaliere M, Mottola G, Iemma M. Monopolar and bipolar radiofrequency thermal ablation of inferior turbinates: 20-month follow-up. Otolaryngol Head Neck Surg 2007;137(2): 256–263
36. Passàli D, Passàli FM, Damiani V, Passàli GC, Bellussi L. Treatment of inferior turbinate hypertrophy: a randomized clinical trial. Ann Otol Rhinol Laryngol 2003;112(8):683–688
37. Yañez C, Mora N. Inferior turbinate debriding technique: ten-year results. Otolaryngol Head Neck Surg 2008;138(2):170–175
38. Bolger WE, Kuhn FA, Kennedy DW. Middle turbinate stabilization after functional endoscopic sinus surgery: the controlled synechiae technique. Laryngoscope 1999;109(11): 1852–1853

35 Functional Rhinoplasty

Sam P. Most

Modern approaches to rhinoplasty must consider function as well as aesthetics. Indeed, the variations of nasal structure among humans from different parts of the globe belie its evolution as a functional apparatus. This is supported by anthropologic studies that purport that features of the human nose developed in response to the need for moisture conservation as activity of the genus *Homo* shifted to more open and arid environments.[1] It is believed that the characteristics that distinguish it from other hominids developed with the emergence of *Homo erectus* 1.6 million years ago.[1] These distinguishing features include the projection of the external nose, the relationship of the pyriform aperture to the nasal bones, and the prominence of the nasal spine, all features that may be altered in conventional aesthetic rhinoplasty. Thus, it is incumbent upon the surgeon to recognize and preserve the function that underlies the form that is the modern human nose. This structural approach to rhinoplasty is a hallmark of modern nasal surgery, both aesthetic and functional.

A thorough understanding of the anatomy of the nose is paramount in rhinoplasty, and herein are described only the essentials. The external contours of the upper third of the nose are the two sidewalls, the dorsum, and the nasofrontal angle. The nasofrontal angle is the external landmark identifying the deepest or posteriormost portion of the nasal dorsum, and may lie several millimeters inferior to the nasion, which is defined here as the bony junction between the frontal and nasal bones (**Fig. 35.1**). The rhinion is the osseocartilaginous junction of the nasal bones inferiorly with the superior edge of the upper lateral cartilages (ULCs).

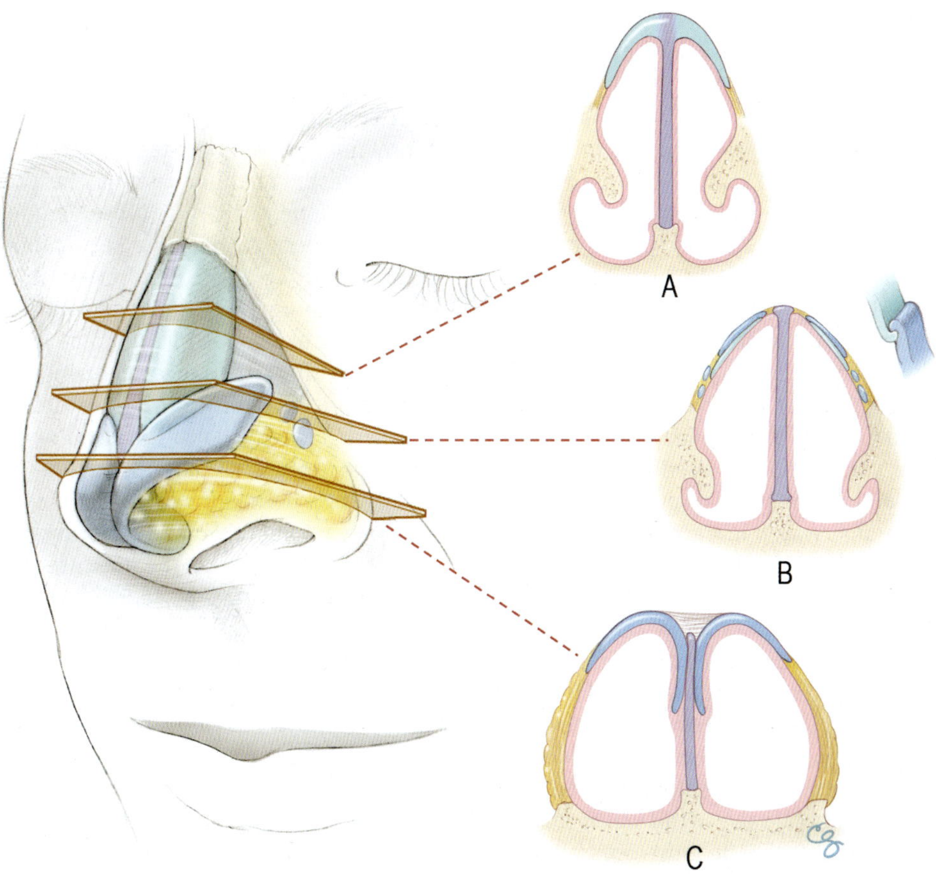

Fig. 35.1 Cross-sectional anatomy of the nose. Note that in the upper and middle cross-section, the upper lateral cartilages (ULCs) are fused to the septum. As shown in the middle cross-section, the ULCs and septum are discontinuous, but the ULCs underlie the lower lateral cartilages (LLCs) in the so-called "scroll." In the most inferior cross-section, note the fibrous tissue between the LLCs and the bony aperture.

The nasal bones are paired structures that attach superiorly to the frontal bone and laterally to the nasal process of the maxillary bones (**Fig. 35.1**). Together, these bones form the bony nasal vault. The perpendicular plate of the ethmoid, a portion of the bony septum, attaches to the undersurface of the nasal bones in the midline. The junction of the quadrangular cartilage and the perpendicular plate of ethmoid typically coincides with the rhinion. This portion of the septum is termed the *keystone area*, and must be preserved during a septoplasty, as it is may be the primary supporting attachment of the septum to the bony skeleton of the face. The septum serves to support the dorsal profile, and loss of this structure can result in a saddle nose deformity. The anterior nasal spine supports the caudal septum.

The paired ULCs are triangular and fused medially to the dorsal septum (**Fig. 35.1**). The cartilages attach to the undersurface of the nasal bones at their superior extent and are connected to the frontal process of the maxilla by dense fibrous connective tissue. The paired lower cartilages support the nasal lobule and nostrils. This fibrocartilaginous arch is supported medially by the caudal septum and nasal spine. Laterally, the arch is supported by the lateral crura and a variable number of small accessory cartilages between the lateral crura and pyriform aperture.

Clinical Evaluation and Classification of Nasal Airway Obstruction

Nasal airway obstruction can be categorized as those causes requiring medical management (e.g., allergic rhinitis) and those requiring surgical management. Although patients often present with mixed etiology and are counseled as such, we focus here on anatomic causes of nasal obstruction. Anatomic nasal airway obstruction has classically been described as due primarily to the following: (1) septal deviation; (2) turbinate hypertrophy; (3) internal valve collapse; and (4) external valve collapse. The first two are covered in Chapter 34 of this book. Herein we focus on internal and external valve collapse.

The internal nasal valve has been alternatively defined as an anatomic angle or as the point of maximal narrowing of the anterior nasal airway.[2,3] In the former definition, the valve is the angle between the ULC and the septum, and with normal being between 10 to 15 degrees. In practice, this angle is examined quite subjectively, and is usually noted to be "narrow" or "normal." The latter definition of the internal nasal valve is perhaps more useful, as it includes examination of all causes of the narrowed airway, including the anterior inferior turbinate and the septum, in addition to the relationship of the ULC and the septum. Further argument for thinking of the internal valve in this way is that the angle is rarely treated alone. Rather, in most cases, all three components are examined and treated as necessary.

The term internal valve collapse also warrants mention. The word collapse conveys a dynamic sense to the cause of the airway obstruction. In practical terms, however, none of the three components of the valve vary dynamically during inspiration. The angle between the ULC and the septum varies little, even with external wall movement (see later); the turbinate and septum do not move. Thus, some (including the author) prefer the term internal valve *narrowing* to describe nasal obstruction due to pathology in this area.

On a physical exam, patients with internal valve narrowing may demonstrate a positive Cottle maneuver.[4] During this maneuver, the examiner expands the nasal sidewall by placing his or her fingers just lateral to the nasal-facial junction and retracting the soft tissue laterally (**Fig. 35.2**). Patients with a positive Cottle sign will experience improved nasal airflow with the maneuver. Alternatively, the examiner may place cotton-tipped applicators in each nostril and expand the lateral nasal wall slightly.

Patients with nasal valve narrowing will often present with a history of prior nasal surgery. One of the most common causes of narrowing of the ULC/septum angle is a prior rhinoplasty, and dorsal hump takedown, in particular. During this procedure, the ULCs are often resected at their attachment to the septum. The remnants of the ULCs are then reattached to the septum or, in some cases, not reattached at all. If the ULCs are left unattached, there is an increased likelihood of retraction of the ULC during healing that may lead to mid-vault narrowing. For this reason, we recommend reattaching the ULC (at the very least) and/or reconstituting the relationship between the ULC and septum by placement of spreader grafts. A newer technique for retaining structural integrity of the ULC/septal complex during aesthetic rhinoplasty is the ULC turn-in.[5,6] With this technique, the ULC is preserved during dorsal hump takedown because only the bony hump and septum are removed. The ULCs are then "turned-in" and sutured to the lowered septum (**Figs. 35.3 and 35.4**). This method is representative of newer *structural rhinoplasty* techniques that recognize the importance of maintaining the structural framework of the nose during aesthetic rhinoplasty.

External valve collapse, on the other hand, is typically a dynamic process (see later discussion of static lateral wall narrowing). Bernoulli's principle states that as the speed of a moving fluid increases, the pressure within the fluid decreases.[7] In the nose, the pressure drops significantly at points of narrowing (**Fig. 35.5**). The lateral nasal wall must withstand the negative forces that are generated by these pressure drops.

In cases of weakening of the lateral wall of the nose, either de novo or due to prior resection of the alar cartilages, the lateral wall cannot withstand negative inspiratory forces. As a result, inward movement of the nasal wall occurs, exacerbating nasal obstruction. Classic external valve collapse primarily involves the ala and is visible externally because the nostril itself closes down (**Fig. 35.6**). For examining such patients, we have found that the "neutral position" Cottle maneuver is effective. In

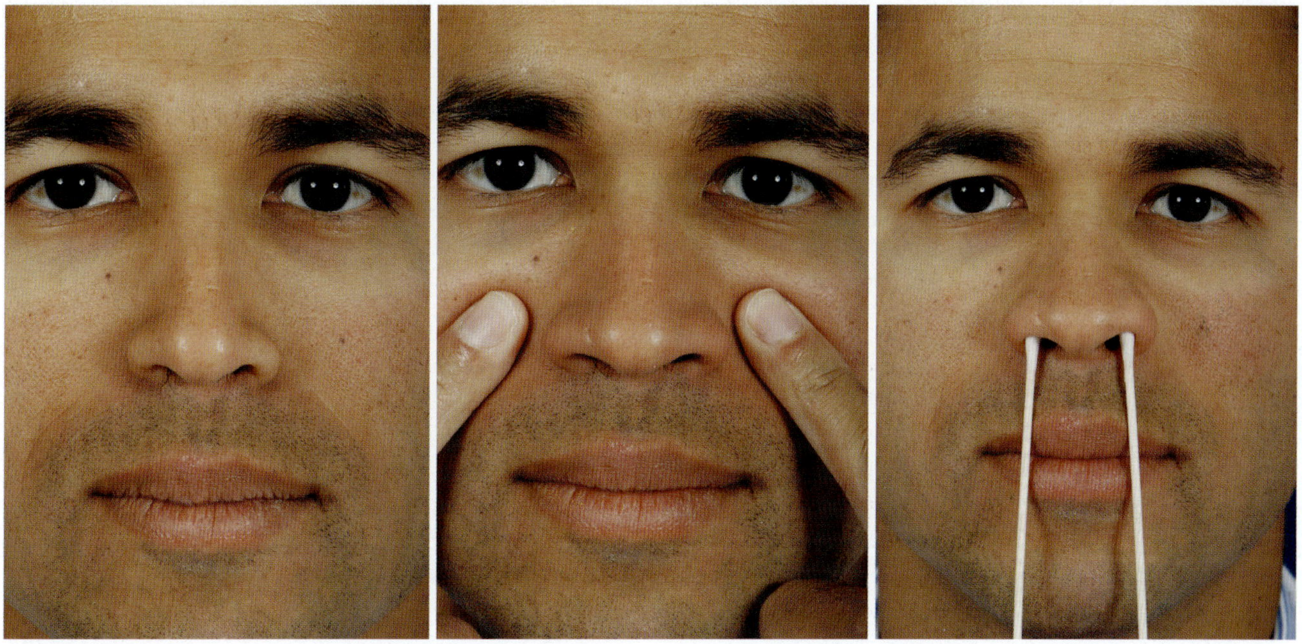

Fig. 35.2 The Cottle maneuver and variations. The left panel depicts the nose at rest. With the traditional technique, the examiner places the thumb and forefinger on each side of the nose and displaces the skin laterally to expand the nasal airway **(middle panel)**. Alternatively, the nasal airway can be expanded intranasally using cotton-tipped applicators **(right panel)**. The author has found these two maneuvers useful in examining patients with internal valve narrowing. The "neutral position" Cottle maneuver involves placement of the thumb and forefinger as in the traditional technique, but *without any lateral displacement*. Rather, the examiner supports the lateral walls during inspiration to determine if lateral wall repair would be of benefit. This is useful in examining a patient with an external wall collapse.

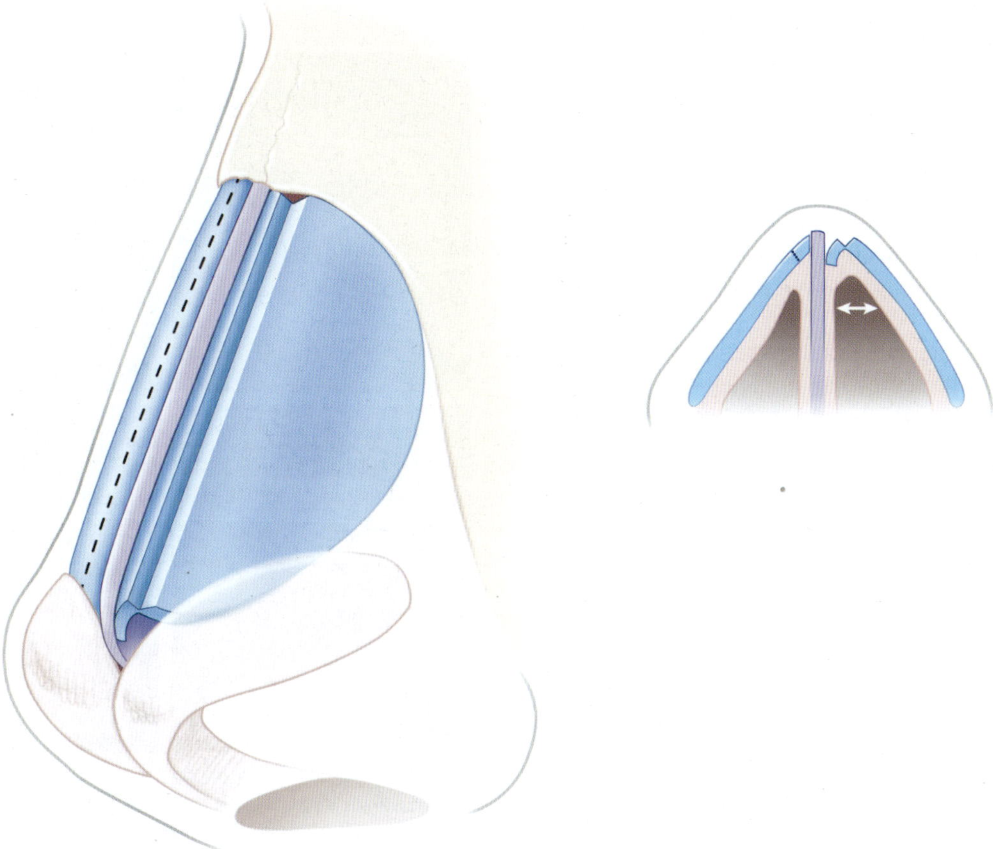

Fig. 35.3 Upper lateral cartilage (ULC) turn-in spreader grafts. To maintain structural support during reductive surgery of the nasal dorsum, the ULCs are released from the septum and "turned-in" to the level of the dorsal septum. The ULCs are then sutured into place using mattressed sutures.

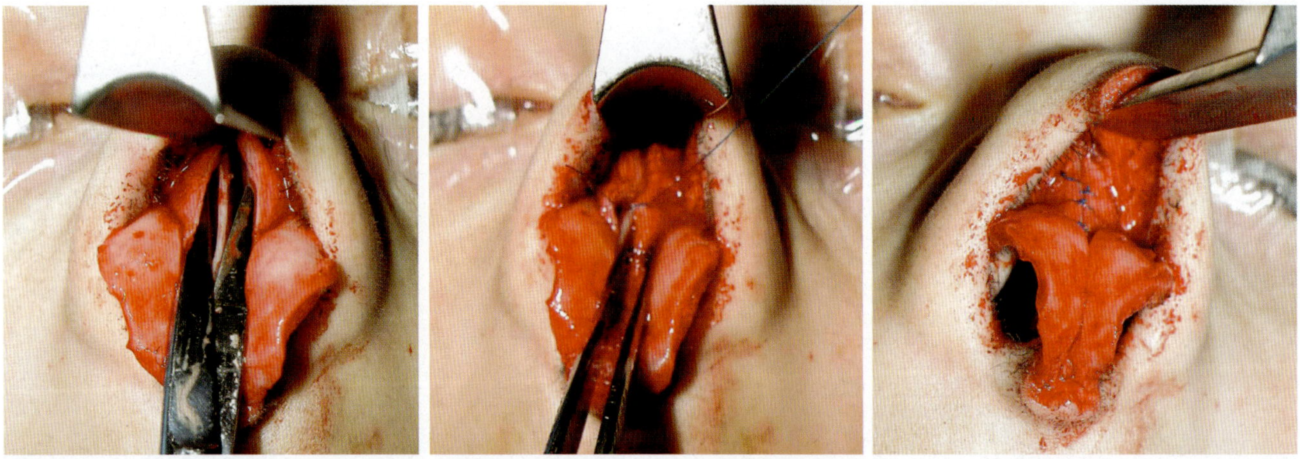

Fig. 35.4 Upper lateral cartilage (ULC) turn-in or "autospreader" graft. Note the composite dorsal reduction **(left panel)**. Following this, the ULCs are incised, turned-in, and sutured to the septum along the dorsum **(middle and right panels)**.

this technique, the examiner does not laterally displace the nasal sidewall but, rather, simply uses pressure to support it and prevent medial collapse during inspiration. The author has found that if a patient experiences improvement in nasal obstruction during inspiration with this maneuver, then they may be a good candidate for external nasal valve repair.

Lateral wall collapse can occur more superiorly in the region of the upper lateral cartilage/lower lateral cartilage complex (or scroll). In such cases, external exam may not demonstrate significant movement of the ala.[8] However, intranasal examination of such patients reveals significant wall movement can occur during inspiration (**Fig. 35.7**). It is useful to grade such collapse as a percentage of airway closure that occurs (**Table 35.1**). Validation studies for this grading system are currently underway. Nonetheless, grading the degree of collapse provides the clinician with a system for documenting movement and efficacy of surgical intervention.

We have found the nomenclature surrounding external valve collapse to be somewhat ambiguous.[8] For this reason, we no longer use the term. Rather, we refer to lateral wall insufficiency, and recognize that it occurs in two zones (**Fig. 35.8**). Zone 1 collapse occurs more superiorly, and is a result of inward movement of the ULC/scroll complex medially during inspiration, as was shown in **Fig. 35.7**. Zone 2 collapse is what is more likely referred to as external valve collapse in the old nomenclature, and occurs at the level of the ala. We have found this nomenclature to be much more suitable to the pathology and treatment paradigms for these patients, and use it in our clinical practice.[8]

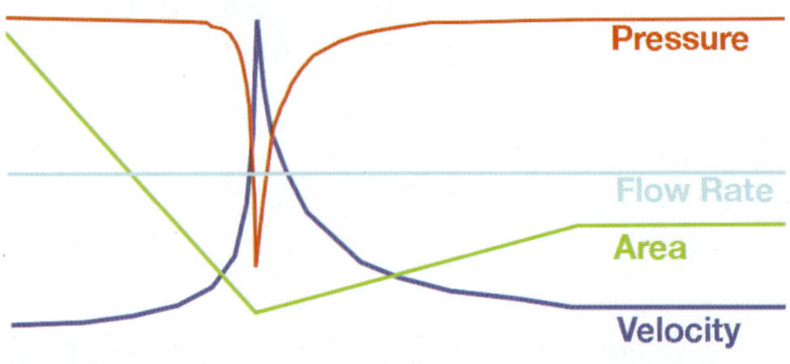

Fig. 35.5 Simulation of the Bernoulli effect. Pressure varies inversely with velocity for a constant flow rate. Thus, as the area decreases, velocity increases and pressure drops significantly.

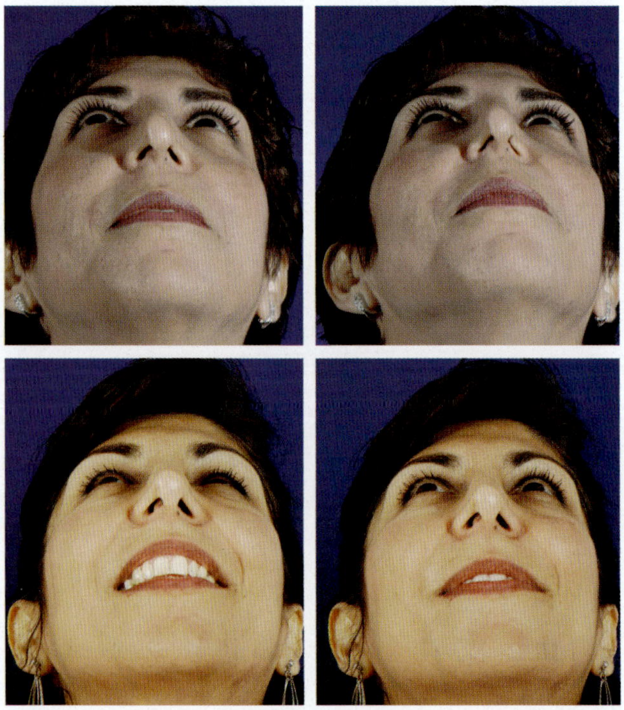

Fig. 35.6 Base view of a patient at rest **(left)** and during normal (nonmaximal) inhalation **(right)**. This patient had undergone aesthetic rhinoplasty at another institution several years earlier, and complained of significant nasal obstruction. Preoperative photos are in the top row and postoperative photos in the bottom row, 1 year after bone-anchored suture technique (BAST) and cartilage grafting.

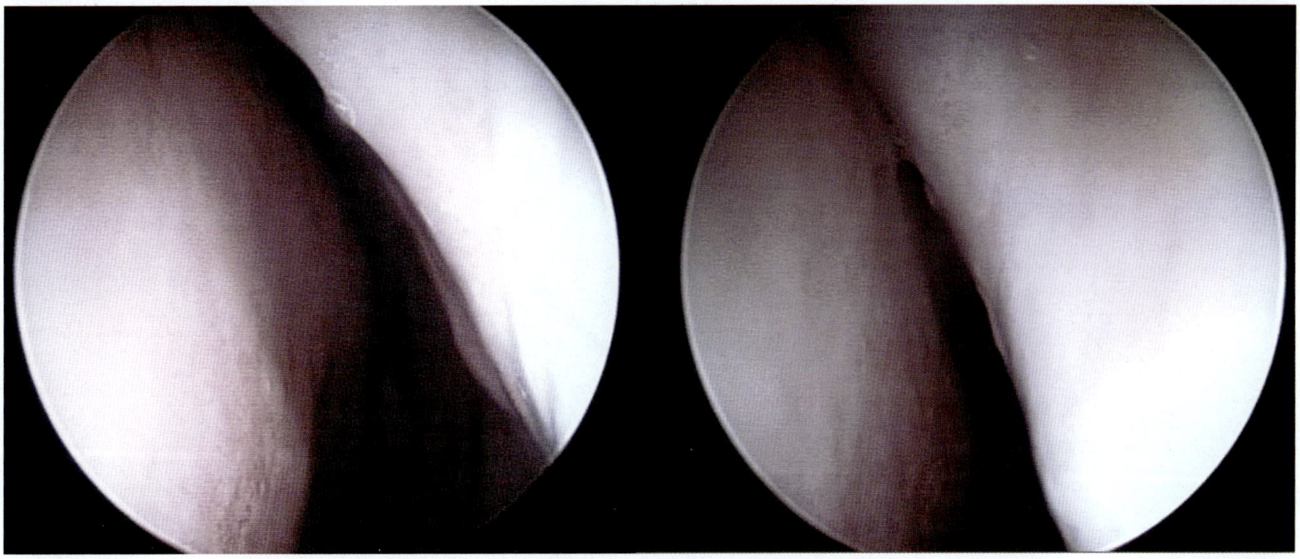

Fig. 35.7 Intranasal view of dynamic wall collapse, using a zero-degree rigid scope without decongestion. Note the position of the lateral wall at rest **(left)** and during inhalation **(right)**.

Bony lateral wall narrowing is a special situation worth mention. In this case, the lateral bony wall is medialized, resulting in a permanently narrow position. Although the bony vault may be congenitally narrow or caused by trauma, in many cases the cause is iatrogenic. Specifically, prior osteotomies during rhinoplasty are a common culprit (**Fig. 35.9**). Indeed, airway obstruction is a recognized complication of rhinoplasty, and lateral osteotomy in particular. For this reason, osteotomy paths have evolved to a so-called “high-low-high” configuration, preserving the lateral wall attachments from the ala to the lower pyriform aperture.[9]

Surgical Management of Nasal Obstruction in Functional Rhinoplasty

Severe Anterior Septal Deviation

Septal deviation is one of the most common findings in patients with symptomatic nasal obstruction. In patients with mild-to-moderate septal deviation, standard or endoscopic septoplasty is often adequate to improve the patient’s nasal airway, and is discussed elsewhere in this text. However, septoplasty is often inadequate in cases of severe anterior septal deviation.[10] Furthermore, in some patients, the cause of nasal airway obstruction includes a narrow valve angle and high septal deflection, which are generally not treated with standard septoplasty techniques. In addition to airway obstruction, crookedness of the dorsal septum can cause contour deformities of the middle third of the nose. Because the anterior L-strut of the septum is vital for structural support, overresection of the anterocaudal septum can lead to loss of tip support. Destabilization of the junction of the quadrangular cartilage and nasal bones (keystone area) can lead to saddle nose deformity. Thus, severe deviations of the anterior septum are a special challenge, and are often best treated via an open approach.

A variety of external rhinoplasty techniques have been described to address this, including septal modifications, crossbar grafts, camouflage grafts, and splinting of the septum with autologous or synthetic materials.[11–14] In the most severe cases of anterior septal deviation, extracorporeal septoplasty may be required.[15–17] One drawback of traditional complete extracorporeal septoplasty, wherein the entire quadrangular cartilage is removed and replaced, is the risk of saddling or notching of the dorsum.[15,16,18] To minimize destabilization of the keystone (and thus preserve dorsal contour), we advocate the anterior septal reconstruction (ASR) as a more conservative approach to extracorporeal septoplasty that preserves dorsal support, which is designed to concomitantly address nasal obstruction and the external contour deformities.[18,19] In this technique, a dorsal strut of the 10 to 15 mm of septal cartilage is left attached to the keystone area. This allows both dorsal continuity and a support structure to which the surgeon attaches the ASR graft (**Fig. 35.10**). This technique improves nasal airflow, while reducing the risk of notching or saddling compared with standard extracorporeal techniques, and can be combined with aesthetic rhinoplasty.

Table 35.1 Grading System for Lateral Nasal Wall Insufficiency

- Grade 0 – No significant lateral wall motion
- Grade 1 – Lateral wall moves <33% of distance to septum
- Grade 2 – Lateral wall moves 33–66% of distance to septum
- Grade 3 – Lateral wall moves >66% of distance to septum

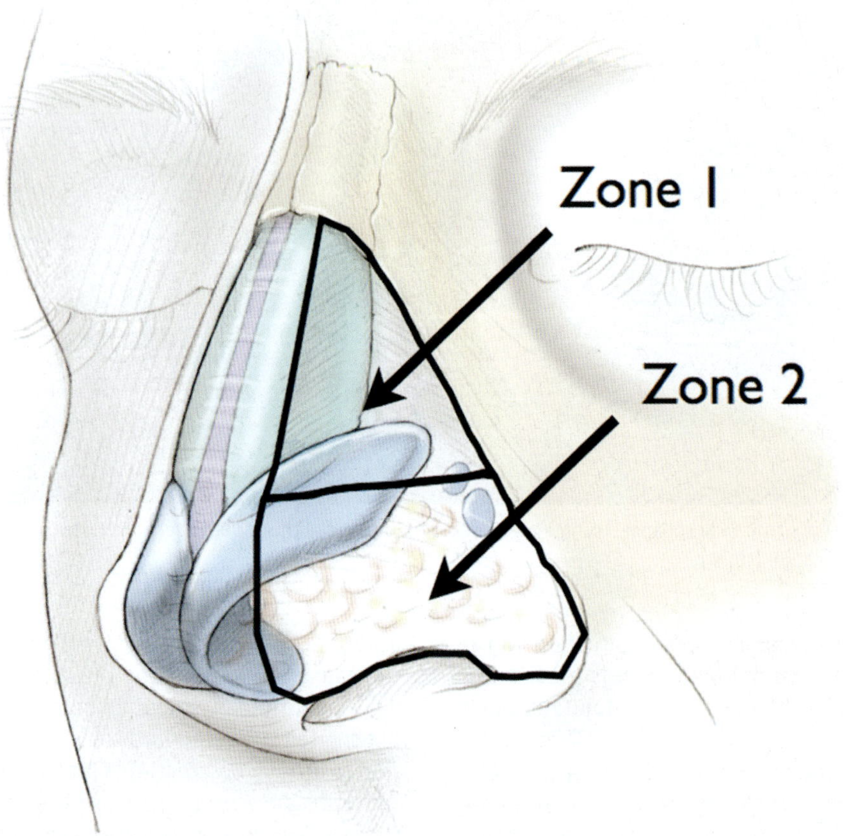

Fig. 35.8 Zones of lateral wall insufficiency (LWI). Zone 1 LWI occurs along the sidewall at the level of the mid vault to the scroll region. Zone 2 LWI occurs more inferiorly, and is often called classic external valve collapse.

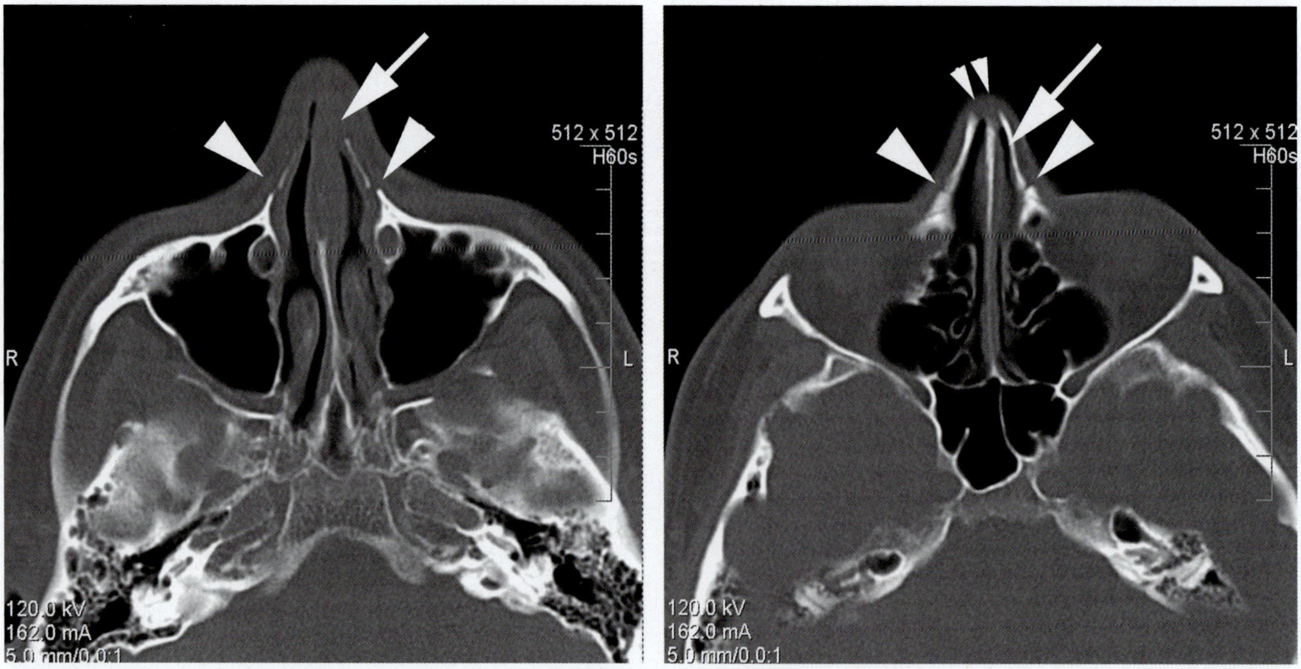

Fig. 35.9 Axial views on computed tomographic scan of patient with primarily left-sided nasal obstruction. The patient had a prior history of dorsal hump takedown (*small double arrowheads*) and osteotomies (*large arrowheads*). Note the worse narrowing of the airway on the left side (*arrows*).

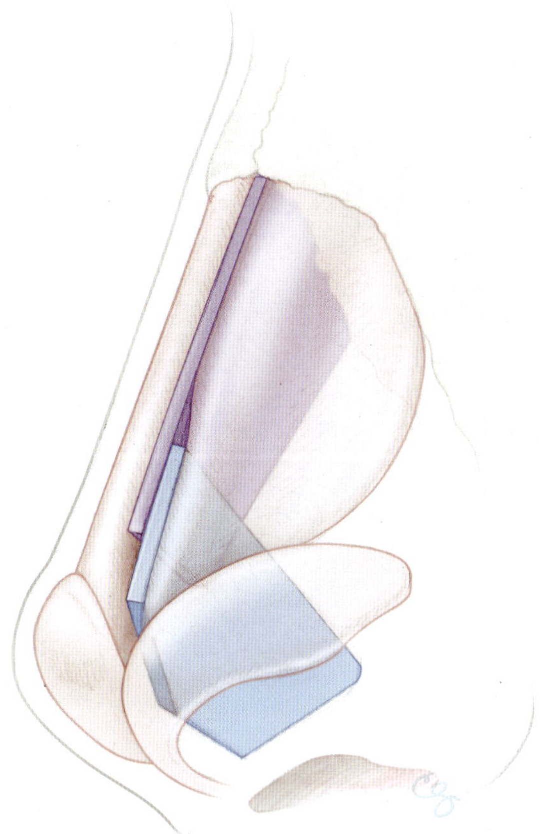

Fig. 35.10 The anterior septal reconstruction. This modified extracorporeal septoplasty technique allows for reconstitution of several anterior septal deviations during open rhinoplasty, and decreases the risk of notching at the rhinion. The septal graft is taken from the native septum.

Techniques for Repair of Internal Valve Collapse

The technique for the repair of internal valve collapse is the spreader graft.[3] In this technique, a long, thin, rectangular piece of cartilage (usually septal) is placed in the space between the ULC and the septum (**Fig. 35.11**). Spreader grafts have also been described as placed intranasally, via a submucosal pocket beneath the ULC/septal junction or externally, the latter approach perhaps more commonly used. The concept of the spreader graft is to increase the cross-sectional area of the nose by increasing the distance from the starting point of the ULC and the septum in the mid vault (**Fig. 35.11**). Multiple variations on the spreader graft have been described, including use of noncartilaginous materials.[13]

One variation of the spreader graft is the so-called onlay-spreader graft.[20] This graft is particularly useful in cases of mid vault collapse associated with a saddle nose deformity. Rather than two separate spreader grafts, one is placed on each side of the septum. A single, wide, rectangular graft is placed from the bony nasal dorsum to the tip, over the septum and sutured to each ULC laterally.

Other options for increasing the angle between the internal nasal valve and the septum include the flaring suture, described by Park, in which a mattressed suture is placed through each ULC and over the dorsum, effectively lifting each ULC and increasing the valve angle.[21] A related technique is the so-called butterfly graft, in which a cartilage graft (usually conchal) is placed in the supratip area.[22]

Techniques for Repair of the External Valve (Lateral Wall Collapse)

Dynamic collapse of the external wall of the nose, or lateral wall insufficiency (LWI), represents a clinical challenge for the facial plastic surgeon for which no clear answer has yet arisen. Iatrogenic dynamic lateral wall collapse is most often caused by overresection of alar cartilages during an aesthetic rhinoplasty.[23] Hence, the technique classically described for repair of such collapse has been augmentation of the lateral wall with cartilage, or alar batten grafts.[24,25] Technically, the procedure involves placement of an elliptical cartilage graft, usually auricular, over the alar remnant. Varying lengths of cartilage have been described. To achieve maximal support, the cartilage would extend from the pyriform aperture to the septum. This is infrequently performed because the external deformity created would be substantial. Instead, the graft is often placed from the pyriform aperture to some point along the midlateral nasal wall. External deformity remains a significant drawback of the technique, even when used in this fashion. Furthermore, as with many facial plastic surgery procedures, there is a paucity of prospective studies examining the efficacy of the technique. However, the method continues to be a mainstay in the treatment of alar collapse.

The lateral crural strut graft is an alternative to batten grafting that has the advantage of supporting the inferior lateral nasal wall with fewer aesthetic drawbacks. In this technique, the lateral crural strut is reinforced on its deep side by the placement of a straight piece of cartilage (usually septal or auricular) between its deep surface and the native cartilage. This technique would seem to be effective for iatrogenic cases of more inferior lateral nasal wall collapse.[26]

In the mid-1990s, the idea of suture suspension of the lateral nasal wall was introduced (bone-anchored suture technique [BAST]).[27,28] As originally described, the technique involves the placement of a permanent suture from the lateral alar cartilage to the bone of the infraorbital rim using a combination of a small intranasal incision and either an external incision on the medial lower lid or a transconjunctival incision. This technique met with limited success initially. However, we have found that when incorporated with the external rhinoplasty approach, the technique is quite effective.[29] Suture suspension (in any surgical procedure) is much more effective when tissue planes are dissected; in this case, the suture acts as a temporary stabilizing force until wound healing generates enough strength in the repositioned tissues. Our experience with this technique has been very positive. During open rhinoplasty,

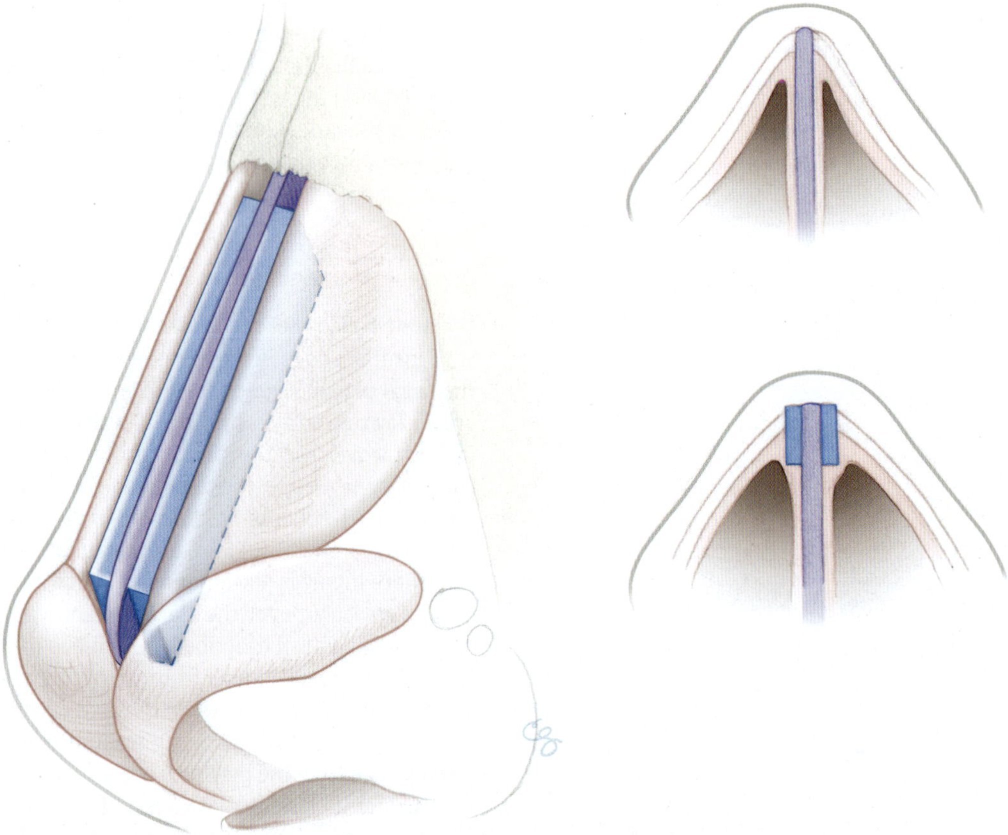

Fig. 35.11 Spreader grafts. The spreader graft (usually composed of septal or auricular cartilage) is placed between the ULC and the septum. Note the increase in the cross-sectional area of the internasal valve area after the placement of the spreader graft.

dissection is carried laterally to the bony aperture of the nose and onto the nasomaxillary buttress and infraorbital rim. A suture-anchor is placed into the infraorbital rim and sutured to the lower ULC and upper LLC (**Fig. 35.12**).

Ideal patients for this technique are those in whom the LWI has occurred de novo, or in post rhinoplasty patients in whom some alar cartilage remains. In patients who have undergone complete division of the alar cartilage, a combination of reconstitution of the lateral cartilaginous strut with suture suspension is warranted. The author's treatment algorithm for LWI is outlined in **Fig. 35.13**.

Outcomes

Studies to measure improvements in the nasal airway have been hampered by several factors, most notably the subjectivity of nasal obstruction symptoms. Determination of improvement in patients' nasal obstruction using quantitative measurement of the nasal air passages has been attempted.[30,31] Anatomic methods measure structural dimensions, such as acoustic rhinometry, which relies on acoustic reflectance to produce an anatomic profile of the cross-sectional area of the nasal cavity.[32] Physiologic methods measure a functional or biological parameter, such as nasal peak inspiratory flow (which measures the rate of inspiratory flow through the nasal passage on inspiration).[33] Discordance between these quantitative measures and patients' subjective symptoms has made studies of methods for improving the nasal airway difficult.[4,31,33,34]

Some groups have studied the efficacy of functional rhinoplasty techniques using patient questionnaires in retrospective analyses.[35] The power of these studies is diminished, however, by their retrospective nature and use of a nonvalidated questionnaire. More recently, validated instruments for evaluation of patients' subjective experiences with nasal obstruction have been developed, such as the Nasal Obstructive Symptoms Evaluation (NOSE) scale.[36] The use of this instrument was first demonstrated in evaluating patients undergoing a septoplasty.[37] Following this, a prospective multicenter trial demonstrated improvement in disease-specific quality of life (QOL) in patients undergoing functional rhinoplasty, although the study consisted of only 20 patients and follow-up was limited to 6 months.[38]

A larger, prospective, single-institution study examined patients undergoing various functional rhinoplasty procedures and found similar results.[39] In this study, patients who underwent spreader grafting for internal valve insufficiency demonstrated improved NOSE scores. Improvement was found in groups who underwent spreader grafting with or

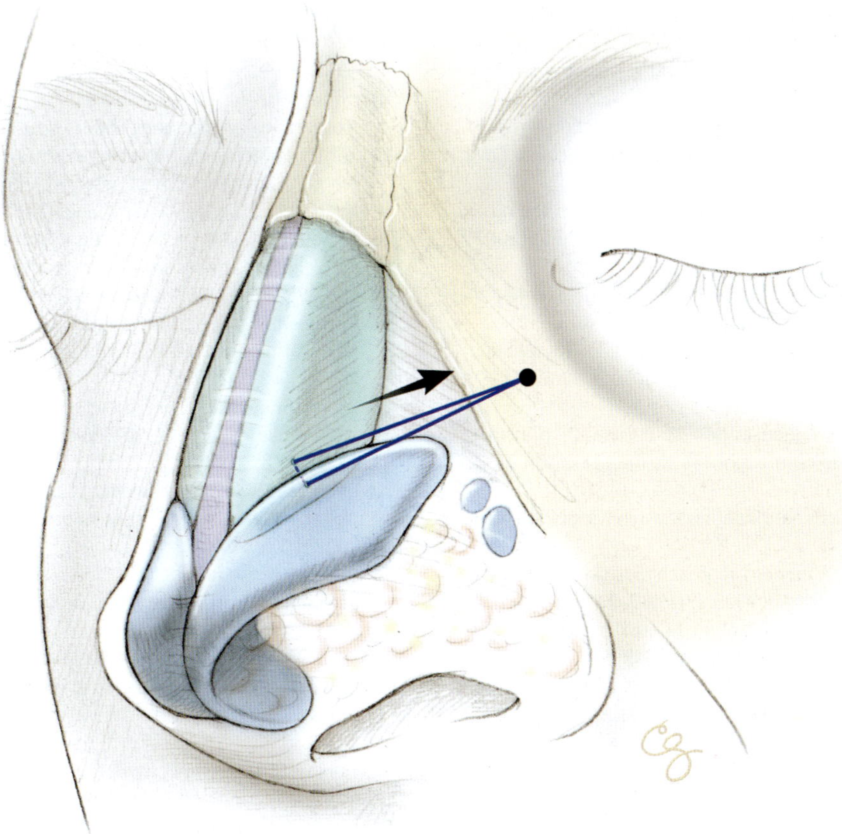

Fig. 35.12 Lateral suture suspension of the nasal wall. The lateral nasal wall is dissected in continuity with a subperiosteal plane on the medial maxilla during an external rhinoplasty. The bone anchor is placed on the infraorbital rim, lateral to the lacrimal apparatus, and sutured to the upper/lower lateral cartilage junction.

without surgical modification of the turbinates. Not surprisingly, the small subset of patients who underwent a septoplasty alone had lower preoperative symptom scores than those who underwent spreader grafting, bone-anchored suturing, or other functional rhinoplasty procedures.

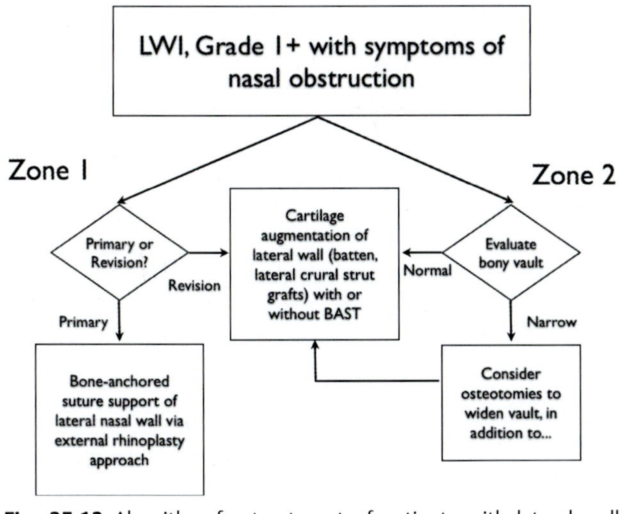

Fig. 35.13 Algorithm for treatment of patients with lateral wall insufficiency.

We now regularly use measures such as the NOSE questionnaire and an accompanying visual analogue scale as one barometer of the efficacy of our functional rhinoplasty procedures. Indeed, we have used it to demonstrate the use of anterior septal reconstruction and bone-anchored suspension of the lateral nasal wall in our technical papers on these topics.[19,29] Use of such measures, in addition to physiologic or anatomic measures, may end up being complementary and necessary for the full evaluation of the efficacy of such techniques.[34]

Conclusion

Preservation or improvement of the physiologic function of the nose requires a thorough understanding of its anatomy. Structural rhinoplasty techniques reinforce, rebuild, or maintain anatomic support of the nose during aesthetic nasal surgery. Similarly, purely functional rhinoplasty techniques are designed to improve nasal airflow while maintaining aesthetic norms for the nose. Although such techniques are evolving, outcome measures, both quantitative and qualitative, are necessary to determine their efficacy, especially as new technical maneuvers emerge.

References

1. Franciscus RG, Trinkaus E. Nasal morphology and the emergence of Homo erectus. Am J Phys Anthropol 1988;75(4):517–527
2. Goode RL. Surgery of the incompetent nasal valve. Laryngoscope 1985;95(5):546–555
3. Sheen JH. Spreader graft: a method of reconstructing the roof of the middle nasal vault following rhinoplasty. Plast Reconstr Surg 1984;73(2):230–239
4. Tikanto J, Pirilä T. Effects of the Cottle's maneuver on the nasal valve as assessed by acoustic rhinometry. Am J Rhinol 2007; 21(4):456–459
5. Byrd HS, Meade RA, Gonyon DL Jr. Using the autospreader flap in primary rhinoplasty. Plast Reconstr Surg 2007;119(6):1897–1902
6. Gruber RP, Park E, Newman J, Berkowitz L, Oneal R. The spreader flap in primary rhinoplasty. Plast Reconstr Surg 2007;119(6): 1903–1910
7. Mitchell M. Animated demonstration of Bernoulli's principle. http://mitchellscience.com/bernoulli_principle_animation. Accessed October 6, 2011
8. Most SP. Trends in functional rhinoplasty. Arch Facial Plast Surg 2008;10(6):410–413
9. Most SP, Murakami CS. A modern approach to nasal osteotomies. Facial Plast Surg Clin North Am 2005;13(1):85–92
10. King ED, Ashley FL. The correction of the internally and externally deviated nose. Plast Reconstr Surg (1946) 1952;10(2):116–120
11. Boccieri A, Pascali M. Septal crossbar graft for the correction of the crooked nose. Plast Reconstr Surg 2003;111(2):629–638
12. Byrd HS, Salomon J, Flood J. Correction of the crooked nose. Plast Reconstr Surg 1998;102(6):2148–2157
13. Mendelsohn M. Straightening the crooked middle third of the nose: using porous polyethylene extended spreader grafts. Arch Facial Plast Surg 2005;7(2):74–80
14. TerKonda RP, Sykes JM. Repairing the twisted nose. Otolaryngol Clin North Am 1999;32(1):53–64
15. Gubisch W. The extracorporeal septum plasty: a technique to correct difficult nasal deformities. Plast Reconstr Surg 1995;95(4):672–682
16. Gubisch W, Constantinescu MA. Refinements in extracorporal septoplasty. Plast Reconstr Surg 1999;104(4):1131–1139, discussion 1140–1142
17. Senyuva C, Yücel A, Aydin Y, Okur I, Güzel Z. Extracorporeal septoplasty combined with open rhinoplasty. Aesthetic Plast Surg 1997;21(4):233–239
18. Gubisch W. Extracorporeal septoplasty for the markedly deviated septum. Arch Facial Plast Surg 2005;7(4):218–226
19. Most SP. Anterior septal reconstruction: outcomes after a modified extracorporeal septoplasty technique. Arch Facial Plast Surg 2006;8(3):202–207
20. Alsarraf R, Murakami C. The saddle nose deformity. Facial Plast Surg Clin North Am 1999;7(3):303–310
21. Park SS. The flaring suture to augment the repair of the dysfunctional nasal valve. Plast Reconstr Surg 1998;101(4):1120–1122
22. Akcam T, Friedman O, Cook TA. The effect on snoring of structural nasal valve dilatation with a butterfly graft. Arch Otolaryngol Head Neck Surg 2004;130(11):1313–1318
23. Ballert JA, Park SS. Functional rhinoplasty: treatment of the dysfunctional nasal sidewall. Facial Plast Surg 2006;22(1): 49–54
24. Millman B. Alar batten grafting for management of the collapsed nasal valve. Laryngoscope 2002;112(3):574–579
25. Toriumi DM, Josen J, Weinberger M, Tardy ME Jr. Use of alar batten grafts for correction of nasal valve collapse. Arch Otolaryngol Head Neck Surg 1997;123(8):802–808
26. Gunter JP, Friedman RM. Lateral crural strut graft: technique and clinical applications in rhinoplasty. Plast Reconstr Surg 1997;99(4):943–952, discussion 953–955
27. Friedman M, Ibrahim H, Syed Z. Nasal valve suspension: an improved, simplified technique for nasal valve collapse. Laryngoscope 2003;113(2):381–385
28. Paniello RC. Nasal valve suspension. An effective treatment for nasal valve collapse. Arch Otolaryngol Head Neck Surg 1996; 122(12):1342–1346
29. Roofe SB, Most SP. Placement of a lateral nasal suspension suture via an external rhinoplasty approach. Arch Facial Plast Surg 2007;9(3):214–216
30. Larsen K, Kristensen S. Peak flow nasal patency indices and self-assessment in septoplasty. Clin Otolaryngol Allied Sci 1990;15(4): 327–334
31. Pirilä T, Tikanto J. Unilateral and bilateral effects of nasal septum surgery demonstrated with acoustic rhinometry, rhinomanometry, and subjective assessment. Am J Rhinol 2001;15(2): 127–133
32. Hilberg O, Jackson AC, Swift DL, Pedersen OF. Acoustic rhinometry: evaluation of nasal cavity geometry by acoustic reflection. J Appl Physiol 1989;66(1):295–303
33. Larsson C, Millqvist E, Bende M. Relationship between subjective nasal stuffiness and nasal patency measured by acoustic rhinometry. Am J Rhinol 2001;15(6):403–405
34. Lam DJ, James KT, Weaver EM. Comparison of anatomic, physiological, and subjective measures of the nasal airway. Am J Rhinol 2006;20(5):463–470
35. Khosh MM, Jen A, Honrado C, Pearlman SJ. Nasal valve reconstruction: experience in 53 consecutive patients. Arch Facial Plast Surg 2004;6(3):167–171
36. Stewart MG, Witsell DL, Smith TL, Weaver EM, Yueh B, Hannley MT. Development and validation of the Nasal Obstruction Symptom Evaluation (NOSE) scale. Otolaryngol Head Neck Surg 2004;130(2):157–163
37. Stewart MG, Smith TL, Weaver EM, et al. Outcomes after nasal septoplasty: results from the Nasal Obstruction Septoplasty Effectiveness (NOSE) study. Otolaryngol Head Neck Surg 2004;130(3):283–290
38. Rhee JS, Poetker DM, Smith TL, Bustillo A, Burzynski M, Davis RE. Nasal valve surgery improves disease-specific quality of life. Laryngoscope 2005;115(3):437–440
39. Most SP. Analysis of outcomes after functional rhinoplasty using a disease-specific quality-of-life instrument. Arch Facial Plast Surg 2006;8(5):306–309

36 Sinonasal Trauma

E. Bradley Strong and Travis T. Tollefson

Facial fractures occur in all age groups and can result in serious functional and aesthetic deformities. The intimate relationships of the paranasal sinuses, brain, orbits, dentition, and lacrimal system make treatment of these injuries quite complex. Traditional surgical approaches to the craniofacial skeleton are the mainstay of fracture repair; however, endoscopic and other minimally invasive techniques have found applicability in the management of selected facial fractures. This chapter presents surgical algorithms and techniques for management of facial fractures involving the nasal bones, frontal sinus, naso-orbito-ethmoid complex, and orbit.

Nasal Fractures

The central location and projection of the nose makes it the most commonly fractured facial bone. The most common etiologies include motor vehicle accidents, sports injuries, and interpersonal altercations. Males are twice as likely as females to sustain nasal fractures. Traumatic disruption of the nasal bones/cartilages can result in significant external deformity and airway obstruction. The type and severity of nasal fracture is dependent on the force, direction, and mechanism of injury.

Anatomy

The paired nasal bones support the upper third of the nose (**Fig. 36.1**). They attach to the frontal process of the maxilla laterally, the frontal bone superiorly, and the perpendicular plate of the ethmoid bone posteriorly. The lower two-thirds of the nose is comprised of the paired upper and lower lateral cartilages, as well as the quadrangular cartilage. The junction of the upper and lower lateral cartilages is termed the scroll region. The angle between the upper lateral cartilage and the nasal septum is termed the internal nasal valve. The internal nasal valve represents the area of greatest resistance to inspiratory airflow. The lower lateral cartilages are thick and have medial and lateral crura. They define the contour of the nasal tip. Major tip support comes from the tripod of the paired medial crus centrally and lateral crus on either side. The caudal septum also provides significant tip support and contour for the columella.

Nasal bone fractures occur most commonly in the thinner inferior portion of the nasal bones, at the junction with the upper lateral cartilages, and can often result in nasal obstruction. A laterally applied force may dislocate the nasal bones, cartilages, and septum, resulting in a "c-shaped" deformity (**Fig. 36.2**). Direct frontal trauma often results in depression and widening of the nasal dorsum. Fractures that involve the caudal septum can result in poor nasal tip support, columellar deviation, and a twisted nose. More severe fractures may extend into the frontal bone, orbit, lacrimal system, or naso-orbital-ethmoid complex.[1]

Diagnosis and Treatment

Accurate diagnosis of nasal fractures is based on a thorough history and physical examination. A complete history

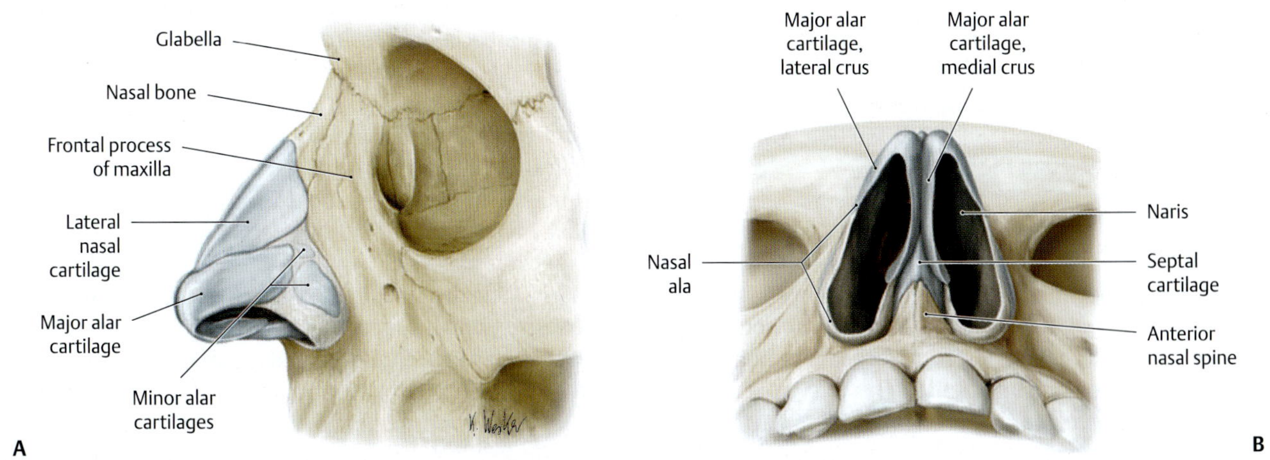

Fig. 36.1 (A,B) Illustrations of the nasal bones and cartilages that provide structural support for the external nose. (Used with permission from Atlas of Anatomy: Head and Neuroanatomy. Thieme 2007.)

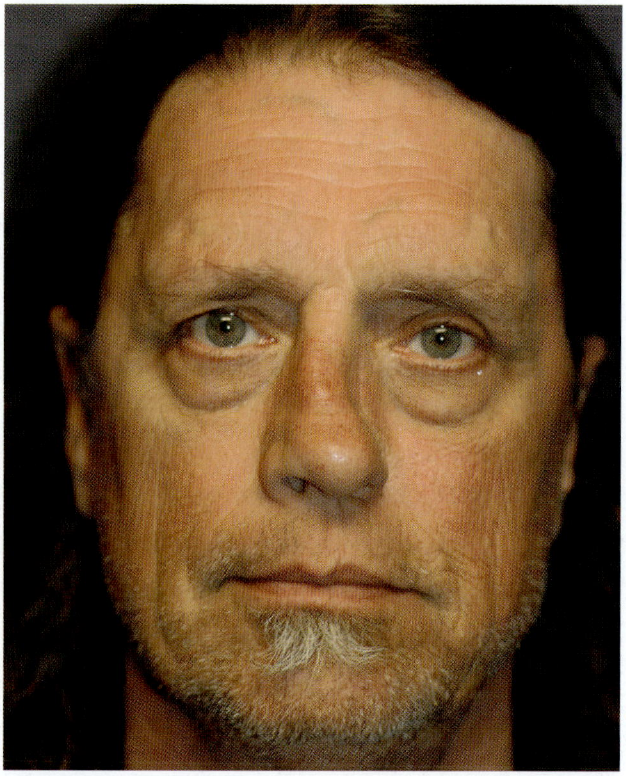

Fig. 36.2 Patient with a "C-shaped" nasal deformity after nasal trauma.

includes documentation of the mechanism of injury, as well as the presence of epistaxis, watery rhinorrhea (suggestive of a cerebrospinal fluid [CSF] leak), nasal obstruction, previous nasal fractures, or nasal surgery. The examination requires a good headlight, suction, and a nasal speculum. Minor bleeding can be controlled with either 4% cocaine or a mixture of oxymetazoline and 1% lidocaine spray. The intranasal examination may reveal mucosal lacerations, septal fractures, or a septal hematoma. Septal hematomas must be evacuated immediately to avoid cartilage necrosis and secondary deformity. Examination of the external nose may show lacerations, bony step-offs, cartilage disruption, mobility, or crepitus. After adequate anesthesia (see Surgical Technique), nasal bone mobility can be assessed by palpating the nasal bones while exerting gentle outward traction with a Boies elevator inserted through the nares.

Radiography

Historically, plain sinus radiographs have been used to evaluate nasal fractures. Although some authors have suggested a medico-legal indication for plain radiographs, studies have shown poor sensitivity and specificity.[2] The authors believe that radiography is not needed for diagnosis of routine nasal fractures; the diagnosis should instead be made on the basis of a thorough history and physical exam.

Timing of Repair

The primary treatment goal in the management of nasal fractures is to reestablish the premorbid function and appearance of the nose. Although the most appropriate timing for fracture reduction remains controversial, several concepts can be applied to most patients. Epistaxis should be controlled immediately, and may require nasal packing. If a septal hematoma is noted, a unilateral 1-cm mucosal incision is used to release the blood. Immediate reduction of nasal fractures can be difficult because soft tissue edema distorts the surgeon's perspective of nasal symmetry. However, an attempt at immediate reduction can be performed with grossly displaced fractures (i.e., fractures that are visible despite the soft tissue edema), or open fractures. Most fractures are more accurately reduced 7 to 10 days after the injury, when the majority of soft tissue edema has resolved. Pediatric fractures will heal more rapidly; however, in the authors' experience, most will remain mobile for at least 7 days. Treatment delays greater than 2–3 weeks will result in callus formation and bone remodeling, making the reduction more difficult. Patients with significant delays in treatment (3 to 12 months) are more likely to require open septorhinoplasty for definitive repair.

Surgical Technique

Appropriate informed consent is obtained prior to treatment. The surgical risks are discussed including bleeding, infection, persistent obstruction, paraesthesias, septal perforation, and poor aesthetic result. Fracture reduction can be accomplished using either an open or closed approach depending on patient and surgeon preference. The majority of repairs can be managed adequately with a closed reduction. Although general anesthesia is required for the pediatric population, local anesthesia is often preferred in adults due to reduced cost and risk. The literature shows a difference in patient tolerance of nasal manipulation, pain, or need for definitive septorhinoplasty when using either a local or general anesthetic.[3] However, each surgeon must take into consideration their level of experience and the patient's tolerance of local anesthesia prior to attempting fracture reduction.

Local anesthesia can be obtained by infiltration of 1% lidocaine with 1:100,000 epinephrine around the supratrochlear and supraorbital foramina. Additional injections along the nasal sidewall, base, dorsum, and columella will complete the regional block. Cocaine (or oxymetazoline and 1% lidocaine) soaked pledgets are placed for intranasal anesthesia. Many surgeons also employ intravenous sedation/analgesia. After allowing 10 to 15 minutes for vasoconstriction and anesthetic effect, the fracture reduction can be performed. The depressed nasal bone is stabilized between a Boies elevator intranasally and the index finger and thumb of the opposite hand externally. As the Boies elevator reduces the depressed nasal bone on one side, the contralateral nasal bone is pushed by the finger or thumb into its premorbid position. Walsh or Asch forceps can be used to reduce septal fractures and dislocations. Once reduced, most fractures will have adequate interfragmentary resistance to maintain the reduction, and intranasal packing can be avoided. However, if the nasal bones become extremely mobile, antibiotic soaked strip gauze can be used to pack the nose and stabilize the fragments. The gauze is packed high into the nasal vault beneath the nasal bones. An oral antibiotic with staphylococcal coverage is used for the duration of the packing placement to minimize the risk of toxic shock syndrome.[4] Moldable external splints (aluminum or heat malleable) are commonly used postoperatively to maintain the reduction. Splints should be contoured to the external nose and kept in place for ~7 days. All patients with significant fractures should be informed that secondary septorhinoplasty may be necessary. These procedures can be challenging and are covered in greater detail in Chapters 34 and 35 of this book.

Frontal Sinus Fractures

Because the frontal sinus is protected by thick cortical bone, fractures are relatively uncommon (5 to 15% of maxillofacial injuries). They are most often the result of high velocity injuries such as motor vehicle accidents, assaults, or sports injuries.[5,6] Concomitant facial fractures are seen in 66% of patients with frontal sinus fractures, and significant mortality rates have been reported for complex through and through fractures.[6,7] Approximately 50 to 60% of frontal sinus fractures involve a combination of the anterior table, posterior table, and/or the nasofrontal recess.[8–11] Isolated anterior table fractures are less common (33%). Isolated posterior table injuries are rare. The treatment of frontal sinus fractures remains one of the most controversial areas of maxillofacial trauma. Improper management can result in aesthetic deformities, chronic sinusitis, pneumocephalus, mucopyocele, meningitis, brain abscess, and death. Unfortunately, the optimal management strategy is difficult to determine because most complications occur months to years after treatment. Prospective, randomized studies comparing treatment strategies do not exist.

Anatomy

The frontal sinus is not present at birth. The anterior ethmoid air cells invade the frontal bone at age 2, and develop into a full size frontal sinus by age 15. Critical structures surrounding the sinus include the orbital roof (sinus floor), the anterior cranial fossa (posterior wall), as well as the forehead and glabella (anterior wall) (**Fig. 36.3**).[12] The size and shape of the adult frontal sinuses are highly variable, commonly asymmetric, and may be divided by one or more septations. Less frequently, patients will have a unilateral (10%), rudimentary (5%), or no frontal sinus (4%).[11] Average frontal sinus dimensions are: height, 30 mm; width, 25 mm; depth, 19 mm; and volume, 10 mL. The anterior table is often much thicker (average 4 mm, but up to 12 mm) than the posterior table (0.1 to 4.8 mm).[13]

Each frontal sinus ostium exits the sinus posteriorly and inferiorly. The true ostia are 3 to 4 mm in diameter, and constitute the narrowest point of an hourglass configuration. The frontal sinus "infundibulum" lies above and the nasofrontal recess below.[14] Neurovascular supply to the frontal sinus is from the supraorbital and supratrochlear arteries, the ophthalmic branch of the trigeminal nerve, and the facial vein. Frontal sinus infections can progress

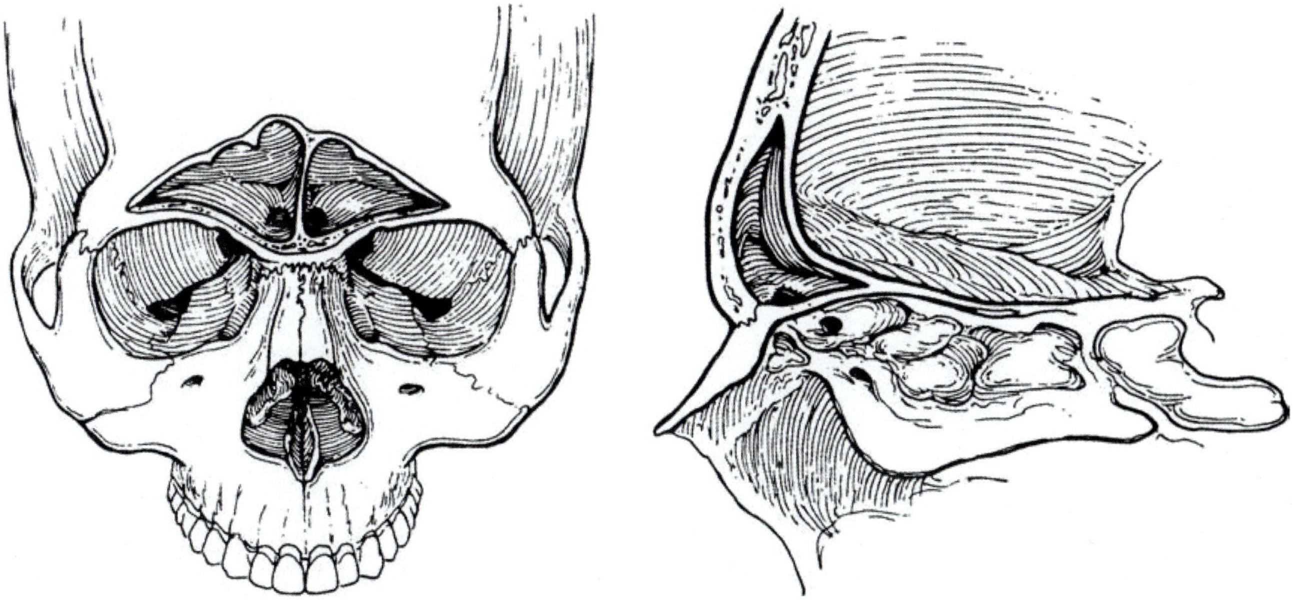

Fig. 36.3 Illustrations of the frontal sinus and its relationship to the orbit, nasal cavity, and intracranial cavity. (Used with permission from Donald PJ. Maxillofacial Trauma: Management of the Difficult Case. Philadelphia: WB Saunders; 1984.)

through the venous system into the cavernous sinus via the ophthalmic vein or foramina of Bruschet.[15]

Diagnosis

The accurate diagnosis of frontal sinus fractures and naso-frontal-recess injuries is crucial. A thorough history should document the presence of: forehead pain, paresthesias, epistaxis, diplopia, epiphora, clear rhinorrhea, or salty postnasal drainage (suggestive of a CSF fluid leak). Clear nasal drainage should be collected and tested for beta-2 transferrin. A complete head and neck examination must be performed. The presence of associated facial fractures must be ruled out, with special attention to examination of the orbits and naso-orbito-ethmoid complex.

Radiography

Plain X-rays are of little use in the diagnosis of frontal sinus fractures. The gold standard is a thin cut (1.0 to 1.5 mm) axial computed tomography (CT) scan. Coronal, sagittal, and three-dimensional (3D) reconstructions should be a routine part of the radiology protocol for all facial fractures. Anterior and posterior table injuries are best viewed with axial cuts. Coronal and sagittal views may demonstrate injuries to the frontal sinus floor and orbital roof. Three-dimensional reconstructions can show fragment orientation, and are also helpful when explaining the injuries to the patient and family.

Treatment Algorithm

Appropriate treatment decisions can be made by assessing injury to four anatomic parameters: anterior table, posterior table, frontal recess, and the dura (CSF leak) (**Fig. 36.4**). The goals of fracture management are protection of the intracranial contents, prevention of early and late complications, and reestablishment of normal sinus contour and function, if possible. Specific treatment options include observation, endoscopic fracture reduction or camouflage, open reduction and internal fixation, sinus obliteration, sinus exenteration (Riedel procedure), and sinus cranialization.

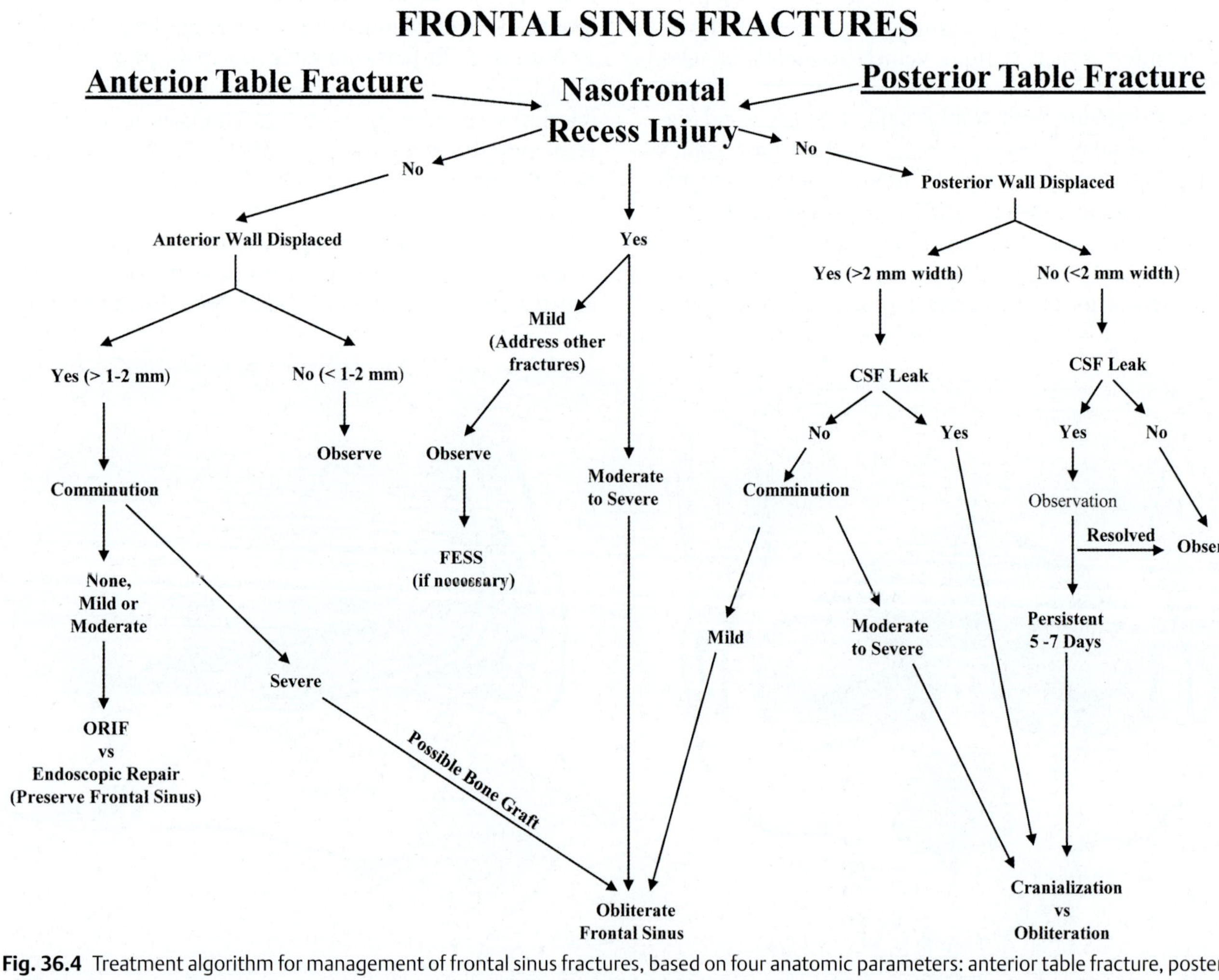

Fig. 36.4 Treatment algorithm for management of frontal sinus fractures, based on four anatomic parameters: anterior table fracture, posterior table fracture, frontal recess injury, and dural integrity. (Adapted with permission from Strong EB. Frontal sinus and naso-orbital-ethmoid complex fractures. In: Papel ID, ed. Facial Plastic and Reconstructive Surgery, 3rd ed. New York: Thieme; 2009, page 980.)

Nasofrontal Recess Injury

Fractures involving the floor of the frontal sinus and medial orbit should raise suspicion for a nasofrontal recess injury (**Fig. 36.4**).[16] Some authors have proposed infusion of dye into the sinus to document frontal recess patency. However, the passage of dye into the nose does not confirm or refute the presence of a fracture and has no documented prognostic value for the ultimate patency of the frontal recess. Therefore, treatment decisions are generally based on thin-cut CT scans. Injuries that result in severe disruption of the frontal recess and outflow tract should undergo frontal sinus obliteration. Fractures that extend into the frontal recess from above, or result in mild bony disruption of the outflow tract, can be more challenging to evaluate.

Recent literature suggests that observation may be an appropriate treatment option for patients with mild-to-moderate nasofrontal injuries.[17] These patients are informed of the signs and symptoms of frontal sinusitis and followed closely. A repeat CT scan is performed 1 month after the injury. If the repeat CT scan reveals opacification of the sinus, an endoscopic frontal sinusotomy is performed. Frontal obliteration is reserved for those patients who fail endoscopic frontal sinusotomy. It must be emphasized that this approach has only recently been described and should be reserved for surgeons with significant experience in both the endoscopic and open management of frontal sinus fractures. Furthermore, patients selected for observation must be compliant with follow-up evaluations.

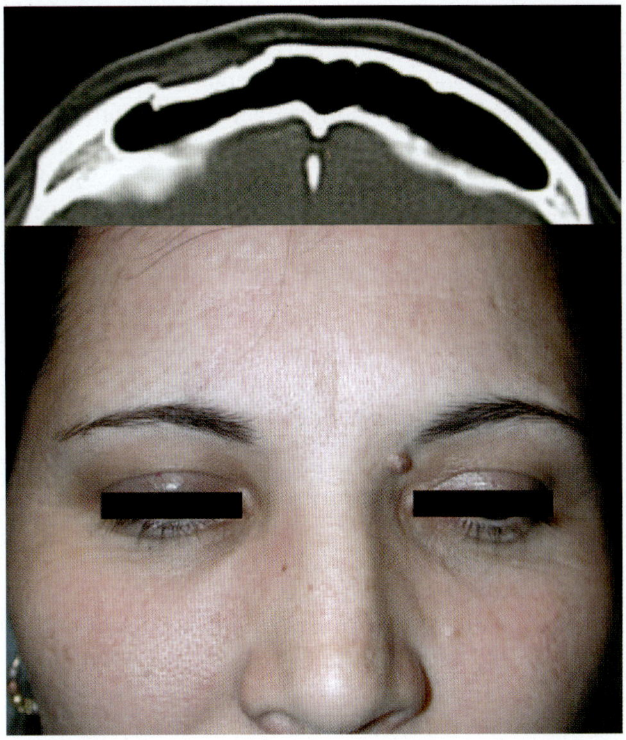
A

B

Fig. 36.5 A patient with a frontal sinus fracture that was untreated and reevaluated at 3 months. A significant bony deformity can be seen on computed tomography scan, but this is not clinically evident on physical examination. (Adapted with permission from Strong EB. Frontal sinus and naso-orbital-ethmoid complex fractures. In: Papel ID, ed. Facial Plastic and Reconstructive Surgery, 3rd ed. New York: Thieme; 2009, page 981.)

Anterior Table Fractures

Minimally displaced anterior table fractures (<1 to 2 mm) pose little risk of mucocele formation or aesthetic deformity (**Fig. 36.4**). These patients should be informed of the risks, signs, and symptoms of frontal sinusitis and observed. Patients with mild to moderately displaced fractures (>2 mm; mild-to-moderate comminution) will likely require some type of surgical intervention. Although open reduction and internal fixation (ORIF) is the gold standard, the associated morbidity of a coronal incision (i.e., alopecia, hypertrophic scarring, paresthesias, and rarely facial nerve injury) may in fact be more severe than the fracture itself. To avoid these undesirable sequelae of a coronal incision, an endoscopic approach for ORIF of anterior table frontal sinus fractures has been described.[18–20] Because endoscopic manipulation of the displaced fragments can be technically challenging, delayed repair using a camouflage technique has also been described.[21] A simple onlay graft is placed to cover the defect. The advantages of a secondary repair are twofold:

1. Resolution of tissue edema allows a more accurate assessment of the aesthetic deformity. In the authors' experience, many patients will opt for no repair once the actual deformity (or lack thereof) is seen (**Fig. 36.5**).
2. The need for endoscopic fracture manipulation is obviated. Disadvantages of secondary frontal fracture repair include the fact that an alloplastic material is typically used for the repair. Fractures that extend over the orbital rim, or have more severe comminution, are extremely difficult or impossible to repair endoscopically.

Posterior Table Fractures

Multiple treatment options exist for management of posterior table fractures (**Fig. 36.4**).[6,7,17,,22] Some surgeons recommend exploration of all posterior table fractures,[23] whereas others suggest careful observation.[24] The authors' decision to surgically intervene is based on several criteria: the degree of fracture displacement, comminution, and presence of a CSF leak. Posterior table fractures that are displaced less than 2 mm (or approximately one table-width) and have no CSF leak may be observed. Long-term follow-up with repeat CT scans at 1 month and 1 year are appropriate to rule out mucocele formation. If a CSF leak is present at time of injury, 1 week of observation is indicated; ~50% of these leaks will resolve spontaneously.[13] If the leak is persistent, then open reduction, dural repair, and sinus obliteration are indicated. In contrast, posterior table fractures, which are displaced greater than one table-width and comminuted, are felt to have a higher rate of complications (dural tears, CSF leak, meningitis, and mucocele formation).[25] Sinus obliteration may be an option for less severe injuries. However, injuries resulting in disruption of more than 25 to 30% of the posterior table should undergo sinus cranialization (particularly if a CSF leak is present).[26] Consultation with a neurosurgical colleague is recommended prior to repair of comminuted posterior table fractures or cranialization of the sinus.

Surgical Technique

Endoscopic Camouflage Technique

This technique is used for isolated anterior table frontal sinus fractures above the orbital rim. The repair is performed 2 to 4 months after the injury, when all forehead swelling has resolved. If the patient is seen acutely, the rationale for a delayed endoscopic repair must be explained (i.e., observation to confirm that an aesthetic deformity is present). The patient must be informed that a traditional open reduction cannot be performed secondarily. Although the risk of mucocele formation is very low, this should also be discussed. Informed consent should include: bleeding, infection, paresthesia, alopecia, poor aesthetic result, and possible need for an open approach.

The surgical approach is similar to an endoscopic brow lift. A 3 to 5 cm parasagittal "working" incision should be placed above the fracture, 3 to 4 cm behind the hairline (**Fig. 36.6**). The actual incision length is dictated by the size of the implant to be inserted. A 1 to 2 cm "endoscope" incision should be placed ~6 cm medial to the working incision. The use of electrocautery should be minimized to prevent alopecia. A "blind" subperiosteal dissection is performed down to the level of the fracture with a brow lift elevator. A 4.0-mm, 30-degree endoscope with endosheath is inserted to visualize the subperiosteal dissection over the defect. The endosheath should have a large guard to elevate and maintain the optical cavity. Under direct visualization, the dissection is then carried over the fracture site. A fibrous scar layer prevents entry into the sinus. The supraorbital and supratrochlear neurovascular pedicles are commonly visualized at the orbital rim. Excessive traction on the pedicles should be avoided, as it can result in postoperative paresthesias. Once the fracture is fully exposed, a 0.85-mm thick porous polyethylene sheet (Medpor, Porex Surgical, Newnan, GA) is trimmed roughly to the size of the defect. The superior edge is marked with a pen to maintain the orientation endoscopically during insertion. The implant is inserted through the working incision and manipulated both internally (with instruments) and externally (with fingers) over the defect. Once the implant is in place, the size and shape are evaluated endoscopically and the implant is removed, trimmed, and refined. The process is repeated until the diameter of the implant is ~2 to 3 mm larger than the defect (**Fig. 36.7**).

Implant fixation is performed through a percutaneous incision. The optimal incision site is determined by passing a 25-gauge needle through the skin over the fracture and endoscopically visualizing the needle tip in the

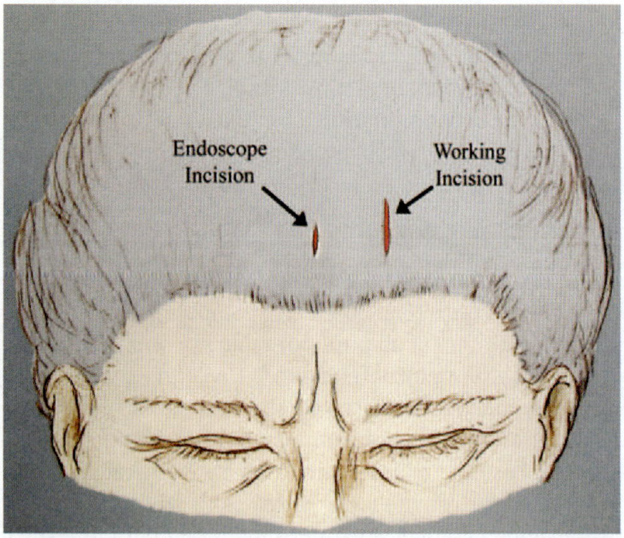

Fig. 36.6 Illustration demonstrating the incisions used for endoscopic repair of anterior table frontal sinus fractures. The working incision is placed 6 cm behind the hairline and directly above the fracture. The endoscope incision is 4 cm medial to the working incision. (Adapted with permission from Strong EB. Frontal sinus and naso-orbital-ethmoid complex fractures. In: Papel ID, ed. Facial Plastic and Reconstructive Surgery, 3rd ed. New York: Thieme; 2009, page 981.)

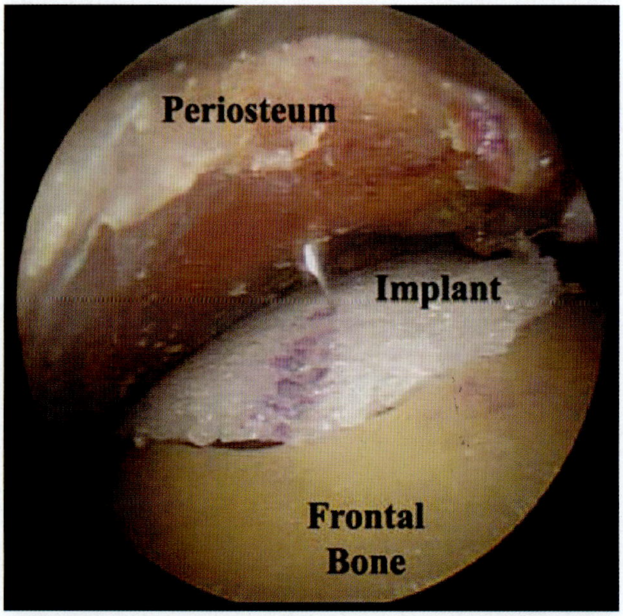

Fig. 36.7 Endoscopic photograph of a porous polyethylene implant being placed over an anterior table frontal sinus fracture. (Used with permission from Strong EB. Frontal sinus and naso-orbital-ethmoid complex fractures. In: Papel ID, ed. Facial Plastic and Reconstructive Surgery, 3rd ed. New York: Thieme; 2009, page 982.)

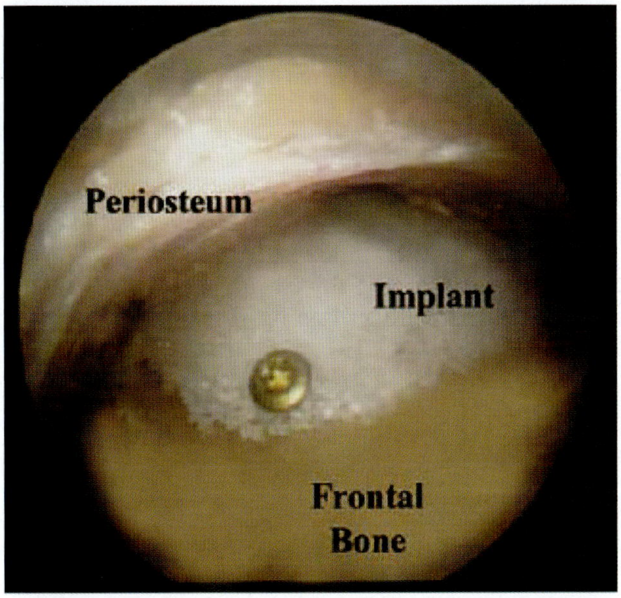

Fig. 36.8 Endoscopic photograph of a porous polyethylene implant stabilized over an anterior table frontal sinus defect with a self-drilling screw holding the implant in place. (Used with permission from Strong EB. Frontal sinus and naso-orbital-ethmoid complex fractures. In: Papel ID, ed. Facial Plastic and Reconstructive Surgery, 3rd ed. New York: Thieme; 2009, page 982.)

subperiosteal plane. Optimal incision placement will allow screws to be placed on either side of the implant through a single incision. Larger implants may require two stab incisions. Once the appropriate site has been determined, a no. 11 blade is used to make a through-and-through stab incision. The implant is then placed and fixated by passing one or two self-drilling micro screws (4 to 6 mm in length) through the incision, through the edge of the implant, and into stable bone peripheral to the fracture edge. The screw must be placed at least 1 mm away from the implant edge or the implant may tear (**Fig. 36.8**). A layered skin closure is performed and a compression dressing is applied.

Open Reduction and Internal Fixation

The patient is consented for the procedure including the risks of bleeding, infection, paresthesia, headache, CSF leak, orbital injury, diplopia, meningitis, external deformity, and late mucocele formation. Large lacerations should be used to assist with the repair, but a coronal incision is generally required for adequate access. The coronal incision is marked out at least 6 cm behind the hairline, and the hair is parted to expose the scalp. The hair need not be shaved. The incision is carried behind each auricle to assist with camouflage. A “zig-zag” incision is used for patients with longer hair (longer than 3 to 4 cm) (**Fig. 36.9**). Postoperatively, when the patient is upright, the “zig-zag” pattern allows gravity to pull the hair inferiorly, covering the transverse arms of the scar. For shorter hair, a straight line widow’s peak incision is used (**Fig. 36.10**). The incision

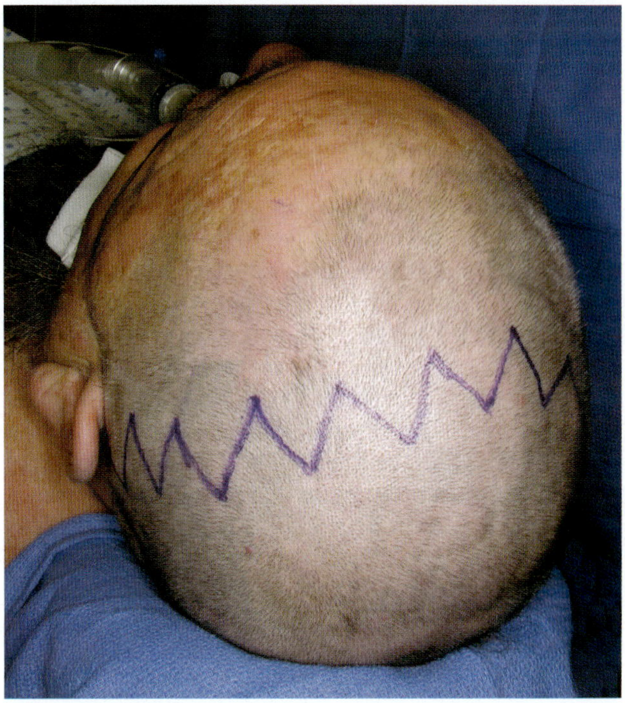

Fig. 36.9 Photograph of a “zig-zag” coronal scalp incision. The zig-zag pattern is used to help camouflage the incision in the hair. (Used with permission from Strong EB. Frontal sinus fractures: current concepts. Craniomaxillofac Trauma Reconstr 2009;2:161–176, page 169, figure 14A.)

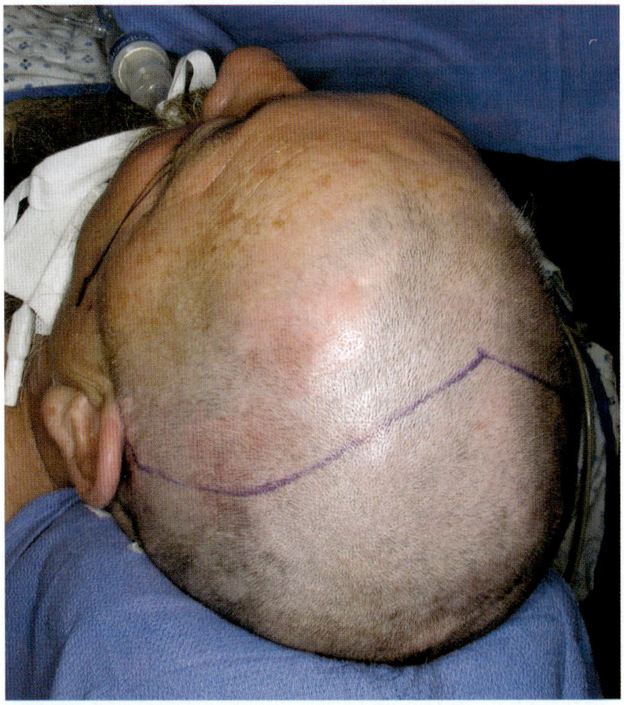

Fig. 36.10 Photograph of a coronal scalp incision with a “widow’s peak.” (Used with permission from Strong EB. Frontal sinus fractures: current concepts. Craniomaxillofac Trauma Reconstr 2009;2: 161–170, page 169, figure 14B.)

can be placed posterior to the vertex in balding patients, but this may require a more extensive lateral dissection to turn the flap anteriorly.

One percent lidocaine with 1:100,000 epinephrine is injected in a subgaleal plane and 10 minutes are allowed for vasoconstriction to take place. The scalp is opened in thirds to minimize blood loss. The skin and subcutaneous tissue are incised from one temporal line to the other. Two opposing double-prong skin hooks are then used to retract the scalp away from the skull, protecting the underlying pericranium. A second pass with the scalpel will incise the galea aponeurosis, allowing air to enter the subgaleal space, and developing an excellent dissection plane. Bleeding from larger vessels should be tied off individually. Electrocautery should be used sparingly to avoid injury to hair follicles. Rainey clips can also be used for hemostasis depending on surgeon preference. The dissection can then be carried anteriorly, taking care to stay within the subgaleal plane. If the dissection is too deep, the pericranium will be violated and bone will be visible. If the dissection is too superficial, hair follicles will become visible, thereby increasing the risk of alopecia.

The lateral scalp dissection demands a thorough understanding of the temporal anatomy. The incision should extend below the temporal line and behind the helix on one side. It should be carried through the temporoparietal fascia (superficial temporal fascia) and onto the temporalis muscle fascia (deep temporal fascia). It will traverse the temporal artery and vein, which should be controlled using a suture ligature or Rainey clips. The flap is then elevated anteriorly using blunt finger dissection or gauze, with limited use of the scalpel. As the temporal flap is elevated forward, it is joined with the midline incision by sharply incising the fibers along the temporal line. A similar technique is then used to elevate the contralateral temporal flap. The entire scalp is then rotated forward and blunt or sharp dissection is used to expose the orbital rims. Care is taken to avoid injury to the supraorbital and supratrochlear neurovascular pedicles. Although periosteal lacerations may exist at the fracture site, a careful dissection will usually maintain an intact vascular supply and provide a lengthy pericranial flap that can be used for repair of any unanticipated CSF leaks or for obliteration of a small frontal sinus. The pericranial flap is incised with a scalpel, extending along both the temporal lines, and back to the skin incision. The flap is easily elevated from the bone, exposing the fractures. If necessary, more extensive inferior dissection can be achieved by releasing the supraorbital and supratrochlear neurovascular pedicles from their foramina and exposing the orbital roof bilaterally. It should be noted that if there is no CSF leak or posterior table injury, the surgeon may choose to elevate the entire central portion of the flap in a subperiosteal plane. This leaves the pericranial flap protected and attached to the scalp flap. With some effort, the pericranial flap can still be separated from the scalp flap after it has been raised.

Anterior table fractures can be difficult to reduce due to interfragmentary resistance between comminuted segments (**Fig. 36.11**). It may be necessary to remove a bone fragment

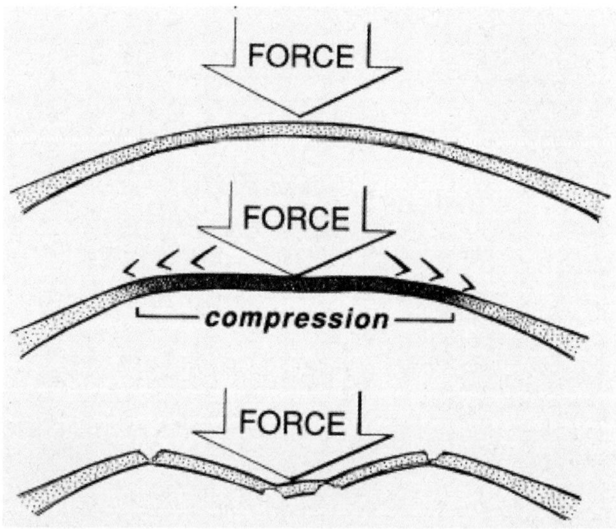

Fig. 36.11 Illustration of the compressive forces on the frontal sinus as it is deformed from a convex to concave shape. Reduction of frontal sinus fractures can be challenging because the bone segments must pass back through this "compressive" phase before they return to their premorbid position. (Used with permission from Strong EB. Frontal sinus and naso-orbital-ethmoid complex fractures. In: Papel ID, ed. Facial Plastic and Reconstructive Surgery, 3rd ed. New York: Thieme; 2009, page 983.)

to release the tension and make room for the reduction. A small bone hook can also be insinuated between the fragments and used for reduction. Another option is placing a small screw (1.5 to 2.0 mm) into a depressed segment to allow external manipulation. Every attempt should be made to keep the majority of the fragments in place. This will allow a more accurate repair. Once the bone fragments are mobilized, the sinus mucosa should be evaluated. If there is concern about injury to the frontal recess, a 30-degree endoscope can be placed through a bone defect and used to inspect the sinus outflow tract. Anterior table bone fragments are then plated with 1.0- to 1.3-mm microplates. Micromesh can be used to cover any small gaps (4 to 10 mm). During wound closure, it is important to resuspend the temporal soft tissues to avoid late ptosis of the forehead and upper midface. Two 2–0 monofilament sutures are passed through the temporoparietal fascia on each side of the flap, and resuspended to the corresponding temporalis muscle fascia (**Fig. 36.12**). A layered skin closure is completed with two Penrose drains and a pressure dressing. The drains are removed on postoperative day one and the dressing is discontinued at 5 to 7 days.

Sinus Obliteration

The consent and surgical approach have been detailed previously (see open reduction and internal fixation). The integrity of the pericranial flap should be maintained, because the risk of dural injury is higher with these injuries. Once the fracture is exposed, all anterior table bone fragments should be removed and kept moist. Arranging the fragments atop a drawing of the fracture helps to maintain the anatomic

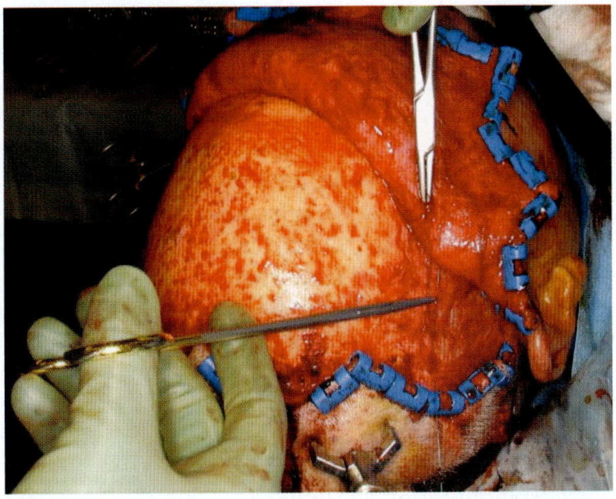

Fig. 36.12 Photograph of a resuspension stitch placed in the temporal region. Resuspension of the soft tissues after a coronal incision is critical to reduce the risk of iatrogenic ptosis of the soft tissues postoperatively. (Used with permission from Strong EB. Frontal sinus fractures: current concepts. Craniomaxillofac Trauma Reconstr 2009;2:161–176, page 171, figure 18.)

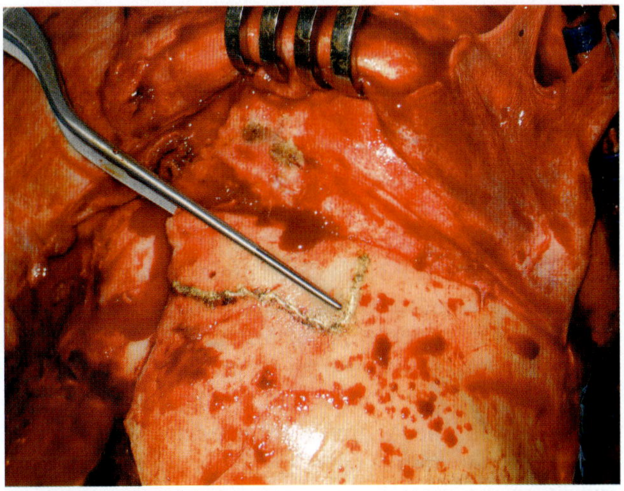

Fig. 36.13 Photograph of bayonet forceps being used to outline the periphery of the frontal sinus. (Used with permission from Strong EB. Frontal sinus and naso-orbital-ethmoid complex fractures. In: Papel ID, ed. Facial Plastic and Reconstructive Surgery, 3rd ed. New York: Thieme; 2009, page 985.)

orientation for the final reconstruction. It may be necessary to osteotomize peripheral anterior table bone to expose the entire sinus. This can be performed in several ways. Historically a "6-foot Caldwell" X-ray was used. However digital radiograph technology has made hard copy X-rays difficult to obtain. Intraoperative navigation can also be used, and is quite accurate. Alternatively, one tine of a bipolar cautery can be placed through the fracture, leaving the other tine externally. The internal tine is then used to "walk" around the periphery of the sinus, whereas the outer tine is used to mark the outline of the sinus on the outer table (**Fig. 36.13**). A third technique uses an endoscope inserted through a fracture line, transilluminating the sinus and delineating the margins.

After the limits of the sinus have been defined, two miniplates are pre-applied, spanning the proposed osteotomy site. This allows the surgeon to accurately reapproximate the bone fragments after the osteotomy. All screws are then removed except one peripheral screw on stable bone outside the sinusotomy. The plate is then rotated around the screw and out of the area of interest (**Fig. 36.14**). The bone flap is cut with a high-speed fluted, side-cutting bit. The surgeon should angle the drill toward the sinus cavity to avoid intracranial penetration and make "postage stamp" perforations around the periphery of the sinus (**Fig. 36.14**).

The perforations are then sequentially joined to completely outline the bone flap. Care should be taken to avoid disruption of the predrilled miniplate holes while performing the osteotomy. The lateral orbital rims and glabella should be osteotomized in a similar fashion, without injuring the supraorbital/supratrochlear neurovascular pedicles or violating the periobita. Next a curved 4-mm osteotome is inserted through the top of the osteotomy and used to gently elevate the bone flap, breaking down any intersinus septations and releasing the anterior table in one piece.

Once the sinus has been fully exposed, the degree of posterior table comminution and/or presence of a CSF leak can be assessed. If the comminution involves less than 25 to 30% of the sinus, an obliteration is indicated. *The key to a successful obliteration is meticulous removal of all sinus mucosa from both the anterior and posterior tables*, first with a cutting burr and then with a diamond burr. Particular attention must be paid to the scalloped areas above the posterior orbit and at the periphery of the sinus. The frontal sinus infundibulum mucosa is elevated inferiorly and a soft tissue plug of either

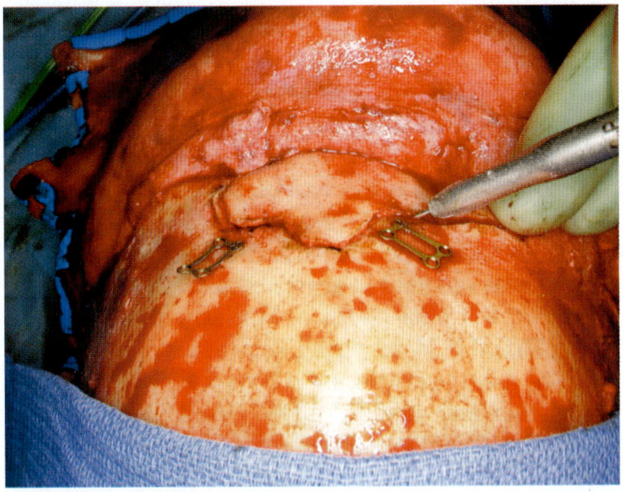

Fig. 36.14 Photograph of a frontal sinusotomy. Note that the hardware is placed prior to the sinusotomy. This ensures that the bone flap returns precisely to its premorbid location. Note also that the burr being used for the osteotomy is placed at an angle to reduce the risk of violating the intracranial cavity. (Used with permission from Strong EB. Frontal sinus fractures: current concepts. Craniomaxillofac Trauma Reconstr 2009;2:161–176, page 172, figure 20.)

pericranium or temporalis fascia is inserted. A small calvarial bone graft can also be harvested from the outer table with a sharp osteotome. This bone graft is wedged into the frontal sinus infundibulum above the fascia graft to complete the separation of the frontal sinus from the nose.

Many different materials have been used for sinus obliteration including abdominal fat, cancellous bone, muscle, pericranium, and spontaneous osteoneogenesis with "auto-obliteration."[11] The authors prefer a fat graft, which is obtained through a left lower quadrant or periumbilical incision using a sterile set of instruments. An attempt should be made to harvest the fat graft in a single piece, with minimal tissue trauma, and avoiding electrocautery when possible. The fat graft is trimmed, inserted into the sinus, and the anterior table fragments are repositioned. The microplates are rotated back into position, screws reapplied, and the scalp is closed as described in open reduction and internal fixation.

Sinus Cranialization

The consent and surgical approach have been detailed previously. Consultation with a neurosurgical colleague is strongly recommended; however, this procedure does not require a formal craniotomy and can be performed through the sinus itself. Lacerations across the inferior pedicle of the pericranial flap are common, but an attempt should be made to preserve the flap for repair of dural tears. All mobile bone fragments from the anterior and posterior table should be removed, drilled free of mucosa, and kept moist for reconstruction of the anterior table. Remaining posterior table bone fragments should be carefully dissected from the dura with Penfield elevators and removed. Any remaining posterior table bone is removed using straight and angled rongeurs. The dura should be elevated from the periphery of the sinus and the brain retracted with a malleable retractor. A drill can then be used to feather the posterior table bone flush with the anterior cranial fossa. The frontal recess is occluded with fascia and bone plugs as previously described (see sinus obliteration section).

Simple lacerations of the dura can be repaired with interrupted 4–0 braided nylon sutures. More complex injuries may require neurosurgical debridement and closure with a pericranial flap. If a pericranial flap is placed intracranially, a 3-mm bone kerf must be generated above the orbital rims. This defect will allow insertion of the pericranial flap without cutting off its blood supply. Reconstruction of the anterior table may require the use of bone fragments from both the anterior and posterior tables. Finally, the incision is closed as described in open reduction and internal fixation.

Naso-Orbito-Ethmoid Complex Fractures

Most naso-orbito-ethmoid fractures are caused by high-velocity injuries associated with motor vehicle accidents, assaults, and sports activities. The complex and intricate anatomy of the central midface makes these injuries the most challenging of all facial fractures to repair. Inadequate treatment can result in: telecanthus, enophthalmos, narrowed palpebral fissure width, as well as deprojection and foreshortening of the nose. Significant functional sequelae can include: CSF fistula, anosmia, epiphora, diplopia, and sinusitis. Treatment goals focus on return of function (orbits, frontal recess, and lacrimal system) followed by restoration of premorbid facial contour (repair of the medial canthus, nasal bones, and frontal bone). The primary repair is critical, because revision surgery is extremely challenging and often unsatisfactory.

Anatomy

The naso-orbito-ethmoid complex encompasses the nasal root (bilateral nasal bones), anterior skull base (frontal bone and cribriform plate), medial orbit (e.g., frontal process of maxilla and lacrimal bones), ethmoid bone (ethmoid air cells and lamina papyracea), nasal septum, and anterior table of the frontal bone. The normal intercanthal distance is ~30 to 35 mm, and is equivalent to the width of the nasal base and each palpebral fissure. The interpupillary distance is normally twice this distance (~60 mm) (**Fig. 36.15**). Intercanthal distances greater than 30 to 35 mm result in telecanthus, which is readily apparent even to the untrained eye. These relationships are maintained by the medial canthal ligament.

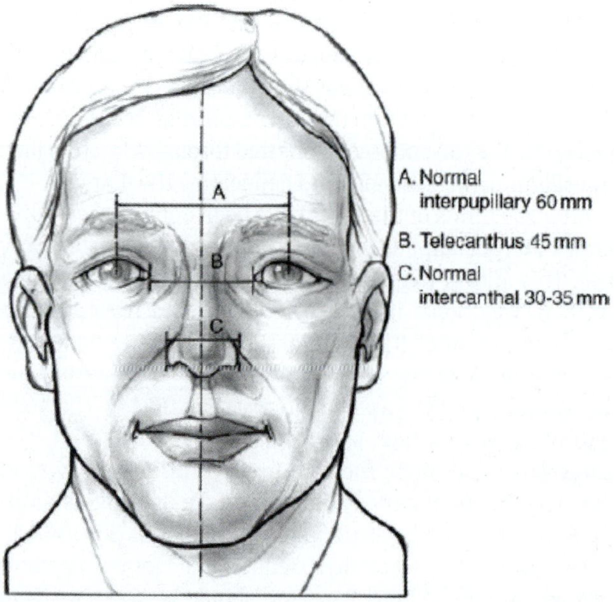

Fig. 36.15 Illustration demonstrating **(A)** normal interpupillary distance, 60 mm; **(B)** widened intercanthal distance (greater than 30 to 35 mm); and **(C)** normal intercanthal distance (30 to 35 mm). Note that the intercanthal distance is normally equivalent to the nasal base width and half the interpupillary distance. (Used with permission from Strong EB. Frontal sinus and naso-orbital-ethmoid complex fractures. In: Papel ID, ed. Facial Plastic and Reconstructive Surgery, 3rd ed. New York: Thieme; 2009, page 987.)

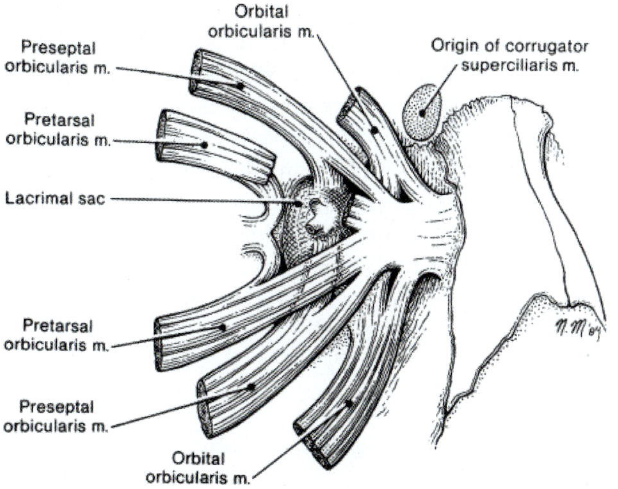

Fig. 36.16 Illustration of the medial canthal ligament. It attaches to the anterior and posterior lacrimal crest. It then diverges to become the pretarsal, preseptal, and orbital orbicularis oculi muscle. (Used with permission from Strong EB. Frontal sinus and naso-orbital-ethmoid complex fractures. In: Papel ID, ed. Facial Plastic and Reconstructive Surgery, 3rd ed. New York: Thieme; 2009, page 987.)

The ligament arises from the tarsal plate and orbicularis oculi muscle. It then splits to surround the lacrimal sac and inserts on the anterior and posterior lacrimal crest, as well as the frontal process of the maxilla (**Fig. 36.16**). The bony horizontal buttresses of the naso-orbito-ethmoid complex are the superior and inferior orbital rims (**Fig. 36.17A**). The vertical buttresses are the frontal process of the maxilla and the frontal bone (**Fig. 36.17B**). The secondary buttresses (nasal septum, ethmoid, and lacrimal bones) provide little structural support. The key anatomic feature of naso-orbito-ethmoid fractures is disruption of the medial orbit (i.e., frontal process of the maxilla and the lacrimal bone) and lateralization of the medical canthal ligament. This ligament-bone complex has been termed the central fragment because it is *central* to both the diagnosis and surgical repair of these injuries (**Fig. 36.18**).

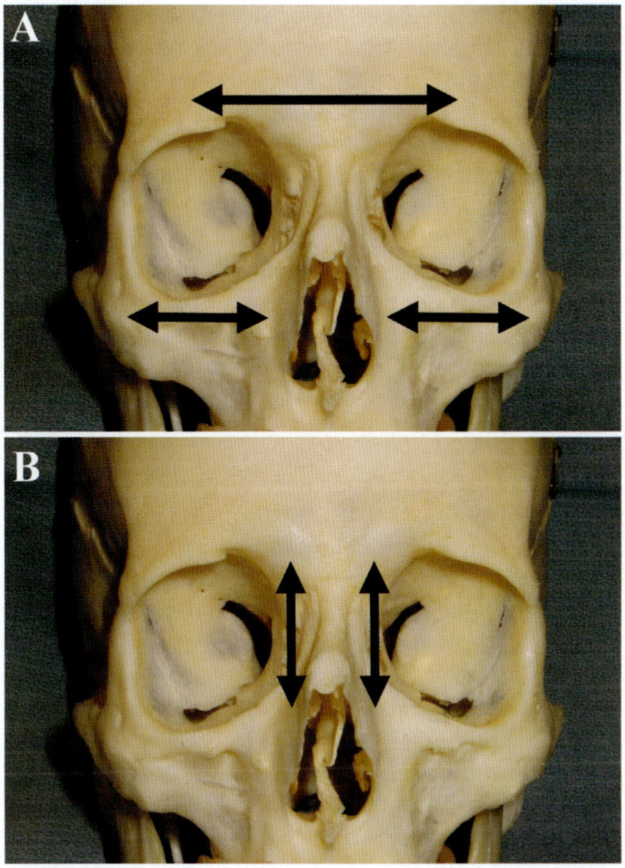

Fig. 36.17 Photograph of the major buttresses supporting the naso-orbito-ethmoid complex. **(A)** The horizontal buttresses include the superior and inferior orbital rims. **(B)** The vertical buttresses include the frontomaxillary buttresses.

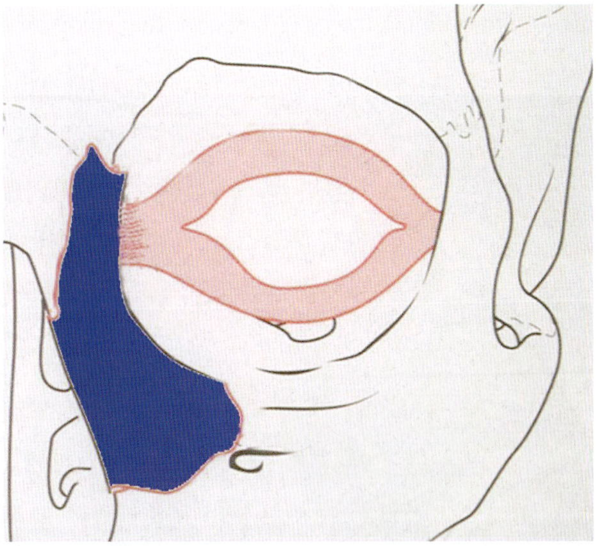

Fig. 36.18 The key to diagnosis and treatment of naso-orbito-ethmoid fractures is the "central fragment" of bone, shown here in blue. The medial canthal ligament normally attaches to this segment of bone.

Diagnosis

Physical Examination

Injuries to the naso-orbito-ethmoid complex can be difficult to diagnose when there is significant facial swelling. A full head and neck examination should be performed including the brain, spine, orbits, and possible CSF leak. Both neurosurgery and ophthalmology consultations are recommended. Physical findings suggestive of a naso-orbito-ethmoid fracture include: (1) widening of the intercanthal distance greater than 30 to 35 mm; (2) narrowing of the palpebral fissure width; (3) widening of the nasal dorsum; and (4) rotation, deprojection, and shortening of the nose. External palpation of the nose may reveal crepitus, mobility, and lack of tip support. Lack of support along the entire nasal dorsum is an indication that bone grafting will be necessary for reconstruction.[27] In sedated or unconscious patients, a “bow string” test can be performed. The medial canthus/eyelid can be grasped with forceps and gently lateralized to evaluate the stability of the medial canthal ligament insertion on the maxillary/lacrimal bones (i.e., central fragment). A “soft” end-point indicates disruption of the naso-orbito-ethmoid complex. A second technique involves insertion of a Boies elevator into the nose and bimanual palpation of the medial canthal insertion. Any mobility of this area indicates a fracture.

Radiography

The gold standard for radiologic diagnosis is a thin-cut (1.0 to 1.5 mm) axial CT, with coronal, sagittal, and 3D reconstructions. Because the nasofrontal recess is just medial to the naso-orbito-ethmoid complex, the frontal sinus outflow tract must be carefully evaluated (see frontal sinus fractures). Characteristic naso-orbito-ethmoid fracture findings include: (1) disruption and widening of the nasal dorsum in the coronal plane; (2) a “Y-sign,” occurring when the frontal process of the maxilla/lacrimal bone fractures is at the insertion of the canthal ligament, resulting in a Y-shaped bone fragment (**Fig. 36.19**); and (3) depression of the nasal root and disruption of the nasofrontal recess. The 3D reconstruction can be quite helpful to determine how many bone fragments are present in the fracture, and to give the patient/family a better understanding of the injury.

Fracture Classification and Incidence

Markowitz et al.[28] devised a classification system for naso-orbito-ethmoid fractures based on the condition of the central fragment.[29] Type I fractures result in a single, noncomminuted central fragment without medial canthal ligament disruption (**Fig. 36.20A**). Type II fractures are characterized by comminution of the bony central fragment, but with maintenance of the medial canthal attachment to a definable segment of bone (**Fig. 36.20B**). Type III fractures demonstrate both severe central fragment comminution and disruption of the medial canthal ligament (**Fig. 36.20C**). Type III fractures are based on soft tissue disruption. The diagnosis is therefore made intraoperatively, not radiographically.

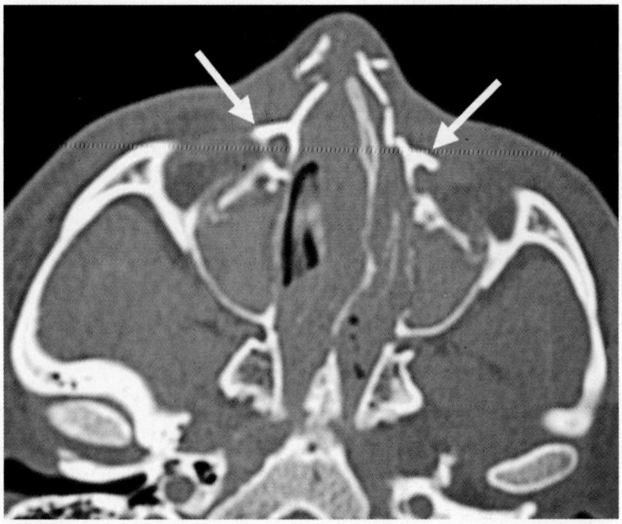

Fig. 36.19 Axial computed tomography scan of a naso-orbito-ethmoid fracture. Note the disruption of the frontal process of the maxilla and the lacrimal system resulting in a Y-sign (*arrows*).

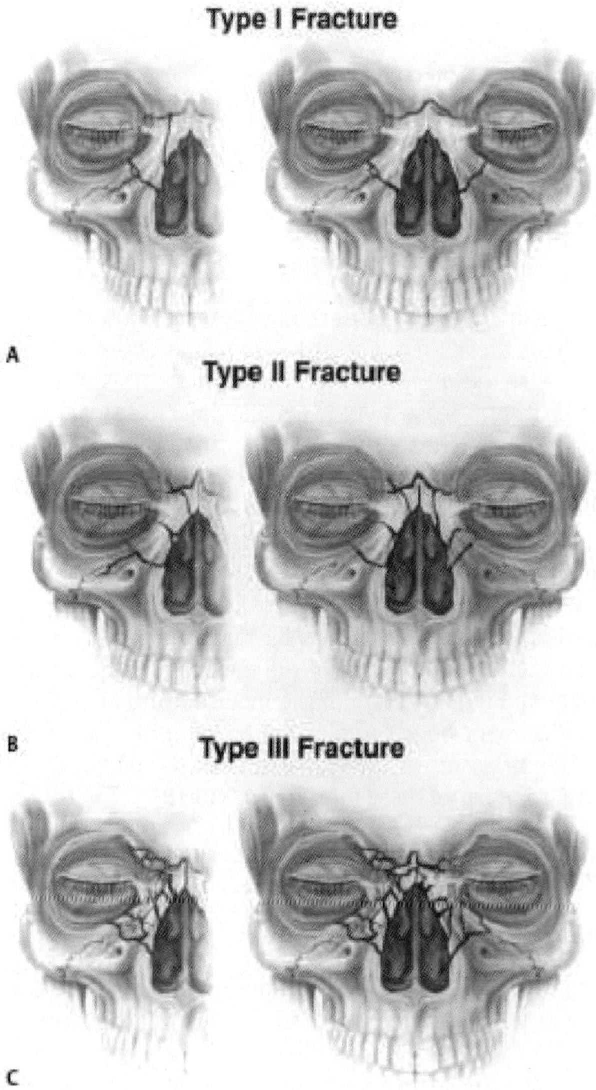

Fig. 36.20 Classification of naso-orbito-ethmoid complex fractures. **(A)** Type I injuries involve a single, noncomminuted central fragment without disruption of the medial canthal tendon; **(B)** type II injuries involve comminution of the central fragment, without disruption of the medial canthal tendon; **(C)** type III injuries involve comminution of the central fragment and disruption of the medial canthal tendon from the bone. (Used with permission from Strong EB. Frontal sinus and naso-orbital-ethmoid complex fractures. In: Papel ID, ed. Facial Plastic and Reconstructive Surgery, 3rd ed. New York: Thieme; 2009, page 988.)

Treatment

Repair of naso-orbito-ethmoid fractures requires an extended surgical exposure, a meticulous bony reconstruction of the central fragment, and careful redraping of the soft tissues in the medial canthal region. Facial fractures peripheral to the naso-orbito-ethmoid complex (maxillary, zygomatic, and frontal sinus) are generally repaired first. This reconstitutes a stable scaffold upon which to base the naso-orbito-ethmoid repair. Although existing lacerations can provide helpful access points for the surgical repair, extended access is generally required for an accurate reduction. The standard surgical approaches used include: a coronal incision for access to the nasal root and application of bone grafts (see frontal sinus fractures treatment); transconjunctival incision(s) for access to the inferior orbital rim and medial orbital wall; and a sublabial incisions for access to the frontal process of the maxilla. Some surgeons prefer a subciliary eyelid incision instead of a transconjunctival incision, because it allows for more direct access to the medial orbital rim and frontal process of the maxilla. The authors prefer to avoid a subciliary eyelid incision to reduce the risk of postoperative ectropion, and to gain direct access to the medial orbit. Instead, the transconjunctival incision is combined with a limited (5 to 10 mm) lower eyelid incision in the "periorbital sulcus" over the frontal process of the maxilla. This limited exposure allows for application of hardware on the frontal process of the maxilla without the risk of ectropion. Incisions across the eyebrows and glabella ("open sky") result in unacceptable scarring/ paresthesias and should be avoided.

Type I Fractures

Nondisplaced fractures can be observed. Significantly displaced fractures (>2 mm) may require open reduction. Because the canthal ligament is intact, caution must be used to ensure that iatrogenic disruption does not occur. Location of the ligament can be determined by passing a 25-gauge needle through the skin just above the medial canthal complex. Subperiosteal elevation from the coronal incision will then expose the needle, alerting the surgeon to stop the dissection prior to reaching the medial canthal ligament. Exposure of the central fragment from above and below is continued until fracture reduction can be achieved. A 3- to 5-hole titanium plate (1.0 to 1.3 mm) is then used to fixate the central fracture to the frontal bone from above. The plate is not placed spanning the central fragment because this exposure would likely result in iatrogenic detachment of the ligament from the central fragment. The width of the plate could also widen the nasal dorsum. A second plate is generally applied inferiorly from the central fragment to the maxilla below, via the sublabial incision and the limited lower eyelid incision. Gross realignment of septal fractures should also be addressed in the acute setting whenever possible because this will improve support for the nasal dorsum and tip.

Type II Fractures

Type II fractures should be treated with ORIF as described for type I fractures. If the central fragment is too small and/or unstable for internal fixation with miniplates, a transnasal wire should be used. Transnasal wires are applied via the coronal approach by drilling two holes in the central fragment: one above and one below the attachment of the medial canthal ligament. One end of a 28-gauge wire is then passed, from lateral to medial, through each of the holes. The free ends are then twisted down tightly onto the internal (nasal) surface of the central fragment. At this point, the central fragment is stable and well controlled with the wire. A 14-gauge needle (or wire passer) is then passed from the contralateral (uninjured) medial canthal region, behind the nasal bones, below the skull base, and exposing the needle tip on the injured side. Accurate needle placement is *critical*. It must be passed below the frontoethmoid suture line (i.e., skull base) to avoid a CSF leak. It must also be passed posterior and superior to the lacrimal fossa to ensure the appropriate angle pull for an accurate reduction (**Fig. 36.21**). Placement anterior to the lacrimal fossa will simply "splay" the canthal ligaments and result in postoperative telecanthus.[30]

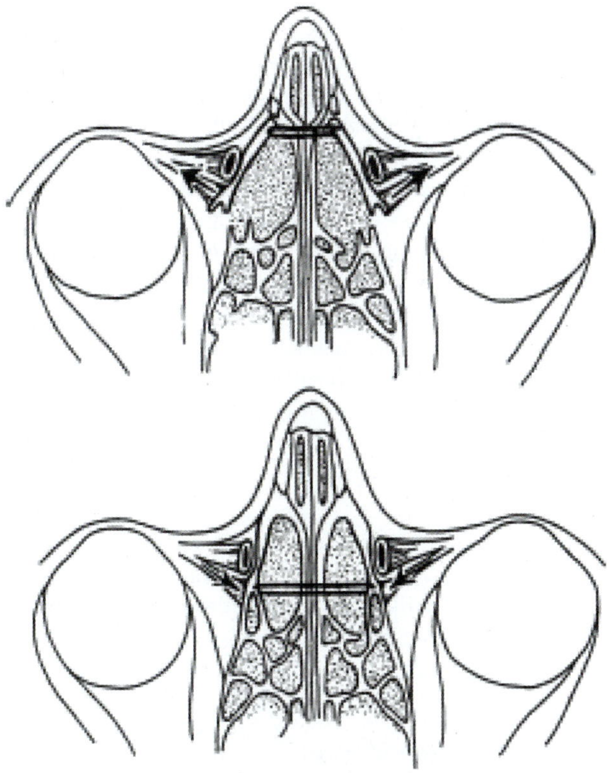

Fig. 36.21 (A) Placement of transnasal wires anterior to the lacrimal fossa results in rotation of the central fragment laterally, resulting in postoperative telecanthus. **(B)** Placement of transnasal wires posterior and superior to the lacrimal fossa provides support for the medial canthal tendon, minimizing the risk of postoperative telecanthus. (Used with permission from Strong EB. Frontal sinus and naso-orbital-ethmoid complex fractures. In: Papel ID, ed. Facial Plastic and Reconstructive Surgery, 3rd ed. New York: Thieme; 2009, page 989.)

The wires are then passed through the needle lumen to the contralateral (uninjured) side, and the needle is removed. The central fragment is then reduced with direct, cutaneous pressure on the medial canthal region. Tension is also applied on the transnasal wire to maintain the reduction. Finally, the wire is fixated to a miniscrew in the glabella region on the contralateral (uninjured) side. Over-reduction of the central fragment reduces the risk of postoperative telecanthus, and excessive narrowing of the intercanthal distance rarely if ever occurs. For bilateral fractures, the technique is identical. However, *both* wires must be passed across the midline prior to fixation.

After closure of the incisions, nasal bolsters are applied to assist with redraping the medial canthal soft tissues. Aquaplast nasal splint material (WFR/Aquaplast Corp., Wyckoff, NJ) is trimmed into two pieces that cover each lateral nasal sidewall. They are not heated, but are used for their rigidity, design (i.e., preexisting holes), and accessibility in the operating room. Each splint is wrapped in iodoform gauze to protect the underlying tissue from pressure necrosis. The bolsters are placed along the lateral nasal side wall and the first of two 14-gauge needles is passed through the holes in the bolster, through the fractured nasal bones just below the nasal root, and through a hole in the opposite bolster. The needle should be passed posterior to the midline of the splint (i.e., away from the nasal dorsum). This will apply pressure preferentially to the nasal base and medial canthus. A second needle is passed through the bolsters in a similar fashion, just below the nasal bones (**Fig. 36.22A**). A 26-gauge wire is then passed through each needle, and the needles are removed. The wires are twisted down simultaneously on each side, helping to redrape the soft tissues of the medial canthal region and lateral nasal sidewall (**Fig. 36.22B**). The wires should be twisted tight enough to apply gentle pressure to the overlying skin, but not result in necrosis. The skin underlying the bolsters should be checked on a daily basis to ensure adequate vascularity. The wires are then cut and the bolsters removed at 1 week. No anesthetic is required for removal.

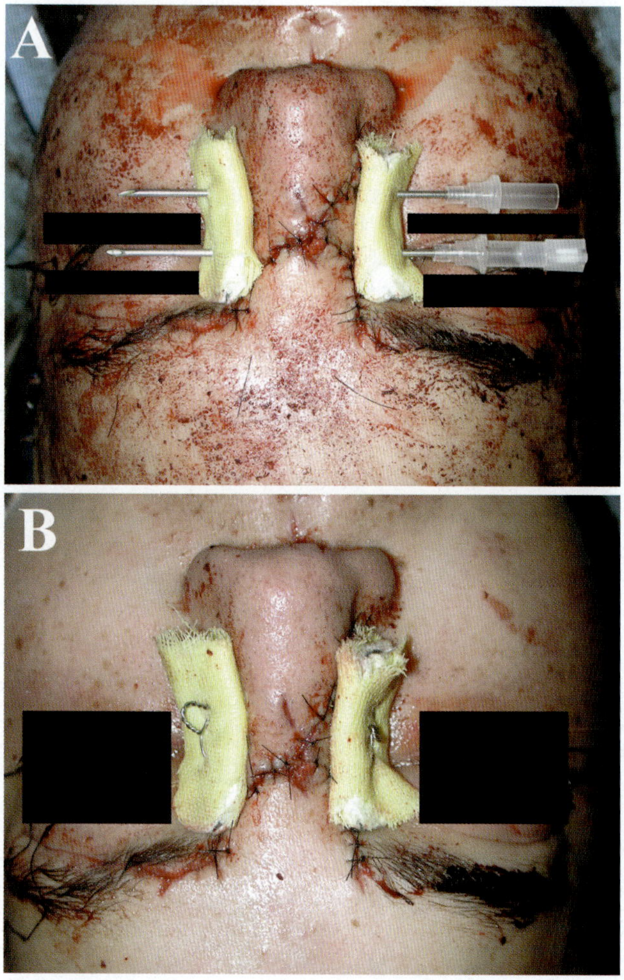

Fig. 36.22 Placement of nasal bolsters. **(A)** Two 14-gauge angiocatheters are placed across the nose and through each of two nasal bolsters. **(B)** A 26-gauge wire is passed through the needles and then twisted down to apply mild pressure to the lateral nasal sidewalls. This will minimize tissue edema and optimize redraping of the soft tissues. Note that nasal bolsters do not play any role in bone reduction. (Used with permission from Strong EB. Frontal sinus and naso-orbital-ethmoid complex fractures. In: Papel ID, ed. Facial Plastic and Reconstructive Surgery, 3rd ed. New York: Thieme; 2009, page 990.)

Type III Fractures

Type III fractures result in disruption of the canthal ligament and comminution of the central fragment. Reconstitution of the medial canthal complex can be performed with one of two techniques: (1) bone graft reconstruction of the central fragment; or (2) use of a "canthal barb."

Bone Graft/Transnasal Wires

Working through the coronal incision, the detached central fragment (or a small bone graft of similar size) is located and two holes are drilled through it to accommodate a transnasal wire. The medial canthal ligament is then located by applying internal traction to the medial canthal soft tissue with forceps, and observing the cutaneous skin movement. The area that results in 1:1 motion of the skin with traction on the soft tissues is the medial canthal ligament. A 28-gauge wire suture is then passed through the internal medial canthal ligament remnant twice. The needle is removed and each end of the wire is passed through one of the holes in the bone graft. The free ends of the wire are twisted down tightly onto the internal (nasal) surface of the bone graft to secure the medial canthal ligament. The medial canthal ligament is now firmly attached to bone, and the injury has been converted from a type III fracture to a type II fracture. This can then be managed as described for type II fractures.

Canthal Barb

A more recently described technique for repair of type III injuries is to use a canthal barb (Synthes Inc., West Chester,

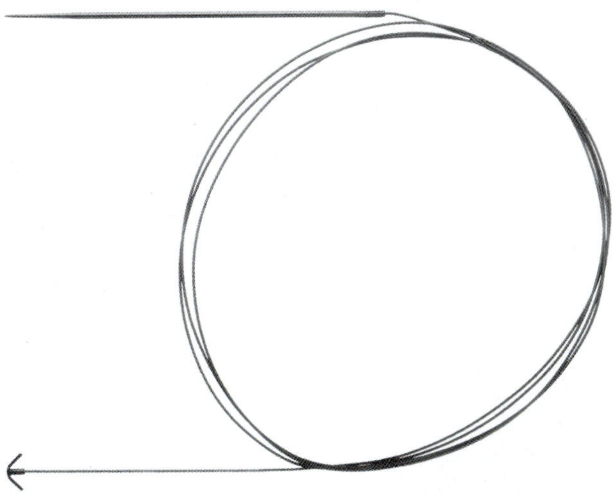

Fig. 36.23 Illustration of a canthal barb consisting of a straight needle with titanium wire and attached barb. (Used with permission from Synthes, Inc. or its affiliates. Copyright 2001. All rights reserved.)

PA). The canthal barb is a 26-gauge wire with a straight 4-cm needle on one end and a v-shaped barb (to "catch" the medial canthal ligament) on the opposite end (**Fig. 36.23**). A small (2-mm) incision is placed just medial to the medial canthus at the area of greatest concavity (**Fig. 36.24**). The needle is passed from superficial to deep through the canthal ligament, and grasped internally through the coronal incision. The wire is pulled through the incision until the barb catches deep in the medial canthal ligament (**Fig. 36.25**). The barb becomes buried in the soft tissue and provides excellent control of the medial canthal complex. A 1.5-mm miniplate is applied to "guide" the barb across the midline in the correct position to anatomically reconstruct the medial canthal complex and allow accurate repositioning of the medial canthus (**Fig. 36.26**). After these steps have been completed, a 14-gauge needle is passed from the contralateral side, below the skull base, exposing the tip on the injured side. The wire barb is then passed through the miniplate and the needle to the contralateral side. It is then fixated to a bone screw in the glabella region. Alternatively, the wire can be threaded through the distal hole in the miniplate before the plate is fixed to the bone. The plate can then be positioned and fixated to pull the canthal barb anatomically into the appropriate position. With this approach, the wire need not be passed across the skull base, but can be fixated to a screw on the ipsilateral glabellar bone.

Patients with type III fractures may have severe comminution of their nasal bones that often requires onlay calvarial bone grafting.[31] The graft must be shaped to mimic the normal nasal length and contour. The cephalic end of the graft is secured to the frontal bone at the glabella with two position screws.[32] An open rhinoplasty

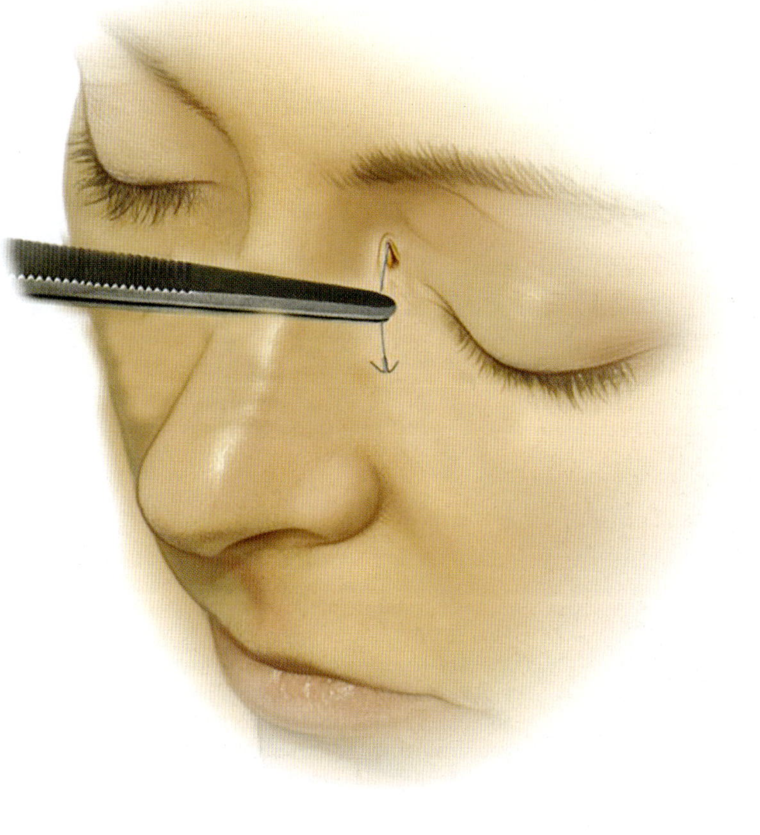

Fig. 36.24 A canthal barb being pulled through a small skin incision. The barb is then fed through the incision and allowed to engage the soft tissue of the medial canthal tendon. (Used with permission from Synthes, Inc. or its affiliates. Copyright 2001. All rights reserved.)

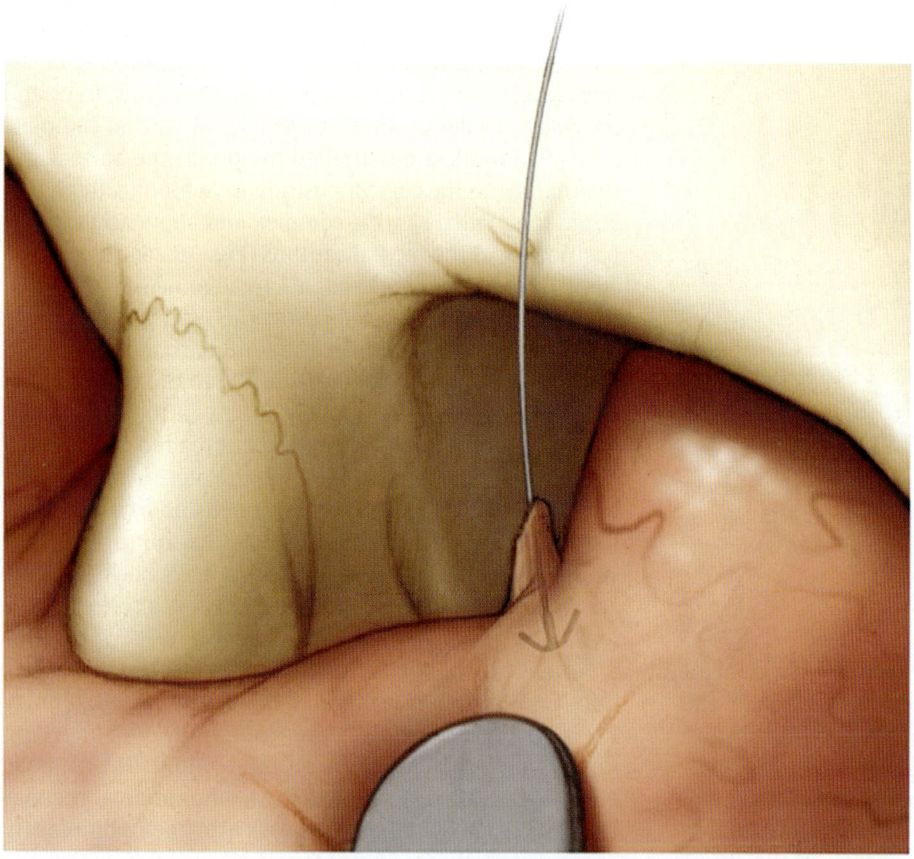

Fig. 36.25 A canthal barb that has engaged the canthal tendon. The surgeon can now control the medial canthal complex with the wire suture. (Used with permission from Synthes, Inc. or its affiliates. Copyright 2001. All rights reserved.)

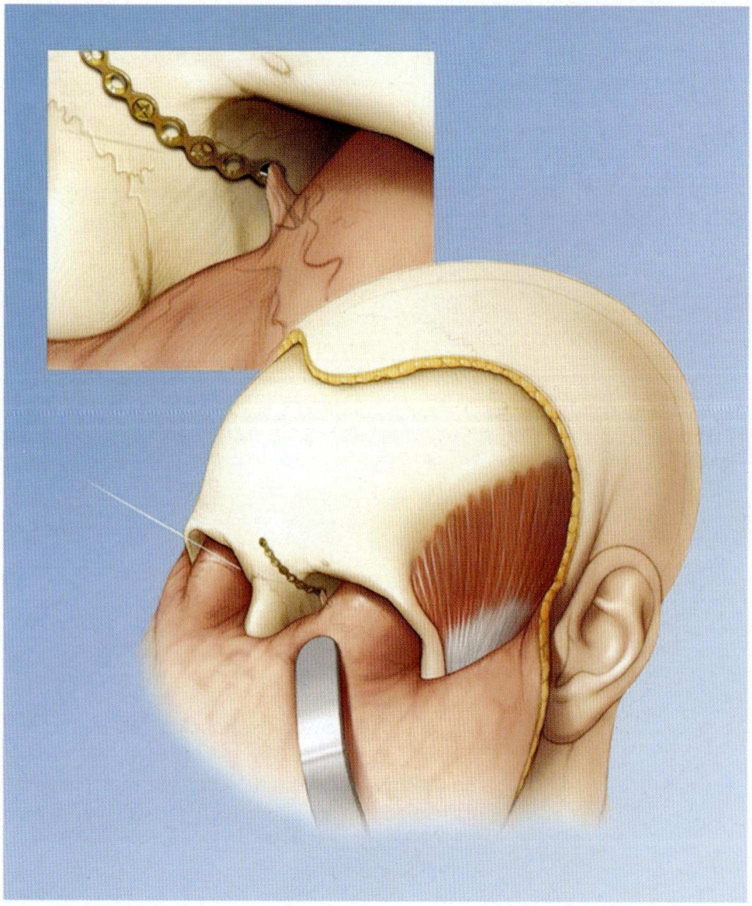

Fig. 36.26 The transnasal wire has been passed across the skull base and is ready to be fixated on the contralateral nasal root. **Inset**: note the medial canthal tendon is controlled by the canthal barb. It is being pulled posterior and superior to the lacrimal fossa. (Used with permission from Synthes, Inc. or its affiliates. Copyright 2001. All rights reserved.)

approach assists in securing the caudal end of the implant between the lower lateral cartilages. Known injuries to the lacrimal system should be managed with stenting at the time of the bony repair.

Orbital Blowout Fractures

Orbital blowout fractures result from direct trauma to the globe or periorbita. The orbital floor and medial orbital wall are most commonly fractured, resulting in the prolapse of orbital contents into the ethmoid and/or maxillary sinuses.[33] Common etiologies include motor vehicle accidents, sports injuries, and interpersonal altercations. Treatment goals include preventing visual loss, diplopia, and enophthalmos. Successful surgical repair of these injuries requires adequate exposure, visualization of the entire fracture, and anatomic repair of the defect.

Diagnosis

Physical Examination

A complete head and neck examination starts by evaluating the ABCs, cervical spine, orbits, and a methodical head and neck examination. Once an orbital injury has been diagnosed, a focused examination should document: the visual acuity, evidence of globe injury (hyphema, globe laceration/rupture), periorbital tenderness or bony "step-offs," extra-ocular muscle function, and infraorbital nerve function. Forced duction testing can be helpful to differentiate extraocular muscle entrapment from edema/contusion. Although this can be done under local anesthesia (tetracaine drops), more accurate results can be obtained under general anesthesia. The rectus muscle is grasped through the sclera at its insertion near the fornix. Upward traction is applied along the arc of globe rotation. Decreased globe mobility, as compared with the contralateral side, is consistent with extraocular muscle entrapment. Limitation of superior gaze suggests inferior rectus entrapment, whereas restriction of lateral gaze suggests medial rectus entrapment. An ophthalmologic consultation is indicated when there is concern for globe injury such as hyphema, retinal detachment, or traumatic optic neuropathy.

Radiography

A thin-cut (1 to 2 mm) axial CT scan is the radiologic gold standard for diagnosis of orbital fractures. Coronal and sagittal reconstructions are essential, whereas 3D reconstructions can be helpful. The coronal cuts provide excellent views of the orbital floor, medial orbital walls, and orbital apex. The bony integrity of the orbit should be evaluated; however, caution must be used when comparing orbital volume between sides. Scans that are taken out of the true orthogonal planes will present slices from different regions of the orbit on each side, giving the false impression that one orbit is larger than the other. Soft tissue findings such as orbital hematoma, emphysema, or extraocular muscle contusion/edema should be documented. Axial views are helpful to evaluate the orbital apex and optic canal. Sagittal views can offer more detailed information about orbital floor integrity and contour. Three-dimensional reconstructions can assist with visualization and orientation of specific bone fragments in complex fractures.

Fracture Classification

Pure orbital blowout fractures can be divided into two main types: lamina papyracea (medial wall) fractures and orbital floor fractures. Lamina papyracea fractures are less common but can incur greater risk of enophthalmos than orbital floor fractures.[34] Orbital floor fractures can be subdivided into two types: trap-door and blowout fractures. Trap-door injuries commonly fracture laterally along the path of the infraorbital nerve and hinge medially from the lamina papyracea (**Fig. 36.27**). This results in prolapse of the orbital contents into the maxillary sinus. Trap-door fractures have a propensity to "snap" closed and strangulate the periobita, particularly in the pediatric population.

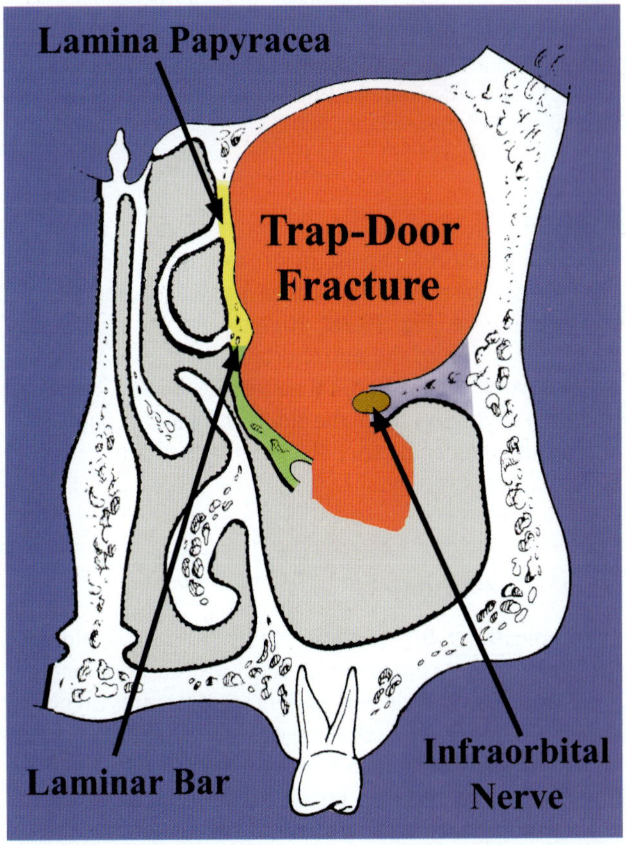

Fig. 36.27 Illustration of a trap-door orbital fracture. (Used with permission from Strong EB, Kim KK, Diaz RC. Endoscopic approach to orbital blowout fracture repair. Otolaryngol Head Neck Surg 2004;131(5):683–695, page 689, figure 10.)

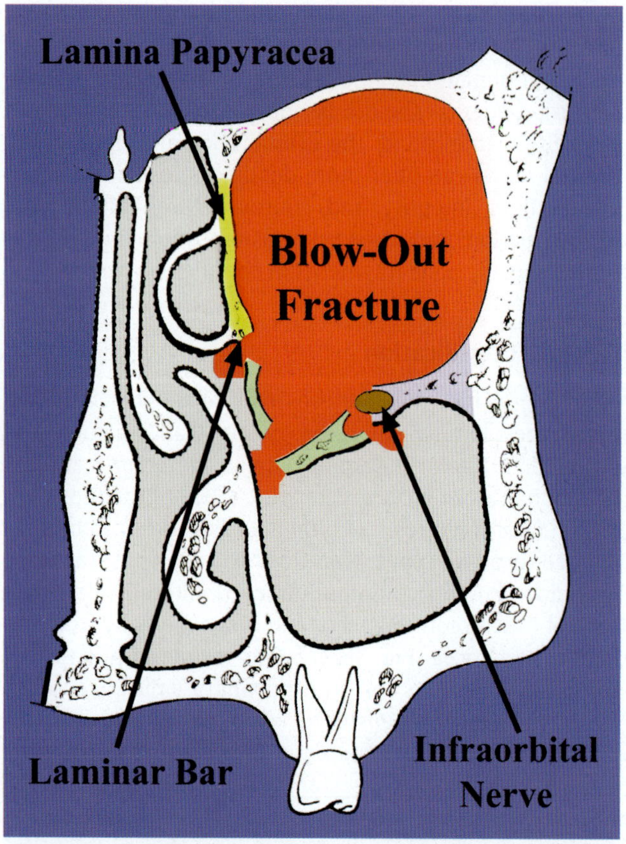

Fig. 36.28 Illustration of an orbital floor blowout fracture. (Used with permission from Strong EB, Kim KK, Diaz RC. Endoscopic approach to orbital blowout fracture repair. Otolaryngol Head Neck Surg 2004;131(5):683–695.)

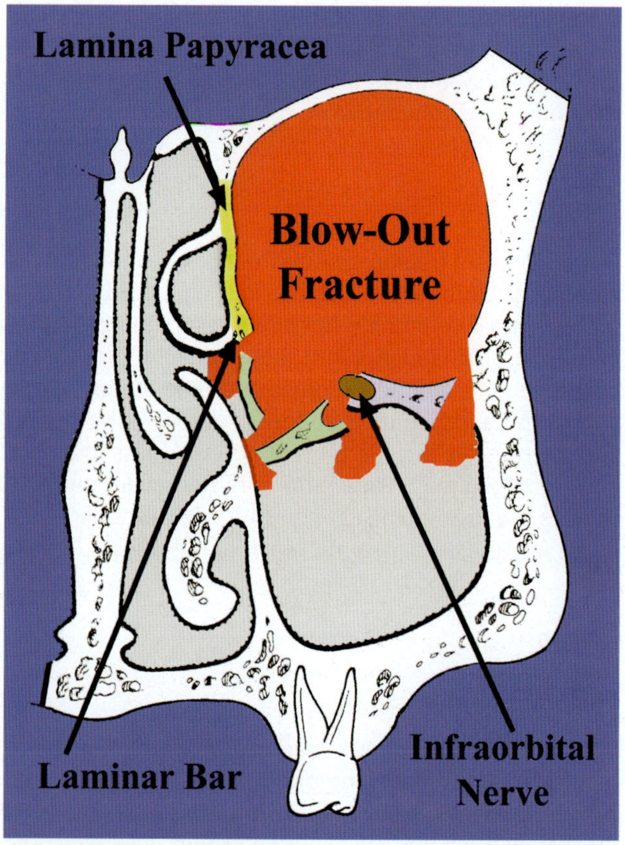

Fig. 36.29 Illustration of a complex orbital floor blowout fracture. (Used with permission from Strong EB, Kim KK, Diaz RC. Endoscopic approach to orbital blowout fracture repair. Otolaryngol Head Neck Surg 2004;131(5):683–695.)

"Blowout fractures" result in greater disruption of the orbital floor between the lamina papyracea and the infraorbital nerve (**Fig. 36.28**). Higher velocity injuries will cause disruption of the entire orbital floor, extending laterally beyond the infraorbital nerve (**Fig. 36.29**). Two-wall fractures involving both the floor and lamina papyracea also occur, and can be very challenging to repair.

Treatment

Surgical Indications

The indications for surgical repair of orbital blowout fractures can be controversial, but most authors include: (1) extraocular muscle entrapment; (2) fractures involving greater than 50% of the orbital floor; and (3) acute enophthalmos in the face of orbital edema. Besides globe immobility and reduced forced duction testing, patients with entrapment may complain of severe pain or nausea with eye motion.

The timing of surgical repair is also controversial. Differentiation between globe restriction secondary to edema, muscle contusion, or frank entrapment can be quite challenging. More recent literature suggests that patients with positive forced duction testing, diplopia within 30 degrees of primary gaze, marked pain or nausea with globe motion, or CT findings suggestive of entrapment will have better outcomes with early intervention. Trap door fractures in the pediatric population should be dealt with urgently to avoid permanent extraocular muscle injury or necrosis.[35]

Surgical Technique (Open Approaches)

All patients are consented for the procedure including the risks of bleeding, infection, diplopia, eyelid malposition, poor aesthetic result, and visual loss. Direct eyelid approaches can be divided into two types: transcutaneous and transconjunctival. The transconjunctival approach can be subdivided into preseptal, postseptal, and transcaruncular. Endoscopic transmaxillary (orbital floor) and transethmoidal (lamina papyracea) approaches have also been described. The choice of surgical approach depends on fracture type, surgeon experience, and patient preference (**Fig. 36.30**).

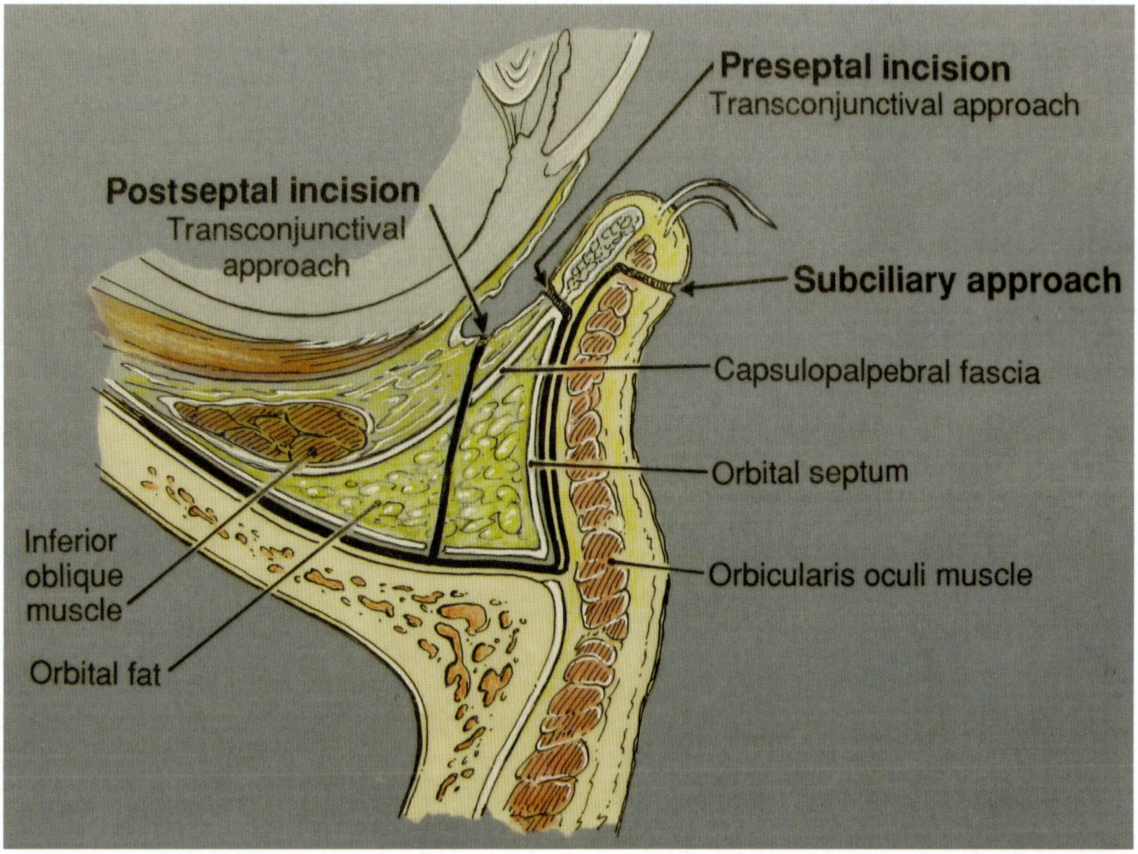

Fig. 36.30 Illustration of the three types of eyelid incisions: (1) transcutaneous; (2) transconjunctival, preseptal; (3) transconjunctival, postseptal. (Used with permission from Strong EB, Sykes JM. Zygoma complex fractures. Facial Plast Surg 1998;14(1):105–115, page 109, figure 7.)

Transconjunctival Preseptal Approach

For the transconjunctival preseptal approach,[36] corneal shields are inserted and the palpebral conjunctiva is injected with ~1 mL of 1% lidocaine with 1:100,000 epinephrine. Retractors are applied to the globe (malleable) and lower eyelid (Desmarres) to expose the fornix of the lower eyelid. If there is significant tension on the lid, a lateral canthotomy and cantholysis can be performed. A semilunar mucosal incision is made 4 to 5 mm inferior to the tarsal plate, through the palpebral conjunctiva. Careful blunt dissection is performed (in a preseptal plane) down to the orbital rim using tenotomy scissors. Cotton-tipped applicators are helpful to assist with blunt dissection. The correct dissection plane is relatively avascular, requiring minimal use of bipolar cautery. If the dissection becomes too deep, orbital fat will be exposed; superficial dissection will expose/disrupt the orbicularis oculi muscle. Once the orbital rim has been exposed, a subperiosteal plane is developed along the orbital floor. The dissection circumferentially exposes the fracture while preserving the infraorbital nerve. Small bone fragments are removed and the orbital contents, including the inferior rectus muscle, are delivered back into the orbital cavity. Excessive traction should not be applied to entrapped tissue. If necessary, a small segment of orbital floor bone can be removed to facilitate reduction of the orbital contents. A sterile piece of X-ray film can be trimmed to ~3 × 4 cm, and inserted into the wound to assist with retraction of orbital fat. The malleable retractor is then inserted below the X-ray film and elevated. This effectively increases the surface area of the retractor to a size much larger than could be accommodated by the incision. After repair of the fracture, interrupted 6–0 fast absorbing gut sutures are used to close the conjunctiva.

Transconjunctival Postseptal Approach

For the transconjunctival postseptal approach,[36] a malleable retractor is inserted to retract the globe and the Desmarres is inserted to retract the lower lid. It is important that the retraction exposes a semilunar incision line ~5 mm anterior to the globe. The orbital fat should be compressed over the rim, between the two retractors. A Colorado Needle (Stryker, Kalamazoo, MI), set on a very low setting, is then used to cut directly onto the orbital rim. The retractors are slid medial and lateral to follow the surgeon. Caution must be used to cut directly onto the leading edge of the rim and to avoid dissection within the bony orbit. A lateral canthotomy and cantholysis can be used if additional exposure is required. The advantages of this technique are ease and rapidity of access, as well as reduced risk of eyelid malposition as the dissection does not violate the eyelid. Wound closure is performed with interrupted 6–0 fast absorbing gut.

Transcaruncular Approach

After injection with local anesthesia, the medial canthal complex is retracted medially with a fine rake, and the globe is retracted laterally with a malleable rake after injection with local anesthesia. A Colorado needle (placed on a low setting) is used to make a 10-mm conjunctival incision through or immediately behind the caruncle (**Fig. 36.31**).[37] The posterior lacrimal crest is then palpated and identified, as the dissection should proceed directly posterior to this landmark. The retractors are advanced into the wound, and pressure is applied on the medial orbital wall compressing the orbital fat posteriorly onto the lamina papyracea. Tenotomy scissors are then used to palpate the posterior lacrimal crest, and moved 1 to 2 mm posteriorly onto the medial orbital wall. Blunt dissection is used to pass between Horner's muscle and the orbital septum, exposing the lamina papyracea (**Fig. 36.32**). The retractors are then advanced and these steps are repeated until the lamina papyracea is well exposed using a Freer elevator (**Fig. 36.33**). A bipolar cautery is used conservatively to control bleeding. The anterior ethmoid artery may need to be ligated to expose the fracture, but this is often disrupted by the fracture and is poorly visualized. After completion of the repair, the caruncle is realigned, but no sutures are necessary for closure.

Implant Placement

Uncommonly, a single large bone fragment can be reduced into its premorbid position, or rotated to fill a small defect. This avoids the need for an implant. However, most fractures will require some type of implant for reconstruction. The majority of surgeons prefer to use alloplastic implants. The most popular materials are titanium mesh, porous polyethylene sheeting, or a composite implant made of titanium mesh surrounded by porous polyethylene sheeting (this composite material combines the malleable properties of titanium, while maintaining the smooth edges of porous polyethylene, allowing the implant to be inserted with ease). The implant may be bent freehand; however, more accurate 3D contouring can be achieved by trimming and bending the implant on a sterilized skull model. The authors currently use "preformed" titanium mesh sheeting that is

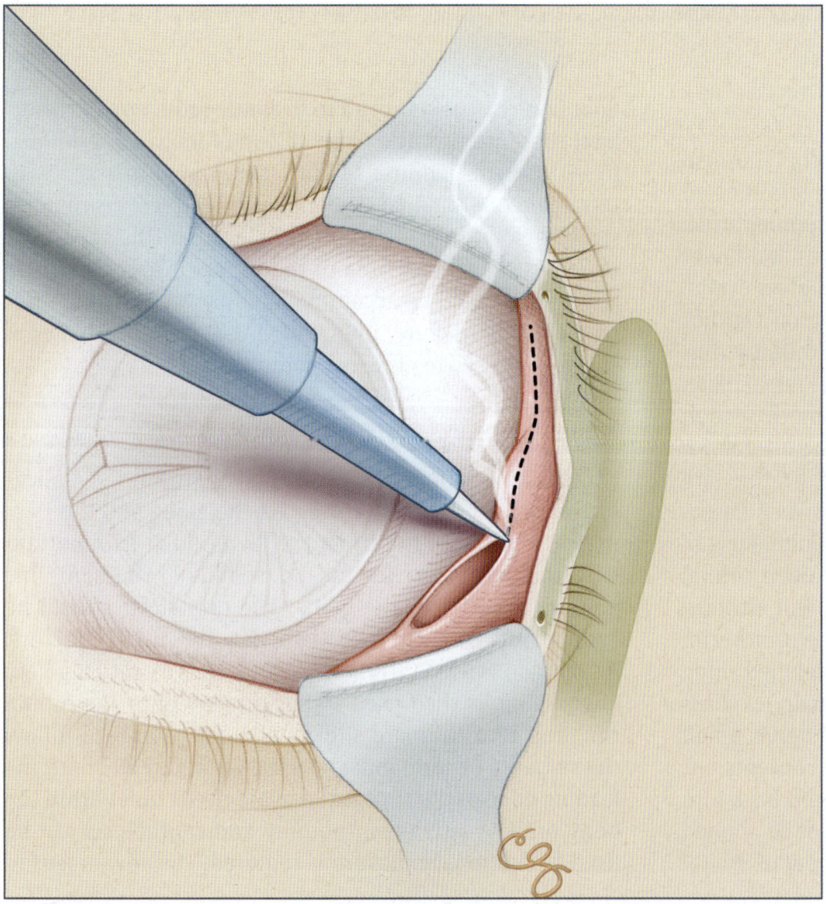

Fig. 36.31 Illustration of transcaruncular eyelid incision (right eye).

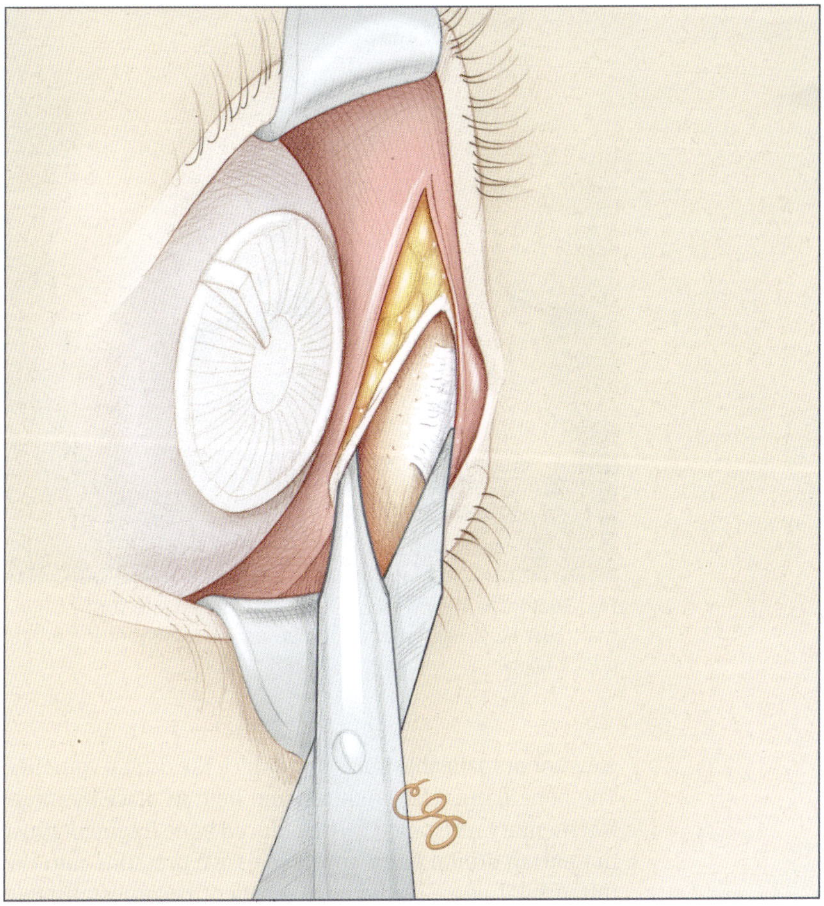

Fig. 36.32 Illustration of the transcaruncular subperiosteal dissection used to expose the lamina papyracea.

fabricated from composite CT data of normal orbital floor contours (Synthes, Paoli, PA).

The *critical step* in implant placement is visualization of the posterior shelf (either floor or medial wall) and placement of the implant on this stable bone (**Fig. 36.34**). Even among experienced orbital surgeons, the most common reason for failure in orbital reconstruction is improper placement of the implant at the posterior shelf, allowing persistent prolapse of the orbital contents into the sinus cavity. A simple way to ensure that the implant is in an acceptable position is to insert a 0-degree endoscope through the incision (or through a defect in the anterior wall of the maxillary sinus) and visualize the position of the implant. The surgeon may choose to secure the implant on the orbital rim with a single miniscrew, depending on the inherent stability of the implant after insertion.

Surgical Technique (Endoscopic Approach)

Endoscopy revolutionized sinus surgery by giving the surgeon an unprecedented view of the sinus cavities. Orbital and sinus surgery have some inherent similarities in that the surgeon is operating in a deep cavity, with limited visualization of the surgical field. Endoscopy allows the surgeon to visualize the posterior orbit, ensuring that there is adequate exposure and that implants are placed in the correct position. Several authors have described techniques for pure endoscopic repair of the orbital fractures using no eyelid incisions.[38–41] The greatest use of the endoscope, however, is that it can be inserted through any incision (i.e., eyelid, sublabial, transnasal, transmaxillary, etc.) to assist with fracture repair.

The endoscopic, transmaxillary approach to fracture repair is most applicable to trap-door and blowout fractures extending between the lamina papyracea and the infraorbital nerve. An "absolute" indication for an endoscopic repair is a trap-door fracture with entrapment and a concomitant hyphema. The hyphema precludes any attempt at anterior exposure, because retraction on the globe may lead to visual loss. But persistent entrapment of the inferior rectus may result in muscle necrosis. The transmaxillary, endoscopic approach allows the surgeon to access the fracture and release the entrapment. Secondary repair after resolution of the hyphema is then at the surgeon's discretion.

The buccal sulcus is injected with 1% lidocaine with 1:100,000 epinephrine. The surgeon stands on the patient's right and the assistant on the left holds the endoscope. A traditional Caldwell-Luc incision is used to expose the maxillary face. The upper lip can be retracted

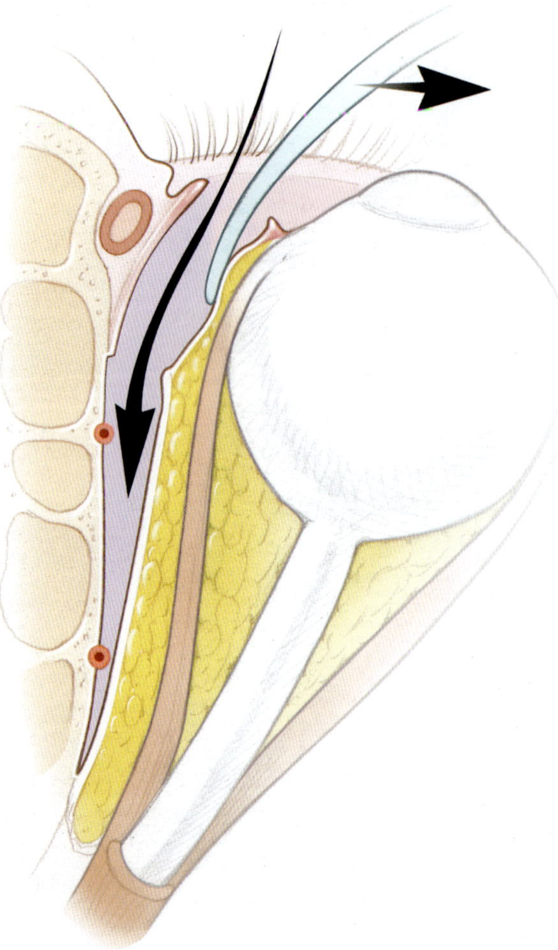

Fig. 36.33 Illustration of subperiosteal dissection used to expose the lamina papyracea fracture. Note that the proper plane of dissection starts behind the posterior lacrimal crest, protecting the lacrimal system from injury.

with a Greenberg retractor. Excessive traction on the infraorbital nerve must be avoided. An approximate 1.5 × 2.0 cm, horizontal antrostomy is placed directly below the infraorbital nerve using an osteotome and Kerrison rongeur (**Fig. 36.35**). A 30-degree endoscope is placed through the antrostomy, blood is suctioned, and the maxillary sinus ostium is identified on the superoposterior medial wall. The infraorbital nerve is identified in the orbital floor. The fracture's dimensions can be localized by applying gentle pressure to the globe while visualizing the orbital floor, looking for areas of mobility or bone loss.[42]

Trapdoor Fractures

Trap-door fractures are typically "hinged" medially and are the easiest to repair endoscopically. No implant is generally required. First, the mucosa is elevated from the lateral aspect of the fracture, maintaining the integrity of the mucosa over the medial "hinge" (**Fig. 36.27**). The lateral edge of the bone flap is distracted inferiorly, and an

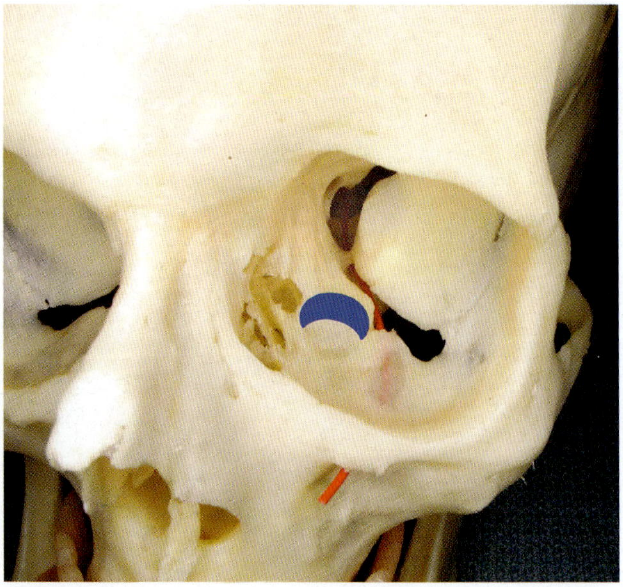

Fig. 36.34 The blue crescent highlights that stable shelf of bone that must be visualized to ensure proper placement of the orbital floor implant.

elevator or malleable is used to reduce the orbital contents. The bone flap is then reduced and held in place by interfragmentary resistance.[41] The reduced bone fragment must not entrap orbital fat or apply excessive pressure onto the infraorbital nerve. If the bone segment becomes unstable or comminuted, the fracture must be managed as a blowout fracture (see later text).

Blowout Fractures

Medial orbital floor blowout fractures are repaired with the same surgical approach as trap-door fractures. Limited circumferential mucosal dissection around the entire defect will provide adequate exposure. The natural ostia should be protected. Visualization of the posterior shelf is critical. Careful removal of all fractured bone fragments will avoid displacement back into the orbit; however, this will result in an expected transient increased prolapse of orbital fat. Once the defect margins are well visualized, a porous polyethylene implant (0.85 × 38 × 50 mm) (Medpor, Porex Surgical, Newnan, GA) is trimmed to approximate the defect. The orbital contents are then reduced using a small malleable retractor while the implant is positioned below the defect. The implant is then removed and trimmed to fit the defect more precisely. This process is repeated until the diameter is slightly (1 to 2 mm) larger than the defect. The implant is then inserted below the malleable retractor and onto the posterior shelf. The instruments are then walked forward along the implant toward the orbital rim. Pressure is applied until the anterior margin of the implant slips above the orbital rim, stabilizing the implant in place. The majority of support should come from the posterior shelf and orbital rim (**Fig. 36.36**). Medial pressure on

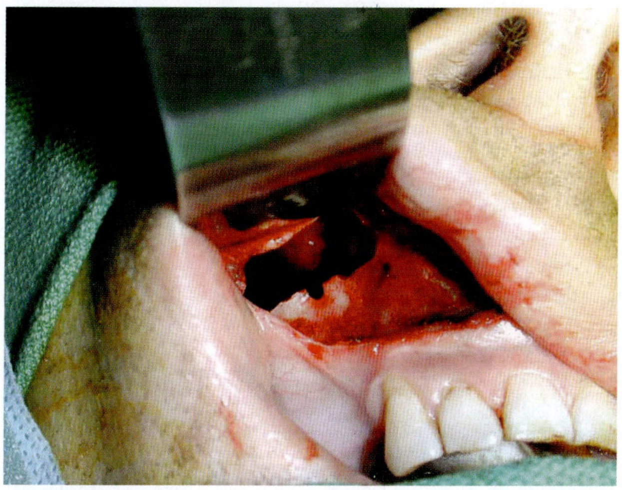

Fig. 36.35 Intraoperative photograph of the maxillary antrostomy used for access to the orbital floor. (Used with permission from Strong EB, Kim KK, Diaz RC. Endoscopic approach to orbital blowout fracture repair. Otolaryngol Head Neck Surg 2004;131(5):683–695.)

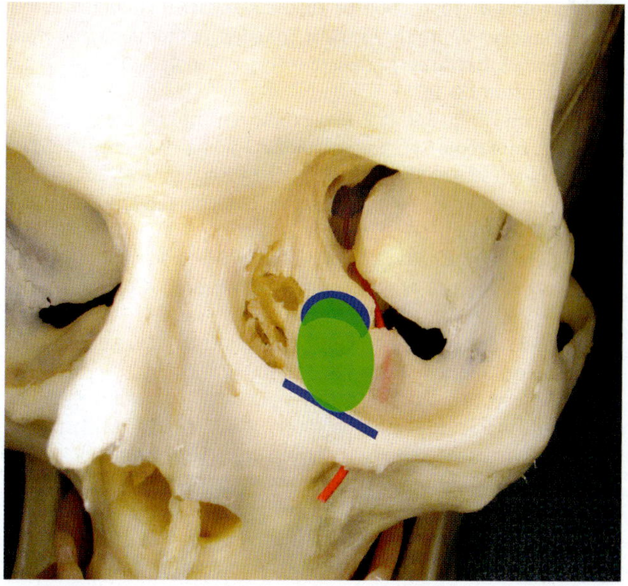

Fig. 36.36 The *blue crescent* and *line* represent the stable bone that the implant rests on. The *green oval* represents proper placement of the implant which avoids excessive pressure on the infraorbital nerve.

the infraorbital nerve should be minimized. The fracture margins are then inspected to ensure there is no fat prolapse or entrapment. A postoperative CT scan is generally obtained to ensure that the reduction is complete and that the implant is in good position.

Conclusion

Facial fractures occur across all ages, genders, races, and social status. These fractures commonly involve the paranasal sinuses. Therefore, a thorough understanding of the anatomy and potential complications (i.e., sinusitis, mucopyocele, meningitis, etc.) is critical. A surgeon who is facile with endoscopy has the advantage of minimally invasive techniques for diagnosis and treatment. Although the management strategies for different types of facial fractures vary, there are common themes. An accurate diagnosis is critical. The indications and timing of surgery should be clear cut and based on accepted physiologic and anatomic principles. Finally, meticulous surgical technique must be used to optimize the potential for a successful outcome.

References

1. Colton JJ, Beekhuis GJ. Management of nasal fractures. Otolaryngol Clin North Am 1986;19(1):73–85
2. Clayton MI, Lesser TH. The role of radiography in the management of nasal fractures. J Laryngol Otol 1986;100(7):797–801
3. Khwaja S, Pahade AV, Luff D, Green MW, Green KM. Nasal fracture reduction: local versus general anaesthesia. Rhinology 2007;45(1):83–88
4. Renner GJ. Management of nasal fractures. Otolaryngol Clin North Am 1991;24(1):195–213
5. Nahum AM. The biomechanics of maxillofacial trauma. Clin Plast Surg 1975;2(1):59–64
6. Wallis A, Donald PJ. Frontal sinus fractures: a review of 72 cases. Laryngoscope 1988;98(6 Pt 1):593–598
7. Donald PJ. Frontal sinus ablation by cranialization. Report of 21 cases. Arch Otolaryngol 1982;108(3):142–146
8. Sataloff RT, Sariego J, Myers DL, Richter HJ. Surgical management of the frontal sinus. Neurosurgery 1984;15(4):593–596
9. Gossman DG, Archer SM, Arosarena O. Management of frontal sinus fractures: a review of 96 cases. Laryngoscope 2006;116(8): 1357–1362
10. Strong EB, Pahlavan N, Saito D. Frontal sinus fractures: a 28-year retrospective review. Otolaryngol Head Neck Surg 2006;135(5):774–779
11. Rohrich RJ, Hollier LH. Management of frontal sinus fractures. Changing concepts. Clin Plast Surg 1992;19(1):219–232
12. Ritter TN. The Paranasal Sinuses: Anatomy and Surgical Technique, 2nd ed. St Louis: CV Mosby; 1978
13. Anon JB, Rontal M, Zinreich SJ. Anatomy of the Paranasal Sinuses. New York: Thieme; 1996
14. Kennedy DW, Stammberger HR. Paranasal sinuses: anatomic terminology and nomenclature. Ann Otol Rhinol Laryngol 1995; 167:7–16
15. Mosher HP, Judd DK. An analysis of seven cases of osteomyelitis of frontal bone complicating frontal sinusitis. Laryngoscope 1933;43:153–212
16. Heller EM, Jacobs JB, Holliday RA. Evaluation of the frontonasal duct in frontal sinus fractures. Head Neck 1989;11(1):46–50
17. Smith TL, Han JK, Loehrl TA, Rhee JS. Endoscopic management of the frontal recess in frontal sinus fractures: a shift in the paradigm? Laryngoscope 2002;112(5):784–790

18. Forrest CR. Application of endoscope-assisted minimal-access techniques in orbitozygomatic complex, orbital floor, and frontal sinus fractures. J Craniomaxillofac Trauma 1999;5(4):7–12, discussion 13–14
19. Graham HD III, Spring P. Endoscopic repair of frontal sinus fracture: case report. J Craniomaxillofac Trauma 1996;2(4):52–55
20. Lappert PW, Lee JW. Treatment of an isolated outer table frontal sinus fracture using endoscopic reduction and fixation. Plast Reconstr Surg 1998;102(5):1642–1645
21. Strong EB, Buchalter GM, Moulthrop TH. Endoscopic repair of isolated anterior table frontal sinus fractures. Arch Facial Plast Surg 2003;5(6):514–521
22. Luce EA. Frontal sinus fractures: guidelines to management. Plast Reconstr Surg 1987;80(4):500–510
23. Sykes JM, Donald PJ. Frontal sinus and nasofrontoethmoidal complex fractures. In: Papel ID, Nachlas N, eds. Facial Plastic and Reconstructive Surgery. Hanover, MD: Mosby-Yearbook, Inc.; 1992: 485–495
24. Heckler FR. Discussion of frontal sinus fractures. Guidelines to Management of Plastic Reconstructive Surgery 1987;80:509
25. McGraw-Wall B. Frontal sinus fractures. Facial Plast Surg 1998;14(1):59–66
26. Donald PJ, Gluckman JL, Rice DH, eds. The Sinuses. New York: Raven Press; 1995
27. Pollock RA. Nasal trauma. Pathomechanics and surgical management of acute injuries. Clin Plast Surg 1992;19(1):133–147
28. Markowitz BL, Manson PN, Sargent L, et al. Management of the medial canthal tendon in nasoethmoid orbital fractures: the importance of the central fragment in classification and treatment. Plast Reconstr Surg 1991;87(5):843–853
29. Leipziger LS, Manson PN. Nasoethmoid orbital fractures. Current concepts and management principles. Clin Plast Surg 1992;19(1):167–193
30. Sargent LA, Rogers GF. Nasoethmoid orbital fractures: diagnosis and management. J Craniomaxillofac Trauma 1999;5(1):19–27
31. Ellis E III. Sequencing treatment for naso-orbito-ethmoid fractures. J Oral Maxillofac Surg 1993;51(5):543–558
32. Hoffmann JF. Naso-orbital-ethmoid complex fracture management. Facial Plast Surg 1998;14(1):67–76
33. Jones DEP, Evans JNG. "Blowout" fractures of the orbit: an investigation into their anatomical basis. J Laryngol Otol 1967;81(10):1109–1120
34. Parsons GS, Mathog RH. Orbital wall and volume relationships. Arch Otolaryngol Head Neck Surg 1988;114(7):743–747
35. Jordan DR, Allen LH, White J, Harvey J, Pashby R, Esmaeli B. Intervention within days for some orbital floor fractures: the white-eyed blowout. Ophthal Plast Reconstr Surg 1998; 14(6):379–390
36. Appling WD, Patrinely JR, Salzer TA. Transconjunctival approach vs subciliary skin-muscle flap approach for orbital fracture repair. Arch Otolaryngol Head Neck Surg 1993;119(9): 1000–1007
37. Goldberg RA, Mancini R, Demer JL. The transcaruncular approach: surgical anatomy and technique. Arch Facial Plast Surg 2007;9(6):443–447
38. Ikeda K, Suzuki H, Oshima T, Takasaka T. Endoscopic endonasal repair of orbital floor fracture. Arch Otolaryngol Head Neck Surg 1999;125(1):59–63
39. Chen CT, Chen YR. Endoscopically assisted repair of orbital floor fractures. Plast Reconstr Surg 2001;108(7):2011–2018, discussion 2019
40. Saunders CJ, Whetzel TP, Stokes RB, Wong GB, Stevenson TR. Transantral endoscopic orbital floor exploration: a cadaver and clinical study. Plast Reconstr Surg 1997;100(3): 575–581
41. Woog JJ, Hartstein ME, Gliklich R. Paranasal sinus endoscopy and orbital fracture repair. Arch Ophthalmol 1998;116(5): 688–691
42. Strong EB, Kim KK, Diaz RC. Endoscopic approach to orbital blowout fracture repair. Otolaryngol Head Neck Surg 2004;131(5): 683–695

37 Epistaxis

Winston Vaughan, Manish Khanna, and Karen Fong

Epistaxis is one of the most common otorhinolaryngologic emergencies and, specifically, the most common nasal emergency. It is estimated that 60% of the general population will suffer from at least one episode and 6% will seek medical intervention for it at some point in their lives.[1] The severity of this condition runs the spectrum from isolated, minor episodes handled in the emergency room or clinic setting to life-threatening instances of near exsanguination requiring definitive management.

There has been a shift in the paradigm for the treatment of refractory epistaxis. Traditional posterior packing with a prolonged hospital course has largely been replaced by early management with either surgery or embolization, and hence, the role of the sinus surgeon has become more critical in the management of recurrent, severe epistaxis. This chapter discusses the evaluation and management of the patient with epistaxis, with a focus on relevant surgical anatomy and surgical treatment options.

Epidemiology

Epistaxis accounts for roughly 1 in 200 emergency room visits in the United States and has a bimodal distribution, most commonly affecting children younger than 10 years and the elderly aged 70 to 79 years.[2] The pediatric population tends to have more recurrent anterior epistaxis involving Kiesselbach's plexus, whereas the posterior epistaxis is more commonly seen in the elderly. Epistaxis is more often encountered in the winter months, when the decreased ambient humidification contributes to a dry environment within the nasal passage, which is conducive to the development of bleeding.[2]

Surgical Anatomy

The recurrent nature of epistaxis is attributed to the rich and redundant blood supply to the nose and paranasal structures. There are multiple anastomoses between vessels from both the internal and external carotid artery systems. The major contributing vessel from the external carotid system is its terminal branch, the internal maxillary artery with a secondary contribution from the facial artery. The internal maxillary artery travels within the pterygopalatine fossa, entering the nose at the sphenopalatine foramen as the sphenopalatine artery (SPA) (**Fig. 37.1**). Along the way, it gives off several branches, including the descending palatine artery, which branches off inferiorly and enters the hard palate through the greater palatine foramen, becoming the greater palatine artery. The vidian and maxillary divisions of the trigeminal nerve travel within the pterygopalatine fossa deep to the internal maxillary artery. This is an important surgical consideration as these structures are at risk during internal maxillary artery ligation.

It is critical for the surgeon to understand that multiple branches of the SPA may exit the sphenopalatine foramen.[3,4] Branches can also exit from accessory foramina in ~10% of cases.[5] The surgeon must recognize these variations to ensure complete ligation of the SPA. The sphenopalatine foramen is located within the superior meatus, between the basal lamella of the middle turbinate and the basal lamella of the superior turbinate, up to 90% of the time, at a distance of roughly 6 cm from the nasal sill.[6] A septal branch of the SPA traverses the anterior face of the sphenoid rostrum inferior to the sphenoid ostium; the artery is thus potentially at risk when extending a sphenoidotomy inferiorly.

This posterior septal division of the SPA supplies the septum through various secondary branches. The superior branch supplies the anterosuperior septum at Little's area, where it forms anastomoses with collaterals from the anterior ethmoid artery from the internal carotid system and alar branches from the superior labial artery, a branch from the facial artery (**Fig. 37.1**).[7] This septal anastomotic complex known as Kiesselbach's plexus is the most common site of anterior epistaxis. Inferior septal branches supply the rest of the septum and form anastomoses with branches of the greater palatine artery through the incisive canal. The posterior lateral nasal branch of the sphenopalatine artery runs along the palatine bone to give off branches that supply the turbinates and the maxillary fontanelle. It forms anastomoses with the anterior and posterior ethmoid arteries superiorly and with the pharyngeal branches (from the internal maxillary artery) inferiorly near the nasal floor. Woodruff's plexus, an aggregation of vessels situated in the posterior aspect of the inferior meatus (also known as the naso-nasopharyngeal plexus), has been thought to be a major source of posterior arterial epistaxis. However, recent anatomic dissections have indicated that Woodruff's plexus is actually a venous plexus.[8] Thus, although Woodruff's plexus may be implicated in posterior epistaxis, its contributions would be expected to be more venous oozing than brisk arterial bleeding.

The contributions from the internal carotid system to the nose are the anterior and posterior ethmoid arteries,

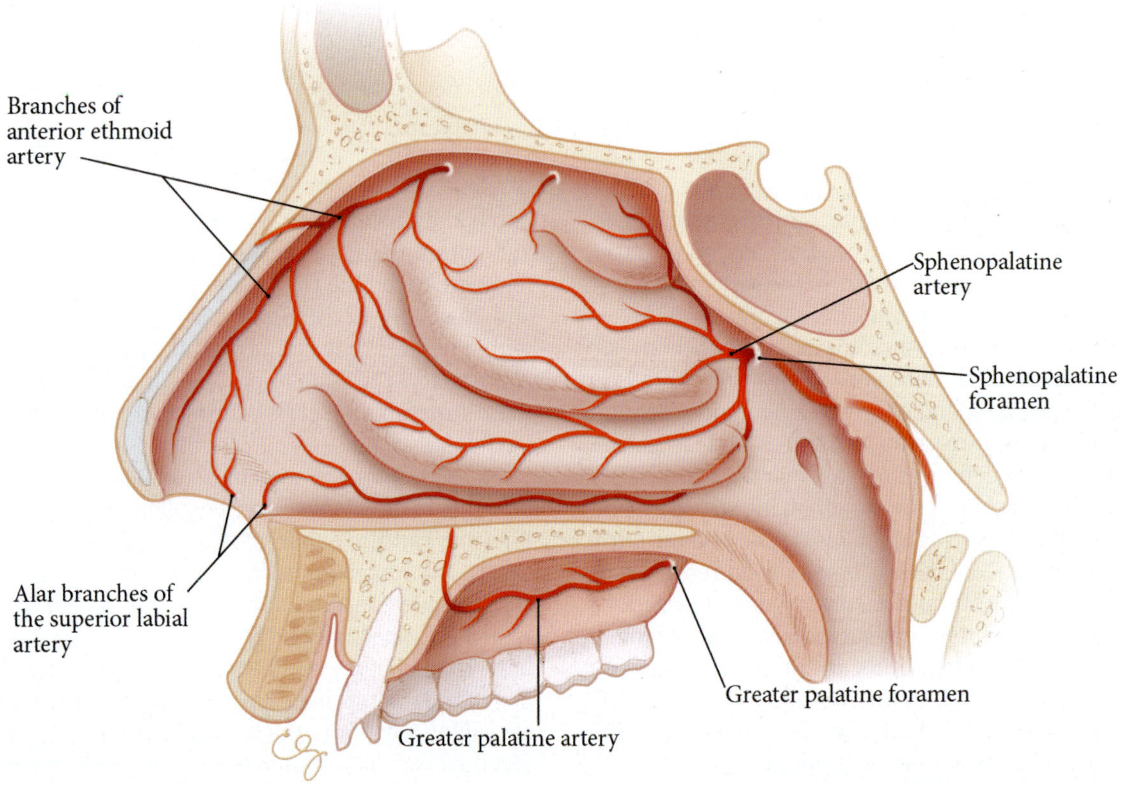

Fig. 37.1 A paramedian sagittal illustration of the nasal passage showing the sphenopalatine artery and its branches as it enters the nasal cavity through the sphenopalatine foramen. Note the anastomoses between multiple vessels, which ultimately emanate from the internal and external carotid artery systems.

which branch from the ophthalmic artery within the orbit (**Fig. 37.2**). Classic anatomic studies by Kirchner et al. helped to delineate the relationship between the ethmoid arteries and other structures of the orbit.[9] A more recent report has demonstrated that the anterior ethmoid artery lies 15 to 23 mm posterior to the frontomaxillolacrimal suture (**Fig. 37.2**).[10] The anterior ethmoid artery enters the nasal cavity at the ethmoid roof, supplies branches to the superior and middle turbinates laterally, and proceeds to the anterior septum where it contributes to Kiesselbach's plexus. The posterior ethmoid artery also enters the nasal cavity at the ethmoid roof, 12 to 15 mm posterior to the anterior ethmoid artery foramen.[11] The posterior ethmoid artery is located only 4 to 7 mm anterior to the optic canal and optic nerve, so the surgeon must use extreme caution when dissecting in close proximity to the vessel.

Diagnostic Evaluation

The causes of epistaxis can be divided into local and systemic factors (**Table 37.1**), and a thorough history and physical examination can help to determine the etiology and to guide appropriate management. The otorhinolaryngologist must be prepared to perform a thorough but streamlined evaluation, especially in the setting of active bleeding.

The history should distinguish between recurrent bleeding versus a solitary episode, because the former may warrant a more extensive workup. Another important historical feature is unilaterality versus bilaterality. Unilateral symptoms may be consistent with an anatomic abnormality or neoplastic process. In a child, unilateral bleeding accompanied by purulent rhinorrhea may indicate a nasal foreign body. A history of trauma is another important clinical feature. Trauma, one of the most common causes of epistaxis, can range from simple digital manipulation causing minor bleeding, to severe skull base fractures causing life-threatening arterial hemorrhaging. Medical conditions such as granulomatous disease, hepatic disease, or hematologic disorders should be elicited. Long-standing or poorly controlled hypertension may predispose one to recurrent epistaxis.[12] A history of prior or recent nasal surgery is clinically relevant. A positive family history may be manifest in patients with hereditary hemorrhagic telangiectasia syndrome, which is transmitted in an autosomal dominant fashion. Medication history is also important, especially with regard to warfarin, aspirin, or newer platelet aggregating inhibitors such as clopidogrel.

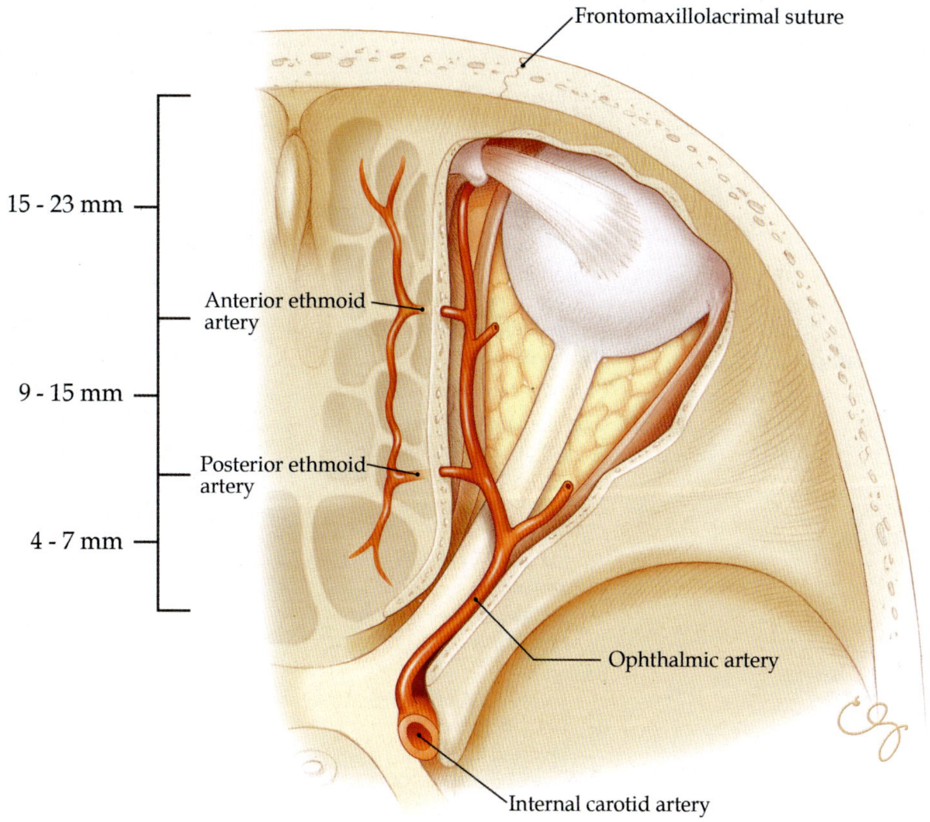

Fig. 37.2 An axial illustration of the orbit showing the anterior and posterior ethmoid arteries as they branch off of the ophthalmic artery. The distances between the arteries and other critical structures of the orbit are noted. Of particular importance is the close proximity of the posterior ethmoid foramen to the optic nerve.

Physical examination can be a challenge in the patient with acute epistaxis, but should not be limited to the nasal passages. The face and neck should be assessed for vascular lesions, such as telangiectasias or other malformations. Brisk epistaxis can cause retrograde blood flow from the nasolacrimal duct through the puncta along the medial portion of the eye. Otologic exam may reveal hemotympanum with subsequent conductive hearing loss resulting from blood egress into the middle ear via the eustachian tube. The oropharynx may demonstrate bleeding or clots, possibly indicative of posterior epistaxis.

Laboratory workup is appropriate in patients with recurrent bleeding. The complete blood count can determine if the patient is anemic or thrombocytopenic. Creatinine levels also should be considered because platelet dysfunction can occur in the setting of uremia. For patients on anticoagulation therapy, coagulation studies to be considered include international normalized ratio (INR) and partial thromboplastin time (PTT). Bleeding time can determine qualitative defects of platelet function. However, because bleeding time is observer-dependent and subjectively measured, it can be subject to wide variability, and thus routine use of bleeding time testing has fallen out of favor. A hematology consultation is warranted in guiding further laboratory evaluations for other coagulopathies such as von Willebrand disease.

Radiologic imaging is not routinely indicated in epistaxis, but may be required in the setting of trauma or for the evaluation of a nasal mass. Maxillofacial computed tomography (CT) scans can determine the extent of traumatic facial fractures; findings of extensive skull base fractures may be an indication for angiography to evaluate the integrity of the carotid circulation.

In the evaluation of nasal masses, magnetic resonance imaging (MRI) provides excellent delineation of soft tissue detail. In adults, neoplastic causes such as squamous cell carcinoma, esthesioneuroblastoma, or nasopharyngeal carcinoma may present with epistaxis, along with other constitutional symptoms. Recurrent, unilateral epistaxis in an adolescent male should raise suspicion for juvenile nasopharyngeal angiofibroma (JNA). Preoperative angiography for JNA can provide important diagnostic information regarding feeding vessels and can allow for therapeutic embolization to reduce surgical blood loss. Angiography with embolization can also be considered for patients with refractory posterior epistaxis as an alternative to surgical ligation of vessels.

Table 37.1 Differential Diagnosis for Epistaxis

Idiopathic	
Local	Trauma • Digital • Maxillofacial Topical nasal steroid sprays Continuous positive airway pressure Foreign body Anatomic • Septal perforation • Septal deviation
Inflammatory	Nasal polyposis Chronic/acute rhinosinusitis Granulomatous conditions • Wegener granulomatosis • Sarcoidosis • Tuberculosis
Neoplastic	Malignant • Squamous cell carcinoma • Melanoma • Esthesioneuroblastoma • Metastasis Benign • Juvenile nasopharyngeal angiofibroma • Hemangioma • Inverted papilloma • Hemangiopericytoma Hematologic • Leukemia • Lymphoma
Systemic	Vascular disorders • Thrombocytopenia • von Willebrand disease • Hemophilia • Hereditary hemorrhagic telangiectasia • Aplastic anemia • Polycythemia vera Malnutrition Vitamin A, C, D, E, or K deficiency Alcoholism Hepatic failure Uremia Medications • Warfarin • Heparin • Nonsteriodal anti-inflammatory drugs • Antiplatelet aggregators • Cocaine
Iatrogenic	Surgery • Functional endoscopic sinus surgery • Septoplasty • Turbinate resection Instrumentation • Nasotracheal intubation • Nasogastric tube

Initial Management

Epistaxis can present as a life-threatening emergency and all patients should be treated with this in mind. Vital signs should be obtained expeditiously and managed appropriately. In the setting of exsanguinating epistaxis, signs of shock, such as tachycardia, tachypnea, and hypotension, may demand aggressive fluid resuscitation and blood transfusion. Hypertension, whether intrinsic or secondary to pain or anxiety, should be controlled because it may be exacerbating the bleeding.

All attempts should be made to determine the site of bleeding and the availability of appropriate equipment helps this process significantly **(Table 37.2)**. Patients who are actively bleeding despite packing that is already in place may need to have the packing removed to evaluate the site of bleeding. The experience of the clinician will determine whether the pack removal and an evaluation for any given patient should be performed in the emergency room, clinic, or in the operating room. When done outside of the operating room, the patient should be seated upright with preprocedure analgesics and/or anxiolytics administered. The blood pressure should be monitored. Topical anesthesia is placed using either 4% cocaine or 4% lidocaine mixed with a decongestant. A greater palatine foramen block can be helpful to control bleeding originating from a sphenopalatine artery source. One and one half to 2 mL of 1% lidocaine with 1:100,000 epinephrine is instilled transpalatally through the greater palatine foramen to infiltrate the pterygopalatine fossa, through which the sphenopalatine artery traverses before entering the nose. A 25-gauge needle bent at 2.5 cm from the tip at a 45-degree angle provides the optimal approach to the foramen, which is located just medial to the alveolar ridge near the junction of the second and third molar.

Identifying the site of bleeding can be a challenging proposition, especially in the setting of clots, new bleeding, and excoriated mucosa that may result from nasal pack placement. The anterior septum and inferior turbinate can be reasonably assessed using a nasal speculum and headlight, but a visualization of posterior structures will be limited. Nasal endoscopy is an essential tool for an examination of the posterior sinonasal passage, including the posterior septum, middle turbinate, nasal floor, and lateral nasal wall. Endoscopy provides excellent visualization of anterior nasal structures as well and should be considered strongly for comprehensive evaluation of the sinonasal anatomy. All attempts should be made to clear clots and debris to help localize the bleeding area. Any septal irregularities, such as deviation, spurs, or perforations, must be documented. In patients who have undergone sinus surgery, angled endoscopes can also help to visualize the frontal recess and maxillary sinus. Angled endoscopes can also help to examine the ethmoid arteries as they traverse the ethmoid roof.

Table 37.2 Equipment Necessary for Optimal Epistaxis Management

Headlight	Nasal speculum
Suction instruments • Frazier • Yankauer • Flexible catheter	Cautery • Silver nitrate • Suction monopolar electrocautery • Bipolar electrocautery
Endoscopes: 0, 30, 45 degree	
Topical vasoconstrictive agents	Nasal packing • Absorbable • Nonabsorbable
Topical lidocaine	
Lidocaine for injection	Bayonet forceps

Epistaxis is typically classified as either anterior or posterior based on the anatomic origin of bleeding and clinical severity. Anterior epistaxis most commonly originates from the anterior septum at Kiesselbach's plexus. The bleeding site can usually be visualized with anterior rhinoscopy (direct or endoscopic) and can be treated using silver nitrate cautery. A useful cautery technique is to apply the silver nitrate applicator circumferentially around the bleeding area initially, then cauterize the bleeding area itself. The contralateral septum adjacent to the cauterized area should be left undisturbed, as cautery to the contralateral side may devascularize the septum and result in a septal perforation. Antibiotic ointment should be applied after chemical cautery to enhance moisture and allow for timely healing. Skin contact with the silver nitrate must be avoided because this may burn and potentially form an unsightly tattoo on the skin. Bipolar or suction monopolar cautery is an alternative if the bleeding is vigorous and refractory to silver nitrate application. Topical anesthetic on a cotton pledget should be applied prior to electrocautery as it may be quite painful for the patient. Extreme care must be taken in using electrocautery because over-aggressive use may also result in septal perforation.

Nasal packing may also be used to control acute bleeding or as a temporizing measure prior to definitive management. Packing can be classified into absorbable and nonabsorbable types. The decision to use either type is dictated by clinician preference. Although absorbable packing may not achieve the same occlusive pressure as expandable nonabsorbable packing, it offers enhanced patient comfort.[13] In patients with thrombocytopenia or coagulopathy, the use of absorbable packing may be more desirable because packing removal may itself be traumatic and may cause recurrence of bleeding. Many types of absorbable packing biomaterials are available—including gelatin, carboxymethyl-cellulose, oxidized cellulose, hyaluronic acid, fibrillar collagen, and starch—and most are manufactured as injectable forms that are simple to place. Some can be combined with thrombin for additional efficacy. Placement of absorbable packing under an endoscopic visualization allows for a precise placement and avoids overpacking. Scheduled follow-up visits are important to debride remnants of packing that can persist and cause sinusitis.

There are a large number of nonabsorbable nasal packs that are commercially available. The advantage of these packs is that they are relatively simple to place and are effective in treating anterior epistaxis. While the pack is in place, patients should be covered with antibiotic prophylaxis against *Staphylococcus aureus* because cases of toxic shock syndrome both with and without nasal packing have been reported.[14] Drawbacks to the use of nonabsorbable packing include the risk of aspiration and patient discomfort. Removal of the nasal packing is recommended between 3 and 5 days.

Posterior epistaxis presents a more daunting challenge because it is usually more profuse and visualization is more difficult. Furthermore, posterior epistaxis tends to be more common in elderly, frail patients. Placement of a posterior nasal pack is typically the first line of treatment and can serve as a temporizing measure or it can be left in for 3 to 5 days as definitive management. The availability of high volume, low pressure balloon packs allows for the simple, rapid control of severe posterior epistaxis and has predominantly replaced the traditional posterior gauze packs and Foley catheter placement.

Once the bichambered pack is in place, the posterior portion is inflated and pulled forward until it contacts the choana. Then, the anterior portion is slowly inflated until no further bleeding is noted in the oropharynx or from the anterior nasal passage. The oropharynx also should be examined to check for inadvertent egress of the pack because it may cause airway obstruction. This can be prevented by securing the packs to the nasal dorsum. Excess pressure from the anterior pack can cause alar necrosis and mucosal trauma. Therefore, the degree of balloon insufflation should be monitored carefully. While the packs are in place, antibiotic prophylaxis is recommended. Patients with posterior packs in place should be hospitalized in a monitored setting as posterior packs may cause hypoxia.[15]

Epistaxis resulting from endoscopic sinus surgery requires immediate endoscopic attention. Bleeding occurring within several hours after surgery usually originates from the anterior ethmoid artery.[16] Orbital manifestations, such as proptosis and visual changes, may accompany ethmoid artery bleeding if the arterial stump retracts into the orbit. If bleeding isolated to the ethmoid arteries cannot be managed endoscopically, then an external approach may be warranted. Bleeding that occurs 1 to 3 weeks after surgery is usually attributed to sphenopalatine arterial branches to the inferior or middle turbinate. Bipolar cautery to the anterior stump of the turbinates after a resection can help control bleeding in those areas. If direct cautery to the turbinates is not effective, then a sphenopalatine artery ligation or embolization procedure should be considered.

Epistaxis can also take hereditary forms. Hereditary hemorrhagic telangiectasia (HHT), also known as Osler-Weber-Rendu disease, is an autosomal dominant condition that commonly presents with epistaxis. It is believed that mutations of the endoglin and ALK-I genes, which code for endothelial receptors of the transforming growth factor (TGF)-beta family, result in systemic development of telangiectasias and arteriovenous malformations. Typically manifesting by adolescence, patients with HHT present with telangiectasias of the mucosal and skin surfaces of the head and neck and digits. Fragile telangiectasias of the nasal mucosa result in frequent epistaxis **(Fig. 37.3)**.

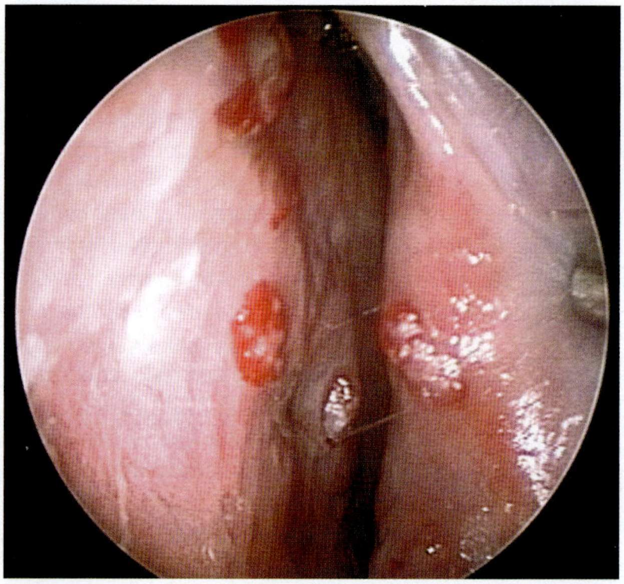

Fig. 37.3 An endoscopic view of a patient with hereditary hemorrhagic telangiectasia. Note the presence of punctate, coalescent lesions along the septum and lateral nasal wall that are amenable to treatment with bipolar cautery or laser photocoagulation.

HHT patients are also susceptible to arteriovenous malformations (AVMs) of the brain, lungs, and gastrointestinal tract. The management of these patients can be a challenge as they may undergo multiple hospitalizations, transfusions, and surgical and medical procedures throughout their lifetimes. Because epistaxis is typically the presenting complaint, the otorhinolaryngologist may be the first clinician to make the diagnosis of HHT. Newly diagnosed patients with HHT should undergo screening for cerebral, pulmonary, and gastrointestinal AVMs, and their family members should be screened for undiagnosed HHT.

Surgical Management

Endoscopic Sphenopalatine Artery Ligation

Initially, the greater palatine foramen is identified along the palate medial to the second maxillary molar and infiltrated with local anesthetic (1.5 to 2 mL of 1% lidocaine with 1:100,000 epinephrine). The nasal cavity is decongested with a topical vasoconstrictive agent. The posterior fontanelle of the maxillary sinus and the perpendicular plate of the palatine bone are palpated. Local anesthetic is infiltrated along the lateral nasal wall ~1 cm anterior to the posteriormost insertion of the middle turbinate on the lateral nasal wall. A maxillary antrostomy is optional and may help to delineate the interface between the fontanelle and the palatine bone by visualizing the posterior maxillary sinus wall because the foramen will be found posterior to it **(Fig. 37.4)**.

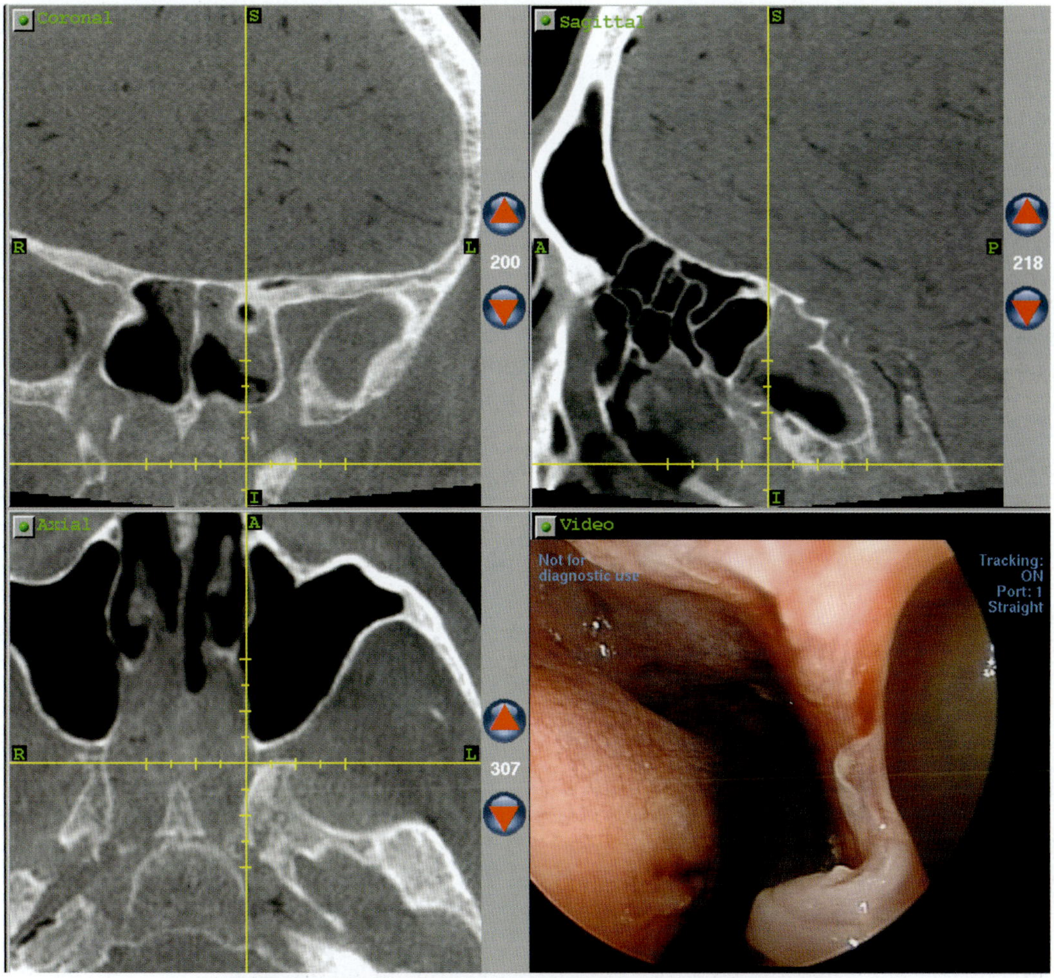

A

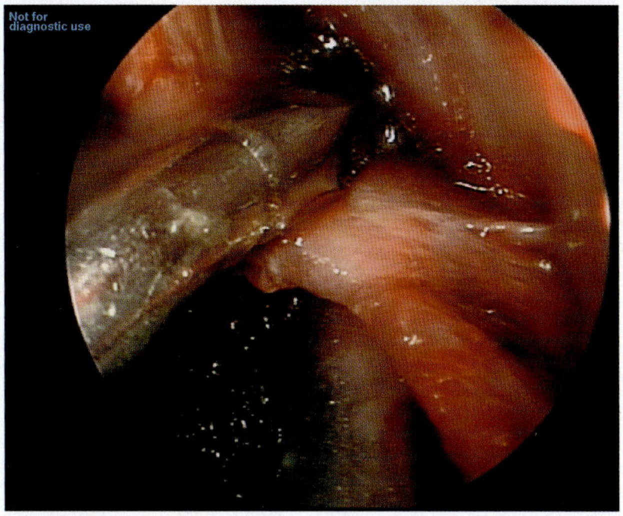

B

Fig. 37.4 Cadaver dissection of the sphenopalatine artery. **(A)** The image guidance probe marks the sphenopalatine foramen, which is best visualized on the axial plane posterior to the posterior wall of the maxillary sinus. **(B)** The sphenopalatine artery is found posterior to the crista ethmoidalis along the lateral nasal wall.

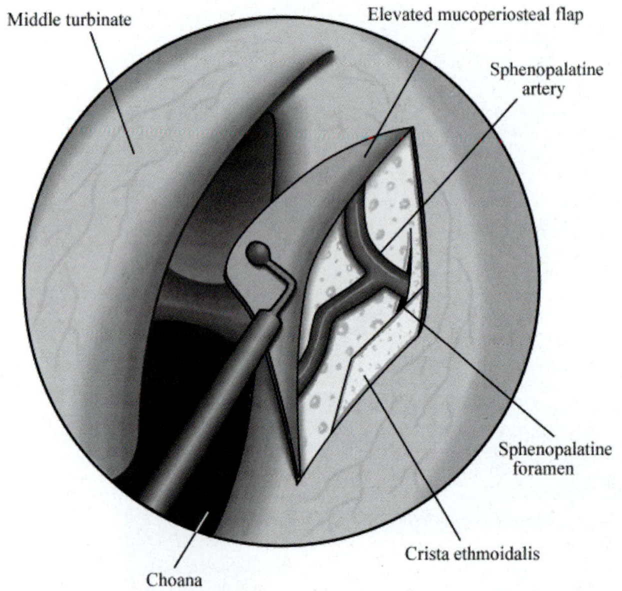

Fig. 37.5 Illustration of the endoscopic view of the sphenopalatine artery after flap elevation.

A vertical incision is then made, and a mucoperiosteal flap is then raised posteriorly toward the sphenopalatine foramen **(Fig. 37.5)**. The crista ethmoidalis, a bony ridge emanating from the perpendicular plate of the palatine bone, is encountered anterior to the sphenopalatine foramen over 95% of the time and is a useful landmark **(Fig. 37.6)**.[5]

There is considerable anatomic variation in the sphenopalatine artery upon entry into the nasal passage as it may exit the foramen as a single vessel or may branch immediately upon exit or within the pterygopalatine fossa. Accessory foramina may be present in up to 12% of cases and can be found in any direction in relation to the sphenopalatine foramen.[5,17] Thus, the lateral nasal wall should be inspected carefully anterior and posterior to the sphenopalatine foramen for additional branches of the artery exiting from separate foramina. If multiple vessels are encountered, each one is then isolated using blunt dissection and cauterized with bipolar forceps. It is prudent to cauterize the vessels as far from the foramen as possible to avoid possible retraction into the pterygopalatine fossa. Alternatively, surgical hemoclips can be used to ligate the vessels. Once ligation is performed to satisfaction, the mucoperiosteal flap is laid back in place and a small strip of absorbable packing may be placed over the flap as a bolster.

The primary complication of sphenopalatine artery ligation is recurrent bleeding, which is mainly a result of failure to recognize and address additional branches of the artery from the sphenopalatine foramen or accessory openings. Rare complications, including septal perforation and inferior turbinate necrosis, have been reported with this procedure.[18]

Ligation of the Ethmoid Arteries

The traditional approach to the anterior and posterior ethmoid arteries is through an external Lynch incision. The curvilinear incision, 3 cm in length, is made medial to the medial canthus, halfway between it and the midline nasal dorsum. The incision is carried through the periosteum of the nasal bone, and the periosteum is then elevated posteriorly along the frontonasal suture

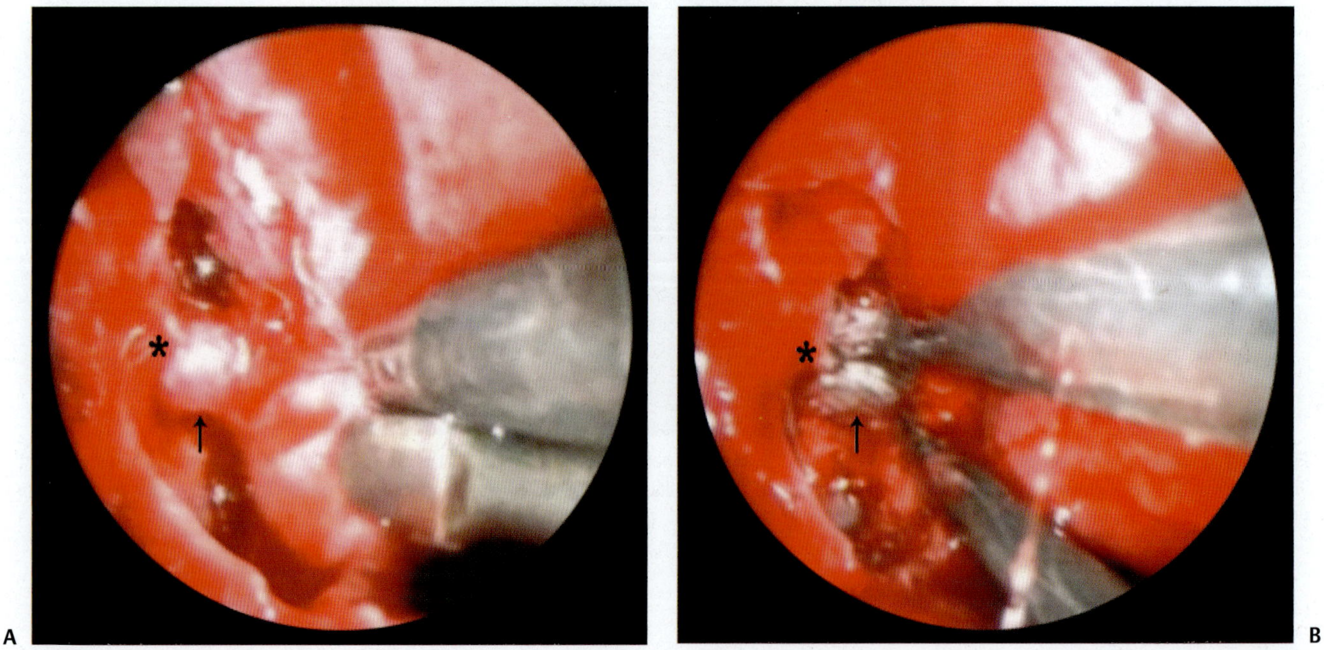

Fig. 37.6 Intraoperative views of the sphenopalatine artery. **(A)** The artery is seen as it exits its foramen as a single branch (*arrow*). The crista ethmoidalis (*asterisk*) is also visualized. **(B)** The artery has been cauterized with bipolar cautery.

line until the posterior lacrimal crest is encountered. The frontomaxillolacrimal suture line serves as an additional landmark, which is found adjacent to the lacrimal crest, marking the conjunction of the frontal, maxilla, and lacrimal bones. Flap elevation is continued 15 to 23 mm posteriorly along the frontoethmoid suture until the anterior ethmoid foramen is encountered. The use of an endoscope has been described to help with visualization and can allow for a smaller Lynch incision.[19] Once the vessel is isolated, it may be ligated with hemoclips, silk ties, or bipolar cautery. The posterior ethmoid artery can be found 9 to 15 mm from the anterior ethmoid foramen **(Fig. 37.2)** and ligated after careful posterior periorbital elevation. The surgeon is warned that the orbital apex is located only 4 to 7 mm from the posterior ethmoid foramen, so extreme care must be used when ligating the artery with the optic nerve in such close vicinity.

A novel endoscopic approach to anterior ethmoid artery ligation has been recently described by Pletcher and Metson.[20] Once the artery or the bony canal in which it lies is identified along the skull base, the lamina is removed around its periphery as it enters the orbit and the exposed vessel is ligated with surgical clips. The close proximity of the anterior ethmoid artery to the orbit and skull base allows for the possibility of cerebrospinal fluid (CSF) leak and orbital injury as potential complications. Additional information with regard to technical points, efficacy, and complication rate will be ascertained as more experience is gained with this approach.

Complications include bleeding secondary to loss of vascular control and orbital injury. This can occur from fat prolapse into the field, thus making reestablishment of vascular control challenging. All attempts to maintain the integrity of the periorbita should be made to avoid this troublesome scenario. Traumatic optic neuropathy and orbital apex syndrome are potentially devastating orbital complications that have been described in the literature.[21,22] They are usually the result of improper clip placement or thermal injury to the structures of the orbital apex. Intravenous steroids and prompt optic nerve decompression are warranted in both situations, with blindness as a potential sequela. If surgical clips were used, orbital exploration with removal of clips must be performed. Meticulous surgical technique and visualization are paramount to help avoid these devastating complications. Lacrimal sac injury is also a possibility and may be addressed with a dacryocystorhinostomy to help relieve the resultant epiphora. Diplopia secondary to superior oblique muscle palsy can occur from direct damage to the trochlear portion of the muscle or its separation from the muscle during flap elevation and globe retraction.[23] Trochlea separation can be prevented by avoiding superior flap elevation up to the level of the orbital roof. Scarring of the external incision is also a potential complication although the incision predominantly heals in a cosmetically acceptable manner. A W-shaped or broken line incision can help to avoid cicatricial wound contracture.

Transantral Internal Maxillary Artery Ligation

Access to the internal maxillary artery within the pterygopalatine fossa allows for ligation of all its contributing branches, including the descending palatine and pharyngeal branches. The upper gingivobuccal sulcus is infiltrated with local anesthesia, and an incision is carried to the anterior wall of the maxillary sinus, with care being taken to avoid the infraorbital nerve. Caldwell-Luc antrostomy is then performed and endoscopic or microscopic examination of the posterior wall is commenced. A laterally or inferiorly based U-shaped flap is raised and the posterior wall is carefully removed using a combination of osteotomes and Kerrison rongeurs. At times, the artery and its branches can be seen pulsating through the outer periosteum of the posterior maxillary sinus wall. If the vessels are not visualized, the periosteum is incised and the fibrofatty contents of the pterygopalatine fossa are inspected for the internal maxillary artery and its branches **(Fig. 37.7)**. Once found, bipolar cautery or hemoclips are used for ligation. All attempts should be made to cauterize or clip as many branches of the artery as possible to help maximize the chance of success.

The procedure may fail if a complete ligation is not performed. Therefore, careful inspection of the fat contained within the pterygopalatine fossa is important to find and ligate the main trunk of the tortuous internal maxillary artery and its branches for maximal results. The pterygopalatine ganglion, as well as the maxillary and vidian divisions of the trigeminal nerve, are all at risk when dissecting within the pterygopalatine fossa. The infraorbital nerve is at risk with

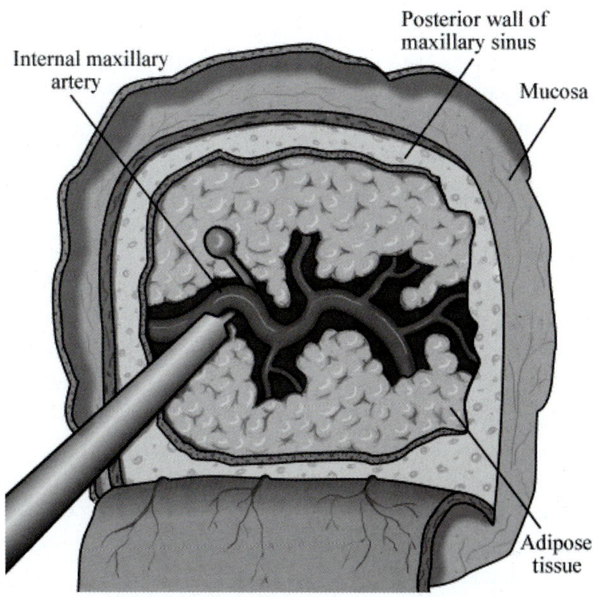

Fig. 37.7 Transantral view of the pterygopalatine fossa after the removal of the posterior wall of the maxillary sinus. The internal maxillary artery and its branches can be found within the adipose tissue. Pulsations of the vessels will help distinguish them from nervous structures.

the Caldwell-Luc approach, and some degree of transient hypesthesia is expected even after uneventful surgery. Oroantral fistula is a rare complication inherent to the Caldwell-Luc approach for exposure and may require local mucosal flaps for repair. Transantral approaches to the internal maxillary artery have been largely replaced by endoscopic approaches to the sphenopalatine artery because the transnasal endoscopic approach allows for specific isolation and targeting of the sphenopalatine branch of the internal maxillary artery.

Surgical Procedures for Hereditary Hemorrhagic Telangiectasia

Surgical treatments for HHT can help to meaningfully improve the quality of life for patients who experience frequent epistaxis. Treatment options include Nd:YAG or KTP laser photocoagulation, bipolar cauterization, systemic hormone therapy, septodermoplasty, and nasal closure (modified Young's procedure); the choice of treatment is often based on the overall severity of bleeding. The nasal vascular pattern in these patients may help to determine the optimal first-line therapy, as those with isolated punctate telangiectasias may be treated with laser photocoagulation or bipolar cautery, whereas those with more diffuse sessile patterns may be candidates for septodermoplasty.[24] The nature of the lesions may also determine the choice of cauterization as some authors have proposed the use of bipolar cautery for larger, more coalescent lesions in place of laser photocoagulation.[25]

For patients who fail to improve with standard cautery or photocoagulation procedures, septodermoplasty is an alternative surgical option. Septodermoplasty involves removal of the involved nasal mucosa and relining of the nasal cavity with a split-thickness skin graft. Using endoscopic guidance, the nasal cavity is gently cleared of any crust and blood clots, and pledgets soaked in a topical vasoconstrictive agent are carefully placed against the septum. Care is taken to avoid disruption of the telangiectasias, which can limit visualization. If severe bleeding occurs, the nose must be packed and the procedure may have to be aborted. Next, local anesthetic is carefully injected into the septum. The microdebrider is then used to remove the septal mucosa with preservation of the perichondrium anteriorly and periosteum posteriorly. A split-thickness skin graft is harvested from the anterior thigh and is shaped in a rectangular manner to approximate the area of lining needed. The graft is then laid over the septum and sutured in place with mattress sutures to the anterior septum or nasal vestibule. A long nasal speculum is then used to push the graft against the septum while antibiotic-impregnated gauze is packed into the nasal cavity just posterior to the graft, acting as a bolster. Alternatively, silastic nasal splints may be used. The lateral nasal wall, including inferior turbinate, may be concurrently treated in similar fashion.[26] Oral antibiotic prophylaxis is given and the packing is removed in 7 to 10 days.

Although this procedure is quite effective for several months to years, a recurrence with ingrowth of abnormal vessels and graft contracture can occur and may necessitate future procedures, including laser, cautery, or revision septodermoplasty. Nasal crusting can be an issue as the mucosal lining is replaced with skin, which sloughs its epithelial surface and can be difficult to clear. Consistent nasal irrigation and humidification can alleviate the burden of chronic crusting.

The most definitive procedure for HHT is complete closure of the nasal airway. The modified Young's procedure is a technique of nasal closure that is an option for the refractory patient, who has failed other modalities. Studies have demonstrated success rates of up to 89%.[27] It is postulated that the efficacy of the procedure is centered on the cessation of turbulent airflow across friable, abnormal blood vessels.[28] Mucocutaneous flaps are raised circumferentially and sutured in a tension-free manner to effectively close the nasal passageway. The disadvantages from a functional and cosmetic standpoint must be weighed against the significant efficacy of the procedure.

Embolization

Arterial embolization is another reasonable option in the patient with recurrent epistaxis with success rates ranging from 71 to 100% based on published reports.[29,30] Embolization is generally reserved for patients with severe posterior epistaxis that has been refractory to local and surgical measures, although it is also used as a primary modality before surgical resection of vascular tumors. It requires the expertise and availability of an interventional neuroradiologist, and these services may not be readily available at all facilities.

One of the advantages of embolization is that it may be performed under local anesthesia and therefore is the procedure of choice in patients who are high-risk candidates for general anesthesia. Transfusions should be given to maintain a hematocrit level above 30 prior to the procedure. A femoral artery catheter is placed, and the external and internal carotid systems are studied under angiography. Once the target artery is identified, several materials can be used for embolization, including polyvinyl alcohol, tris-acryl gelatin microspheres, ethanol, and platinum coils. Bilateral embolization is considered in cases where the bleeding site cannot be clearly ascertained.

There are certain risks and limitations with arterial embolization. The ethmoid arteries are not accessible for embolization due to the risk of compromise to the ophthalmic artery, which may lead to blindness. Complications can be divided into major and minor complications (**Table 37.3**). The most common minor complication is recurrent bleeding, which can be managed with repeat embolization or surgery.[30]

Table 37.3 Complications of Embolization

Major	Minor
Myocardial infarction	Groin hematoma
Blindness	Transient ischemic attack
Cerebrovascular accident	Recurrent bleeding
Carotid injury	Facial pain
Palatal necrosis	Jaw claudication
Alar/columella necrosis	Headache
Facial nerve palsy	Sialadenitis

Outcomes

Over the years, the management of posterior epistaxis has changed as instrumentation has evolved. The placement of posterior packing with hospital admission was considered the appropriate conservative approach to these patients. Recent studies have demonstrated the first-line management for patients with recurrent posterior epistaxis with either surgery or embolization is superior to posterior packing in terms of efficacy, complication rates, and cost-effectiveness.[31]

Sphenopalatine artery ligation has become a popular modality for the treatment of refractory posterior epistaxis. Success rates of 93 to 98% have been reported, which is comparable, if not superior, to both internal maxillary artery ligation and embolization.[32] A theoretical advantage of sphenopalatine artery ligation over internal maxillary ligation is that the most distal branch and, thus, the vessel closest to the bleeding, is addressed. This helps prevent unnecessary ligation of collateral vessels. Proponents also cite the avoidance of the complications associated with the Caldwell-Luc approach.

A published report by Cullen and Tami demonstrated similar complication rates between surgical ligation and embolization of the internal maxillary artery. However, the embolization group suffered from more severe complications, including carotid artery injury and myocardial infarction.[33] In a literature review done by the same authors, the overall complication rate was higher in the surgery group in comparison to the embolization group (26% versus 14%), whereas failure rates were higher with embolization (20% versus 12%). Failure of either surgery or embolization is seen more commonly in elderly patients. This may be attributed to more extensive collateral circulation.[34] Proponents of sphenopalatine artery ligation feel that the use of a direct examination of the affected area provides important diagnostic information that embolization fails to provide.[35] An additional advantage of sphenopalatine artery ligation is that external ethmoid artery ligation can be performed concurrently. Cost comparisons between sphenopalatine artery ligation and embolization have demonstrated conflicting conclusions regarding relative cost-effectiveness.

Ethmoid artery ligation is more commonly used in the setting of maxillofacial trauma or iatrogenic causes, where bleeding originates in the superior portion of the nasal cavity. It is also performed in conjunction with sphenopalatine artery ligation in patients with severe, refractory epistaxis in whom the bleeding site cannot be identified. Ligation of the posterior ethmoid artery has a more limited role due to its close proximity to the optic canal and because of its absence in many cases.[32] As discussed earlier, the endoscopic approach to ethmoid artery ligation has been reported. Floreani and colleagues studied its feasibility in a cadaver model.[36] They discovered that clip ligation was possible in only 20% of the vessels, which were clearly visualized within the mesentery and in cases of partial bony canal dehiscence. Possible risks include significant hemorrhage and orbital hematoma secondary to inadequate control of the vessel, as well as CSF leak. They conclude that endoscopic ligation may be considered in select cases, but the external approach is safer, especially in cases of trauma. It is clear that endoscopic anterior ethmoid artery ligation requires further investigation to assess technical and safety parameters, as well as efficacy.

Conclusion

Key points of this chapter include the following:

- Epistaxis has a bimodal distribution pattern. Anterior epistaxis is more commonly seen in the pediatric population below the age of 10, whereas posterior epistaxis is encountered more commonly in the elderly.
- The etiology of epistaxis can be divided into idiopathic, local, inflammatory, systemic, iatrogenic, and neoplastic causes.
- All attempts should be made to localize the site of bleeding. Appropriate equipment is necessary to effectively examine and treat patients with acute epistaxis. The endoscopic exam is an important modality to isolate and treat the affected areas.
- Several surgical procedures are available to treat epistaxis depending on the site of bleeding.
- Endoscopic sphenopalatine artery ligation is considered a safe, effective treatment for recurrent, severe epistaxis. It should be considered as first-line surgical treatment.
- The sphenopalatine artery exhibits much anatomic variation as it enters the nasal passage. Accessory foramina and multiple branches may be present and, thus, the lateral wall should be carefully inspected and additional branches should be addressed.
- Extreme caution must be used when addressing the posterior ethmoid artery due to its close proximity to the optic nerve and other structures of the orbital apex.
- The endoscopic approach to ethmoid artery ligation is recently described, novel technique. Future

studies and more experience with this procedure will determine its efficacy and will bring technical refinement.

- Careful inspection of the structures within the pterygopalatine fossa is critical in avoiding complications and maximizing success when performing transantral internal maxillary artery ligation.
- Hereditary hemorrhagic telangiectasia is an autosomal dominant disorder causing severe, recurrent epistaxis. Treatment options include bipolar cautery, laser photocoagulation, septodermoplasty, and nasal closure (modified Young's procedure).
- Embolization requires specialized expertise and is comparable to sphenopalatine artery ligation in terms of efficacy. Although overall complication rates may be higher in sphenopalatine artery ligation, major complications occur more commonly with embolization, and embolization cannot be used to address the ethmoid arteries due to the risk of blindness.

References

1. Small M, Murray JA, Maran AG. A study of patients with epistaxis requiring admission to hospital. Health Bull (Edinb) 1982;40(1):20–29
2. Pallin DJ, Chng YM, McKay MP, Emond JA, Pelletier AJ, Camargo CA Jr. Epidemiology of epistaxis in US emergency departments, 1992 to 2001. Ann Emerg Med 2005;46(1):77–81
3. Simmen DB, Raghavan U, Briner HR, Manestar M, Groscurth P, Jones NS. The anatomy of the sphenopalatine artery for the endoscopic sinus surgeon. Am J Rhinol 2006;20(5): 502–505
4. Schwartzbauer HR, Shete M, Tami TA. Endoscopic anatomy of the sphenopalatine and posterior nasal arteries: implications for the endoscopic management of epistaxis. Am J Rhinol 2003;17(1):63–66
5. Pádua FG, Voegels RL. Severe posterior epistaxis-endoscopic surgical anatomy. Laryngoscope 2008;118(1):156–161
6. Lee HY, Kim HU, Kim SS, et al. Surgical anatomy of the sphenopalatine artery in lateral nasal wall. Laryngoscope 2002;112(10): 1813–1818
7. Babin E, Moreau S, de Rugy MG, Delmas P, Valdazo A, Bequignon A. Anatomic variations of the arteries of the nasal fossa. Otolaryngol Head Neck Surg 2003;128(2):236–239
8. Chiu TW, Shaw-Dunn J, McGarry GW. Woodruff's plexus. J Laryngol Otol 2008;122(10):1074–1077
9. Kirchner JA, Yanagisawa E, Crelin ES Jr. Surgical anatomy of the ethmoidal arteries. A laboratory study of 150 orbits. Arch Otolaryngol 1961;74:382–386
10. Akdemir G, Tekdemir I, Altin L. Transethmoidal approach to the optic canal: surgical and radiological microanatomy. Surg Neurol 2004;62(3):268–274, discussion 274
11. Han JK, Becker SS, Bomeli SR, Gross CW. Endoscopic localization of the anterior and posterior ethmoid arteries. Ann Otol Rhinol Laryngol 2008;117(12):931–935
12. Lubianca Neto JF, Fuchs FD, Facco SR, et al. Is epistaxis evidence of end-organ damage in patients with hypertension? Laryngoscope 1999;109(7 Pt 1):1111–1115
13. Douglas R, Wormald PJ. Update on epistaxis. Curr Opin Otolaryngol Head Neck Surg 2007;15(3):180–183
14. Jacobson JA, Kasworm EM. Toxic shock syndrome after nasal surgery. Case reports and analysis of risk factors. Arch Otolaryngol Head Neck Surg 1986;112(3):329–332
15. Lin YT, Orkin LR. Arterial hypoxemia in patients with anterior and posterior nasal packings. Laryngoscope 1979;89(1): 140–144
16. Stankiewicz JA. Nasal endoscopy and control of epistaxis. Curr Opin Otolaryngol Head Neck Surg 2004;12(1):43–45
17. Wareing MJ, Padgham ND. Osteologic classification of the sphenopalatine foramen. Laryngoscope 1998;108(1 Pt 1):125–127
18. Moorthy R, Anand R, Prior M, Scott PM. Inferior turbinate necrosis following endoscopic sphenopalatine artery ligation. Otolaryngol Head Neck Surg 2003;129(1):159–160
19. Douglas SA, Gupta D. Endoscopic assisted external approach anterior ethmoidal artery ligation for the management of epistaxis. J Laryngol Otol 2003;117(2):132–133
20. Pletcher SD, Metson R. Endoscopic ligation of the anterior ethmoid artery. Laryngoscope 2007;117(2):378–381
21. Yeh S, Yen MT, Foroozan R. Orbital apex syndrome after ethmoidal artery ligation for recurrent epistaxis. Ophthal Plast Reconstr Surg 2004;20(5):392–394
22. Brouzas D, Charakidas A, Androulakis M, Moschos M. Traumatic optic neuropathy after posterior ethmoidal artery ligation for epistaxis. Otolaryngol Head Neck Surg 2002;126(3):323–325
23. Couch JM, Somers ME, Gonzalez C. Superior oblique muscle dysfunction following anterior ethmoidal artery ligation for epistaxis. Arch Ophthalmol 1990;108(8):1110–1113
24. Mahoney EJ, Shapshay SM. New classification of nasal vasculature patterns in hereditary hemorrhagic telangiectasia. Am J Rhinol 2006;20(1):87–90
25. Ghaheri BA, Fong KJ, Hwang PH. The utility of bipolar electrocautery in hereditary hemorrhagic telangiectasia. Otolaryngol Head Neck Surg 2006;134(6):1006–1009
26. Fiorella ML, Ross D, Henderson KJ, White RI Jr. Outcome of septal dermoplasty in patients with hereditary hemorrhagic telangiectasia. Laryngoscope 2005;115(2):301–305
27. Lund VJ, Howard DJ. Closure of the nasal cavities in the treatment of refractory hereditary haemorrhagic telangiectasia. J Laryngol Otol 1997;111(1):30–33
28. Gluckman JL, Portugal LG. Modified Young's procedure for refractory epistaxis due to hereditary hemorrhagic telangiectasia. Laryngoscope 1994;104(9):1174–1177
29. Sadri M, Midwinter K, Ahmed A, Parker A. Assessment of safety and efficacy of arterial embolisation in the management of intractable epistaxis. Eur Arch Otorhinolaryngol 2006;263(6):560–566
30. Christensen NP, Smith DS, Barnwell SL, Wax MK. Arterial embolization in the management of posterior epistaxis. Otolaryngol Head Neck Surg 2005;133(5):748–753
31. Klotz DA, Winkle MR, Richmon J, Hengerer AS. Surgical management of posterior epistaxis: a changing paradigm. Laryngoscope 2002;112(9):1577–1582
32. Kumar S, Shetty A, Rockey J, Nilssen E. Contemporary surgical treatment of epistaxis. What is the evidence for sphenopalatine artery ligation? Clin Otolaryngol Allied Sci 2003;28(4):360–363
33. Cullen MM, Tami TA. Comparison of internal maxillary artery ligation versus embolization for refractory posterior epistaxis. Otolaryngol Head Neck Surg 1998;118(5):636–642
34. Metson R, Lane R. Internal maxillary artery ligation for epistaxis: an analysis of failures. Laryngoscope 1988;98(7):760–764
35. Miller TR, Stevens ES, Orlandi RR. Economic analysis of the treatment of posterior epistaxis. Am J Rhinol 2005;19(1):79–82
36. Floreani SR, Nair SB, Switajewski MC, Wormald PJ. Endoscopic anterior ethmoidal artery ligation: a cadaver study. Laryngoscope 2006;116(7):1263–1267

38 Rhinologic Aspects of Sleep-Disordered Breathing

Shannon S. Sullivan, Oscar Carrillo, and Robson Capasso

The relationship between sleep-disordered breathing (SDB) and nasal function has been the subject of attention for over a century. In 1898, renowned otorhinolaryngologist Walter Wells reviewed and presented his experience with nasal obstruction and described symptoms of "melancholy, drowsiness, disturbed sleep causing difficulty attending to household and other duties" that greatly improved after treatment of "nasal stenosis."[1] Indeed, although it would be over 70 years until the term obstructive sleep apnea syndrome (OSAS) was coined,[2] clinical descriptions of nasal and upper airway obstruction associated with sleepiness have existed for much longer.

The terms obstructive sleep apnea (OSA), and more broadly, SDB, involve a spectrum of respiratory abnormalities occurring during sleep, which can be associated with an array of daytime symptoms. These are commonly secondary to increased upper airway resistance and repetitive upper airway narrowing (hypopneas) and/or closure (apneas) during sleep that can result in sleep fragmentation with or without recurrent oxygen saturation drops. OSA, defined by an Apnea Hypopnea Index (AHI) of greater than five events per hour, has an estimated population prevalence of 24% of middle-aged men and 9% of middle-aged women[3]; ~1 to 3% of children are also thought to be affected. It is a highly prevalent, although underdiagnosed, condition. Moderate and severe OSA has increasingly been demonstrated to be an independent risk factor for increased rates of hypertension, myocardial infarction, stroke, and overall mortality. It has also been associated with decreased quality of life, neurocognitive impairment, mood disorders, and increased rates of motor vehicle accidents.

In addition to distinct apneas and hypopneas, increased upper airway resistance may lead to other disturbances. When progressive increases in airway resistance result in an increased respiratory effort terminating in brief arousals from sleep with typically little oxygen desaturation, the term respiratory effort related arousals (RERAs) is used. These events are frequent in upper airway resistance syndrome (UARS), a term used to describe patients with chronic daytime sleepiness in the absence of actual apneas or hypopneas. In UARS, airflow is only mildly reduced, but increased respiratory effort is required to maintain the flow of air. RERAs in UARS are detectable by the measurement of pressure changes in the esophagus, a surrogate for the increased frequency of negative intrathoracic pressures associated with increased respiratory effort.

Snoring, which has an estimated prevalence of ~40% in the United States,[4] is one of the most common symptoms associated with obstructed breathing during sleep. Whether snoring exists in isolation as a primary condition is debated. Although snoring per se has not been definitively associated with increased morbidity or mortality, it may be a source of significant social and psychological distress to the patient and bed partner. Importantly, it is not possible to distinguish between OSA and "simple" snoring by history alone, and sleep testing is recommended to ascertain the magnitude of respiratory abnormalities during sleep. The continuum of SDB conditions is summarized in **Table 38.1**.

The prevalence of nasal obstruction is unknown. Extrapolating from data on the prevalence of allergic rhinitis and inflammatory/infectious rhinosinusitis, conditions in which congestion is the most frequently described symptom, the prevalence of inflammatory nasal obstruction might be roughly estimated to be 20%.[5] Although the connection between nasal obstruction and snoring is widely accepted, if only as evidenced by the wide availability of nasal strips, clips, medications, and other targeted nasal interventions, the relationship between increased nasal resistance and obstruction and SDB is less well universally accepted. Data from the Wisconsin Cohort, a large, longitudinal, population-based study, suggest that all-cause nocturnal nasal congestion is associated with a threefold increase in the likelihood of habitual snoring.[4] Furthermore, those with symptomatic allergic rhinitis

Table 38.1 Sleep-Disordered Breathing Diagnoses of Interest to the Rhinologist

Primary Snoring	Sound produced by vibration of the soft tissues of the upper airway during sleep, not associated with apneas or hypopneas
Upper Airway Resistance Syndrome	Chronic daytime sleepiness in the absence of actual apneas or hypopneas, associated mostly with RERAs and snoring
Obstructive Sleep Apnea	Subject presents five or more episodes of apneas or hypopneas per hour of sleep (AHI >5)
Obstructive Sleep Apnea Syndrome	Patient presents five or more episodes of apneas or hypopneas per hour of sleep (AHI >5) and has symptoms (i.e., excessive daytime sleepiness)

Abbreviations: AHI, Apnea Hypopnea Index; RERA, respiratory effort related arousals.

were 1.8 times more likely to have moderate-to-severe SDB independent of sex, age, body mass index (BMI), smoking, and asthma.[6] Udaka et al. reported data on 7980 workers demonstrating a significant association between observed apnea and nasal obstruction of unspecified etiology.[7] These data likely include those with both variable and fixed nasal obstruction in adults. However, in children, too, nasal abnormalities are thought to be significant risk factors for at least mild SDB.[8]

The coexistence of these two highly prevalent conditions is an evolving area of investigation and a subject of great interest to those practicing sleep medicine and rhinology. Many have proposed a causal and/or contributory relationship between nasal obstruction and SDB; but defining the pathophysiologic features and mechanisms, the relationship between nasal findings and symptoms and polysomnogram (PSG) findings, the selection of appropriate nasal interventions for appropriate patients, and the impact of nasal interventions across a field of metrics are all the subject of ongoing research and clinical effort. This chapter summarizes relevant advances in this area and outlines new directions in the field of nasal contributions to OSA.

Pathophysiology

The pathophysiology of OSA is complex and incompletely understood. Functional abnormalities in neuromuscular modulation of upper airway dilators, possible abnormalities in ventilatory control, anatomic abnormalities of the upper airway, and arousability are all understood to be important in this disorder. Although the relationship between the nasal airway and SDB is not fully understood, partial and total nasal occlusion during sleep in normal subjects increases awakenings, induces frequent sleep stage changes, reduces deep sleep, and increases apneas and hypopneas as well as oxygen desaturation.[9,10] Mechanistically, dynamic changes in nasal resistance, sleep-related breathing route alterations, and nasal reflexes have been implicated in SDB, and are discussed later.

Nasal Resistance

It is understood that nasal resistance (NR) to airflow is responsible for approximately one half of total airway resistance in upright, awake, normal individuals, with the main contribution coming from the anterior part of the nose including the nasal valve.[11] NR is greatest during infancy and decreases with age. The primary sites of NR include the nasal vestibule, the nasal valves, and the middle and inferior turbinates in the setting of vascular engorgement. The nasal valve complex, which encompasses the minimal cross-sectional area of the nasal cavity, contributes to most of total NR. This functional complex of compliant and dynamic tissues, whose detailed anatomic components are described elsewhere in this volume, is modulated laterally by the tone of alar muscles, and stabilized by bone and cartilage and has a lumen that is regulated by nasal erectile mucosa.[9,12]

Beyond the structure of the nose itself, there are important dynamic components of nasal resistance as well. The nasal cycle is an important physiologic variation in nasal patency, mediated by changes in the engorgement of the submucosal capacitance vessels in the middle and lower turbinates, with a frequency of every 2 to 4 hours in the majority of individuals. The nasal cycle not only continues during sleep, but has been proposed to influence overall airflow through the nasal cavity during sleep (**Fig. 38.1**).

Position is another important dynamic modifier of nasal resistance and probably interacts synergistically with the nasal cycle to heighten recumbent nasal resistance during sleep periods. Specifically, the nose becomes significantly more resistive when the patient moves from upright to supine, and during the nasal cycle, nasal resistance may greatly increase in the ipsilateral nasal passage in the lateral recumbent position.[9,13,14]

Of great importance to airway resistance is the sleep-wake status and, more specifically, stage-specific alterations in upper airway resistance and size. With sleep, the muscle tone in the oropharynx and its responsiveness to stimuli decrease. At sleep onset, therefore, total upper airway resistance increases. Traditionally, it has been held that the sites of increased resistance are palatal or hypopharyngeal; little attention has been placed on the nasal component of sleep-induced increased resistance. It has been noted, however, that patients with OSA have higher nasal airway resistance.[15] Interestingly, in one study, there is evidence that in rapid eye movement (REM) sleep, the nose becomes most congested, and in non-REM sleep, the nose is least congested, less so even than in wakefulness.[16] Although studies of sleep-related and position-related changes in nasal resistance are relatively few in number, the Starling resistor model of OSA can help explain why the concept of heightened nasal resistance (whether from fixed or dynamic sources, or sleep stage-related changes) is so intriguing in the pathophysiology of OSA.[17,18] Using this conceptual model, the pharynx is represented as a collapsible part of a tube with stable upstream (nasal airway) and downstream (tracheal airway) segments. Maximal airflow through the collapsible segment may be reduced by a narrow or resistive upstream segment. Therefore, according to this model, increased nasal resistance increases pharyngeal collapsibility.

Sleep and Breathing Route

In those with nasal obstruction and SDB, oral breathing may also impose instability in respiration and sleep. In one study of sleep in normal subjects, upper airway resistance was shown to be lower with imposed nasal breathing than with imposed oral breathing, in contrast to the supine and

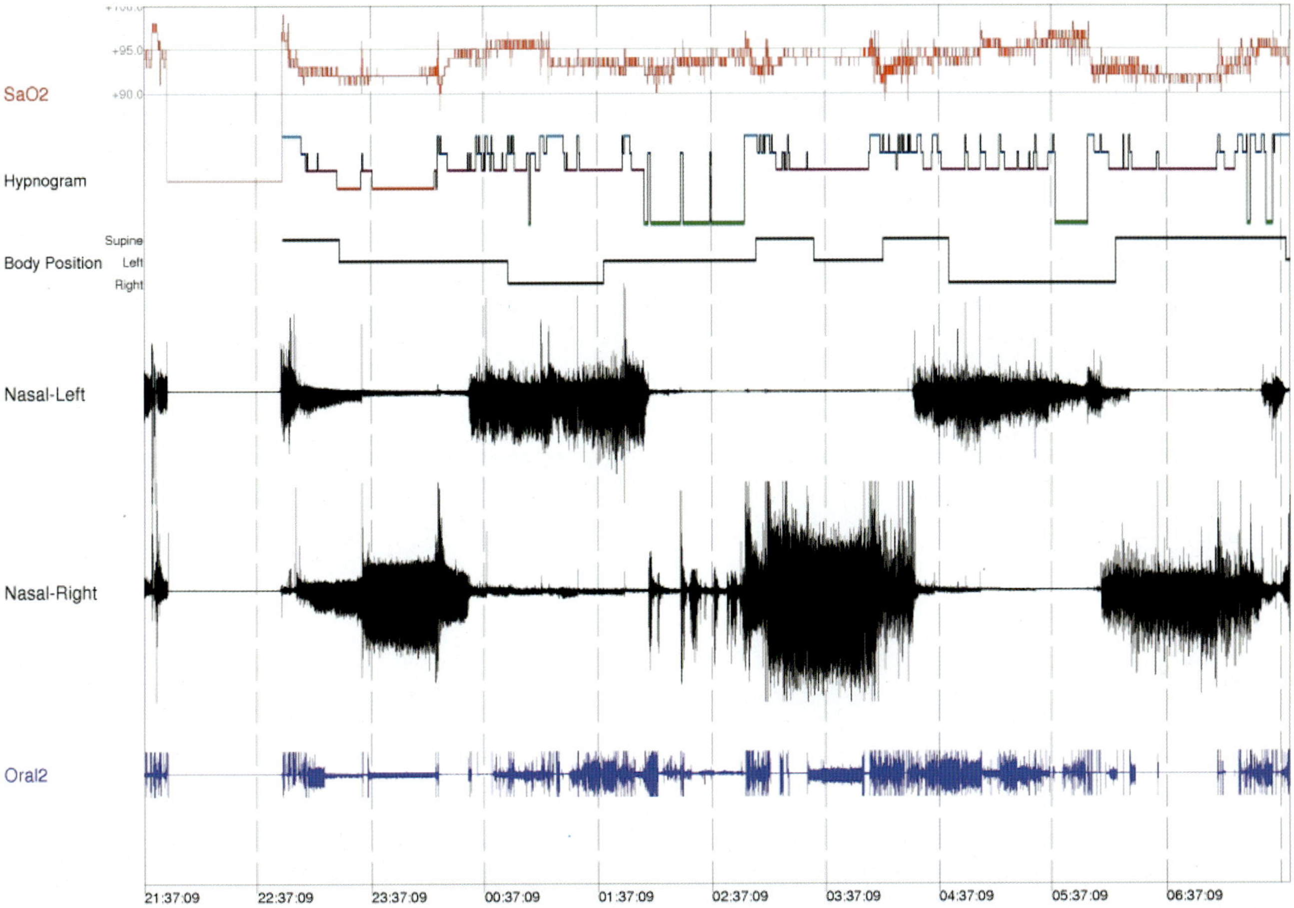

Fig. 38.1 The nasal cycle during sleep. A FloCHANNEL (Chad Therapeutics, Chatsworth, CA) nasal pressure transducer was used to measure airflow through each naris independently. Airflow transitions substantially between the right and left naris over the 9-hour sleep period; the transitions may be gradual or abrupt. Mouth breathing occurs intermittently. On the hypnogram, green bars represent rapid eye movement sleep; orange bars represent slow wave sleep; purple bars represent stage 2 sleep; light blue bars represent wake. SaO_2, oxygen saturation; Oral2, oral thermocouple.

upright awake states, where nasal resistance is higher than oral resistance.[19,20] In normal sleeping subjects, nasal breathing is expected to be the preferred route, unless it is impaired and associated with increased work of breathing or destabilized ventilation, in which case a switch to the oral route may be seen.

Oral breathing may in itself contribute to SDB because it narrows the pharyngeal lumen secondary to posterior displacement of the mandible, with consequent posterior displacement of the tongue, leading to decreased upper airway muscle tension.[21] In OSA patients but not in normal subjects, resistance of the posterior nasal airway is decreased with tongue protrusion.[22] Furthermore, in PSGs of sleep clinic patients using a specialized oral scoop to detail oral and nasal breathing routes, frequent transitions between nasal and oral breathing have been demonstrated to be associated with the increased work of breathing as well and arousals near the point of oral-nasal and nasal-oral transition. As **Fig. 38.2** demonstrates, it is possible to study the bidirectional transitions between breathing route in normal and OSA subjects with characterized nasal resistance and volume, but this work has not substantially been performed yet.

Nasal Reflexes

Another mechanism by which impaired nasal airflow may lead to SDB involves local nasal receptors and reflex responses. There is evidence to suggest that receptors in the nasal cavity and nasopharynx affect muscle tone in the oropharynx. Nasal breathing augments both minute ventilation and flow rate compared with mouth breathing[23,24] and this effect seems to be putatively mediated by local nasal reflexes. Such nasal reflexes would serve to decrease both nasal and total upper airway collapsibility. In one experiment, ablation of nasal neural reflexes by topical nasal cavity anesthesia with 4% lidocaine resulted in increased nasal and pharyngeal resistance and was associated with a fourfold increase in SDB events. This finding suggests that nasal neural receptors are sensitive to airflow and may be important in maintaining respiratory rate and upper airway patency.[21]

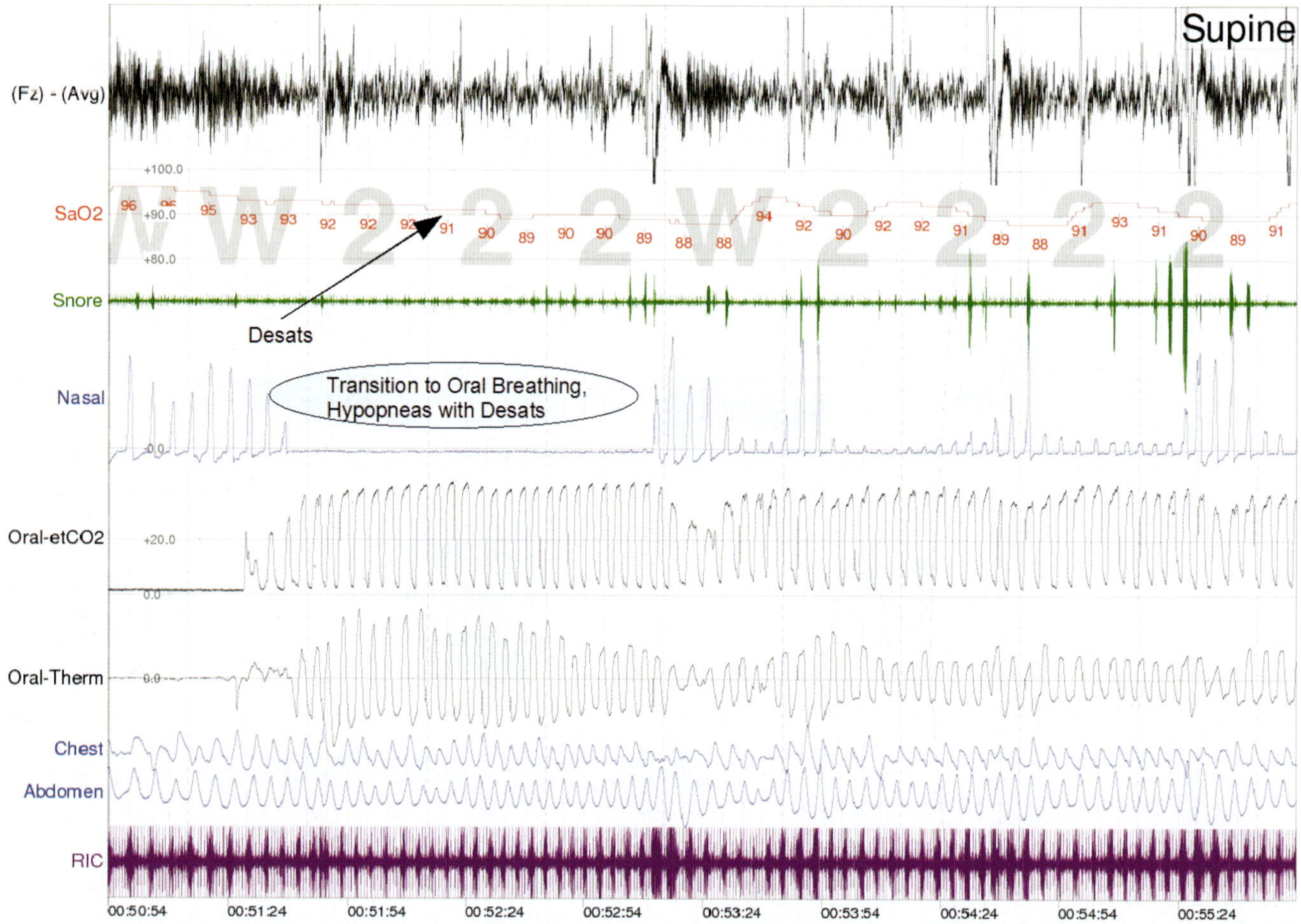

A

Fig. 38.2 Nasal-oral breathing route transitions, oxygenation, and sleep. A modified canula with an oral scoop (PureFlow Duo, Braebon, Ontario, Canada) was used to separately detect nasal and oral breathing routes. Oral airflow is sampled from the oral scoop, and measured via a thermistor suspended within the scoop. **(A)** Dynamic breathing route changes occur during sleep. In this patient, snoring increases as oral airflow decreases in the absence of nasal airflow. Note the repetitive oxygen desaturation with oral breathing. Resaturation occurs after brief arousals. *(continued)*

Clinical Presentation

The clinical evaluation of nasal patency and flow and comorbid sleep complaints can be quite challenging, and requires an upper airway specialist who has adequate knowledge of clinical and diagnostic sleep medicine. First, as confirmed in many reports, subjective symptoms of nasal obstruction measured by symptom scores may not correlate with objective examination findings or actual resistance to airflow (as measured by rhinomanometry and acoustic rhinometry).[25,26] In a classic example, patients who have undergone extensive turbinate resection may perceive nasal obstruction despite objective evidence of excellent nasal patency; in the other extreme, some patients may have significant nasal mucosal edema or nasal anatomic abnormalities but report no symptoms of nasal congestion. Similarly, in sleep apnea, the intensity of complaints does not correlate with objective measurements of OSA severity.[27]

To evaluate symptoms of nasal congestion, a detailed investigation and correlation of daytime, nighttime, positional and sleep/wake patterns, and fluctuations of nasal obstruction are of utmost importance. Associated nasal symptoms and previous nasal surgeries should be investigated, as well as topical and systemic medications that may change nasal patency. Age and gender are important variables because OSA prevalence increases with age and is more prevalent in males; however, postmenopausal women have an increased incidence of OSA, nearing that of men. Treatment approaches may have age-related differences in compliance and efficacy as well.

The clinical evaluation for OSA requires a careful history, including an assessment of daytime sleepiness, which may be measured using a validated psychometric tool such as the Epworth Sleepiness Scale or Stanford Sleepiness Scale. A history of unrefreshing sleep despite adequate sleep time, frequent nocturnal awakenings and/or nocturia, snoring, gasping, choking, dry mouth, excessive movements, or parasomnias should also be elicited. Daytime expressions of OSA may include sleepiness, fatigue, low energy, neurocognitive dysfunction, mood changes, or cardiovascular health problems such as hypertension. Motor vehicle and/or work-related accident risk must be assessed in someone

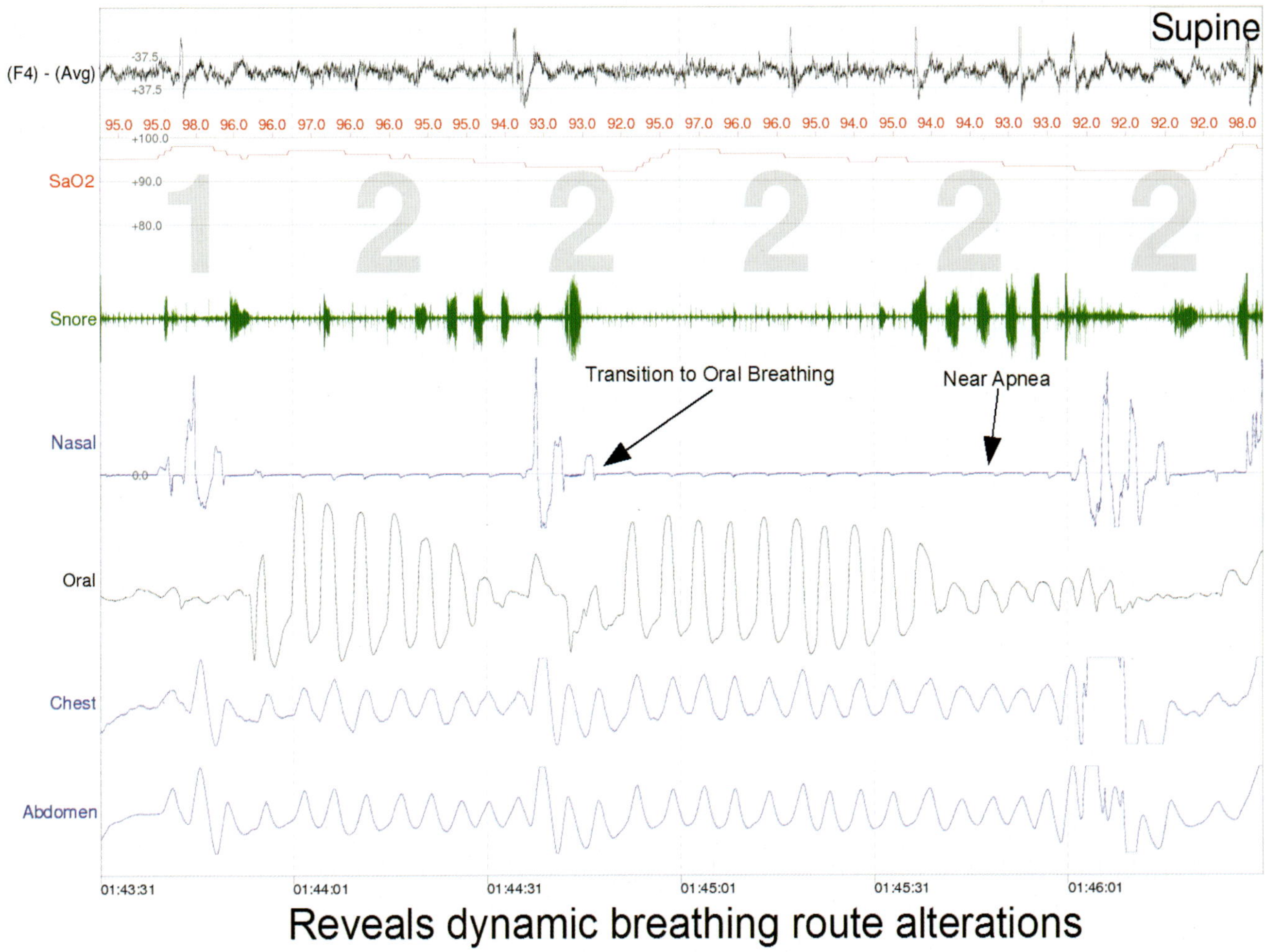

B

Fig. 38.2 *(continued)* **(B)** This individual rapidly transitions from nasal to oral breathing with sleep onset. Oxygen desaturation with oral breathing and increased respiratory effort just before arousal can be seen. *(continued)*

suspected of OSA. Close analysis of the patient's bed habits, and the use of alcohol, tobacco, illicit drugs, hypnotics, and other medications that can potentially interfere with sleep quality and architecture is mandatory. Furthermore, one must consider medical, psychiatric, and sleep disorders that have a high incidence of comorbidity with sleep apnea, such as hypothyroidism, insomnia, circadian rhythm disorders, insufficient or inadequate sleep, narcolepsy, or mood disorders. Close familiarity with sleep disorders is thus important for the rhinologist whose focus may lie in the surgical management of upper airway problems.

Diagnostic Workup

Physical examination is the cornerstone of the evaluation of anatomic predisposition for OSA. However, it is important to note that in-office techniques performed in awake and upright patients do not reflect the changes that occur during supine sleep. This presents a challenge: How best can one evaluate the upper airway in suspected OSA patients? The nasal examination for OSA initiates with the inspection of the nasal pyramid and nostrils, with special attention to the often neglected nasal valves. Although some degree of collapsibility on inspiration is expected, narrowed, surgically or traumatically distorted, or extremely collapsible nasal valves are very important findings. Anterior rhinoscopy and fiberoptic nasal endoscopy allow for the detection of nasal abnormalities such as septal deviation, turbinate hypertrophy, inflamed nasal mucosa, purulent or watery rhinorrhea, nasal polyps, and other masses.

Beyond the nasal exam, oral cavity and pharyngeal examination may reveal an enlarged and/or elevated tongue position in relation to other craniofacial elements; enlarged tonsils; oropharynx luminal narrowing by the lateral pharyngeal walls; an elongated, enlarged uvula; or an elongated soft palate. Dental malocclusion or other maxillary or mandibular deficiencies are likely to be associated with a narrowed airway column. Increased neck circumference—greater than 44 cm (or 17 inches) in males—and the presence of submental lipomatosis are common findings associated with OSA.

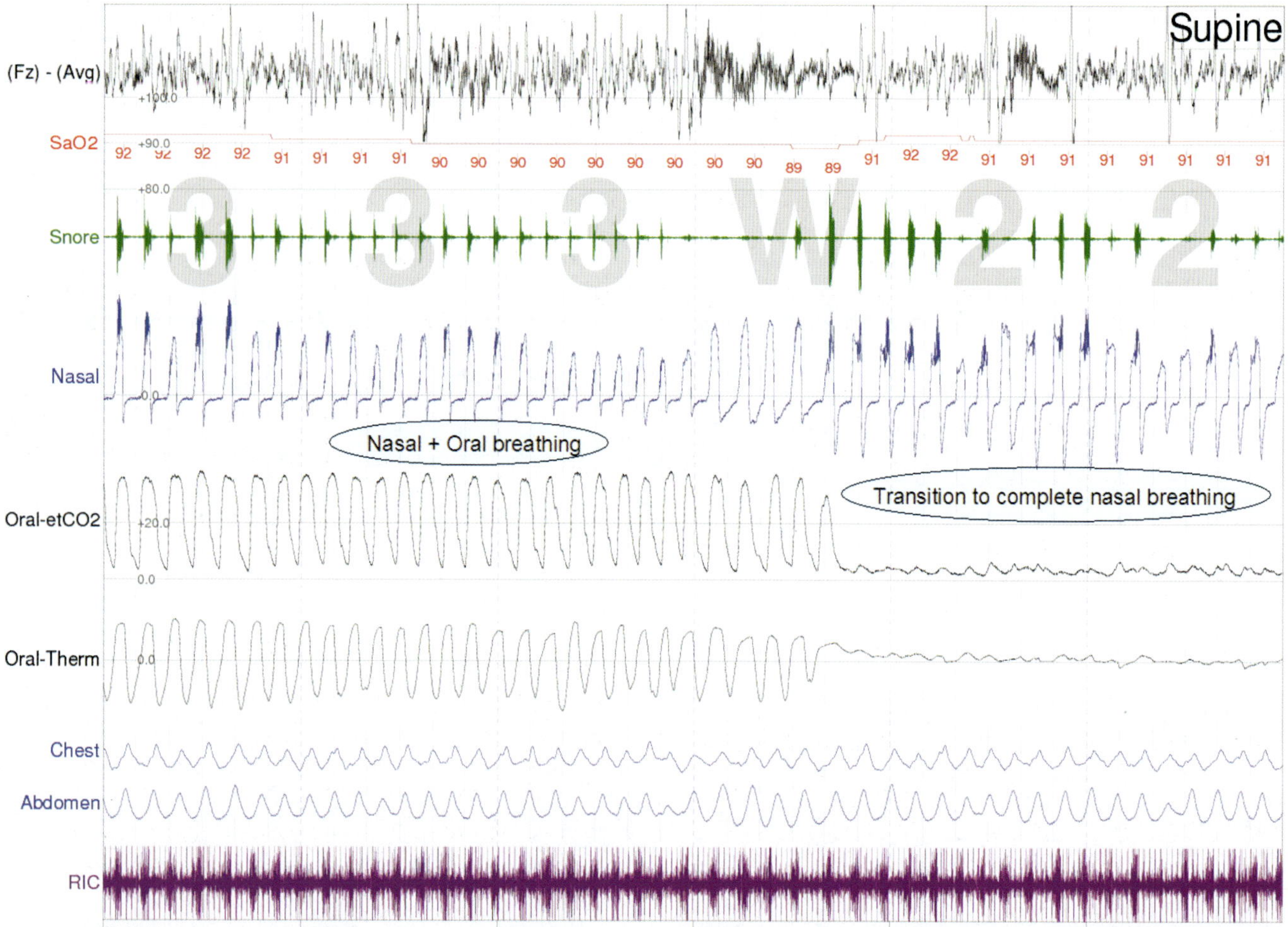

C

Fig. 38.2 *(continued)* **(C)** Mixed nasal and oral breathing. Increased snoring with nasal-only breathing in this individual. **(B,C)** End-tidal carbon dioxide measurement confirmed by oral airflow. SaO_2, oxygen saturation; Fz-Avg, frontal EEG signal; W, stage wake; 2, stage 2 sleep; 3, stage 3 sleep; RIC, right intercostal muscle activity.

Several diagnostic techniques have been described to evaluate dynamic upper airway collapsibility during wakefulness (pharyngeal critical pressure and negative expiratory pressure techniques) and sleep (acoustic reflection, fluoroscopy). Fixed anatomic upper airway abnormalities may be evaluated by cephalometric radiographs, computed tomography (CT) scans, and magnetic resonance imaging (MRI).[28] What follows is a description of techniques used to assess nasal contributions to OSA.

Nasopharyngoscopy can be a helpful adjunct in evaluating patients for OSA. Although dynamic collapsibility may be better measured using other techniques, a direct visualization can offer a distinct and necessary perspective on anatomic contributions to the narrowed airway. This is particularly true if a surgical modification of the airway is being considered. Nasopharyngoscopy is most often performed while the patient is awake, when muscle tone, respiratory drive, and head position are different than during sleep, and thus results of this examination should be considered with this in mind. General anesthesia with agents such as propofol has been used to perform drug-induced sleep endoscopy (DISE) to understand anatomic changes in the upper airway during sleep. However, some have pointed out that this technique does not emulate the changes in ventilatory drive, neuromuscular responsiveness, and dynamic airway changes that occur during various stages of natural sleep.

Another potential limitation of nasopharyngoscopy is that the presence of an instrument in the nasal cavity can distort the evaluation of the upper airway. Nonetheless, a recent report has indicated reasonably good inter-rater reliability for identifying the level of obstruction (e.g., palate versus hypopharynx) though somewhat lower inter-rater reliability for identifying specific structures contributing to obstruction. Reliability of assessment of nasal structures, per se, was not tested in this study.[29]

Acoustic rhinometry and rhinomanometry are not widely used clinically, but they may be a promising and helpful way to bypass the difficulty of examining the upright awake patient. It has been used both during the awake state, to measure nasal cross-sectional area at baseline and with position change from upright to supine; and serially during sleep, to measure sleep- and stage-related dynamic changes in nasal obstruction. Studies using supine acoustic rhinometry to measure nasal volume found a significant correlation with AHI, and demonstrated an average 18% decrease of nasal airway volume from supine positioning (awake) in one study.[13] Work has demonstrated that in nonobese individuals (BMI <25), nasal obstruction as measured by acoustic rhinometry significantly correlates with OSA severity as measured by the respiratory disturbance index and continuous positive air pressure (CPAP2) requirement.[30] More recently, acoustic rhinometry performed during sleep has demonstrated a significant decrease in nasal patency during REM sleep, suggesting another etiology for the worsening of OSA during this sleep stage.[16]

Nonetheless, the interpretation of data using acoustic rhinometry data remains somewhat controversial. For example, although data obtained anterior to the maxillary sinus ostia are considered to be accurate, there is not agreement regarding the accuracy of measurements posterior to the ostia, and thus care must be taken when interpreting results.[31,32] Although some data suggest that acoustic rhinometry measurements do not correlate with subjective complaints of nasal obstruction, other reports support a connection.[30,33] Studies using real-time dynamic MRI and sleep monitoring may also hold promise in understanding the roles of anatomy as well as functional and sleep-related changes in upper airway dynamics.

The diagnosis of OSA is definitively established using functional measures of breathing while asleep; an overnight clinical PSG is the gold standard. This test provides an AHI, or number of apneas and hypopneas seen per hour of sleep; a respiratory disturbance index (RDI) is a more inclusive measure of respiratory abnormalities that is used at many centers. Interestingly, definitions of hypopnea rely on amplitude of the nasal flow signal (as measured by an intranasal differential pressure), without consideration of oral airflow, which heightens the impact of nasal blockage in hypopnea scoring. Additionally, PSG does not identify the site(s) of airway obstruction.

To date, measuring nasal-oral and oral-nasal transitions has not been part of mainstream polysomnography. However, the use of an oral scoop to separate nasal and oral airflows more accurately (compared with the currently used oronasal thermistor for combined airflow) allows improved resolution of these breathing route transitions, and increased work of breathing and arousals may be detected at these transition points in some patients (**Fig. 38.2**). Also of interest is the measurement of the nasal cycle during sleep, which may be inferred from single-naris measures of flow using specialized equipment.

Interventions and Outcomes

The nose plays a key role in almost all available treatment options for OSA. CPAP is considered first-line therapy for OSA and is almost always applied via the nasal or oronasal route. Although CPAP is efficacious, effectiveness may be limited by poor adherence to therapy. Nasal-related complaints of excessive nasal pressure, obstruction, dryness, or rhinorrhea are commonly reported causes of decreased patient compliance.[34] Heated humidification is usually recommended with CPAP use to minimize nasal dryness, and the use of nasal pillows may be an acceptable alternative to facial masks for patients with claustrophobic tendencies.

Patients who require high CPAP to maintain airway patency (as determined by CPAP titration) may be intolerant of CPAP due to the discomfort of high applied pressure. For patients with evidence of structural nasal airway compromise, procedures such as septoplasty and inferior turbinate reduction may lower CPAP requirements and thus make CPAP more tolerable. Studies have shown improved compliance with CPAP when upper airway obstruction has been surgically relieved.[35]

Nasal obstruction may also limit the efficacy of non-CPAP treatments for OSA as well. Oral appliances are a treatment option for mild-to-moderate OSA, and one analysis of possible outcome predictors suggests that increased nasal resistance (in addition to elevated BMI) were one of the main factors that negatively influenced treatment outcomes.[15] A new disposable expiratory positive airway pressure (EPAP) nasal device has been developed that uses mechanical valves over each naris with an adhesive collar to form a seal. The valve produces increased resistance during expiration with minimal resistance during inspiration. Application of this device has had partial success in reducing AHI and improving sleepiness across a wide range of OSA severity.[36] This therapy, however, requires a patent nasal airway.

Randomized, placebo-controlled studies indicate that intranasal steroids reduce AHI in children and adults with OSA and comorbid rhinitis.[37–39] Mechanisms may include the reduction of nasal resistance and the suppression of adenotonsillar hypertrophy, among others.[40] The clinical impact of nasal airway surgery on OSA has been explored through a growing body of literature, but relatively few studies employ rigorous study designs and objective outcome measures (PSG, rhinometry, etc.). Classifying a nasal obstruction rigorously is another understudied area and is the necessary starting point for understanding the important issue of subject selection for potential intervention. There are few well-designed studies that have evaluated the impact of nasal surgery on AHI in OSA patients, but available data suggest that nasal surgery as a monotherapy is incompletely effective or ineffective at reducing AHI in most patients. Subjects are more likely to respond well if they were oral breathers preoperatively and are converted to nasal breathing postoperatively.[41–43] Milder OSA, lower BMI, and normal preoperative cephalometry have also been proposed to be factors favoring improvement in OSA severity from nasal surgery.[44] Negative prognostic indicators include obesity, abnormal craniofacial features, and pharyngeal tissue enlargement or redundancy.

Yet, AHI should not be considered the only important outcome when considering nasal surgery in OSA patients. Surgically decreasing nasal resistance has been shown to improve sleep quality, decrease snoring, and reduce daytime sleepiness despite no significant changes in AHI.[45] Nasal airway surgery for improved CPAP adherence also remains an important indication. Additionally, future research directions should include studying changes in stability of sleep in subjects before and after relief of nasal obstruction, relationships to work of breathing during sleep and nasal-oral transitions, and understanding the impact of nasal obstruction on daytime symptoms and subjective sleep quality in OSA patients.

Conclusion

Although the relationship between nasal function and sleep quality have been described extensively, notably for most patients reporting improvement in nasal and sleep symptoms after correction of nasal airway obstruction. However, clinical and surgical management of nasal obstruction alone does not consistently improve OSA when the measurement is based on AHI alone, but has been demonstrated to contribute to a CPAP efficacy and compliance.

While there is a long path to clarify the exact relationship between nasal function and sleep, correction of the obstructed nasal airway should certainly be included in the overall treatment plan for patients with SDB.

References

1. Wells W. Some nervous and mental manifestations occurring in the connection with nasal disease. Am J Med Sci 1898;116: 677–692
2. Bao G, Guilleminault C. Clinical Neurophysiology of Sleep Disorders, Handbook of Clinical Neurophysiology. Vol 6. Phildelphia: Elsevier; 2005: 91
3. Young T, Palta M, Dempsey J, Skatrud J, Weber S, Badr S. The occurrence of sleep-disordered breathing among middle-aged adults. N Engl J Med 1993;328(17):1230–1235
4. Young T, Finn L, Palta M. Chronic nasal congestion at night is a risk factor for snoring in a population-based cohort study. Arch Intern Med 2001;161(12):1514–1519
5. Stewart M, Ferguson B, Fromer L. Epidemiology and burden of nasal congestion. Int J Gen Med 2010;3:37–45
6. Young T, Finn L, Kim H; The University of Wisconsin Sleep and Respiratory Research Group. Nasal obstruction as a risk factor for sleep-disordered breathing. J Allergy Clin Immunol 1997;99(2):S757–S762
7. Udaka T, Suzuki H, Fujimura T, et al. Relationships between nasal obstruction, observed apnea, and daytime sleepiness. Otolaryngol Head Neck Surg 2007;137(4):669–673
8. Bixler EO, Vgontzas AN, Calhoun S. The Penn state child cohort: diagnostic criteria and possible etiologic factors of sleep apnea based on objective clinical outcomes. Sleep Med Clin 2009; 4(1):1–8
9. Rappai M, Collop N, Kemp S, deShazo R. The nose and sleep-disordered breathing: what we know and what we do not know. Chest 2003;124(6):2309–2323
10. Armengot M, Hernández R, Miguel P, Navarro R, Basterra J. Effect of total nasal obstruction on nocturnal oxygen saturation. Am J Rhinol 2008;22(3):325–328
11. Ferris BG Jr, Mead J, Opie LH. Partitioning of respiratory flow resistance in man. J Appl Physiol 1964;19:653–658
12. Kasperbauer JL, Kern EB. Nasal valve physiology. Implications in nasal surgery. Otolaryngol Clin North Am 1987;20(4):699–719
13. Virkkula P, Maasilta P, Hytönen M, Salmi T, Malmberg H. Nasal obstruction and sleep-disordered breathing: the effect of supine body position on nasal measurements in snorers. Acta Otolaryngol 2003;123(5):648–654
14. Lal D, Gorges ML, Ungkhara G, Reidy PM, Corey JP. Physiological change in nasal patency in response to changes in posture, temperature, and humidity measured by acoustic rhinometry. Am J Rhinol 2006;20(5):456–462
15. Zeng B, Ng AT, Qian J, Petocz P, Darendeliler MA, Cistulli PA. Influence of nasal resistance on oral appliance treatment outcome in obstructive sleep apnea. Sleep 2008;31(4):543–547
16. Morris LG, Burschtin O, Setlur J, et al. REM-associated nasal obstruction: a study with acoustic rhinometry during sleep. Otolaryngol Head Neck Surg 2008;139(5):619–623
17. Gold AR, Schwartz AR. The pharyngeal critical pressure. The whys and hows of using nasal continuous positive airway pressure diagnostically. Chest 1996;110(4):1077–1088
18. Egan K, Kezirian E, Kim D. Nasal obstruction and sleep-disordered breathing. Operative Techniques in Otolaryngology 2006;17:268–272
19. Fitzpatrick MF, McLean H, Urton AM, Tan A, O'Donnell D, Driver HS. Effect of nasal or oral breathing route on upper airway resistance during sleep. Eur Respir J 2003;22(5):827–832
20. Wheatley JR, Amis TC, Engel LA. Nasal and oral airway pressure-flow relationships. J Appl Physiol 1991;71(6):2317–2324
21. White DP, Cadieux RJ, Lombard RM, Bixler EO, Kales A, Zwillich CW. The effects of nasal anesthesia on breathing during sleep. Am Rev Respir Dis 1985;132(5):972–975
22. Coste A, Lofaso F, d'Ortho MP, et al. Protruding the tongue improves posterior rhinomanometry in obstructive sleep apnoea syndrome. Eur Respir J 1999;14(6):1278–1282
23. McNicholas WT, Coffey M, Boyle T. Effects of nasal airflow on breathing during sleep in normal humans. Am Rev Respir Dis 1993;147(3):620–623
24. Douglas NJ, White DP, Weil JV, Zwillich CW. Effect of breathing route on ventilation and ventilatory drive. Respir Physiol 1983;51(2):209–218
25. Stewart MG, Smith TL. Objective versus subjective outcomes assessment in rhinology. Am J Rhinol 2005;19(5):529–535
26. Lam DJ, James KT, Weaver EM. Comparison of anatomic, physiological, and subjective measures of the nasal airway. Am J Rhinol 2006;20(5):463–470
27. Weaver EM, Woodson BT, Steward DL. Polysomnography indexes are discordant with quality of life, symptoms, and reaction times in sleep apnea patients. Otolaryngol Head Neck Surg 2005;132(2):255–262
28. Togeiro SM, Chaves CM Jr, Palombini L, Tufik S, Hora F, Nery LE. Evaluation of the upper airway in obstructive sleep apnoea. Indian J Med Res 2010;131:230–235
29. Kezirian EJ, White DP, Malhotra A, Ma W, McCulloch CE, Goldberg AN. Interrater reliability of drug-induced sleep

endoscopy. Arch Otolaryngol Head Neck Surg 2010;136(4):393–397

30. Morris LG, Burschtin O, Lebowitz RA, Jacobs JB, Lee KC. Nasal obstruction and sleep-disordered breathing: a study using acoustic rhinometry. Am J Rhinol 2005;19(1):33–39
31. Tarhan E, Coskun M, Cakmak O, Celik H, Cankurtaran M. Acoustic rhinometry in humans: accuracy of nasal passage area estimates, and ability to quantify paranasal sinus volume and ostium size. J Appl Physiol 2005;99(2):616–623
32. Cakmak O, Tarhan E, Coskun M, Cankurtaran M, Celik H. Acoustic rhinometry: accuracy and ability to detect changes in passage area at different locations in the nasal cavity. Ann Otol Rhinol Laryngol 2005;114(12):949–957
33. Morris LG, Burschtin O, Setlur J, et al. REM-associated nasal obstruction: a study with acoustic rhinometry during sleep. Otolaryngol Head Neck Surg 2008;139(5):619–623
34. Morris LG, Setlur J, Burschtin OE, Steward DL, Jacobs JB, Lee KC. Acoustic rhinometry predicts tolerance of nasal continuous positive airway pressure: a pilot study. Am J Rhinol 2006;20(2):133–137
35. Chandrashekariah R, Shaman Z, Auckley D. Impact of upper airway surgery on CPAP compliance in difficult-to-manage obstructive sleep apnea. Arch Otolaryngol Head Neck Surg 2008;134(9):926–930
36. Rosenthal LC, Massie CA, Dolan DC, Loomas B, Kram J, Hart RW. A multicenter, prospective study of a novel nasal EPAP device in the treatment of obstructive sleep apnea: efficacy and 30-day adherence. J Clin Sleep Med 2009;5(6):532–537
37. Kiely JL, Nolan P, McNicholas WT. Intranasal corticosteroid therapy for obstructive sleep apnoea in patients with co-existing rhinitis. Thorax 2004;59(1):50–55
38. Brouillette RT, Manoukian JJ, Ducharme FM, et al. Efficacy of fluticasone nasal spray for pediatric obstructive sleep apnea. J Pediatr 2001;138(6):838–844
39. Kheirandish-Gozal L, Gozal D. Intranasal budesonide treatment for children with mild obstructive sleep apnea syndrome. Pediatrics 2008;122(1):e149–e155
40. Kheirandish-Gozal L, Serpero LD, Dayyat E, et al. Corticosteroids suppress in vitro tonsillar proliferation in children with obstructive sleep apnoea. Eur Respir J 2009;33(5):1077–1084
41. Koutsourelakis I, Georgoulopoulos G, Perraki E, Vagiakis E, Roussos C, Zakynthinos SG. Randomised trial of nasal surgery for fixed nasal obstruction in obstructive sleep apnoea. Eur Respir J 2008;31(1):110–117
42. Sériès F, St Pierre S, Carrier G. Effects of surgical correction of nasal obstruction in the treatment of obstructive sleep apnea. Am Rev Respir Dis 1992;146(5 Pt 1):1261–1265
43. Virkkula P, Bachour A, Hytönen M, et al. Snoring is not relieved by nasal surgery despite improvement in nasal resistance. Chest 2006;129(1):81–87
44. Sériès F, St Pierre S, Carrier G. Surgical correction of nasal obstruction in the treatment of mild sleep apnoea: importance of cephalometry in predicting outcome. Thorax 1993;48(4):360–363
45. Li HY, Lee LA, Wang PC, Fang TJ, Chen NH. Can nasal surgery improve obstructive sleep apnea: subjective or objective? Am J Rhinol Allergy 2009;23(6):e51–e55

39 External Approaches to the Paranasal Sinuses

Andrew H. Murr and Andrew N. Goldberg

It is fascinating to consider the speed of technological advancement that has occurred in the field of endoscopic sinus surgery. Only 20 years ago, papers and presentations concentrated on disseminating the anatomy of the paranasal sinuses and on securing the appropriate place of the new endoscopic surgical technology in the clinical armamentarium. Ironically, the anatomy was rediscovered from astute work that occurred over a century ago. Instrument development, the application of computer technology for use in the operating room, and powered instrumentation have created a revolution in the widespread application of endoscopic sinus surgery throughout otorhinolaryngology–head and neck surgery and now into other fields such as neurosurgery. New research concerning the underlying causes of sinusitis has helped to more accurately define the surgical candidacy of patients with specific problems. The current generation of young otorhinolaryngologists is so familiar with the endoscopic approach that many have never even seen traditional external approaches to the sinuses. This chapter describes the current place of external sinus surgery approaches in the modern decision-making process for the care of patients with surgical sinus disease.

Specifically, this chapter reviews the Caldwell-Luc approach to the maxillary sinus, the external ethmoidectomy, the external frontoethmoidectomy or Lynch procedure, the Lynch procedure with Sewall-Boyden flap reconstruction, frontal sinus trephination, and the osteoplastic approach to the frontal sinus.

The Caldwell-Luc Approach

Description

The Caldwell-Luc operation is typically performed under general anesthesia, although it can be performed under a local anesthesia with or without intravenous sedation if the situation demands. With the patient in a supine position, a local anesthetic is injected into the gingivobuccal sulcus on the side of the operation. An incision is made in the gingiva 1 cm from the fixed gingival margin to leave a cuff of mucosa to allow for the facile closure at the end of the procedure. Electrocautery can then be used to divide the muscle and to approach the periosteum of the anterior face of the maxilla, which forms the anterior wall of the maxillary sinus. The incision through the periosteum is made either with electrocautery or a knife. At this point, a Freer elevator or Cottle elevator is used to raise the cheek flap in a subperiosteal plane up to the level of the infraorbital foramen, being careful to preserve the infraorbital nerve as it exits the foramen. A Frazier suction is usually used to suction any blood from the dissection field, although if the subperiosteal plane is used, the dissection proceeds with minimal bleeding. Army-Navy retractors are used by the assistant to retract the cheek soft tissue to help with visualization (**Fig. 39.1**). Once the cheek is fully elevated, a 4 mm chisel is used to enter the anterior maxilla in the canine fossa, making certain that the entry point preserves the canine tooth root, which is the longest root. Alternatively, a 3-mm cutting burr can be used to outline the limits of the anterior wall window, and the bone of the anterior wall can be removed in one piece.

Once this window is opened, a Kerrison rongeur is used to remove the remaining anterior wall of the maxilla from the piriform aperture to the lateral maxillary wall while preserving the infraorbital nerve and the infraorbital foramen and the maxillary tooth roots. An opening through the anterior maxillary wall ~2 × 3 cm results from the full removal of bone and the direct visualization of the maxillary sinus results (**Fig. 39.2**). Historically, Takahashi forceps and Coakley curettes were used to completely remove the lining of the maxillary sinus. This resulted in a denuded sinus cavity. At the end of the procedure, the inferior turbinate was fractured medially and a curved rat tail rasp was levered through the lateral nasal wall beneath the inferior turbinate to create a nasal-antral window in the inferior meatus for dependent drainage. In modern times, the Caldwell-Luc approach to gain access to the maxillary sinus is still used, but with preservation of as much mucosa as possible. At the end of the procedure, the cheek is replaced. Closure consists of a single layer of dissolvable suture, usually a 3–0 or 2–0 chromic gut in a running, running-locking, or interrupted fashion. Antibiotic coverage is typically recommended for 1 week after the procedure depending on the indications and pathology being treated. Ice is recommended for the cheek to help decrease swelling.

Discussion

In around 1893 and 1897, respectively, Drs. Caldwell and Luc separately described a surgical approach to the maxillary sinus that used a gingivobuccal sulcus incision, an anterior bone trephination through the thin anterior maxillary wall, and an aggressive surgical curettage of the lining of the maxillary sinus. The approach also espoused an inferior meatus antrostomy or nasal-antral window that theoretically

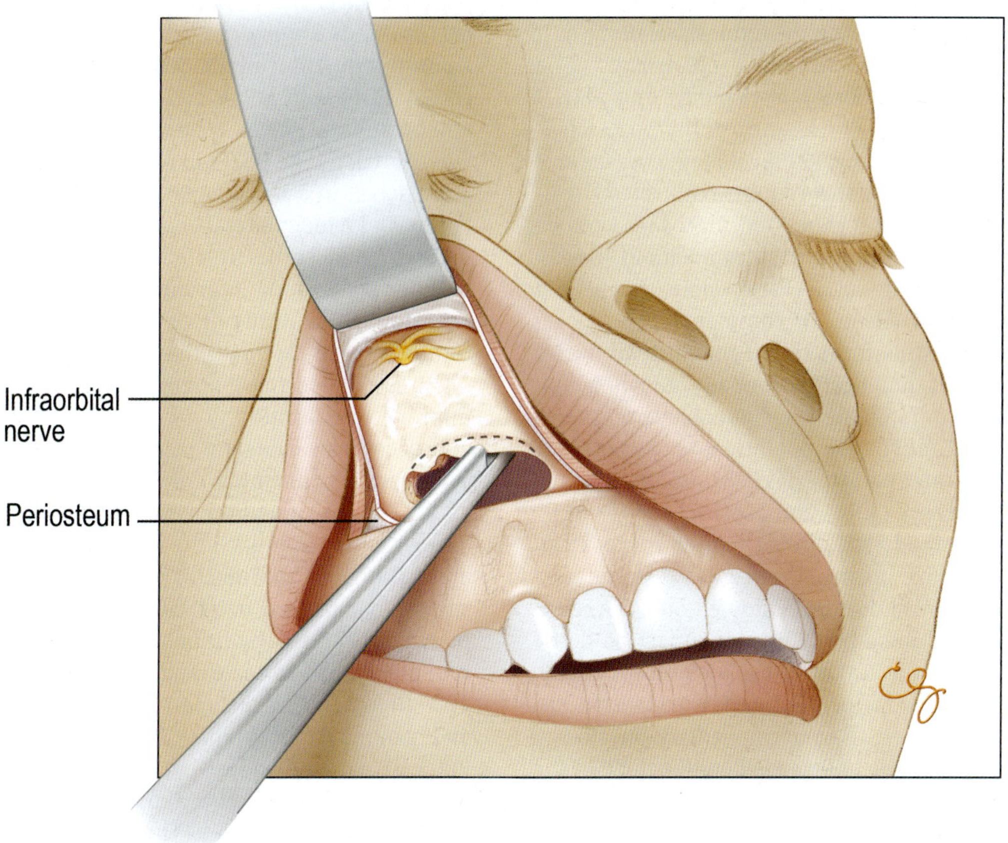

Fig. 39.1 During a Caldwell-Luc approach, the cheek is retracted and a Kerrison rongeur is used to take down the anterior maxillary sinus wall. The second division of the trigeminal nerve is pictured just beneath the retractor at the superior limit of the cheek flap close to the orbital rim.

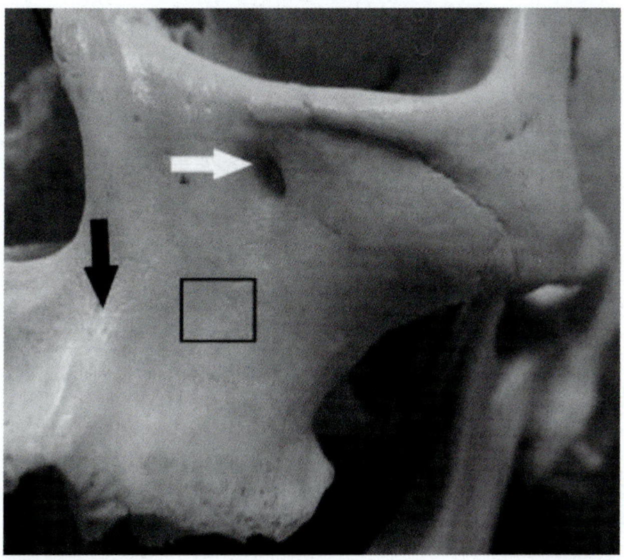

Fig. 39.2 The anterior maxilla. The *white arrow* delineates the infraorbital foramen, the *black arrow* points to the long canine tooth root, and the *box* shows the area of the anterior wall that can be entered with a chisel to allow complete and unhindered access to the maxillary sinus.

allowed for the dependent drainage for the sinus. This was the mainstay of surgical approaches to the maxillary sinus for the next 85 years.[1,2] There were problems with this approach. First, the inferior meatus antrostomy is actually not physiologically optimal for sinus drainage. Work by Messerklinger in the 1960s described the ciliary physiology of the maxillary sinus, and it is now established that the mucus flow of the maxillary sinus transports mucus to the middle meatus through the natural ostium of the maxillary sinus, through the infundibulum, and to the hiatus semilunaris.[3] Widening a surgical window inferior to the inferior turbinate ignores this ciliary organization which preferentially transports mucus to the site of the natural ostium. Nonphysiologic drainage of this kind may fail to resolve mucus stasis and thus perpetuate chronic infection.

Second, the curettage of the maxillary sinus lining with Coakley curettes and other instruments could injure the second division of the trigeminal nerve and create cheek numbness. The maxillary nerve traverses the floor of the orbit and is often covered only by thin bone, which may render the nerve vulnerable to injury. The superior alveolar nerves, which derive from the maxillary nerve and supply sensation to the teeth, can also be injured during maxillary sinus curettage. Traction on the infraorbital nerve as it exits the anterior maxillary wall also can create anesthesia of the cheek, typically temporary, lasting days or weeks.

Third, traditional Caldwell-Luc antrostomy poses challenges for satisfactory healing. Removal of mucosa creates large areas of exposed bone that require a protracted healing time. In addition, the regenerated mucosa is notable for increased fibrosis and reduced seromucinous glands. Contracture of the post–Caldwell-Luc sinus cavity and obliteration with scar tissue are common. There is also a risk of oroantral fistula formation if the gingival buccal sulcus incision does not heal, potentially allowing oral flora and food to contaminate the sinus. Modern studies of a large series of Caldwell-Luc operations showed a fairly high complication rate: paresthesias (9%), oroantral fistula (1%), wound dehiscence (1.5%), and dacryocystitis (2.5%).[4]

It is now understood that diseased sinus mucosa can largely normalize once optimal drainage is restored, and thus removal of mucosa during a Caldwell-Luc procedure is not necessary and in some cases may in fact be detrimental. The role of the Caldwell-Luc operation in current practice is thus extremely limited. It may have use in situations where a return to normal ciliary physiology is not expected. Examples to be considered include cystic fibrosis, where chromosome 7 mutations affect the chloride channel of the mucosal lining and cause mucus stasis, chronic mucosal inflammation, and *Pseudomonas aeruginosa* overgrowth. It would not be expected for the patient to develop physiologic recovery in this genetic disorder. Another possible example is primary ciliary dyskinesia or Kartagener syndrome, where there is a genetic ciliary disorder causing generalized, permanent mucosal dysfunction. In these two disorders, because ciliary physiology is fundamentally altered, removal of diseased sinus lining with an inferiorly placed drainage port has some theoretical chance of improving the patient's condition. On the other hand, a comparable surgery could also be accomplished endoscopically, avoiding the gingival incision and the risk of oroantral fistula, especially if complete sinus lining removal was not a goal of the surgery.

The role of the Caldwell-Luc approach in current practice is more applicable. The word "approach" here is used to mean that the maxillary sinus is surgically accessed through an anterior direct surgical incision in the gingival buccal sulcus and through the anterior wall of the maxilla. However, curettage of the lining is not done and an inferior meatus nasal antral window is not created; rather, a standard middle meatus antrostomy is created. This approach was popularized in the late 1980s by several investigators using a trephine through the anterior maxillary wall with a trocar. The 4-mm trocar allowed endoscopic examination of the maxillary sinus and the natural ostia and also allowed some limited instrumentation of the sinus.[5,6] In today's practice, a wide middle meatus antrostomy viewed with 45- and 70-degree endoscopes provides excellent visualization of most of the maxillary antrum, thus largely obviating the need for a maxillary sinus trephination or Caldwell-Luc approach. However, certain disease locations and certain types of disease may still be appropriate to access through the open Caldwell-Luc approach (**Fig. 39.3**). Examples of lesions that may be approached in a more facile manner through a sublabial approach include: lateral and inferiorly positioned fungus balls; foreign bodies related to endodontic tooth treatment or penetrating injury; tumors based on the anterior or anterolateral walls of the maxillary sinus; and bony tumors such as osteomas that may require extensive drilling. It is noteworthy that endoscopes can still be used to improve visualization and access by using the external approach as a channel for passage of the endoscope.

Current instrumentation is still quite rudimentary in its ability to turn around the corner of a wide middle meatus antrostomy to approach the anterior and inferior and lateral aspects of the maxillary sinus. Several endoscopic sinus surgeons have noted the use of the Caldwell-Luc approach for certain conditions, including a series of articles by Peter-John Wormald and his coauthors published in 2005 that espouse a technique called canine fossa puncture and canine fossa trephination.[7–9] In one study reported in 2005, 25 patients underwent canine fossa puncture for an indication that included "extensive radiologic opacification of their maxillary sinuses." Disease was further defined in this study based upon pathology to be due to chronic rhinosinusitis, nonallergic eosinophilic fungal sinusitis, and

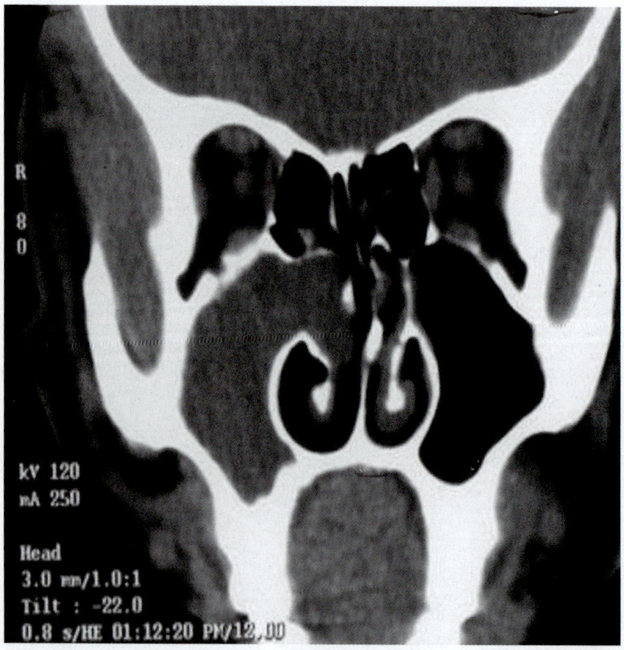

Fig. 39.3 Masses that are incompletely treated and recur after an endoscopic attempt at excision are potentially accessible via a Caldwell-Luc approach, such as an antral choanal polyp, which may have a difficult-to-access point of attachment.

allergic fungal sinusitis.[7,9] One of the key benefits advocated was a more complete removal of sinus polyps and inspissated secretions. The complications of canine fossa puncture appeared to be mostly transient, with facial tingling, facial numbness, and facial pain persisting in a small group of the patients studied.[9] Finally, a transantral balloon dilation procedure performed through a canine fossa puncture technique has been described recently. The advantages offered by this Caldwell-Luc approach include improved visualization and more direct access to the natural ostium of the maxillary sinus to effect dilation of the ostium with balloon technology.[10]

In summary, a Caldwell-Luc approach to the maxillary sinus with mucosal preservation is compatible with functional sinus surgery concepts. It is a reasonable approach to remove maxillary sinus disease, especially in the anterior, inferior, and lateral corner of the sinus. It allows direct instrumentation and visualization of otherwise inaccessible corners. The approach has had a resurgence in interest and has an acceptably low complication rate.

External Ethmoidectomy

Description

The external ethmoidectomy is performed through a curvilinear incision midway between the nasion and the medial canthus, inferior to the eyebrow and anterior to the lacrimal sac. The incision can include a Z-plasty or notch to limit scar contracture (**Fig. 39.4**). The surgeon will typically encounter a branch of the facial artery called the angular artery deep to the incision. The angular artery and its branches should be ligated and divided to prevent troublesome bleeding throughout the case. Once these branches are divided, dissection continues directly to bone through the periosteum, which is also sharply divided. A Cottle elevator is used to carefully elevate the periosteum posteriorly along the medial orbital wall across a wide front. The lacrimal sac is identified and elevated in toto from its fossa in the lacrimal bone without disruption. Use of a zero-degree nasal endoscope and a suction Freer elevator can facilitate this dissection and provide excellent visualization.

Care is taken to preserve the integrity of the orbital periosteum (periorbita) and prevent fat herniation into the field, which may interfere with the dissection. The Sewall retractor and malleable ribbon retractors are useful to gently retract the orbital contents to allow access to the medial orbital wall without violating the periosteum. The frontoethmoid suture line, which demarcates the relative position of the skull base, is identified as an important landmark. Dissection should be kept inferior to this suture line to allow for safe surgery without a violation of the skull base. Both the anterior and posterior ethmoid arteries exit the orbit at the frontoethmoid suture line. The anterior ethmoid artery is identified and a surgical clip may be placed upon it or it can be ligated and divided for added exposure (**Figs. 39.5 and 39.6**).

A Frazier suction is used to evacuate pooled blood, which can obstruct the view. It should be noted that the medial canthal tendon attachment is elevated with the subperiosteal dissection, but will reattach if the periosteum is preserved. Consistent measurements are made to alert the surgeon to the impending landmarks of the external ethmoidectomy. The anterior ethmoid artery is ~22 to 25 mm

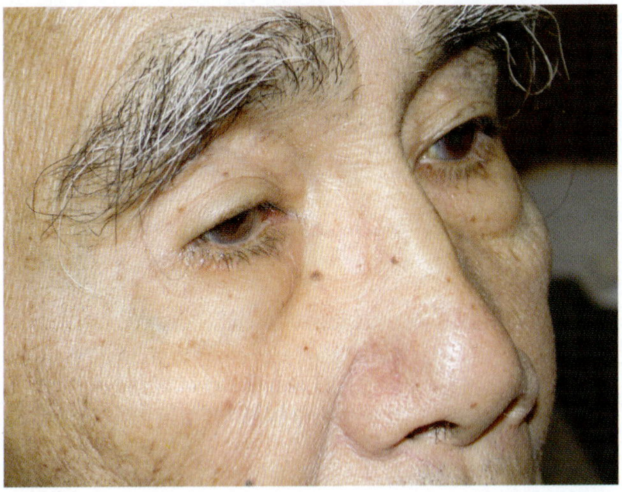

Fig. 39.4 This postsurgical wound is shown 12 years after a right medical maxillectomy. The incision is nearly invisible when healed.

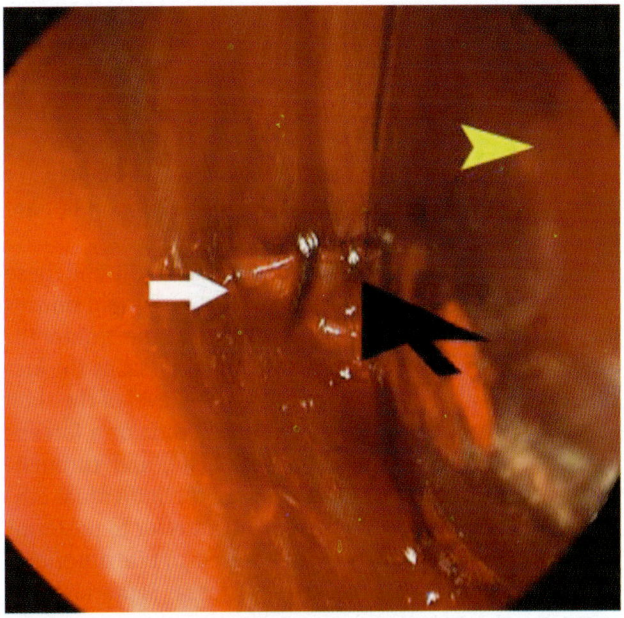

Fig. 39.5 Surgical clips are easily applied on the anterior ethmoid artery via an external ethmoidectomy approach. The *white arrow* shows the patient's left-sided anterior ethmoid artery foramen at the frontoethmoid suture line. The *black arrow* shows a surgical clip on the artery, and the *yellow arrow* shows a retractor holding the periorbita.

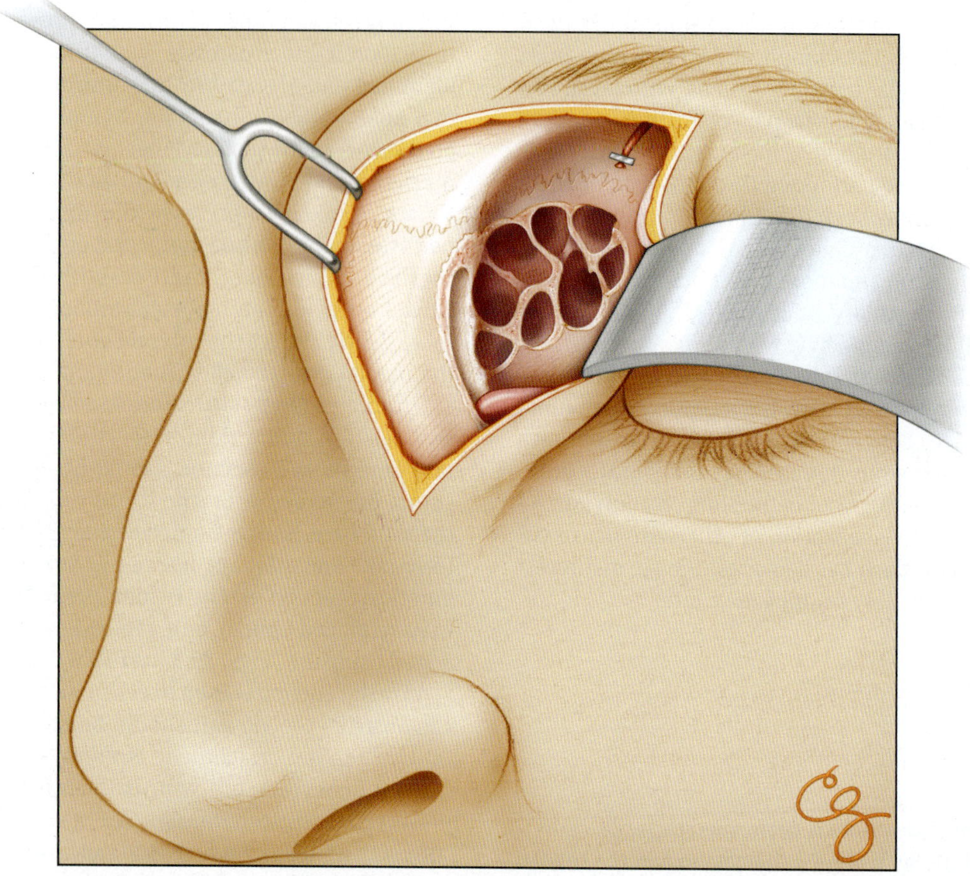

Fig. 39.6 The external ethmoidectomy approach affords excellent direct exposure to the ethmoid cells and anterior ethmoid artery, which can be seen with a clip placed from the surgeon's viewpoint. The lacrimal sac is depicted inferiorly, dissected and retracted free from the lacrimal fossa.

posterior to the anterior lacrimal crest. The distance from the anterior ethmoid artery to the posterior ethmoid artery is ~14 mm along the frontoethmoid suture line, and 7 mm posterior to the posterior ethmoid artery lies the optic nerve (**Fig. 39.7**). These measurements vary slightly depending on individual patient variation but are good guides to these landmarks.

Once the orbital contents are elevated laterally and these landmarks identified, it is safe to enter the ethmoid sinuses through the lamina papyracea inferior to the frontoethmoid suture line or through the lacrimal fossa, as the lacrimal fossa is always found inferior to the level of the skull base. The ethmoid is entered with the Cottle or a forceps and then a Blakesley forceps, Takahashi, and through-cutting instruments are used to enter the individual ethmoid cells and exenterate them in an anterior to posterior direction. Kerrison rongeur can be used to bite anteriorly into the hard bone of the lacrimal fossa. Septations are taken down under direct visualization. The sphenoid can be entered if desired, but the maxillary sinus is difficult to enter from this approach. The middle turbinate can be preserved or removed depending on the surgeon's preference and the patient's pathology. If the middle turbinate is to be removed, the middle turbinate lamina should be

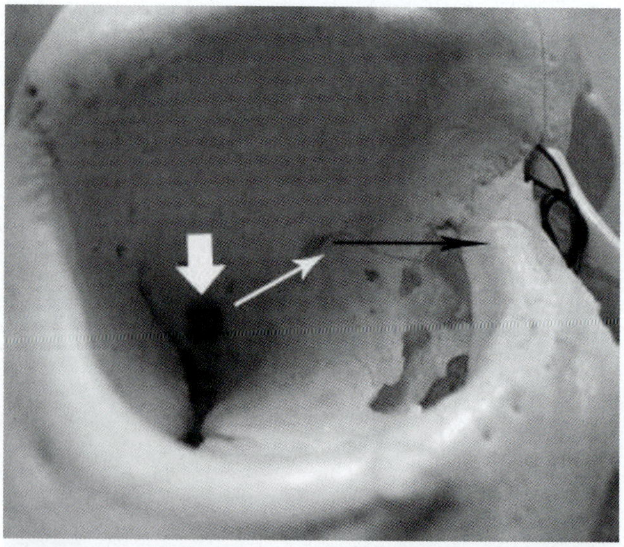

Fig. 39.7 The distance from the anterior ethmoid artery to the anterior lacrimal crest is typically ~21 mm as shown by the *black arrow*. The distance from the posterior ethmoid artery to the anterior ethmoid artery is typically ~14 mm as shown by the *white arrow*. The *wide white arrow* points to the optic foramen.

cut sharply at its anterior attachment preserving ~1 cm of vertical attachment. This is done to avoid avulsion of the cribriform plate anteriorly where the skull base is thin and violation is possible. A complete ethmoidectomy can be accomplished. Closure consists of allowing the orbital contents to return to their normal position. The orbital periosteum is ideally kept intact as noted previously to prevent orbital fat from herniating into the sinus. Care must be taken to position the medial canthus in its presurgical position with a tacking suture such as a 5–0 monofilament suture. Subcutaneous chromic or other absorbable suture is used to close the periosteum and subcutaneous tissue followed by 6–0 fast absorbing gut or nylon sutures in the skin. Nasal packing can be used if desired but is not absolutely necessary. Perioperative antibiotics are typically used for a variable amount of time depending on the patient's pathology and surgeon's preference.

Discussion

In the surgeon's current armamentarium, the role for the external ethmoidectomy approach to the sinuses is limited, but the current indications, while rare, are important. The external ethmoidectomy or external ethmoidectomy approach is still useful in the treatment of complications of acute sinusitis, in epistaxis, and in trauma such as nasoethmoid complex and medial orbital wall fractures. Because the external ethmoidectomy incision brings the dissection directly onto the periosteum, the orbital contents can be directly retracted to allow access to the lacrimal bone, lacrimal sac, lamina papyracea, the orbit, the ethmoid bone, the nasal process of the frontal bone, the frontal process of the maxilla, the skull base, and the anterior and posterior ethmoid arteries. Although this approach allows access to both the sphenoid sinus and the frontal sinus, it does not allow direct maxillary sinus access. Extension of this approach to the frontal sinus can be useful even for skilled endoscopic surgeons and is discussed in the section on the frontoethmoidectomy, or Lynch procedure.

External ethmoidectomy seems to have had its major application in the 1930s, 1940s, and 1950s. It was this era that straddled the discovery and more widespread use of antibiotics. It was also in this time period that Harris P. Mosher observed that the transnasal sphenoethmoidectomy was a potentially dangerous operation.[11,12] Mosher was influential in popularizing the external ethmoidectomy as a safer surgical choice when ethmoid surgery was necessary. Because the technique involved an external incision and because plain X-ray sinus studies did not show ethmoid sinusitis in an accurate way, it seems that the indications for the procedure were more conservative and were not recommended as frequently as current functional endoscopic sinus surgery procedures are recommended today. It is fair to say that the primary role of the ethmoid in the pathophysiology of sinus disease was underappreciated and certainly not as widely accepted in the heyday of external ethmoid surgery.

In circumstances where acute ethmoid sinusitis has caused a subperiosteal abscess or an orbital abscess, the external ethmoidectomy approach to the drainage of the abscess has several advantages versus endoscopic drainage. The approach is a direct approach to the subperiosteal space to allow for the efficient and complete exploration of the abscess. Although computed tomography (CT) scans with contrast are suggestive of abscess, the differentiation between abscess and phlegmon is not as accurate as to be infallible.[13] When using the external ethmoidectomy approach, there is no doubt about the thoroughness of the exploration of this space without the need to remove the lamina papyracea to allow for a complete examination as the endoscopic approach requires. Certainly, an endoscopic approach to subperiosteal abscess drainage is feasible, but the acuity of the infection causes inflammation, which makes hemostasis more challenging. The basic tenet of endoscopic techniques involves superior visualization, and the ability to achieve this in a bloody, edematous field will take patience. The external ethmoidectomy approach has the advantage of speed, direct access without necessarily removing the lamina papyracea, and the ability to perform a thorough and complete drainage operation. The external scar is cosmetically acceptable, as it is in an area that is easily camouflaged (**Fig. 39.8**). To further this point, numerous facial plastic surgeons have described external osteotomy approaches to the lateral osteotomies sometimes required in cosmetic rhinoplasty.[14,15] An osteotome is positioned through the skin in several locations lateral to the dorsum to perforate the nasal bone and accomplish the lateral osteotomy in a controlled fashion. These few skin perforations (between one and three) heal invisibly enough to allow this technique in a cosmetic population, and the incision for an external ethmoidectomy, if closed

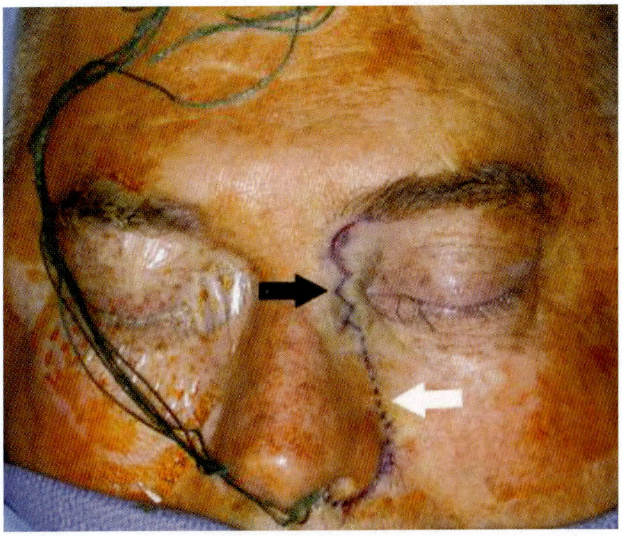

Fig. 39.8 The *black arrow* shows a running W-plasty incorporated into an external frontoethmoidectomy incision. The *white arrow* shows an extension of the incision to become a medial maxillectomy, if needed.

in an attentive fashion, should be acceptable to the physician and patient as well.

The external ethmoidectomy approach may also be used in decompression of Graves' ophthalmopathy. Although endoscopic techniques are typically favored in primary decompression, the external ethmoidectomy technique may still be appropriate on occasion, especially in revision surgery. Certain types of tumor extirpation surgery where extensive drilling is required, such as for fibro-osseous tumors, is a persisting indication for an external ethmoidectomy approach, albeit rarely. The external approach allows for good access for using an otologic drill in the surgical cavity. Finally, the external ethmoidectomy approach is still a reasonable approach to the anterior and posterior ethmoid artery in the treatment of refractory epistaxis, especially that which persists after ligation or transvascular occlusion of the branches of the internal maxillary artery.

Complications of the external ethmoidectomy approach include all of the potential complications associated with endoscopic surgery. Cerebrospinal fluid leak can occur, particularly if the surgeon strays superior to the frontoethmoid suture line. Direct orbital injury is possible, but because the orbit is retracted under direct visualization, orbital injury or eye muscle injury is unlikely. However, deep orbital retraction in the external ethmoidectomy approaches can potentially place traction on the optic nerve with blindness as a result in rare cases. Prolapse of the orbit into the ethmoid cavity causing obstruction or sinusitis is a theoretical concern in the external ethmoidectomy approach. As a practical matter, this is rarely the case and maintaining an intact periosteum should minimize the chance of this problem. Diplopia related to superior oblique muscle manipulation is another potential concern in external ethmoidectomy. Diplopia of short duration is not uncommon if the periosteum deep to the trochlea is elevated, and in rare situations, can last up to 6 weeks. However, if the periosteum is elevated from the underlying medial and superior orbit intact, it will reattach the trochlea to the bone without incident. Cosmetic deformity of malposition of the medial canthal tendon can be minimized by meticulously reattaching the medial canthal tendon with a permanent suture at the same level as its original attachment. Finally, an external scar is a most obvious difference between techniques. By incorporating a notch in the incision line, webbing will be minimized. In general, the incision will heal well and will be quite imperceptible in long-term follow-up.

External Frontoethmoidectomy

Description

The external frontoethmoidectomy procedure, or Lynch procedure, is an extension of the external ethmoidectomy technique. A curvilinear incision is made midway between the nasion and the medial canthus. A notch can be incorporated into the incision to reduce the chance of webbing. Angular vessel branches should be controlled and individually ligated. Periosteum is sharply incised and a Cottle elevator or Freer is used to elevate the periorbita from the medial orbital wall while preserving the integrity of the orbital periosteum. The anterior ethmoid artery is identified and surgical clips are placed upon it. It can be divided if necessary for access, which is not always required. A complete ethmoidectomy can be accomplished beginning in the lacrimal fossa, which is always below the skull base. A Kerrison rongeur can be used to remove the medial orbital wall anterior to the anterior ethmoid artery continuing superiorly to the frontal sinus, even including the floor of the frontal sinus. This removal of bone gives wide access to the inferior medial aspect of the frontal sinus, agger nasi, and anterior ethmoid cells and allows wide and direct instrumentation of the frontal recess. After extirpation of the obstructing cells, a stent or drain can be left in this space and wound closure consists of reapproximating the medial canthal tendon to the presurgical location with a 5–0 monofilament suture. The incision line is closed in a meticulous plastic fashion.

Sewall-Boyden Modification

The Sewall-Boyden modification might more accurately be termed the Sewall-Boyden-McNaught-Baron-Dedo-Henry modification, based on those physicians who advocated its use. Sewall practiced at what is now Stanford University and Boyden practiced in Oregon but they both recognized the use of trying to reconstruct the drainage tract of the frontonasal recess. This discussion was particularly pertinent in the 1960s when the principal controversy in frontal sinus surgery was whether osteoplastic fat obliteration was appropriate or whether the frontal sinus should be preserved as an aerated space.[16] The Sewall-Boyden modification was a sinus preservation technique. In essence, this technique allowed a septal mucosal flap from the superior aspect of the nasal septum to be developed to re-line either the medial or lateral aspect of the surgically enlarged frontal sinus drainage tract (**Figs. 39.9 and 39.10**).[17] Ironically, the flap is partially created from part of the nasal septum mucosa that is typically removed during an endoscopic Lothrop procedure. This technique of flap reconstruction of the frontal recess is purported to decrease stenosis rates in the postoperative period.

Discussion

With the development and refinement of the endoscopic modified Lothrop technique or Draf III operation, the need for an external frontoethmoidectomy with or without a Sewall-Boyden flap reconstruction is highly limited.[18] Development of these endoscopic procedures, however, occurred years after the initial description of the external techniques and was dependent on concomitant instrument

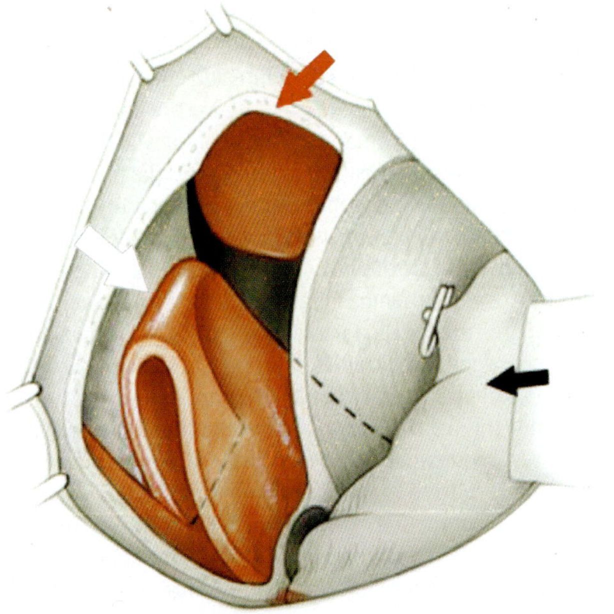

Fig. 39.9 The Sewall-Boyden flap is created through an external ethmoidectomy incision after the nasal bone is removed and a frontoethmoidectomy is accomplished. The flap is created from septal mucosa and from the mucosa on the inner surface of the nasal bone as shown in the figure. The *red arrow* shows the cut edge of nasal bone, the *black arrow* shows the orbital contents in retraction, and the *white arrow* shows the development of a laterally based septal mucosal flap. (Used with permission from Dedo HH, Broberg TG, Murr AH. Frontoethmoidectomy with Sewall-Boyden reconstruction: alive and well, a 25-year experience. American Journal of Rhinology. Volume 12, Number 3, May-June 1998, pp. 191-198[8].)

improvements to allow for an endoscopic visualization and instrumentation of the area. One remaining advantage of external frontoethmoidectomy is that it can be accomplished with common instrumentation available in almost every operating room setting in the United States. Sophisticated endoscopes, special instruments, drills, computerized image guidance, and microdebriders are not absolutely necessary for the technique. The frontoethmoidectomy allows for the treatment of lateral frontal sinus pathology such as inverted papilloma while maintaining aeration of the sinus to facilitate a prolonged follow-up.

The main criticism of frontoethmoidectomy is that it has a tendency to stenose the surgically manipulated frontal recess. The extensive bone removal and removal of anterior ethmoid mucosa creates a circumferentially raw surface area that may cicatrize and contract. Soft tissue prolapse can further narrow the frontal recess and impede frontal sinus drainage. Despite decades of surgical innovation, the stenosis rate of the Lynch procedure remained in the general neighborhood of 33%, regardless of the type of stent used (**Fig. 39.11**).[19] Nevertheless, in the modern era of endoscopic frontal sinus surgery, a stenosis of the surgically altered recess is still a key issue. A review of the stenosis rates reported in the endoscopic literature show a variety of results, but stenosis rates approaching 33% are published in some series.[18,20] Although the Sewall-Boyden flap is now mainly an historical concept, this flap technique addressed some of the stenosis problems associated with standard Lynch surgery by introducing a mucosal rotation flap to cover critical raw areas; some proponents reported a 100% postoperative patency rate. However, many of the results were reported before endoscopes and high-resolution CT imaging, so the determination of patency was not nearly as accurate as it is today. Unfortunately, this flap technique is difficult to describe, difficult to draw, and difficult to teach. A modern version of this concept using endoscopic surgical approaches is called the frontal sinus rescue technique, where a mucosal flap is used to line a previously obliterated recess.[21]

Other adverse sequelae of the Lynch frontoethmoidectomy may include scarring, webbing, orbital prolapse, diplopia, and numbness from injury to the supratrochlear or supraorbital neurovascular bundle. As in external ethmoidectomy, orbital prolapse is unusual, and the external scar is cosmetically acceptable. Diplopia is a valid concern as the more extensive bone removal encompassed in this technique can hinder reattachment of the trochlea. Numbness can be avoided through respectful identification and preservation of the supratrochlear and supraorbital neurovascular structures.

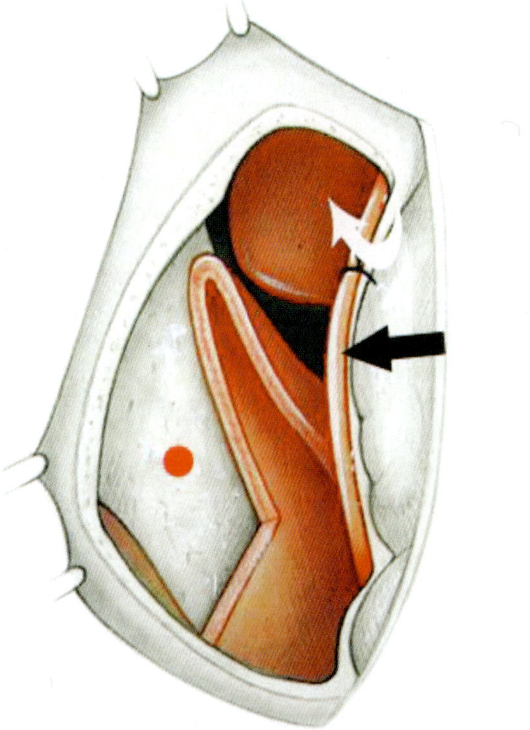

Fig. 39.10 The flap is in place to line the frontal tract. The *white arrow* shows the opened frontal sinus, the *black arrow* shows the flap sutured to orbital periosteum, and the *red dot* shows a denuded septum where the flap was elevated. The concept of the frontal sinus rescue procedure is nearly identical to this Sewall-Boyden flap design. (Used with permission from Dedo HH, Broberg TG, Murr AH. Frontoethmoidectomy with Sewall-Boyden reconstruction: alive and well, a 25-year experience. American Journal of Rhinology. Volume 12, Number 3, May-June 1998, pp. 191-198[8].)

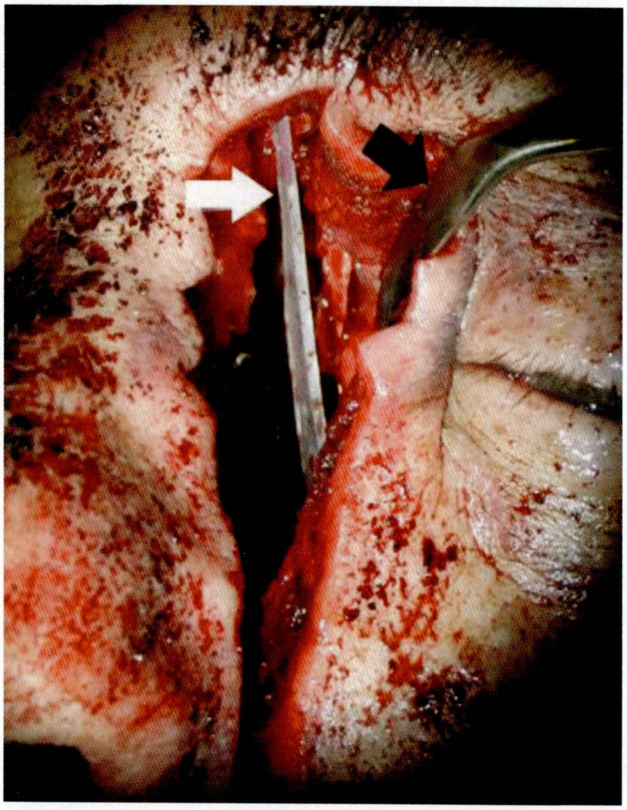

Fig. 39.11 A stent can be used in conjunction with an external frontoethmoidectomy approach to try to decrease the 33% stenosis rate. The *white arrow* shows a silicone sheet, and the *black arrow* points to a Sewall retractor retracting the orbital contents.

Indications of the procedure in the modern era are few, but real. Because wide access is afforded by the technique, it is a good technique when drills are needed to approach lesions in the lateral frontal sinus. It is still a reasonable approach for complications of acute sinusitis such as periorbital abscess, epidural abscess, brain abscess, and for when both the frontal sinus and the orbit must be drained. It is a potential revision procedure for a failed endoscopic transnasal approach to the frontal sinus and when the frontal recess is unfavorable due to severe scarring and osteoneogenesis or due to an unusually narrow anatomic configuration.

Frontal Sinus Trephination

Description

Frontal sinus trephination can be accomplished under general or local anesthesia. A 1-cm incision is outlined just medial to the medial end of the eyebrow, and below the eyebrow hairline. The incision is typically curvilinear or can incorporate a notch. Small, double-pronged skin hooks can be used to tent up the underlying tissue to allow a layered dissection down to the periosteum. Image guidance can be used to be assured of the optimal location for the trephination or a 6-foot Caldwell view plain X-ray at a 1:1 magnification can be used as a template. In the latter case, the frontal sinus contour can be outlined on a piece of film and cut out, brought to the operating room, sterilized, and used in the operating field to have a close approximation of the frontal sinus shape and extent. With the best position for entry into the frontal sinus accurately delineated, a 5-mm round diamond burr mounted on an otologic drill can be used to create a shallow entry in a gradual fashion through the bone (**Fig. 39.12**). The frontal sinus mucosa will then be identified. Entry into the sinus can first be confirmed with a needle, which should return air or purulence, depending on the pathology in the sinus. A Freer or Cottle elevator can be used to elevate the mucosa, and an entry into the frontal sinus can then be made. Attention to plastic techniques should be used to close the wound.

As an alternative to the open approach described previously, a percutaneous system exists for trephination and irrigation of the frontal sinus. A trocar and drill with appropriate stops to prevent intracranial entry can be used to enter the frontal sinus and irrigate in cases of acute infection or for endoscopic identification of the frontal recess, as described later.

Discussion

The frontal sinus trephination technique is a valuable adjunct to today's endoscopic armamentarium with renewed importance in direct access to the frontal sinus. It uses a small incision that should heal to a nearly invisible level. It can be a time-saving procedure in conjunction with endoscopic frontal sinus approaches, especially during Draf II A, II B, or III surgery where the identification of an obscured or a diseased frontal recess is needed.[22] Its adjunctive use resides in the ability to use direct access to the frontal sinus to help

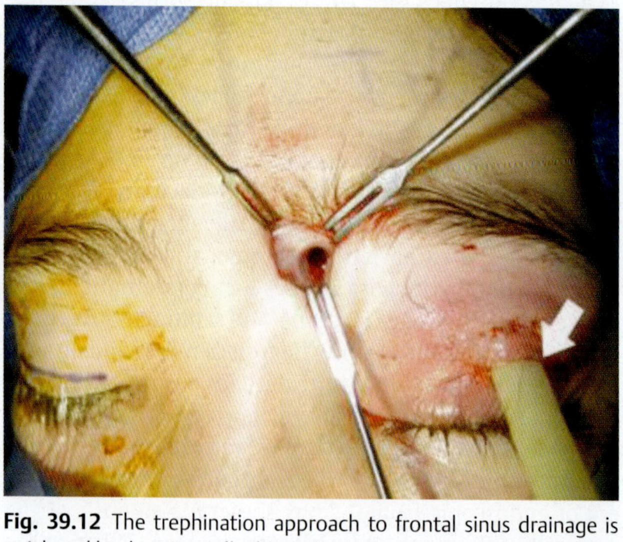

Fig. 39.12 The trephination approach to frontal sinus drainage is quick and heals quite well. This patient has a computed tomography scan shown in **Fig. 39.8**. The *white arrow* points to a Penrose drain that was placed into the orbit through a superior lid incision.

guide surgical decision making from below. For instance, saline can be instilled in the frontal sinus, allowing the surgeon to visualize the fluid trickle while dissecting the recess to definitively orient and direct the removal of the anterior ethmoid cells. It is also possible to pass a Fogarty catheter, sinus dilation balloon, or other instruments from above to help direct surgery in revision or difficult cases. Additionally, for some pathology that is laterally located in the frontal sinus, such as an obstructing type IV frontal cell, an expanded trephination offers direct access through this route. The minimal disruption to mucosa and minimal removal of bone at a location distant from the frontal recess decreases the possibility of a stricture or stenosis.

As a stand-alone procedure, frontal sinus trephination may be indicated in severe acute bacterial frontal sinusitis, or complications of ethmoid and frontal sinusitis such as subperiosteal abscess (**Fig. 39.13**).[23] A frontal sinus trephination technique takes ~30 minutes to accomplish and can be a very quick and direct method for surgical drainage. If indicated, after trephination, the sinus is irrigated and cultures are taken. After the pathology has been addressed, closure over a drain or red rubber catheter for irrigation can occur. Some use a double lumen catheter or place two catheters side by side to allow for irrigation to be instilled in one and egress from the other in the days after surgery. When edema has lessened and the patient can taste irrigation when injected into the frontal sinus, the drainage pathway is open and catheter removal can be considered.

Complications of the operation should be minimal, but numbness from injury to the supratrochlear or supraorbital neurovascular bundle and scarring can occur. Careful selection of the point of entry is important to avoid intracranial entry.

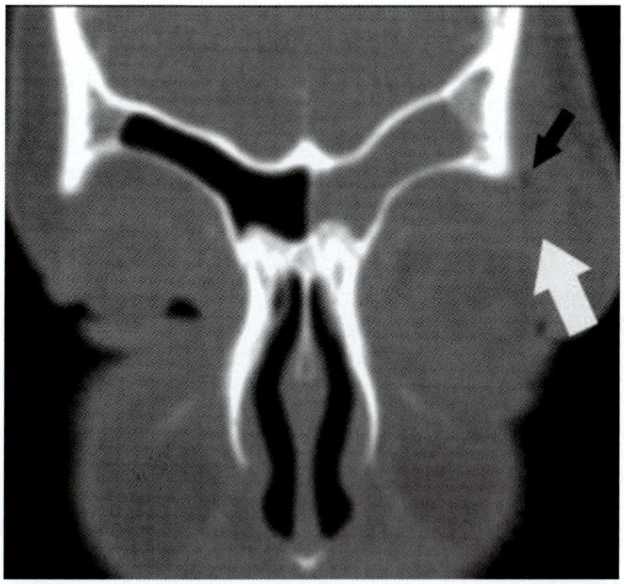

Fig. 39.13 A computed tomogrpahy shows a superior orbital abscess from an acute frontal sinusitis. The *white arrow* shows the abscess and the *black arrow* shows air in the orbit. Orbital and frontal sinus drainage must be accomplished. A frontal sinus trephination is a quick and facile approach that usually heals quite well.

Frontal Sinus Osteoplastic Flap

Description

The osteoplastic flap procedure can be performed on one or both frontal sinuses to address unilateral or bilateral pathology. It is performed under general anesthesia with the patient in the supine position with the head stabilized on a donut pillow or Mayfield head holder. The table can be rotated 180 degrees. Typically, the abdomen is prepped to allow for the harvest of a fat graft from the subcutaneous abdominal fat pad. An incision in the patient's left lower quadrant can be used for harvest to avoid potential confusion later with an appendectomy scar. Alternatively, a periumbilical incision can be used, which is cosmetically acceptable. It is standard to have a template cut out of a 6-foot Caldwell 1:1 magnification plain X-ray in the operating room and on the field to outline the frontal sinus saw cuts that will need to be made. Alternatively, image guidance with the array fixed on a bone pin can be used. The surgical approach can be through a bicoronal incision, through a midforehead incision, or through a brow incision. Although a midforehead or brow incision has the advantage of direct access, the patient suffers permanent anesthesia in the supraorbital nerve distribution distal to the incision. The coronal incision can be brought back far posteriorly near the vertex if need be and can include a running W-plasty if desired. It is the coronal incision that is typically considered to be the workhorse for this technique. The flap can be raised in the subperiosteal or subgaleal plane down to the brow with careful preservation of the branches of the first division of the trigeminal nerve. Modern surgical experience has found that the bone flap will survive despite full elevation of the periosteum. As such, it is probably more appropriate to preserve a pericranial flap during this operation. The pericranial flap can be used for either obliteration or for dural repair either at the time of the current surgery or in the future. With the pericranial flap preserved and the forehead flap held by surgical hooks, the entire frontal bone should be exposed. At this point, the template is used to outline an anterior osteotomy approach to the anterior table of the frontal sinus (**Fig. 39.14**).

The supraorbital rims serve as a guide to placement. A marker can be used to outline the bone cuts just inside of the template. A sagittal saw is then used to make cuts into the frontal sinus beveled from the periphery toward the center of the sinus. Once these cuts are completed, a horizontal osteotomy through the glabella is made with the sagittal saw, which can be extended to the inferior cuts on each side of the frontal flap. Alternatively, after the glabellar cut, the osteoplastic flap can be levered up with osteotomes. The inferior border of the flap superior to the supraorbital rims will hinge forward and fracture and will allow the anterior frontal table

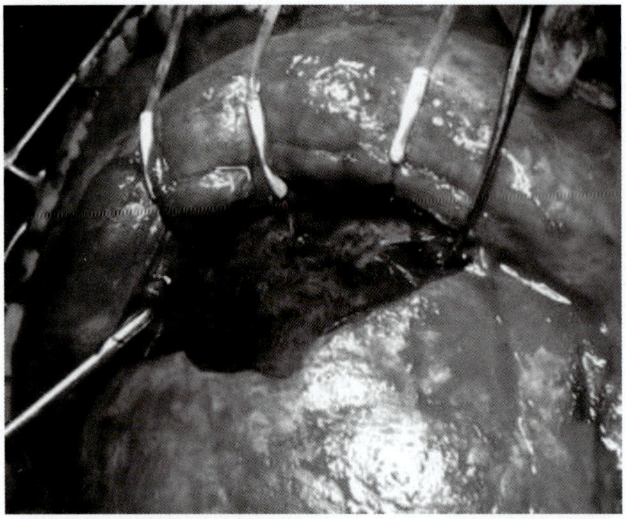

Fig. 39.14 A template of the outline of the anterior wall of the frontal sinus can be created from a 1:1 magnification Caldwell plain X-ray taken at a focal distance of exactly 6 feet. The template can be used during surgery to outline the bone cuts necessary to turn the anterior table bone flap.

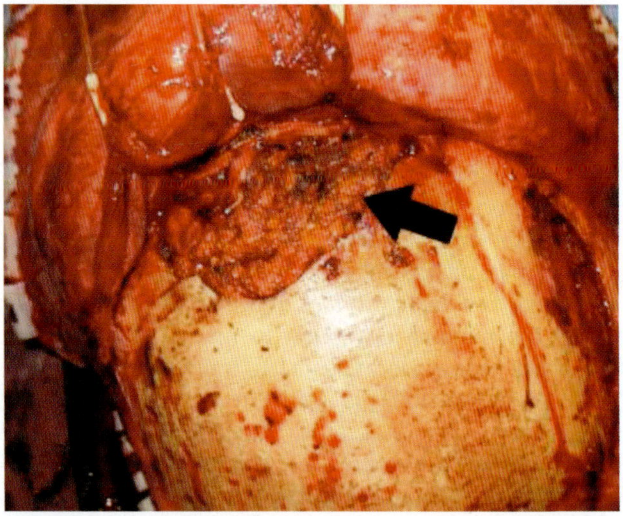

Fig. 39.15 Fat is placed in the sinus after removing the mucosa and drilling the bone with a diamond burr. The *black arrow* shows the abdominal wall fat packed into the sinus.

to hinge forward. Before removing the osteoplastic flap, any residual attachments of the intersinus septum or other bony attachments that may remain tethered should be removed. This approach allows direct, wide access to the frontal sinus and to the frontal recess from above. The pathology is then addressed and the decision is made if the frontal sinus is to be obliterated, cranialized, or left aerated.

If an obliteration is to be done, a Freer, curettes, and a Cottle can be used to remove the mucosal lining of the frontal sinus and the frontal recess. Bone septations can be removed as well. The mucosa on the inside of the anterior table must also be removed. Once gross removal is accomplished, a diamond burr is used on an otologic drill to remove mucosal remnants and to polish the surface of the bone. On a microscopic level, the foramina of Breschet allow invaginations of mucosa to become entrapped and the purpose of the diamond burr is to sand down the surface of the posterior table to remove mucosa as completely as possible. A microscope is commonly used to assist in drilling. Once this is completed, the frontal recess must be occluded. Many different materials can be used including fat, muscle, fascia, pericranium, bone pate, or absorbable gelatin or cellulose packing. Combinations of these autologous materials are often used depending on the surgeon's preference. This can be sealed with a small amount of tissue glue if desired. Obliteration can be accomplished with these autologous tissues as well, but fat is the most commonly used material. Strips of fat are placed into the sinus, and the sinus is slightly overfilled (**Fig. 39.15**).

The bone flap is returned to its usual anatomic position, and secured in place with either titanium or absorbable plates or suture, passed through holes drilled in the bone flap and frontal bone (**Fig. 39.16**). Closure of the wound must be done meticulously to reapproximate pericranium, galea, subcutaneous tissue, and skin. Staples may be used with good effect on the skin closure. Usually, two Jackson-Pratt suction drains are used to remove fluid that is expected to accumulate postoperatively. Antibiotic ointment can be used on the incision line.

If a cranialization is to be performed, the bone of the posterior wall of the frontal sinus is removed along with its mucosal lining. Mucosa of the anterior table and of the remaining sinus is removed and drilled with a diamond burr, and the frontal recess is occluded as described previously. As the brain will be allowed to herniate forward into the frontal sinus space, sharp edges of the frontal bone are drilled with a cutting and diamond burr. Any cerebrospinal fluid (CSF) leak that may be present is repaired. The bone flap is replaced as described previously.

Lastly, if the sinus is to be left aerated, frontal recesses are not occluded but rather opened widely from above

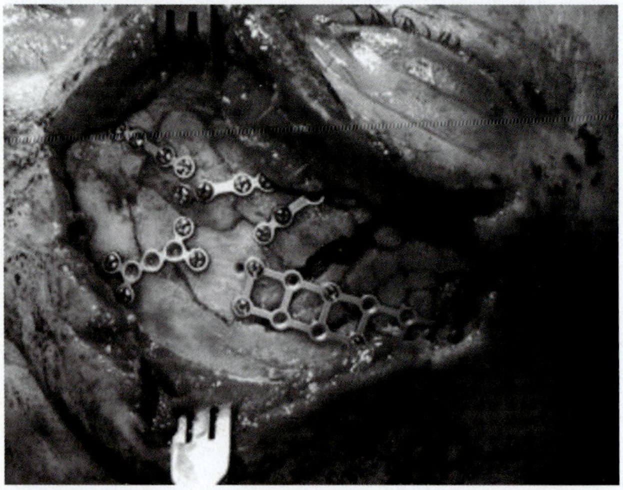

Fig. 39.16 A comminuted anterior table frontal sinus fracture approached through a preexisting laceration. To accomplish open reduction and internal fixation, an open sinus approach is required.

and below to provide a common drainage pathway for the right and left frontal sinuses. In cases where the mucosa has been removed from apposing surfaces of the sinus, a flexible silicone sheet may be cut to fit the sinus and placed between the raw surfaces. The frontal recess will need to be sufficiently patent to allow the flexible sheet to be delivered through the nose, typically 3 to 6 weeks after surgery.

Discussion

Osteoplastic fat obliteration of the frontal sinus was long considered to be the gold standard for safe handling of frontal sinus disease. It was popularized by Bergara and then Montgomery in the 1950s and 1960s. Montgomery published a landmark paper with Hardy showing good results with long-term follow-up of patients treated with this technique, but their series also showed a fairly high total complication rate approaching 10%.[24] Complications include numbness due to injury to the first division of the trigeminal nerve, infection, flap failure, disease persistence, CSF leak, and all the other potential complications of sinus surgery. One major concern about this technique regarded the long-term follow-up. It was felt that late mucocele formation could occur even decades after the surgery with potentially devastating results. A follow-up of 20 years or more was felt to be necessary to truly assess the success of the procedure. Dr. Montgomery died in 2003, but he probably had the single largest practice with regard to the osteoplastic flap procedure. Dr. Montgomery also practiced in a single location from 1955 to 2002. He did not feel it necessary to update the complication rates reported in his landmark 250 patient series, but indicated that the procedure still had a role in the modern era of endoscopic surgery. His wisdom should not be underestimated; Montgomery wrote his final publication on the subject, delineating a continued place for the procedure in the modern armamentarium.[25] Current indications in his article included failed endoscopic surgery, treatment of CSF leaks, benign tumor surgery, and treatment of depressed fractures.

A valid criticism of osteoplastic obliteration is that it is difficult to follow the patient for evidence of persistent or recurrent disease after surgery. Certainly, ascertainment of frontal patency is much easier in patients who have undergone endoscopic frontal sinusotomy, with the advantage of direct endoscopic visualization and follow-up. Nevertheless, MRI can be used to provide surveillance postoperatively for patients who have had osteoplastic fat obliteration to look for mucocele development or tumor recurrence.[26] Disadvantages of the flap procedure include the extensive coronal incision or a forehead incision required for the exposure and the need for several days of hospitalization to recover from the procedure. The procedure is also nonphysiologic in nature, with the goal of removing the sinus from participation as a functional aerated space.

Indications for the frontal sinus obliteration are much narrower today than during the peak of its popularity. Chronic frontal sinusitis can be treated effectively with endoscopic surgery including Draf I, Draf IIA, and Draf IIB procedures. For failures of this type of recess surgery, the Draf III or endoscopic modified Lothrop procedure has an impressive track record in a difficult patient group that has failed other methods.[27] If Draf III procedure fails, a frontal sinus osteoplastic flap procedure would be a reasonable next step when treating refractory chronic rhinosinusitis. The osteoplastic flap approach, with or without obliteration, still has use in tumor surgery where drilling within the frontal sinus itself is required. Typically, it would be considered as a first-line approach in cases where the tumor is located laterally in the frontal sinus. However, a postoperative office endoscopic inspection with an aerated sinus is valuable as a method of follow-up, making obliteration unattractive. Finally, the osteoplastic approach still has primary use in circumstances of frontal sinus trauma where plating of displaced fractures will be necessary from both a cosmetic and functional standpoint.[28] In general, if a CSF leak is present or if a displaced posterior table frontal sinus fracture is present, an osteoplastic flap approach may be needed during the surgical approach to reduce and stabilize the fractures, followed by cranialization. (**Figs. 39.17**

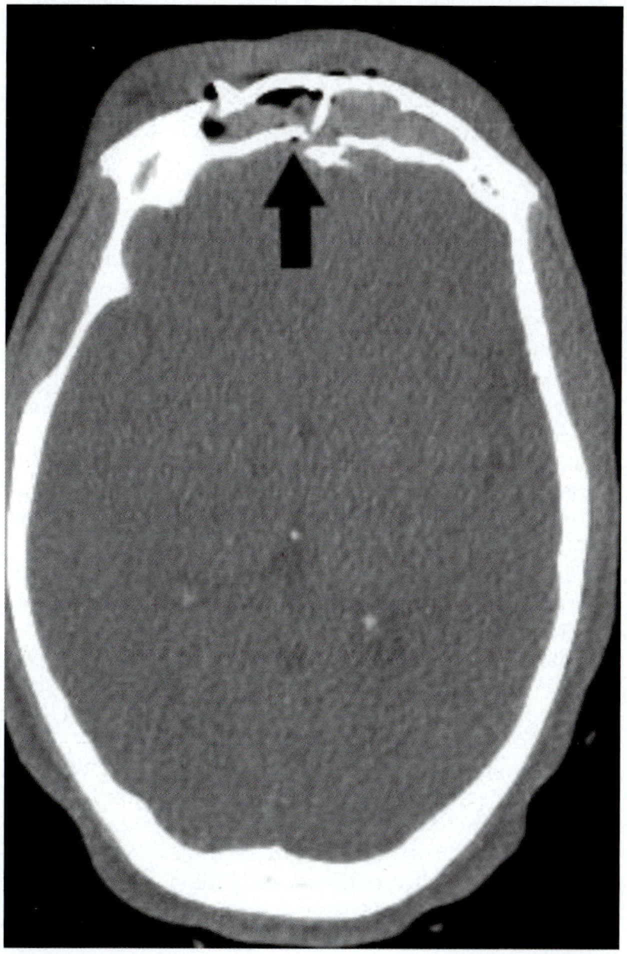

Fig. 39.17 An anterior and posterior table frontal sinus fracture is present. The *black arrow* points to intracranial air and a posterior table that is displaced. This fracture must be approached in such a way as to enable open reduction and internal fixation of the fracture while at the same time preventing distant complications such as mucocele formation.

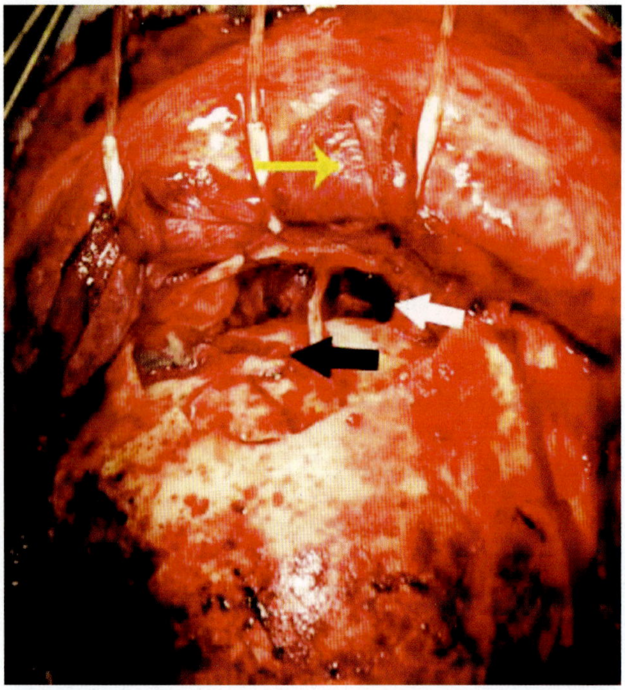

Fig. 39.18 The same patient in Fig. 39.17 at the time of surgery. The *black arrow* points to a minimally displaced posterior table fracture with a cerebral spinal fluid leak. The *white arrow* shows the frontal recess from above. The *yellow arrow* shows a preserved pericranial flap retracted by surgical hooks.

and 39.18). Obliteration is also a reasonable option if the frontal recess is involved in the fracture and is unlikely to function normally after healing is completed. It should be noted that the frontal sinus osteoplastic fat obliteration technique is not an optimal procedure for treatment of acute infection. If infection of the bone flap or fat graft were to occur, bone flap necrosis or loss might follow. Rather, temporizing the situation with a trephination and parenteral antibiotics would take precedence over an osteoplastic flap operation in this risk-laden setting.

Conclusion

Although endoscopic techniques have been developed to address the vast majority of sinus pathology, external approaches are valuable in select situations. Significant advantages of the external approaches in these situations mandate that the techniques be taught and mastered to complete the surgical armamentarium. It is likely that with a significantly reduced volume of external sinus surgery being performed and taught in training programs, external approaches will increasingly be referred to centers of excellence where the volume and expertise in these approaches is maintained.

References

1. Caldwell G. Diseases of nasal sinuses. NY Med J 1893;58:527
2. Macbeth R. Caldwell-Luc operation 1952-1966. Arch Otolaryngol 1968;87(6):630–636
3. Messerklinger W. Endoscopy of the Nose. Baltimore: Urban and Schwarzenberg; 1978
4. DeFreitas J, Lucente FE. The Caldwell-Luc procedure: institutional review of 670 cases: 1975-1985. Laryngoscope 1988;98(12): 1297–1300
5. May M, Sobol SM, Korzec K. The location of the maxillary os and its importance to the endoscopic sinus surgeon. Laryngoscope 1990;100(10 Pt 1):1037–1042
6. Kennedy DW, Zinreich SJ, Rosenbaum AE, Johns ME. Functional endoscopic sinus surgery. Theory and diagnostic evaluation. Arch Otolaryngol 1985;111(9):576–582
7. Robinson S, Wormald PJ. Patterns of innervation of the anterior maxilla: a cadaver study with relevance to canine fossa puncture of the maxillary sinus. Laryngoscope 2005;115(10): 1785–1788
8. Sathananthar S, Nagaonkar S, Paleri V, Le T, Robinson S, Wormald PJ. Canine fossa puncture and clearance of the maxillary sinus for the severely diseased maxillary sinus. Laryngoscope 2005;115(6):1026–1029
9. Robinson SR, Baird R, Le T, Wormald PJ. The incidence of complications after canine fossa puncture performed during endoscopic sinus surgery. Am J Rhinol 2005;19(2):203–206
10. Stankiewicz J, Tami T, Truitt T, Atkins J, Liepert D, Winegar B. Transantral, endoscopically guided balloon dilatation of the ostiomeatal complex for chronic rhinosinusitis under local anesthesia. Am J Rhinol Allergy 2009;23(3):321–327
11. Mosher HP. Surgical anatomy of the ethmoid labyrinth. Arch Otolaryngol 1929;38:869–901
12. Lawson W. The intranasal ethmoidectomy: evolution and an assessment of the procedure. Laryngoscope 1994;104 (6 Pt 2):1–49
13. Noordzij JP, Harrison SE, Mason JC, Hashisaki GT, Reibel JF, Gross CW. Pitfalls in the endoscopic drainage of subperiosteal orbital abscesses secondary to sinusitis. Am J Rhinol 2002;16(2): 97–101
14. Murakami CS, Larrabee WF Jr. Comparison of osteotomy techniques in the treatment of nasal fractures. Facial Plast Surg 1992;8(4):209–219
15. Goldfarb M, Gallups JM, Gerwin JM. Perforating osteotomies in rhinoplasty. Arch Otolaryngol Head Neck Surg 1993;119(6):624–627
16. Baron SH, Dedo HH, Henry CR. The mucoperiosteal flap in frontal sinus surgery. (The Sewall-Boyden-McNaught operation.). Laryngoscope 1973;83(8):1266–1280
17. Dedo HH, Broberg TG, Murr AH. Frontoethmoidectomy with Sewall-Boyden reconstruction: alive and well, a 25-year experience. Am J Rhinol 1998;12(3):191–198
18. Weber R, Draf W, Kratzsch B, Hosemann W, Schaefer SD. Modern concepts of frontal sinus surgery. Laryngoscope 2001;111(1): 137–146
19. Neel HB III, McDonald TJ, Facer GW. Modified Lynch procedure for chronic frontal sinus diseases: rationale, technique, and long-term results. Laryngoscope 1987;97(11):1274–1279
20. Tran KN, Beule AG, Singal D, Wormald PJ. Frontal ostium restenosis after the endoscopic modified Lothrop procedure. Laryngoscope 2007;117(8):1457–1462

21. Kuhn FA, Javer AR, Nagpal K, Citardi MJ. The frontal sinus rescue procedure: early experience and three-year follow-up. Am J Rhinol 2000;14(4):211–216
22. Bent JP III, Spears RA, Kuhn FA, Stewart SM. Combined endoscopic intranasal and external frontal sinusotomy. Am J Rhinol 1997;11(5):349–354
23. McIntosh DL, Mahadevan M. Frontal sinus mini-trephination for acute sinusitis complicated by intracranial infection. Int J Pediatr Otorhinolaryngol 2007;71(10):1573–1577
24. Hardy JM, Montgomery WW. Osteoplastic frontal sinusotomy: an analysis of 250 operations. Ann Otol Rhinol Laryngol 1976;85(4 Pt 1):523–532
25. Montgomery WW. State-of-the-art for osteoplastic frontal sinus operation. Otolaryngol Clin North Am 2001;34(1):167–177
26. Loevner LA, Yousem DM, Lanza DC, Kennedy DW, Goldberg AN. MR evaluation of frontal sinus osteoplastic flaps with autogenous fat grafts. AJNR Am J Neuroradiol 1995;16(8):1721–1726
27. Schulze SL, Loehrl TA, Smith TL. Outcomes of the modified endoscopic Lothrop procedure. Am J Rhinol 2002;16(5):269–273
28. Smith TL, Han JK, Loehrl TA, Rhee JS. Endoscopic management of the frontal recess in frontal sinus fractures: a shift in the paradigm? Laryngoscope 2002;112(5):784–790

40 Evidence-Based Medicine in Rhinology and Skull Base Surgery

Michael G. Stewart

Evidence-based medicine is an increasingly important topic in contemporary medicine. Although the basic concept—patient treatment decisions should be based on results from good-quality studies—has been implicitly assumed for generations of medical practice, the explicit techniques of "evidence-based medicine" have only recently been described and popularized.[1] Evidence-based medicine (EBM) has been defined as "the conscientious, explicit, and judicious use of the current best evidence in making decisions about the care of individual patients."[2] However, proponents of EBM always point out that the practice of EBM includes integrating *individual clinical expertise* with the *best available evidence* from systematic research.[2]

The fundamental concept in EBM is that not all evidence is equal. Studies are given different strength and "weight" based on the quality of the methodology, using the following guidelines: randomized studies are better than nonrandomized, prospective studies are better than retrospective, and controlled studies are better than noncontrolled. So, results from studies with stronger methodology are given preference over results from studies with weaker methodology. Also, by definition, only clinical studies using human subjects are considered in EBM; basic laboratory research results are not included.

Understanding Evidence-Based Medicine

There are five steps in EBM[1]:

1. Ask an answerable clinical question.
2. Search for the best available external evidence.
3. Critically appraise the quality of the evidence.
4. Understand the findings from the best evidence and create a summary/recommendation.
5. Integrate the best evidence with clinical expertise and unique patient factors (desires, values, special circumstances).

Step 1: Ask an Answerable Clinical Question

This might seem easy, but in fact can be more difficult than anticipated. Many questions of interest are actually quite nonspecific; for example, "Is endoscopic sinus surgery effective for chronic rhinosinusitis?" There will often be no evidence that directly addresses such a broad question. Missing are the following important issues: How is "effective" defined, and for what time period? In which patients? And compared with what? Although it is *possible* to practice EBM when starting with a very general question, experts know that focusing the question makes all the subsequent steps easier—particularly the search for evidence.

Step 2: Search for the Best Available External Evidence

This should be a rigorous search for the most contemporary evidence—not simply finding a textbook chapter or other nearby reference. Some available databases such as the Cochrane Library have already identified and graded pertinent literature on many clinical topics, using rigorous methodology, and are usually updated regularly. Also, evidence-based literature reviews might have been performed and published, or posted on Web sites, etc. So it may be possible to identify the best evidence without doing the search yourself. However, to perform a comprehensive search, some sort of electronic search engine must be used, with comprehensive but focused search criteria. The steps used in the search, including search terms, must be reported. MEDLINE is a database of the published biomedical literature from around the world and is perhaps the most useful tool for literature searches. The details of performing a literature search using MEDLINE have been reported.[3]

Searching for the best evidence is an iterative process. For example, MEDLINE is quite comprehensive and your search might yield a very large number of articles that are not pertinent to your question. So, the list should be manually searched to identify the pertinent articles. In addition, the references from appropriate articles should be reviewed because many times, one or more pertinent articles were missed by the initial search. Although MEDLINE includes most of the published literature, articles are indexed by people (librarians) and occasionally some are not indexed correctly and are missed by the search criteria. Also, MEDLINE includes only articles published after ~1950, and not *all* medical journals are indexed into MEDLINE. Nevertheless, MEDLINE is a very powerful tool for searching the biomedical literature and is a key part of a search strategy. There are proprietary and other Internet-based search tools; however, many of them simply use the MEDLINE index, or they use less rigorous tools for searching, and therefore identify items that were not peer-reviewed, for example.

After the search is completed, all articles that address the focused question should be pulled for further review.

Table 40.1 Evidence Levels for Therapy/Etiology Studies and Prognosis Studies

Evidence Level	Therapy/Etiology	Prognosis
1a	Systematic review (SR) of randomized controlled trials	SR of inception cohort studies
1b	Single randomized controlled trial	Individual cohort study
1c	"All or none" study	"All or none" case series
2a	SR of cohort studies	SR of either retrospective cohort studies or untreated control groups in randomized trials
2b	Individual cohort study	Retrospective cohort studies or untreated control groups in randomized trials
2c	Outcomes research	Outcomes research
3a	SR of case-control studies	
3b	Individual case-control study	
4	Case series (with or without comparison)	Case series
5	Expert opinion	Expert opinion

Source: Data from Sackett DL, Straus SE, et al. Evidence-based Medicine: How to Practice and Teach EBM, 2nd ed. Edinburgh, England: Wolfe Pub Ltd.; 2000: 1–261.

Step 3: Critically Appraise the Quality of the Evidence

Individual studies are assigned a *level* based on the quality of the methodology. The standard hierarchy of levels, which is widely used (originally proposed by Sackett), is shown in **Table 40.1**. After studies are given a level, they should be organized from highest level to lowest for further review. Often, it is easiest to create a table for this purpose. If there are minor flaws in methodology or reporting, for example a missing power analysis, the study can be given a "minus" level; for example, level "2−." If a study has methodologic flaws that are major, it should either be excluded, or preferably should be reclassified according to the actual methods used. For example, if a study is reported as a "prospective controlled study," but in fact there was no randomization or treatment assignment and in fact the study is a retrospective comparison of patients who received different treatments, then the study should be classified as a retrospective case-control study, or perhaps a "case series (with or without comparison)."

It is important to repeat that, at this point, you are simply evaluating the study design/methodology, not reviewing results or outcomes. After the studies are grouped by level, then the evidence is reviewed further.

Step 4: Understand the Findings from the Best Evidence and Create a Summary/Recommendation

Once individual studies have been rated, then the overall results and findings are reviewed for evidence quality and the consistency of results. Individual studies are given *levels*, but the overall evidence is given a *grade*. Grades of evidence are based on the majority of the studies, and are shown in **Table 40.2**. There is some judgment involved in assigning an evidence grade, which should be based on the best quality evidence, and the consistency of evidence and results, not just the level of evidence with the most papers. For example, there are often multiple case series (level 4 evidence) reported, but if there are a large number of randomized controlled trials (level 1 evidence) with consistent results, that would be considered grade A evidence even if there are numerically more level 4 studies. On the other hand, having one or two randomized controlled trials does not automatically mean that the evidence is grade A. If the few studies show conflicting results or have methodological problems, and the rest of the studies are case series, then the overall evidence might actually be grade C. Again, this requires some interpretation and judgment by the reviewer.

Step 5: Integrate the Best Evidence with Clinical Expertise and Unique Patient Factors (Desires, Values, Special Circumstances)

This is an important last step in practicing EBM. After the clinician has reviewed the recommendation based on the best external evidence, that recommendation should be then integrated with the patient's unique circumstances and the clinician's experience and judgment. Even in

Table 40.2 Grades of Overall Evidence

Evidence Grade	Levels of Evidence
Grade A	Consistent level 1 studies
Grade B	Consistent level 2 or 3 studies
Grade C	Level 4 studies
Grade D	Level 5 studies

Source: Data from Sackett DL, Straus SE, et al. Evidence-Based Medicine: How to Practice and Teach EBM, 2nd ed. Edinburgh, England: Wolfe Pub Ltd.; 2000:1–261.

circumstances where consistent grade A evidence exists, there may be compelling reasons to choose a different treatment based on individual factors. So the practice of EBM should include awareness of the best external evidence, but just not automatic or mandatory treatment guidelines.

Relying only on published high-level studies or relying only on clinical intuition and personal experience represent two extremes in medical decision making. It is unrealistic to think that every clinical problem has been addressed by well-done prospective clinical studies. So, clinicians must rely on their experience in many circumstances. However, if clinicians only rely on experience and opinion and do not use results from well-done clinical research, their practice can quickly become out of date or even inappropriate. In fact, some studies may challenge the conventional thinking, but as believers in the scientific process, physicians should be willing to accept that and make treatment decisions accordingly.

Evidence-Based Medicine in Surgical Fields

Acquiring high-level evidence for surgical treatments has two main barriers: practicality, and the approval process. The highest level evidence requires randomization and blinding. From a practical standpoint, when comparing surgical to nonsurgical treatments, randomization takes on added complexity, and of course blinding is impossible unless the study can be designed so that some patients undergo sham surgery, which is a large ethical barrier to overcome. Obviously when comparing, say, an active oral medication versus placebo or versus another medication, it is much easier to create a placebo or alternative treatment that is visually identical to the active treatment, which allows blinding. Comparing two different surgical treatments would be more feasible from the standpoint of study implementation, but to be able to randomize patients, the researcher/participant must have true clinical equipoise between different treatment options, and as standards of care evolve, such equipoise is not always possible.

The approval process for new surgical treatments or devices is quite different from the approval process for new medications. New and modified surgical treatments are reported based on clinicians' experience, but do not require level 1 evidence before introduction. Again, depending on the question being asked, a study to obtain level 1 evidence might be impractical or unethical to design. For surgical devices, the U.S. Food and Drug Administration (FDA) requires only the demonstration of equivalence to existing approved technology. In contrast, before a new medication can be released, it must demonstrate efficacy—and often improved efficacy compared with existing medications—in randomized controlled trials (RCTs). Drug companies know this of course, and fund RCTs demonstrating efficacy before drugs can be introduced. Surgical devices, however, are currently not required by the FDA to demonstrate efficacy; therefore, the device companies typically do not fund RCTs before introduction. As a device is introduced and surgeons begin using it, it may then be difficult to randomize patients away from the surgical "advance" to perform an RCT, and even if a trial could be ethically designed, accrual might be very low. Furthermore, even if those barriers could be overcome, such trials are expensive and are unlikely to be funded by industry when their device has already been approved.

In medical fields, when comparisons are between, say, classes of medication used to treat hypertension or two different chemotherapy protocols, opinion leaders can debate evidence from level 1 studies (required and funded before the drugs were introduced) to make treatment recommendations. In surgical fields, this level of evidence is often not available. This is not because surgeons do not value high-level evidence, but rather is often due to the fundamental issues with study design and blinding, as well as the level of evidence required for the federal approval process. Having said that, the surgical community should be more proactive about collecting the highest level evidence possible, and fortunately that seems to be happening to a greater extent.

The Evidence Level for Rhinology and Skull Base Surgery

Endoscopic Sinus Surgery

The initial reports describing the efficacy of functional endoscopic sinus surgery (ESS) for the treatment of chronic sinusitis were based on many years of experience and thousands of patients with prospective data collection and careful outcome analysis. Comparisons were made with open sinus surgery in terms of sinus function, but these comparisons were based on historical or simultaneously treated series, not a randomized design. This is an excellent example of rigorous prospective evidence, which nevertheless was not level 1.

Subsequent studies on ESS addressed many types of outcome analyses, including the development and validation of the first quality of life instruments for rhinosinusitis,[4,5] and the development of staging systems based on computed tomography (CT) scans and endoscopy findings.[6–8] Patient-based outcome assessment tools, such as the Chronic Sinusitis Survey, Sino-Nasal Outcome Tool (SNOT)-20, and Rhinosinusitis Disability Index, have been used in many studies to assess the changes in quality of life after sinus surgery.

Smith et al., working as part of the American Academy of Otolaryngology-Head and Neck Surgery's "Evidence Machine" project assessing the quality of existing evidence in the specialty, performed a systematic evidence-based review of the evidence supporting ESS in the management of adult chronic rhinosinusitis.[9] The specific question was the following: "In adults with chronic rhinosinusitis who have failed medical management, does ESS improve symptoms and/or quality of life?" Articles were reviewed up until January 2004. The authors identified 886 potential articles, reviewed 75 articles, and included 45 articles in their review. Almost all the articles were level 4 (case series) evidence; two were level 5 and one was level 2. The outcome measure in the majority of studies was symptom improvement, although some studies did use a validated outcomes instrument. The studies all found that ESS improved symptoms and/or quality-of-life (QOL) in patients with chronic rhinosinusitis (CRS), and the authors concluded that "there is substantial level 4 evidence with supporting level 2 evidence that ESS is effective in improving symptoms and/or QOL in adult patients with CRS." The authors also recommended that future research efforts should focus on prospective studies with a comparison group.

Later, in 2004, after the systematic review was completed, an RCT in CRS was reported.[10] Ninety patients who had failed the initial treatment for CRS (6 weeks of nasal steroid/decongestant combination twice a day [BID], with nasal alkaline irrigation) were then randomized to receive either intensive medical therapy or ESS. The intensive medical regimen included 12 weeks of erythromycin (500 mg BID for 2 weeks, then 250 mg BID for 10 weeks), alkaline irrigation, and nasal steroids BID. Patients with polyposis received a different nasal steroid at a higher dose, and a few patients with polyps had a taper of oral corticosteroids as well. The surgical group underwent ESS, then after surgery had 2 weeks of erythromycin 500 mg BID, and nasal corticosteroids for 12 weeks. Patients completed the SNOT-20 disease-specific QOL instrument and the SF-36 global QOL instrument, and a visual analogue scale for symptom severity, and they also had objective assessment of the nasal airway performed. Follow-up was performed at 6 and 12 months. The authors found that disease-specific QOL and seven of eight domains of global QOL showed statistically significant improvement after treatment, but there was no significant difference between medical and surgical treatment groups. Similarly, there were significant improvements in symptom burden as well as objective measures, and no differences between medical and surgical treatment groups. The authors point out that erythromycin also has anti-inflammatory properties, and that the treatment protocol was extensive and prolonged and not entirely standardized. In addition, the surgical group received fairly extensive medical therapy. Nevertheless, this level 1 evidence is an important contribution to the literature and raises issues for future studies directly comparing medical and surgical therapy.

Prospective studies have also been performed to address the factors that predict outcome after surgery.[6,11,12] A large part of the question here is what is the primary outcome being measured? Some studies have addressed outcomes from the standpoint of eventual cure and, therefore, revision surgery was considered a failure. But, in many patients, inflammatory rhinosinusitis is best considered a chronic disease, and eventually, surgical management will be required again. That does not mean a poor outcome, especially if the surgery resulted in improved QOL, and the treatment course (including intermittent surgery) caused overall improvement in, say, symptoms, functional status, or the severity of a comorbid disease. Similarly, the need for medications should not necessarily be considered a poor outcome because medical therapy is part of the treatment of CRS.

A large multidisciplinary group[13] studied this issue—optimal outcomes and study designs for different questions in rhinosinusitis—with the eventual goal of standardizing future research and accumulating improved evidence. For CRS, the recommended primary outcome assessment was symptoms. Symptoms drive health care use and are correlated with QOL. Currently, there is no standardized symptom score tool for CRS, although there is general consensus on which symptoms are most important, and furthermore, disease-specific QOL instruments measure symptom severity, and seem to correlate well with symptom score tools. Symptoms are more short term and directed, and QOL tends to be assessed from a longer temporal period and also includes broader concepts. Nevertheless disease-specific QOL is certainly affected by symptom severity and is a reasonable proxy.

One prospective study[14] looked at two primary outcomes: endoscopic findings and disease-specific QOL. They found significant improvement in both outcomes after ESS. They found that similar factors predicted a poorer outcome: patients with worse CT scans and no aspirin intolerance had better outcomes (than patients with better CT scans and aspirin intolerance). For the endoscopic primary outcome, patients with worse endoscopic findings at presentation were more likely to have a greater improvement after surgery. For the QOL primary outcome, patients with poorer QOL at presentation were more likely to have larger improvement in QOL after surgery. Although this might seem counterintuitive (worse severity at presentation predicts better outcome), in fact, those patients likely have more room for improvement. In addition, it is not only magnitude of change that is greater, but actually proportional (relative) change that is larger. So, it is not a simple mathematical phenomenon (larger number on the scale means larger improvement) but actually larger relative improvement as well.

Another study[6] found that poorer endoscopic findings after the first surgery predicted a greater probability of needing further surgery in the future, although the primary outcome was revision surgery rather than, say, symptoms or QOL. Other studies[12,15] have found that greater symptomatic improvement is predicted by higher stage of CT scan at presentation. Again, apparently greater burden of mucosal disease or greater anatomic extent of disease seems to predict larger improvement after surgical treatment. However, not every study looking at CT has found stage to be predictive of outcome. Other studies looking at surgical success (i.e., symptom improvement, need for revision surgery) have found conflicting results on the impact of factors such as nasal polyposis, allergies, asthma, and even smoking. This is a bit surprising because many have assumed that factors such as polyposis or allergy would definitely be poor prognostic indicators. Further studies in this area are definitely needed, with clearly defined primary outcomes and prospective assessment of predictive factors.

Even if symptoms are a primary outcome, then other outcomes are still important, such as CT scan findings and endoscopic findings. However, asymptomatic patients are less likely to seek medical attention than symptomatic patients. Abnormal CT scan and endoscopic findings are important, but probably not a primary outcome. Furthermore, we know that CT scan findings do not correlate well with symptoms or QOL.[16,17]

Another important outcome is the effect on other diseases. There is some limited but consistent evidence that treatment of CRS results in improvement in symptoms of asthma.[18] Interestingly, objective measures—such as peak flow or forced expiratory volume—do not necessarily improve, but symptoms, severity, use of rescue medications, unexpected admissions, and other subjective measures of health status do improve. There is increasing evidence of the connection between the upper and lower airways (the "unified airway model") giving physiologic underpinning to this clinical phenomenon. In other diseases such as cystic fibrosis, improvement in sinus disease status results in improvement in overall QOL and in pulmonary disease status.

Image-Guided Surgery

Image-guidance technology is an example of technology that was developed and widely adopted before randomized trials were performed. It is clearly a useful surgical device that has gained widespread acceptance. And, it is an excellent example of where requiring only the highest level evidence is unrealistic.

In an evidence-based review, Smith et al.[14] systematically reviewed the evidence concerning the use of image-guidance technology in endoscopic sinus surgery looking at two focused questions: does image-guidance reduce complications or improve outcomes? There were many published articles on the use of image guidance; however, many articles only described the technology, or were "how I do it" reviews. Five articles were identified that addressed the pertinent questions. These were case series (level 4 evidence) with very limited data on outcomes assessment and generally very low complication rates. The studies found that image-guidance technology was feasible, and allowed access to a greater number of sinuses, with good outcomes and no apparent increase in complications. Because there were no randomized controlled trials on image-guided surgery, the authors further discussed the problems of performing a randomized trial. First, it would probably be unethical at the time to randomize patients away from a treatment that has become available and widely used. Second, complication rates are already very low in ESS and, based on calculations and reported complication rates, it would require a huge study (at least 2200 patients per group) to achieve statistical significance and power to detect differences in complication rates between groups. Therefore, given the ethical and methodological issues in conducting a randomized trial, the authors concluded that in the area of image-guidance technology, case series evidence and expert opinion *were* the best available evidence and were likely to remain so. It is impractical to demand level 1 evidence on this topic.

Skull Base Surgery

The level of evidence reporting for skull base surgery is also less than optimal. However, there are significant issues limiting the level of evidence in these cases. First, these are very rare cases, and even tertiary centers do not accumulate large numbers of similar cases. Because of their often delayed presentation at advanced stages, and multiple different manifestations and behavior, it is very difficult—even within a larger series—to generate a series of similar lesions with which to prognosticate or compare. Second, endoscopic skull base surgery techniques are still fairly new, and in many cases, current manuscripts are in the "how to do it best" stage of development—minimizing complications, improving access and visualization, how to reconstruct, etc. Other papers report on new classification schemes for tumors, anatomic location, surgical approach, or reconstruction.

For surgery performed for neoplasms, obviously, tumor control and mortality are pivotal outcomes. However, if tumor control and mortality are equivalent between different treatment methods, then QOL (which can be combined with mortality and reported as quality-adjusted life years [QALY]) is an important outcome that should be a key decision point for patients and clinicians. If two treatments have the same mortality and tumor control, then the treatment with better QOL should be chosen.

A review of the level of evidence in skull base surgery shows that there are several studies available; however, almost all are case series, some with comparisons between techniques but many with no comparisons. Some series were all the same pathology (i.e., chordoma, meningioma) or the same location (i.e., clivus, petrous apex). Some series reported on a variety of low-grade and high-grade tumors. Series varied in size from small (n = 7) to large (n = 183). In addition to the heterogeneity in staging, severity, and technique, there is also substantial variety in pathology. One of the largest series included ~65% of patients with malignancy, 25% benign pathology, and the rest were congenital lesions, inflammatory lesions, and even some traumatic defects. Other series included transsphenoidal pituitary surgery as skull base surgery. So, there is a tremendous amount of heterogeneity in the literature on endoscopic skull base surgery, even including the definition of "skull base surgery."

In the few studies that compared open and endoscopic techniques, the authors generally recognized and addressed the selection bias inherent in such nonrandomized comparisons; generally, more extensive tumors with invasion and other unfavorable features are more likely to have an open procedure performed, which could make outcomes of endoscopic techniques look artificially better than the open procedures. Nevertheless, it does seem that skull base surgery is an oncologically sound technique with comparable survival outcomes and perhaps improved QOL, but there are almost no comparative data on that topic.

Issues with Evidence-Based Medicine in Everyday Practice

It is important to remember that lack of evidence does *not* mean lack of effectiveness. In many cases, lack of evidence means that the trials have not been performed, not that the results of trials showed no effectiveness. As discussed earlier, even when evidence is lacking and is desired, it may be very difficult to perform trials of the highest level, for methodological and ethical reasons.

We should reiterate that practicing EBM does *not* require use of only randomized clinical trials; there is an important difference between using the "best available" evidence versus "only the best" evidence. If findings from a randomized clinical trial are available, then that is strong, high-quality evidence, and should be used. If, however, randomized trials have not been performed, and therefore that type of evidence is not available, you can still practice EBM by using the best available evidence. Some proponents of EBM take a "top down" approach saying they will only review the best (level 1) evidence, because the time taken to review lower level evidence is not worthwhile in terms of strength of the eventual recommendation. This approach is logical, but in this writer's opinion is impractical for many clinical questions, particularly involving surgery or new technology.

Furthermore, the developers of EBM stress that practicing EBM does *not* eliminate the physician's own experience or knowledge base. Physicians should integrate their own clinical experience with the patient's desires and with the current best clinical evidence when deciding on the best treatment for an individual patient. The practice of EBM has been likened to a three-legged stool, which would be unstable if one leg were missing.[2] The three "legs" of the stool are best evidence, clinical experience, and the patient's wishes. Along those lines, it would not be practical or reasonable for a physician to rely only on results from high-quality evidence to make clinical decisions because there are many questions and issues that have not been addressed with experimental studies. On the other hand, if a physician relies only on personal experience, their practice could become out of date or inappropriate. So, the thoughtful and appropriate combination of experience and evidence is a goal to emulate.

Next Steps for Evidence-Based Medicine and Rhinology

We have a large amount of evidence supporting the efficacy of surgical treatment of sinus disease under the appropriate circumstances. However, the quality of the evidence is not as high as would be desired by the medical community. Future studies should focus on clearly defined outcome measures, and controlled or at least comparative study designs, to improve the overall level of evidence in these important diseases. For skull base surgery, it will always be more difficult to collect the highest level evidence, given the small number of cases and the wide variety in presentation, severity, etc. Because it seems, however, that oncologic and survival outcomes may be similar or identical between endoscopic and open approaches, then QOL and functional status outcomes become very important to guide clinicians and patients. Although larger series with controlled designs would be optimal, at a minimum, systematic assessment of QOL should give important insight into the potential benefits of endoscopic skull base surgery.

References

1. Sackett DL, Straus SE, Richardson WS, et al. Evidence-based Medicine: How to Practice and Teach EBM, 2nd ed. Edinburgh, England: Wolfe Pub Ltd.; 2000:1–261
2. Sackett DL, Rosenberg WMC, Gray JAM, Haynes RB, Richardson WS. Evidence based medicine: what it is and what it isn't. BMJ 1996;312(7023):71–72
3. Stewart MG, Kuppersmith RB, Moore AS. Searching the medical literature on the Internet. Otolaryngol Clin North Am 2002;35(6):1163–1174, v–vi
4. Gliklich RE, Metson R. Techniques for outcomes research in chronic sinusitis. Laryngoscope 1995;105(4 Pt 1):387–390
5. Piccirillo JF, Merritt MG Jr, Richards ML. Psychometric and clinimetric validity of the 20-item Sino-Nasal Outcome Test (SNOT-20). Otolaryngol Head Neck Surg 2002;126(1):41–47
6. Kennedy DW, Wright ED, Goldberg AN. Objective and subjective outcomes in surgery for chronic sinusitis. Laryngoscope 2000;110(3 Pt 3, Suppl 94):29–31
7. Lund VJ, Kennedy DW. Staging for rhinosinusitis. Otolaryngol Head Neck Surg 1997;117(3 Pt 2):S35–S40
8. Kennedy DW. Prognostic factors, outcomes and staging in ethmoid sinus surgery. Laryngoscope 1992;102(12 Pt 2, Suppl 57):1–18

9. Smith TL, Batra PS, Seiden AM, Hannley M. Evidence supporting endoscopic sinus surgery in the management of adult chronic rhinosinusitis: a systematic review. Am J Rhinol 2005;19(6):537–543
10. Ragab SM, Lund VJ, Scadding G. Evaluation of the medical and surgical treatment of chronic rhinosinusitis: a prospective, randomised, controlled trial. Laryngoscope 2004;114(5):923–930
11. Smith TL, Mendolia-Loffredo S, Loehrl TA, Sparapani R, Laud PW, Nattinger AB. Predictive factors and outcomes in endoscopic sinus surgery for chronic rhinosinusitis. Laryngoscope 2005;115(12):2199–2205
12. Bradley DT, Kountakis SE. Correlation between computed tomography scores and symptomatic improvement after endoscopic sinus surgery. Laryngoscope 2005;115(3):466–469
13. Meltzer EO, Hamilos DL, Hadley JA, et al; Rhinosinusitis Initiative. Rhinosinusitis: Developing guidance for clinical trials. Otolaryngol Head Neck Surg 2006;135(5, Suppl):S31–S80
14. Smith TL, Stewart MG, Orlandi RR, Setzen M, Lanza DC. Indications for image-guided sinus surgery: the current evidence. Am J Rhinol 2007;21(1):80–83
15. Stewart MG, Donovan DT, Parke RB Jr, Bautista MH. Does the severity of sinus computed tomography findings predict outcome in chronic sinusitis? Otolaryngol Head Neck Surg 2000;123 (1 Pt 1):81–84
16. Bhattacharyya T, Piccirillo J, Wippold FJ II. Relationship between patient-based descriptions of sinusitis and paranasal sinus computed tomographic findings. Arch Otolaryngol Head Neck Surg 1997;123(11):1189–1192
17. Stewart MG, Johnson RF. Chronic sinusitis: symptoms versus CT scan findings. Curr Opin Otolaryngol Head Neck Surg 2004; 12(1):27–29
18. Stewart MG. Evidence-based medicine in rhinology. Curr Opin Otolaryngol Head Neck Surg 2008;16(1):14–17

41 Endoscopic Anatomy of the Skull Base and Parasellar Region

Luigi Maria Cavallo, Paolo Cappabianca, Felice Esposito, Isabella Esposito, Domenico Solari, and Manfred Tschabitscher

The entire skull base area is one of the most complex regions of the human body as a result of the many different anatomic structures from which it is constituted. Due to its frontline position between the brain and the extracranial compartment (i.e., nasofacial structures anteriorly and vertebral joints posteriorly), a variety of lesions, neoplastic or otherwise, may be present, the management of which can be very difficult. Several different extensive transcranial and/or nasofacial approaches, such as the anterior, anterolateral, and posterolateral routes, have been adopted to access this area.[1–17] However, these surgical techniques often require a certain degree of tissue disruption with brain retraction and neurovascular manipulation, which can be aesthetically disfiguring and, furthermore, can provide a higher rate of surgical morbidity and mortality.

During the past few decades, technological progress and continuous surgical advances have led otorhinolaryngologists–head and neck surgeons and neurosurgeons to consider the possibility of ways to reduce the invasiveness of such approaches and, at the same time, to evaluate access to the areas through a different surgical corridor, namely transsphenoidally. Although (due its high versatility) the transsphenoidal route provides the possibility to access the skull base from the nose, it was initially reserved for the treatment of intrasellar tumors. It should be considered the less traumatic route to the sella, because it avoids any brain retraction and provides an excellent visualization of the pituitary gland and related pathology, thus offering at the same time a lower morbidity and mortality rate as compared with the transcranial procedures. In 1987, Weiss[18] termed and originally described the extended transsphenoidal approach, intending a transsphenoidal approach with removal of additional bone along the tuberculum sella and the posterior planum sphenoidale between the optic canals, with subsequent opening of the dura mater above the diaphragma sella. This approach, initially performed by microscopic technique, grants a midline access and direct visualization of the suprasellar space without brain manipulation, thus offering the possibility to treat small midline suprasellar lesions traditionally approached transcranially. More recently, due to the contribution provided by the otorhinolaryngologists' experience in functional endoscopic sinus surgery (FESS),[19–21] the endoscope has been gradually introduced side by side with the microscope during traditional transsphenoidal surgery.[22,23] Finally, the "pure" endoscopic endonasal approach was defined, with the endoscope as the sole visualizing tool along the whole procedure.[24–26] In fact, it was the widespread use of the endoscope that shed new interest on the transsphenoidal technique, thereby affording the extension of such an approach. The wider and more panoramic view offered by the endoscope pushed the development of a variety of modifications of the transsphenoidal approach targeted primarily at the entire midline skull base, from the anterior fossa to the craniovertebral junction and adjacent areas.

Credit for this last systematic innovation with described approaches to the skull base on the sagittal and coronal planes goes to Kassam's prior Pittsburgh group, with their strictly anatomic methodology and rigorous team approach.[27] Through several anatomic studies and clinical reports that have been performed to better detail the anatomy of the endoscopic endonasal approach, the potential offered by this approach has been clarified. The endonasal technique offers a direct and minimally invasive approach that permits excellent midline access with direct exposure of the suprasellar, retrosellar, and retroclival space, obviating brain retraction. Moreover, the use of the endoscope in such a technique has offered the surgeon the opportunity to visualize the surgical field safely and effectively, thus providing the possibility to pass through a physiologically neutral structure (the nasal cavity) to reach a physiologically critical one (the brain, with its neurovascular structures).

Endoscopic Anatomy of the Skull Base

To best describe the anatomy of the skull base from the endoscopic endonasal point of view, it can be divided into four areas according to the different surgical approaches:

1. The anterior midline skull base, from the frontal sinus to the posterior ethmoidal artery (for olfactory groove lesions)
2. The middle skull base, inside the sphenoid sinus cavity (for sellar/suprasellar lesions and upper clival lesions)
3. The posterior midline skull base, from the lower clivus to the craniovertebral junction (for posterior cranial fossa lesions)
4. The parasellar region (for cavernous sinus lesions)

First, however, it is important to describe the surgical anatomy of the standard endoscopic approach to the sellar region. As a matter of fact, it is through achieving great confidence with this approach that surgeons already experienced in such fields become boosted to explore the possibility of reaching the surrounding areas by the means of an endoscopic technique.

Standard Endoscopic Endonasal Approach to the Sellar Region

To access the sellar region,[28] the endoscope is usually introduced through one nostril, following the floor of the nasal cavity. As the nose is entered, the inferior turbinate and the middle turbinate become visible laterally, and the nasal septum is seen medially.

The head of the middle turbinate is pushed laterally to enlarge the space between the middle turbinate and the nasal septum to create an adequate surgical corridor in the posterior part of the nasal cavity. As the endoscope slides posteriorly, following the tail of the inferior turbinate, it reaches the choana, limited medially by the vomer (which is a midline marker) and, superiorly, by the floor of the sphenoid sinus; lateral to the choana lies the posterior end of the inferior turbinate. Then the endoscope is angled upward along the roof of the choana ~1.5 cm, until it reaches the sphenoid ostium (**Fig. 41.1**).

Sometimes, the sphenoid ostium is covered by either the superior or the supreme turbinate; these can be gently lateralized or removed to protect the lateral lamella of the cribriform plate on which they are inserted. Nevertheless, it is not mandatory to see the sphenoid ostium once the choana is identified; after ascending along the sphenoethmoid recess for ~1 to 1.5 cm, access to the sphenoid cavity can be achieved as well by using a blunt instrument.

After the identification of the sphenoid cavity, the nasal septum is separated from the sphenoid rostrum. The whole anterior wall of the sphenoid sinus is enlarged circumferentially, taking care to not enlarge the sphenoidotomy too much in the inferolateral direction where the sphenopalatine artery or its major branches lie.

Sometimes, the removal of the posterior part of the nasal septum is performed to obtain a wider space in which to maneuver, thus facilitating a two-nostril, four-handed approach.[27,29] It is crucial to widely expose and open the anterior face of the sphenoid to gain a proper working angle for all the instruments to be passed readily across the sphenoid with their tips in the sella.

Once the anterior sphenoidotomy has been performed, one or more septa inside the sphenoid sinus need to be removed (**Fig. 41.2A**); thereafter, the posterior and lateral walls of the sphenoid sinus are visible, with the sellar floor at the center, the sphenoethmoid planum above it, and the clival indentation below. Lateral to the sellar floor, the bony prominences of the intracavernous carotid artery (ICA) and the optic nerve can be seen, and between them the opticocarotid recess, molded by the pneumatization of the optic strut of the anterior clinoid process (**Fig. 41.2B**).[30,31]

Basic Concepts for Extended Endoscopic Approaches

In contrast to the standard endoscopic approach, in which the sphenoid sinus itself creates a surgical room to gain access to the sellar region, the extended approaches require the creation of a wider surgical corridor to expose and to work with the instruments in the different areas around the sella. Referring to the concept introduced by Perneczky[32] of the "keyhole" procedure, the sphenoid sinus cavity could be considered the "main entrance" to many areas of the skull base.

A

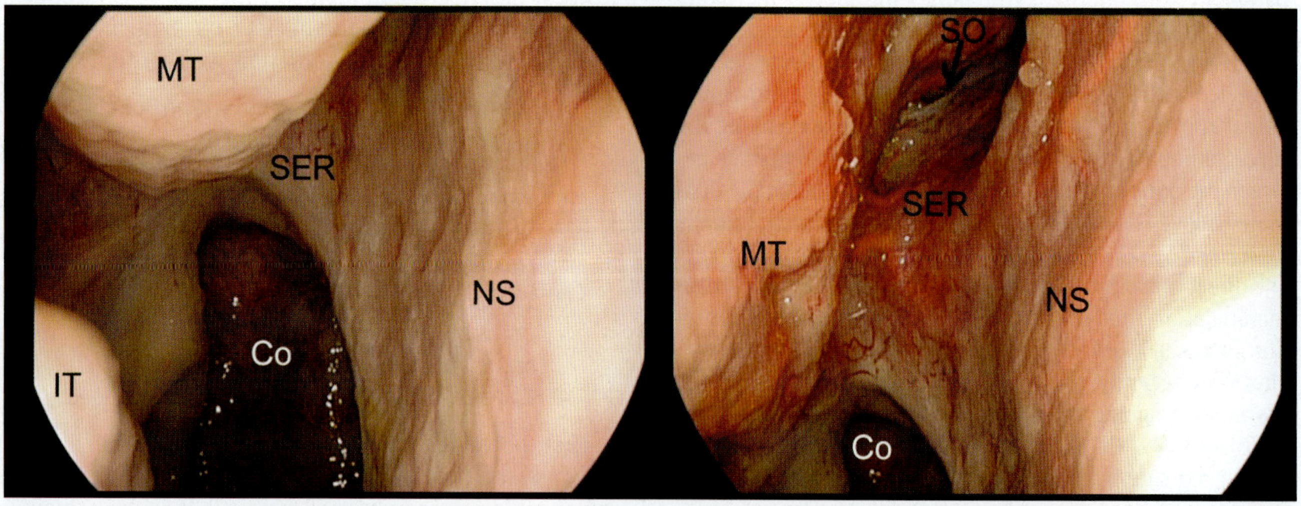

B

Fig. 41.1 Endoscopic view obtained in a cadaver showing the nasal aspects of the standard approach (right nostril). **(A)** Exploration of the posterior part of the nasal cavity and identification of the choana. **(B)** Localization of the sphenoid sinus. Starting from the choana and angling the endoscope along the sphenoethmoid recess, the sphenoid sinus is reached. Note the branches of the septal artery along the sphenoethmoid recess. *NS*, nasal septum; *MT*, middle turbinate; *SER*, sphenoethmoid recess; *Co*, choana; *IT*, inferior turbinate; *SO*, sphenoid ostium.

A 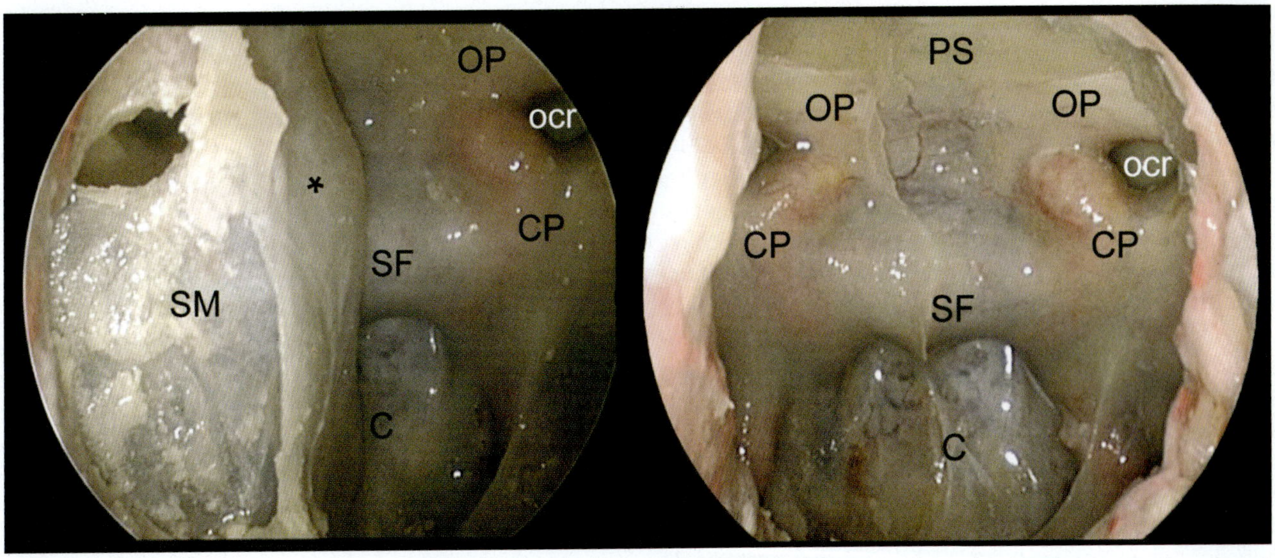 B

Fig. 41.2 Sphenoid phase of the procedure. **(A)** In this specimen, a median septum divides the sphenoidal sinus into two compartments. **(B)** Identification of the landmarks inside the sphenoid sinus after removal of the intersinus septum. *SF*, sellar floor; *CP*, carotid protuberance; *C*, clivus; *PS*, planum sphenoidale; *OP*, optic protuberance; *ocr*, opticocarotid recess; *SM*, sphenoidal mucosa; *asterisk*, median sphenoid septum.

As a matter of fact, to increase the working space and the maneuverability of instruments in the areas surrounding the sella, we have to apply the basic rules for extended approaches to the skull base introduced by Kassam and his earlier Pittsburgh group; that is, the removal of the middle turbinate on one side (usually the right one), the lateralization of the middle turbinate in the other nostril (sometimes even this turbinate can be removed), and the removal of the posterior portion of the nasal septum. In this way, it is possible to create the necessary access to use two or three instruments plus the endoscope through both nostrils. The procedure begins with removing the right middle turbinate and with a homolateral ethmoidectomy.

The head of the middle turbinate is cut with nasal scissors and pushed downward, then upward to expose its tail, and after hemostasis has been achieved around it, the turbinate is removed (**Fig. 41.3**). It is not mandatory to completely remove the tail of the middle turbinate because it does not affect the surgical trajectory and removal

A 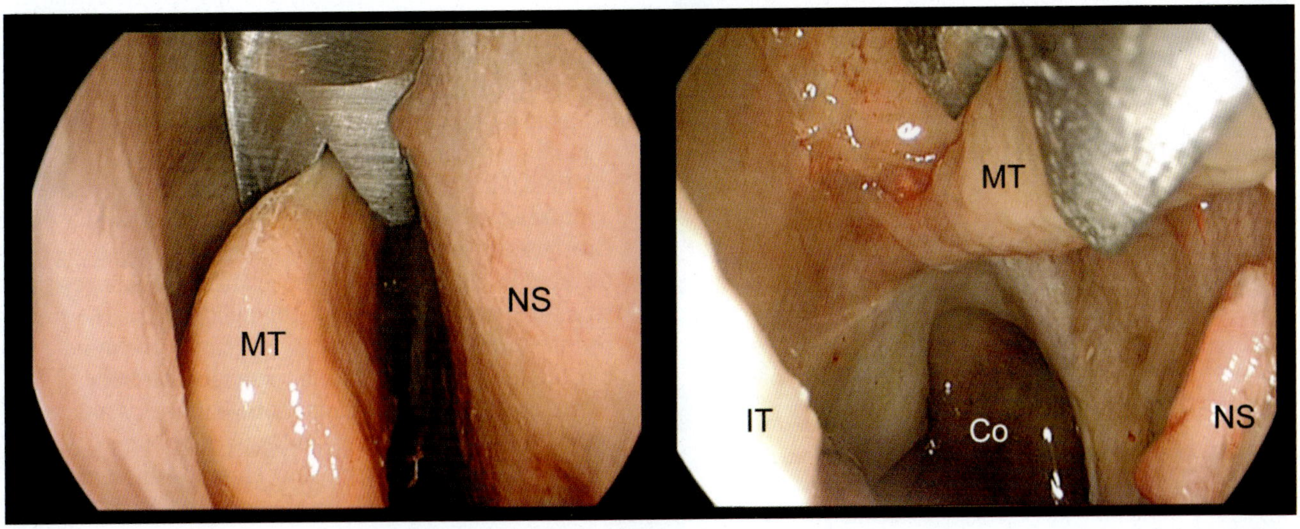 B

Fig. 41.3 Right middle turbinectomy. **(A)** The head of the middle turbinate is cut with nasal scissors following a superior to inferior trajectory to avoid injury to the ethmoidal roof. **(B)** Pushing downward and medially, the tail of the middle turbinate is exposed and cut. *NS*, nasal septum; *MT*, middle turbinate; *Co*, choana; *IT*, inferior turbinate.

of this area may increase the risk of sphenopalatine artery bleeding.[33] Then, the posterior nasal septum is detached from the sphenoid prow with a microdrill and removed with a retrograde bone punch. The mucosal edges are carefully coagulated with the bipolar forceps. Finally, the middle turbinate of the opposite nostril is pushed laterally or removed, according to the width of the nasal cavities. Such maneuvers provide a wider view because the other instruments (e.g., a suction tube) can be inserted through the other nostril.

In this situation, the extent of the anterior sphenoidotomy needed is wider than in the standard approach; therefore, it is useful to remove the superior turbinate and the posterior ethmoid air cells (bilaterally) so as to create sufficient space. All of the septa inside the sphenoid sinus are removed, including those attached on bony protuberances and depressions on the posterior wall of the sphenoid sinus cavity. It has to be said that each single irregularity of the bone and/or either of the mucosa covering the limit between sphenoidal and ethmoidal planum should be flattened to allow for better maneuverability of the endoscope and of the surgical instruments while working above the sella. Once a complete exposure of the posterior wall of the sphenoid sinus is achieved, a series of protuberances and depressions (according to the degree of pneumatization) again become visible[28]; the precise knowledge of such anatomic landmarks is of great importance for the correct orientation and subsequent bone removal (**Fig. 41.4**).

From now on, the surgeon has the possibility of performing a bimanual dissection while the co-surgeon holds the endoscope, moving it dynamically and, if needed, inserting another surgical instrument.[29] The endoscope can also be fixed to an endoscope holder that can be adjusted by a single surgeon, although most surgeons find the dynamic scope movement afforded by a co-surgeon to be markedly advantageous.

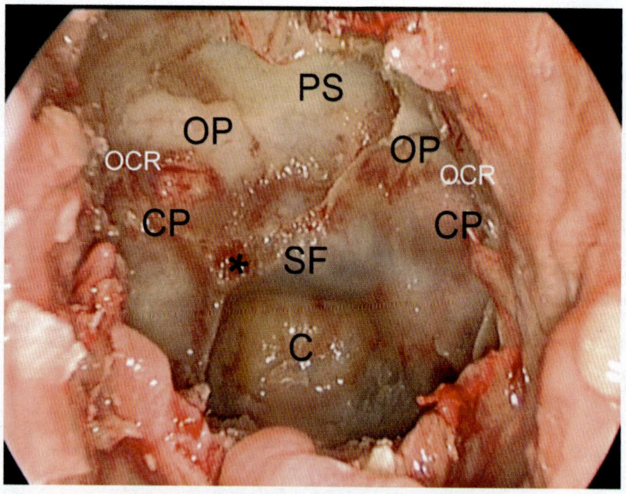

Fig. 41.4 After a wide anterior sphenoidotomy, the posterior and lateral walls of the sphenoid sinus became visible, with the sellar floor at the center, the sphenoid planum above it, and the clival region below. *SF*, sellar floor; *CP*, carotid protuberance; *C*, clivus; *PS*, planum sphenoidale; *OP*, optic protuberance; *OCR*, opticocarotid recess; *asterisk*, sphenoid septum flattened.

Anterior Skull Base

As seen from below, in the endoscopic endonasal view, the midline anterior skull base represents the roof of the nasal cavity. To expose it, both middle turbinates are removed together with the bulla ethmoidalis, the anterior and posterior ethmoid cells, and the superior part of the nasal septum until a rectangular area of the cranial base is exposed, which is limited by the lamina papyracea (orbital walls) laterally, the planum sphenoidale posteriorly, and the frontal recesses anteriorly (**Fig. 41.5A,B**). Such an area results in two symmetrical parts divided by the lamina perpendicularis of the ethmoid; each side is made up of the lamina cribrosa medially and the ethmoidal labyrinth laterally. The lamina cribrosa is a thin osseous layer pierced by the small nerves that arise from the olfactory bulbs lying on it. The ethmoidal labyrinth is made up of the anterior ethmoidal complex represented by the bullar and suprabullar recesses and the posterior complex, the two of which are separated by the basal lamella of the middle turbinate.[34]

Above this area, the blood supply to the dura mater is provided by the anterior and posterior ethmoidal arteries, which are both branches of the ophthalmic artery; over the cribriform plate many small branches of such vessels exchange with nasal branches of sphenopalatine artery. The anterior ethmoidal artery runs along the medial part of the optic nerve, between the lateral part of the superior and medial rectus muscles, and passes into the anterior ethmoidal foramen of the lamina papyracea. At this point, it immediately curves posteriorly and then anteriorly, moving in a slight anteromedial direction inside the anterior ethmoidal canal toward the lamina cribrosa (**Fig. 41.5C,D**).[35–37] The position of the anterior ethmoidal artery within the ethmoidal planum is variable: it can run within or below it in its bony canal, usually between the second and third ethmoidal lamellae. Because it is a crucial point during the approach to the anterior part of the skull base, it has to be clearly recognized. It is therefore useful to expose the frontal recesses because of the close relationship between these structures and the anterior ethmoidal canals. The frontal recesses are limited by the anterior part of the middle turbinate medially and the lamina papyracea laterally.

Posteriorly, the posterior ethmoidal artery passes between the superior rectus and superior oblique muscles, to emerge from the orbit and enter the posterior ethmoidal canal, which crosses the ethmoidal roof horizontally. This artery runs anterior to the opticocarotid recess, only a few millimeters from the anterior boundary of the sphenoidal sinus roof. It is mandatory to consider this

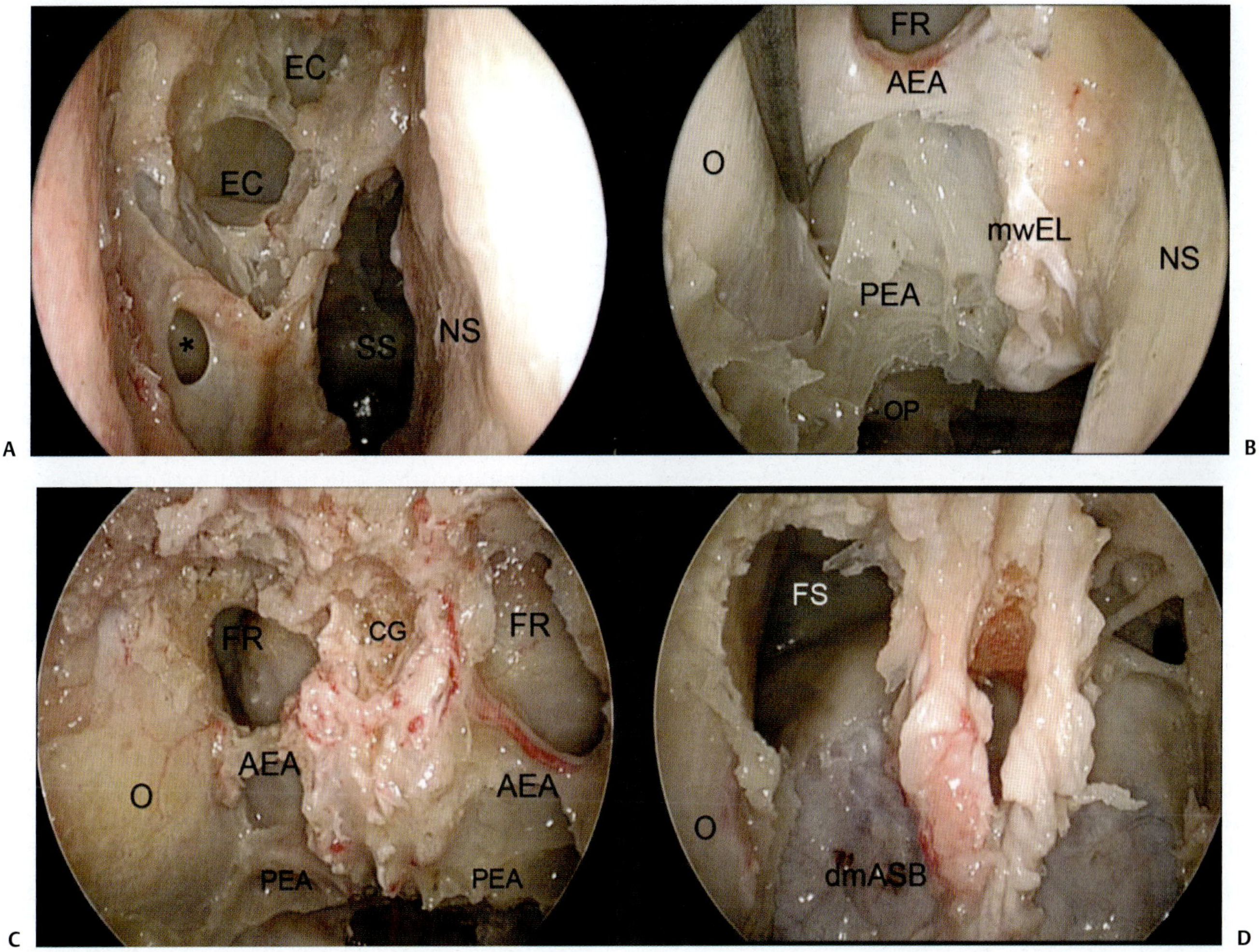

Fig. 41.5 Endoscopic endonasal anatomy of the anterior skull base. **(A)** The right middle and superior turbinates and the anterior wall of the sphenoid sinus have been removed. The right ethmoid complex and the ostium of the maxillary sinus are visible. **(B)** After the right ethmoidectomy and the removal of the lamina papyracea, the anterior and posterior ethmoidal arteries are identified. **(C)** The superior portion of the nasal septum has been removed and the same steps of the procedure have been repeated in the left nostril, thus exposing the entire cribriform plate. **(D)** The cribriform plate and the crista galli have been removed, taking care to avoid injury to the underlying dura. *EC*, ethmoid cells; *NS*, nasal septum; *SS*, sphenoid sinus; *OP*, optic protuberance; *O*, orbit; *AEA*, anterior ethmoidal artery; *PEA*, posterior ethmoidal artery; *mwEL*, medial wall of the ethmoidal labyrinth; *FR*, frontal recess; *FS*, frontal sinus; *CG*, inferior aspect of the crista galli; *dmASB*, dura mater of the anterior skull base; *asterisk*, ostium of the right maxillary sinus.

anatomic landmark when performing an anterior suprasellar transsphenoidal approach such as the transplanum transtuberculum route.

When an endoscopic endonasal approach is performed to manage lesions arising from or involving this area, the superior portion of the lamina papyracea has to be removed, and the anterior and posterior ethmoidal arteries are isolated on both sides. The bone of the anterior skull base between the two orbits is then removed, thus creating a wide surgical corridor, which can be extended laterally between the two medial orbital walls, and anteroposteriorly from the frontal recess to the sella (**Fig. 41.6**). The dura is then opened, thus allowing the exposure of the intracranial contents.

Middle Skull Base

Through the endoscopic endonasal route, the middle skull base coincides with the superior, posterior, and lateral walls of the sphenoid sinus; although a wider opening of the anterior wall of the sphenoid sinus, with the removal of the superior and/or supreme turbinates and of the posterior ethmoid cells, is crucial to achieve a better exposure of such areas (**Fig. 41.7A**). Particular attention must be paid to avoid injuries to the posterior ethmoidal artery (**Fig. 41.7B**). It is also important not to extend the removal of the nasal septum and the ethmoid too anteriorly to avoid damaging the olfactory nerve and/or the *lamina cribrosa*.

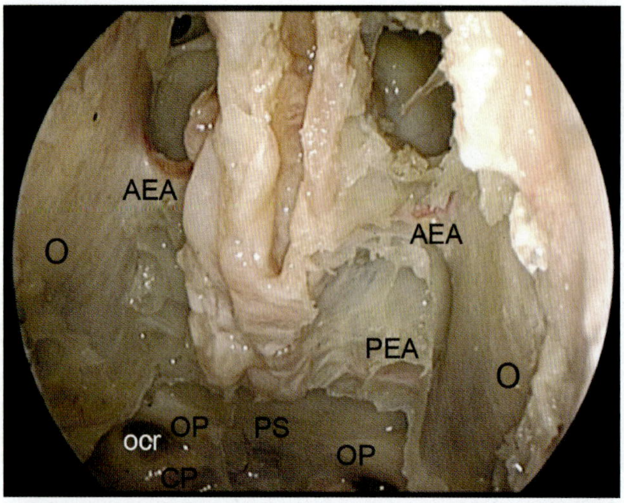

Fig. 41.6 Endoscopic endonasal anatomy of the anterior skull base. Through the endoscopic endonasal approach to the ethmoidal planum, the part of the anterior skull base enclosed between the medial wall of the two orbits has been exposed. *PS*, planum sphenoidale; *CP*, carotid protuberance; *OP*, optic protuberance; *ocr*, opticocarotid recess; *O*, orbit; *AEA*, anterior ethmoidal artery; *PEA*, posterior ethmoidal artery.

Thus, when the sphenoid cavity has been entirely exposed and all the septa within are removed, a series of protuberances and depressions becomes visible on its posterior wall. The sellar floor occupies a central position, the sphenoid planum is above, and the clival indentation is below. On both sides, lateral to the sellar floor, the two bony prominences of the intracavernous carotid arteries can be seen with the optic nerves slightly superiorly and, between these two protuberances, depending on sphenoid sinus pneumatization, the course of the optic strut of the anterior clinoid process creates the lateral opticocarotid recess (**Fig. 41.8A**).[31]

The superior boundary adjacent to the carotid recess is covered by a thickening of the dura mater and periosteum, which represent the distal dural ring, which divides the optic nerve from the clinoidal segment of the internal carotid artery. The inferior margin of the lateral opticocarotid recess is covered as well by a thickening of the dura mater and periosteum, which is identified as the proximal dural ring that covers the third cranial nerve from the cavernous sinus because it pierces the superior orbital fissure. The bony protuberances of the optic nerve and the intracavernous carotid artery, together with the lateral opticocarotid recess, also represent useful landmarks to recognize the medial opticocarotid recess; this structure represents the lateral limit of bone removal above the sella.[38]

Moving further laterally, other relevant anatomic structures such as the cavernous sinus apex, the trigeminal maxillary, and the trigeminal mandibulary protuberances can be identified through the bony thin layer with which they are clothed. Again, between such bony protuberances, some depressions are formed; the first one is limited by the cavernous sinus apex and the V_2 protuberances, whereas the second is enclosed by the protuberances of V_2 and V_3.[39,40] Further, on the floor of the sphenoid sinus cavity, it is possible to identify the protuberance of the vidian nerve,[41] which courses along the middle cranial fossa and the foramen lacerum through the pterygoid canal to reach

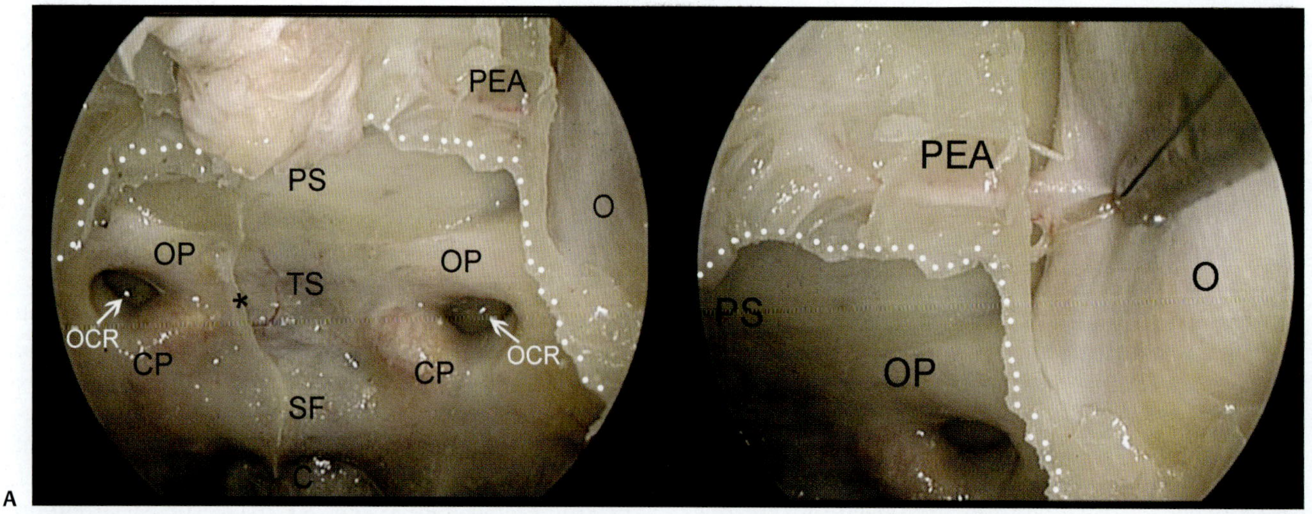

Fig. 41.7 An endoscopic view of the endonasal anatomy of the middle skull base. **(A)** The main landmarks on the posterior wall of the sphenoid sinus are identified. The posterior ethmoidal artery represents the anterior limit of the planum sphenoidale opening. **(B)** Further lateralization of the periorbita allows the identification of the posterior ethmoidal artery, where it leaves the orbit to enter its osseous canal. At this point, it can be isolated and coagulated. The dotted line borders the limit of the anterior wall of the sphenoid sinus. Note the close relationship between the posterior ethmoidal artery and the anterior wall of the sphenoid sinus. *SF*, sellar floor; *CP*, carotid protuberance; *C*, clivus; *TS*, tuberculum sella; *PS*, planum sphenoidale; *OP*, optic protuberance; *O*, orbit; *OCR*, lateral opticocarotid recess; *PEA*, posterior ethmoidal artery; *asterisk*, sphenoid septum flattened; *dotted line*, border of the anterior sphenoidotomy.

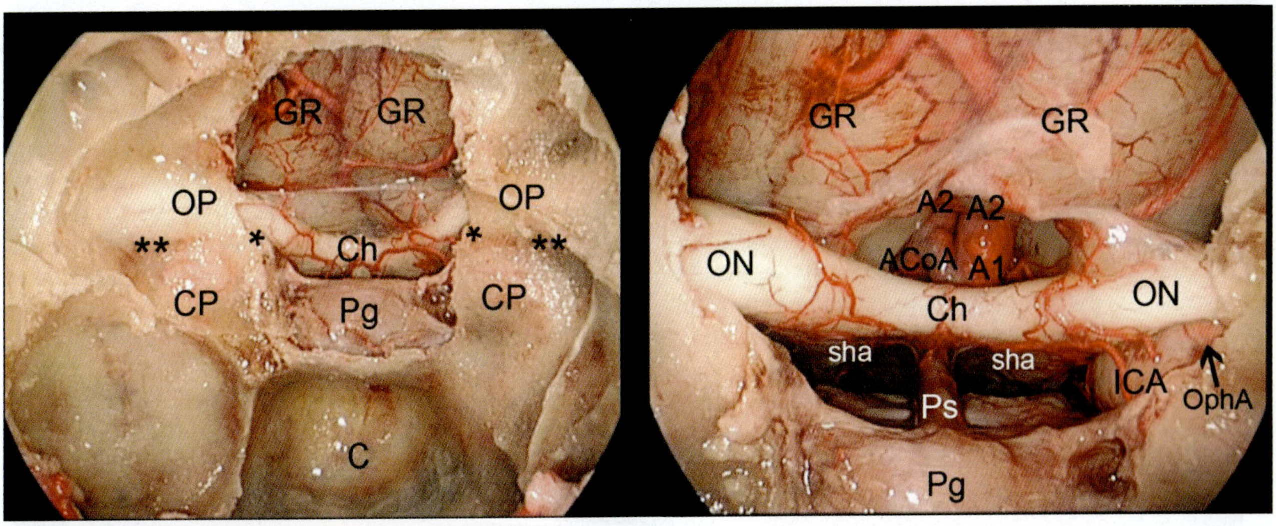

A B

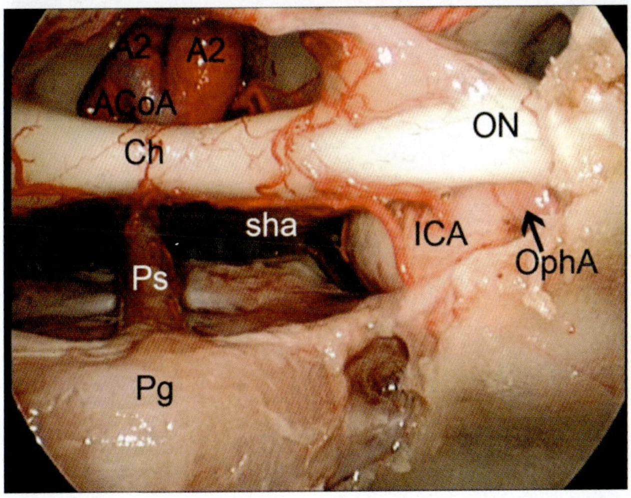

C

Fig. 41.8 Endoscopic endonasal anatomy of the sellar-suprasellar area. Intradural exploration. **(A)** In the transtuberculum-transplanum sphenoidale approach, the bone opening extends laterally between the two medial opticocarotid recesses. **(B)** View of the suprachiasmatic and subchiasmatic areas. **(C)** The complete removal of the medial opticocarotid recess allows for the exposure of the origin of the ophthalmic artery from the clinoidal segment of the internal carotid artery. *GR*, gyrus rectus; *OP*, optic protuberance; *CP*, carotid protuberance; C, clivus; asterisk, medial opto-carotid recess; double asterisk, lateral opto-carotid recess; *Ch*, chiasm; *ON*, optic nerve; *Ps*, pituitary stalk; *Pg*, pituitary gland; *ICA*, internal carotid artery; *ACoA*, anterior communicating artery; *A1*, precommunicating tract of the anterior cerebral artery; *A2*, postcommunicating tract of the anterior cerebral artery; *OphA*, ophthalmic artery; *sha*, superior hypophyseal artery.

the pterygopalatine ganglion inside the pterygopalatine fossa.[42–45]

Finally, moving the endoscope in a more anterior trajectory, immediately above the sellar floor, it is possible to observe the angle formed by the convergence of the sphenoid planum with the sellar floor; this area corresponds, on the intracranial compartment side, to the tuberculum sella. In a slightly anterior direction, the sphenoid planum is identified, which is limited on both sides by the protuberances of the optic nerves as they diverge anteriorly toward the apices of the orbits.[30,45,46]

The removal of the upper half of the sella, the tuberculum sellae, and the posterior portion of the planum sphenoidale offers the possibility to explore the suprasellar region.

The extent of removal of the tuberculum sella and/or of the sphenoid planum should be 1.5 to 2 cm in a posteroanterior direction, where it is naturally limited by the protuberances of the optic nerves in a lateral direction.

After the bone has been removed, the dura over the sellar floor, the tuberculum sella, and planum sphenoidale are opened and the main suprasellar neurovascular structures become visible.

The entire suprasellar region has been divided into four areas by two imaginary planes—one passing through the inferior surface of the chiasm and the mammillary bodies and another passing through the posterior margin of the chiasm and the dorsum sellae.[30,31,46] These imaginary planes allow for the best conceptualization of the suprachiasmatic region, the subchiasmatic region, the retrosellar region, and the ventricular region.

In the suprachiasmatic region, as soon as the dura is opened, the chiasmatic and the lamina terminalis cisterns appear. In the chiasmatic cistern, the anterior margin of the chiasm and the medial portion of both optic nerves are observed. The whole spectrum of anterior cerebral arteries, A1 and A2 segments of both sides, the anterior communicating artery, and the recurrent Heubner arteries, together with the gyri recti of the frontal lobes, are identified after the lamina terminalis cistern is opened (**Fig. 41.8B**). The lamina terminalis can be exposed by enlarging the space between the anterior communicating artery and the chiasm.

In the subchiasmatic space, immediately after breaching the arachnoid between the optic nerves, the pituitary stalk is encountered below the chiasm. In the surrounding space, the inferior and superior hypophyseal artery with its perforating branches can be identified, providing blood supply to the inferior surface of the chiasm and the optic nerves. The origin of the ophthalmic artery under the optic nerve can also be seen, and more laterally and deeply, the internal carotid artery, its bifurcation, and the first A1 segment (**Fig. 41.8C**). As a matter of fact, the superior aspect of the pituitary gland and the dorsum sellae are also visible (**Fig. 41.9A**).

In the retrosellar area, by passing the endoscope between the pituitary stalk and the internal carotid artery (**Fig. 41.9B**) above the dorsum sellae, we gain access to the upper third of the basilar artery, the pons, the superior cerebellar arteries, the oculomotor nerves, the posterior cerebral arteries, and lastly the mammillary bodies and the floor of the third ventricle.[47] To gain a wider exposure of the retroinfundibular space, it is possible to elevate the

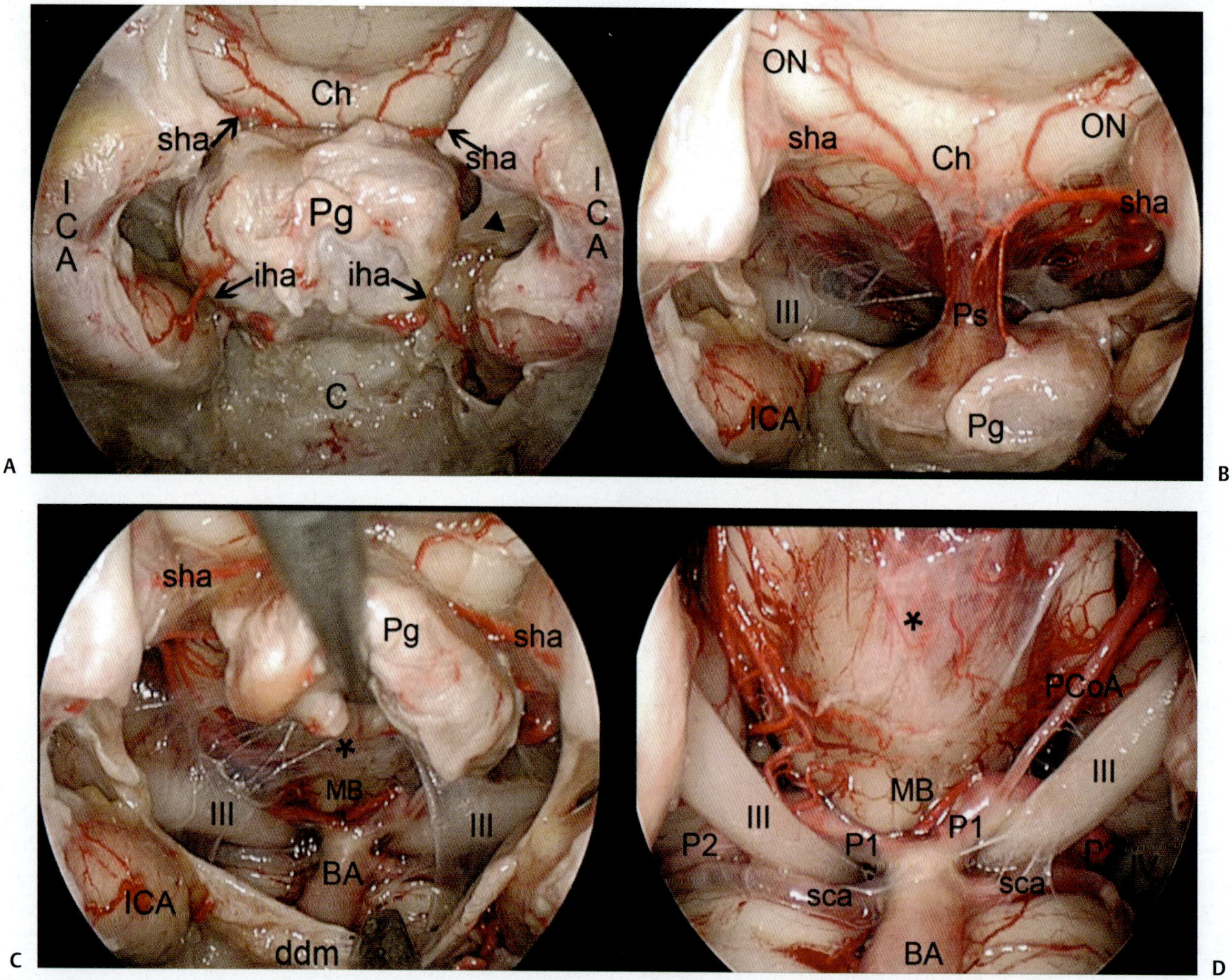

Fig. 41.9 Endoscopic endonasal anatomy of the sellar and retrosellar areas. Intradural exploration. **(A)** The sellar meningo-periosteal layers have been removed, thus highlighting the vascular relationships of the pituitary gland. The sellar floor has been completely removed to mobilize the gland during dissection maneuvers. **(B)** In this anatomic exposure, the inferior hypophyseal arteries have been cut to allow for the elevation of the gland. The diaphragma sellae has been removed and the third cranial nerve entering the cavernous sinus comes into view. **(C)** After dorsum sellae drilling, posterior clinoids removal, and the retrosellar dura opening, the pituitary gland is elevated to expose the retrosellar neurovascular structures. **(D)** Endoscopic retrosellar exploration showing the floor of the third ventricle, the basilar tip, and the third cranial nerves. *ICA*, internal carotid artery; *sha*, superior hypophyseal artery; *iha*, inferior hypophyseal artery; *Ch*, chiasm; *ON*, optic nerve; *Ps*, pituitary stalk; *Pg*, pituitary gland; *C*, clivus; *III*, third cranial nerve; *MB*, mammillary bodies; *PCoA*, posterior communicating artery; *P1*, precommunicating tract of the posterior cerebral artery; *P2*, postcommunicating tract of the posterior cerebral artery; *sca*, superior cerebellar artery; *BA*, basilar artery; *IV*, fourth cranial nerve; *ddm*, dura mater of the dorsum sellae; *arrowhead*, diaphragma sellae; *asterisk*, floor of the third ventricle.

pituitary gland in the supradiaphragmatic area and remove the bone of the dorsum sellae (**Fig. 41.9C**).[48]

In the retrosellar area, the floor of the third ventricle can be widely exposed (**Fig. 41.9D**); it is opened at level of the tuber cinereum and the endoscope can be advanced inside the ventricular cavity, obtaining a panoramic view of the ventricular area (**Fig. 41.10**). The thalami, which represent its lateral walls and the *massa intermedia* among them, the foramina of Monro anteriorly, the pineal and the suprapineal recesses, the posterior commissure, the habenular commissure, the habenular trigone, and the beginning of the aqueduct, are visualized posteriorly.

Posterior Skull Base

From an endonasal point of view, the anterior surface of the clivus, which extends from the dorsum sellae to the craniovertebral junction, represents the posterior cranial fossa. Access is possible by the means of endoscopic techniques by using a lower trajectory, as compared with that necessary for the sellar region.

The clivus is divided by the sphenoid sinus inferior wall in two portions—that is, the sphenoid (upper clivus) and the rhino-pharyngeal (lower clivus) segment. As a matter of fact, the degree of pneumatization of the sphenoid sinus influences the measure of each segment; therefore, entry into the posterior cranial fossa through the clivus is most easily gained in a retrosellar type sphenoid sinus due to a reduced bone thickness, as opposed to the case in a conchal type of the sphenoid sinus.

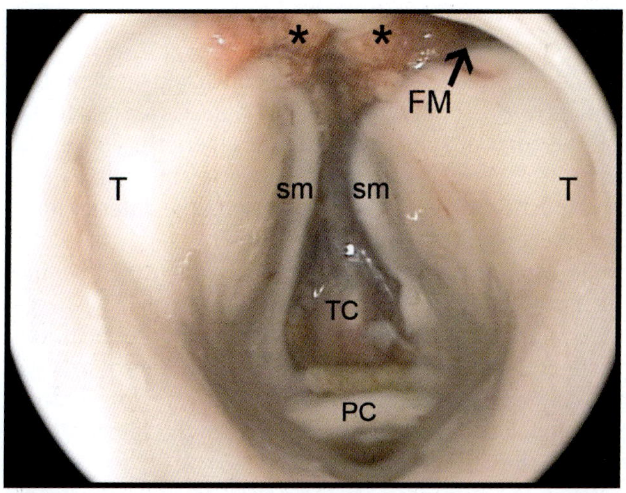

Fig. 41.10 An endoscopic endonasal view inside the cavity of the third ventricle. After exposure of the retrosellar area, the floor of the third ventricle has been opened at the level of the tuber cinereum. Advancing the endoscope through this opening and under the *massa intermedia*, the posterior part of the third ventricle is visualized. *T*, thalamus; *sm*, striae medullaris; *TC*, tela choroidea; *PC*, posterior commissure; *FM*, foramen of Monro; *asterisk*, choroid plexus.

The nasal mucosa is detached from the vomer, along the inferior wall of the sphenoid sinus, and bilaterally and superiorly to identify the vidian nerves that represent the lateral limits of the surgical corridor.

The vomer and the inferior wall of the sphenoid sinus have to be removed completely in an anteroposterior direction to allow the exposure of both the sphenoidal and rhinopharyngeal parts of the clivus.[49,50] The removal of the inferior wall is permitted up to the point where the vidian nerves are identified (**Fig. 41.11A**).[40,51] These nerves can be identified laterally to the vomer-sphenoid junction. The vidian nerves, after crossing the intrapetrous carotid artery from above, reach the pterygopalatine fossa at a level inferior to that of the intrapetrous carotid artery. For this reason, they represent a useful landmark during the bone removal of the inferior wall of the sphenoid sinus because, by remaining medial to these nerves, the risk of injuries to the intrapetrous portion of the carotid artery is avoided.[41] The vidian nerve should be considered the lowest limit while removing the bone in this area to avoid the risk of injury of the intrapetrous carotid artery.

Inside the sphenoid sinus cavity, the lateral limit of the sphenoid portion of the clivus is represented by the paraclival tracts of the intracavernous carotid artery, which are clearly visible (**Fig. 41.11B**).

The clival bone contains the most extensive series of intercavernous venous connections across the midline (i.e., the basilar plexus). Once it is removed, the periosteum-dural layer becomes visible. By removing more bone up to the carotid protuberances, it becomes possible to recognize the sixth cranial nerve (**Fig. 41.11C**). This nerve enters the cavernous sinus by passing through the basilar sinus close to the paraclival tract of the intracavernous carotid in close contact to the dorsal meningeal artery. The latter is a branch of the meningohypophyseal artery and provides arterial blood supply to the dura of the clival region.[45]

After the opening of the dura, the basilar artery and its branches are well seen, in addition to the upper cranial nerves, as they course in the posterior cranial fossa (**Fig. 41.12A**). Furthermore, extending the clival bone opening downward, the anterior surface of the craniovertebral junction is reached. To provide a wider exposure of this area, however, the nasopharynx and the vomer can be completely removed up to the hard palate.

Removing the lower third of the clivus up to the occipital condyles enables both *foramina lacera* to be exposed. The anterior third of the occipital condyles can also be removed along with the anterior and middle third of the condyles. Indeed, it is important to remember that the articular surface of the condyles lies on its lateral portion, hence the removal of the anterior inner aspect does not affect the joint functioning.[45,49,52] The mucosa of the nasopharynx is then reflected and the atlanto-occipital membrane, the

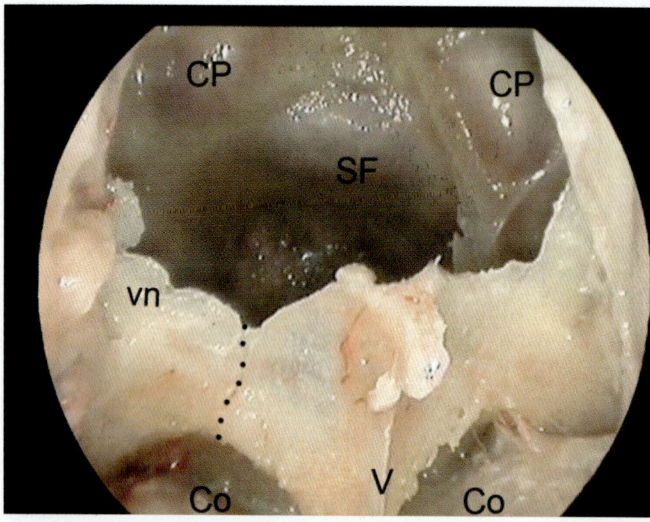

A

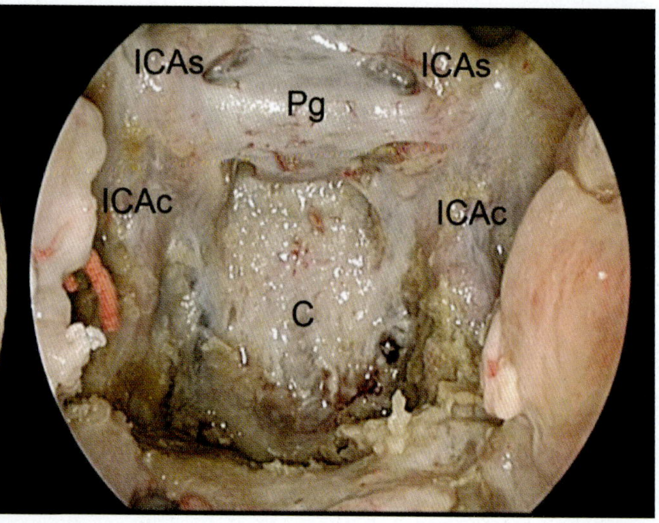

B

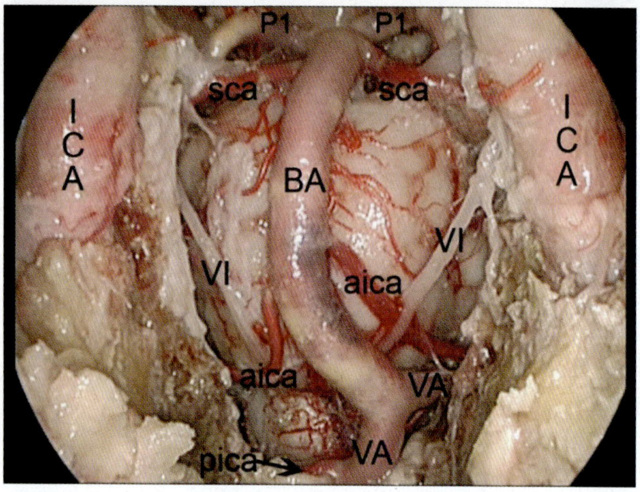

C

Fig. 41.11 An endoscopic view of the endonasal anatomy of the posterior skull base. **(A)** During vomer removal, the sphenoid-vomer junction is exposed and, further laterally, also the vidian nerve, which represents the lateral limit of the bone removal. **(B)** After removal of the bone, the periosteum-dural layer is exposed. **(C)** After dura opening, the ventral surface of the brain stem and the surrounding neurovascular structures are exposed. *CP*, carotid protuberance; *SF*, sellar floor; *vn*, vidian nerve; dotted line, sphenoid-vomer junction; *Co*, choana; *V*, vomer; *C*, clivus; *Pg*, pituitary gland; *ICAs*, parasellar segment of the internal carotid artery; *ICAc*, paraclival segment of the internal carotid artery; *ICA*, internal carotid artery; *P1*, posterior cerebral artery; *sca*, superior cerebellar artery; *BA*, basilar artery; *aica*, anteroinferior cerebellar artery; *pica*, posteroinferior cerebellar artery; *VI*, abducent nerve; *VA*, vertebral artery.

longus capitis and *longus colli* muscles, the atlas, and axis come into view.

After dissecting the muscular structures, the anterior arch of the atlas is removed and the dens is exposed. By using the microdrill, the dens can be thinned, separated from the apical and alar ligaments, dissected from the transverse ligament, and then removed.[50,53] Opening the dura offers the potential to observe all the neurovascular structures running through the anterior part of the foramen magnum (**Fig. 41.12B**).

The first vascular structures to be identified are the vertebral arteries, which can be explored from their entrance in the vertebral canal up to the basilar artery. The intradural segment of the vertebral artery, after emerging from the fibrous dural canal, ascends in front of the rootlets of the hypoglossal nerve to reach the anterior aspect of the medulla oblongata where it unites near the junction of the pons and medulla with its homologue to form the basilar artery. During its intradural course, two arterial branches can be identified through an anterior approach—the posterior inferior cerebellar artery (PICA), which courses backward around the lateral surface of the medulla and between the rootlets of glossopharyngeal, vagus, and accessory nerves; and the anterior spinal artery. More superiorly, above and behind the vertebral artery, the lower cranial nerves and the acoustic-facial bundle (VII-VIII) with the anterior inferior cerebellar artery (AICA) are visible.

The hypoglossal nerve can be clearly identified behind the first tract of the intradural vertebral artery. This nerve arises along the front of the inferior olive anterior to the origin of the cranial accessory fibers as a series of rootlets that converge on the dural orifice of the hypoglossal canal. The hypoglossal nerve passes anterior to the spinal root of the accessory nerve.

Below the entrance of the vertebral artery in the canal, the dentate ligament is attached to the pia mater between the dorsal and ventral rootlets of the spinal cord and presents a series of triangular toothlike processes on each side that are attached at intervals to the dura mater. At the craniocervical junction, the dentate ligament is located behind the vertebral artery and the ventral rootlets of C1 and C2.

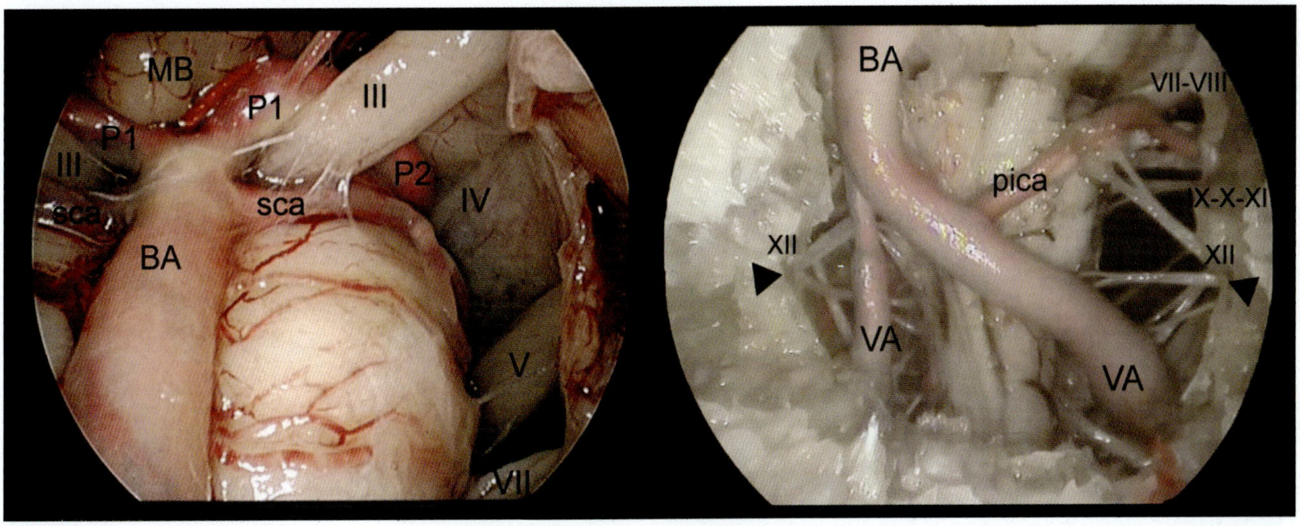

A B

Fig. 41.12 Endoscopic endonasal anatomy of the posterior skull base. Intradural exploration. **(A)** The ventral surface of the pons, the basilar artery with its branches, and the higher cranial nerves are highlighted. **(B)** Angling the endoscope downward, the ventral surface of the medulla oblongata, the lower cranial nerves, and the vertebral arteries are exposed. The lateral extension of the bone removal is restrained by the hypoglossal canal. *MB*, mammillary bodies; *III*, oculomotor nerve; *P1*, posterior cerebral artery; *P2*, posterior cerebral artery; *sca*, superior cerebellar artery; *BA*, basilar artery; *VA*, vertebral artery; *pica*, posteroinferior cerebellar artery; *IV*, trochlear nerve; *V*, trigeminal nerve; *VII-VIII*, acoustic-facial bundle; *IX-X-XI*, glossopharyngeal, vagus, and accessory nerves; *XII*, hypoglossal nerve; *arrowhead*, hypoglossal canal.

The Parasellar Region

Because the endoscope offers the opportunity to clearly explore the midline of the skull base, it provides access to the lateral sellar compartment,[54] represented mainly by the cavernous sinus.[39,40,51,55–57] This area remains accessible also through the sphenoid sinus, but in this case, through its lateral wall (**Fig. 41.13A**). To allow a better exposure of such areas, as already previously described, the anterior sphenoidotomy has to be extended more laterally and then superiorly, the supreme turbinates must be removed, and the posterior ethmoid cells must be opened. Alternatively, a more direct trajectory, which passes laterally to the middle turbinate, could be performed to expose the lateral wall of the sphenoid sinus. In such a transethmoid approach, the first structure to be removed is the uncinate process, then the bulla ethmoidalis is opened, and finally the access is gained through the anterior and posterior ethmoid cells.[51,55,58,59] To widely expose the lateral recess of the sphenoid sinus through the pterygopalatine fossa,[40,60,61] the portion of the medial pterygoid process enclosed between the pterygoid canal and the foramen rotundum has to be removed (**Fig. 41.13B**).[41–44]

Once anatomic landmarks have been identified, the bone covering the lateral wall of the sphenoid sinus and the carotid protuberances is removed to expose all of the neurovascular structures enclosed within the anterior part of the cavernous sinus (**Fig. 41.13C**). Its medial wall is constituted by a fibrous trabecular structure that separates the cavernous sinus from the outer periosteal layer of the pituitary gland. The opening of such structure immediately sheds light on the C-shaped segment of the intracavernous carotid artery (**Fig. 41.14A**).

Displacing the carotid artery laterally, it is possible to visualize the meningohypophyseal artery and its branches, the dorsal meningeal, the inferior hypophyseal, and the tentorial arteries. On the other hand, the inferolateral trunk, with its branches to the intracavernous cranial nerves, lies laterally to the carotid artery and embedded in the lateral wall of the cavernous sinus. Furthermore, moving the endoscope superiorly, the oculomotor and trochlear nerves are seen coming up from the C-shaped tract toward the superior orbital fissure.

Lateral to the intracavernous carotid artery, the oculomotor, the abducent, and the maxillary nerves can be detected lying in a more medial plane when compared with that occupied by the trochlear and the ophthalmic nerves (**Fig. 41.14B**). In actual fact, from the endoscopic standpoint, the oculomotor nerve partially covers the trochlear nerve, whereas the V_1 branch of the trigeminal nerve is partially hidden behind the sixth nerve. The sixth cranial nerve usually receives sympathetic fibers from the internal carotid artery adventitia,[62] while passing laterally to the C-shaped tract of the vessel. Inferiorly, after crossing the lower paraclival tract of the carotid artery, the trochlear nerve runs parallel to the oculomotor nerve. Both nerves, together with the ophthalmic nerve, course in a slight lateral superior direction toward the superior orbital fissure, while the maxillary nerve runs inferiorly to reach the foramen rotundum.

Nevertheless, a better anatomic description could be achieved by analyzing each area separately as separated

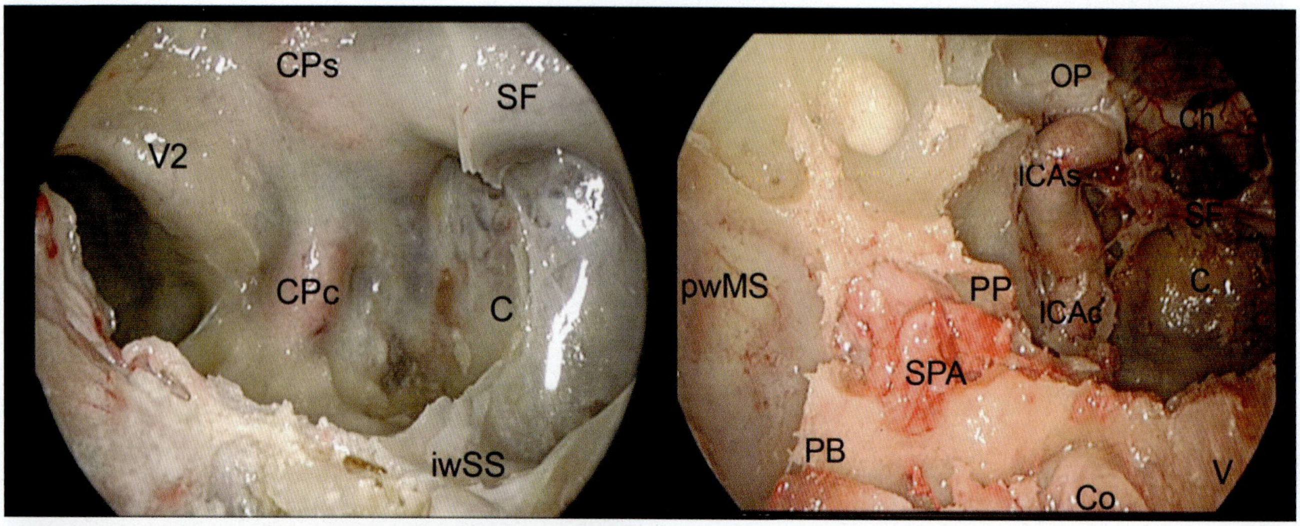

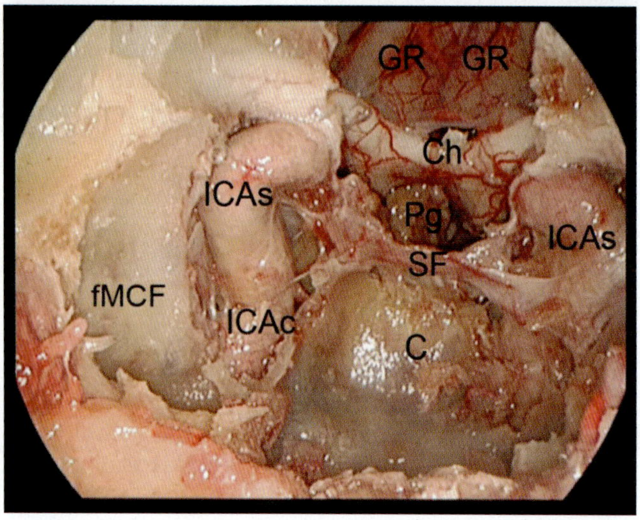

Fig. 41.13 Endoscopic endonasal approach to the cavernous sinus. **(A)** A case of well-pneumatized sphenoid sinus lightens the exposure of the parasellar area. Note the bone covering of the maxillary branch of the trigeminal nerve, which is well outlined in this specimen. **(B)** After a maxillary antrostomy, the posterior wall of the maxillary sinus is exposed and the sphenopalatine foramen enlarged. **(C)** The superomedial part of the pterygoid process has been drilled, thus enlarging the surgical corridor to the lateral recess of the sphenoid sinus. *CPs*, parasellar segment of the carotid protuberance; *CPc*, paraclival segment of the carotid protuberance; *C*, clivus; *SF*, sellar floor; *iwSS*, inferior wall of the sphenoid sinus; *V2*, bone covering of the second branch of the trigeminal nerve; *pwMS*, posterior wall of the maxillary sinus; *PB*, orbital process of the palatine bone; *PP*, medial pterygoid process; *Co*, choana; *V*, vomer; *SPA*, sphenopalatine artery; *OP*, optic protuberance; *SF*, sellar floor; *C*, clivus; *GR*, gyri recta; *fMCF*, floor of the middle cranial fossa; *Ch*, chiasma; *Pg*, pituitary gland; *ICAs*, parasellar segment of the internal carotid artery; *ICAc*, paraclival segment of the internal carotid artery.

by the main anatomic structures.[51] The oculomotor nerve superiorly and the abducent inferiorly form the limits of a triangular area whose base is represented by the lateral loop of the carotid artery. The lateral aspect of this area contains the fourth cranial nerve and a portion of the V_1 branch of the trigeminal nerve. The abducent nerve superiorly and V_2 inferiorly enclose a quadrangular area, which is limited laterally by the bony surface of the lateral wall of the sphenoid sinus extending from the superior orbital fissure to the foramen rotundum and medially by the carotid artery. The ophthalmic branch of the trigeminal nerve and arteries to the inferior cavernous sinus pass through this area. Finally, especially in cases of well-pneumatized sinuses, an inferior quadrangular area can be identified. It is limited superiorly by V_2 and inferiorly by the vidian nerve, whereas its anterior and posterior margins are represented respectively by the bony surface of the lateral wall of the sphenoid sinus from the foramen rotundum to the pterygoid canal and the intrapetrous segment and caudal portion of the carotid artery. This last area seems to offer the safest entry into the lateral compartment of the cavernous sinus.[51]

As for any surgical procedure, but particularly in this area where we are dealing with evolving technical procedures in critical areas reached through selected and narrow corridors, a perfect understanding and conceptualization of the anatomy is fundamental. The numerous studies produced in recent years on anatomic themes related to navigating the transsphenoidal route with an endoscope bear witness to the vitality, rapid evolution, and progress of these types of contemporary surgery.

Conclusion

The endoscopic endonasal route is a very versatile approach that provides direct visualization of the entire midline skull base extending from crista galli to the

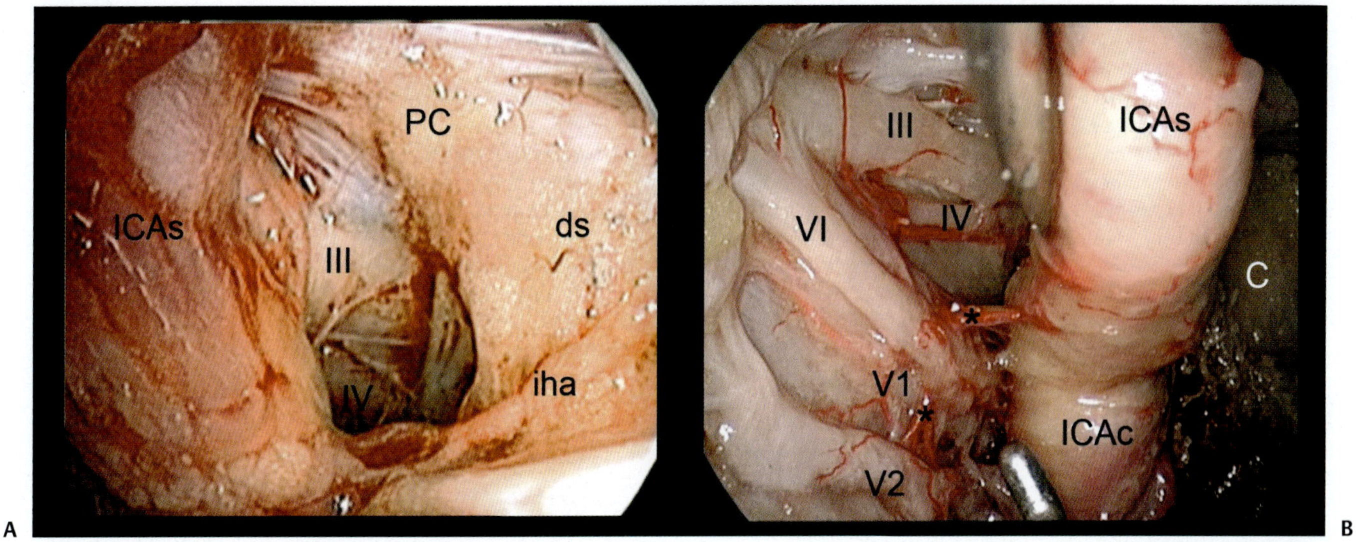

Fig. 41.14 Endoscopic endonasal anatomy of the right cavernous sinus. **(A)** Approach to the medial compartment of the cavernous sinus. After the removal of the medial wall of the cavernous sinus, the third and fourth cranial nerves, running laterally to the intracavernous carotid artery, are recognizable. **(B)** Approach to the lateral compartment of the cavernous sinus. After the removal of the lateral wall of the cavernous sinus, displacing the internal carotid artery medially, are exposed the third, fourth, sixth, ophthalmic, and maxillary nerves and the inferolateral trunk, the tiny branches of which supply the cavernous segment of these nerves. *PC*, posterior clinoid; *ICAs*, parasellar segment of the internal carotid artery; *ICAc*, paraclival segment of the internal carotid artery; *III*, oculomotor nerve; *IV*, trochlear nerve; *VI*, abducent nerve; *V1*, ophthalmic branch of the trigeminal nerve; *V2*, maxillary branch of the trigeminal nerve; *iha*, inferior hypophyseal artery; *ds*, dorsum sellae; *C*, clivus; *asterisk*, inferolateral trunk.

craniovertebral junction; as a matter of fact, through the sphenoid sinus chamber, it is possible to gain a wide exposure of the portion of the skull base extending from the posterior planum sphenoidale to the upper two-thirds of the clivus. Also, around the sphenoid sinus it is possible to explore the more anterior portion of the cranial base via the ethmoid sinuses, whereas the posterior cranial base is exposed through the nasopharynx.

The authors definitely think that laboratory cadaveric dissection remains undefeated in anatomic study, as it offers a unique experience of a wide range of sensorial inputs; however, it has to be reminded that the study of surgical anatomy recently changed. It has been evolving continuously, being integrated and upgraded by the modern imaging systems, lately with the development of three-dimensional computed tomography–based models.[63–66] This latter innovation tremendously eases the identification and the understanding of surgical anatomy, and provides a realistic depiction of the spatial relationships of the structures dealt with.

References

1. Javed T, Sekhar LN. Surgical management of clival meningiomas. Acta Neurochir Suppl (Wien) 1991;53:171–182
2. Fahlbusch R, Schott W. Pterional surgery of meningiomas of the tuberculum sellae and planum sphenoidale: surgical results with special consideration of ophthalmological and endocrinological outcomes. J Neurosurg 2002;96(2):235–243
3. al-Mefty O, Ayoubi S, Smith RR. The petrosal approach: indications, technique, and results. Acta Neurochir Suppl (Wien) 1991;53:166–170
4. Goel A, Muzumdar D, Desai KI. Tuberculum sellae meningioma: a report on management on the basis of a surgical experience with 70 patients. Neurosurgery 2002;51(6):1358–1363, discussion 1363–1364
5. Goel A, Desai K, Muzumdar D. Surgery on anterior foramen magnum meningiomas using a conventional posterior suboccipital approach: a report on an experience with 17 cases. Neurosurgery 2001;49(1):102–106, discussion 106–107
6. Chanda A, Nanda A. Partial labyrinthectomy petrous apicectomy approach to the petroclival region: an anatomic and technical study. Neurosurgery 2002;51(1):147–159, discussion 159–160
7. Hakuba A, Liu S, Nishimura S. The orbitozygomatic infratemporal approach: a new surgical technique. Surg Neurol 1986;26(3): 271–276
8. Hakuba A, Tanaka K, Suzuki T, Nishimura S. A combined orbitozygomatic infratemporal epidural and subdural approach for lesions involving the entire cavernous sinus. J Neurosurg 1989; 71(5 Pt 1):699–704
9. James D, Crockard HA. Surgical access to the base of skull and upper cervical spine by extended maxillotomy. Neurosurgery 1991;29(3):411–416

10. Kawase T, Shiobara R, Toya S. Anterior transpetrosal-transtentorial approach for sphenopetroclival meningiomas: surgical method and results in 10 patients. Neurosurgery 1991;28(6):869–875, discussion 875–876
11. Lang DA, Neil-Dwyer G, Iannotti F. The suboccipital transcondylar approach to the clivus and cranio-cervical junction for ventrally placed pathology at and above the foramen magnum. Acta Neurochir (Wien) 1993;125(1–4):132–137
12. MacDonald JD, Antonelli P, Day AL. The anterior subtemporal, medial transpetrosal approach to the upper basilar artery and ponto-mesencephalic junction. Neurosurgery 1998;43(1):84–89
13. Miller E, Crockard HA. Transoral transclival removal of anteriorly placed meningiomas at the foramen magnum. Neurosurgery 1987;20(6):966–968
14. Nakamura M, Samii M. Surgical management of a meningioma in the retrosellar region. Acta Neurochir (Wien) 2003;145(3): 215–219, discussion 219–220
15. Seifert V, Raabe A, Zimmermann M. Conservative (labyrinth-preserving) transpetrosal approach to the clivus and petroclival region—indications, complications, results and lessons learned. Acta Neurochir (Wien) 2003;145(8):631–642, discussion 642
16. Sepehrnia A, Knopp U. The combined subtemporal-suboccipital approach: a modified surgical access to the clivus and petrous apex. Minim Invasive Neurosurg 2002;45(2):102–104
17. Reisch R, Bettag M, Perneczky A. Transoral transclival removal of anteriorly placed cavernous malformations of the brainstem. Surg Neurol 2001;56(2):106–115, discussion 115–116
18. Weiss MH. The transnasal transsphenoidal approach. In: Apuzzo MLJ, ed. Surgery of the Third Ventricle. Baltimore: Williams & Wilkins; 1987: 476–494
19. Messerklinger W. [Endoscopy technique of the middle nasal meatus (author's transl)]. Arch Otorhinolaryngol 1978;221(4): 297–305
20. Kennedy DW. Functional endoscopic sinus surgery. Technique. Arch Otolaryngol 1985;111(10):643–649
21. Stammberger H, Posawetz W. Functional endoscopic sinus surgery. Concept, indications and results of the Messerklinger technique. Eur Arch Otorhinolaryngol 1990;247(2):63–76
22. Jankowski R, Auque J, Simon C, Marchal JC, Hepner H, Wayoff M. Endoscopic pituitary tumor surgery. Laryngoscope 1992;102(2): 198–202
23. Gamea A, Fathi M, el-Guindy A. The use of the rigid endoscope in trans-sphenoidal pituitary surgery. J Laryngol Otol 1994; 108(1):19–22
24. Cappabianca P, Alfieri A, de Divitiis E. Endoscopic endonasal transsphenoidal approach to the sella: towards functional endoscopic pituitary surgery (FEPS). Minim Invasive Neurosurg 1998;41(2):66–73
25. Carrau RL, Jho HD, Ko Y. Transnasal-transsphenoidal endoscopic surgery of the pituitary gland. Laryngoscope 1996;106(7): 914–918
26. Jho HD, Carrau RL, Ko Y. Endoscopic pituitary surgery. In: Wilkins H, Rengachary S, eds. Neurosurgical Operative Atlas, Vol. 5. Park Ridge, IL: American Association of Neurological Surgeons; 1996:1–12
27. Kassam A, Snyderman C, Carrau R. An evolving paradigm to the ventral skull base. Skull Base 2004;14(suppl 1):23
28. Cappabianca P, Cavallo LM, de Divitiis E. Endoscopic endonasal transsphenoidal surgery. Neurosurgery 2004;55(4):933–940, discussion 940–941
29. Castelnuovo P, Pistochini A, Locatelli D. Different surgical approaches to the sellar region: focusing on the "two nostrils four hands technique." Rhinology 2006;44(1):2–7
30. Cappabianca P, Alfieri A, de Divitiis E, Tschabitscher M. Atlas of Endoscopic Anatomy for Endonasal Intracranial Surgery. New York: Springer-Verlag; 2001
31. Tschabitscher M, Galzio RJ. Endoscopic anatomy along the transnasal approach to the pituitary gland and the surrounding structures. In: de Divitiis E, Cappabianca P, eds. Endoscopic Endonasal Transsphenoidal Surgery. Wien: Springer-Verlag; 2003:21–39
32. Perneczky A, Muller-Forell W, van Lindert E, Fries G. Keyhole Concept in Neurosurgery. Stuttgart: Thieme; 1999
33. Laws ER Jr. Vascular complications of transsphenoidal surgery. Pituitary 1999;2(2):163–170
34. Stammberger H, Hosemann W, Draf W. [Anatomic terminology and nomenclature for paranasal sinus surgery]. Laryngorhinootologie 1997;76(7):435–449
35. White DV, Sincoff EH, Abdulrauf SI. Anterior ethmoidal artery: microsurgical anatomy and technical considerations. Neurosurgery 2005;56(2, Suppl):406–410, discussion 406–410
36. Erdogmus S, Govsa F. The anatomic landmarks of ethmoidal arteries for the surgical approaches. J Craniofac Surg 2006; 17(2):280–285
37. Moon HJ, Kim HU, Lee JG, Chung IH, Yoon JH. Surgical anatomy of the anterior ethmoidal canal in ethmoid roof. Laryngoscope 2001;111(5):900–904
38. Kassam A, Snyderman CH, Mintz A, Gardner P, Carrau RL. Expanded endonasal approach: the rostrocaudal axis. Part I. Crista galli to the sella turcica. Neurosurg Focus 2005;19(1):E3
39. Alfieri A, Jho HD. Endoscopic endonasal cavernous sinus surgery: an anatomic study. Neurosurgery 2001;48(4):827–836, discussion 836–837
40. Magro F, Solari D, Cavallo LM, et al. The endoscopic endonasal approach to the lateral recess of the sphenoid sinus via the pterygopalatine fossa: comparison of endoscopic and radiological landmarks. Neurosurgery 2006;59(4, Suppl 2):ONS237–ONS242, discussion ONS242–ONS243
41. Kassam AB, Vescan AD, Carrau RL, et al. Expanded endonasal approach: vidian canal as a landmark to the petrous internal carotid artery. J Neurosurg 2008;108(1):177–183
42. Alfieri A, Jho HD, Schettino R, Tschabitscher M. Endoscopic endonasal approach to the pterygopalatine fossa: anatomic study. Neurosurgery 2003;52(2):374–378, discussion 378–380
43. Solari D, Magro F, Cappabianca P, et al. Anatomical study of the pterygopalatine fossa using an endoscopic endonasal approach: spatial relations and distances between surgical landmarks. J Neurosurg 2007;106(1):157–163
44. Cavallo LM, Messina A, Gardner P, et al. Extended endoscopic endonasal approach to the pterygopalatine fossa: anatomical study and clinical considerations. Neurosurg Focus 2005;19(1):E5
45. Cavallo LM, Messina A, Cappabianca P, et al. Endoscopic endonasal surgery of the midline skull base: anatomical study and clinical considerations. Neurosurg Focus 2005;19(1):E2
46. Cavallo LM, de Divitiis O, Aydin S, et al. Extended endoscopic endonasal transsphenoidal approach to the suprasellar area: anatomic considerations - part 1. Neurosurgery 2007;61:ONS-24–ONS-34
47. Figueiredo EG, Zabramski JM, Deshmukh P, Crawford NR, Preul MC, Spetzler RF. Anatomical and quantitative description of the transcavernous approach to interpeduncular and prepontine cisterns. Technical note. J Neurosurg 2006;104(6):957–964
48. Kassam AB, Prevedello DM, Thomas A, et al. Endoscopic endonasal pituitary transposition for a transdorsum sellae approach to the interpeduncular cistern. Neurosurgery 2008;62(3, Suppl 1): 57–72, discussion 72–74
49. Cavallo LM, Cappabianca P, Messina A, et al. The extended endoscopic endonasal approach to the clivus and cranio-vertebral junction: anatomical study. Childs Nerv Syst 2007;23(6):665–671
50. Messina A, Bruno MC, Decq P, et al. Pure endoscopic endonasal odontoidectomy: anatomical study. Neurosurg Rev 2007; 30(3):189–194, discussion 194

51. Cavallo LM, Cappabianca P, Galzio R, Iaconetta G, de Divitiis E, Tschabitscher M. Endoscopic transnasal approach to the cavernous sinus versus transcranial route: anatomic study. Neurosurgery 2005;56(2, Suppl):379–389, discussion 379–389
52. Wen HT, Rhoton AL Jr, Katsuta T, de Oliveira E. Microsurgical anatomy of the transcondylar, supracondylar, and paracondylar extensions of the far-lateral approach. J Neurosurg 1997;87(4):555–585
53. Kassam AB, Snyderman C, Gardner P, Carrau R, Spiro R. The expanded endonasal approach: a fully endoscopic transnasal approach and resection of the odontoid process: technical case report. Neurosurgery 2005;57(1, Suppl):E213, discussion E213
54. Parkinson D. Extradural neural axis compartment. J Neurosurg 2000;92(4):585–588
55. Frank G, Pasquini E. Approach to the cavernous sinus. In: de Divitiis E, Cappabianca P, eds. Endoscopic Endonasal Transsphenoidal Surgery. Wien: Springer-Verlag; 2003: 159–175
56. Kassam AB, Gardner P, Snyderman C, Mintz A, Carrau R. Expanded endonasal approach: fully endoscopic, completely transnasal approach to the middle third of the clivus, petrous bone, middle cranial fossa, and infratemporal fossa. Neurosurg Focus 2005;19(1):E6
57. Prevedello DM, Kassam AB, Snyderman C, et al. Endoscopic cranial base surgery: ready for prime time? Clin Neurosurg 2007;54:48–57
58. Cappabianca P, Cavallo LM, Esposito F, et al. Extended endoscopic endonasal approach to the midline skull base: the evolving role of transsphenoidal surgery. In: Pickard JD, Akalan N, Di Rocco C, et al, eds. Advances and Technical Standards in Neurosurgery. Wien, New York: Springer; 2008: 152–199
59. de Divitiis E, Cappabianca P, Cavallo LM. Endoscopic transsphenoidal approach: adaptability of the procedure to different sellar lesions. Neurosurgery 2002;51(3):699–705, discussion 705–707
60. Bolger WE. Endoscopic transpterygoid approach to the lateral sphenoid recess: surgical approach and clinical experience. Otolaryngol Head Neck Surg 2005;133(1):20–26
61. Al-Nashar IS, Carrau RL, Herrera A, Snyderman CH. Endoscopic transnasal transpterygopalatine fossa approach to the lateral recess of the sphenoid sinus. Laryngoscope 2004;114(3): 528–532
62. Mariniello G, Annecchiarico H, Sardo L, Buonamassa S, de Divitiis E. Connections of sympathetic fibres inside the cavernous sinus: a microanatomical study. Clin Neurol Neurosurg 2000;102(1):1–5
63. de Notaris M, Solari D, Cavallo LM, et al. The use of a three-dimensional novel computer-based model for analysis of the endonasal endoscopic approach to the midline skull base. World Neurosurg 2011;75(1):106–113, discussion 36–40
64. de Notaris M, Prats-Galino A, Cavallo LM, et al. Preliminary experience with a new three-dimensional computer-based model for the study and the analysis of skull base approaches. Childs Nerv Syst 2010;26(5):621–626
65. Petersson H, Sinkvist D, Wang C, Smedby O. Web-based interactive 3D visualization as a tool for improved anatomy learning. Anat Sci Educ 2009;2(2):61–68
66. Wiet GJ, Stredney D. Update on surgical simulation: the Ohio State University experience. Otolaryngol Clin North Am 2002; 35(6):1283–1288, viii

42 Pathology of the Sinonasal Region and Anterior and Central Skull Base

Michael J. Kaplan, Griffith R. Harsh IV, Benzion Joshua, Deborah J. Chute, and Gerald J. Berry

Although epithelial tumors predominate in the paranasal sinuses and the anterior and central skull base, markedly diverse histopathology is seen. Benign and malignant primary tumors may originate from the different cellular constituents, such as the respiratory mucosa and minor salivary glands of the paranasal sinuses, the olfactory epithelium of the olfactory bulb, arachnoid, dura, bone, and cartilage. This chapter provides an overview of the complex pathology that might be considered in a differential diagnosis based on the clinical and radiologic information available prior to biopsy. Facility with and an understanding of both radiologically and histologically pertinent information provides the highest likelihood of streamlined, cost-effective evaluation with a minimum of patient discomfort and delay.

Respiratory mucosa lining the nose and paranasal sinuses, along with specialized olfactory epithelium at the cribriform plate, give rise to tumors of epithelial origin. The most common of these is squamous cell carcinoma (SCC), the histology of 65 to 70% of paranasal sinus malignancies. Sinonasal undifferentiated carcinoma (SNUC) and malignant melanoma are also believed to be of sinonasal mucosal origin, and tumors of neural crest origin, such as esthesioneuroblastoma (olfactory neuroblastoma) and neuroendocrine carcinoma, are common. About 20% of paranasal sinus malignancies are of minor salivary gland origin, of which adenoid cystic carcinomas and adenocarcinomas are most common. Lymphomas, such as B cell lymphoma and the rarer CD56-positive natural killer (NK)-T cell lymphomas represent ~10% of paranasal sinus malignancies. Matrix-producing sarcomas, such as osteosarcoma and chondrosarcomas, are not uncommon here, and other sarcomas, such as rhabdomyosarcoma and synovial sarcoma, may also occur. Rare mesenchymal neoplasms, such as solitary fibrous tumor, may be difficult to diagnose both clinically and histologically. Metastases to the skull base from remote primary tumors are uncommon, but must be considered, especially when the lesion is predominantly within the bony structures in a patient with a prior known malignancy. Meningiomas and tumors of neural origin, such as schwannomas, also are encountered frequently, as are chordomas, which originate from notochordal remnants. In addition, several benign proliferations, such as angiofibroma, inverted papilloma, fibrous dysplasia, and pituitary adenomas, warrant discussion.

Radiologic evaluation begins with an appropriate magnetic resonance image (MRI). An MRI-skull base protocol is superior to computed tomography (CT) scanning in determining tumor extent, orbital involvement, and dural extension. CT imaging is a useful complementary study in evaluating apparent fibrous dysplasia, possible Paget disease, or involvement of the cribriform plate.

Following thorough radiologic evaluation, tissue for definitive histologic diagnosis is often, but not always, the next step in evaluation. When accessible, tissue should be obtained transnasally, usually with an endoscope. Frozen section evaluation prior to definitive surgical resection is indicated in thoughtfully selected situations. Surgical excision will be a significant component of the treatment of many of the pathologic entities seen at the skull base, but not all. The role of surgery is generally limited to obtaining diagnostic tissue in cases of malignant lymphoma and selected pediatric tumors such as rhabdomyosarcomas. Hence, before therapeutic resection is undertaken in the absence of prior diagnostic biopsy, a comprehensive step-wise analysis, informed by appropriate radiologic and oncologic consultation, should be completed. Often, this includes a metastatic evaluation, usually with positron emission tomography (PET)-CT (except for sarcomas, where CT of the neck, chest, abdomen, and pelvis may be a better screen).

An initial diagnostic biopsy is not indicated when (1) the differential diagnosis includes only histologies for which the mode of treatment would be unchanged (e.g., surgery only, or clinical monitoring only); (2) the tumor's location confers to the biopsy procedure either significant risk (e.g., adjacent to the internal carotid artery) or invasiveness and patient discomfort (e.g., inaccessible by a simple transnasal approach); or (3) the tumor is very vascular and other studies are diagnostic (e.g., angiofibroma).

Separate chapters of this book address endoscopic and external surgical approaches that may be warranted for selected pathologic entities.

Benign Tumors

Angiofibroma

Accounting for 0.5% of all head and neck tumors, juvenile nasal angiofibromas (JNAs) occur almost exclusively in males between age 11 and young adulthood. Rarely is there a presentation over age 25, and there are only a few case reports of lesions interpreted as a JNA in women (which perhaps should be reevaluated in light of the later discussion of solitary fibrous tumors). They invariably begin at the lateral basisphenoid at the junction of the sphenoid sinus and pterygopalatine fossa near the sphenopalatine artery, from which they can expand in all directions to disrupt adjacent structures. Extension laterally bows the posterior maxillary

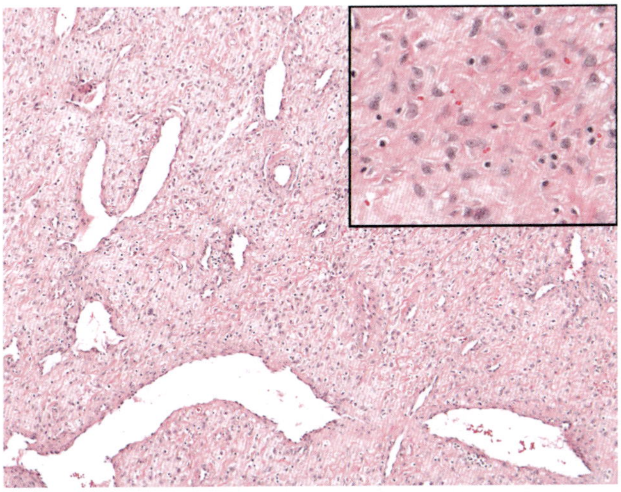

Fig. 42.1 Angiofibroma is composed of an admixture of delicate, branching blood vessels and small muscularized vessels and a fibrocollagenous stroma (H&E ×100). **Inset**: High-power magnification showing round and oval nuclei with small central nucleoli (H&E ×400).

sinus wall forward, a common finding (Holman Miller sign) reported in the days of plain roentgenology. Today, the flow voids seen on MRI in the context of an otherwise healthy young man with nasal obstruction and epistaxis is rarely confused with any other diagnosis, although in the cachectic patient, one must consider malignancies in this age group, such as embryonal rhabdomyosarcoma.

Typical histopathologic findings include a polypoid mass with smooth or bosselated edges, and characteristically irregular delicate, thin-walled "staghorn" blood vessels embedded in a variably hyalinized collagenous stroma containing plump, stellate, or spindled fibroblasts (**Fig. 42.1**). Inflammatory cells are rare, including mast cells. Pleomorphism, mitotic activity, and necrosis are uncommon, except in cases of infarction following preoperative embolization. The stromal cells and endothelial cells are immunoreactive with antibodies for androgen, estrogen, and progesterone receptors. Beta-catenin mutations have been reported in the stroma of JNAs.[1,2] Although additional information on genetic alterations in JNAs is accumulating, much remains to be learned.[3]

Treatment is resection. Although some advocate surgery without embolization in selected cases, preoperative embolization significantly reduces intraoperative bleeding to the point that transfusion is rarely required. Various staging systems exist, but careful evaluation of the preoperative MRI will ultimately determine the approach and extent of surgery. Even for the 10 to 20% that extend to the cranial base, endoscopic resection is usually indicated. Recurrence rates are low. Irradiation is reserved for surgically inaccessible tumor remnants that progressively enlarge on serial MRI scans. Even in recurrent cases, growth usually stops after adolescence. Thus, if the patient is near adulthood and the tumor is asymptomatic and slow growing, observation may be preferable to irradiation. The prognosis is excellent.

Inverted Papilloma and Other Papillomas

The histopathologic review of papillomas by Hyams remains fully valid today,[4] as discussed anew by Batsakis.[5] Inverted papillomas represent an epithelial inversion of the ectodermally derived respiratory sinonasal mucosa into a polypoid, edematous stroma, sometimes with fibromyxomatous features. Of the three types of Schneiderian papillomas, inverted papilloma (IP) is the most common and it is the one that may occasionally pose surgical challenges at the skull base. This is particularly true for the 5 to 10% of IPs that at presentation or thereafter harbor an SCC. Microscopically, islands of thickened epithelial cells are surrounded by edematous and inflamed stroma. The invaginated nests are composed of mature nonkeratinized squamous cells admixed with mucinous cells and mucous cysts and enveloped by a thin basement membrane (**Fig. 42.2**). Atypia is mild,

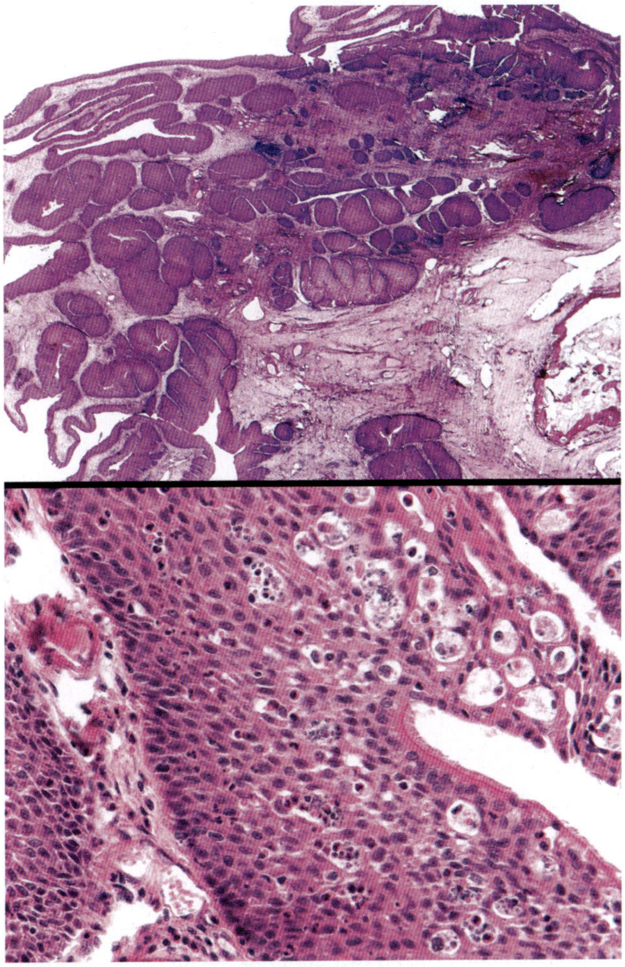

Fig. 42.2 Upper panel: Schneiderian papilloma, inverted type is characterized by an endophytic growth pattern. The rounded nests are enveloped by basement membranes and lack a desmoplastic host response (H&E ×20). **Lower panel**: High-power magnification showing a proliferation of uniform, bland nonkeratinized squamous cells admixed with chronic inflammatory cells and intraepithelial mucous microcysts. Note the preservation of cellular polarity, lack of cytologic atypia, and absence of division figures. Ciliated columnar cells are retained at the surface (H&E ×400).

mitotic figures are restricted to the basal layer, and normal cellular maturation is noted from the basal layer to the surface. Although histopathologic features associated with the risk for malignant transformation have been sought, none have been found consistently. Nonetheless, increased cellularity, keratinization in the superficial aspect, and loss of normal maturation of the squamous proliferation should prompt a thorough examination of the specimen and vigilant subsequent clinical surveillance for SCC, including serial endoscopic examinations and periodic MRI.

When the tumor is confined to the nasal cavity, ethmoid sinus, and medial maxillary wall, endoscopic surgical resection of inverted papilloma has a low recurrence rate (less than 5%). Busquets and Hwang conducted a meta-analysis, which revealed that endoscopic resection of IPs had lower rates of recurrence than external approaches (no significant selection bias for larger tumors was noted in the external group).[6] Landsberg emphasizes that subperiosteal resection of the mucosal tumor attachment site is important in reducing the rate of recurrence.[7] Cannady reviewed the recent literature and staging systems.[8] When involvement originates in or extends to the sphenoid sinus, frontal sinus, or lateral maxillary antrum, the recurrence rate rises to 20%. Whether this increase reflects underlying tumor biologic predisposition or the technical difficulty of completely resecting the attachment site is difficult to discern. The recurrence rate is ~35% for the few cases (10%) that extend beyond the paranasal sinuses, such as through the anterior skull base. Surgical resection of these, especially when recurrent, can be challenging, even with supplemental external approaches.

Cylindrical Cell or Oncocytic Papilloma

Less common than the inverted type, oncocytic papillomas share similar clinical and prognostic features, including a small propensity for malignant degeneration. Its cells are organized in a multilayered columnar fashion with abundant granular eosinophilic cytoplasm. Endophytic and exophytic growth is seen. Their behavior and treatment is the same as for IPs and a careful follow-up is essential.

Septal Papilloma

Septal papilloma occurs as an exophytic mass on the anterior nasal septum. The papillary fronds are composed of up to 20 cell layers and display normal squamous maturation toward the surface epithelium. Variable areas of ciliated columnar cells, mucocytes, and inflammatory cells are present. With practically no malignant potential, it is less aggressive than the other types. Complete surgical excision is curative. It is distinguishable from a nasal vestibular squamous papilloma, which is derived from adjacent epidermal skin.

Pituitary Adenoma

The pituitary gland develops embryologically from Rathke's pouch (anterior lobe) and the diverticulum of the diencephalons (posterior lobe). As the anterior lobe migrates posteriorly to fuse with the infundibulum, small islands may remain along the path. These ectopic foci may give rise to ectopic adenomas adjacent to the gland or within the sphenoid bone.

Pituitary adenomas account for 10% of intracranial tumors (**Fig. 42.3**). They become symptomatic by causing either overproduction or underproduction of pituitary hormones or by compressing nearby structures. About half secrete active forms of adrenocorticotropin (ACTH), growth hormone, thyroid-stimulating hormone (TSH), or, in women, prolactin, and usually present with symptoms and signs of hypercortisolism (Cushing syndrome), gigantism or acromegaly, hyperthyroidism, and oligo/amenorrhea and galactorrhea, respectively. Many of these are discovered as microadenomas (<10 mm in diameter). The remaining half of tumors either secrete no hormone, or may secrete a luteinizing hormone (LH), follicle-stimulating hormone (FSH), or inactive fragments of any of the six anterior pituitary hormones, or, in men, prolactin. Hence, without hormonally associated symptoms, these usually present instead with symptoms that occur secondary to compression of adjacent structures, such as the remaining pituitary gland (hypopituitarism), dura (headache), optic nerve or chiasm (visual field loss), oculomotor nerves (diplopia), and trigeminal divisions (facial numbness). MRI usually clearly defines tumor extension beyond the sella: superiorly toward the suprasellar optic nerve or chiasm, laterally toward the

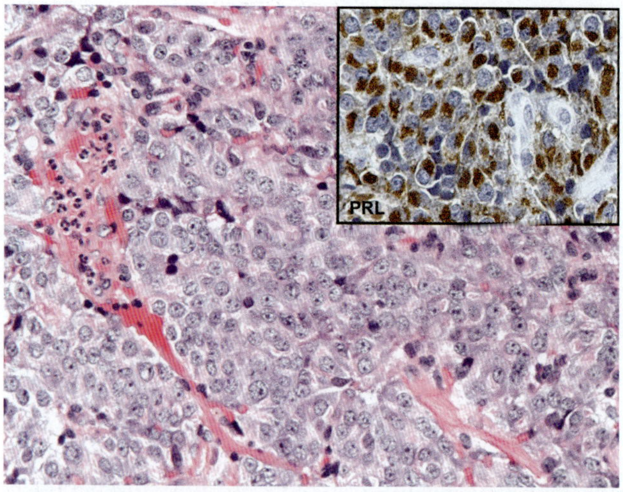

Fig. 42.3 Pituitary adenomas are arranged as sheets or nests of uniform cells with small central nuclei. The appearance of the cytoplasm is helpful in subclassification (H&E ×400). **Inset**: Formalin-fixed paraffin embedded immunohistochemistry is routinely performed for definitive classification. Prolactin-secreting tumors are the most common type (×600).

cavernous sinus containing the internal carotid artery and sixth cranial nerve, posteriorly toward the brainstem, or inferiorly into the sphenoid sinus.

The classification and histopathology of pituitary adenomas is a vast topic, combining light microscopy, electron microscopy ultrastructural findings, and immunoelectron microscopy supplemented with immunohistochemical (IHC) staining for selected hormones.[9,10] Microscopically, adenomas are composed of sheets, nests, ribbons, trabeculae, and papillary arrangements of uniform round cells within a delicate fibrovascular network. One often sees elongated small cells forming pseudorosettes around dilated capillaries. The cytoplasm of the cells ranges from acidophilic, amphophilic, basophilic, to clear (chromophobic). IHC staining is routinely used to further characterize the secretory product. Prolactinomas, for example, are typically predominantly chromophobic, containing only prolactin by IHC.

Choice of treatment options depends on several factors. Small endocrinologically inactive tumors found incidentally may be observed with serial scans; 10% will regress, 40% will remain stable, but 50% will progress over 5 years.[11] Prolactin-secreting tumors are often initially managed pharmacologically with dopamine-receptor agonists such as bromocriptine or cabergoline.[12] Cabergoline and the somatostatin analogue, pasireotide, are under investigation in Cushing disease when surgery has unsuccessfully reduced adrenocorticotropin levels. Endoscopic transsphenoidal adenomectomy is the treatment of choice for tumors secreting other anterior pituitary hormones (ACTH, TSH, growth hormone [GH], LH, FSH), for prolactinomas refractory to dopaminergic suppression, and for larger endocrinologically inactive tumors that cause symptoms of compression. The extent of resection achieved varies with tumor type, size, invasiveness, direction of extension, and adjacent structures involved. Recurrence rates vary between 6 and 46% among these almost exclusively benign tumors, reflecting these same factors.

Benign Fibro-Osseous Lesions

The spectrum of benign bone-containing lesions of the paranasal sinuses shares the common feature of replacement of normal bone by fibroblasts and a variably mineralized collagen matrix. With the exception of fibrous dysplasia, they can have overlapping histologic features. Hence, definitive diagnosis incorporates clinical history (e.g., the age of the patient, the location and progression of growth), radiologic appearance, and histopathology. Among the more commonly encountered benign fibro-osseous lesions along this spectrum are fibrous dysplasia (with the least bone), ossifying fibroma, and osteoma (which contains the most bone). As the spectrum contains rare aggressive lesions, such as juvenile ossifying fibroma, some familiarity with the radiologic and histopathologic findings is important.

Osteomas

Osteomas are dense, well-delineated radiopaque lesions that histologically resemble normal compact cancellous lamellar bone that contains variable amounts of marrow (**Fig. 42.4**). They require surgical intervention if they produce pain and sinusitis associated with blocked drainage of a sinus, typically the frontal sinus or the ethmoid sinus. They may, on occasion, present as a craniofacial deformity or be noted solely as an incidental radiologic finding. Rarely, a secondary mucocele can extend intracranially.[13] Most sinonasal osteomas are solitary. Multiple osteomas raise the possibility of Gardner syndrome (familial adenomatous polyposis, characterized by gastrointestinal polyposis prone to malignant degeneration). The classical radiologic finding is a dense, well-delineated radiopaque lesion. Osteoid osteomas, a variant often producing pain said to be exquisitely sensitive to aspirin, have typical CT features, and may occur solely within the frontal bone, and thus is inaccessible to endoscopic approaches.

Fibrous Dysplasia

Fibrous dysplasia is an osseous proliferation of the mandible and maxilla characterized by excessive production of immature bone. It usually presents in adolescent and young women as an asymmetric, painless swelling, but may occur in older adults. Much has been learned about it in the past 20 years.[14] It is caused by missense mutations in the alpha subunit of the stimulatory G-protein, Gs, in the GNAS (guanine nucleotide binding, alpha stimulating) complex whose gene is in chromosome 20q13.[15] Bone involvement can be polyostotic or confined to one bone (monostotic). When associated with endocrine dysfunction (typically, precocious puberty) and cutaneous pigmented lesions (café-au-lait spots), McCune-Albright syndrome is diagnosed, but this is present in fewer than 5% of cases.

The CT appearance of fibrous dysplasia can vary, but the typical ground glass appearance is most common and highly suggestive of the diagnosis. When this typical appearance is present in an asymptomatic patient, histologic confirmation is not required and serial CT suffices for follow-up.

Histologically, one sees an expanded intramedullary space containing immature spindle fibroblast like cells in parallel or in whorls embedded in poorly mineralized collagen fibrils, often with interspersed trabeculae of woven bone, and the cortical bone may be thinned secondary to surrounding osteoclasts.[16] The classic histologic findings are geometrically shaped (C- and S-shaped) trabeculae of woven bone lacking osteoblasts along their peripheral edges. It has been remarked by some that the shapes made by the irregular woven bony spicules resemble Chinese characters.[17] These aggregates of immature bone merge with the uninvolved cancellous bone at the periphery of the lesion (**Fig. 42.4**). Malignant transformation to aggressive osteosarcoma is rare.

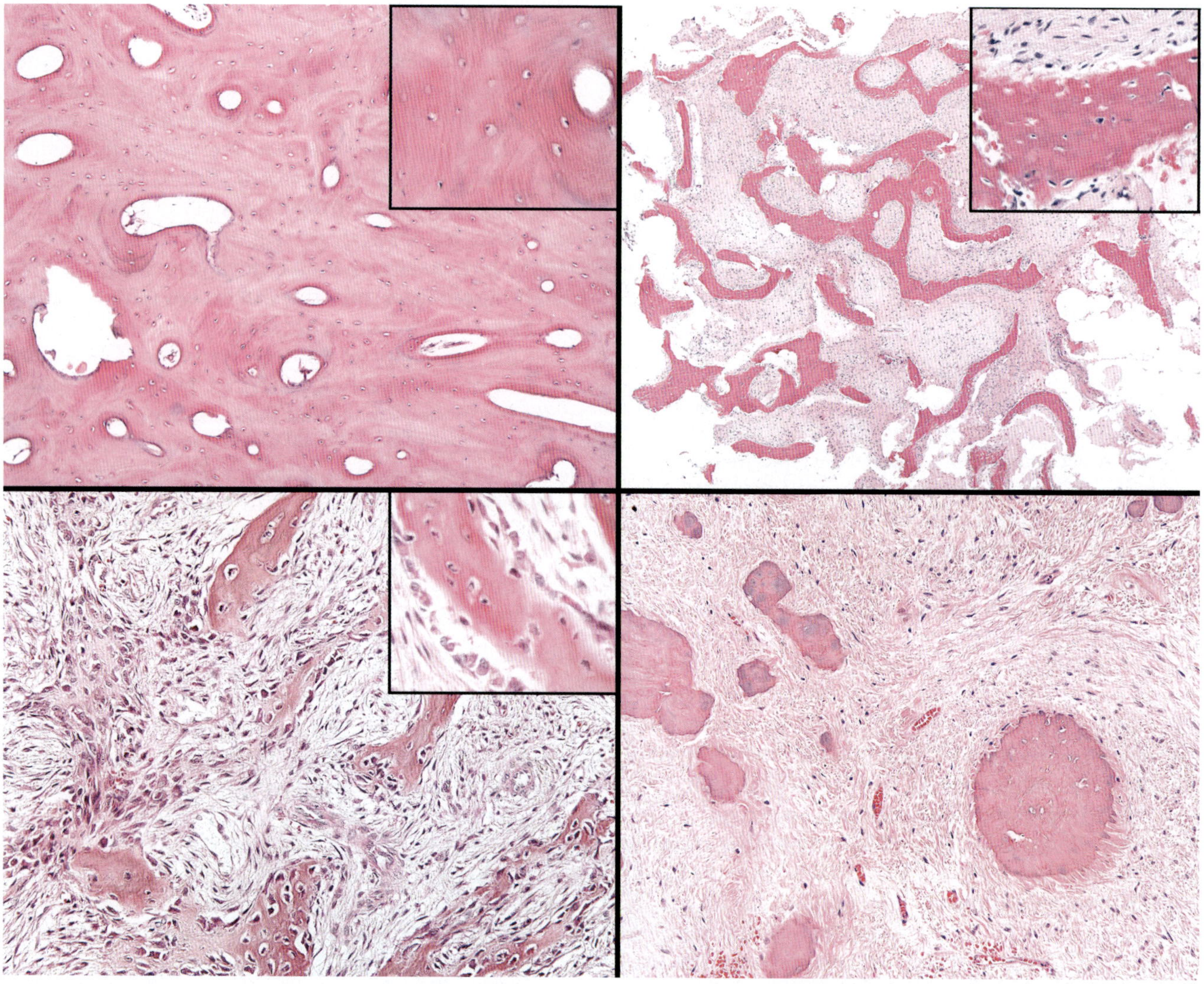

Fig. 42.4 Benign fibro-osseous lesions of the base of skull region. **Upper left**: Osteoma is a bland osseous proliferation composed of mature cancellous bone (H&E ×100). **Inset**: High-power magnification showing normal compact or lamellar bone (H&E ×400). **Upper right**: Fibrous dysplasia is composed of irregularly shaped bony trabeculae arranged haphazardly. The fibrous stroma contains bland spindled cells (H&E ×40). **Inset**: High-power magnification showing immature woven bone lacking a rim of osteoblasts (H&E ×400). **Lower left**: Ossifying fibroma is composed of scattered bony trabeculae embedded in a richly cellular stroma (H&E ×100). **Inset**: The central portions contain woven or immature bone lined by a prominent osteoblastic layer (H&E ×400). **Lower right**: Some fibro-osseous lesions are difficult to classify (H&E ×100). Radiologic-pathologic correlation is essential for all osseous lesions.

Surgery is indicated for disfiguring fibrous dysplasia, such as can occur in the maxilla or to alleviate compression causing neurologic deficit, such as visual loss. Sculpting involved bone, such as that of an expanded superior orbital rim or an anteriorly enlarged maxilla, may be considered for esthetic indications. Although usually asymptomatic, fibrous dysplasia can cause significant pain, a problem often managed with bisphosphonates. Serial CT and monitoring for loss of color vision (which may antedate decreased visual acuity as a manifestation of optic canal compromise) is important.

Ossifying Fibroma

Ossifying fibromas are radiologically and surgically well-demarcated osseous lesions, distinct from fibrous dysplasia.[18] They usually present in a slightly older population than does fibrous dysplasia. Although more common in the mandible and maxilla (where they may be referred to using older terms such as cementifying fibroma and cemento-ossifying fibroma), they can occur in the orbit, paranasal sinuses, and anterior skull base, where they may come to the attention of the rhinologist. They may be noted as incidental radiologic findings or as symptomatic swelling. Their radiologic appearance depends in large part on the maturity of the lesion and can range from radiolucent to radiopaque.

Recognizing the confusing terminology of ossifying fibromas in the literature, the World Health Organization (WHO) attempted to provide some clarification in 2005.[19] Histologically, there is a surrounding outer border of cellular fibrous tissue, within which there is relatively avascular fibrous tissue that may range in the same tumor from highly cellular to almost acellular collagen. The mineralized tissue is composed of unoriented woven and lamellar bony trabeculae that are usually rimmed by osteoblasts, and acellular spherical calcified deposits resembling the cementum that cover dental roots. In the stroma, a cellular storiform pattern, with or without giant cells, is seen in about half of cases (**Fig. 42.4**).

Unlike for fibrous dysplasia, it is best to resect ossifying fibromas completely because their growth rate can be unpredictable. As the lesions are generally well demarcated, this can be done with narrow margins (similar to curettage in the mandible) unless clinically aggressive behavior or recurrence has been noted.

Juvenile (Aggressive) Ossifying Fibroma

Juvenile (aggressive) ossifying fibroma, occurring in adolescents, may grow aggressively and with a propensity for recurrence if incompletely resected. In the paranasal sinuses, the psammomatoid variant is more common than the trabecular. Given its rarity, the clinical and pathologic challenge is making the diagnosis so that effective resection can be planned. Radiologically it is well demarcated, often with central lucent zone, and may initially be misdiagnosed as a mucocele if the lack of an associated blocked sinus is not appreciated. Histologically, one sees spherical ossicles with irregular seams of osteoid within a highly cellular fibrous background.[20–22] Division figures are often present.

Other Benign Fibro-Osseous Lesions

Other benign fibro-osseous lesions occurring in the skull base region include both nonneoplastic and neoplastic lesions. In a small number of cases, the small biopsy samples preclude a definitive diagnosis and a descriptive diagnosis is rendered. The evaluation of any fibro-osseous lesion requires careful radiologic and pathologic correlation. Osteoradionecrosis develops as a complication of radiation treatment and can mimic a neoplastic process.

Meningioma

Meningiomas[23] are common (15 to 25% of all intracranial tumors) benign tumors that arise from arachnoid cap cells, are more common in women, and usually grow slowly. They typically are seen in older patients, and may be diagnosed as incidental findings on an MRI done for other reasons. Exposure to irradiation (20 to 30 years prior to the presentation of a meningioma), and the deletion of the neurofibromatosis type 2 (NF2) gene are established risk factors. The paranasal sinuses may be the site of true extracranial meningiomas,[24] which account for 4% of meningiomas, or meningiomas may extend to the anterior or central skull base directly from adjacent dura, such as from

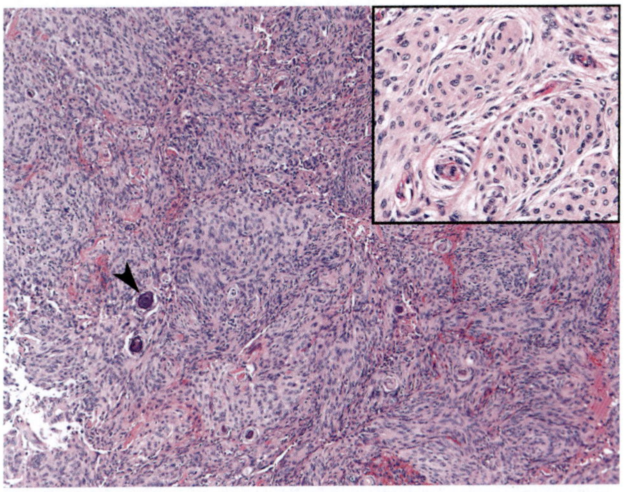

Fig. 42.5 Meningiomas may display a variety of growth patterns. The meningotheliomatous pattern is characterized by a syncytium of lobules and scattered psammoma bodies (*arrowhead*) (H&E ×100). **Inset**: High-power magnification showing lobules of bland epithelioid cells with abundant eosinophilic cytoplasm and lacking distinct cell borders or cytologic atypia (H&E ×400).

the olfactory groove.[25–27] Hyperostotic adjacent bone is not uncommon. Their radiologic appearance may include a dural tail (which is not pathognomonic) or a speckled calcification pattern within a soft tissue mass. This calcification pattern correlates with the presence of the psammoma bodies on histologic sections (**Fig. 42.5**).

Histologically, the typical arrangement is nests and lobules of uniform cells separated by delicate fibrovascular structures. The neoplastic cells display indistinct cell borders, abundant eosinophilic cytoplasm, and nuclei with central clearing and nuclear pseudoinclusions. This whorled growth pattern and psammoma bodies, combined with immunohistochemical staining for epithelial membrane antigen (EMA) and vimentin, are typically seen in most meningiomas and establish the diagnosis. Immunoreactivity for progesterone receptor and, less commonly, an estrogen receptor is reported. Atypical meningioma (WHO grade II) is characterized by high mitotic activity or three of the following: increased cellularity, high nucleus; cytoplasm ratio, prominent nucleoli, patternless sheet-like growth; and foci of necrosis. Atypical (WHO grade II) meningiomas represent less than 10% of meningiomas, and malignant meningiomas less than 1%. Papillary and hemangiopericytic patterns, negative staining for progesterone receptors, and deletions or loss of heterozygosity also correlate with worse prognosis in some studies.[28]

Because meningiomas usually grow slowly, neurologic and radiographic observation is often appropriate. Intervention is indicated for progressive growth that threatens neurologic deficit, or for alleviation of such a deficit. Treatment is generally surgical,[29] with the optimal approach guided by the surgeon's technical experience and the location and anatomic extent of the tumor as assessed by

MRI. The long-term control rates for completely resected WHO grade I[30] in patients under 65 years is 70 to 80%. The control rate is ~50 to 60% in older patients and is less than 50% for atypical meningiomas. Remnants of incompletely removed grade I meningiomas should be followed closely radiographically as significant growth warrants irradiation. Small tumors distant from radiosensitive structures can be treated initially or at recurrence after surgery with stereotactic radiosurgery (14 to 18 Gy to the tumor margin).[31] Large tumors, those involving radiosensitive structures, or those occurring in a patient whose medical condition precludes surgery can be treated with fractionated radiotherapy (50 to 54 Gy). Rates of long-term tumor control can exceed 90%. Most agree that postoperative radiation (56 to 60 Gy) is indicated for remnants of grade II meningiomas and all grade III meningiomas, even those completely resected.

Peripheral Nerve Sheath Tumors[32,33]

Schwannomas (neurolemmomas) and neurofibromas are the most common benign peripheral nerve sheath tumors. They are usually suspected on the basis of clinical and MRI findings. Perineurinomas and malignant peripheral nerve sheath tumors (MPNST) are rare, although it is estimated that patients with neurofibromatosis 1 (NF1) have a 10% chance of developing an MPNST.

Peripheral nerves consist of three layers, the surrounding epineurium, the perineurium (a continuum from the pia-arachnoid, forming concentric layers around nerve fascicles), and the endoneurium. Peripheral nerve tumors are classified by their features of cellular differentiation, and may occur sporadically or as part of NF1 or NF2. Schwannomas, whether sporadic or associated with NF2, often have a deletion of the NF2 gene locus 22q12.2, which encodes schwannomin (or merlin). Neurofibromas often have a deletion of the tumor suppressor gene NF1 on 17 g12.41, which encodes neurofibromin, an activating protein for K-ras.

Schwannomas

Schwannomas (or neurilemmomas) derive from the myelinating cell (Schwann cell) cylinders that surround individual axons. They arise most commonly as a solitary, sporadic lesion (95%). They may occur as multiple tumors in the setting of NF2 (5%). As they expand within a capsule, they eccentrically compress adjacent axons. Schwannomas commonly involve the vestibular nerve and dorsal roots of the spinal cord. They commonly may involve other sensory nerves in the head and neck, such as the trigeminal nerve, presenting as a parapharyngeal or skull base mass.

Neurofibromas

Neurofibromas contain perineural cells, axons, and fibroblasts in addition to Schwann cells. They usually present as painless masses in the skin and soft tissue. The solitary neurofibroma occurs without gender predilection, usually in the third and fourth decades of life. Distinct from that of schwannoma, the intraneural growth pattern of neurofibroma results in radial expansion of the nerve within a thickened perineurium, entrapping otherwise uninvolved axons. When multiple fascicles or multiple branches of a nerve plexus are involved, one sees plexiform growth, as in NF1.[34] Neurofibromas are circumscribed but unencapsulated masses are composed of Schwann cells, fibroblasts, and perineural like cells and are less organized than schwannomas, and the stroma contains inflammatory cells.

Classic histopathologic features are the Antoni A and Antoni B areas, the relative proportion of which may affect radiologic imaging characteristics. Antoni A areas are highly cellular; the cells are stacked in fusiform clusters with tapered ends such that their nuclei appear aligned (nuclear palisading). Such areas may be absent in vestibular schwannomas. When palisading areas alternate with acellular clear areas high in laminin, the pattern is referred to as Verocay bodies (although these can be seen in tumors other than schwannoma). Antoni B areas contain loosely organized myxomatous and microcystic regions of basophilic mucin (that may coalesce into radiographically demonstrated macrocysts), lipid-containing histiocytes, hyalinized vessel walls, and lymphocytes. These biphasic fusiform or globular masses, with densely cellular areas containing Verocay bodies, Antoni A alternating with hypocellular Antoni B areas, and thick-walled blood vessels are demonstrated in **Fig. 42.6**. The spindled tumor cells show strong diffuse immunoreactivity for the S100 protein.

Treatment of schwannomas and neurofibromas is aimed toward the preservation of function (e.g., hearing and facial nerve function threatened by an acoustic schwannoma)

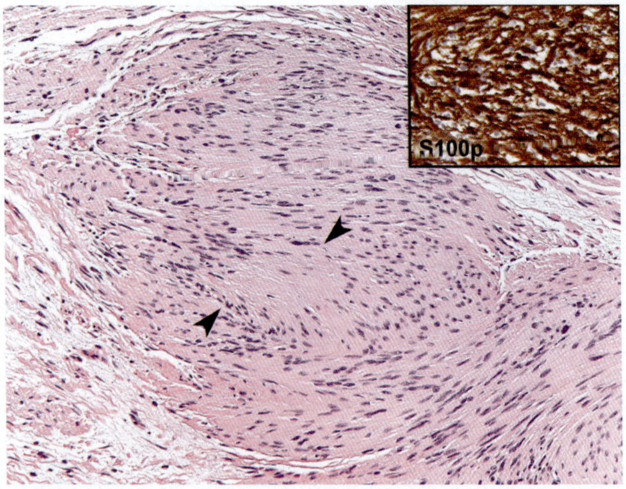

Fig. 42.6 Schwannoma or neurilemmoma is composed of cellular Antoni A regions containing Verocay bodies alternating with the less cellular Antoni B zones (H&E ×200). **Inset**: The bland spindled cells have elongated nuclei and finely fibrillar, eosinophilic cytoplasm, and show strong immunoreactivity for the S100 protein (H&E ×400).

and/or control of pain (e.g., face pain caused by a trigeminal schwannoma). Schwannomas and neurofibromas of the anterior skull base are very rare and more likely to arise from intraorbital branches of the trigeminal nerve than from the olfactory, optic, or oculomotor nerves. As with meningiomas, clinical and radiographic observation is often preferred. Surgery is indicated to relieve symptoms from compression, and surgery or irradiation (stereotactic radiosurgery or fractionated radiotherapy, in doses similar to those for meningioma) is indicated when progressive growth threatens neurologic function or cosmesis.

Glomangiopericytoma

Glomangiopericytoma, also named sinonasal hemangiopericytoma and hemangiopericytoma like tumor, is a rare neoplasm. The clinical behavior and immunophenotypic profile warrant its distinction from the soft tissue counterpart, hemangiopericytoma (see section on solitary fibrous tumor). Glomangiopericytomas are currently classified as borderline neoplasms and more closely resemble glomus tumors. They present as polypoid or circumscribed masses. Microscopically, the cells show oval to spindled nuclei and are arranged in storiform packets and whorls separated by delicate vascular channels, including "staghorn" vessels (**Fig. 42.7**). Diffuse strong immunoreactivity for actins, factor XIIIa, and vimentin and lack of staining for CD34 are typical. Most glomangiopericytomas behave in a benign manner; local recurrences are reported in up to 30% of cases. Aggressive clinical behavior has been associated with larger tumors (>5 cm), tumor cell necrosis, pleomorphism, and high mitotic rates and local tissue invasion.[35]

Solitary Fibrous Tumor/"Hemangiopericytoma"

Solitary fibrous tumor (SFT) is another mesenchymal neoplasm that is classified with glomangiopericytoma (see earlier) in the borderline group of soft tissue tumors of the head and neck. Appropriately, it is discussed here straddling the sections on benign and malignant tumors. In the nasal cavity and nasopharynx they are uncommon, with fewer than 30 reports in the literature.[36–40] In recent years, however, they are increasingly being recognized; we have seen several cases in the past few years.

Clinically, SFTs are usually well demarcated but their growth may affect adjacent structures, such as cranial nerves. At the time of presentation, distinguishing "benign" from "malignant" is difficult, although the sparse literature states that 10 to 15% are malignant. Both histologically and clinically, they can resemble paragangliomas.[41] Treatment is surgical with generally excellent results; postoperative radiation may be considered for recurrences or those behaving aggressively. Although the clinical course is usually fairly indolent, this is not always the case, and there are rare reports of metastases.

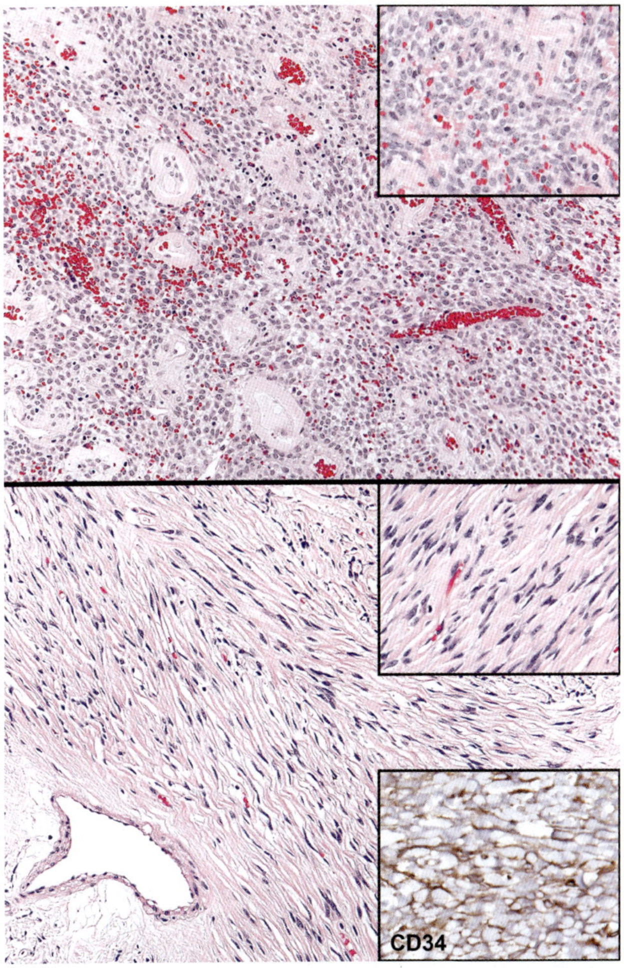

Fig. 42.7 Upper panel: Glomangiopericytoma or hemangiopericytoma like tumor is characterized by a cellular proliferation arranged in nests, whorls, or fascicles admixed with delicate vascular spaces. Dense, perivascular, or peritheliomatous hyalinization is conspicuous in this tumor (H&E ×200). **Inset**: The neoplastic cells display uniform, small oval to spindled nuclei, and are often admixed with mast cells and eosinophils (H&E ×400). **Lower panel**: Solitary fibrous tumor showing a variably cellular but uniform proliferation of bland spindled cells arranged either haphazardly or in fascicles and embedded in a collagenous stroma (H&E ×200). **Upper inset**: The neoplastic cells demonstrate a fine chromatin pattern and are separated by collagen fibers (H&E ×400). **Lower inset**: Strong immunoreactivity against CD34 is characteristic of SFT (×400).

Histologically, the concept of solitary fibrous tumor has evolved from the nonspecific "hemangiopericytoma," and establishing a diagnosis of solitary fibrous tumor remains challenging. Most mesenchymal tumors that were once called hemangiopericytoma are today classified as SFTs.[42] SFTs are found throughout the body, well beyond the pleura where they were initially described. There is a spectrum of appearances, ranging from highly cellular with thin-walled vessels to quite heterogeneous and fibrotic with hyalinized thick-walled vessels; with variants such as giant cell angiofibroma (which may account for the misunderstanding of JNA when apparently encountered outside the usual adolescent male) and lipomatous hemangiopericytoma, and an overlap with variants of fibrous histiocytoma.[37] In fibrous SFTs, one sees alternating fibrous and hypercellular regions, with round to spindle bland-appearing cells within a fascicular or storiform pattern. Nuclei show a vesicular appearance with open chromatin, and sometimes have pseudo inclusions. There are generally ramified vessels with thick hyalinized walls (**Fig. 42.7**). Less common cellular SFTs have a more monotonous pattern with monomorphic oval nuclei; there is little fibrosis, and vessels have thinner walls and are arrayed in staghorn branching patterns.[37] They may demonstrate pericytic, fibroblastic, or myofibroblastic differentiation, and often express CD34 (>80% of fibrous SFT; less frequent and more focal in cellular variants) and CD99 (70%), and may express bcl-2 (30%) and EMA (30%).

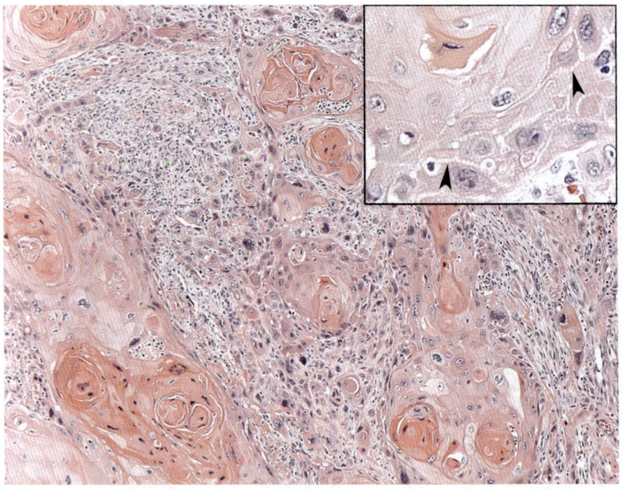

Fig. 42.8 Squamous cell carcinoma is characterized by nests of tumor cells associated with a desmoplastic inflamed stromal response. Keratin formation within the tumor nests is conspicuous at low-power magnification (H&E ×100). **Inset**: The tumor cells demonstrate intercellular bridges between tumor cells (H&E ×400).

Malignant Tumors

Squamous Cell Carcinoma

The most common malignancy of the paranasal sinuses is SCC. The maxillary sinus is the most common site, but extension posteriorly toward the pterygopalatine fossa and greater wing of the sphenoid, and superomedially to the ethmoid and cribriform plate, may compel a skull base resection as part of planned surgery and postoperative irradiation or cisplatin-based chemotherapy. Occasionally, one sees SCC arise within an inverted papilloma, as discussed earlier. Thin-section MRI to evaluate for lymphadenopathy and the possibility of perineural spread along the course of V2 assists in treatment planning. About 10% of patients present with cervical nodal metastases, and another 20% develop cervical nodal metastases if elective neck irradiation is not included in the treatment plan.[43–45]

Histologically, SCC arising within the paranasal sinus is often a bulky exophytic mass with necrotic and friable surfaces. In the nasal cavity, the tumors are generally well differentiated and display cytoplasmic keratinization, intercellular bridges, and squamous pearls (**Fig. 42.8**). Nuclear pleomorphism and mitotic figures are usually inconspicuous. In the paranasal sinuses, the tumors are arranged in large nests, often with central necrosis, and lack abundant keratin pearls or cytoplasmic keratinization ("nonkeratinizing"). They are generally graded as moderately or poorly differentiated based on these features. This distinction does not correlate with natural history, and it determines neither suggested treatment nor expected response to treatment. Nasopharyngeal carcinoma, discussed next, is a very different tumor, although it can resemble poorly differentiated sinus SCC.

Surgery and postoperative intensity-modulated radiation therapy (IMRT) is usually the best intervention for resectable paranasal epithelial carcinomas such as SCC. In advanced sinonasal malignancies, the adequacy of resection generally correlates with the likelihood of obtaining local control.[46] Although the overall cure rates have improved only minimally over the past years, IMRT has reduced the toxicity associated with irradiation.[47–49] Retrospective single institution series, of which the literature is replete, often combine tumors with different histology with a limited number of patients, and include patients treated over intervals of years during which there were changes in staging systems, indications for choice of therapy, surgical techniques, and dose and method of irradiation.[50] Nevertheless, meta-analyses do appear to suggest that the combination of skull base surgery combined with current postoperative cisplatin-based chemoradiation with IMRT has improved the overall local control and cure rates from less than 50% to <60%.

Nasopharyngeal Carcinoma

Although the optimal treatment of nasopharyngeal carcinoma (NPC) continues to evolve, there is clear consensus that IMRT is part of the mainstay of initial intervention when disease is limited to the primary site and neck nodes. For early stage disease, this alone may suffice. For most NPCs, however, cisplatin-based chemoradiation offers local control rates in excess of 90%, as well as good control of cervical nodal involvement. The role of induction chemotherapy or adjuvant chemotherapy is under active investigation in several phase II and phase III trials, with at times conflicting results, but it is clear that chemoradiation is superior to radiation alone.

The most recent WHO classification (2005) retains three types of NPC: keratinizing SCC, nonkeratinizing carcinoma, and basaloid SCC. The numeric grades have been eliminated. Nonkeratinizing carcinomas are the most common type and is further divided into differentiated and undifferentiated subtypes. These subtypes do not differ in their response to therapy or overall survival rates. The undifferentiated category is the most common pattern and includes neoplasms previously classified as lymphoepithelioma. The nonkeratinizing types are associated with Epstein-Barr virus (EBV) and are more prevalent in patients of southern Chinese ancestry.

Histologically, the neoplastic cells are arranged as sheets and syncytial aggregates and exhibit medium to large nuclei with vesicular chromatin, conspicuous nucleoli, and scant cytoplasm. A variable lymphocyte and plasma cell response is present. EBV genome is readily demonstrated by in situ hybridization. The neoplastic cells are strongly positive for cytokeratin and fail to react against antibodies for hematolymphoid differentiation. The differentiated form of nonkeratinizing NPC resembles transitional cell carcinomas of the urinary tract (**Fig. 42.9**). Necrosis and an inflammatory response can be present. The keratinizing form of NPC resembles other SCCs of the aerodigestive tract in having the cellular features of intercellular bridges and cytoplasmic or extracellular keratinization in most of the tumor cells. Basaloid SCC is the least common type and resemble its counterpart in the larynx and hypopharynx.

Following appropriate IMRTs or chemotherapy with concomitant IMRT (with or without induction or adjuvant chemotherapy), long-term cancer surveillance is necessary. A baseline postintervention MRI is helpful in interpreting subsequent positron emission tomography (PET)-CT scans, begun no earlier than 3 months following completion of IMRT. Local recurrences in the absence of distant metastases (and nodal recurrences) are reevaluated by MRI. A modified radical neck dissection is recommended for resectable nodal recurrences. Local recurrences amenable to endoscopic skull base resection with intraoperative navigation (or an open approach, depending on surgeon

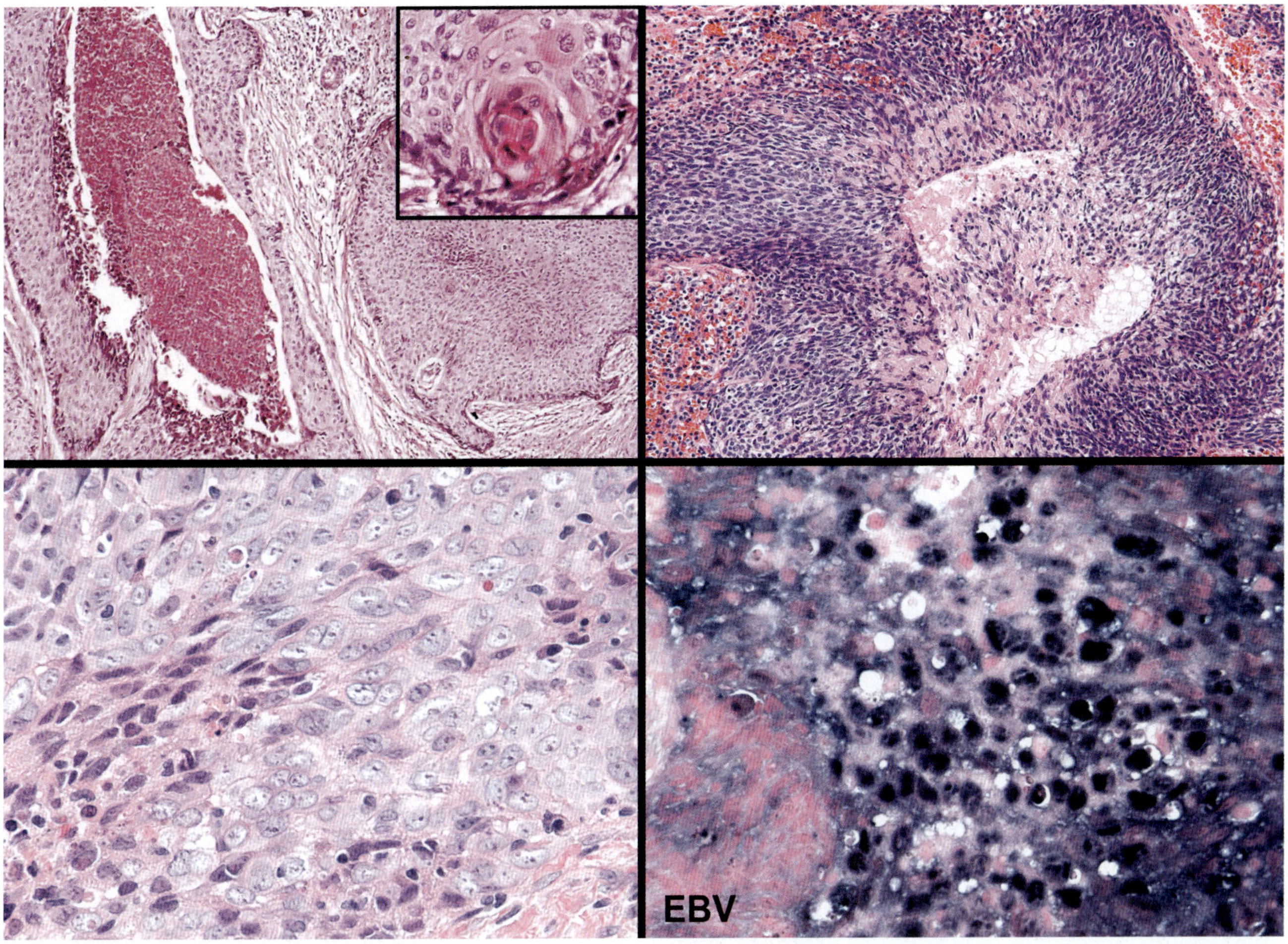

Fig. 42.9 Nasopharyngeal carcinoma (NPC) is currently classified by World Health Organization into three major types. **Upper left panel**: Keratinizing NPC is similar to squamous cell carcinoma in other sites of the aerodigestive tract. Nests of tumor cells often display central necrosis (H&E ×100). **Inset**: Whorling of tumor cells and keratinization of the cytoplasm is present (H&E ×400). **Upper right panel**: Nonkeratinizing NPC, differentiated type exhibit nesting and cellular stratification resembling transitional cell carcinoma (H&E ×100). **Lower left panel**: Nonkeratinizing NPC of an undifferentiated type displays syncytial arrangements of tumor cells with indistinct cell borders and vesicular chromatin patterns (H&E ×600). **Lower right panel**: In situ hybridization for EBER-1 genome is strongly nuclear labeling of most of the tumor cells (×600). Basaloid squamous carcinoma is a rare type of NPC.

experience and extent of tumor) should be considered, with reirradiation reserved for more extensive recurrences. Resection may be selectively indicated for re-recurrences following reirradiation as well, despite greater risk of wound healing problems.

Chordoma

As chordomas arise from remnant (or ectopic) notochord tissue, the embryologic origin of the vertebral column, it is not surprising that chordomas can develop anywhere from the sella turcica superiorly, to the sacrococcygeal area inferiorly. About one-third of all of these rare (1:1,000,000) lesions occur near the spheno-occipital synchondrosis of the clivus, usually in patients between the ages of 50 to 70 years.

Three histologic patterns of chordoma can be seen: classic, chondroid, and dedifferentiated. It may be difficult to distinguish the classic variant from the chondroid variant (with foci of cartilaginous matrix). The de-differentiated form is exceedingly rare in the skull base, exhibits more cytologic atypia and mitotic activity, and behaves as a high-grade sarcoma, with commensurate prognosis. In the classic type, a lobulated growth pattern is present. Epithelioid cells are distributed in a myxoid or mucoid matrix. These cells range from small, uniform oval cells with scant eosinophilic cytoplasm to cells with abundant glycogen-rich vacuolated cytoplasm (so-called physaliphorous cells) with dense chromatin (**Fig. 42.10**). Mucoid microcysts and fibrovascular strands and cords of eosinophilic syncytial cells are commonly seen. In some cases, numerous mitotic figures and nuclear atypia can be found. There is immunoreactivity with antibodies to cytokeratins. Like chondrosarcomas, chordoma shows immunoreactivity with antibodies for vimentin and S100, and these two tumors may at times be difficult to distinguish from each other.[51] Brachyury (a transcription factor involved in notochord developmental regulation) has been recently shown to be a biomarker of chordoma.[52,53]

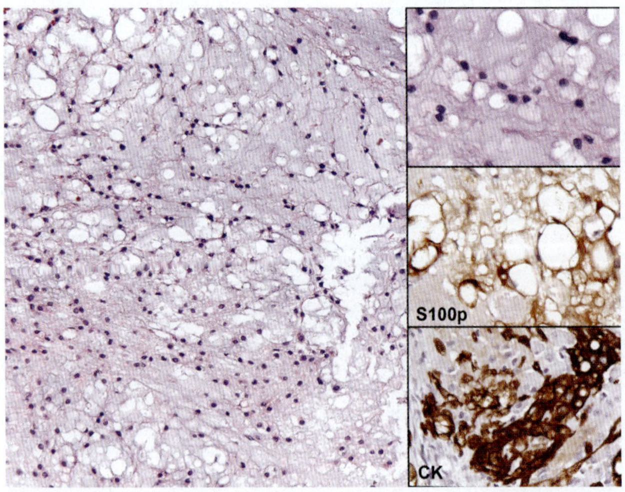

Fig. 42.10 Chordoma is arranged as lobules of pale, myxoid stroma showing variable cellularity (H&E ×200). **Inset**: The neoplastic cells are arranged in cords and single cells and exhibit vacuolated cytoplasm. The multivacuolated cells are called physaliphorous cells (H&E ×400). The tumor cells express the S100 protein and react against antibodies to cytokeratin (×400).

Chordomas are often suspected by the symptoms, such as headache and sixth nerve palsy causing diplopia, and by sensory trigeminal deficits, when a radiologically consistent location and appearance are seen on MRI. Typically, the MRI shows very high T2-weighted signal with heterogeneous gadolinium enhancement in a midline location. MRI is essential in assessing the extent of disease and planning for surgery. The tumor may be quite large at presentation and may abut or encase the cavernous segment of the internal carotid artery, or abut the basilar artery. Although imaging is sufficiently characteristic that a presumptive diagnosis can be suspected, a confirmatory intraoperative biopsy is obtained early in a planned endoscopic resection. The clinical differential diagnosis may include several other entities (e.g., metastasis, plasmacytoma, lymphoma, nasopharyngeal carcinoma, and certain benign lesions such as Langerhans histiocytosis).

Treatment is as complete a resection as possible by an appropriate approach, usually transsphenoidal (endoscopic[54,55] or sublabial[56]), or transoral or subfrontal (depending on extent) with intraoperative navigation, followed by high-dose irradiation. Surgery and postoperative charged particle irradiation[57] to 65 to 70 Gy is associated with 5-year control rates of ~75% in previously untreated tumors smaller than 75 cm^3, depending in part on the extent of resection. About 90% of tumors at the skull base are in this favorable group. Larger tumors, de-differentiated tumors, and recurrences predict a worse outcome, with a 5-year control rate of ~35%. The possibility of stereotactic radiosurgery (e.g., 35 Gy in five sessions) has also been explored as an alternative to charged particles.[58] Chemotherapy does not usually have a role except in dedifferentiated chordoma. Recurrences may occur at the original tumor site or along routes of surgical access of the initial resection, and there is a low rate of metastases to neck nodes and the lungs.

Sarcomas

Chondrosarcoma

Chondrosarcomas of the skull base are cartilaginous malignancies that represent ~5 to 15% of all skull base tumors. Radiographically and morphologically, they may be difficult to distinguish from chordomas. Unlike chordomas that typically arise in the clival midline, chondrosarcomas characteristically originate from the paramedian petroclival synchondrosis and often involve the petrous apex. Almost all skull base chondrosarcomas are well differentiated and not high-grade or dedifferentiated types.

It may be difficult morphologically to distinguish a chondrosarcoma (**Fig. 42.11**) of the skull base from a chordoma,

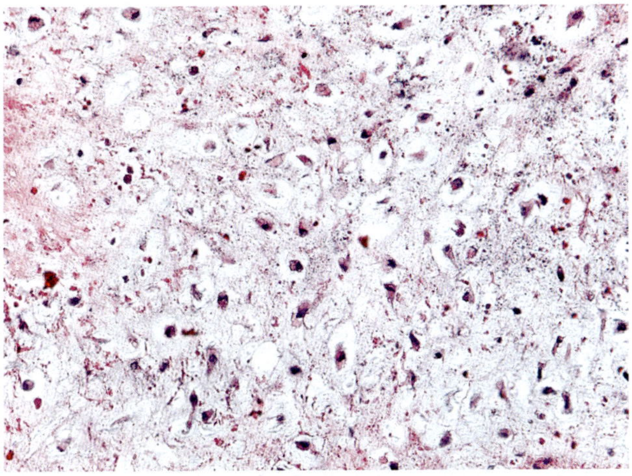

Fig. 42.11 Chondrosarcoma arises in the bones of the skull base and is composed of malignant cells embedded in an extracellular chondroid matrix. The cellularity and nuclear atypia are used to grade the neoplasm (grade 1) (H&E ×200).

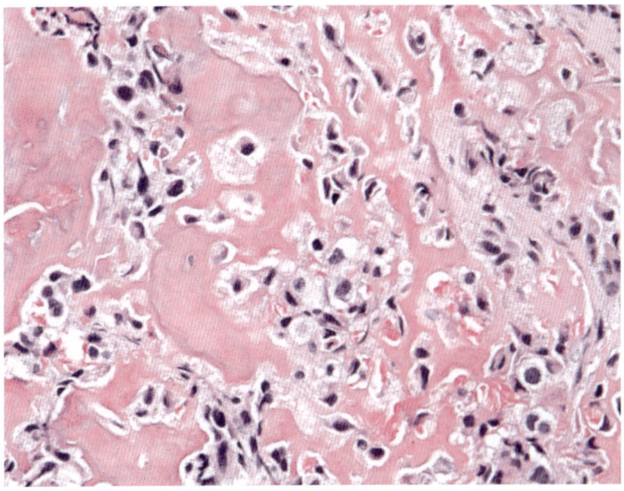

Fig. 42.12 Osteosarcoma arises in the skull bones and is characterized by malignant mesenchymal cells producing eosinophilic/basophilic osteoid ("tumor bone") (H&E ×400).

especially a chondroid chordoma. Immunohistochemical staining can be helpful in making this distinction. Cytokeratins and epithelial membrane antigen staining are not seen in chondrosarcomas but are present in chordomas. Podoplanin, on the other hand, may serve as a marker of chondrosarcoma; it was present in <80% of chondrosarcomas, but only 5% of conventional chordomas, and 21% of chondroid chordomas.[59]

As with chordomas, treatment is cytoreductive surgery, usually with postoperative irradiation. Several lateral skull base[60] and anterior endoscopic transsphenoidal approaches are available, sometimes in sequential combination, depending on tumor extent and surgeon's experience.[61–64] For tumors limited to the petrous apex, an endoscopic approach may be appropriate.[65] The most appropriate approach for any patient is best chosen after review of the tumor extent on MRI, and will take into consideration the experience of the surgical team. Postoperative stereotactic radiosurgery or proton beam irradiation is usually recommended, similar to that in chordomas (see previous text), especially for incomplete resections as is common. Long-term survival is the norm, albeit with complications associated with surgery in difficult areas, especially in recurrent cases.[66]

Osteosarcoma

Osteosarcoma (**Fig. 42.12**) is the most common primary bone malignancy in children and young adults. Although far more common in metaphyses of long bones, in the head and neck region, the mandible, maxilla, and occasionally the bones of the ethmoid or sphenoid sinuses are sites of origin. The most common type of osteosarcoma is a central osteosarcoma, a high grade malignancy with frequent lung metastases. The primary osteosarcomas of the mandible and paranasal sinuses, in older adults or in children,[67] which are not associated with prior irradiation or retinoblastoma, behave as low- or intermediate-grade malignancies and are treated by primary surgical resection. This group may not benefit from irradiation or chemotherapy, and hence may warrant a careful review of histologic grade and margin status. Other retrospective reports, however, suggest a poor prognosis, warranting consideration of irradiation and chemotherapy.[68,69] Because of their rarity,[70] however, definitive postsurgical recommendations are difficult to make, and a thorough discussion of postsurgical options in a multidisciplinary tumor board setting is recommended.

It is far from clear that the treatment of osteosarcomas of the mandible, maxilla, or sphenoethmoid area in adults should be the same as for children. Treatment in children for osteosarcomas of long bones is focused on neoadjuvant chemotherapy followed by resection of the primary and metastases (lung metastases are the most common; 10 to 15% of patients have lung metastases at the time of primary evaluation), and then additional chemotherapy based on evaluation of initial response.[71,72] Ongoing multi-institutional trials continue to investigate the role of common chemotherapeutic drugs such as cisplatin, doxorubicin, and methotrexate, and the role of interferon-alpha-2b in maintenance chemotherapy in patients who demonstrate a good response to initial chemotherapy. The 5-year control rate of 70% for nonmetastatic disease has not improved in the past two decades. Patients with metastases or recurrent disease have less than a 20% 5-year control rate.[73] Sarcomas that arise following prior irradiation or in patients with a prior retinoblastoma (either within and or outside the initial irradiation field) fare worse.[74] The rare childhood primary osteosarcoma of the maxilla or mandible, however, is often *not* high grade, and hence has a better prognosis, such that surgery alone may be sufficient.

The most common type of osteosarcoma is a conventional osteosarcoma, a high-grade malignancy with frequent metastases, especially to the lung. Irregularly distributed pale osteoid "tumor bone" is intermingled with malignant cells with hyperchromatic, large nuclei (**Fig. 42.12**). Rare juxtacortical osteosarcomas include intermediate-grade periosteal and low-grade parosteal variants. Recognizing these rare variants is important as the prognosis is far better and surgery alone may suffice. Low-grade osteosarcomas, including parosteal and periosteal osteosarcoma,[75] of the paranasal sinuses are exceedingly rare.[76–78] Taken together with the MRI and CT appearance that lacks the typical invasive features, a diagnosis of low grade osteosarcoma may be suggested.

Rhabdomyosarcoma: Embryonal, Alveolar, Other Subtypes

The treatment of childhood rhabdomyosarcoma (RMS) continues to evolve, with progressively improving survival rates in risk-adapted therapies administered through the Intergroup Rhabdomyosarcoma Group I-V. The overall 5-year survival rate for embryonal rhabdomyosarcoma (ERMS) has improved to 80%, and the survival rate for alveolar RMS (ARMS) has increased to 52%.[79] RMS that involves parameningeal sites (as is often present with tumors of the nose, nasopharynx, and paranasal sinuses) do notably worse. More favorable sites include the nasopharynx, nasal cavity, and middle ear/mastoid, with a 46% failure-free 10-year survival (FFT). Less favorable sites include the paranasal sinuses, infratemporal fossa and pterygopalatine fossa with an FFT of 18%. Patients with ERMS had a 37% FFT compared with a 19% FFT in non-ERMS.[80]

RMSs occasionally present in the paranasal sinuses in adults, with a higher proportion of these being ARMS than at other locations. The prognosis in adults appears worse than that in children.[81] Treatment should include 50 Gy local intensity modulated radiation therapy (IMRT) and prolonged VAC (vincristine, actinomycin D, and cyclophosphamide) chemotherapy in accordance with sarcoma study group recommendations.[82]

There are well-established histopathologic, immunohistochemical, and molecular criteria for the diagnosis of RMS.[83,84] Rhabdomyoblasts of various shapes and sizes and degrees of differentiation are seen on hematoxylin and eosin (H&E) sections and display eccentrically placed, round-oval nuclei, and a bright eosinophilic cytoplasm. Cross-striations may be difficult to identify in many cases. The botryoid type is a special variant of ERMS. ARMS shows fibrovascular septa outlining clusters of primitive neoplastic cells mimicking pulmonary alveolar like spaces. In some cases, the neoplastic cells are arranged as solid sheets. IHC antibodies that detect myogenic differentiation, such as MyoD1 (myogenic determination factor), desmin, muscle specific actin, myoglobulin, and nuclear myogenin are helpful in distinguishing RMS from other small round blue cell tumors (**Fig. 42.13**).

Distinguishing the various types of RMS by histologic criteria alone is difficult in some cases.[85] The Children's Oncology Group has recently suggested a gene expression molecular classification, recognizing that the associated genotypes may refine the correlation with prognosis, and hence affect risk-adapted intervention strategies.[86] ERMS is associated with loss of heterozygosity at 11p15.5. In 75% of ARMS, there is a chimeric Pax-Fox (P-F) fusion product of a translocation that fuses FOXO1 (or FHKR, on chromosome 13q14) with PAX3 (on chromosome 2q35) or PAX7.[87] These fusion products, t(2;13)(q35;q14) or t(1; 13)(p36;q14) can be identified by molecular analysis routinely used in clinical molecular laboratories. Patients with the PAX 7 translocation have a better prognosis than those with the PAX3 translocation. IHC in formalin-fixed tissue can be used indirectly to identify P-F products; TFAP2 is highly expressed in P-F (+) RMS tumors, whereas HMGA2 (transcription factor encoding gene) is up regulated in P-F (−) RMS, and thus is a marker of ERMS.

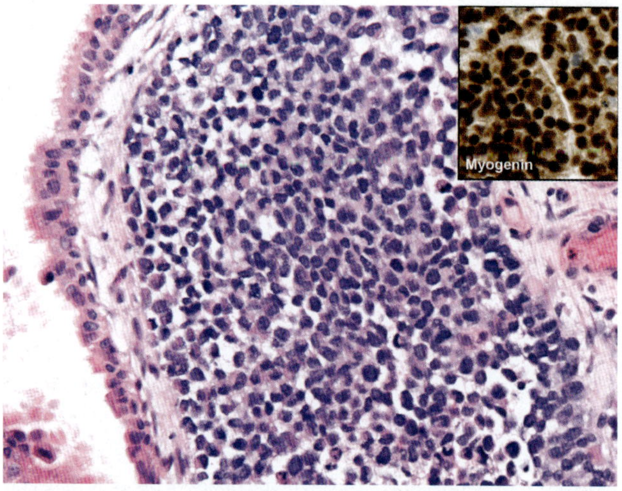

Fig. 42.13 Rhabdomyosarcoma arises in the nasopharynx and sinonasal tracts. In the alveolar type, the tumor cells are arranged in cohesive groups and display eccentric eosinophilic cytoplasmic globules (H&E ×400). **Inset**: Strong nuclear reactivity with myogenin supports muscular differentiation (×400).

Other Soft Tissue Sarcomas

Other soft tissue sarcomas that may be encountered in this region from time to time include malignant fibrous histiocytoma, synovial sarcoma, clear cell sarcoma, leiomyosarcoma, liposarcoma, and extraosseous peripheral neuroectodermal tumor (PNET/Ewing sarcoma). PNET tumors arise in the differential diagnosis of small round undifferentiated tumors, but cytogenetic or reverse transcriptase-PCR demonstration of the fusion of the EWS gene with the FLI or ERG gene resulting from the reciprocal translocation of 11:22 (q24;q12) specifically and reliably identifies this family of tumors.[88,89]

Sarcomas arising in the head and neck often have a worse outcome than those originating at other sites. Some of the factors that correlate with a poorer prognosis include positive surgical margins, size (>10 cm), high grade, and recurrence. The 5- and 15-year control rates for the entire group of soft tissue sarcomas in adults is good, ranging from 70 to 90% for those with good prognostic parameters to <50% for those, such as in the head and neck, with poor prognostic parameters.[90] Surgery and irradiation are the mainstay of treatment, sometimes with adjuvant chemotherapy.

Definitive treatment recommendations are based on the specific tumor type, grade, and numerous patient factors.[91]

Malignancies of Minor Salivary Gland Origin

Adenoid Cystic Carcinoma

Adenoid cystic carcinoma (ACC) was first reported by Billroth in 1856 when he described a "cylindroma" of the sinuses. ACC accounts for <10% of sinonasal malignancies in the United States. The maxillary sinus and nasal cavity are the most common sites, but perineural extension along V_2 to the foramen rotundum and extension toward or through the foramen ovale is not uncommon. Detailed evaluation of a preoperative MRI skull base protocol to evaluate for perineural extension is imperative prior to planning both surgical intervention and subsequent IMRT.[92,93] Histologically, the subtypes of ACC carry prognostic significance but do not affect treatment recommendations.[94] The cribriform subtype (**Fig. 42.14**) is the most common pattern and is characterized by fused glands with "microcystic" spaces, and the tubular subtypes are associated with a better prognosis. The solid subtype behaves more aggressively. The spaces in the cribriform and tubular patterns contain pale basophilic or bright eosinophilic mucopolysaccharide-rich material. The duct like structures are composed of a biphasic population of tumor cells. Perineural invasion is easily identified. Varying proportions of the three patterns can be found in the same tumor, and the classification is based on the predominant pattern. In addition to histologic subtype, other factors such as anatomic site, margin status, clinical extent, and the presence of metastases affect prognosis significantly.

Surgery[95] and postoperative IMRT, possibly boosted with proton irradiation[96] or stereotactic radiosurgery, is the treatment of choice, with local control rates greater than 70%. However, 30 to 40% develop distant metastases

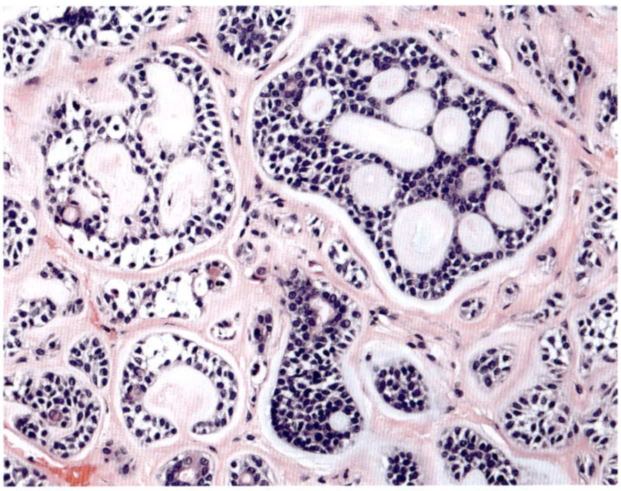

Fig. 42.14 Adenoid cystic carcinoma of salivary gland origin exhibits a distinctive cribriform architecture. The tumor cells show small angulated nuclei and are arranged around invaginations of pale eosinophilic basement membrane material (H&E ×300).

(lung and liver are the most common sites) over time.[97] The indolent growth of the primary tumor (particularly, tubular and cribriform subtypes) and lung metastases account for the high 5-year overall survival, usually reported at ~75 to 80% despite the fact that the disease-free survival rate is 20% lower.

Surgical treatment for recurrent disease is often indicated. Limited lung metastases are best removed via video-assisted thoracoscopic resection. Local recurrences may be re-resected endoscopically, sometimes with supplemental irradiation such as stereotactic radiosurgery. There are fair 5-year survival rates even after the development of distant metastasis or local recurrence, reported to be <20% and 60%, respectively,[98] although the development of bone metastasis is associated with a shorter median survival than that which follows lung metastases (21 versus 54 months).[99] As the response rate to chemotherapy is low and duration of response is brief, the role of chemotherapy for metastatic disease remains poorly defined.[100] Cisplatin-based regimens have been used in the management of recurrent disease. Similar to SCC and malignant melanoma, perineural spread is common and should be investigated by high-quality thin-section MRI, both initially and in subsequent surveillance examinations. Radiosurgery along the trigeminal nerve branches and to Meckel's cave and the cavernous sinus is effective in both reducing pain and controlling disease progression.

Adenocarcinoma

Nasoethmoid adenocarcinomas are seen less frequently in the United States than in Europe, where instead of accounting for 10% of sinonasal malignancies, they represent 25 to 75%.[50,101] An association with the dust encountered by woodworkers and in the leather industry is noted.[102,103] Adenocarcinoma of the sinonasal region is classified as intestinal (ITAC) and nonintestinal (NITAC) types. ITAC is graded as well, moderately, or poorly differentiated papillary types or as mucinous/goblet cell/signet ring cell types. The well differentiated papillary intestinal type (ITAC), which is uncommon in the United States, displays a papillary growth pattern and has a favorable prognosis. Moderately and poorly differentiated papillary types resemble colonic adenocarcinoma of similar grade and display increased cellular pleomorphism and mitotic activity (**Fig. 42.15**). The mucinous type of ITAC resembles its counterpart in the gastrointestinal (GI) tract and is associated with an overall poor prognosis. The immunohistochemical staining profile for ITAC is similar to tumors of the gastrointestinal tract, including immunoreactivity for pancytokeratins, CK20, CDX2, villin, and/or CK7 (variable reactivity).[104,105]

Sinonasal NITAC is a rare form of adenocarcinoma involving the ethmoid or maxillary sinuses, or nasal cavity. It is classified into low grade and high grade types. The low grade variant has an excellent prognosis and is treated by surgical resection. Five-year disease-specific survival around 85 to 90% are reported, with ~95% for selected tumors, such as those amenable to endoscopic resection.[106]

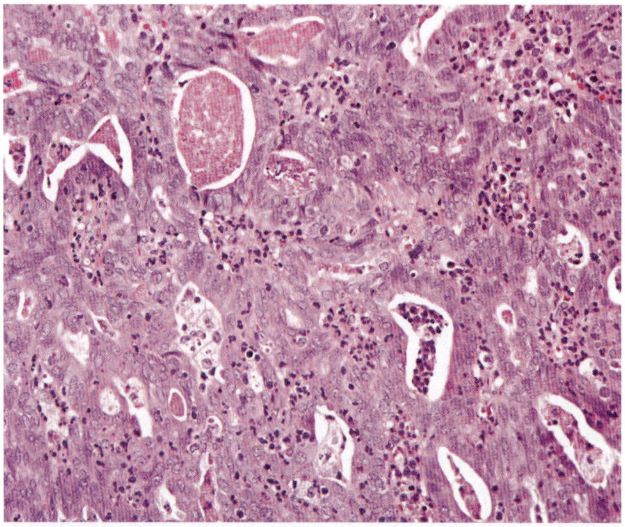

Fig. 42.15 Adenocarcinoma of intestinal type (moderately differentiated) is composed of fused glands containing luminal necrotic debris (H&E ×400).

Neuroectodermal Tumors

Tumors that exhibit neuroectodermal differentiation occur commonly in the sinonasal region, and can be confusing to an otorhinolaryngologist and pathologist alike. Many sinonasal tumors appear on light microscopy as small round blue-cell tumors that are largely undifferentiated. The differential diagnosis includes not only the broad group of neuroectodermal tumors and malignant melanoma, but also some carcinomas, sarcomas, lymphomas, and plasmacytoma. IHC staining, cytogenetic studies, and molecular analysis have improved the diagnostic accuracy considerably in recent years, allowing for directed risk-adapted intervention strategies.[104] As additional cytogenetic and molecular techniques become available, further refinement of classification will be possible.[105]

In addition, tumors such as an ectopic pituitary adenoma or macroadenoma (discussed earlier) may have neuroendocrine features and may come to the initial attention of the rhinologist without advance radiologic or clinical suspicion of a hypophyseal mass. Routine morphology may show an overlap of histopathologic features between basaloid SCC and small cell neuroendocrine carcinoma. In an effort to provide a structural framework, we will follow the construct of Mills,[107–109] dividing neuroectodermal tumors into two groups:

- Group I: those with *epithelial differentiation*, including well, moderately, and poorly differentiated neuroendocrine carcinomas, with the poorly differentiated ones further subdivided into small cell and large cell types; and
- Group II: the more diverse tumors *without epithelial features but with neural features*, which include olfactory neuroblastoma (or esthesioneuroblastoma), malignant melanoma, and peripheral neuroectodermal tumor (PNET, Ewing sarcoma). (The second group also includes neurofibroma, schwannoma, malignant peripheral nerve sheath tumor [all discussed earlier], and paraganglioma.)

Poorly Differentiated Small Cell Neuroendocrine Carcinoma/Small Cell Undifferentiated Carcinoma

By any of its names, this is a very rare sinonasal tumor, but it can be confused with other apparently "undifferentiated" sinonasal tumors, such as SNUC, and has a poor prognosis.[110] Unlike in the larynx, where moderately differentiated neuroendocrine carcinoma (NEC) is reported to be the most common nonsquamous cell carcinoma malignancy, major and minor salivary NEC is usually of the small cell poorly differentiated type. A *large* cell poorly differentiated NEC has not been definitely described in the head and neck, but SNUC is a likely candidate (see later text). A moderately well differentiated NEC has the typical nest and cords with peripheral nuclei palisading, and, by IHC, are positive for synaptophysin and chromogranin (as well as carcinoembryonic antigen, calcitonin, and cytokeratin), but with more nuclear pleomorphism and mitoses than seen in well differentiated NEC (**Fig. 42.16**).

Poorly differentiated NEC of the small cell subtype (often referred to as small cell undifferentiated carcinoma or small cell NEC) is indistinguishable from "oat cell" or small cell lung carcinomas, with sheets of spindle or ovoid cells with little cytoplasm, high mitotic activity, and areas of necrosis. Like lung small cell carcinoma, it has variable immunoreactivity for NEC markers (such as NSE, chromogranin, or synaptophysin) and punctate perinuclear cytokeratin staining. It is usually negative for S100, vimentin, desmin, and myogenin, and is rarely positive for CD99.

Sinonasal Undifferentiated Carcinoma/Large Cell Neuroendocrine Carcinoma

SNUC is probably synonymous with poorly differentiated large cell NEC. SNUCs are biologically very aggressive and have very poor prognoses. They arise in the nose and ethmoid sinuses, and frequently invade the orbit and skull base. Nodal and distant metastases are present in 20% of patients at presentation. Multimodality therapy is generally applied with functionally noncompromising surgery to the extent feasible; there is currently no consensus on specific irradiation fractionation or chemotherapy protocols. Aggressive surgery, chemotherapy, and IMRTs have resulted in longer disease-free intervals than in the past, but prognosis remains poor. Use of proton beam radiotherapy in conjunction with cisplatin and VP-16, often with surgery, has been reported in 13 patients to yield a 3-year overall survival rate of 59%.[111] The goal of treatment is control of local disease, to preserve vision and limit significant intracranial extension.

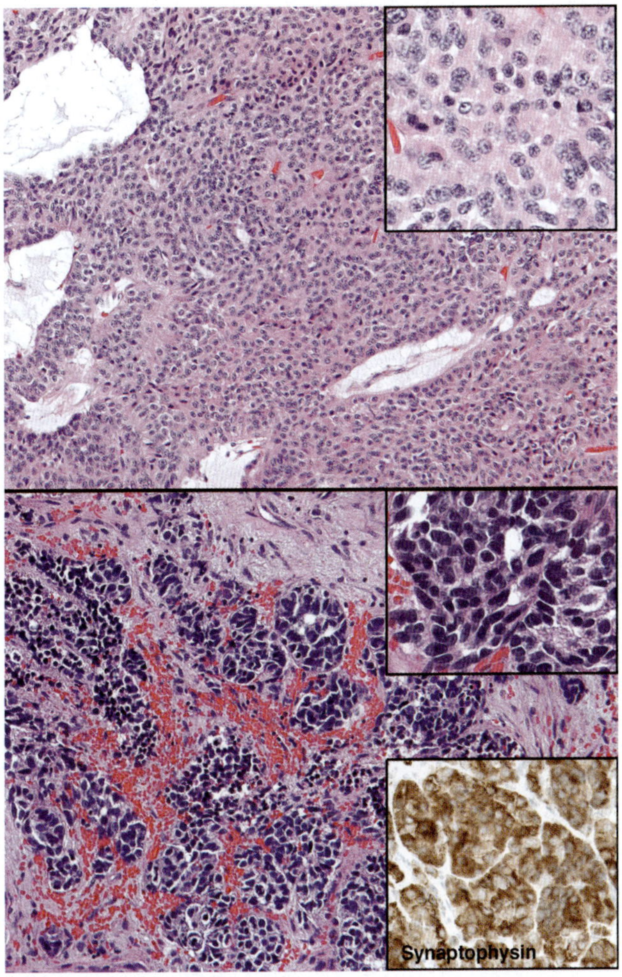

Fig. 42.16 Neuroendocrine carcinoma (NEC) demonstrates a range of differentiation from well-differentiated NEC (carcinoid tumor), moderately differentiated NEC (atypical carcinoid), and small cell undifferentiated/poorly differentiated NEC. **Upper panel**: Well differentiated tumor resembles its pulmonary counterpart with nests of uniform cells (H&E ×200). **Inset**: The epithelioid cells display a stippled chromatin pattern and eosinophilic cytoplasm (H&E ×400). **Lower panel**: Moderately differentiated NEC showing irregular groups of hyperchromatic cells admixed with hemorrhage and necrosis (H&E ×200). **Upper inset**: High-power magnification showing malignant cells with neuroendocrine differentiation (H&E ×400). **Lower inset**: Strong immunoreactivity against synaptophysin supports neuroendocrine differentiation (×400).

Histologically, one sees intermediate-to-large (although occasionally smaller) polygonal undifferentiated cells with large ovoid nuclei and prominent nucleoli, numerous and often aberrant mitotic figures, and vascular invasion (**Fig. 42.17**). Nests of cells may show central necrosis. Fewer than half of SNUCs have IHC reactivity other than strong immunoreactivity for cytokeratin, although some express neuron specific enolase, EMA, or beta-tubulin (consistent with abortive neuroendocrine differentiation), but not the usual NEC marks of synaptophysin and chromogranin.[112] Similarly, SNUCs lack the morphologic features of neuronal differentiation (see olfactory neuroblastoma section).

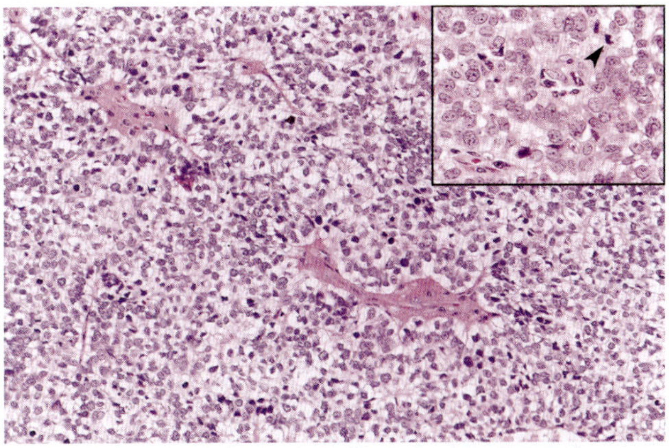

Fig. 42.17 Sinonasal undifferentiated carcinoma grows in sheets and nests containing numerous apoptotic bodies (H&E ×200). **Inset**: High-power magnification showing round to oval nuclei with conspicuous nucleoli and small amounts of eosinophilic to clear cytoplasm. Mitotic figures are easily discernible (H&E ×400).

Olfactory Neuroblastoma/Esthesioneuroblastoma

Olfactory neuroblastoma (or esthesioneuroblastoma) is the most common of the group II tumors. It is seen almost exclusively in the superior nasal cavity medial to the middle turbinate along the cribriform plate. Radiologic imaging (MRI, sometimes with complementary coronal CT to assess subtle erosion of the cribriform plate) will often demonstrate extension through the anterior skull base, a finding that is usually present. There are reports of olfactory neuroblastoma occurring outside the superior third of the nasal septum, but without full availability of pathologic review, these represent another type of neuroectodermal tumor.

On light microscopy, the cells of olfactory neuroblastomas form well demarcated nests or sheets, with high nuclear cytoplasmic ratios, small round nuclei with punctate chromatin, and small or absent nucleoli. The Hyams' grading scheme (**Fig. 42.18**) indicates grade of tumor according to the following criteria: the presence or size of nucleoli; mitotic figures; degree of pleomorphism and necrosis; and presence of neural features such as a fibrillary cytoplasmic background (that are neuronal cell processes) and Homer Wright rosettes (nuclei surrounding a central fibrillary aggregate). Immunohistochemical reactivity with the neural marker synaptophysin is common; staining with neuron-specific enolase and chromogranin is more variable. S100 protein staining of the sustentacular cells at the periphery of cellular nests is characteristic, rather than diffuse S100 staining of malignant melanoma. About a third of olfactory neuroblastomas may also have IHC reactivity for low-molecular weight keratin, but it is usually weak and patchy. Occasionally, an extraosseous peripheral neuroectodermal tumor (PNET/Ewing sarcoma) may mimic an olfactory neuroblastoma, but CD99 (also called MIC2; positive in 95% of PNET, and negative in olfactory neuroblastoma) can help distinguish the two entities.

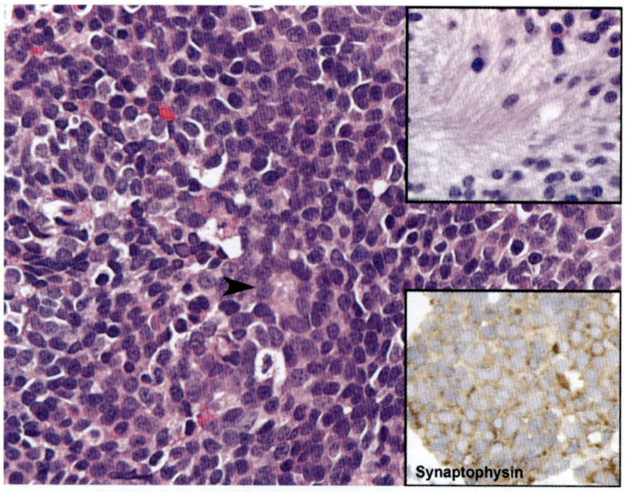

Fig. 42.18 Olfactory neuroblastoma is characterized by sheets of small round blue cells. Homer Wright rosettes are found especially in grade 1 and 2 lesions (H&E ×600). **Upper inset**: A fine fibrillary stroma is also seen in the better differentiated tumors (H&E ×400). **Lower inset**: Immunoreactivity with antibodies to the neuroendocrine marker; synaptophysin is usually noted (×400).

Treatment of olfactory neuroblastoma is resection, with most agreeing that postoperative IMRT (or proton beam irradiation[113]) is indicated.[114–118] Classically, an open anterior skull base resection has been performed, but selectively these tumors, including dura and the olfactory bulb, can be resected endoscopically, and the skull base repaired with a large mucoperichondrial nasal septal flap based on the posterior nasal artery of the sphenopalatine artery. An endoscopically harvested pericranial flap is a recently described alternative repair.[119]

Although cisplatin-based chemotherapy has been used, there is no conclusive evidence it is helpful.[120] As these are rare tumors, and the prognosis is quite good, it is understandable that it is difficult to prove efficacy. Chemotherapy is reserved for advanced tumors (involvement of brain or orbit), for local recurrences after re-resection if feasible, or when the histopathologic diagnosis is not definitive. Confining the definition of olfactory neuroblastoma to the type II neuroectodermal tumors discussed herein, the 5-year local control rate is in excess of 75%, and possibly as high as 90 to 94%. Although metastases are uncommon at presentation, ~10 to 15% will develop cervical nodal metastases. A neck dissection and irradiation would thus be indicated as they provide excellent tumor control. Distant metastases do occur rarely, and can be seen as late as a decade following the initial intervention. Local recurrences can be along dura and are amenable to stereotactic radiosurgery.

Sinonasal Melanoma

Sinonasal melanomas represent <1% of all melanomas, and are more commonly seen in the anterior nasal cavity and maxillary sinus than in the sphenoethmoid area. They are generally not seen more superiorly where olfactory neuroblastomas occur, a fact that helps resolve those cases with overlapping histopathologic or immunohistochemical findings. The light microscopic appearance of melanoma can be more variable than cutaneous malignant melanoma, ranging from the common small round blue-cell tumor resembling NEC or malignant lymphoma, to rhabdoid cells suggestive of sarcoma. Solid, fascicular, and nesting architectural patterns are common. About one-third do not have cytoplasmic melanin pigment on light microscopy. As noted previously, the diffuse strong S100p reactivity of malignant melanoma differs from the S100 reactivity of sustentacular cells in the periphery of olfactory neuroblastoma. In addition, malignant melanomas usually show strong immunohistochemical reactivity for melanA, tyrosinase, and HMB45 (**Fig. 42.19**).

Clinically, sinonasal melanoma is associated with a poor prognosis, with most single institution retrospective series

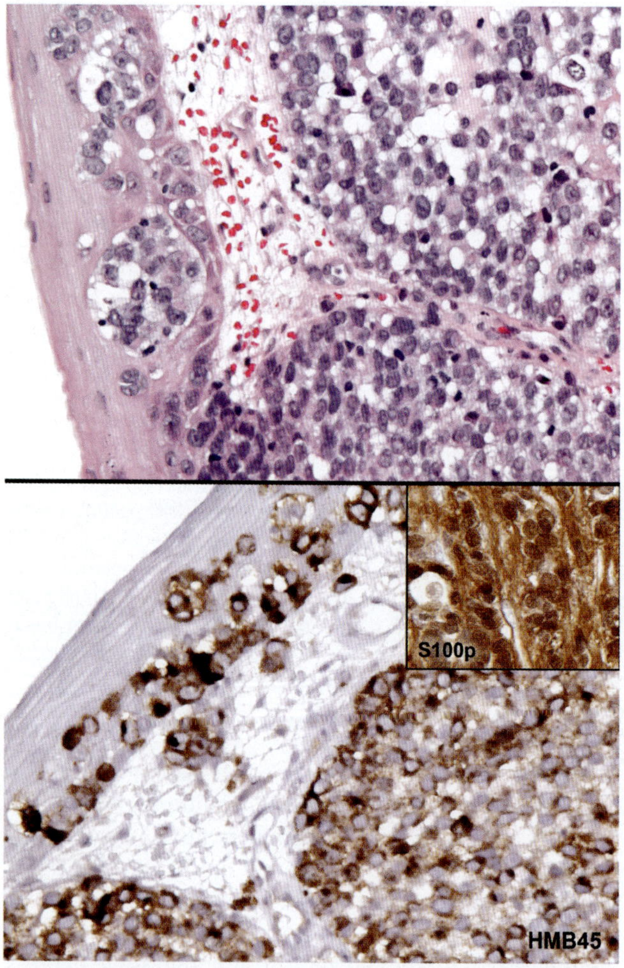

Fig. 42.19 Malignant melanoma of the sinonasal tract is typically arranged in sheets and nests of the submucosal layer with involvement of the mucosal layer (H&E ×400). The cytologic patterns include epithelioid, plasmacytoid, and peritheliomatous types. Intranuclear inclusions, mitotic figures, and cytoplasmic pigment can be variable. **Lower panel**: Immunohistochemical markers of melanocytic differentiation include HMB-45 and S100p (×400).

reporting a 20 to 25% 5-year survival, and some as low as 14%.[121,122] Surgical resection, conservative so as to avoid functional loss, and postoperative IMRT is recommended. Over 90% recur locally within 5 years. Re-resection is warranted if it can be achieved with limited morbidity, as this may help to maintain a patent nasal airway, reduce epistaxis, and lengthen, sometimes significantly, quality survival. Distant metastases are also common, and initial staging studies are warranted. Protocols involving interferon and chemotherapy are available. In most cases, local recurrence precedes the development of subsequent nodal and distant metastases. This fact, plus the lack of highly effective systemic therapy, may diminish the zeal with which systemic tumor surveillance is pursued.

Extramedullary Plasmacytoma

Extramedullary plasmacytoma (EMP)[123–127] is a rare indolent extraosseous monoclonal plasma cell proliferation with light chain restriction, and no radiologic or marrow evidence of multiple myeloma (or malignant lymphoma).[128] It is less common than solitary plasmacytoma of bone and accounts for <4% of all plasma cell disorders. About 80% occur in the upper aerodigestive tract, with the majority in the sinonasal area. They present as a solitary polypoid or submucosal mass. Histologically, EMP is indistinguishable from other plasma cell dyscrasias of nonosseous origin.[129] Sheets of plasma cells in varying degrees of maturation or differentiation are seen within a vascular matrix containing minimal fibrous stroma (**Fig. 42.20**), and occasionally with amyloid deposits. A monoclonal expansion of kappa or lambda light chains is demonstrated by IHC or in situ hybridization. Delineation from immunoblastic lymphoma or other plasmacytoid lymphomas requires careful histopathologic and immunohistochemical delineation.

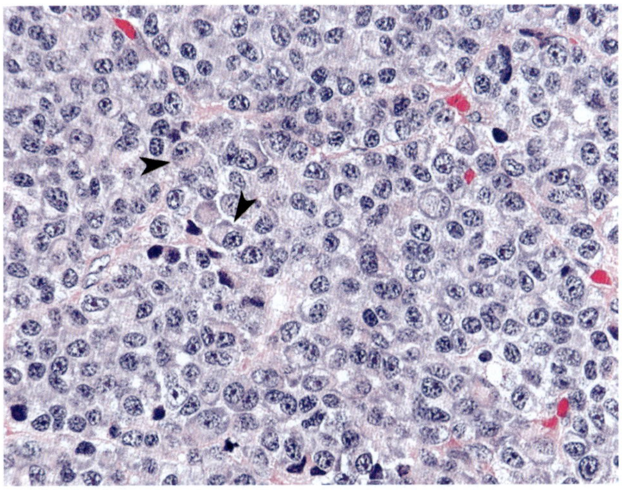

Fig. 42.20 Plasmacytoma is arranged in sheets and nests. The tumor cells display stippled chromatin and nucleoli and often have eccentrically placed collections of cytoplasm (H&E ×600). Immunohistochemical staining for kappa or lambda light chain, not shown, shows a monoclonal proliferation, further assisting in diagnosis.

It is likely that the sinonasal biopsy will be the first, and at times, only manifestation of the disease. Subsequent hematologic evaluation (complete blood count [CBC], erythrocyte sedimentation rate [ESR], serum and urine immunoelectrophoresis, quantitative immunoglobulin titers), skeletal survey with plain films and MRI, and bone marrow biopsy are then performed to investigate for systemic involvement. If isolated, treatment of EMP is 35 to 60 Gy (usually in the lower range) of irradiation. Five-year local recurrence-free survival is ~80%. Unlike solitary plasmacytoma of bone, in which 60% progress to multiple myeloma, only 23 to 37% of EMP progress, with the interval to myeloma between 4.5 months to 8.6 years. Hence, long-term follow-up, both at the primary site and systemically, is important.

Lymphoma: B cell and CD 56 (+) NK/T Cell

Paranasal lymphomas are not rare, and are in the differential diagnosis of small round tumors of childhood and adults. Malignant lymphoma represents <10% of nonepithelial malignancies of the paranasal sinuses. Diffuse large cell B cell lymphoma is most common,[130] and usually presents as stage 1E. With the current multimodality therapy, two-thirds of these patients are cured. Extranodal CD56 (+) natural killer (NK)/T cell lymphoma represents about a third of lymphomas with nasal involvement predominance. These have been previously classified as polymorphic or malignant midline reticulosis or lethal midline granuloma. The histopathologic features include a polymorphous population of atypical small and large lymphocytes, tumor cell necrosis, and numerous apoptotic bodies (**Fig. 42.21**). Infiltration and destruction of blood vessels by lymphoid cells is observed (angiocentric/

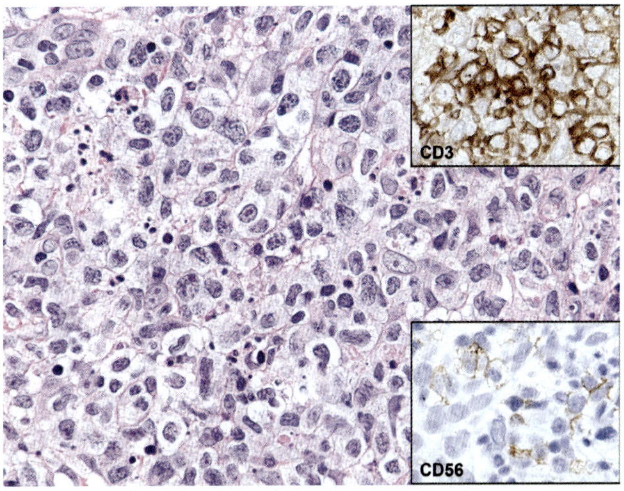

Fig. 42.21 Extranodal natural killer (NK)/T cell lymphoma of the nasal type is common in the sinonasal region. The polymorphous admixture of lymphoid cells includes atypical large cells with abundant pale eosinophilic to clear cytoplasm (H&E ×400). Vascular invasion (angiocentricity and destruction) is observed in 50 to 60% of cases. **Inset:** Strong immunoreactivity with the antibody to the T cell marker, CD3, and the NK/cytotoxic-related marker. CD56 is seen (×600).

angiodestructive). Most (>95%) cases demonstrate the presence of EBV genome. The diagnosis requires a panel of T cell antibodies including CD2, CD3, CD43, CD45RO, and CD56 and lack of reactivity for B cell antibodies. Although some studies from Asia suggest a poorer prognosis, most patients survive.

Conclusion

The pathology of the nose and paranasal sinuses is diverse. Familiarity with the pitfalls, nuances, areas of controversy, and clinical correlations of difficult dilemmas should improve accurate patient care.

References

1. Abraham SC, Montgomery EA, Giardiello FM, Wu TT. Frequent β-catenin mutations in juvenile nasopharyngeal angiofibromas. Am J Pathol 2001;158(3):1073–1078
2. Zhang PJ, Weber R, Liang HH, Pasha TL, LiVolsi VA. Growth factors and receptors in juvenile nasopharyngeal angiofibroma and nasal polyps: an immunohistochemical study. Arch Pathol Lab Med 2003;127(11):1480–1484
3. Coutinho-Camillo CM, Brentani MM, Nagai MA. Genetic alterations in juvenile nasopharyngeal angiofibromas. Head Neck 2008;30(3):390–400
4. Hyams VJ. Papillomas of the nasal cavity and paranasal sinuses. A clinicopathological study of 315 cases. Ann Otol Rhinol Laryngol 1971;80(2):192–206
5. Batsakis JG, Suarez P. Schneiderian papillomas and carcinomas: a review. Adv Anat Pathol 2001;8(2):53–64
6. Busquets JM, Hwang PH. Endoscopic resection of sinonasal inverted papilloma: a meta-analysis. Otolaryngol Head Neck Surg 2006;134(3):476–482
7. Landsberg R, Cavel O, Segev Y, Khafif A, Fliss DM. Attachment-oriented endoscopic surgical strategy for sinonasal inverted papilloma. Am J Rhinol 2008;22(6):629–634
8. Cannady SB, Batra PS, Sautter NB, Roh HJ, Citardi MJ. New staging system for sinonasal inverted papilloma in the endoscopic era. Laryngoscope 2007;117(7):1283–1287
9. Osamura RY, Kajiya H, Takei M, et al. Pathology of the human pituitary adenomas. Histochem Cell Biol 2008;130(3):495–507
10. Asa SL. Practical pituitary pathology: what does the pathologist need to know? Arch Pathol Lab Med 2008;132(8):1231–1240
11. Dekkers OM, Pereira AM, Romijn JA. Treatment and follow-up of clinically nonfunctioning pituitary macroadenomas. J Clin Endocrinol Metab 2008;93(10):3717–3726
12. Colao A, Di Sarno A, Guerra E, De Leo M, Mentone A, Lombardi G. Drug insight: Cabergoline and bromocriptine in the treatment of hyperprolactinemia in men and women. Nat Clin Pract Endocrinol Metab 2006;2(4):200–210
13. Nabeshima K, Marutsuka K, Shimao Y, Uehara H, Kodama T. Osteoma of the frontal sinus complicated by intracranial mucocele. Pathol Int 2003;53(4):227–230
14. Chapurlat RD, Orcel P. Fibrous dysplasia of bone and McCune-Albright syndrome. Best Pract Res Clin Rheumatol 2008;22(1):55–69
15. Riminucci M, Robey PG, Bianco P. The pathology of fibrous dysplasia and the McCune-Albright syndrome. Pediatr Endocrinol Rev 2007;4(Suppl 4):401–411
16. Greco MA, Steiner GC. Ultrastructure of fibrous dysplasia of bone: a study of its fibrous, osseous, and cartilaginous components. Ultrastruct Pathol 1986;10(1):55–66
17. Waldron CA. Fibro-osseous lesions of the jaws. J Oral Maxillofac Surg 1993;51(8):828–835
18. Brannon RB, Fowler CB. Benign fibro-osseous lesions: a review of current concepts. Adv Anat Pathol 2001;8(3):126–143
19. Slootweg PJ, El-Mofty SK. Ossifying fibroma. In: Barnes L, Eveson JW, Reichart P, et al, eds. Pathology and Genetics of Head and Neck Tumors: World Health Organization Classification of Tumors. Lyon, France: IARC Press; 2005: 319–322
20. Smith SF, Newman L, Walker DM, Papadopoulos H. Juvenile aggressive psammomatoid ossifying fibroma: an interesting, challenging, and unusual case report and review of the literature. J Oral Maxillofac Surg 2009;67(1):200–206
21. Johnson LC, Yousefi M, Vinh TN, Heffner DK, Hyams VJ, Hartman KS. Juvenile active ossifying fibroma. Its nature, dynamics and origin. Acta Otolaryngol Suppl 1991;488:1–40
22. Wenig BM, Vinh TN, Smirniotopoulos JG, Fowler CB, Houston GD, Heffner DK. Aggressive psammomatoid ossifying fibromas of the sinonasal region: a clinicopathologic study of a distinct group of fibro-osseous lesions. Cancer 1995;76(7):1155 –1165
23. Campbell BA, Jhamb A, Maguire JA, Toyota B, Ma R. Meningiomas in 2009: controversies and future challenges. Am J Clin Oncol 2009;32(1):73–85
24. Thompson LD, Gyure KA. Extracranial sinonasal tract meningiomas: a clinicopathologic study of 30 cases with a review of the literature. Am J Surg Pathol 2000;24(5):640–650
25. Hentschel SJ, DeMonte F. Olfactory groove meningiomas. Neurosurg Focus 2003;14(6):e4
26. Spektor S, Valarezo J, Fliss DM, et al. Olfactory groove meningiomas from neurosurgical and ear, nose, and throat perspectives: approaches, techniques, and outcomes. Neurosurgery 2005;57(4, Suppl):268–280, discussion 268–280
27. Nakamura M, Struck M, Roser F, Vorkapic P, Samii M. Olfactory groove meningiomas: clinical outcome and recurrence rates after tumor removal through the frontolateral and bifrontal approach. Neurosurgery 2008;62(6, Suppl 3):1224–1232
28. Marosi C, Hassler M, Roessler K, et al. Meningioma. Crit Rev Oncol Hematol 2008;67(2):153–171
29. Kryzanski JT, Annino DJ, Gopal H, Heilman CB. Low complication rates of cranial and craniofacial approaches to midline anterior skull base lesions. Skull Base 2008;18(4):229–241
30. Louis DN, Scheithauer BW, Budka H, von Deimling HA, Kepes JJ. Meningiomas. In: Kleihues P, Cavenee WK, eds. Pathology and Genetics. Tumors of the Nervous System, WHO Classification of Tumors. Lyon, France: IARC Press; 2000: 176–184
31. Debus J, Wuendrich M, Pirzkall A, et al. High efficacy of fractionated stereotactic radiotherapy of large base-of-skull meningiomas: long-term results. J Clin Oncol 2001;19(15):3547–3553
32. Ferner RE, O'Doherty MJ. Neurofibroma and schwannoma. Curr Opin Neurol 2002;15(6):679–684
33. Mrugala MM, Batchelor TT, Plotkin SR. Peripheral and cranial nerve sheath tumors. Curr Opin Neurol 2005;18(5):604–610
34. Wippold FJ II, Lubner M, Perrin RJ, Lämmle M, Perry A. Neuropathology for the neuroradiologist: Antoni A and Antoni B tissue patterns. AJNR Am J Neuroradiol 2007;28(9):1633–1638
35. Thompson LDR, Fanburg-Smith JC, Wenig BM. Borderline and low malignant potential tumors of soft tissues. In: Barnes L, Eveson JW, Reichart P, Sidransky D. Pathology and Genetics of Head and Neck Tumors. Lyon, France: IARC Press; 2005: 43–45

36. Catalano PJ, Brandwein M, Shah DK, Urken ML, Lawson W, Biller HF. Sinonasal hemangiopericytomas: a clinicopathologic and immunohistochemical study of seven cases. Head Neck 1996;18(1):42–53
37. el-Naggar AK, Batsakis JG, Garcia GM, Luna ML, Goepfert H. Sinonasal hemangiopericytomas. A clinicopathologic and DNA content study. Arch Otolaryngol Head Neck Surg 1992;118(2):134–137
38. Compagno J, Hyams VJ. Hemangiopericytoma-like intranasal tumors. A clinicopathologic study of 23 cases. Am J Clin Pathol 1976;66(4):672–683
39. Thompson LD, Miettinen M, Wenig BM. Sinonasal-type hemangiopericytoma: a clinicopathologic and immunophenotypic analysis of 104 cases showing perivascular myoid differentiation. Am J Surg Pathol 2003;27(6):737–749
40. Zeitler DM, Kanowitz SJ, Har-El G. Malignant solitary fibrous tumor of the nasal cavity. Skull Base 2007;17(4):239–246
41. Tse LLY, Chan JKC. Sinonasal haemangiopericytoma-like tumour: a sinonasal glomus tumour or a haemangiopericytoma? Histopathology 2002;40(6):510–517
42. Gengler C, Guillou L. Solitary fibrous tumour and haemangiopericytoma: evolution of a concept. Histopathology 2006; 48(1):63–74
43. Le QT, Fu KK, Kaplan MJ, Terris DJ, Fee WE, Goffinet DR. Lymph node metastasis in maxillary sinus carcinoma. Int J Radiat Oncol Biol Phys 2000;46(3):541–549
44. Paulino AC, Fisher SG, Marks JE. Is prophylactic neck irradiation indicated in patients with squamous cell carcinoma of the maxillary sinus? Int J Radiat Oncol Biol Phys 1997;39(2):283–289
45. Cantù G, Bimbi G, Miceli R, et al. Lymph node metastases in malignant tumors of the paranasal sinuses: prognostic value and treatment. Arch Otolaryngol Head Neck Surg 2008;134(2):170–177
46. Resto VA, Chan AW, Deschler DG, Lin DT. Extent of surgery in the management of locally advanced sinonasal malignancies. Head Neck 2008;30(2):222–229
47. Chen AM, Daly ME, Bucci MK, et al. Carcinomas of the paranasal sinuses and nasal cavity treated with radiotherapy at a single institution over five decades: are we making improvement? Int J Radiat Oncol Biol Phys 2007;69(1):141–147
48. Daly ME, Chen AM, Bucci MK, et al. Intensity-modulated radiation therapy for malignancies of the nasal cavity and paranasal sinuses. Int J Radiat Oncol Biol Phys 2007;67(1):151–157
49. Madani I, Bonte K, Vakaet L, Boterberg T, De Neve W. Intensity-modulated radiotherapy for sinonasal tumors: Ghent University Hospital update. Int J Radiat Oncol Biol Phys 2009;73(2):424–432
50. Cantù G, Riccio S, Bimbi G, et al. Craniofacial resection for malignant tumours involving the anterior skull base. Eur Arch Otorhinolaryngol 2006;263(7):647–652
51. Almefty K, Pravdenkova S, Colli BO, Al-Mefty O, Gokden M. Chordoma and chondrosarcoma: similar, but quite different, skull base tumors. Cancer 2007;110(11):2457–2467
52. Vujovic S, Henderson S, Presneau N, et al. Brachyury, a crucial regulator of notochordal development, is a novel biomarker for chordomas. J Pathol 2006;209(2):157–165
53. Romeo S, Hogendoorn PC. Brachyury and chordoma: the chondroid-chordoid dilemma resolved? J Pathol 2006;209(2):143–146
54. Schwartz TH, Fraser JF, Brown S, Tabaee A, Kacker A, Anand VK. Endoscopic cranial base surgery: classification of operative approaches. Neurosurgery 2008;62(5):991–1002, discussion 1002–1005
55. Fatemi N, Dusick JR, Gorgulho AA, et al. Endonasal microscopic removal of clival chordomas. Surg Neurol 2008;69(4):331–338
56. Al-Mefty O, Kadri PA, Hasan DM, Isolan GR, Pravdenkova S. Anterior clivectomy: surgical technique and clinical applications. J Neurosurg 2008;109(5):783–793
57. Nguyen QN, Chang EL. Emerging role of proton beam radiation therapy for chordoma and chondrosarcoma of the skull base. Curr Oncol Rep 2008;10(4):338–343
58. Henderson FC, McCool K, Seigle J, Jean W, Harter W, Gagnon GJ. Treatment of chordomas with CyberKnife: Georgetown University experience and treatment recommendations. Neurosurgery 2009;64(2, Suppl):A44–A53
59. Oakley GJ, Fuhrer K, Seethala RR. Brachyury, SOX-9, and podoplanin, new markers in the skull base chordoma vs chondrosarcoma differential: a tissue microarray-based comparative analysis. Mod Pathol 2008;21(12):1461–1469
60. Brackmann DE, Teufert KB. Chondrosarcoma of the skull base: long-term follow-up. Otol Neurotol 2006;27(7):981–991
61. Sekhar LN, Pranatartiharan R, Chanda A, Wright DC. Chordomas and chondrosarcomas of the skull base: results and complications of surgical management. Neurosurg Focus 2001; 10(3):E2
62. Tzortzidis F, Elahi F, Wright DC, Temkin N, Natarajan SK, Sekhar LN. Patient outcome at long-term follow-up after aggressive microsurgical resection of cranial base chondrosarcomas. Neurosurgery 2006;58(6):1090–1098, discussion 1090–1098
63. Wanebo JE, Bristol RE, Porter RR, Coons SW, Spetzler RF. Management of cranial base chondrosarcomas. Neurosurgery 2006;58(2):249–255, discussion 249–255
64. Lustig LR, Sciubba J, Holliday MJ. Chondrosarcomas of the skull base and temporal bone. J Laryngol Otol 2007;121(8):725–735
65. Zanation AM, Snyderman CH, Carrau RL, Gardner PA, Prevedello DM, Kassam AB. Endoscopic endonasal surgery for petrous apex lesions. Laryngoscope 2009;119(1):19–25
66. Nguyen-Huynh A, Blevins NH, Jackler RK. The challenges of revision skull base surgery. Otolaryngol Clin North Am 2006;39(4):783–799, viii
67. Gadwal SR, Gannon FH, Fanburg-Smith JC, Becoskie EM, Thompson LD. Primary osteosarcoma of the head and neck in pediatric patients: a clinicopathologic study of 22 cases with a review of the literature. Cancer 2001;91(3):598–605
68. Canadian Society of Otolaryngology-Head and Neck Surgery Oncology Study Group. Osteogenic sarcoma of the mandible and maxilla: a Canadian review (1980-2000). J Otolaryngol 2004;33(3):139–144
69. Huber GF, Dziegielewski P, Wayne Matthews T, Dort JC. Head and neck osteosarcoma in adults: the province of Alberta experience over 26 years. J Otolaryngol Head Neck Surg 2008;37(5):738–743
70. Wanebo HJ, Koness RJ, MacFarlane JK, et al; Society of Head and Neck Surgeons Committee on Research. Head and neck sarcoma: report of the Head and Neck Sarcoma Registry. Head Neck 1992;14(1):1–7
71. Bielack SS, Carrle D, Hardes J, Schuck A, Paulussen M. Bone tumors in adolescents and young adults. Curr Treat Options Oncol 2008;9(1):67–80
72. Bielack SS, Carrle D. State-of-the-art approach in selective curable tumors: bone sarcoma. Ann Oncol 2008;19(Suppl 7):vii155–vii160
73. Chou AJ, Geller DS, Gorlick R. Therapy for osteosarcoma: where do we go from here? Paediatr Drugs 2008;10(5):315–327
74. Maghami EG, St-John M, Bhuta S, Abemayor E. Postirradiation sarcoma: a case report and current review. Am J Otolaryngol 2005;26(1):71–74
75. Hewitt KM, Ellis G, Wiggins R, Bentz BG. Parosteal osteosarcoma: case report and review of the literature. Head Neck 2008;30(1): 122–126
76. Vlychou M, Ostlere SJ, Kerr R, Athanasou NA. Low-grade osteosarcoma of the ethmoid sinus. Skeletal Radiol 2007;36(5):459–462
77. Park YK, Ryu KN, Park HR, Kim DW. Low-grade osteosarcoma of the maxillary sinus. Skeletal Radiol 2003;32(3):161–164

78. Koka V, Vericel R, Lartigau E, Lusinchi A, Schwaab G. Sarcomas of nasal cavity and paranasal sinuses: chondrosarcoma, osteosarcoma and fibrosarcoma. J Laryngol Otol 1994;108(11):947–953
79. Crist WM, Anderson JR, Meza JL, et al. Intergroup rhabdomyosarcoma study-IV: results for patients with nonmetastatic disease. J Clin Oncol 2001;19(12):3091–3102
80. Raney B, Anderson J, Breneman J, et al; Soft-Tissue Sarcoma Committee of the Children's Oncology Group, Arcadia, California, USA. Results in patients with cranial parameningeal sarcoma and metastases (Stage 4) treated on Intergroup Rhabdomyosarcoma Study Group (IRSG) Protocols II-IV, 1978-1997: report from the Children's Oncology Group. Pediatr Blood Cancer 2008;51(1):17–22
81. Simon JH, Paulino AC, Ritchie JM, Mayr NA, Buatti JM. Presentation, prognostic factors and patterns of failure in adult rhabdomyosarcoma. Sarcoma 2003;7(1):1–7
82. Curtis AE, Okcu MF, Chintagumpala M, Teh BS, Paulino AC. Local control after intensity-modulated radiotherapy for head-and-neck rhabdomyosarcoma. Int J Radiat Oncol Biol Phys 2009;73(1):173–177
83. Newton WA Jr, Gehan EA, Webber BL, et al. Classification of rhabdomyosarcomas and related sarcomas. Pathologic aspects and proposal for a new classification—an Intergroup Rhabdomyosarcoma Study. Cancer 1995;76(6):1073–1085
84. Qualman SJ, Coffin CM, Newton WA, et al. Intergroup Rhabdomyosarcoma Study: update for pathologists. Pediatr Dev Pathol 1998;1(6):550–561
85. Parham DM, Ellison DA. Rhabdomyosarcomas in adults and children: an update. Arch Pathol Lab Med 2006;130(10):1454–1465
86. Davicioni E, Anderson MJ, Finckenstein FG, et al. Molecular classification of rhabdomyosarcoma—genotypic and phenotypic determinants of diagnosis: a report from the Children's Oncology Group. Am J Pathol 2009;174(2):550–564
87. Parham DM, Qualman SJ, Teot L, et al; Soft Tissue Sarcoma Committee of the Children's Oncology Group. Correlation between histology and PAX/FKHR fusion status in alveolar rhabdomyosarcoma: a report from the Children's Oncology Group. Am J Surg Pathol 2007;31(6):895–901
88. Sandberg AA, Bridge JA. Updates on cytogenetics and molecular genetics of bone and soft tissue tumors: Ewing sarcoma and peripheral primitive neuroectodermal tumors. Cancer Genet Cytogenet 2000;123(1):1–26
89. Thacker MM, Temple HT, Scully SP. Current treatment for Ewing's sarcoma. Expert Rev Anticancer Ther 2005;5(2):319–331
90. Zagars GK, Ballo MT, Pisters PW, et al. Prognostic factors for patients with localized soft-tissue sarcoma treated with conservation surgery and radiation therapy: an analysis of 1225 patients. Cancer 2003;97(10):2530–2543
91. Sturgis EM, Potter BO. Sarcomas of the head and neck region. Curr Opin Oncol 2003;15(3):239–252
92. Hanna E, Vural E, Prokopakis E, Carrau R, Snyderman C, Weissman J. The sensitivity and specificity of high-resolution imaging in evaluating perineural spread of adenoid cystic carcinoma to the skull base. Arch Otolaryngol Head Neck Surg 2007;133(6):541–545
93. Maroldi R, Farina D, Borghesi A, Marconi A, Gatti E. Perineural tumor spread. Neuroimaging Clin N Am 2008;18(2):413–429, xi
94. Batsakis JG, Luna MA, el-Naggar A. Histopathologic grading of salivary gland neoplasms: III. Adenoid cystic carcinomas. Ann Otol Rhinol Laryngol 1990;99(12):1007–1009
95. Pitman KT, Prokopakis EP, Aydogan B, et al. The role of skull base surgery for the treatment of adenoid cystic carcinoma of the sinonasal tract. Head Neck 1999;21(5):402–407
96. Pommier P, Liebsch NJ, Deschler DG, et al. Proton beam radiation therapy for skull base adenoid cystic carcinoma. Arch Otolaryngol Head Neck Surg 2006;132(11):1242–1249
97. Lupinetti AD, Roberts DB, Williams MD, et al. Sinonasal adenoid cystic carcinoma: the M. D. Anderson Cancer Center experience. Cancer 2007;110(12):2726–2731
98. Rhee CS, Won TB, Lee CH, et al. Adenoid cystic carcinoma of the sinonasal tract: treatment results. Laryngoscope 2006;116(6): 982 –986
99. Sung MW, Kim KH, Kim JW, et al. Clinicopathologic predictors and impact of distant metastasis from adenoid cystic carcinoma of the head and neck. Arch Otolaryngol Head Neck Surg 2003;129(11):1193–1197
100. Dodd RL, Slevin NJ. Salivary gland adenoid cystic carcinoma: a review of chemotherapy and molecular therapies. Oral Oncol 2006;42(8):759–769
101. Knegt PP, Ah-See KW, Velden LA, Kerrebijn J. Adenocarcinoma of the ethmoidal sinus complex: surgical debulking and topical fluorouracil may be the optimal treatment. Arch Otolaryngol Head Neck Surg 2001;127(2):141–146
102. Bimbi G, Saraceno MS, Riccio S, Gatta G, Licitra L, Cantù G. Adenocarcinoma of ethmoid sinus: an occupational disease. Acta Otorhinolaryngol Ital 2004;24(4):199–203
103. Roux FX, Behm E, Page P, Laccourreye O, Pages JC, Brasnu D. [Adenocarcinomas of the ethmoid sinuses. Epidemiological data]. Ann Otolaryngol Chir Cervicofac 2002;119(5):271–280
104. Iezzoni JC, Mills SE. "Undifferentiated" small round cell tumors of the sinonasal tract: differential diagnosis update. Am J Clin Pathol 2005;124(Suppl):S110–S121
105. Cordes B, Williams MD, Tirado Y, et al. Molecular and phenotypic analysis of poorly differentiated sinonasal neoplasms: an integrated approach for early diagnosis and classification. Hum Pathol 2009;40(3):283–292
106. Nicolai P, Battaglia P, Bignami M, et al. Endoscopic surgery for malignant tumors of the sinonasal tract and adjacent skull base: a 10-year experience. Am J Rhinol 2008;22(3):308–316
107. Mills SE. Neuroectodermal neoplasms of the head and neck with emphasis on neuroendocrine carcinomas. Mod Pathol 2002;15(3):264–278
108. Iezzoni JC, Mills SE. "Undifferentiated" small round cell tumors of the sinonasal tract: differential diagnosis update. Am J Clin Pathol 2005;124(Suppl):S110–S121
109. Bellizzi AM, Bourne TD, Mills SE, Stelow EB. The cytologic features of sinonasal undifferentiated carcinoma and olfactory neuroblastoma. Am J Clin Pathol 2008;129(3):367–376
110. Babin E, Rouleau V, Vedrine PO, et al. Small cell neuroendocrine carcinoma of the nasal cavity and paranasal sinuses. J Laryngol Otol 2006;120(4):289–297
111. Chan AW, Pommier P, Deschler DG, et al. Combined proton radiotherapy with chemotherapy for advanced sinonasal neuroendocrine carcinoma [abstract]. Proceedings of the Sixth International Conference on Head and Neck Cancer. August 10, 2004
112. Cerilli LA, Holst VA, Brandwein MS, Stoler MH, Mills SE. Sinonasal undifferentiated carcinoma: immunohistochemical profile and lack of EBV association. Am J Surg Pathol 2001;25(2):156–163
113. Nishimura H, Ogino T, Kawashima M, et al. Proton-beam therapy for olfactory neuroblastoma. Int J Radiat Oncol Biol Phys 2007;68(3):758–762
114. Dias FL, Sa GM, Lima RA, et al. Patterns of failure and outcome in esthesioneuroblastoma. Arch Otolaryngol Head Neck Surg 2003;129(11):1186–1192
115. Bradley PJ, Jones NS, Robertson I. Diagnosis and management of esthesioneuroblastoma. Curr Opin Otolaryngol Head Neck Surg 2003;11(2):112–118
116. Lund VJ, Howard D, Wei W, Spittle M. Olfactory neuroblastoma: past, present, and future? Laryngoscope 2003;113(3): 502–507

117. Loy AH, Reibel JF, Read PW, et al. Esthesioneuroblastoma: continued follow-up of a single institution's experience. Arch Otolaryngol Head Neck Surg 2006;132(2):134–138
118. Zafereo ME, Fakhri S, Prayson R, et al. Esthesioneuroblastoma: 25-year experience at a single institution. Otolaryngol Head Neck Surg 2008;138(4):452–458
119. Zanation AM, Snyderman CH, Carrau RL, Kassam AB, Gardner PA, Prevedello DM. Minimally invasive endoscopic pericranial flap: a new method for endonasal skull base reconstruction. Laryngoscope 2009;119(1):13–18
120. Klepin HD, McMullen KP, Lesser GJ. Esthesioneuroblastoma. Curr Treat Options Oncol 2005;6(6):509–518
121. Brandwein MS, Rothstein A, Lawson W, Bodian C, Urken ML. Sinonasal melanoma. A clinicopathologic study of 25 cases and literature meta-analysis. Arch Otolaryngol Head Neck Surg 1997;123(3):290–296
122. Patel SG, Prasad ML, Escrig M, et al. Primary mucosal malignant melanoma of the head and neck. Head Neck 2002;24(3):247–257
123. Sulzner SE, Amdur RJ, Weider DJ. Extramedullary plasmacytoma of the head and neck. Am J Otolaryngol 1998;19(3):203–208
124. Dimopoulos MA, Kiamouris C, Moulopoulos LA. Solitary plasmacytoma of bone and extramedullary plasmacytoma. Hematol Oncol Clin North Am 1999;13(6):1249–1257
125. Mendenhall WM, Mendenhall CM, Mendenhall NP. Solitary plasmacytoma of bone and soft tissues. Am J Otolaryngol 2003;24(6):395–399
126. Ozsahin M, Tsang RW, Poortmans P, et al. Outcomes and patterns of failure in solitary plasmacytoma: a multicenter Rare Cancer Network study of 258 patients. Int J Radiat Oncol Biol Phys 2006;64(1):210–217
127. Bachar G, Goldstein D, Brown D, et al. Solitary extramedullary plasmacytoma of the head and neck—long-term outcome analysis of 68 cases. Head Neck 2008;30(8):1012–1019
128. Bink K, Haralambieva E, Kremer M, et al. Primary extramedullary plasmacytoma: similarities with and differences from multiple myeloma revealed by interphase cytogenetics. Haematologica 2008;93(4):623–626
129. Batsakis JG, Medeiros JL, Luna MA, El-Naggar AK. Plasma cell dyscrasias and the head and neck. Ann Diagn Pathol 2002;6(2):129–140
130. Vega F, Lin P, Medeiros LJ. Extranodal lymphomas of the head and neck. Ann Diagn Pathol 2005;9(6):340–350

43 The Nasopharynx

Dharmbir S. Sethi and Hin Ngan Tay

Located posterior to the nasal cavity, the nasopharynx is a unique structure involved both in deglutition and respiration. It connects with the nasal cavity anteriorly and with the oropharyngeal cavity inferiorly. It is related superiorly with the sphenoid sinus, laterally with the parapharyngeal space (PPS) and infratemporal fossa, and posteriorly with the middle and the lower clivus. Its inner surface is lined by various types of epithelium: keratinized and nonkeratinized squamous, pseudostratified, ciliated, and columnar. The epithelium contains glandular and lymphoid tissues. Pathology involving the nasopharynx is not common. Diverse benign tumors arising from the epithelia, lymphoid, glandular, and connective tissue are occasionally encountered. Primary malignancy of the nasopharynx is even rarer. Although rare in the West, nasopharyngeal carcinoma (NPC) is endemic in Asia and Africa, especially in southern China and among those of southern Chinese descent.[1] Often, pathology may extend into the nasopharynx from the surrounding regions, such as the sphenoid sinus, clivus, nasal cavity, paranasal sinuses, and the pterygopalatine fossa or sphenopalatine foramen.

Anatomy of the Nasopharynx

Embryology

The nasopharynx is a derivative of the foregut. Like the rest of the primitive gut, it is an endoderm-lined tube. The cephalic part ends blindly at the buccopharyngeal membrane, which separates it from the ectodermally lined stomatodeum. Development of the pharyngeal arches and pouches has been extensively described and will not be fully elaborated here. Nasopharyngeal structures are largely derived from the first pharyngeal arch and pouch, with the eustachian tubes being the most recognizable feature. The eustachian tube is formed by the invagination of the first pharyngeal pouch laterally, which forms the middle ear cavity, terminating at the tympanic membrane by constituting its innermost layer. From the nasal cavity to the nasopharynx and the oropharynx, there is a gradual transition from Schneiderian membrane derived mucosa to the transitional zone and then endodermally derived squamous mucosa. Mesenchymal condensations associated with infiltrating lymphocytes develop into the Waldeyer's ring, the most cephalad formation being the adenoids, which appear in the third month of gestation. The characteristic sagittal folds start appearing by the fifth month, and the adenoids are fully formed by the seventh month. Pharyngeal endoderm is closely associated with the notochord as it develops up to the fifth week. In later stages, connective tissue interposes between them except at an area caudal to the future position of the adenoids. This area of close contact or persistent attachment becomes the pharyngeal bursa as the notochord becomes incorporated into the skull base.[2] This process is important in the formation of nasopharyngeal cysts.

Boundaries

The boundaries of the nasopharynx, as defined in the American Joint Committee on Cancer (AJCC) Cancer Staging Manual,[3] are anteriorly at the posterior choana, following the plane of the airway to the level of the free border of the palate (**Fig. 43.1A**). The anterior boundary is a fixed air boundary, whereas the inferior boundary is variable, depending on the position of the soft palate, which lies lower at rest than on swallowing. The roof and posterior wall is a slope defined by the floor of the sphenoid sinus continuing onto the clivus and the craniocervical junction. The lateral wall is divided into two parts: the anterior part is limited by the medial pterygoid plate, whereas the posterior part is a soft tissue interface where the pharyngobasilar fascia separates the nasopharynx from the paranasopharynx.

Bony Relations

The nasopharynx is related to the sphenoid bone, the occipital bone, the ethmoid bone, and the palatine bones. Of these, its relationship with the sphenoid bone is the most intimate. In the midline, the body of the sphenoid and the clivus form the sloping roof and posterior wall, separating the nasopharynx from the sphenoid sinus and the posterior cranial fossa (**Fig. 43.1A**).

Anatomically, the clivus can be divided into three zones. The upper third is formed by the basisphenoid. The middle clivus is formed by the rostral part of the basiocciput and the lower clivus by the caudal part of the basiocciput. Located in the midline at the junction of the middle and lower clivus ~1 cm above the foramen magnum is a small bony elevation termed the pharyngeal tubercle, which serves as the site of attachment of the pharyngeal raphe of the superior pharyngeal constrictor muscle. The bones of the nasopharynx above the pharyngeal tubercle are covered by mucosa, minimal submucosal tissue, and periosteum. Below the pharyngeal tubercle, the intervening soft

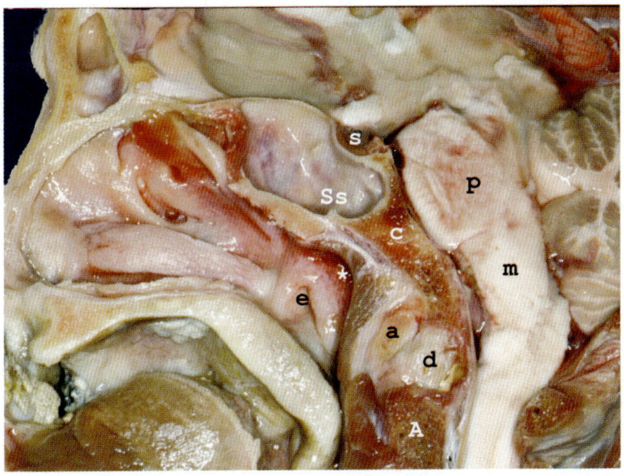

A

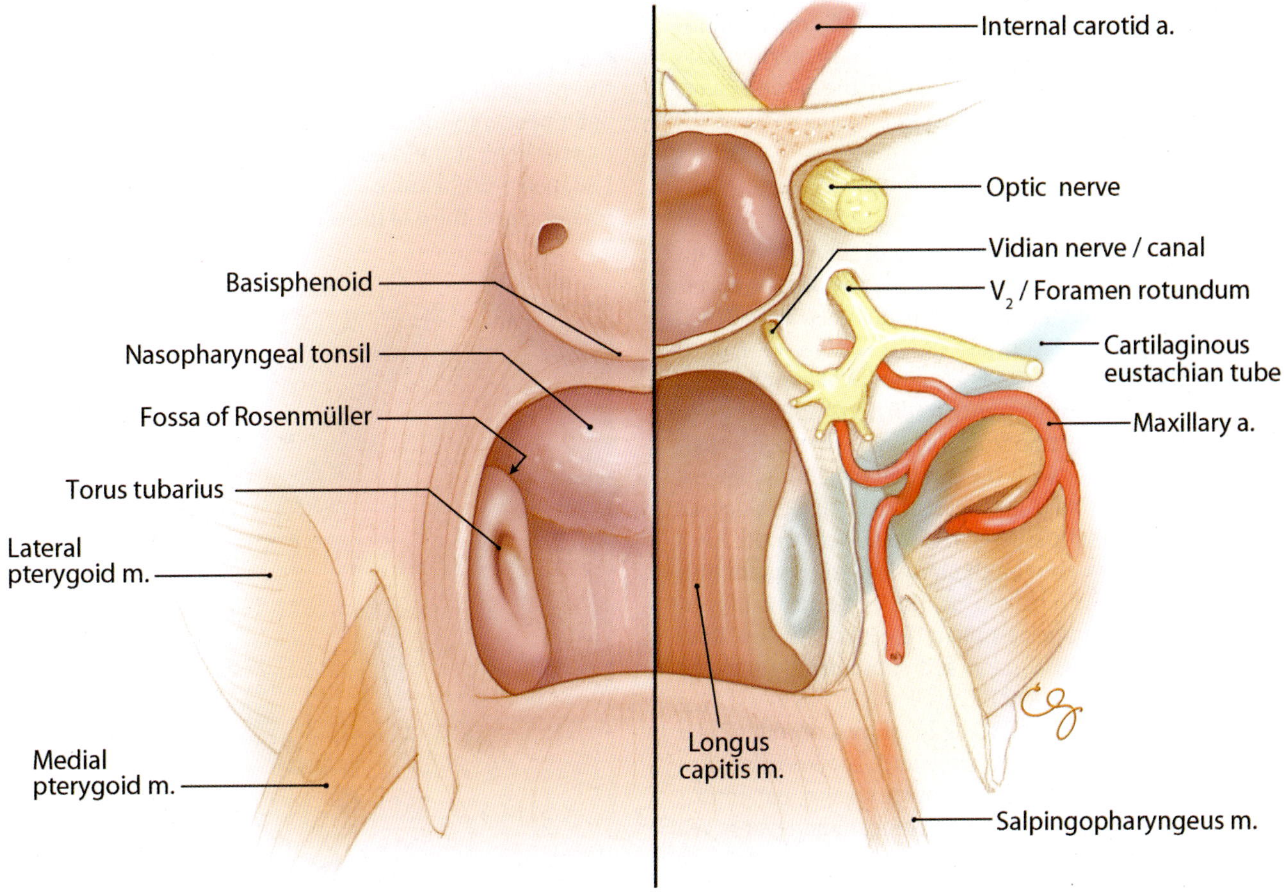

B

Fig. 43.1 (A) Midline sagittal section of cadaver head showing the nasopharynx and its relationship to the surrounding structures. The nasopharynx is bordered above by the posterior part of the sphenoid (*Ss*) and upper to middle clivus (*c*) and posteriorly by the lower clivus, atlas (*a*), and axis (*A*). The eustachian tube (*e*) opens into the lateral wall of the nasopharynx. The pons (*p*) faces the upper and middle clivus. The medulla (*m*) faces the lower clivus, the foramen magnum, and upper part of the dens (*d*). The *white asterisk* indicates the location of the lateral pharyngeal recess (fossa of Rosenmüller). **(B)** Drawing of a coronal section of the nasopharynx at the level of the cavernous sinus. The nasopharynx is bounded above by the sphenoid sinus and laterally by the eustachian tube and is separated from the oropharynx by the soft palate. Laterally, the infratemporal fossa located below the greater wing of the sphenoid bone. The medial pterygoid and lateral pterygoid muscles occupy the infratemporal fossa. On the left side, the medial and lateral pterygoids have been removed to expose the internal maxillary artery and the mandibular nerve (V_1) as it exits from the foramen ovale. Also seen are the internal carotid artery, the tensor veli palatini, levator veli palatini, and the muscles of the eustachian tube.

tissue increases in thickness over the lower portion of the clivus and the anterior arch of the atlas (**Fig. 43.1A**). Laterally, the medial pterygoid plates form the lateral boundaries of the nasopharynx. Attached to the posterior margins of the medial pterygoid plates is the thick dense pharyngobasilar fascia. The bony orifice of the posterior choana is formed by the vomer, the perpendicular plate of the ethmoid, and the palatine bone.

The numerous bony foramina located within and near the nasopharynx are important routes of extension or invasion of both benign and malignant lesions. Anteriorly, the sphenopalatine foramen transmits the sphenopalatine artery and is commonly the site of origin of juvenile nasopharyngeal angiofibromas, which often expand the foramen and extend into the pterygopalatine fossa laterally (**Fig. 43.1B**). Following the middle cranial fossa laterally, there are multiple potential avenues for intracranial extension of tumors that have invaded the PPS and infratemporal fossa: foramen rotundum (maxillary nerve [V2]), foramen ovale (mandibular nerve [V3]), the carotid canal, and the jugular foramen.

Soft Tissue

The mucosal surfaces include the vault, the lateral walls (including the fossae of Rosenmüller and the mucosa covering the torus tubarius), the posterior pharyngeal wall, and the superior/pharyngeal surface of the soft palate. Associated with this mucosa is a variable amount of lymphoid tissue, known as the nasopharyngeal tonsils or adenoids. The adenoids are typically trapezoidal in shape with deep vertical furrows. Together with the palatine tonsils and lingual tonsils, these lymphoid aggregates form the Waldeyer's ring. Some lymphoid tissue is also found within the fossa of Rosenmüller and even on the torus tubarius where they are referred to as the tubal tonsils. The first echelon of lymphatic drainage from the nasopharynx is to the node of Rouviere or retropharyngeal node and subsequently into the deep cervical chain of nodes, levels II and V.

The nasopharynx can be thought of as a fibromuscular sling suspended from the basisphenoid. The inner longitudinal layer consists of the salpingopharyngeus, palatopharyngeus, and stylopharyngeus. The tensor and levator veli palatini, which are muscles of the soft palate, also contribute to this layer at their superior ends. The outer circular layer at the level of the nasopharynx is formed by the superior constrictor, with the superior aspect of the middle constrictor overlapping it inferiorly. The median raphe of the superior constrictor is attached to the pharyngeal tubercle superiorly. Lateral to the pharyngeal tubercle on each side, the longus capitis muscle is attached to the middle and the lower clivus. The anterior surface of this muscle, which is convex forward on each side of the midline, also furnishes attachment to the pharyngobasilar fascia and the prevertebral fascia on the middle clivus. The border between the roof and posterior wall of the nasopharynx is sited at the pharyngeal tubercle in the midline and along an anterior margin of attachment of the longus capitis muscle laterally. Thus, the nasopharyngeal roof extends down to the middle clivus in the midline, but is confined to the upper clivus by the longus capitis muscle on either side.

The configuration of the nasopharynx is determined by the very tough pharyngobasilar fascia, which attaches to the base of the skull from the posterior margin of the medial pterygoid plate to the petrous part of the temporal bone immediately in front of the carotid foramina. Its fibers are continuous with that of the foramen lacerum (**Fig. 43.2**). The fascia forms an entirely closed and very resistant fibrotic chamber, which is perforated only by the passage of the eustachian tube. This aperture is the sinus of Morgagni.

Eustachian Tube System and Soft Palate

The eustachian tube is a prominent anatomic feature on the lateral nasopharyngeal wall (**Fig. 43.1A,B**). It connects the nasopharynx to the middle ear, is ~3 to 4 cm long, and opens into the lateral wall of the nasopharynx immediately behind the medial pterygoid plate by an inverted J-shaped protuberance called the torus tubarius. The posterolateral one-third of the eustachian tube is bony, whereas

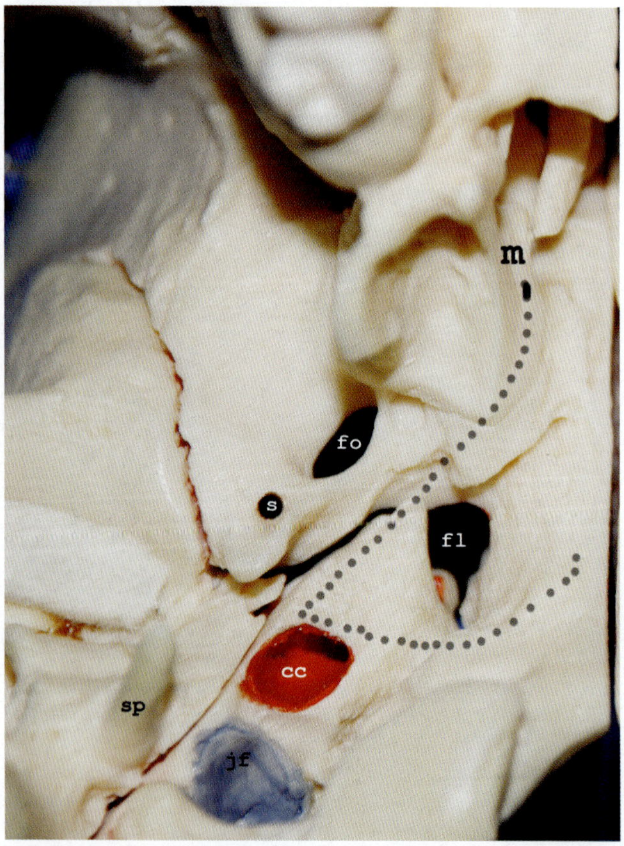

Fig. 43.2 Photograph of normal skull base (*right half*) showing bone landmarks and foramina. The insertion of the pharyngobasilar fascia (*dotted line*). *m*, medial pterygoid; *fo*, foramen ovale; *cc*, carotid canal; *jf*, jugular foramen; *sp*, styloid process; *s*, foramen spinosum.

the anteromedial two-thirds is composed of cartilage and connective tissue. The torus tubarius is formed by the medial end of the cartilaginous tube elevating the overlying mucosa. The medial or posterior limb of the cartilage is longer than the lateral or anterior limb. The eustachian tube is bounded anteriorly and laterally by the tensor veli palatini and posteriorly and inferiorly by the levator veli palatini. The levator veli palatini originates from the quadrate area of the petrous bone and partly from the short limb of the cartilaginous eustachian tube and runs almost parallel to it. Along with the cartilaginous portion of the eustachian tube, the levator veli palatini passes directly to the soft palate through the sinus of Morgagni. Isotonic contraction of this muscle elevates the soft palate and expands the tubal orifice as it splays open the medial and lateral limbs. The tensor veli palatini originates from the scaphoid fossa of the sphenoid bone anterolateral to the levator veli palatini muscle. The tensor veli palatini muscle reaches the palate indirectly by hooking around the hamulus of the medial pterygoid and inserts into the median raphe. It opens the tube by traction on the lateral tubal membrane and the lateral limb of the cartilage. The lateral pharyngeal recess (fossa of Rosenmüller) is located at the junction of the lateral and posterior walls of the nasopharynx, projecting laterally behind the orifice of the eustachian tube. The recess is bounded anteriorly by the levator veli palatini, posteriorly by the longus capitis muscle, and its roof is attached to the thick connective tissue covering the foramen lacerum above. The posterolateral depth of the recess is separated from the cervical internal carotid artery by only a layer of fibroconnective tissue. It is in this recess that most nasopharyngeal carcinomas arise.

Blood Supply

The nasopharynx is mainly supplied by the external carotid system. The majority of its supply is from the ascending pharyngeal artery, which arises in the proximal external carotid artery (ECA). Branches are given off to supply the pharyngeal wall as it ascends, with a palatine branch passing over the superior edge of the superior constrictor, which supplies the soft palate and mucosa. Another small branch gives off a branch to supply the eustachian tube. The ascending palatine branch of the facial artery and the greater palatine and pterygoid branches of the internal maxillary artery also contribute. The sphenopalatine artery and its posterior septal branch contribute to the blood supply of the roof and choanal aspects of the nasopharynx.

Venous drainage of the nasopharynx consists of two layers of venous plexuses, namely the submucous layer and the external pharyngeal plexus. These plexuses are continuous from the nasopharynx inferiorly into the oropharynx. The pharyngeal plexus of the nasopharynx drains laterally into the pterygoid plexus and downward into the internal jugular vein.

Innervation

The neural network around the nasopharynx is also known as the pharyngeal plexus, which is located in the buccopharyngeal fascia. Components of this plexus include motor, sensory, and autonomic systems. The motor supply is derived from the nucleus ambiguous, by way of the pharyngeal branch of the vagus nerve, which supplies all pharyngeal muscles except the stylopharyngeus, which is the only muscle controlled by the glossopharyngeal nerve. Sensory innervation is supplied by the glossopharyngeal nerve, with the exception of a small patch behind the eustachian tube, which is supplied by the pharyngeal branch of V_2. The cell bodies of these afferent fibers are located in their respective ganglia, with central connections to the nucleus of the tractus solitarius and the spinal tract of V. The parasympathetic secretomotor supply arise from the superior salivary nucleus, whose fibers travel from the brainstem via the nervus intermedius, through the geniculate ganglion, proceeding anteriorly in the greater superficial petrosal nerve, and reaching the pterygopalatine ganglion via the nerve of the pterygoid canal. Postganglionic axons travel to the pharynx via the pharyngeal branch. Sympathetic fibers, as in the rest of the body, travel together with the blood vessels. The preganglionic cell bodies arise from the lateral column of T1 through T3, traveling up the sympathetic trunk to synapse in the superior cervical ganglion.

Histology

The epithelium of the nasopharynx is mainly pseudostratified ciliated columnar type near the choanae and adjacent part of the roof of the nasopharynx, becoming stratified squamous in the lower and posterior regions. Almost 60% of the nasopharynx is lined by stratified squamous epithelium derived from endoderm. Areas of transitional epithelium are encountered in the junctional zone of the roof and lateral walls. The transitional zone between the nasopharynx and oropharynx is lined by stratified columnar epithelium, which changes to the nonkeratinizing stratified squamous epithelium of the oropharynx. Typical of respiratory mucosa, mucus production is by goblet cells, although there are seromucinous glands in the submucosa. Deep to the mucosa lies the lamina propria, which is frequently infiltrated by lymphoid tissue, which, in the child, forms a midline aggregation posteriorly of varying size, termed the adenoid (nasopharyngeal tonsil).

Mucosa-associated lymphoid tissue (MALT) forms the Waldeyer's ring. These lymphoid aggregates, although found mainly in the lamina propria, may extend into the submucosa if hypertrophic.

Imaging

Radiologic Anatomy

Conventional radiographs yield limited information about the nasopharynx. Cross-sectional imaging (e.g., computed tomography [CT] scan or magnetic resonance imaging [MRI]) are the modalities of choice in evaluation of the nasopharynx. CT is ideal for outlining the bony architecture, whereas MRI provides soft tissue details. These modalities are complementary and are often used together to demonstrate the full disease extent (**Fig. 43.3A,B**)

Radiologic Boundaries of the Nasopharynx

As a prelude to understanding the radiologic anatomy of the nasopharynx, it is important to identify its radiologic boundaries. A line connecting the posterior wall of the maxillary sinus bilaterally is taken as a landmark for the posterior choana, which forms the anterior boundary of the nasopharynx. The medial pterygoid plates (**Fig. 43.3A,** *m*) and a line extrapolated posteriorly to the internal carotid artery (**Fig. 43.3A,** *c*) delineate the lateral limits of the nasopharynx. The PPS (**Fig. 43.3A,** *p*) is readily identified as a pad of fat but, for purposes of standardization, is taken to be lateral to the line described earlier, up to a line extrapolated from the lateral pterygoid plate (**Fig. 43.3A,** +) to the styloid process (**Fig. 43.3A,** *s*). Lateral to the PPS is the infratemporal fossa or the masticator space.

The retropharyngeal and prevertebral spaces lie anterior to the arch of the atlas and the body of the axis. The fossa of Rosenmüller (**Fig. 43.3A,** *white asterisk*) is located superior and posterior to the torus tubarius (**Fig. 43.3A,** *t*). The inverted J configuration of the torus tubarius results in the fossa appearing posterior (on axial images) and superior (on coronal images) to the eustachian tube orifice.[4] The bilaterally paired recesses of the upper nasopharynx are a characteristic finding; however, the shape of the fossa may show wide variations. The opening of the eustachian tube (**Fig. 43.3A,** *e*), however, is usually symmetrical and any asymmetry should be treated with suspicion. A discrepancy of more than 5 mm between sides should prompt suspicion of a lesion (**Fig. 43.3B**).[5] The node of Rouviere, which is a retropharyngeal lymph node and the first echelon of lymphatic drainage from the nasopharynx, is often enlarged in NPC and can be identified on CT scan and may be the first sign of nasopharyngeal carcinoma (**Fig. 43.3C**).

Although CT offers an excellent study of the bony details of the nasopharynx, MRI is the superior study for soft tissue structures (**Fig. 43.3D**). The cartilaginous end of the eustachian tube is usually of similar or lower signal intensity than surrounding muscle. Tubular tonsillar tissue present in this area may give a fairly intense signal depending on the amount of lymphoid tissue present and the effects of volume averaging (**Fig. 43.3D,** *t*). Lymphoid tissue in the nasopharynx is most prominent along the roof. The signal of lymphoid tissue is always more intense than that of muscle because it is normally located submucosally and it never obliterates the deeper tissue planes of the nasopharynx (**Fig. 43.3E**). The muscles of the nasopharynx are routinely visible on the MRI as bands of intermediate signal intensity (**Fig. 43.3E,** *M*). The PPS appears as a loose network of high-signal fibrofatty tissue and is always symmetrical. Lateral to the parapharyngeal space is the infratemporal fossa. The medial and the lateral pterygoid muscles fill the bulk of the infratemporal fossa. The pharyngobasilar fascia may be identified on MRI as a low-intensity line extending from the medial pterygoid plate to the carotid foramen. From

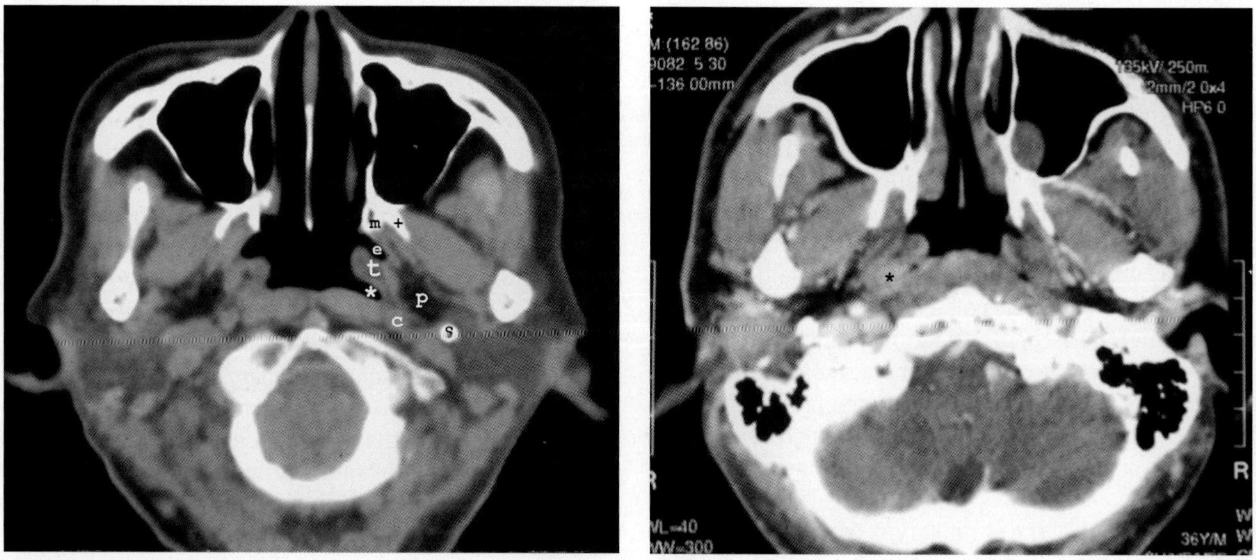

A B

Fig. 43.3 **(A)** Computed tomography (CT) scan of the nasopharynx. A line from the medial pterygoid plate (*m*) to the internal carotid artery (*c*) defines the lateral limits of the nasopharynx. The infratemporal fossa is lateral to a line drawn from the lateral pterygoid plate (+) to the styloid process (*s*). The torus (*t*) is a prominent feature on the lateral wall. The eustachian tube (*e*) opens anterior to the torus tubarius, whereas the lateral pharyngeal recess (*white asterisk*), also known as the fossa of Rosenmüller, is seen posteriorly. The parapharyngeal space (*p*) is lateral to the eustachian tube. **(B)** CT scan of the nasopharynx showing asymmetry caused by a small enhancing lesion (*asterisk*). A biopsy of this lesion confirmed an undifferentiated nasopharyngeal carcinoma. *(continued)*

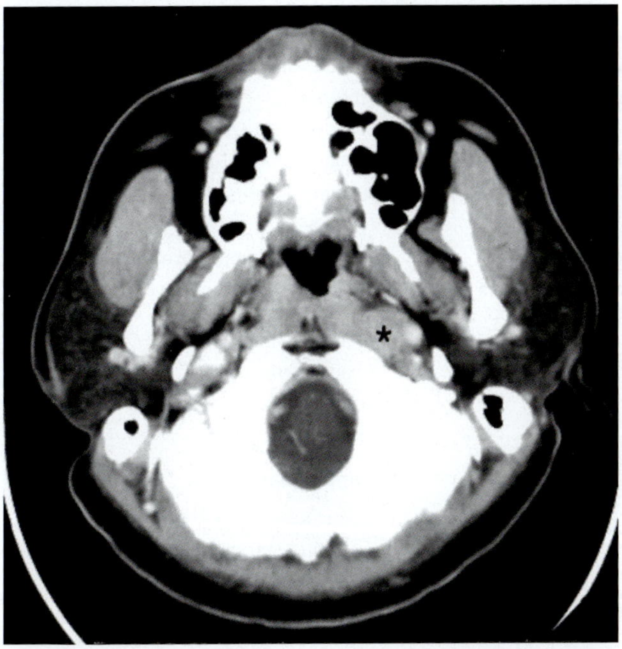

C

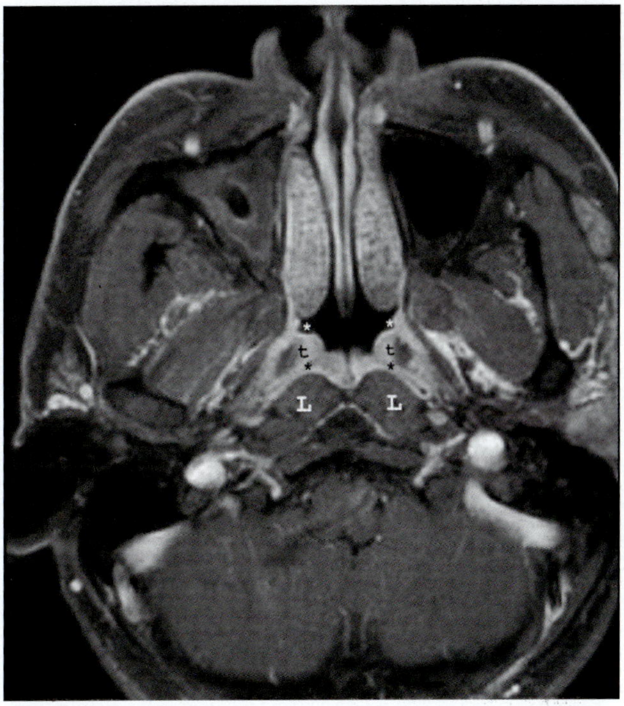

D

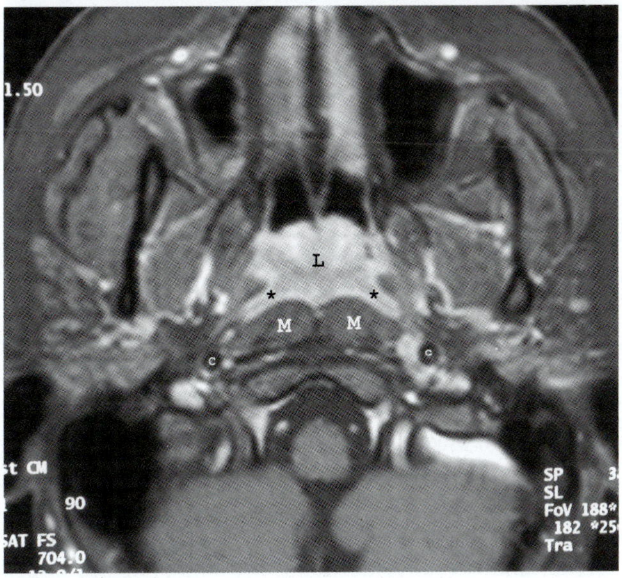

E

Fig. 43.3 *(continued)* **(C)** Axial CT showing an enlarged left retropharyngeal lymph node shown by the asterisk (node of Rouviere) in a patient with an early detected nasopharyngeal carcinoma. **(D)** Axial T-1 weighted postcontrast magnetic resonance image (MRI) of the nasopharynx. The MRI provides superior information of the surrounding soft tissue on the nasopharynx. The torus tubarius (*t*) and the fossa of Rosenmüller (*asterisk*) show smooth mucosal enhancement. Note the tissue interface between the mucosa and the underlying longus capitis (*L*) muscle situated immediately deep to the mucosa of the posterior nasopharyngeal wall. The white asterisk indicates the eustachian tube orifice on the lateral wall of the nasopharynx. **(E)** Axial T-1 weighted postcontrast image of the nasopharynx. Lymphoid tissue (*L*) enhances well demonstrating the "crypt enhancement pattern" and shows good demarcation from the prevertebral muscles (*M*). The *asterisk* indicates the lateral pharyngeal recess which shows good symmetry bilaterally. The internal carotid artery (*c*) is seen as a signal void due to high flow. Together with the internal jugular vein and the vagus nerve, it lies within the carotid sheath, which forms the posterolateral compartment of the nasopharynx. (B and E, courtesy of Dr. Tan Tiong Yong, Chief of Radiology, Changi General Hospital, Singapore.)

the carotid foramina the fascia reflects medially over the longus colli and rectus capitis muscles.

The pterygopalatine fossa appears on axial and sagittal MRI as a flat space filled with high-signal fat. The cortical margins of the clivus and the basisphenoid show no signals; however, the fatty marrow within gives a characteristic high signal. Any infiltration of these marrow spaces will be delineated on MRI.

Pathology of the Nasopharynx

Pathology in the nasopharynx may arise from any of its constituents, including the epithelium, soft tissue, neural, vascular, etc., and even metastatic disease from anywhere else in the body. **Table 43.1** lists the wide spectrum of pathologies encountered in the nasopharynx; however, most of them are rare and beyond the scope of this chapter. Some common and significant lesions encountered in the authors' practice are elaborated in this chapter.

Epithelial

Nasopharyngeal Carcinoma

NPC, although rare in the West, is endemic in East Asia. NPC is the most common type of malignancy of the nasopharynx encountered in our practice. It has a distinctive geographic distribution, clustering in the south of China and southeast Asia, with increased incidence also

Table 43.1 Pathologies in the Nasopharynx

Inflammatory	**Neoplastic epithelial**	**Fibrous and fibrohistiocytic**
Nasopharyngitis/Adenoiditis	Schneiderian papilloma	Fibroma
Granulomatosis	Nasopharyngeal carcinoma	Fibromatosis (Desmoid tumor)
Tuberculosis	Sinonasal undifferentiated carcinoma	Benign fibrous histiocytoma
Sarcoidosis	Salivary-type tumors	Malignant fibrous histiocytoma
Leprosy	Low-grade adenocarcinoma	Fibrosarcoma
Rhinoscleroma	Intestinal type adenocarcinoma	Myxoma and fibromyxoma
Fungal	Small cell neuroendocrine carcinoma	**Muscle**
Nonneoplastic	Carcinoid tumor	Rhabdomyoma
Lymphoid hyperplasia	**Neuroectodermal**	Rhabdomyosarcoma
Mucus retention cyst	Paraganglioma	Leiomyoma
Tornwaldt cyst/pharyngeal bursa	Schwannoma	Leiomyosarcoma
Wegener's granulomatosis	Neuroma	**Lymphoplasmacytic**
Glial heterotopia and meningo/encephalocele	Ectopic pituitary adenoma	Non-Hodgkin lymphoma
Dermoid cyst	Malignant melanoma	T cell and natural killer cell lymphoma
Respiratory epithelial adenomatoid hamartoma	**Vascular**	Plasmacytoma
Nasal chondromesenchymal hamartoma	Juvenile nasopharyngeal angiofibroma	**Miscellaneous**
Necrotizing sialometaplasia	Hemangioma	Lipoma/sarcoma
Rosai-Dorfman disease	Lobular capillary hemangioma	Meningioma
Amyloidosis	Intravascular papillary endothelial hyperplasia	Craniopharyngioma
	Hemangiopericytoma	Teratoma/carcinoma
	Angiosarcoma	Metastasis
	Kaposi sarcoma and bacillary angiomatosis	

noted in North Africa and in the Inuit. The highest rates are found in Hong Kong, followed by Singapore and Chinese-Americans.[6] In Singapore, NPC occurs in 7% of all malignancies in males and 4.1% of all malignancies in females. It is the fifth and seventh most common cancer in males and females, respectively. NPC affects children, adolescents, and the middle aged. The peak incidence is between 40 and 60 years with a two to three times male predilection.[7]

The etiology of NPC is based on the interaction among genetic susceptibility and environmental factors including carcinogens and the Epstein-Barr virus (EBV).[8] Evidence for a possible oncogenic role for EBV includes ethnic heterogeneity, tumor load dependent elevation in IgA against viral capsid antigen (VCA) and early antigen (Ea), presence of EBV DNA or RNA in all tumor cells, presence of EBV in clonal episomal form (indicating that virus was present before clonal expansion), and/or presence of EBV in the precursor lesion of NPC but not in normal nasopharyngeal epithelium.

Environmental factors have been extensively studied in Hong Kong and China. An association with preserved foods like salted fish, particularly when exposure is very early in life (e.g., in the weaning diet), carries an odds ratio from 2 to 7.5 in various studies.[9]

The nasopharynx is a relatively silent area and many symptoms occur due to either ulceration, mass effect, or by direct infiltration to the surrounding structures. This accounts for the late stage of the disease at initial diagnosis in most cases.

Cervical lymphadenopathy is common in NPC. Often, it is the enlarged neck nodes that prompt initial medical consultation. Seventy-five percent of patients have enlarged cervical nodes at presentation (**Fig. 43.4A**). About 80% of these patients may present with bilateral lymphadenopathy. Nodal metastasis shows an orderly inferior spread, and the affected nodes are larger in the upper neck.[10]

NPC tends to spread submucosally with early infiltration of the palatal muscles, particularly the levator veli palatini, which runs parallel to the eustachian tube. Because this muscle is responsible for opening the eustachian tube orifice during swallowing, dysfunction leads to disequilibrium in the air pressure within the middle ear and the nasopharynx. The eustachian tube orifice may also be obstructed by the tumor itself. These factors commonly result in serous otitis media, which is the second most common presentation of NPC (**Fig. 43.4B**).[11] Bloodstained postnasal discharge is a more frequent symptom, as opposed to frank epistaxis. Unilateral or bilateral nasal obstruction may result from a large nasopharyngeal tumor obstructing the nasal airway (**Fig. 43.4C**). Diplopia due to sixth cranial nerve palsy may be the presenting symptom in some patients. With locally advanced tumors, other problems may arise due to invasion of surrounding structures, such as cranial nerve palsies, facial pain due to trigeminal nerve involvement, and headaches due to meningeal involvement.

Examination of the nasopharynx with flexible or rigid endoscopes often reveals the diagnosis. Most tumors originate in the fossa of Rosenmüller, and obliteration of the fossa is an early sign of malignancy (**Fig. 43.4D**). NPC presents unilaterally in the nasopharynx in 80% of cases with almost equal frequency between right and left. Forty percent occur on the lateral wall, especially in the fossa of Rosenmüller and 30% in the posterior superior wall and the rest on the anterior and inferior aspects of the nasopharynx.

The neoplasm may appear as a polypoidal, ulcerative, or an infiltrative lesion. Rarely, the disease may be a submucosal lesion, and the overlying mucosa may appear normal. Any mucosal irregularity in this situation is treated with deep suspicion, and a biopsy of the region performed.

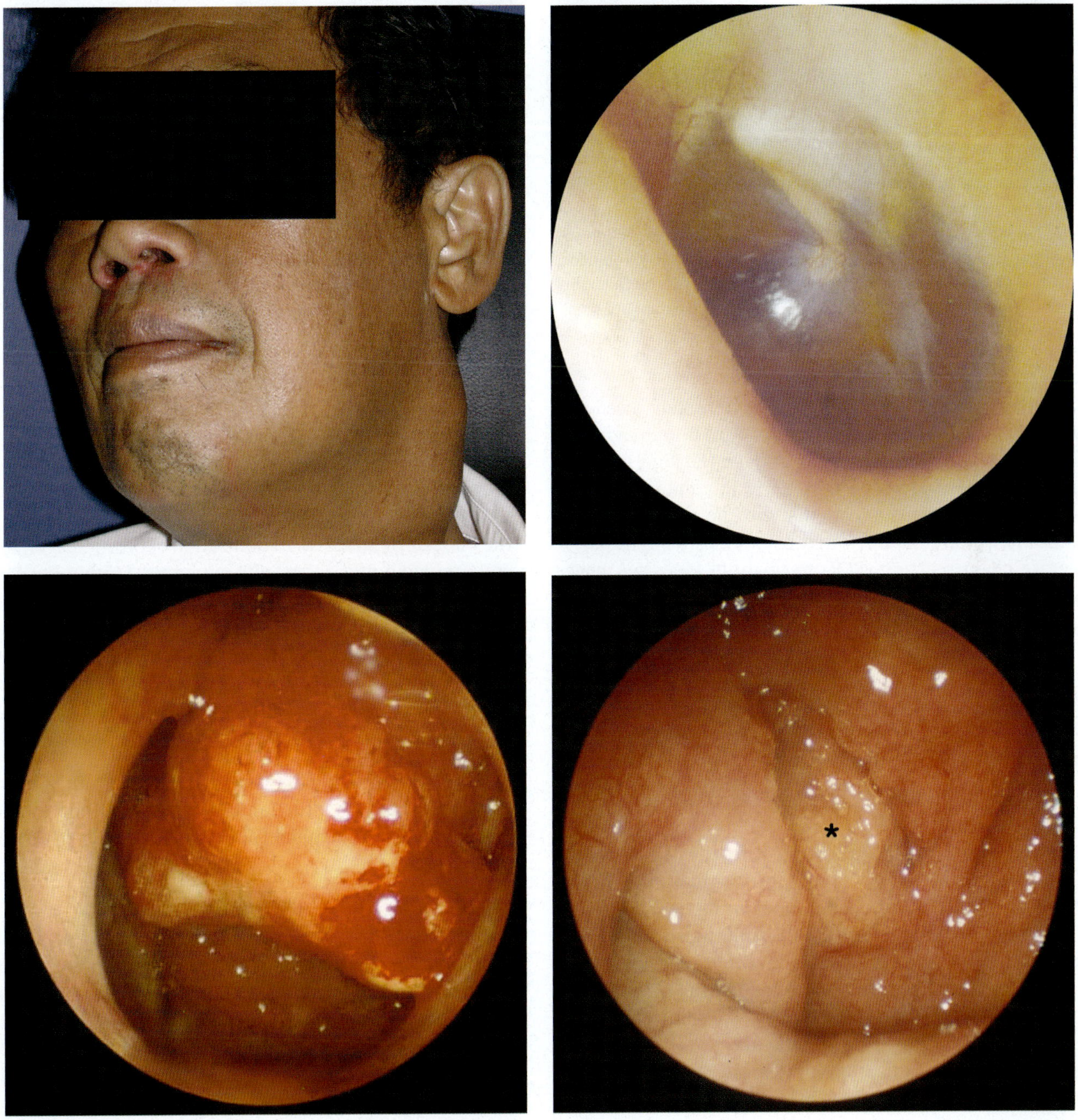

A B C D

Fig. 43.4 A 52-year-old Chinese man presenting with **(A)** left cervical lymphadenopathy and **(B)** left middle ear effusion noted to have **(C)** an exophytic nasopharyngeal mass on endoscopic examination. Histology of the lesion was reported as undifferentiated carcinoma. **(D)** Endoscopic examination showing effacement of the right lateral pharyngeal recess. Biopsy revealed an undifferentiated carcinoma. *(continued)*

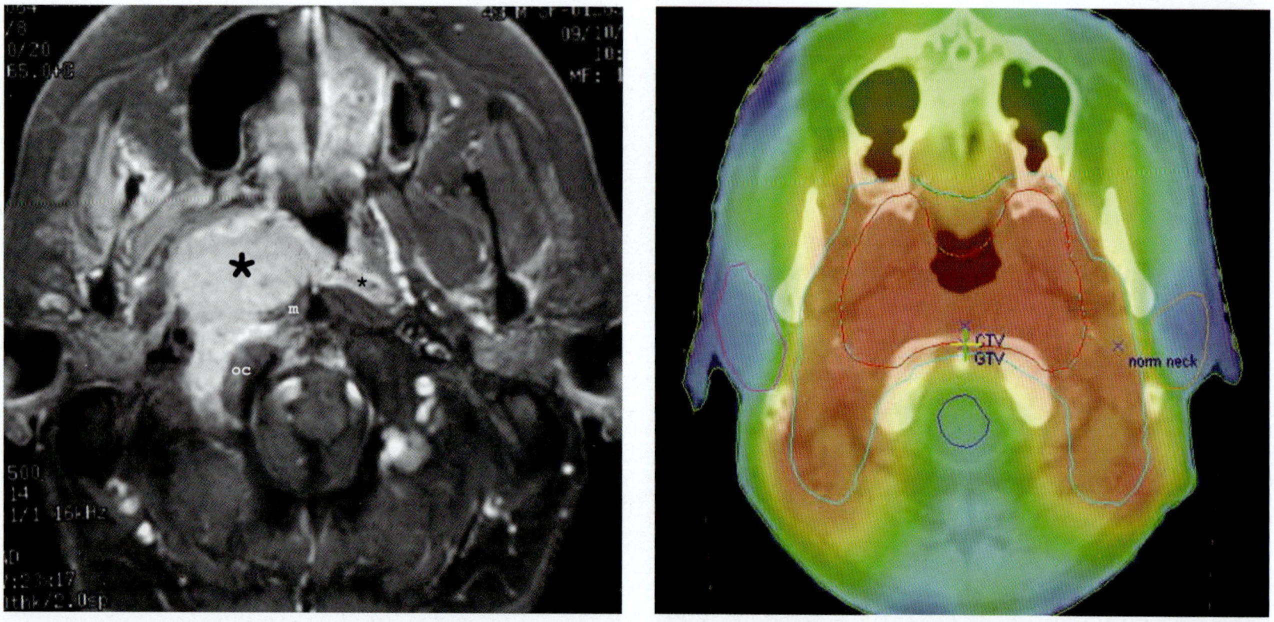

E F

Fig. 43.4 *(continued)* **(E)** Axial postcontrast T-1 weighted magnetic resonance image showing lateral and posterior extension of nasopharyngeal carcinoma. Note the normal fossa of Rosenmüller on the left (*small asterisk*). The lateral pharyngeal recess on the right is effaced by a large tumor extending laterally to the parapharyngeal space and posteriorly to the prevertebral muscles (*m*) and around the occipital condyle (*oc*). **(F)** Intensity modulated radiotherapy for NPC. (E, courtesy of Dr. Tan Tiong Yong, Chief of Radiology, Changi General Hospital, Singapore; F, courtesy of Dr. Joseph Wee, Department of Radiation Oncology, National Cancer Center, Singapore.)

Serologic markers for EBV are extensively used in endemic areas. Viral capsid antigen (VCA) immunoglobulin A (IgA) is sensitive but early antigen (EA) IgA is more specific, so both are used frequently in combination for screening of suspicious patients with no definite lesion clinically.[12] More sophisticated techniques using a polymerase chain reaction (PCR) to quantify EBV DNA have been found to be useful for diagnosis and posttreatment surveillance, as titers are related to tumor load.[13]

Spread of Nasopharyngeal Carcinoma

NPC spreads along well-defined routes. The following pattern of spread may be observed in various combinations.

Anterior Spread

Tumors often spread anteriorly into the nasal fossa. The tumor may infiltrate the pterygopalatine fossa (PPF) through the sphenopalatine foramen. The earliest sign of involvement of the PPF is obliteration of the normal fat content. This can be readily observed on CT and MRI. Once the tumor is in the PPF, the tumor may extend in all directions. Posteriorly, the tumor may extend along the foramen rotundum and the vidian canal, laterally into the infratemporal fossa, and superiorly to the inferior orbital fissure, superior orbital fissure, and the orbital apex. From the superior orbital fissure, tumor spread may continue posteriorly into the cavernous sinus.

Lateral Spread

Lateral spread results in infiltration of PPS. This is the most common direction of spread. This can be recognized by the partial or complete effacement of the fat-filled PPS (**Fig. 43.4E**). Further lateral spread takes the tumor into the masseteric space (MS). Infiltration of the medial or lateral pterygoid muscles results in trismus. Within the MS, the mandibular nerve is vulnerable to perineural infiltration and subsequent intracranial extension. Posterolateral spread into the retrostyloid compartment may result in the infiltration of the carotid space.

Posterior Spread

NPC not infrequently infiltrates the prevertebral muscles (**Fig. 43.4E**). Destruction of the vertebral bodies and involvement of the spinal canal is occasionally observed in late cases.

Superior Spread

Skull base erosion may be detected in up to one-third of patients.[14] The most common route of intracranial spread is through the foramen ovale and not foramen lacerum as previously thought.[14] Dural thickening along the floor of the middle cranial fossa may be the first sign of intracranial infiltration. Tumor may also infiltrate the mandibular nerve, gasserian ganglion, trigeminal nerve, and pons. This often results in denervation atrophy of the muscles of mastication. All these ways of spread can lead to infiltration of the cavernous sinus, placing cranial nerves III, IV, ophthalmic division of V, and VI at risk. When tumor spreads posterolaterally into the jugular foramen and posterior cranial fossa, palsies of cranial nerves IX, X, and XI cranial nerves may become evident.

Distant Metastasis

NPC shows a high frequency of distant metastasis compared with other tumors of the head and neck. The most common site of metastasis is bone (20%), followed by lung (13%) and liver (9%).[15]

There are three histologic types of NPC according to the classification of the World Health Organization (WHO): type 1 is keratinizing squamous cell carcinoma (SCC); type 2 is nonkeratinizing SCC; and type 3 is undifferentiated carcinoma. WHO type 3 is the predominant type found among Asians.

Histologically, nonkeratinizing tumors comprise solid sheets, irregular islands, dyscohesive sheets, and trabeculae of carcinoma intermingled with lymphocytes and plasma cells. In the undifferentiated subtype, syncytial-appearing large cells with indistinct borders and vesicular nuclei may be crowded with overlapping. In the differentiated subtype, there is cellular stratification and pavementing, often with a plexiform growth pattern. An abundance of infiltrating lymphocytes and plasma cells may appear to break up the epithelial component into small clusters, aptly termed in these cases, lymphoepithelial carcinoma. The prognosis for both the differentiated and undifferentiated subtypes is similar. Keratinizing tumors are similar histologically to SCC of the other head and neck sites. Their association with EBV is controversial and association with human papillomavirus has been proposed. Their prognosis is worse than nonkeratinizing tumors with poorer response to radiation with or without chemotherapy.

Staging of Nasopharyngeal Carcinoma

Staging is according to the AJCC TNM system. It is based on both clinical and radiologic criteria. Cross-sectional imaging with either CT scans or MRI is the mainstay for primary staging workup of NPC. MRI is superior in being able to detect the tumor, and its use is slowly becoming more widespread. The role of positron emission tomography (PET) scans is currently still investigational. A little more than half of patients will have stage III and IV disease at diagnosis and ~5% of patients will have distant metastases at initial presentation. Metastatic screen is performed with an X-ray or CT for the lungs, ultrasound or CT of the liver, and a bone scan.

Treatment of Nasopharyngeal Carcinoma

The primary treatment of NPC is radiotherapy. Radiosensitivity of NPC is dependent on histologic type. The WHO type 1 or keratinizing SCC is less sensitive and holds a poorer prognosis.[16,17] Endemic NPC in East Asia or the undifferentiated type carries a better prognosis with 5-year survivals in the range of 60%.[18] The use of chemotherapy concurrent with radiotherapy (RT) has been a major advancement in the treatment of NPC. Prospective randomized trials of chemo-RT have shown superior results when RT is administered with concurrent cisplatin. Overall 5-year cure rates are now in the region of 70%. Chemo-RT is now the standard of care for patients with stage III and IV NPC.

The acute side effects of radiotherapy include xerostomia, mucositis, and dermatitis. Late effects of irradiation may include endocrine sequelae, radiation caries, and soft tissue fibrosis. The most severe complications of radiation are the neurologic sequelae, including cranial nerve palsies and temporal lobe necrosis. The median reported incidence of these severe complications is ~1 to 5%. Primary tumor control, after conventional radiotherapy techniques, is ~72%.[19] Several strategies are available to improve these results. These include intracavitary brachytherapy, the use of a "parapharyngeal boost" for tumors that have infiltrated into the parapharyngeal space, and stereotactic radiosurgery as a boost following conventional RT.

The use of intensity modulated radiotherapy (IMRT) and inverse treatment planning has revolutionized RT for NPC and other head and neck cancers (**Fig. 43.4F**). Excellent tumor control with the added advantage of sparing normal tissues like the parotid glands have been consistently reported. Surgical salvage nasopharyngectomy is reserved for highly selected subpopulations of recurrent NPC.

Nasopharyngeal Adenocarcinomas (Fig. 43.5)

Primary nasopharyngeal adenocarcinomas (NPACs) are a rare but generally recognized category of neoplasms, constituting only 0.38 to 0.48% of all malignant nasopharyngeal neoplasms and 0.70% of all NPCs. They may be classified by their morphologic features and clinical behavior into two main categories: the mucosal surface origin type[20] and the salivary gland type.[21] Most NPACs of mucosal surface origin have a papillary configuration, are of low grade rather than high grade, and can be identified by their light microscopic appearance. The mean age of patients is 38 years and incidences are higher in females than males. Treatment is usually surgery and prognosis is excellent.

Salivary gland type of NPACs arise in the submucosal seromucous salivary glands and are more aggressive than low-grade papillary NPACs. Patients with these tumors are generally older (mean age of 51 years), and incidence is slightly higher in males than in females. Examples include adenoid cystic carcinomas, mucoepidermoid carcinomas, and adenocarcinomas not otherwise classified. The behavior of this tumor entity is unpredictable, which makes an individually tailored therapeutic approach difficult.

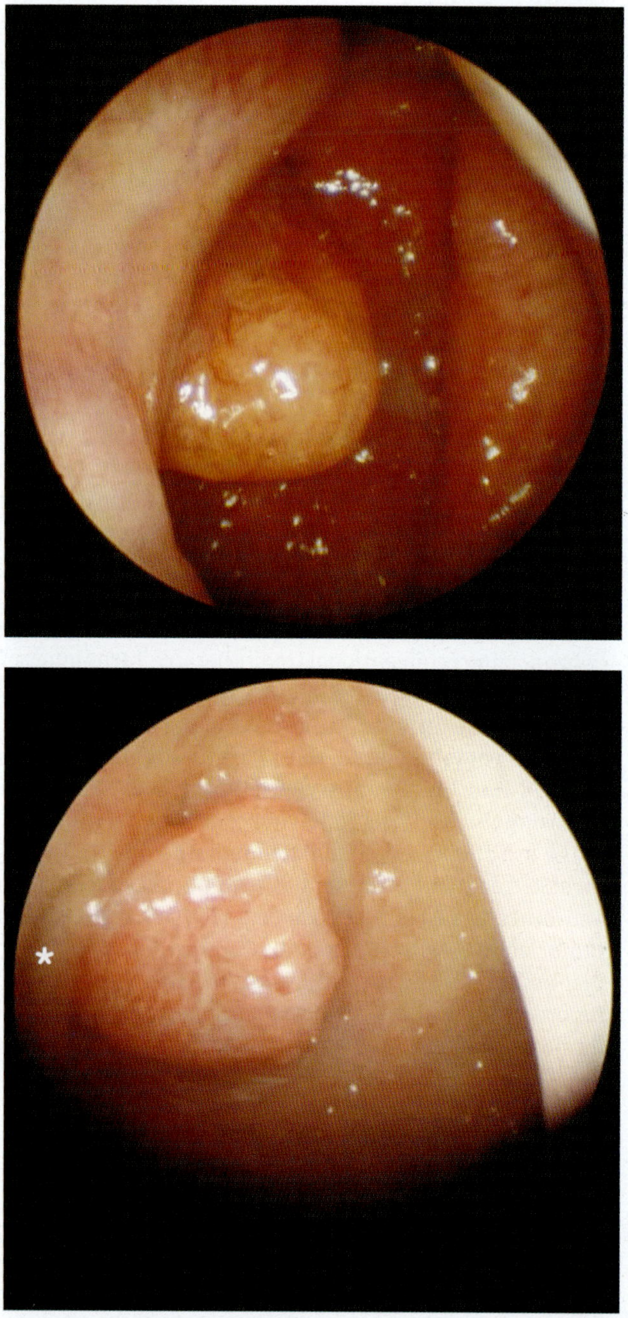
A
C

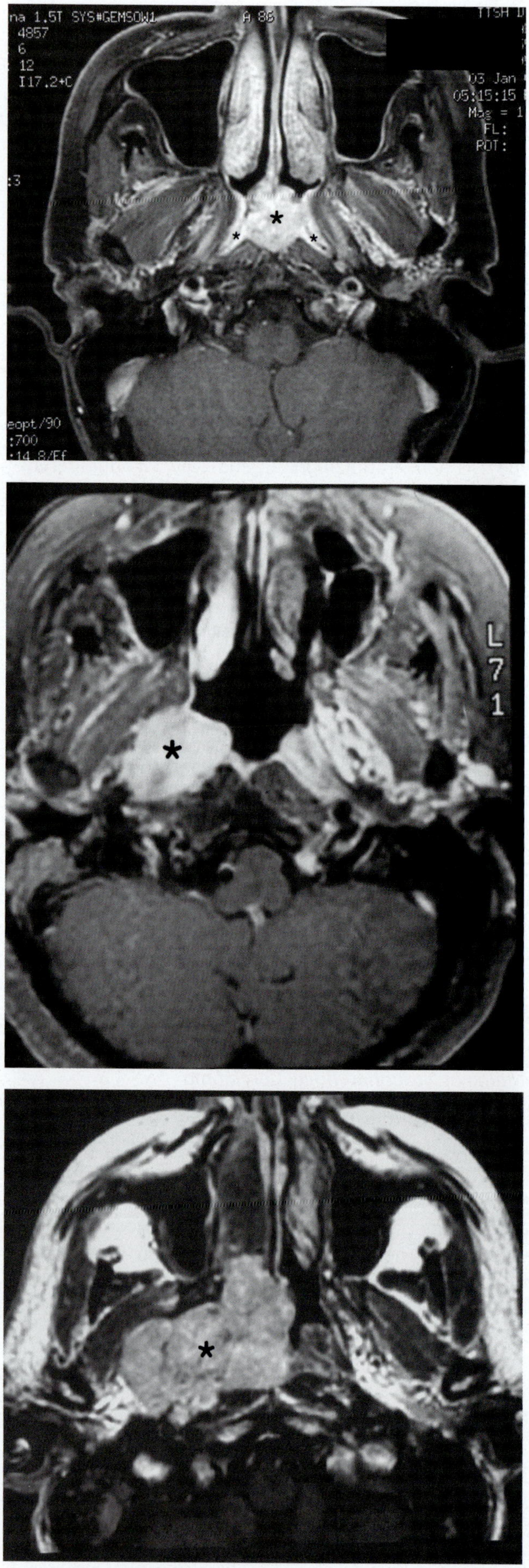

B
D
E

Fig. 43.5 **(A)** Nasopharyngeal mass in a patient complaining of nasal obstruction that arises from the right wall of the nasopharynx (endoscopic view from the left side). Biopsy revealed a low-grade adenocarcinoma. This patient underwent an endoscopic nasopharyngectomy. **(B)** Axial T-1 weighted postcontrast magnetic resonance image showing an enhancing midline mass (*large asterisk*), bilaterally sparing the fossa of Rosenmüller (*small asterisk*). **(C)** A fleshy tumor seen arising from the right lateral pharyngeal recess in a patient complaining of throat discomfort. Nasopharyngeal carcinoma (NPC) was suspected. Biopsy revealed an adenoid cystic carcinoma. *White asterisk* indicates the right eustachian tube orifice. **(D)** The mass (*asterisk*) enhances postcontrast and is indistinguishable from NPC. Note that the mass, however, is not infiltrating the surrounding tissue. This patient underwent an endoscopic nasopharyngectomy with adjuvant postoperative radiotherapy. **(E)** Axial T1-weighted postcontrast scan showing an enhancing mass (*asterisk*) extending laterally to the parapharyngeal space, anteriorly to the nasal cavity, and posteriorly to the carotid space. (B and E courtesy of Dr. Tan Tiong Yong, Chief of Radiology, Changi General Hospital, Singapore.)

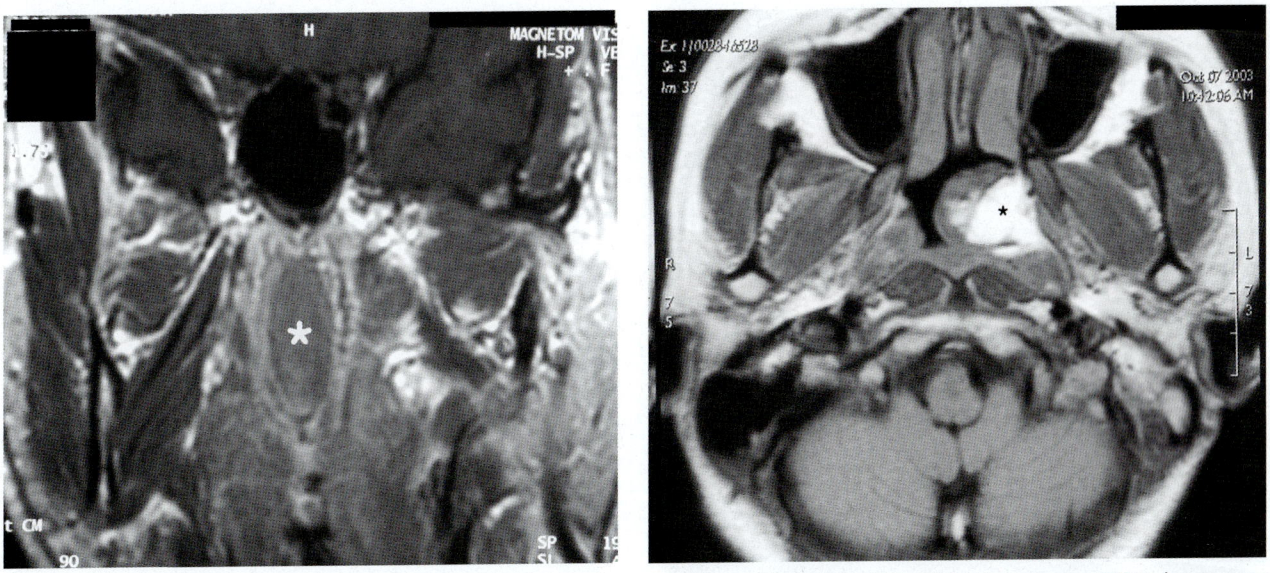

Fig. 43.6 (A) Coronal T-1 weighted postcontrast magnetic resonance image (MRI) of the nasopharynx showing a low signal intensity, nonenhancing midline mass (*asterisk*). The cyst was marsupialized endoscopically. **(B)** This 32-year-old Chinese woman was noted to have an incidental nasopharyngeal mass. Outpatient biopsy of the mass was reported as chronic inflammation. A subsequent MRI study was done. Axial T-1 weighted noncontrast MRI shows a mass arising from the left lateral wall of the nasopharynx. Note the high signal area (*asterisk*) indicating the fatty component of the lesion. Patient underwent endoscopic nasopharyngectomy. Histology of the mass was reported as immature teratoma. (Courtesy of Dr. Tan Tiong Yong, Chief of Radiology, Changi General Hospital, Singapore.)

The treatment options of these tumors may vary depending on clinical stage, histologic grade, and histomorphology. These tumors exhibit aggressive local invasion with perineural and vascular spread distant from the primary tumor. Surgery is the treatment of choice when possible. Tumor-free margins are an important prognostic factor. Often, this is not possible due to diffuse infiltration and perineural spread. Postoperative radiation is generally recommended in such situations.

Nasopharyngeal Cysts

Nasopharyngeal cysts are an uncommon entity, often encountered as an incidental finding. These may occur in the midline or may have lateral origin.

Tornwaldt's cyst occurs in the midline bursa of the nasopharynx, and represents the notochord remnants communicating with the pharyngeal endoderm. They occur on the upper border of the superior constrictor muscle. These cysts may remain asymptomatic or may cause symptoms like nasal obstruction, headaches, postnasal discharge, and eustachian tube dysfunction when the cyst is inflamed. MRI is the imaging modality of choice for Tornwaldt's cysts (**Fig. 43.6A**). The signal intensity is bright on both T1- and T2-weighted images because of either high protein content of the cyst or a hemorrhage within the cyst.[22] Treatment of the cyst involves excision or wide marsupialization of the cyst under general anesthesia.

Nasopharyngeal teratomas (**Fig. 43.6B**) and dermoids are very rare congenital tumors that most commonly arise from the midline or lateral nasopharyngeal wall.

Inverted Papillomas

Inverted papillomas (IPs) are benign epithelial growths arising from the underlying stroma of the nasal cavity or paranasal sinuses. The majority of IPs originate in the lateral nasal wall or sinuses and may extend to the nasopharynx. The nasopharynx as the primary site for origin of IP is extremely rare. The senior author has encountered only one case. Diagnosis was made following a biopsy of a nasopharyngeal mass (**Fig. 43.7**). Treatment is surgical removal with a wide margin. This patient underwent an endoscopic partial nasopharyngectomy.

Vascular

Juvenile Nasopharyngeal Angiofibroma

Juvenile nasopharyngeal angiofibroma (JNA) is a highly vascular and locally invasive tumor that has a high incidence of persistence and recurrence. These tumors are believed to arise in the fibrovascular stroma present in the posterolateral wall of the nasal roof where the sphenoidal process of the palatine bone meets the horizontal ala of the vomer and the pterygoid process. Initially, the tumor grows in the submucosa of the nasopharyngeal roof, reaching the septum and posterior aspect of the nasal space, and creating a mass effect that may cause nasal airway obstruction. As the process continues, the anterior face of the sphenoid sinus is eroded and invaded. The tumor may grow forward into the nasal fossa and may expand the posterior end of the middle turbinate, which

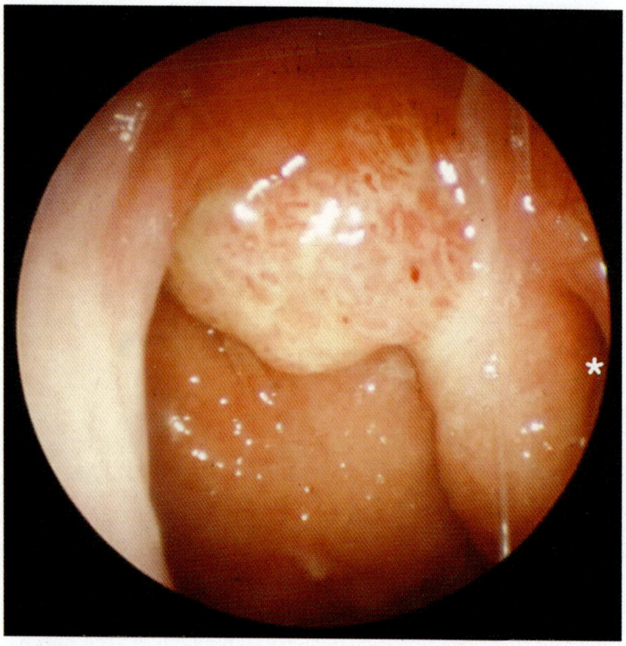

Fig. 43.7 A papillomatous lesion arising from the roof of the nasopharynx. Endoscopic view shown is from the left side of the nasal cavity. Clinically, a nasopharyngeal carcinoma was suspected. *White asterisk* indicates a left eustachian tubal orifice. Biopsy was reported as an inverting papilloma. No other papillomatous lesion was found in the nasal cavity or paranasal sinuses. This lesion was isolated to the nasopharynx. An endoscopic wide excision (partial nasopharyngectomy) was performed for this patient.

A

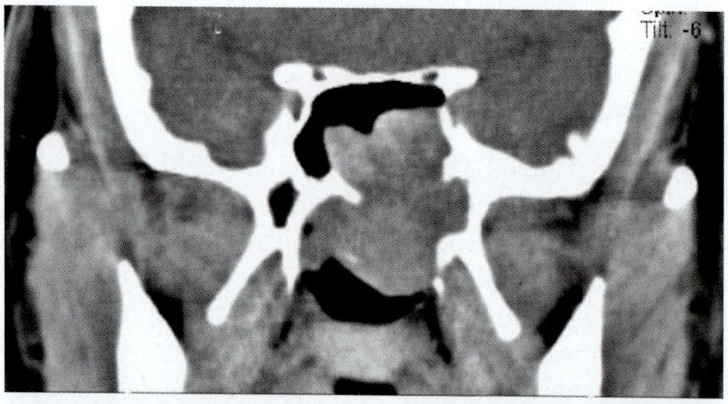

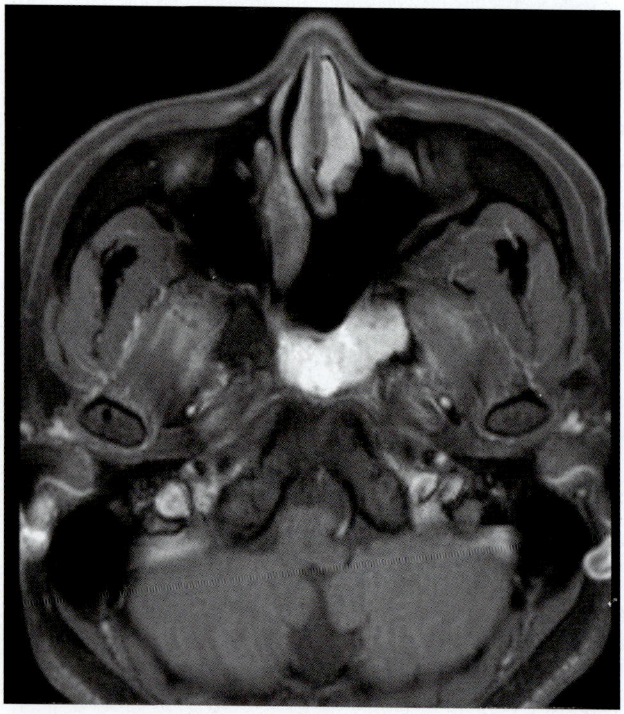

B

C

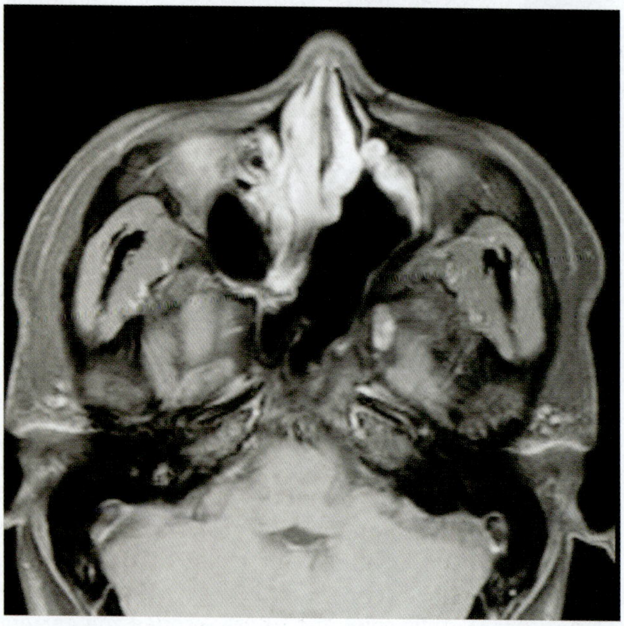

Fig. 43.8 **(A)** Coronal computed tomography scan shows residual mass eroding the roof of the nasopharynx and effacing the sphenoid sinus, following a lateral rhinotomy approach for the removal of juvenile nasopharyngeal angiofibroma (JNA). **(B)** Axial T1-weighted postcontrast magnetic resonance image (MRI) showing a brightly enhancing mass in the nasopharynx. **(C)** Axial T-1 weighted postcontrast MRI scan following endoscopic nasopharyngectomy for recurrent JNA in Fig. 43.8B.

thereby becomes continuous with the mass of tumor. Laterally, angiofibroma may extend to the pterygomaxillary fossa and may cause bowing of the posterior wall of the maxillary sinus and distortion and posterior displacement of the pterygoid plates. Eventually, the tumor may involve the infratemporal fossa, orbit, and middle cranial fossa.

Patterns of spread to local structures may be widely unpredictable and do not always follow a stepwise progression. During initial evaluation, contrast CT and MRI reliably assess tumor extent. Angiography is useful as an adjunct to diagnosis but, more importantly, to decrease tumor vascularity during surgery by embolization. Surgery remains the treatment of choice for JNA. Many surgical approaches have been used, including transpalatal, transzygomatic, transmandibular, transhyoid, and transantral approaches; lateral rhinotomy; midface degloving; and concomitant craniotomy. In the past decade, endoscopic transnasal surgery for confined lesions has generated interest. Whether the approach is open or endoscopic, the complete surgical resection should be attempted. **Figure 43.8** shows an example of a patient who had residual angiofibroma in the roof of the nasopharynx following a lateral rhinotomy approach. This patient underwent an endoscopic nasopharyngectomy for the removal of the residual angiofibroma.

Lymphoplasmacytic

Non-Hodgkin Lymphoma

Nasopharyngeal non-Hodgkin lymphoma (NHL) accounts for 2.5% of all extranodal NHLs (**Fig. 43.9**). There is frequently concomitant involvement of the nasal cavity or the rest of Waldeyer's ring. In the West, the majority of cases are B cell lymphomas with a median age of 63 years and a male to female ratio of 1.2:1. Unlike the T cell lymphomas, there is only a weak association between diffuse large B cell lymphoma (DLBCL) with EBV. DLBCL has a propensity for lymph node spread from extranodal sites. The differential diagnosis is NPC, especially when the lymphocytes form tight clusters. Differentiation is with immunohistochemistry, with positive CD20 for DLBCL and cytokeratin for NPC. Treatment is with chemotherapy and/or RT. Results are better than for T cell lymphomas.

Sinonasal T Cell and Natural Killer Cell Lymphoma (Angiocentric Lymphoma, Polymorphic Reticulosis)

As opposed to in the West, in Asia, only 50 to 60% of NHL are from the B cell lineage. There is a higher incidence of T cell and NK cell lymphomas. More than 95% are associated with EBV regardless of the ethnic background. The median age is lower at 53 years, with a male predilection of 3:1. There is a higher tendency to disseminate to skin, gastrointestinal (GI) tract, liver, lymph nodes, and the testes compared with DLBCL. Prognosis is worse than with B cell lymphomas. Treatment is with RT, which achieves a survival of 30 to 50%.

Plasmacytoma: Extramedullary Plasmacytoma

Extramedullary plasmacytomas (EMPs) are isolated neoplasms that represent less than 10% of all plasma cell tumors (**Fig. 43.10**). An EMP originates from a submucosal plane and may be associated with bone destruction from an advancing margin. EMPs manifest in the head and neck in more than 80% of all cases.[23] Approximately 18% of head and neck extramedullary plasmacytomas occur in the nasopharynx. It is the second most common site. They usually occur in patients between 50 and 60 years of age, and they are more common in men. Both CT and MRI provide valuable information for the diagnosis of these lesions. The primary radiographic differential diagnosis for EMP is that of lymphoma. Plasmacytomas are associated with homogeneous, high-signal intensity on both T1- and T2-weighted MRI scans. Treatment of skull base plasmacytomas relies on the radiosensitivity of the tumor. When complete removal is possible, surgical intervention is an excellent treatment option. For patients with a diagnosis of multiple myeloma and skull base plasma cell tumors, chemotherapy for systemic disease takes precedence.

Bone and Cartilage Tumors: Chordoma

Chordomas are low grade malignant tumors associated with the primitive notochord (**Fig. 43.11**). They account for 4% of malignant bone tumors. About one-third involve the skull base, including the clivus. There is a male predilection with presentation usually in adulthood. Radiology demonstrates lytic destruction of the clivus and patients may have nonspecific symptoms like a headache and nasal obstruction and, with involvement, cranial nerve palsies. Treatment is with resection where possible and radiation for residual or unresectable disease.

Neuroectodermal Tumors: Paraganglioma

Paragangliomas include schwannomas, neurofibromas, and glomus tumors. These tumors rarely arise within the nasopharynx. Paragangliomas more commonly involve the structures within the carotid sheath and may extend to the nasopharynx. Although benign, paragangliomas may cause significant local morbidity due to mass effect and erosion. Small lesions may be an incidental finding on routine examination or imaging. Patients may present with cranial nerve palsies due to skull base involvement caused by the erosive nature of these tumors. Glomus

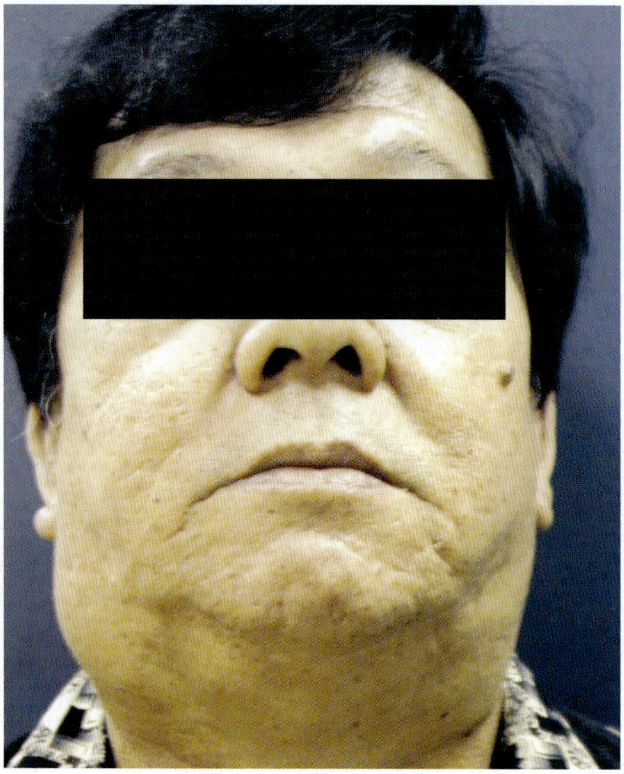

A

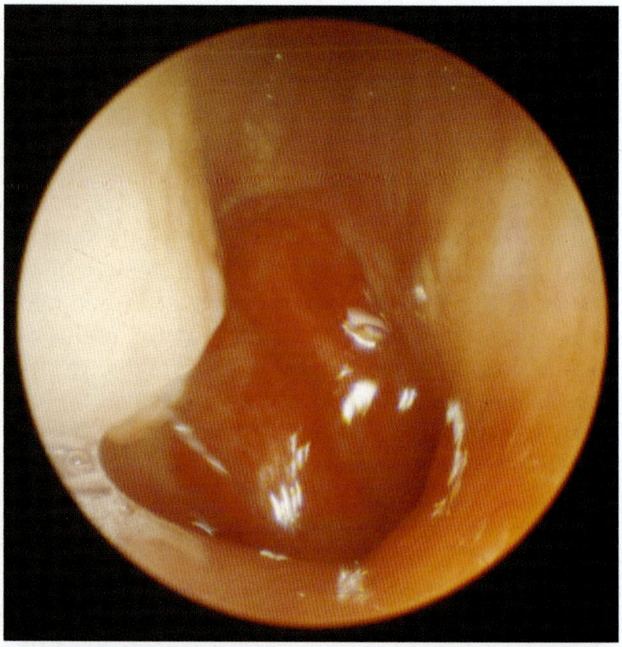

B

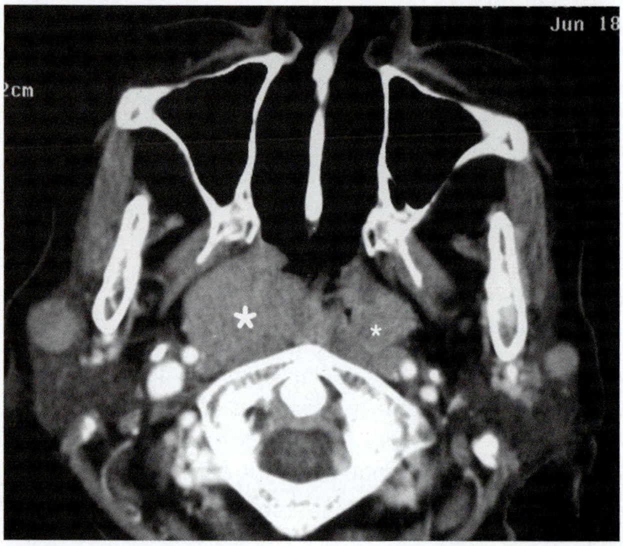

C

Fig. 43.9 **(A)** A chronic smoker of 30 years presented with nasal obstruction and bilateral cervical lymphadenopathy. **(B)** Endoscopic examination of the patient in Fig. 43.9A showed a large smooth surfaced mass occupying the entire nasopharynx and obstructing the posterior choanae bilaterally. Biopsy revealed this mass to be malignant lymphoma. **(C)** Axial computed tomography scan of the patient showing an enhancing mass in the nasopharynx larger (*large asterisk*) on the right than on the left (*small asterisk*). (C, courtesy of Dr. Tan Tiong Yong, Chief of Radiology, Changi General Hospital, Singapore.)

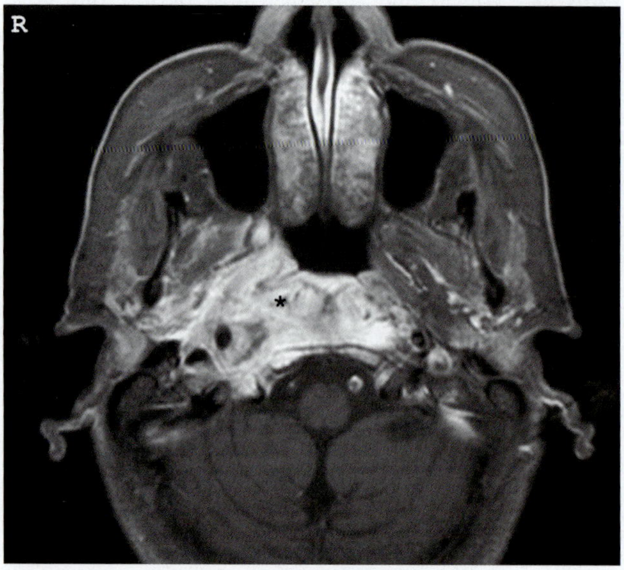

Fig. 43.10 Axial T-1 weighted postcontrast magnetic resonance image shows a diffusely enhancing lesion involving the right nasopharynx, prevertebral muscles, and skull base. Histology was reported as a plasmacytoma. (Courtesy of Dr. Tan Tiong Yong, Chief of Radiology, Changi General Hospital, Singapore.)

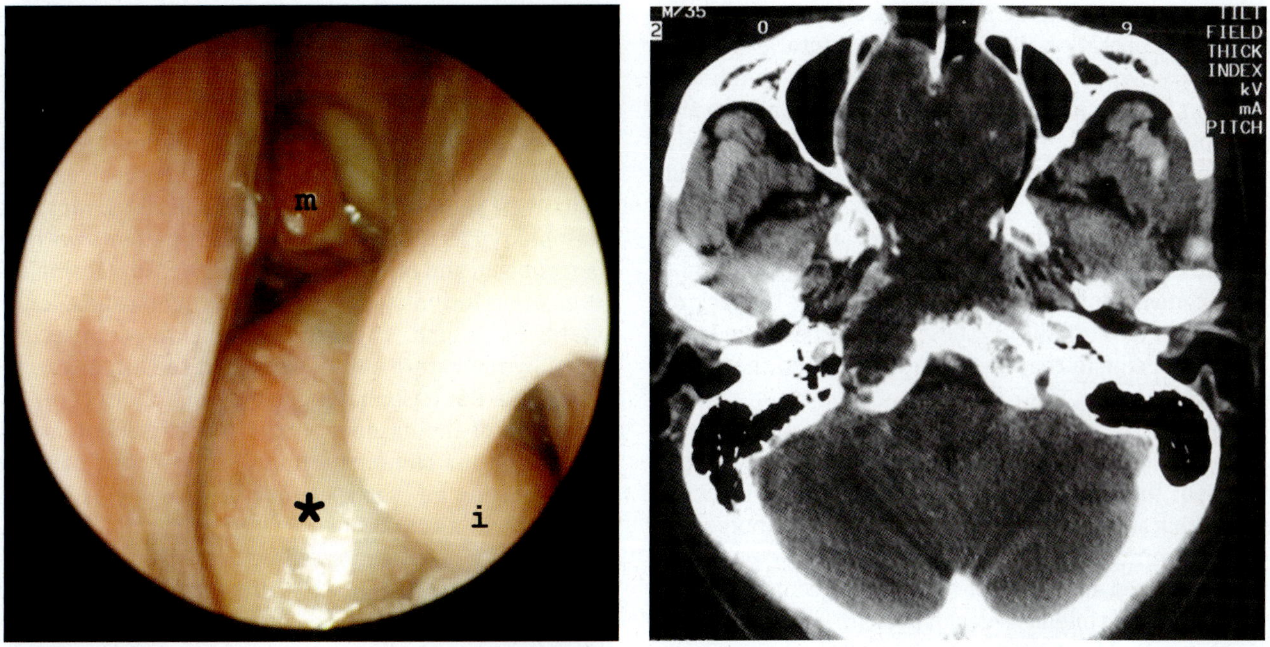

A B

Fig. 43.11 (A) A 35-year-old man presented with bilateral nasal obstruction of a few months' duration. Endoscopic examination showed a large cystic mass (*asterisk*) obstructing the posterior choanae bilaterally and extending anteriorly into the nasal cavity. *m*, middle turbinate; *i*, inferior turbinate. **(B)** Axial computed tomography scan shows an extensive mass lesion involving the clivus and extending anteriorly into the nasal fossa bilaterally. Speckled calcification is seen within the mass. Histology reported as clival chordoma.

tumors typically show a permeative pattern of destruction in contrast to neurofibromas or schwannomas that produce characteristic smooth and scalloped erosions. On MRI, glomus tumors enhance intensely following the administration of contrast material. Complete resection is the treatment of choice.

Fibrous Fibrohistiocytic and Muscle Tumors

This category of tumors is extremely rare and includes benign fibrous histiocytoma, fibromatosis, fibrosarcoma, malignant fibrous histiocytoma, rhabdomyoma, and rhabdomyosarcoma.

Miscellaneous Tumors

Craniopharyngioma

These tumors are believed to arise from the obliterated craniopharyngeal duct of Rathke's pouch, although some have proposed origin from misplaced odontogenic epithelium.

Ectopic Pituitary Adenoma

These tumors are most commonly found in the sphenoid sinus and sphenoid bone. They are believed to arise from the remnants of the embryonic adenohypophysis left along the path of the developing Rathke's pouch. Females are affected more commonly, and 58% of these tumors are functional with hyperactivity. Histology of these adenomas is similar to typical sellar pituitary adenomas. Complete surgical excision is the treatment of choice.

Metastatic Tumors

Metastasis to the nasopharynx is extremely rare. Reported primaries include malignant melanomas and kidney, lung, breast, colon, and cervical cancers. The clinical presentation is dependent on the size and surface integrity. Metastasis naturally implies poor prognosis.

Surgical Approaches to the Nasopharynx

The nasopharynx is situated in an inaccessible location almost right in the middle of the head. The orifice leading most directly to it is the nasal cavity, with access limited largely by the size of the piriform aperture and intranasal protuberances like the inferior and middle turbinates. A further limiting factor is the presence of the nasal septum, which divides half the narrow access. The mouth is the other natural orifice connected with the nasopharynx, but the hard and soft palates present barriers to direct line of sight and instrumentation. Several surgical approaches have been described to overcome this inaccessibility, and they can be classified according to the direction of approach. In the open midline approach, the most direct are transseptal approaches and midfacial degloving with bilateral medial maxillectomies[24,25] or the Denker operation.[26] For improved lateral exposure, a maxillary swing[27] may be performed. From an inferior direction, a transpalatal approach[28] may be adopted if the tumor is largely confined to the midline. This may be combined with a transcervico-mandibulo-palatal or mandibular swing[29,30] if the tongue or mandible is obstructing (e.g., with trismus). The lateral infratemporal fossa approach is technically feasible, but is not a first choice approach due to the difficulty, the lack of exposure, and morbidity.[31] These approaches have been well described and their discussion is beyond the scope of this chapter.

In our practice, indications for a nasopharyngectomy mainly include recurrent NPC, and other benign and malignant tumors such as JNA, IPs, adenocystic carcinomas, adenocarcinomas, and certain skull base tumors such as clival chordomas.

The preferred approach for nasopharyngectomy, in our institution, is the midfacial degloving with bilateral medial maxillectomy. Maxillary swing approach is reserved for tumors with an extensive parapharyngeal component or for tumors that have infiltrated below the level of the hard palate. For recurrent NPC or tumors with minimal lateral extension, we have been performing endoscopic resection since 1997, which will be discussed in the following text (**Fig. 43.12**).

Endoscopic Approach for Nasopharyngectomy

Built on the foundation of endoscopic sinus surgery, endoscopes have been used to perform surgery on most of the regions surrounding the nasopharynx. These include transsphenoidal surgery of the sella and the parasellar region, endoscopic approaches to the pterygopalatine fossa, and the transpterygoid approach to the lateral recess of the sphenoid sinus. More recently, there have been reports on the use of endoscopes to perform surgery on tumors of the nasopharynx.[31,32]

An excellent panoramic view of the nasopharynx may be obtained by removing the entire posterior bony nasal septum. Removal of the entire posterior nasal septum does not cause any external cosmetic deformity because the cartilaginous septum is preserved. Removal of the bony nasal septum allows a better visual angle for resection, facilitates improved lateral reach of the instruments, and allows two surgeons to work together, critical in skull base surgery. One surgeon maintains visualization by navigating the endoscope and controlling the suction, while the second surgeon performs the resection with a retracting instrument and a cutting instrument or drill as necessary. It is possible to extend the operative field superiorly or laterally, as the pathology requires, by removing the floor of the sphenoid sinus or even the clivus and laterally and by removing the posterior maxillary wall and the pterygoid process.

Criticism of this approach is frequently focused on violation of the principle of en bloc resection for cancer, but even with the open approach, a true en bloc resection without breaching the tumor at all is difficult except for small lesions. Tumors that can be removed in a truly en bloc fashion with the open approach can also usually be removed en bloc endoscopically. Endoscopic nasopharyngectomy may be used for patients with recurrent NPC and minimal parapharyngeal extension and even other lesions such as adenocarcinoma and adenoid cystic carcinoma. The extent of the resection is dictated by the nature and the extent of the tumor varying from a partial nasopharyngectomy to a more complete resection of the nasopharynx. Tissue dissection is performed with a combination of diathermy and coblator. The resulting en bloc specimen is the same as in open surgery.

In addition to posterior septectomy, which is routinely done for this approach, exposure to the nasopharynx, if necessary, may be enhanced by bilateral removal of inferior turbinates, the lower aspect of the middle turbinates, and the lateral nasal wall. The posterior wall of the maxillary sinus may be removed to expose the pterygopalatine and infratemporal fossae, often necessary in large JNAs. This enables ligation of the internal maxillary artery and vascular control. The parapharyngeal space can be reached with a transpterygoid approach using a combination of drill and diathermy or coblator. The safety of the internal carotid artery may be enhanced by image guidance.

In a typical endoscopic nasopharyngectomy, we perform a posterior septectomy with bilateral inferior turbinectomies for exposure. We also typically resect widely the anterior face of the sphenoid together with the floor, first as an additional margin of resection but also to decrease the risk of posterior choanal stenosis because the patients are typically radiotherapy failures or recurrences and have a correspondingly increased risk. The limits of resection follow the open approach, taking the ipsilateral eustachian tube across to the contralateral fossa of Rosenmüller. The extent of the lateral resection depends on the tumor.

We have performed endoscopic nasopharyngectomies for tumors of the nasopharynx for selected cases since 1997 (**Table 43.2**). The degree of nasopharyngectomy was dictated by the extent and nature of the tumor. For recurrent NPC a near-complete nasopharyngectomy was attempted sparing the contralateral eustachian tube, whereas for other lesions in **Table 43.2**, a partial nasopharyngectomy and wide excision of the tumor was performed.

Pointers for Tumor Resection and Resurfacing the Nasopharynx

Techniques of resection of tumors in the nasopharynx depend on the site and extent of origin of the lesion.

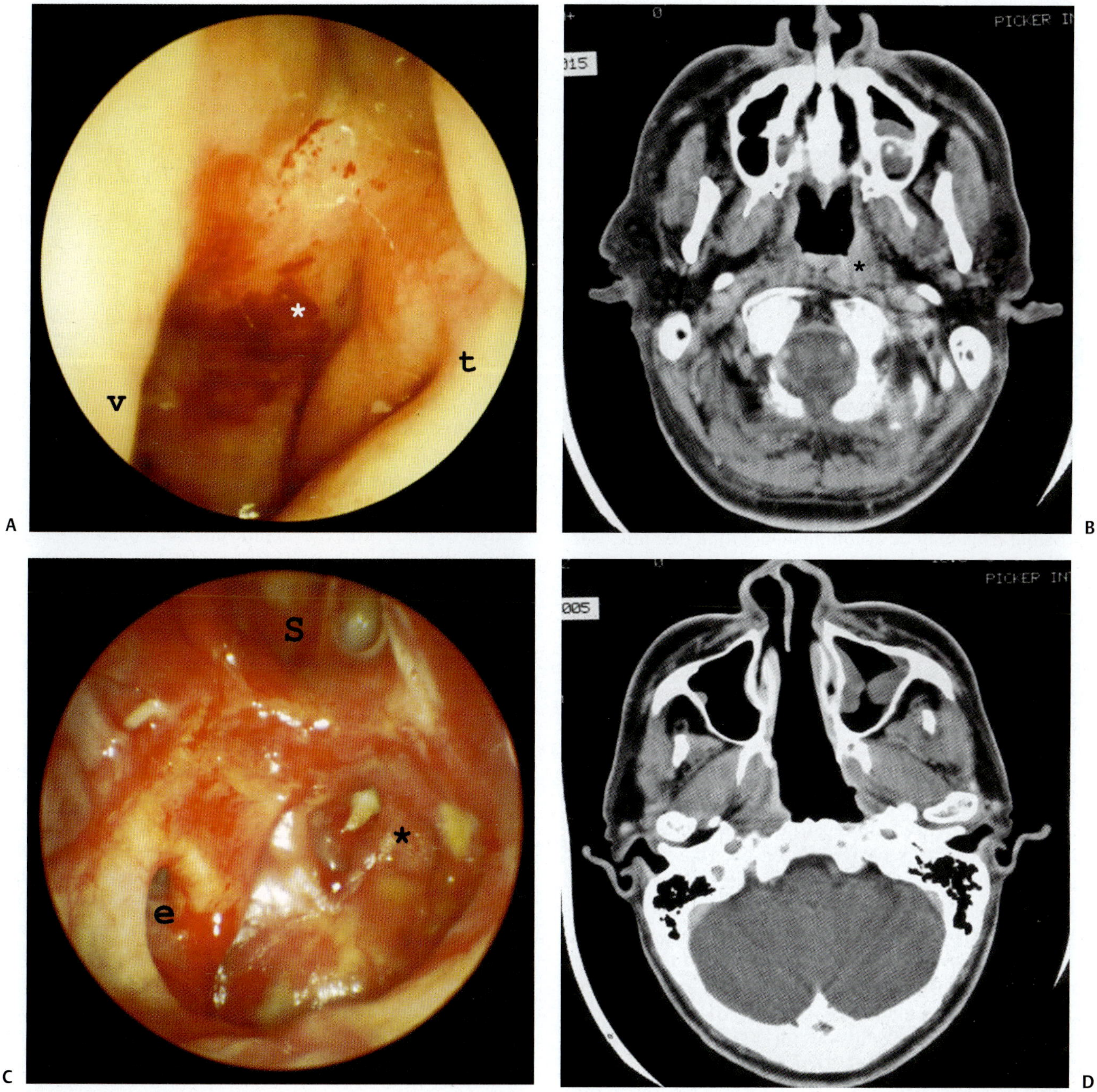

Fig. 43.12 **(A)** Endoscopic view of the twice recurrent nasopharyngeal carcinoma confirmed with a positive histology of undifferentiated carcinoma. Note the bulge of the tumor (*white asterisk*) on the left side of the nasopharynx, the left eustachian tubal orifice (*t*), and the nasal septum (*v*). **(B)** Computed tomography (CT) scan of the patient showing the tumor (*asterisk*) as an enhancing lesion, which is confined to the nasopharynx and does extend to the paranasopharynx. This patient underwent an endoscopic nasopharyngectomy in 1997. **(C)** Postendoscopic nasopharyngectomy 1 year after the surgery. The right eustachian tube (*e*) was preserved. Removal of the posterior nasal septum provided excellent view of the nasopharynx, enabling endoscopic visualization and instrumentation. Resection margins were similar to that with an open approach. Note the sphenoid sinus(*s*) has been opened and roof of the nasopharynx has been removed with a drill. *Asterisk* indicates the site where the tumor was located. **(D)** Postoperative CT scan showing that the tumor has been completely removed. This patient survived 10 years and died of unrelated causes in 2007.

Table 43.2 Endoscopic Nasopharyngectomy

Age (years)	Sex	Diagnosis	Disease-Free Period (Months)	Adjuvant Therapy	Status
65	Female	Adenoid cystic carcinoma	101	RT	NED
46	Male	Inverting papilloma	12	None	NED
70	Male	Adenocarcinoma (low grade)	76	None	NED
23	Male	Juvenile nasopharyngeal fibroma	7	None	NED
45	Male	Recurrent nasopharyngeal carcinoma	120*	None	Deceased*
44	Male	Recurrent nasopharyngeal carcinoma	66	None	Recurred

*Patient died of unrelated causes 10 years after the endoscopic nasopharyngectomy.
Abbreviations: NED, no evidence of disease; RT, radiotherapy.

For lesions like NPC or inverting papilloma, the mucosa obviously cannot be spared. Resection thus would necessitate mucosal removal. In malignant disease, the depth of resection is at least until the clivus is left bare. In benign disease, the depth of resection is determined by the disease, and margins may be controlled with frozen sections. Coverage of the bare clivus is preferred, if possible. This may be accomplished with a free mucosal graft, either harvested from the septum or the inferior turbinate. A better alternative to this would be a vascularized posterior pedicled septal mucosal flap based on the posterior septal branch of the sphenopalatine artery. This needs to be harvested before the septectomy and may be tucked unobtrusively into the sphenoid or maxillary sinuses.[33] A pedicled mucosal flap from the inferior turbinate has been described, but this may not be ideal due to its tendency to stay folded and its relative thickness.[34] The caveat for both pedicled flaps is that the margins of the resection must not encroach on the flap or pedicle, which is posteriorly based. This may be an issue in NPC involving the roof of the nasopharynx or the posterior choana.

Postoperatively, the nasopharynx may be packed in a variety of ways. We typically use flavine-soaked roller gauze or bismuth iodoform paraffin paste (BIPP) pack for open approaches and Gelfoam (Baxter Healthcare, Hayward, CA) with sponge packs like Merocel (Medtronic, Mystic, CT) for endoscopic surgery. To retain a free mucosal graft or free flap, a urinary catheter balloon may be used in the nasopharynx, taking care not to excessively compress the flap with overinflation.

Complications

Complications may arise from the approach and the resection. Generic complications like cerebrospinal fluid (CSF) leak and orbital injury are addressed in other chapters and will not be repeated here. Intraoperative bleeding may occur from vascular trauma. This will be discussed briefly.

Vascular Injury

The sphenopalatine or internal maxillary arteries may be injured both during the access or tumor resection. Avoidance is an exercise in preoperative preparation. The proximity of the lesion to the sphenopalatine foramen or pterygopalatine fossa should be identified on preoperative scans. If there is significant encroachment into these territories, it is prudent to widen the access laterally and ligate the artery proximal to the tumor. This decreases the vascularity of the tumor during surgery and also allows the vessel to be addressed under controlled conditions. An alternative is preoperative intra-arterial embolization.

Injury of the internal carotid artery is the most feared complication in nasopharyngectomy. In the open approach, digital palpation is possible, but this is not so in the endoscopic approach. If there is no oncologic necessity to skeletonize the internal carotid artery (ICA), image guidance may be used to control the lateral extent of resection. If it is necessary, the ICA may be protected with a blunt malleable retractor medially after dissection from the neck. In these cases, coverage of the ICA is necessary. Traditionally, we have used a free radial forearm flap for coverage, but this requires a maxillary swing to allow insetting and anastomosis. A good alternative now is the posteriorly based septal flap, which can even be used in the endoscopic setting.

Osteoradionecrosis

With the exception of cases with free flap coverage, there will be some exposed bone in the nasopharynx after nasopharyngectomy. As these patients have undergone radiotherapy or even chemoradiation, healing is impaired and the underlying bone may have an element of radionecrosis. Re-epithelialization is slow and crusting and infection is common. Osteomyelitis of the clivus may occur, occasionally spreading intracranially to present as meningitis. Routine coverage of the bare clivus would probably decrease the incidence of this complication. This is now easily accomplished, at least partially, with a posterior septal flap, which compares favorably to a free radial forearm flap.

Conclusion

The nasopharynx presents a challenge to access. Pathology involving this area is varied but uncommon in the West. However, nasopharyngeal carcinoma is endemic in East Asia, where nasopharyngectomies are routinely performed for primary site recurrence. Traditionally, surgery of the nasopharynx requires wide, invasive access, but with development of advanced endoscopic techniques, nasopharyngectomy can be accomplished transnasally without compromising oncologic principles. Lateral extension may be reached via a transpterygoid approach. Although image guidance is useful, a good understanding of the three-dimensional surgical anatomy of this region is important. The advent of the nasoseptal flap has further enhanced the repertoire of the endoscopic surgeon, allowing for the resurfacing of exposed vessels and, potentially, osteonecrotic bone (e.g., internal carotid artery, clivus) after tumor resection, without the need for a free radial forearm flap.

References

1. Young LS, Rickinson AB. Epstein-Barr virus: 40 years on. Nat Rev Cancer 2004;4(10):757–768
2. Babić MS. Development of the notochord in normal and malformed human embryos and fetuses. Int J Dev Biol 1991;35(3): 345–352
3. Edge S, Byrd D, Compton C, Fritz A, Greene F, Trotti A, eds. American Joint Committee on Cancer Staging Manual, 7th ed. New York: Springer; 2010
4. Silver AJ, Mawad ME, Hilal SK, Sane P, Ganti SR. Computed tomography of the nasopharynx and related spaces. Part I: Anatomy. Radiology 1983;147(3):725–731
5. Chong VF, Khoo JB, Fan YF. Imaging of the nasopharynx and skull base. Neuroimaging Clin N Am 2004;14(4):695–719
6. Parkin DM, Whelan DL, Ferley J, et al, eds. Cancer Incidence in Five Continents, Vol VII. Lyon, IARC No 143, 1997
7. Chia KS, Lee HP, Seow A, et al. Trends in Cancer Incidence in Singapore 1968–1992. Singapore: Singapore Cancer Registry; 1996
8. Choi PHK, Suen MW, Huang DP, Lo KW, Lee JC. Nasopharyngeal carcinoma: genetic changes, Epstein-Barr virus infection, or both. A clinical and molecular study of 36 patients. Cancer 1993;72(10):2873–2878
9. Yu MC, Ho JH, Lai SH, Henderson BE. Cantonese-style salted fish as a cause of nasopharyngeal carcinoma: report of a case-control study in Hong Kong. Cancer Res 1986;46(2):956–961
10. Chong VFH, Fan YF, Khoo JBK. MRI features of cervical nodal necrosis in metastatic disease. Clin Radiol 1996;51(2):103–109
11. Hsu MM, Young YH, Lin KL. Eustachian tube function of patients with nasopharyngeal carcinoma. Ann Otol Rhinol Laryngol 1995; 104(6):453–455
12. Low WK, Leong JL, Goh YH, Fong KW. Diagnostic value of Epstein-Barr viral serology in nasopharyngeal carcinoma. Otolaryngol Head Neck Surg 2000;123(4):505–507
13. Lo YM, Chan LY, Chan AT, et al. Quantitative and temporal correlation between circulating cell-free Epstein-Barr virus DNA and tumor recurrence in nasopharyngeal carcinoma. Cancer Res 1999;59(21):5452–5455
14. Chong VFH, Fan YF, Khoo JBK. Nasopharyngeal carcinoma with intracranial spread: CT and MR characteristics. J Comput Assist Tomogr 1996;20(4):563–569
15. Sham JST, Cheung YK, Chan FL, Choy D. Nasopharyngeal carcinoma: pattern of skeletal metastases. Br J Radiol 1990;63(747):202–205
16. Hoppe RT, Williams J, Warnke R, Goffinet DR, Bagshaw MA. Carcinoma of the nasopharynx—the significance of histology. Int J Radiat Oncol Biol Phys 1978;4(3-4):199–205
17. Shanmugaratnam K, Chan SH, de-Thé G, et al. Histopathology of nasopharyngeal carcinoma: correlations with epidemiology, survival rates and other biological characteristics. Cancer 1979;44(3): 1029–1044
18. Lee AW, Sze WM, Au JS, et al. Treatment results for nasopharyngeal carcinoma in the modern era: the Hong Kong experience. Int J Radiat Oncol Biol Phys 2005;61(4):1107–1116
19. Fong KW, Chua EJ, Chua ET, et al. Patient profile and survival in 270 computer tomography-staged patients with nasopharyngeal cancer treated at the Singapore General Hospital. Ann Acad Med Singapore 1996;25(3):341–346
20. Wenig BM, Hyams VJ, Heffner DK. Nasopharyngeal papillary adenocarcinoma. A clinicopathologic study of a low-grade carcinoma. Am J Surg Pathol 1988;12(12):946–953
21. Schramm VL Jr, Imola MJ. Management of nasopharyngeal salivary gland malignancy. Laryngoscope 2001;111(9):1533–1544
22. Christmas DA Jr, Yanagisawa E, Mirante JP. Endoscopic view of obstructing nasopharyngeal cysts (Tornwaldt's cysts). Ear Nose Throat J 2007;86(10):591–592
23. Miller FR, Lavertu P, Wanamaker JR, Bonafede J, Wood BG. Plasmacytomas of the head and neck. Otolaryngol Head Neck Surg 1998;119(6):614–618
24. Browne JD. The midfacial degloving procedure for nasal, sinus, and nasopharyngeal tumors. Otolaryngol Clin North Am 2001;34(6): 1095–1104, viii
25. To EWH, Teo PML, Ku PKM, Pang PCW. Nasopharyngectomy for recurrent nasopharyngeal carcinoma: an innovative transnasal approach through a mid-face deglove incision with stereotactic navigation guidance. Br J Oral Maxillofac Surg 2001;39(1): 55–62
26. Hardillo JA, Vander Velden LA, Knegt PP. Denker operation is an effective surgical approach in managing juvenile nasopharyngeal angiofibroma. Ann Otol Rhinol Laryngol 2004;113(12): 946–950
27. Wei WI, Ho CM, Yuen PW, Fung CF, Sham JS, Lam KH. Maxillary swing approach for resection of tumors in and around the nasopharynx. Arch Otolaryngol Head Neck Surg 1995;121(6): 638–642
28. Enepekides DJ, Donald PJ. Transoral approaches to the clivus and nasopharynx. Otolaryngol Clin North Am 2001;34(6): 1105–1121, ix
29. Morton RP, Liavaag PG, McLean M, Freeman JL. Transcervico-mandibulo-palatal approach for surgical salvage of recurrent nasopharyngeal cancer. Head Neck 1996;18(4):352–358

30. Moreira-Gonzalez A, Pieper DR, Cambra JB, Simman R, Jackson IT. Skull base tumors: a comprehensive review of transfacial swing osteotomy approaches. Plast Reconstr Surg 2005;115(3):711–720
31. Yoshizaki T, Wakisaka N, Murono S, Shimizu Y, Furukawa M. Endoscopic nasopharyngectomy for patients with recurrent nasopharyngeal carcinoma at the primary site. Laryngoscope 2005; 115(8):1517–1519
32. Chen MK, Lai JC, Chang CC, Liu MT. Minimally invasive endoscopic nasopharyngectomy in the treatment of recurrent T1-2a nasopharyngeal carcinoma. Laryngoscope 2007;117(5): 894–896
33. Hadad G, Bassagasteguy L, Carrau RL, et al. A novel reconstructive technique after endoscopic expanded endonasal approaches: vascular pedicle nasoseptal flap. Laryngoscope 2006;116(10): 1882–1886
34. Fortes FSG, Carrau RL, Snyderman CH, et al. The posterior pedicle inferior turbinate flap: a new vascularized flap for skull base reconstruction. Laryngoscope 2007;117(8):1329–1332

44 Cerebrospinal Fluid Leaks and Encephaloceles

Bradford A. Woodworth and Rodney J. Schlosser

Over 20 years ago, neurologic surgeons were primarily responsible for managing cerebrospinal fluid (CSF) leaks and meningoencephaloceles extending into the nasal cavity from the anterior and middle cranial fossae. Neurosurgeons performed skin incisions with craniotomies, retracting the brain to seal defects from above the cranial base. Subsequently, widespread experience with endoscopic instrumentation has allowed minimally invasive operations on the skull base through the nose with decreased morbidity. Now, skull base defects and encephaloceles of the sinus and nasal cavities have been repaired with high success rates using these accepted endoscopic techniques for nearly 20 years. Success rates of over 90% are quoted in multiple patient series, where it has truly become the standard of care in routine CSF leaks of the anterior skull base.[1-3]

Classification, Etiology, and Pathophysiology

Most CSF leaks can be broadly classified into site of CSF leak and etiology. Although the etiology will influence the size and structure of the bony defect, degree and nature of the dural disruption, intracranial pressure, and meningoencephalocele formation, the site of skull base defect will determine the surgical approach. These factors greatly influence medical and surgical treatment and predict long-term success.

Trauma (Accidental and Iatrogenic)

Traumatic CSF leaks may result from blunt or penetrating trauma. Traumatic disruption of the skull base can create an obvious CSF leak or may present years later with meningitis, delayed leak, or encephaloceles. Projectile injuries from bullets, shotgun blasts, or shrapnel can result in significant comminution of the skull base, and are more likely to involve intracranial injury.[4] Although conservative, nonsurgical measures are often adequate for limited injuries to the skull base, such as closed head trauma, there is a reported 29% incidence of meningitis with long-term follow-up of CSF leaks that are managed nonsurgically.[5]

Functional endoscopic sinus surgery (FESS) and neurologic surgery are the two most common surgeries leading to iatrogenic skull base defects. Bone resection near the skull base, especially with powered instrumentation, can create significant defects. Areas of the skull base that are particularly vulnerable include the lateral lamella of the cribriform plate and the posterior wall of the frontal sinus, which are less than 1 mm thick. An expansile mucocele or tumor can also create a dehiscence in the skull base that is more susceptible to iatrogenic CSF leak during instrumentation.

CSF leak following neurologic surgery can occur during a craniotomy if the superior or lateral recess of the frontal sinuses is entered upon removal of the bony plate. Individuals with extensive pneumatization are at higher risk. Furthermore, skull base defects secondary to intracranial tumor removal can develop anywhere along the skull base.

Spontaneous

In this subset of patients, successful repair rates are dismal with recurrences reported anywhere from 25 to 87% over time.[6] Fortunately, knowledge and experience with idiopathic/spontaneous CSF leaks has increased dramatically over the last decade.[4,7-11] The majority of these patients exhibit clinical symptoms and radiographic signs of elevated intracranial pressure (ICP). Normal ICP is ~10 to 15 cm H_2O pressure. Woodworth et al. found elevated ICPs via lumbar drains or lumbar puncture in 45 out of 48 patients with available ICP measurements (average ICP of 27 cm H_2O) in the largest series to date of surgically repaired spontaneous CSF leaks ($n = 56$).[12]

Elevated ICP most commonly manifests itself in the syndrome of benign intracranial hypertension (BIH), also known as pseudotumor cerebri. Patients with BIH will present clinically with pulsatile tinnitus, balance problems, headache, and visual disturbances. Prior studies have indicated that the "spontaneous" etiology of patients most often represents a variant of BIH according to modified Dandy criteria.[10] Evaluating radiographic, clinical, and ICP data for the most rigid diagnosis of BIH reveals that more than 70% of spontaneous leak patients meet these diagnostic criteria. Radiographically, many of these patients have total or partial empty sella syndrome (ESS) caused by dural herniation through the sellar diaphragm into the sella turcica up to 85% of the time.[12,13] The sella has the radiographic appearance of an absent pituitary gland because it fills with CSF (**Fig. 44.1**). Other radiologic findings associated with elevated ICP include encephaloceles, arachnoid pits, abnormalities of the optic nerve sheath complex, dilated Meckel's caves, and dural ectasia.[12]

There are several clinical similarities between patients with high-pressure spontaneous CSF leaks and those with

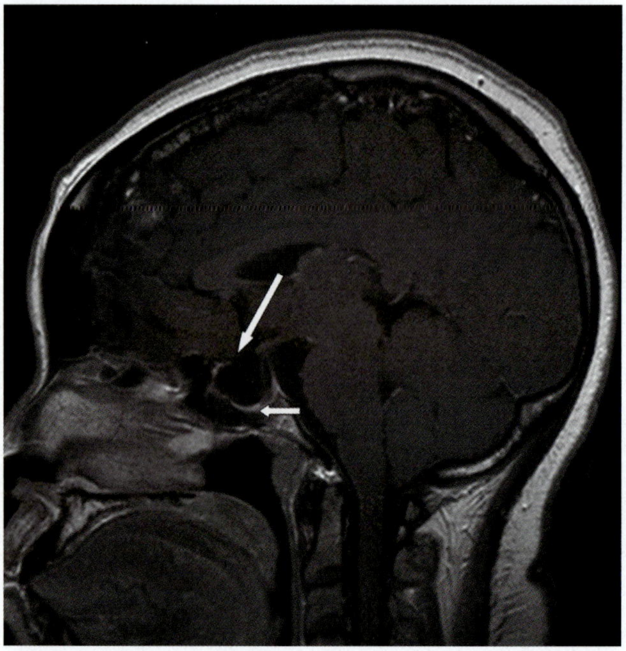

Fig. 44.1 Sagittal T1-weighted magnetic resonance image demonstrating an empty sella identified in a spontaneous cerebrospinal fluid (CSF) leak patient. The *long arrow* indicates the CSF-filled sella, whereas the *short arrow* points to the compressed sliver of remnant pituitary gland.

BIH. In terms of demographics, the majority of patients who develop the diagnosis of BIH are obese, middle-aged women. In one study, 77% of patients with spontaneous CSF leaks were women.[12] Furthermore, the average body mass index (BMI) was 36.2 with 46 of 55 patients considered obese with a BMI >30. The association of obesity with BIH has been reported in many studies.[14,15] Radhakrishnan et al.[14] calculated an increase in incidence to 21.4 per 100,000 for obese females with a BMI of 30, ~10- to 20-fold of the incidence in the total population. Thus, the large body habitus seen in patients with spontaneous CSF leaks indicates a potential role for obesity in the underlying pathophysiology and suggests that this patient population is a likely variant of BIH.

Although there are several theories postulated to explain the relationship between obesity and elevated ICP, the pathophysiology of the disease is currently unknown. One common theory behind the association of obesity and elevated ICP is that excess weight in the central compartment of the body leads to high intra-abdominal pressures. An increase in intra-abdominal pressure raises ICP by decreasing cerebral venous return to the heart. This obstructs cerebral venous outflow, thereby raising cerebral blood volume and increasing ICP by preventing normal CSF absorption. This theory is supported by several studies showing that morbidly obese patients have both higher intra-abdominal pressures and a higher incidence of BIH than nonobese patients.[16] Furthermore, these morbidly obese patients likely have a higher propensity for sleep apnea. Thus, altered respiratory mechanics associated with hypoxemia during sleep may trigger cerebral vasodilation and increases in cerebral blood volume. These changes could potentially create sustained elevations in ICP.[17]

Obesity may also cause neuroendocrine disturbances from extraovarian production of estrone in adipose tissue. Androstenedione conversion to estrone increases exponentially when body weight exceeds 50% over the ideal body weight.[18] A relative hypoadrenalism could then alter the drainage channels and vacuolar transport across the arachnoid villi and increase resistance to CSF outflow.

Given that the prevalence of obesity is as high as 16% in the population, one would expect spontaneous CSF leaks to be much more common if obesity were the major inciting factor in elevated ICP.[12] Given the current epidemic of obesity in the developed world, it is possible that we may also see a significant increase in the incidence of spontaneous CSF rhinorrhea. Ultimately, an additional etiologic factor, such as an underlying anatomic abnormality of the arachnoid villi, must be present to account for this discrepancy.

Regardless of the underlying mechanism leading to an elevated ICP, constant pulsatile pressure applied to the skull base over time ultimately leads to erosion at sites of inherent structural weakness. Examples of this include the dura of the sellar diaphragm, perforations in the cribriform plate, and adjacent to natural foramina of the skull base. Although spontaneous leaks rarely occur in the frontal sinus, they are more likely to occur immediately adjacent to the frontal recess in thin areas of the ethmoid roof or anterior cribriform plate. The most common area for spontaneous CSF leaks and encephaloceles is in the lateral recess of the sphenoid sinus.[12] Arachnoid villi in the lateral skull base provide another site of inherent weakness, leading to arachnoid pits and thinning of the skull base (**Fig. 44.2**). Until recently, these latter areas were relatively undocumented.[11] Herniation of temporal lobe tissue often occurs through a middle cranial fossa defect lateral to the foramen rotundum and vidian canal. These patients have excessive pneumatization of the pterygoid process with an attenuated sphenoid sinus recess roof and skull base, thus increasing the likelihood of defects developing in the floor of the middle fossa.[19] It is possible that individuals with a thicker skull base could manifest as BIH, whereas those who have developed thinning of the skull base in areas such as these result in CSF rhinorrhea.

Neoplasms

Sinonasal and skull base tumors can create CSF leaks directly through erosion of the anterior cranial fossa or middle cranial fossa, or indirectly secondary to therapeutic treatments for the tumor. Persistent malignant tumor following resection and repair will continue to erode the skull base and create a CSF leak. Developing a watertight seal between the sinonasal and intracranial cavities after tumor removal can be challenging. If the tumor is

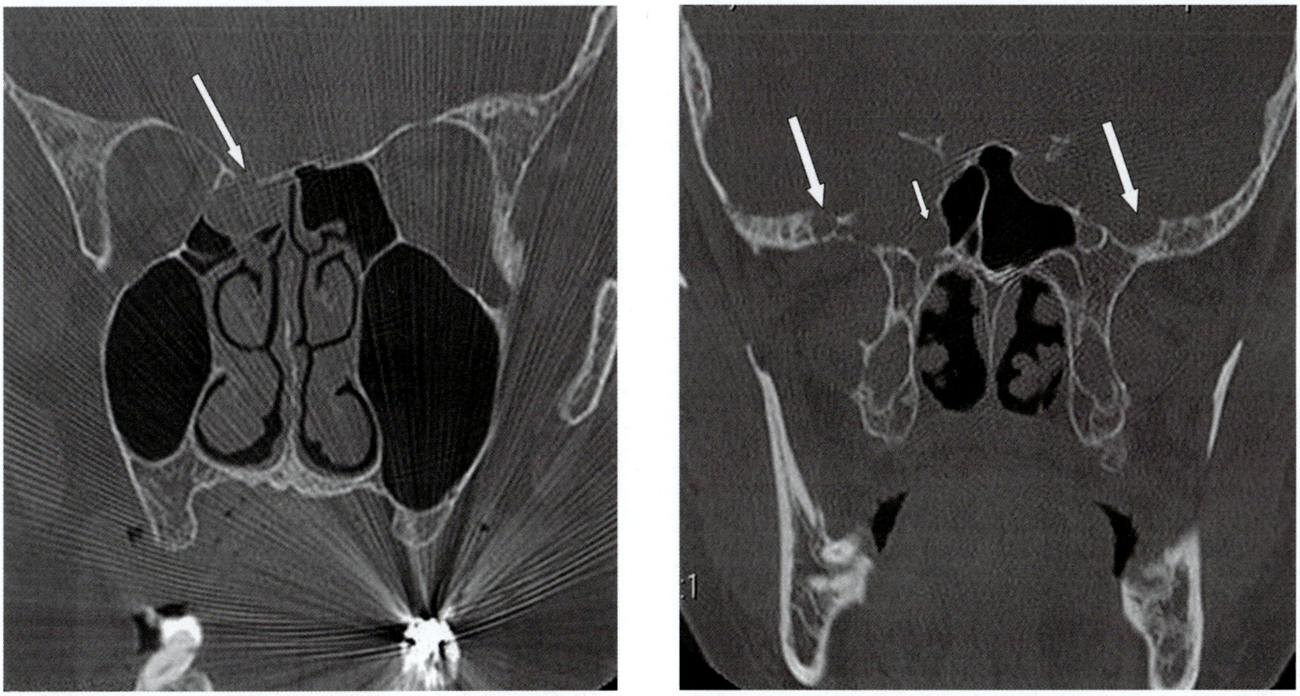

A B

Fig. 44.2 Coronal computed tomography scan images of an obese man with cerebrospinal fluid (CSF) rhinorrhea and elevated intracranial pressure. This patient has multiple spontaneous CSF leaks and encephaloceles. An encephalocele is visualized within the right posterior ethmoid where there is thinning and attenuation around the skull base defect (*arrow* **[A]**). In the middle cranial fossa **(B)**, he has multiple erosions in the lateral skull base (*large arrows*) and a large lateral encephalocele (*small arrow*). Arachnoid pits in the middle cranial fossa represent weaknesses for focal erosions secondary to chronic elevated intracranial pressure. Meningeal diverticula can occur next to the natural foramina, such as foramen rotundum lateral to the sphenoid sinus.

approached intracranially, a pericranial flap is often used to create a barrier. CSF leaks may still occur due to tears in the flap that occur during elevation, devascularization, and necrosis, or from inadequate coverage. Posterior table defects and frontal sinus floor defects (after cranialization) may still be present after coverage and contribute to a CSF leak. Fortunately, very large defects can still be repaired via an endoscopic approach (**Fig. 44.3**). Prior chemotherapy or radiation can lead to significant healing difficulties due to poor vascularity of the wound bed.

Congenital

Congenital encephaloceles were initially divided by Suwanwela and Suwanwela[20] into sincipital (also referred to as anterior or frontoethmoidal) and basal encephaloceles. The basal type encephaloceles are intranasal in location and have been variously described as transethmoidal, sphenoethmoidal, sphenomaxillary, spheno-orbital, transsphenoidal, and transtemporal.[21] Clinically, the cribriform niche adjacent to the vertical attachment of the middle turbinate anteriorly and the superior and lateral walls of the sphenoid appear to be the most common sites for these congenital defects.[22]

Transsphenoidal encephaloceles are the only congenital type found in the sphenoid sinus, of which there are two main varieties: the intrasphenoidal and the true transsphenoidal.[11] The former describes those extending into the sphenoid sinus but confined by its floor. The latter represents encephaloceles that traverse the floor of the sphenoid sinus and protrude into the nasal cavity or nasopharynx. The true transsphenoidal-type encephaloceles that are transmitted through the sphenoid bone correspond to the median cleft face syndrome and will most commonly have coexisting abnormalities of the face, optic system, and brain.[23] In addition, these encephaloceles may be associated with hypothalamic-pituitary dysfunction. High surgical risks may be encountered with transsphenoidal encephaloceles in the early infantile period because the pituitary-hypothalamic structures are usually incorporated in the herniated encephalocele of this age group.[24] Congenital facial anomalies are subtle or absent and diagnosis may be delayed until rhinorrhea occurs, a visual field defect becomes evident, hormonal deficiency is noted, or an epipharyngeal mass is discovered. In adults, the intrasphenoidal type of congenital encephalocele has reportedly had a good outcome with transsphenoidal repair, but a true transsphenoidal meningoencephalocele must be viewed with caution, because of the involvement of vital structures and complexity of distorted anatomy.[11]

Transethmoidal encephaloceles usually originate at the foramen cecum and typically have a deviated crista galli and variable posterior extension into the cribriform or ethmoid roof (**Fig. 44.4**). These are thought to be secondary to failure of closure of the fonticulus frontalis during development.[22] The second type is typically an isolated ethmoid roof defect with a normal foramen cecum. The skull base in these patients is extremely low-lying and they often have a funnel shaped bony defect. The anterior location of these defects and small nasal cavities due to presentation at a young age makes surgical repair more difficult.

Although it can be helpful to separate congenital encephaloceles into categories for research and descriptive purposes, it is important to note that bony dehiscences are found in 14% of ethmoid bones in anatomic studies,[22] and congenital defects can occur at any point in the skull base. Although these defects are present since birth, they may not be diagnosed clinically until the patient presents with CSF leak, meningitis, facial deformity, or nasal obstruction.

Diagnosis and Preoperative Tests

The current diagnostic studies and preoperative imaging that are available for the localization of CSF leaks permit accurate identification with minimal operative morbidity. Preoperative tests should be individualized for each patient and tailored toward the clinical picture. Furthermore, the invasiveness of the diagnostic test and the risks to the patient should be taken into account.

Beta-2 Transferrin

Prior to any surgical intervention, it is important to firmly establish the diagnosis of CSF leak to differentiate CSF rhinorrhea from other causes of rhinorrhea. The most commonly accepted method of differentiating CSF from nasal secretions is testing for beta-2 transferrin. This is a very reliable, accurate, and noninvasive method to establish the diagnosis of an active CSF leak with a low incidence of

A

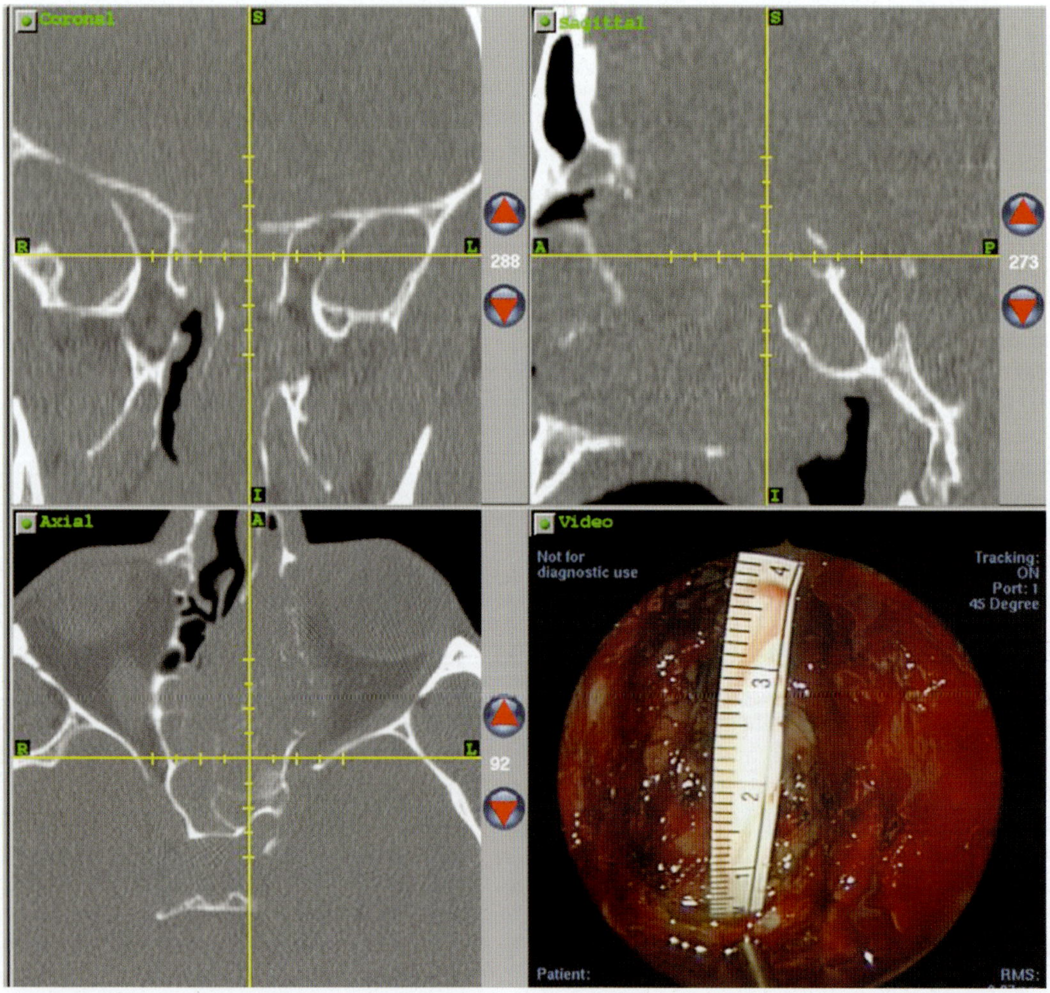

Fig. 44.3 Image-guided triplanar computed tomography imaging **(A)** of a large skull base defect following endoscopic resection of an esthesioneuroblastoma. This defect extended from the posterior table of the frontal sinus to the planum sphenoidale in an anteroposterior direction and from the junction of the medial orbital wall and skull base bilaterally. *(continued)*

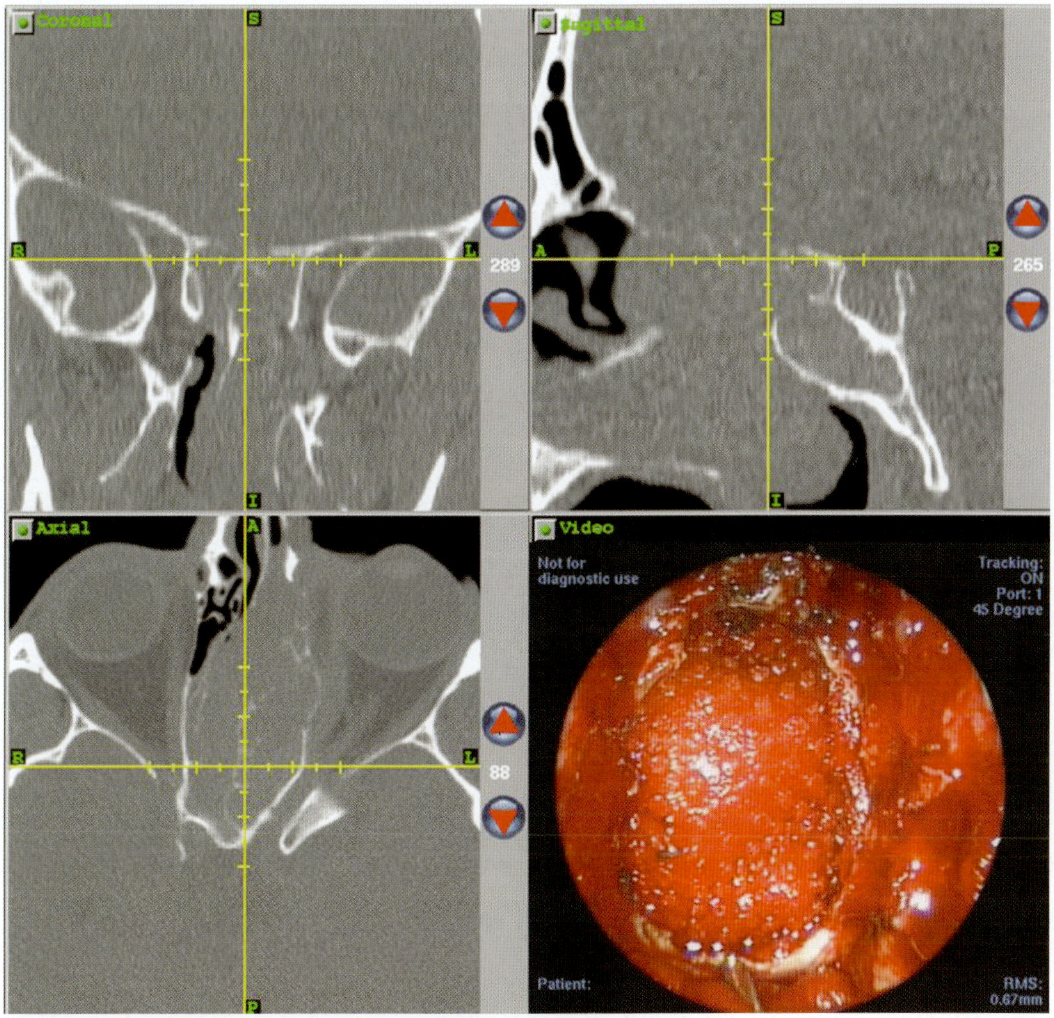

B

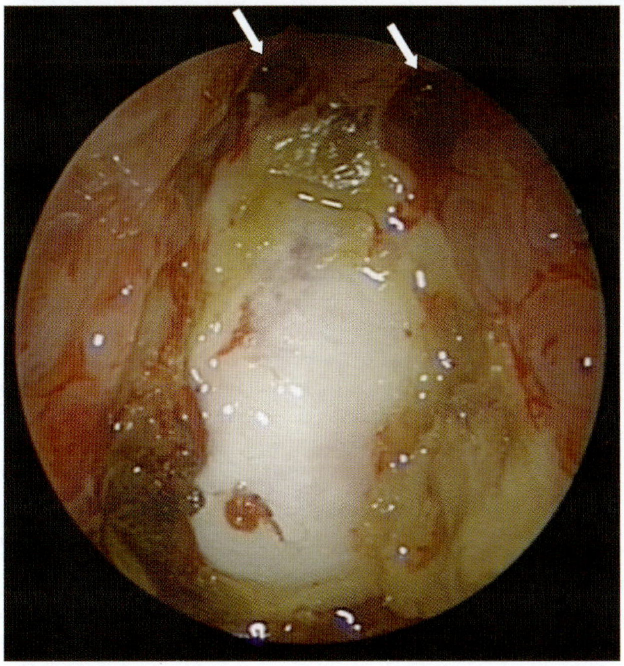

C

Fig. 44.3 *(continued)* A DuraGen graft is placed in an underlay fashion. **(B)**. A cadaveric pericardial overlay graft was also used to seal this defect. A 70-degree endoscopic view of the pericardial graft at 6 weeks postoperative **(C)**. The frontal sinusotomies are open anteriorly with no iatrogenic scarring (*arrows*).

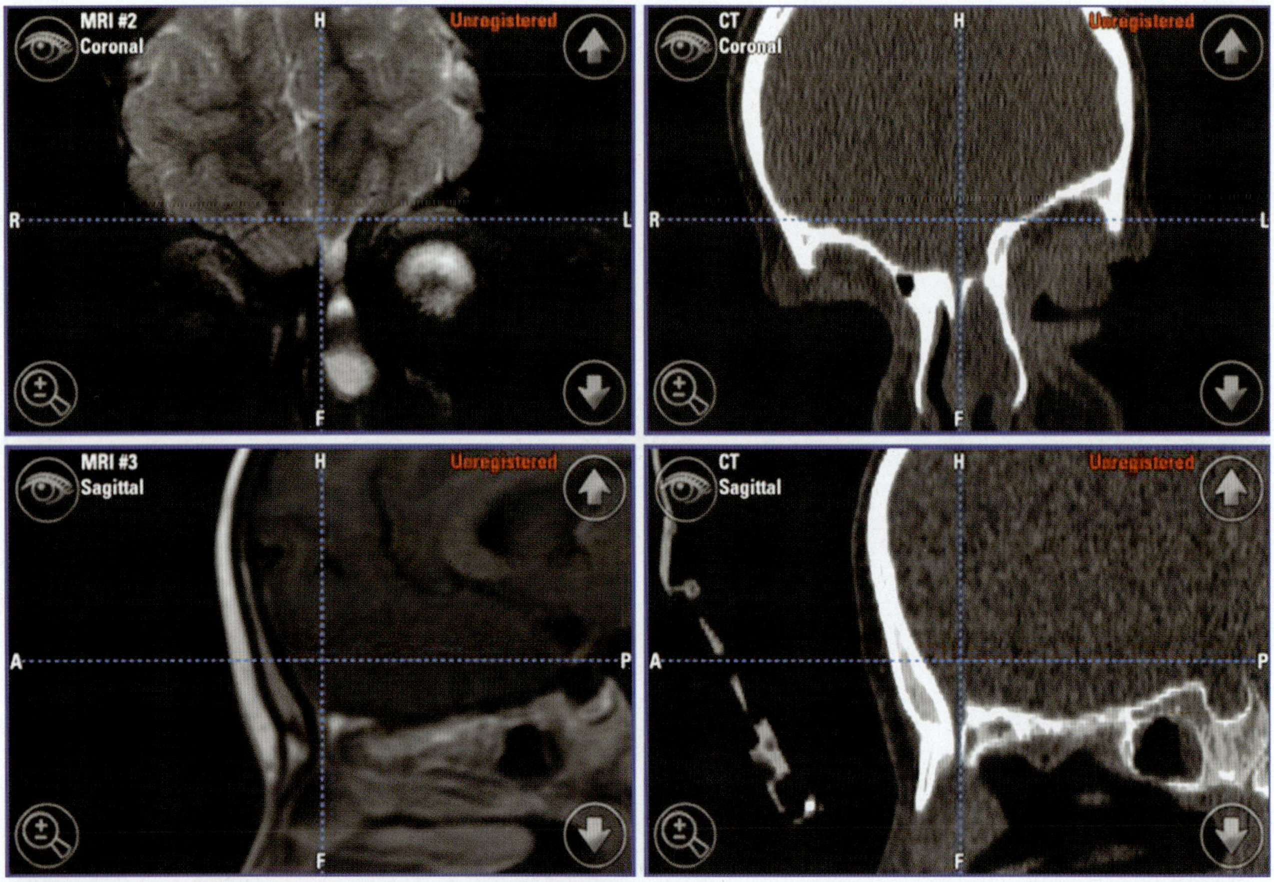

A

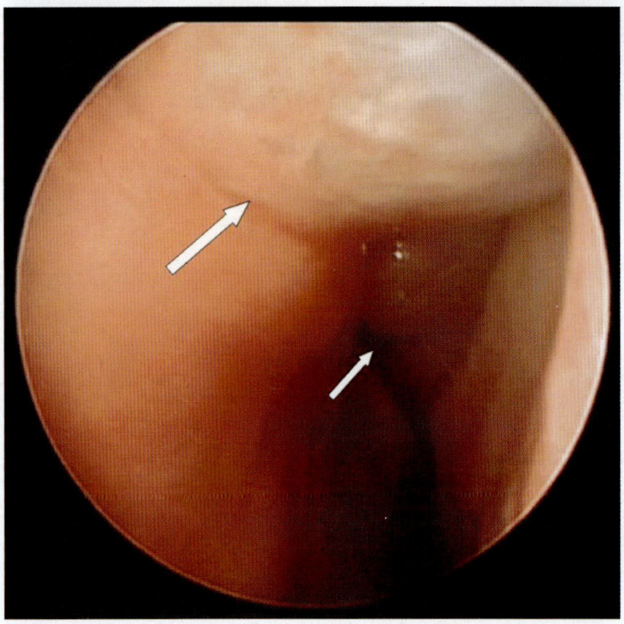

B

Fig. 44.4 (A) Magnetic resonance image (*left*) and computed tomography scan (*right*) coronal and sagittal views of a congenital meningoencephalocele in a 3-year-old child are demonstrated in the region of the foramen cecum. Note the displacement of surrounding normal structures. **(B)** Transnasal endoscopy verified the position of the encephalocele with anterior submucosal extension of the sac below the nasal bones (*large arrow*) anterior to the normal middle turbinate (*small arrow*). *(continued)*

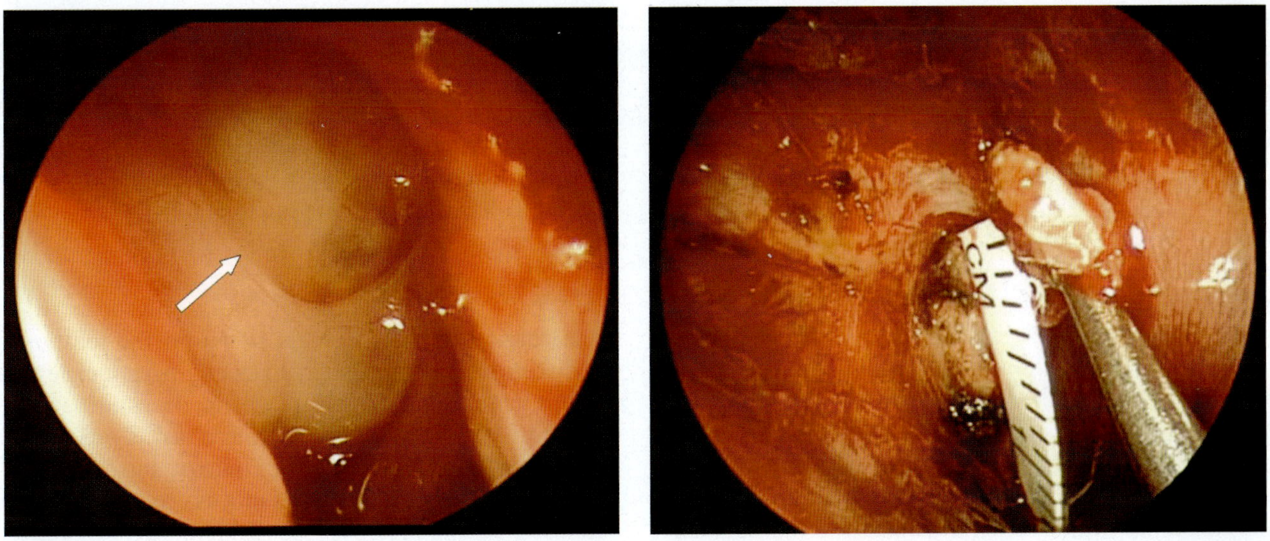

C D

Fig. 44.4 *(continued)* **(C)** Rather than "resect" or ablate the encephalocele, the sac was entered and the bony defect at the skull base within the neck of the encephalocele was easily identified (*arrow*). **(D)** The submucosal extensions of the encephalocele and surrounding normal structures were left alone to minimize collateral damage. The defect was prepared and a laterally based mucosal flap was rotated in preparation for closing the defect.

false positives and false negatives.[25] Beta-trace protein is another noninvasive marker that is used most commonly in Europe and is very specific for CSF.[4]

Computed Tomography

Imaging studies for CSF leaks and encephaloceles generally consist of both coronal and axial computed tomography (CT) scans to identify any dehiscences in the skull base. These also provide important bony detail that is useful in the surgical approach. The walls of the frontal and sphenoid sinuses have contributions from the skull base in multiple planes. In particular, the unique orientation of the skull base in the sphenoid sinus with both anterior and middle cranial skull base contributing to the superior and posterolateral walls, respectively, necessitates both coronal and axial imaging to evaluate these areas. Unfortunately, the inability to distinguish CSF from other soft tissue limits CT in its diagnostic accuracy. In addition, it cannot firmly establish the location of the leak because defects may not be actively leaking and defects may be present without a leak.

Computed Tomography Cisternogram

CT scans can localize an active leak if intrathecal contrast material is administered prior to the scan. A CT cisternogram may be the only test required if it positively identifies contrast material within a specific paranasal sinus or meningoencephalocele sac. It is particularly helpful for identifying sphenoid sinus leaks because the sphenoid acts as a reservoir for contrast material. This test may miss intermittent leaks because it represents only one point in time and the sensitivity is reported anywhere from 48 to 96% in several studies.[25]

Radiolabelled Cisternogram

Another type of cisternogram uses intrathecal injection of a radioactive marker instead of contrast material. The radiolabelled cisternogram requires endoscopic placement of intranasal pledgets for several hours, followed by measurement of radioactivity within the pledgets. Low volume or intermittent leaks can continuously collect CSF if a leak is present because the pledgets remain in place for several hours. Because CSF and nasal secretions mix to collect on all the pledgets on a given side, this test can only localize the defect to a side (right versus left) of the leak. The sensitivity of this study is reported anywhere from 62 to 76% and is used infrequently due to its invasiveness, a significant false positive rate, and low use.[4,25]

Magnetic Resonance Imaging

Magnetic resonance imaging (MRI) is particularly useful for identifying brain parenchyma and CSF that have herniated through the skull base in a meningoencephalocele. In addition, intermittent and low-flow CSF leaks can be imaged using a fast spin-echo sequence with fat suppression and image reversal to highlight CSF.[26] An MRI/magnetic resonance angiography (MRA) study may also be helpful for avoiding potential complications, such as an aneurysm of a dehiscent, cavernous carotid artery in an opacified lateral recess of the sphenoid sinus. MRI also can detect the presence of empty sella, which should be evaluated in all spontaneous CSF leaks as it is representative of elevated ICP. Thus, this study is not only a diagnostic test for CSF leak, but can also indicate underlying pathophysiology. Unfortunately, MRI lacks fine bony detail of the skull base, which limits its accuracy in localizing CSF leaks. Sensitivity has been reported at 85 to 92% with 100% specificity.[4,25]

Intrathecal Fluorescein

One of the most useful advancements in diagnosing and localizing CSF leaks has been the use of intrathecal fluorescein with a thorough endoscopic examination. For those patients with an unclear diagnosis, a thorough endoscopic exam following the administration of intrathecal fluorescein can be particularly helpful in establishing the preoperative diagnosis. This test is more useful in individuals who have had prior sinus surgery and have an exposed, skeletonized skull base. For this reason, fluorescein is more commonly administered intraoperatively, so that complete skeletonization of the skull base may permit accurate diagnosis and localization. Preoperative injection of intrathecal fluorescein is useful for localizing defects, identifying multiple CSF leaks, and inspecting for a watertight closure at the conclusion of the case. If it is not readily apparent where the fluorescein is originating from, thorough skull base exposure must be obtained intraoperatively for evaluation. The fluorescein may be significantly diluted or excreted by the time skull base exposure is attained depending on the rate of CSF turnover, the rate of the leak, and the timing of the intrathecal injection. A blue light filter improves the detection of diluted fluorescein when needed.

Fluorescein is not U.S. Food and Drug Administration (FDA) approved for intrathecal injection because seizures and neurotoxicity have been reported when using higher concentrations or more rapid injections. A mixture of 0.1 mL of 10% fluorescein diluted in 10 mL of the patient's CSF slowly injected over 10 to 15 minutes has resulted in only one minor complication in over 15 years of use—an arrhythmia that resolved within 24 hours.[12]

Surgical Anatomy and Principles

Preoperative Evaluation

A preoperative evaluation of all patients should consist of a thorough history and physical examination, a nasal endoscopic exam, and radiographic imaging. At the least, coronal and axial CT scans of the sinuses should be obtained before surgery. Imaging, such as computer-aided or image-guided surgical navigation CT scans and MRI studies, is performed on a case-by-case basis, as previously mentioned. Frameless, stereotactic surgical navigation is useful for intraoperative localization and orbital and skull base navigation and recommended for CSF leak repair. Three-dimensional CT scans and triplanar reconstructions are helpful for preoperative planning and for visualization of the skull base defects, but not required.[27]

General Principles of CSF Leak Repair

The surgical approach differs based on the location of the skull base defect, but the underlying principles and philosophy regarding repair remain the same and are illustrated in **Fig. 44.5**. The recipient bed is prepared by removing several millimeters of mucosa surrounding the bony defect. Because the sinus mucosa contains exocrine mucus glands, this step is essential for decreasing the risk of mucus lifting the graft from the recipient bed. Stripping mucosa also leads to osteoneogenesis around the defect and can aid with the future strength of the repair. After preparation of the recipient site, any encephaloceles are reduced or ablated using bipolar cautery as much as possible. Meticulous hemostasis is mandatory while ablating the encephalocele to avoid retracting the sac into the cranial cavity with subsequent intracranial hemorrhage.

If the defect is large or if the patient has elevated intracranial pressure, bone or fascia grafts may be placed in an underlay fashion in the epidural space after gently elevating the dura above the bony skull base defect. This gives an added layer of support to decrease the chance of encephalocele recurrence. Bone grafts are not recommended following skull base tumor resection if the patient will undergo postoperative radiation due to the risk of osteoradionecrosis. Delicate otologic elevators are useful in defining the epidural space. An overlay soft tissue graft is then placed with or without the presence of the underlay bone graft. A variety of soft tissue materials may be used for an overlay graft, including temporalis fascia, cadaveric dermis or fascia, or free mucosal or mucoperichondrial grafts. Unilateral or bilateral pedicled septal or inferior turbinate mucosal flaps based on the posterior septal branch of the sphenopalatine artery can also be used (**Fig. 44.6**). These are very useful for patients with a history of prior radiation and potential healing difficulties.

Surgical Approach

Sphenoid Sinus

A standard transnasal parasagittal endoscopic approach with a wide sphenoidotomy is standard for simple defects involving the central sphenoid sinus. The sphenoid ostium is opened widely with sphenoid and Kerrison punch instruments. If additional lateral exposure is needed, a complete endoscopic ethmoidectomy is performed with the identification of the natural ostium of the sphenoid sinus

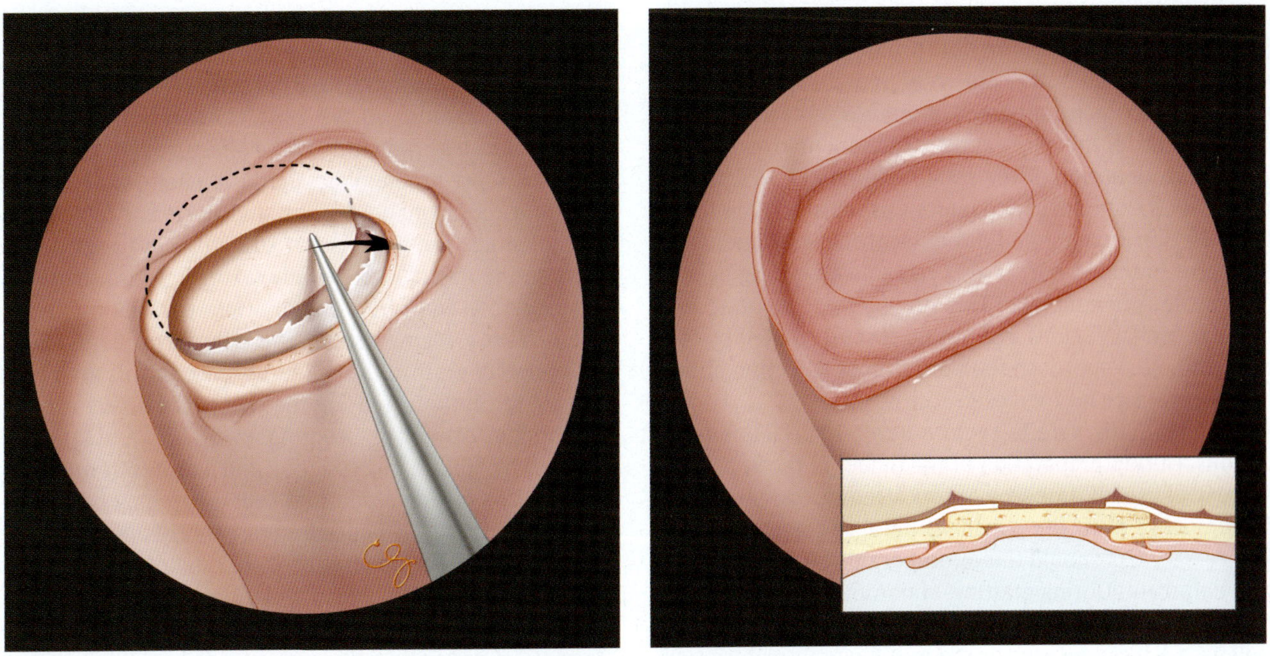

A B

Fig. 44.5 Illustrations demonstrating the proper technique in the placement of an underlay bone graft **(A)** and an overlay mucosal graft **(B)**.

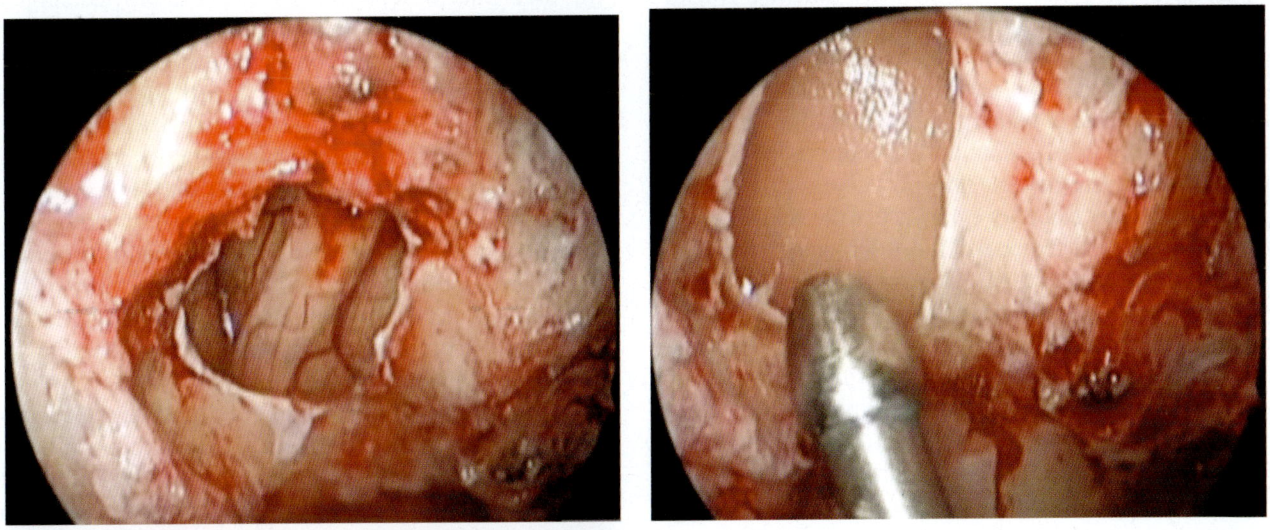

A C

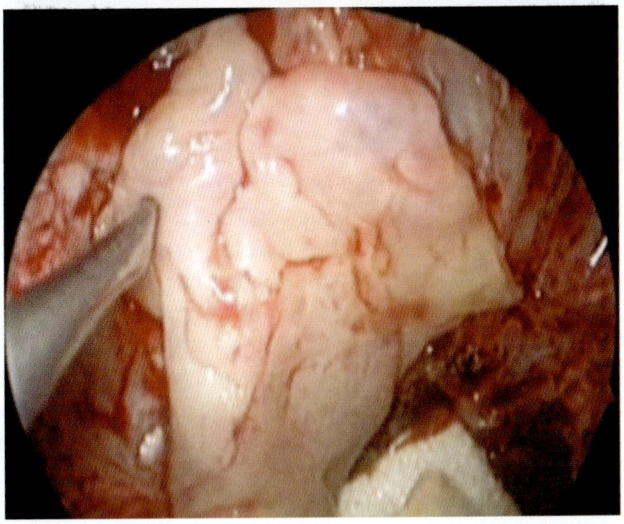

B

Fig. 44.6 Skull base defect after resecting recurrent adenocarcinoma up to olfactory bulb in a previously radiated patient **(A)**. The site is meticulously prepared stripping all mucosa around the defect. A DuraGen underlay graft is tucked over the edges of the defect in the subdural plane, **(B)** and a pedicled inferior turbinate mucosal graft is rotated **(C)**.

following perforation of the basal lamella and resection of the inferior third of the superior turbinate.

Alternatively, an endoscopic transseptal approach with nasal septectomy and sphenoid intersinus septectomy may be performed for increased access. The sphenoid ostium on one side is identified in the sphenoethmoidal recess. The rostrum of the sphenoid and intersinus septum is removed with Kerrison punches and through cutting instruments. A 15-degree diamond burr is also valuable for enlarging the hole in the sphenoid face. This provides excellent access to the perisellar regions and can be complemented by the transethmoidal approach with or without resection of the middle turbinate for increased access.

Sphenoid sinus defects require several special considerations. During preparation of the defect in the sphenoid sinus, it is usually unnecessary to attempt to remove all sinus mucosa from the sphenoid because this creates an unnecessary risk should the carotid or optic nerve be clinically dehiscent. During grafting, abdominal fat can be useful in the sphenoid sinus as opposed to other areas of the skull base. Fat can be used as the primary graft material, or a piece of fascia can be placed over the defect and abdominal fat can serve a secondary supportive function. The fat is also useful for obliterating dead space after resection of sellar or suprasellar tumors. The nasoseptal flap is also a useful technique for large, skull base defects involving this region.[28] Regardless of which graft or flap is used, multiple layers of absorbable packing are then placed within the sphenoid sinus. A removable finger cot contained in a nonlatex gloved finger placed over the face of the sphenoid will prevent inadvertent removal of the absorbable packing.

Skull base defects of the middle cranial fossa in the lateral recess of the sphenoid sinus are difficult to access by the midline transeptal or transethmoidal approaches and ultimately may require an endoscopic transpterygoid approach.[29] Here, a complete ethmoidectomy, wide maxillary antrostomy, and wide sphenoidotomy are performed first. To gain access to the pterygopalatine fossa, the posterior wall of the maxillary sinus is removed. The internal maxillary artery and its branches are identified and transposed inferiorly or clipped and divided. In the deeper areas of the pterygopalatine fossa, meticulous dissection of the maxillary division of cranial nerve V and the vidian nerve will decrease morbidity. The anterior face of the sphenoid sinus that has pneumatized into the pterygoid plates is drilled away to gain exposure of the lateral recess of the sphenoid sinus. Full exposure of this recess is possible through this approach, and repair of the defect is performed as described earlier. This provides the exposure required to reduce the encephalocele and repair the skull base defect with bone and fascia grafts.

The Ethmoid Roof/Cribriform Plate

The posterior ethmoid roof and lateral lamella of the middle turbinate are two of the most common areas for iatrogenic CSF leaks.[25] In general, these are the easiest areas to repair because they only require an ethmoidectomy for exposure of the defect. The mucosa is easily elevated around the defect for preparation of the graft. However, CSF leaks and encephaloceles originating in the olfactory cleft/cribriform plate are more problematic. Unlike other areas, such as the ethmoid roof, sphenoid sinus, and posterior table of the frontal sinus, the bone is not smooth. Elevating the mucosa on the defect is extremely taxing because the cleft is very narrow and often has multiple perforations where the olfactory filaments exit the cribriform plate. Placing an underlay graft in the epidural space in this area without significantly increasing the size of the defect is nearly impossible. Instead of elevating mucosa here, ablating the mucosa by bipolar cauterization and placing a simple overlay graft or raising a pedicled septal flap may be a better option. However, if high intracranial pressure is evident, then an underlay bone graft can be helpful for support. One must weigh the risks of enlarging a small defect with long-term consequences of subsequent encephalocele formation and CSF leak recurrence. The middle turbinate should be resected up to the skull base to gain access to this area, but the septum is left intact to provide support for packing materials.

In the management of congenital encephaloceles of the ethmoid sinuses, precise surgical technique that minimizes trauma to surrounding tissues and sinuses that may otherwise result in "collateral damage" is recommended.[30] This will help minimize any impact on the growth and development of the nose and paranasal sinuses. Small defects that originate at the foramen cecum can be repaired without even performing an uncinectomy or turbinectomy. Furthermore, encephaloceles that originate at the foramen cecum often dissect submucosally along the anterosuperior septum, the nasal bones, and even to the upper lateral cartilages. Identifying the bony skull base defect at the neck of the encephalocele without resecting these extensions will decrease the risk of nasal stenosis. Preserving mucosa over peripheral components of the encephalocele sac does not appear to compromise the skull base repair.[22]

The Frontal Sinus

CSF leaks originating from the frontal sinus must be approached with two major goals in mind. First is the successful repair of the skull base defect. The second goal is either maintaining patency of the frontal sinus or successfully obliterating/ablating the sinus with meticulous removal of all mucosa. Endoscopic repairs of frontal sinus CSF leaks may result in iatrogenic mucoceles if graft material and/or packing obstruct the frontal sinus outflow tract or contribute to synechiae formation and subsequent frontal sinusitis. The approach will also depend on the overall health of the patient, associated intracranial or intraorbital injuries, and other skull base or facial fractures. Both objectives must be kept in mind when deciding on a specific surgical approach and repair for each skull base defect.

Another factor that greatly influences the surgical approach and repair is the anatomic site of the CSF leak. Based on the authors' experience, frontal sinus CSF leaks can be divided into three anatomic sites: (1) those just adjacent to the frontal recess; (2) those with direct involvement of the frontal recess; and (3) those located within the frontal sinus proper.[31] Although most leaks are limited to one of these distinct sites, some defects encompass multiple anatomic areas.

Repairing frontal sinus CSF leaks via an endoscopic approach requires a thorough knowledge of frontal recess anatomy and its variants and that the patient has appropriate anatomy to provide intranasal access. All air cells encroaching on the frontal sinus outflow tract, such as agger nasi cells anterolaterally or suprabullar cells posteriorly, must be removed to increase the chance of long-term frontal patency. At the same time, careful attention to preserving the mucosa surrounding the outflow tract is also essential. Stripping the mucosa will ultimately lead to scar tissue formation and osteitic bone and increase failure rates. Therefore, expertise with angled scopes and frontal giraffe instruments is indispensable for operating efficiency and adequate visualization.

After wide exposure of the skull base defect through a wide frontal sinusotomy, an intraoperative judgment must be made regarding the ability to perform a successful CSF leak repair while maintaining patency of the frontal recess. Attempting endoscopic repair initially does not burn any bridges, because an open procedure can be performed at a later time if failure occurs or if outflow tract obstruction develops. When the defect approaches the midline, a modified endoscopic Lothrop or Draf III procedure will increase surgical access and provide bilateral frontal sinus drainage if ipsilateral stenosis of the frontal recess is expected from the repair. The nasoseptal flap is also useful for repairing skull base defects involving the frontal sinus and can cover up to 3 cm of the posterior table depending on the orientation of the defect (**Fig. 44.7**).[32] Likewise, a frontal trephine can provide access to the superior limits of a defect, and endoscopes may be used through the trephine as well as from below.[33]

Although we discourage the use of hard stents to maintain frontal sinus patency secondary to an increased probability of reactive scar formation and osteitic bone formation, we have found soft silastic stents useful in maintaining patency if the mucosa is preserved and the stent is gently placed in the frontal sinus outflow tract. This stent has the added advantage of helping maintain placement of the soft tissue overlay graft, especially when the skull base defect is located in the vertical plane of the posterior table.

Although the limits of endoscopic approaches continue to expand with improved equipment and experience, posterior table defects located beyond the reach of frontal sinus instruments superiorly or laterally to the sinus outflow tract may require an open approach.[31] For example, CSF leaks located within the lateral recess are difficult to repair endoscopically and may need an osteoplastic flap or trephine approach. The method most often used is an osteoplastic flap with thorough removal of all mucosa and unilateral or bilateral obliteration (depending on the size of the frontal sinus). Repairing a posterior table defect via an osteoplastic flap can be performed without obliteration if the defect is sufficiently superior or lateral to avoid compromising the sinus outflow tract. Alternatively, placement of grafts over defects limited to the lateral recess via a frontal trephine may preserve the frontal recess and avoid the need for frontal obliteration. Because the potential for mucocele formation is significant regardless of surgical approach, close follow-up is essential and must be emphasized to the patient.

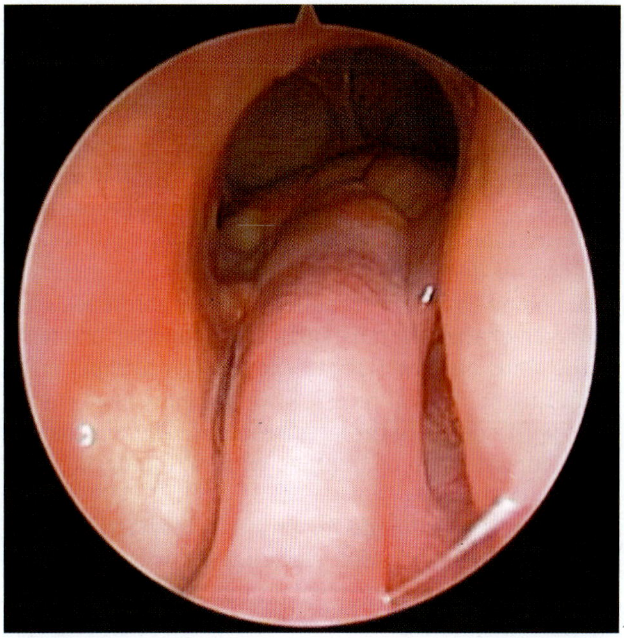

Fig. 44.7 A 70-degree nasal endoscopic view of a right frontal sinus posterior table cerebrospinal fluid leak repair with a nasoseptal flap at 1 year postoperatively. The flap extends 1 cm up the posterior table here, but can reach 3 cm for certain defects.

Defects in the posterior table of the frontal sinus are often not amenable to a strict endoscopic approach. Leaks that are particularly difficult to repair are those that extend to the isthmus of the frontal sinus outflow tract. It is this site where the skull base transitions from the horizontal (axial) orientation of the ethmoid roof/cribriform plate to the vertical (coronal) orientation of the posterior table. Depending on the amount of experience of the surgeon, this area may require a combined approach because it is at the limit of an external osteoplastic approach from above and an endoscopic approach from below. A frontal trephine can provide access to the superior limits of the defect and endoscopes may be used through the trephine as well as from below, but if meticulous removal of mucosa from the entire frontal sinus with subsequent obliteration is needed, an osteoplastic flap, rather than a trephine, is recommended.

Posterior table defects that are superior to the sinus outflow tract can be repaired with an external, extracranial approach using a traditional osteoplastic flap with or without frontal sinus obliteration. Attempts at repairing a posterior table defect without obliteration is not recommended for defects in the frontal sinus, unless there is a concomitant Draf III procedure with wide anteroposterior diameter or the defect is sufficiently superior or lateral to the sinus outflow tract to allow repair without compromising the frontal recess. A well-pneumatized frontal sinus with a defect in the lateral recess can be repaired via an osteoplastic flap or trephine without interfering with the outflow tract.

The specific technique for raising osteoplastic flaps is described elsewhere. After elevating the osteoplastic flap with direct access to the frontal sinus, preparation of the recipient bed and grafting is performed in a similar fashion as endoscopic management if the surgeon feels the frontal sinus outflow tract is not compromised, and the frontal drainage pathway is left open. Fat obliteration should be performed if there is a question about the feasibility of a patent drainage pathway after repair. After all mucosal remnants are stripped and meticulously drilled with a diamond burr, underlay bone and overlay fascia grafts are placed as needed to close the defect. Bilateral obliteration must be performed for relatively small frontal sinuses or involvement of both posterior tables. Finally, the mucosa of the frontal recess is stripped and abdominal fat packed in the sinus.

Repair of large defects in the posterior table, as seen in severe facial trauma or tumors, via cranialization of the frontal sinus and pericranial flap may be preferable in some cases. This approach provides excellent exposure of the defect and allows better access for removal of the mucosa, but does require a craniotomy and retraction on the frontal lobe with possible sequelae such as anosmia, intracranial hemorrhage or edema, epilepsy, and memory and concentration deficits.[34]

Lumbar Drain Management

Lumbar drains are a useful adjunctive treatment in the management of CSF leaks because they can aid a questionable diagnosis with the preoperative injection of intrathecal fluorescein, lower elevated ICP, and facilitate graft placement. In general, lumbar drains are opened at the time of graft placement, and the height of the collection chamber is adjusted to maintain drainage at 5 to 10 mL per hour. Patients with high opening pressure on initial tap or with suspected elevated ICP will likely have even more elevation in their ICP postoperatively due to overproduction against a closed defect. In these individuals, lumbar pressure drainage and pressure measurements are useful to dictate therapeutic interventions for elevated ICP. All patients are kept on strict bedrest while lumbar drains are in place.

To obtain lumbar pressure measurements, the drain is clamped on the morning of postoperative day 2, and 3 to 6 hours is allowed to pass to replenish the patient's CSF volume. A standardized pressure transducer is connected and zeroed with the patient lying perfectly flat and at rest. The pressure monitor displays dynamic waveforms and CSF pressure measurements. A Queckenstedt test (compression of both jugular veins resulting in increased ICP) will confirm that the catheter is in the lumbar cistern and actually recording the intracranial CSF pressure. If pressure is elevated, intravenous acetazolamide (500 mg) is administered and read again in 3 to 4 hours to assess the diuretic's effect. Acetazolamide is a carbonic anhydrase inhibitor diuretic that can decrease CSF production up to 48% and may decrease CSF leak recurrence.[25]

If CSF pressure is elevated over 15 cm H_2O on initial lumbar puncture or according to this protocol, medical treatment with a diuretic, primarily acetazolamide, is recommended to decrease ICP.[9] Acetazolamide is also recommended in those cases with radiographic signs of increased ICP, but normal pressure on protocol. In patients with significantly elevated ICP (generally >35 cm H_2O at baseline) or an inadequate response to medical therapy with diuretics (generally <10 cm H_2O decrease), neurosurgical consultation should be obtained for permanent ventriculoperitoneal shunting. All others, including patients who refuse a ventriculoperitoneal (VP) shunt, are started on oral acetazolamide 500 mg twice a day (BID) or furosemide (Lasix) if a sulfa allergy is present. Electrolytes are checked periodically to ensure no life-threatening abnormalities. Because the underlying etiology of elevated CSF pressure (either obesity or decreased arachnoid granulations) is likely to not change over time, we generally recommend lifelong use of the diuretic.

Management of elevated ICP in spontaneous CSF leaks is critical to successful treatment through the use of acetazolamide and VP shunts. Although weight loss therapies are promoted in these individuals, significant weight loss appears to be required for this to become an effective treatment of elevated ICP.[14] Thus, important factors for a successful repair in these patients are decreasing their ICP through nutritional, medical, or surgical means.

Postoperative Care

After the lumbar drain is removed, patients gradually resume ambulation. Patients are instructed on movement techniques to avoid Valsalva maneuvers and breath holding and are encouraged to continuously inhale or exhale when changing positions. A stool softener is prescribed for every patient and light activity is mandatory for 6 weeks after surgery. Patients are placed on an antistaphylococcal antibiotic until the packing is removed at the first postoperative visit, usually 5 to 7 days after the surgical repair. Patients are seen every 1 to 2 weeks postoperatively for a conservative endoscopic debridement.

Complications

Potentially disastrous complications may occur during skull base reconstruction, including significant intracranial and orbital injury. Meticulous bipolar cautery of the encephalocele sac will decrease the chances of intracranial bleeding after repair. Visualization must be kept at an optimum level by minimizing excessive bleeding during the procedure. Providing careful topical and infiltrative vasoconstriction early in the case and minimizing mucosal trauma, especially to the nasal mucosa anteriorly in the nose, is recommended. Avoiding trauma to the anterior ethmoid artery and limiting dissection in the region of the sphenopalatine artery and its branches will reduce bleeding. If during surgery, bleeding persists so that it interferes with visualization, it is safer to stop the procedure and if necessary, return at a later time. The use of an EndoScrub (Medtronic Inc., Jacksonville, FL) device to clear the endoscope lens of blood is extremely helpful in maintaining good visualization and thereby reducing complications from bleeding.

Outcomes

Outcomes with endoscopic repair of CSF leaks are generally over 90% according to multiple studies.[4] The highest failure rates occur in individuals with spontaneous leaks and intracranial hypertension. However, management of this subset of patients is successful in over 90% at 3 years when intracranial hypertension is appropriately managed.[12] Unfortunately, CSF pressure cannot be checked periodically due to the invasive nature of lumbar punctures. Medical treatment with acetazolamide or frequent monitoring by neurosurgeons of implanted VP shunts is the best option at this time. Decreasing the underlying intracranial hypertension is essential for increasing success rates in patients with spontaneous CSF leaks.

Conclusion

Management of CSF leaks has evolved over the last 10 to 20 years as a result of advancements in technology and expertise. Comprehensive knowledge of diagnostic testing, understanding underlying pathophysiology, and expertise with a variety of surgical techniques are critical for successful outcomes in CSF leak repair.

References

1. Mattox DE, Kennedy DW. Endoscopic management of cerebrospinal fluid leaks and cephaloceles. Laryngoscope 1990;100(8): 857–862
2. Schick B, Ibing R, Brors D, Draf W. Long-term study of endonasal duraplasty and review of the literature. Ann Otol Rhinol Laryngol 2001;110(2):142–147
3. Banks CA, Palmer JN, Chiu AG, O'Malley BW Jr, Woodworth BA, Kennedy DW. Endoscopic closure of CSF rhinorrhea: 193 cases over 21 years. Otolaryngol Head Neck Surg 2009;140(6): 826–833
4. Woodworth BA, Schlosser RJ. Repair of anterior skull base defects and CSF leaks. Oper Tech Otolaryngol Head Neck Surg 2006;18:111–116
5. Bernal-Sprekelsen M, Bleda-Vázquez C, Carrau RL. Ascending meningitis secondary to traumatic cerebrospinal fluid leaks. Am J Rhinol 2000;14(4):257–259
6. Hubbard JL, McDonald TJ, Pearson BW, Laws ER Jr. Spontaneous cerebrospinal fluid rhinorrhea: evolving concepts in diagnosis and surgical management based on the Mayo Clinic experience from 1970 through 1981. Neurosurgery 1985;16(3):314–321
7. Schlosser RJ, Bolger WE. Spontaneous nasal cerebrospinal fluid leaks and empty sella syndrome: a clinical association. Am J Rhinol 2003;17(2):91–96
8. Schlosser RJ, Bolger WE. Significance of empty sella in cerebrospinal fluid leaks. Otolaryngol Head Neck Surg 2003;128(1):32–38
9. Schlosser RJ, Wilensky EM, Grady MS, Palmer JN, Kennedy DW, Bolger WE. Cerebrospinal fluid pressure monitoring after repair of cerebrospinal fluid leaks. Otolaryngol Head Neck Surg 2004;130(4):443–448
10. Schlosser RJ, Woodworth BA, Wilensky EM, Grady MS, Bolger WE. Spontaneous cerebrospinal fluid leaks: a variant of benign intracranial hypertension. Ann Otol Rhinol Laryngol 2006;115(7): 495–500
11. Woodworth BA, Neal JG, Schlosser RJ. Sphenoid sinus cerebrospinal fluid leaks. Oper Tech Otolaryngol Head Neck Surg 2006; 17:37–42
12. Woodworth BA, Prince A, Chiu AG, et al. Spontaneous CSF leaks: a paradigm for definitive repair and management of intracranial hypertension. Otolaryngol Head Neck Surg 2008;138(6): 715–720
13. Schlosser RJ, Wilensky EM, Grady MS, Bolger WE. Elevated intracranial pressures in spontaneous cerebrospinal fluid leaks. Am J Rhinol 2003;17(4):191–195
14. Radhakrishnan K, Thacker AK, Bohlaga NH, Maloo JC, Gerryo SE. Epidemiology of idiopathic intracranial hypertension: a prospective and case-control study. J Neurol Sci 1993;116(1):18–28
15. Wilson DH, Gardner WJ. Benign intracranial hypertension with particular reference to its occurrence in fat young women. Can Med Assoc J 1966;95(3):102–105
16. Bloomfield GL, Ridings PC, Blocher CR, Marmarou A, Sugerman HJ. A proposed relationship between increased intra-abdominal, intrathoracic, and intracranial pressure. Crit Care Med 1997;25(3):496–503
17. Lee AG, Golnik K, Kardon R, Wall M, Eggenberger E, Yedavally S. Sleep apnea and intracranial hypertension in men. Ophthalmology 2002;109(3):482–485
18. Edman CD, Aiman EJ, Porter JC, MacDonald PC. Identification of the estrogen product of extraglandular aromatization of plasma androstenedione. Am J Obstet Gynecol 1978;130(4):439–447
19. Reynolds JM, Tomkinson A, Grigg RG, Perry CF. A Le Fort I osteotomy approach to lateral sphenoid sinus encephalocoeles. J Laryngol Otol 1998;112(8):779–781

20. Suwanwela C, Suwanwela N. A morphological classification of sincipital encephalomeningoceles. J Neurosurg 1972;36(2):201–211
21. David DJ, Sheffield L, Simpson D, White J. Fronto-ethmoidal meningoencephaloceles: morphology and treatment. Br J Plast Surg 1984;37(3):271–284
22. Woodworth BA, Schlosser RJ, Faust RA, Bolger WE. Evolutions in the management of congenital intranasal skull base defects. Arch Otolaryngol Head Neck Surg 2004;130(11):1283–1288
23. Moore MH, Lodge ML, David DJ. Basal encephalocoele: imaging and exposing the hernia. Br J Plast Surg 1993;46(6):497–502
24. Peter JC, Fieggen G. Congenital malformations of the brain—a neurosurgical perspective at the close of the twentieth century. Childs Nerv Syst 1999;15(11-12):635–645
25. Schlosser RJ, Bolger WE. Nasal cerebrospinal fluid leaks: critical review and surgical considerations. Laryngoscope 2004;114(2):255–265
26. Eljamel MS, Pidgeon CN, Toland J, Phillips JB, O'Dwyer AA. MRI cisternography, and the localization of CSF fistulae. Br J Neurosurg 1994;8(4):433–437
27. Schlosser RJ, Faust RA, Phillips CD, Gross CW. Three-dimensional computed tomography of congenital nasal anomalies. Int J Pediatr Otorhinolaryngol 2002;65(2):125–131
28. Hadad G, Bassagasteguy L, Carrau RL, et al. A novel reconstructive technique after endoscopic expanded endonasal approaches: vascular pedicle nasoseptal flap. Laryngoscope 2006;116(10): 1882–1886
29. Bolger WE. Endoscopic transpterygoid approach to the lateral sphenoid recess: surgical approach and clinical experience. Otolaryngol Head Neck Surg 2005;133(1):20–26
30. Woodworth BA, Schlosser RJ. Endoscopic repair of a congenital intranasal encephalocele in a 23 months old infant. Int J Pediatr Otorhinolaryngol 2005;69(7):1007–1009
31. Woodworth BA, Schlosser RJ, Palmer JN. Endoscopic repair of frontal sinus cerebrospinal fluid leaks. J Laryngol Otol 2005;119(9):709–713
32. Virgin F, Barañano CF, Riley K, Woodworth BA. Frontal sinus skull base defect repair using the pedicled nasoseptal flap. Otolaryngol Head Neck Surg 2011;145(2):338–340
33. Purkey MT, Woodworth BA, Hahn S, Palmer JN, Chiu AG. Endoscopic repair of supraorbital ethmoid cerebrospinal fluid leaks. ORL J Otorhinolaryngol Relat Spec 2009;71(2):93–98
34. McCormack B, Cooper PR, Persky M, Rothstein S. Extracranial repair of cerebrospinal fluid fistulas: technique and results in 37 patients. Neurosurgery 1990;27(3):412–417

45 Endoscopic Approaches to the Anterior Cranial Fossa

Jean Anderson Eloy, Belachew Tessema, and Roy R. Casiano

Anterior skull base surgery is a relatively young discipline, existing for approximately half a century.[1] Purely endoscopic skull base resection remains in its infancy since its first description in 2001.[2] Most early skull base surgery literature concentrated on anterior skull base resection.[3] Anterior cranial fossa tumors were traditionally resected using external surgical approaches, such as the anterior craniofacial resection (ACFR) with the addition of postoperative radiotherapy with or without chemotherapy. During the past 50 years, ACFR was widely considered the gold standard for anterior skull base resection by most oncologic head and neck surgeons and was shown to have positive treatment results for paranasal sinus tumors extending to the anterior skull base.[4–7] Although successful in experienced hands, ACFR has several limitations and is associated with significant morbidity.[8] Many reports quote a 30 to 40% major complication rate and postoperative mortality approaching 5%.[4,9–11] Furthermore, en bloc resection, a primary proposed benefit of AFCR, is now called into question due to limited visualization of key areas such as the orbital apex, frontal recess, and sphenoid sinus.[12–14]

With continuous advances in surgical instrumentation, optical aids, and more accurate image guidance systems, multiple minimally invasive endoscopic approaches to the anterior cranial fossa have been described.[15] Since the initial description of endoscopic anterior skull base resection by Casiano[2] in 2001, many centers have adopted this method as the primary treatment method for small, benign lesions of the anterior cranial fossa.[16] Others have extended its use to larger and more extensive anterior skull base malignancies.[2,17–26] The advantages of this approach include pristine visualization, improved cosmesis, decreased major and minor complications, decreased blood loss, and shorter hospital stays, while maintaining proper oncologic principles.

This chapter briefly explains appropriate patient selection for each approach, reviews diagnostic workup of patients with anterior skull base tumors, discusses the most common minimally invasive endoscopic surgical approaches to the anterior cranial fossa and nasal vault, and expands on surgical outcomes and complications of endoscopic anterior skull base resection. It is not our intention to discuss any specific approach extensively because in the majority of situations, a combination of different routes is used to achieve optimal surgical access. External surgical approaches to the anterior cranial fossa are discussed in Chapter 50 and will not be covered here.

Patient Selection and Indications

Appropriate patient selection is important for all anterior skull base tumor resections and remains paramount for endoscopic approaches. Evaluation for possible total endoscopic tumor resection must be made through careful preoperative endoscopic evaluation and review of available imaging. If complete resection cannot be achieved by this technique, other approaches must be considered. Likewise, if it is realized intraoperatively that surgical margins cannot be cleared endoscopically, the surgeon must be prepared to either stage the procedure for a later date or convert to an open approach. Neurosurgical support must be available at all times in case an open craniotomy is even a remote possibility. Currently, absolute contraindications for transnasal endoscopic resection of anterior skull base tumors include lesions with orbital extension necessitating orbital exenteration (**Fig. 45.1**), recurrent tumor with fibrosis and intracranial extension (**Fig. 45.2**), tumors with lateral extension over the orbital roof, and tumors with anterior extension involving facial soft tissue (**Fig. 45.3**). Relative contraindications include tumors with large intracranial extension (**Fig. 45.4**), tumors with significant extension to the floor of the nose with palatal involvement (**Fig. 45.5**), and tumors extending to the pterygomaxillary space (**Fig. 45.6**) or infratemporal fossa (**Fig. 45.7**). In these cases, although a purely endoscopic resection may be attempted at first, the surgeon should be prepared for possible open conversion or start with an endoscopic-assisted craniofacial resection. Apart from the previous exceptions, significant bleeding disorders, and other significant medical comorbidities precluding general anesthesia, almost all anterior skull base tumors are candidates for endoscopic resection.

Diagnostic Workup

Nasal obstruction, epistaxis, facial pain, headache, and visual disturbances represent the most common presentations of patients with anterior skull base tumors. Accordingly, patients presenting with these symptoms should have complete otorhinolaryngologic, ophthalmologic, and neurologic evaluations to rule out an anterior skull base lesion. The otorhinolaryngologic evaluation should include a complete head and neck examination (including cranial nerves) as well as flexible or rigid nasopharyngoscopy. Imaging studies include a triplanar (axial, coronal,

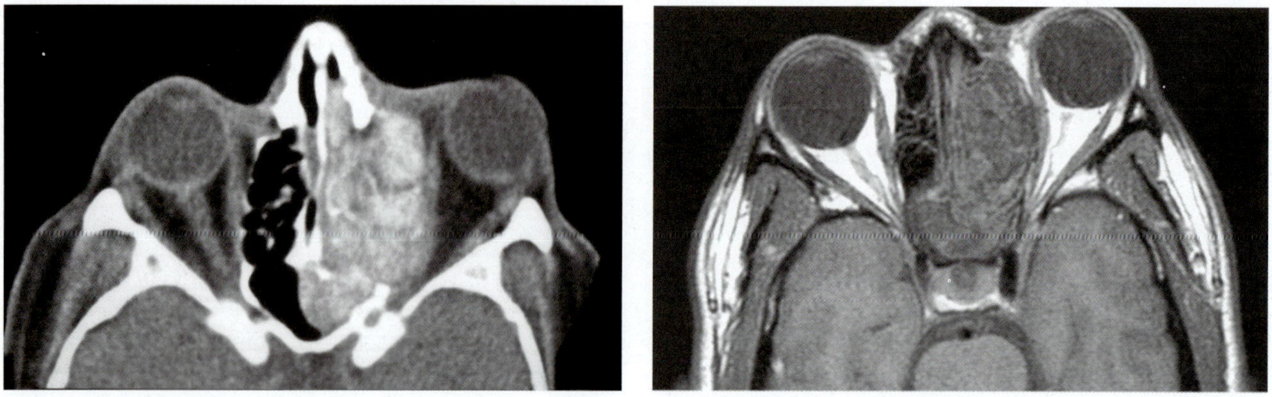

A B

Fig. 45.1 (A) Axial computed tomography and **(B)** T1-weighted magnetic resonance image of a patient with a left sinonasal malignancy extending to the orbit. The intraorbital extension made this patient a poor candidate for a purely transnasal endoscopic approach. This case was approached via an endoscopic-assisted anterior craniofacial resection.

and sagittal) computed tomographic (CT) scan and magnetic resonance imaging (MRI) of the paranasal sinuses, orbits, and brain. These two imaging modalities are complementary to each other and should both be available for appropriate interpretation. Although MRI is very accurate at evaluating soft tissue structures, CT scan is very sensitive and necessary to assess bony destruction. A nonvascular appearing lesion can be biopsied in the office. Any suspicion of increased vascularity warrants radiographic confirmation prior to biopsy. If a lesion is revealed to be an aggressive malignancy after biopsy, a total body positron emission tomography (PET)/CT scan should be considered to evaluate regional and distant metastasis. After appropriate workup, all of these patients should have a neurologic evaluation in case surgical resection is considered. Chapters 31 and 32 provide a concise review on the presentation, diagnosis, and treatment of the different types of benign and malignant sinonasal tumors, respectively. Accordingly, different tumor histopathologies will not be covered in this chapter.

Surgical Anatomy

See Chapter 41 on endoscopic anatomy of the skull base and parasellar region.

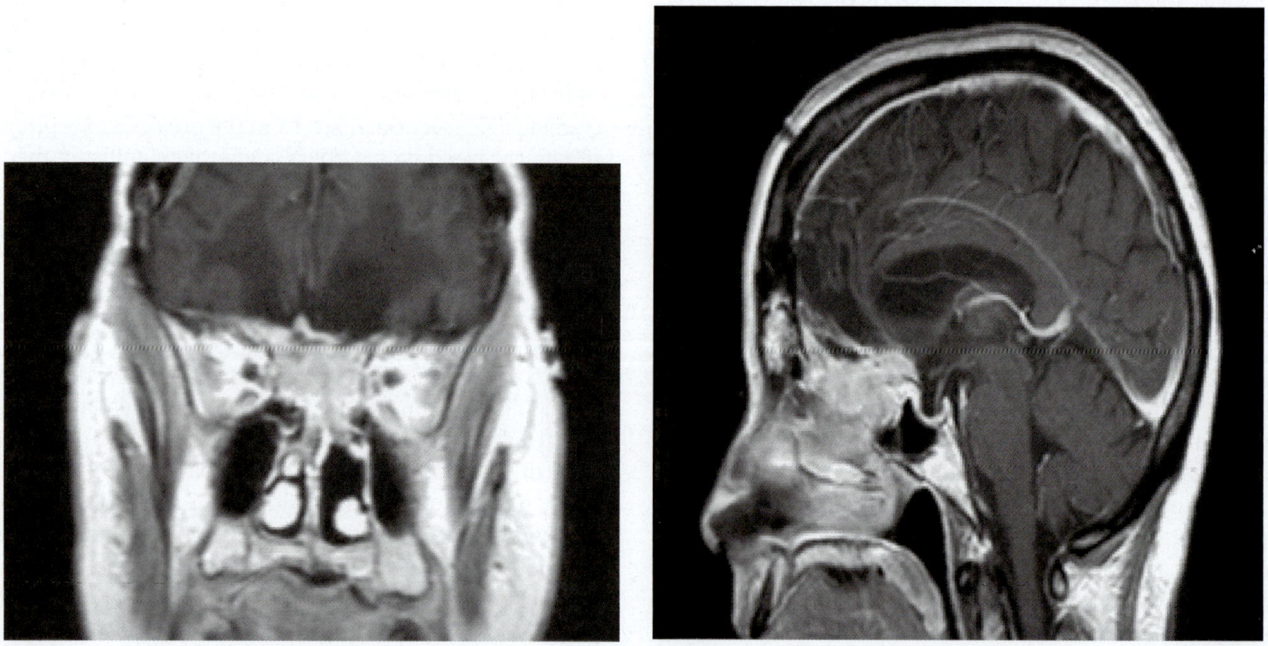

A B

Fig. 45.2 (A) Coronal and **(B)** sagittal gadolinium-enhanced T1-weighted magnetic resonance image of a patient with recurrent bilateral anterior skull base malignancy. Due to the expected intracranial fibrosis, an endoscopic-assisted anterior craniofacial resection was performed.

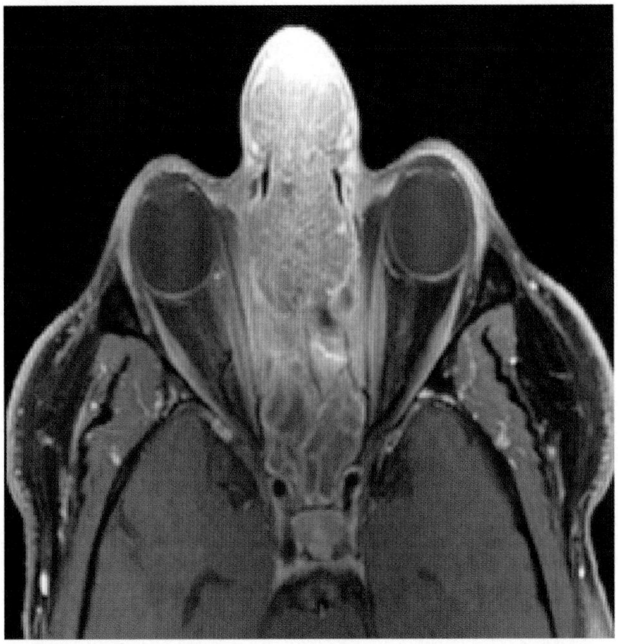

Fig. 45.3 Axial fat-suppressed gadolinium-enhanced T1-weighted magnetic resonance image of a patient with anterior skull base malignancy with involvement and destruction of nasal bones and dermal enhancement. This patient underwent endoscopic-assisted anterior craniofacial resection and rhinectomy.

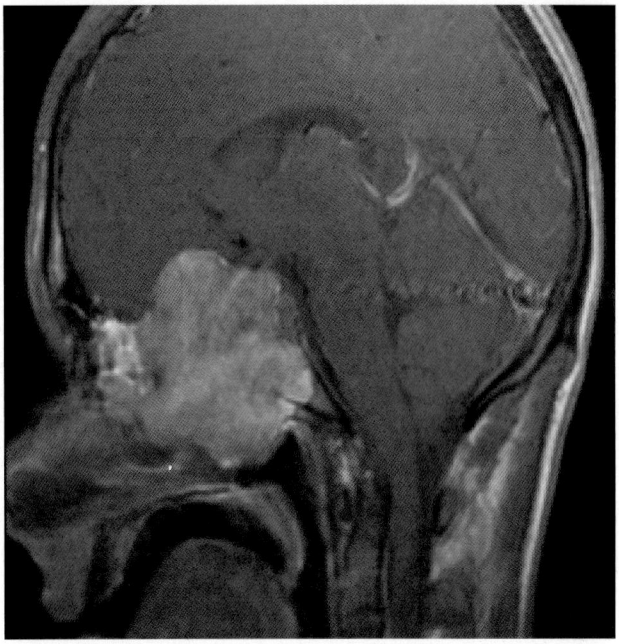

Fig. 45.4 Sagittal gadolinium-enhanced T1-weighted magnetic resonance of a patient with anterior skull base tumor with significant intracranial extension. A benign lesion in this location can be resected endoscopically. For malignant sinonasal tumors, intracranial involvement of this extent is a relative contraindication to a purely endoscopic resection.

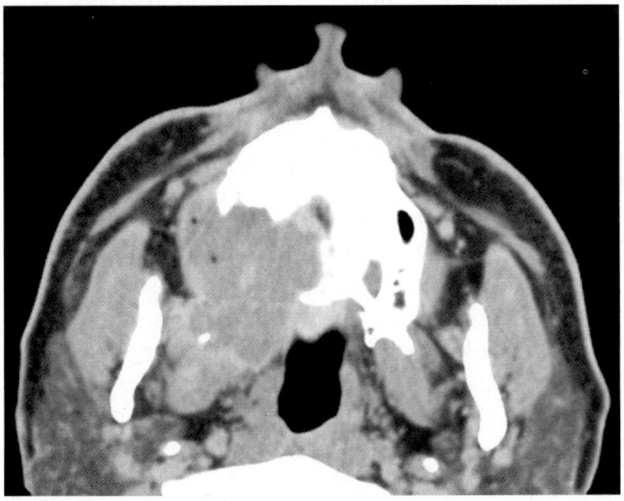

Fig. 45.5 Axial computed tomography scan of a patient with right sinonasal squamous cell carcinoma with extension and destruction of the hard palate. The palatal involvement rendered this patient a poor candidate for a purely endoscopic approach.

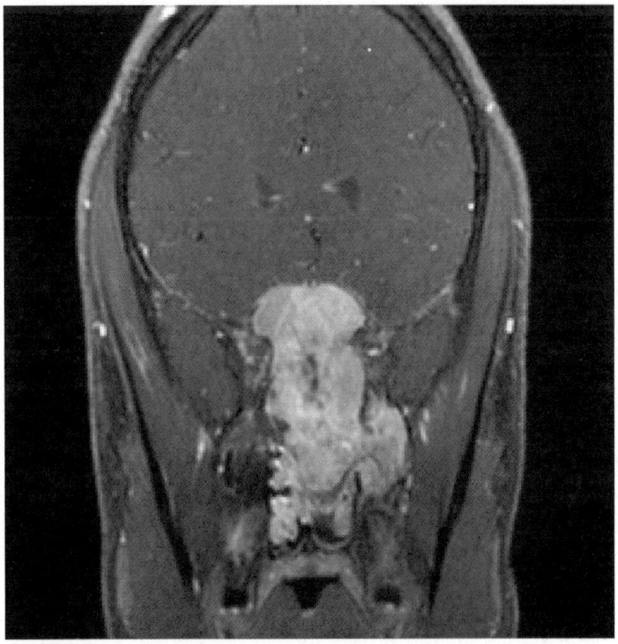

Fig. 45.6 Coronal gadolinium-enhanced T1-weighted magnetic resonance image of a patient with anterior skull base malignancy extending to the left pterygomaxillary space. A benign lesion in this location can be resected endoscopically. For malignant sinonasal tumors, the pterygomaxillary space extension observed in this patient represents a relative contraindication to a purely endoscopic resection.

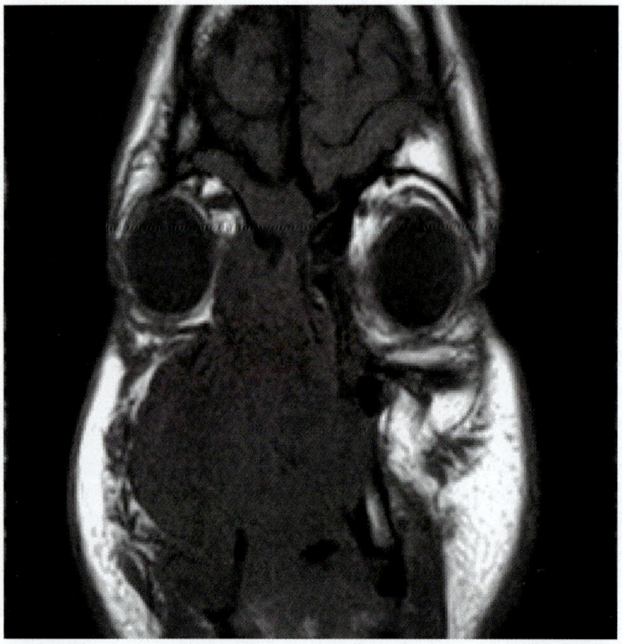

Fig. 45.7 Coronal T1-weighted magnetic resonance image of a patient with right anterior skull base malignancy, lateral maxillary wall destruction, and infratemporal fossa extension. The infratemporal fossa extension represents a relative contraindication to a purely endoscopic resection.

Surgical Technique

Although many methods of classification exist to describe approaches and techniques for removal of anterior cranial fossa tumors, a nonambiguous classification of these approaches includes: (1) external anterior craniofacial resection; (2) endoscopic-assisted anterior craniofacial resection; and (3) purely endoscopic anterior skull base resection without craniotomy or external incision. Each of these techniques contains many variations used to improve visualization and access based on tumor location and surgeon's preference.

External Anterior Craniofacial Resection

External anterior craniofacial resection is the gold standard for anterior skull base tumor extirpation.[3–7] Although the popularity of this procedure has declined since the advent of endoscopic-assisted ACFR and purely endoscopic anterior skull base resection, it still remains a key component in the armamentarium of the anterior skull base surgeon. As mentioned previously, intraorbital involvement and large intracranial parenchymal extension remain important indications for this procedure. Likewise, tumors with dermal involvement, tumors with lateral extension over the orbit, recurrent tumors with increased fibrosis, and adherence to intracranial vascular structures or brain parenchyma may require this approach. Involvement of the sphenoid sinus, the orbital apex, the nasopharynx, and the optic canal represent relative contraindication to this technique due to limited access and visualization. External skull base surgeries including external anterior craniofacial resection are discussed in Chapter 54 and will not be covered further in this chapter.

Endoscopic-Assisted Anterior Craniofacial Resection

Endoscopic-assisted anterior craniofacial resection was first described by Thaler et al. in 1999.[12] This approach was initially used for tumors without significant inferior extension to the nasal floor or significant lateral extension to the maxillary sinus. During this procedure, patients undergo standard intracranial exposure through a bicoronal incision with frontal craniotomy or subcranial approach. The tumor is removed through the external incisions (cranial side of the skull base) instead of endoscopically via the nasopharynx. The nasal endoscope is used to perform safer, more accurate osteotome cuts through the external incision under direct endoscopic visualization. The direction, orientation, and proximity of the septal and ethmoid cuts to the tumor can be assessed under superior visualization to ensure safer margins without sacrificing vital structures. If needed, certain inferior septal and lateral nasal wall cuts that would be difficult and potentially unsafe to perform externally can be achieved transnasally. The anterior skull base defect is then routinely repaired with a pericranial flap or vascularized free tissue transfer as is performed in the standard ACFR procedure. According to its proponents, this technique allows en bloc resection of many large anterior skull base tumors with achievable clear margins while significantly reducing associated morbidity.

Currently, many oncologic head and neck surgeons not yet comfortable with a purely endoscopic anterior craniofacial resection for malignant anterior skull base tumors favor this technique for the improved visualization offered during tumor resection.[27,28] This procedure is also frequently performed and praised by these experts because an en bloc resection can still be achieved.

Endoscopic Anterior Skull Base Resection Without Craniotomy

Purely endoscopic anterior craniofacial resection (without craniotomy or external incision) was initially described by Casiano[2,14] in 2001 in a group of patients with olfactory neuroblastomas. This procedure stemmed from observations and successful reports by Steiner that en bloc resection is not necessary to achieve oncologic cure in patients with laryngeal cancer.

After the induction of general anesthesia, patients are usually given an intravenous antibiotic that crosses the blood-brain barrier, a glucocorticoid, and an anticonvulsant

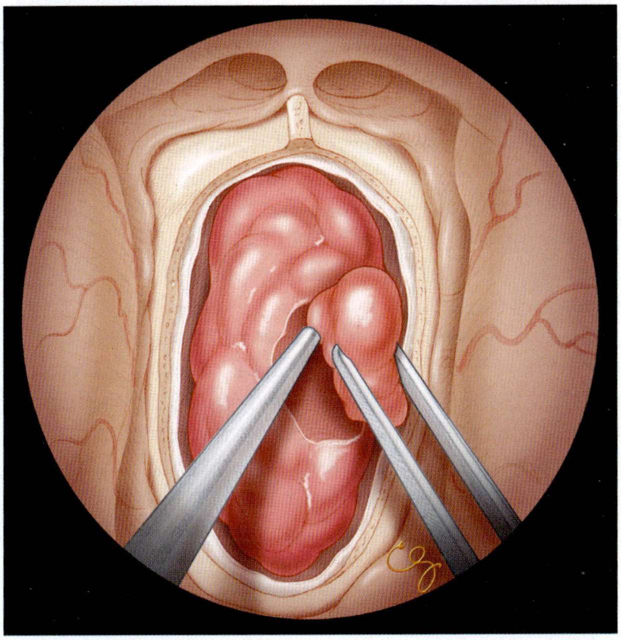

Fig. 45.8 Diagram depicting the endoscopic view of the anterior skull base prior to tumor resection. Note the circumferential clearance around the tumor prior to resection.

(i.e., cefuroxime, dexamethasone or hydrocortisone, and phenytoin). A prophylactic lumbar drain, an arterial line, and Foley catheter are routinely placed. The nasal mucosa is vasoconstricted with oxymetazoline-soaked Cottonoids. The patient is then positioned with the head turned slightly to the right and elevated ~30 degrees. Rigid head fixation may or may not be used and is based on surgeon's preference and type of navigation system used. A clear disadvantage of using rigid fixation is the commitment to keep the patient's head in one position throughout the case. Many endoscopic skull base surgeons prefer to keep the patient's head mobile throughout the procedure to maintain a dynamic state of visualization. After final preparation and draping, the navigation system is calibrated and tested prior to incision.

The typical endoscopic anterior skull base resection starts with endoscopic transnasal debulking of the tumor with a 4-mm microdebrider blade with the objective of identifying the stalk of the tumor. The microdebrider suction is attached to a filter/collector (sock) for each side to collect the tissue removed. Key structures such as the nasal septum, lateral nasal wall, and posterior nasal choanae are localized. In case of ethmoidal involvement, endoscopic medial maxillectomy is performed with removal of involved lamina papyracea, medial maxillary wall, and total ethmoidectomy with or without lacrimal duct resection.

The anterior margin of resection is exposed by performing an extended frontal sinusotomy (modified Lothrop procedure). This section of the procedure starts by localizing the frontal recess and ostea bilaterally. A superior/anterior septectomy is performed anterior to the cribriform plate (anterior to the tumor). C-spine curettes (SSI Ultra Specialty Surgical Instruments; Nashville, TN) are then used to make and enlarge the common frontal sinusotomy by removing the intersinus and intrasinus septations, thereby exposing the posterior frontal sinus wall. The nasofrontal beak is subsequently thinned using large cutting burrs once the posterior wall of the common frontal cavity is visualized.

The posterior margin of resection is exposed with an extended sphenoid sinusotomy by removing the intersinus septum, sphenoid rostrum, and the common wall between the most posterior ethmoid cells and sphenoid as far lateral as the lamina papyracea. Vital structures, such as the optic nerves and carotid artery, are identified bilaterally and left undisturbed. The fovea ethmoidalis and sphenoid roof anterior to the optic chiasm are thinned with large diamond burrs and are removed with rongeurs to expose the underlying dura circumferentially around the remaining bony septum, middle and superior turbinate remnants, lamella lateralis, and the olfactory cleft bilaterally (**Fig. 45.8**). The dura is elevated off the orbital roof laterally by bluntly pushing a neurologic Cottonoid between the bone and dura to facilitate placement of graft material at the end of the procedure. The anterior and posterior ethmoidal arteries are identified and cauterized with monopolar or bipolar cautery. Adherence of the dura to the orbital roof may signify more extensive tumor invasion, potentially necessitating an open neurosurgical approach. Dural resection begins at the posterior frontal region and extending as far posterior as the optic chiasm (**Fig. 45.9**).

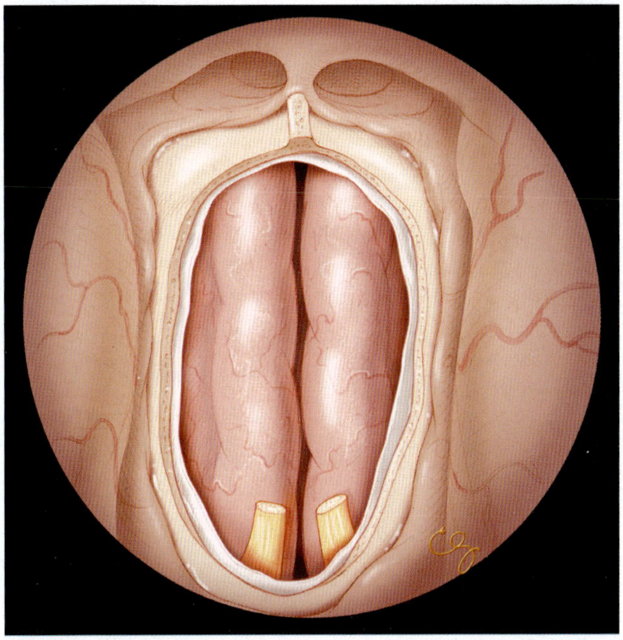

Fig. 45.9 Diagram depicting the endoscopic view of the anterior skull base after bilateral endoscopic anterior skull base resection. Dural resection starts just posterior to the frontal region, and extends as far posterior as the optic chiasm. The lateral dural margin is initially resected a few millimeters medial to the junction of the lamina papyracea or medial orbital wall periosteum and the fovea ethmoidalis.

The lateral dural margin is initially resected a few millimeters medial to the junction of the lamina papyracea or medial orbital wall periosteum and the fovea ethmoidalis. En bloc removal of the entire specimen is performed in an anterior-to-posterior direction with the specimen gradually dropping inferiorly into the nose as one proceeds posteriorly. The excised specimen includes the dura, bilateral cribriform plates with olfactory bulbs, middle and superior turbinate remnants, perpendicular plate of the ethmoid, and the inferior aspect of the crista galli (**Fig. 45.10**).

This removal allows direct visualization, access to any vessels adjacent to the structures, and avoidance of undue trauma to any cortical vessels or brain parenchyma. Bipolar cautery is used to control any intracranial bleeding vessels. Adjacent brain parenchyma and the intracranial cavity are meticulously inspected for the presence of neoplasm, and frozen-section diagnoses of specimens from the dural margins, olfactory nerve endings, septum, and nasopharynx are obtained. Although not widely available, in patients with intracranial extension, intraoperative MRI may be used to assist with tumor resection and to assess for completeness of tumor removal. Endoscopic marsupialization of the lacrimal duct and sac is performed to minimize the chance of stenosis and epiphora. About 15 to 20 specimens from specific anatomic areas (right and left anterior ethmoid, posterior ethmoid, sphenoid, medial maxillary wall, maxillary sinuses, turbinates, septum, frontal recess, and nasopharynx, among others) are obtained at the conclusion of the procedure. These specimens allow accurate pathologic mapping of the tumor in case a second procedure is required and for postoperative planning of radiation therapy. In patients with smaller unilateral lesions, resection is performed in a similar fashion but with sparing of the contralateral septal mucosa, cribriform plate, and sinuses.

Many different techniques and graft materials can be used for reconstruction. Acellular dermal allografts[29] (LifeCell Corporation; Branchburg, NJ), septal cartilage or bone,[15] mucoperichondrial/mucoperiosteal vascularized rotational flaps,[30] fascia lata, dural substitutes, and numerous other synthetic materials have been used alone or in combination with success. The extent of reconstruction depends on the size of the defect. Larger defects require more rigid reconstruction with cartilage, bone, thick acellular dermal allograft, or two- to three-ply lyophilized dura (Dura-Guard; Synovis; St. Paul, MN). With the exception of the mucoperichondrial/mucoperiosteal nasoseptal pedicled flap, graft material usually acts merely as a scaffold for ingrowth of granulation tissue and fibroblasts. Unfortunately, due to the disease process and location,

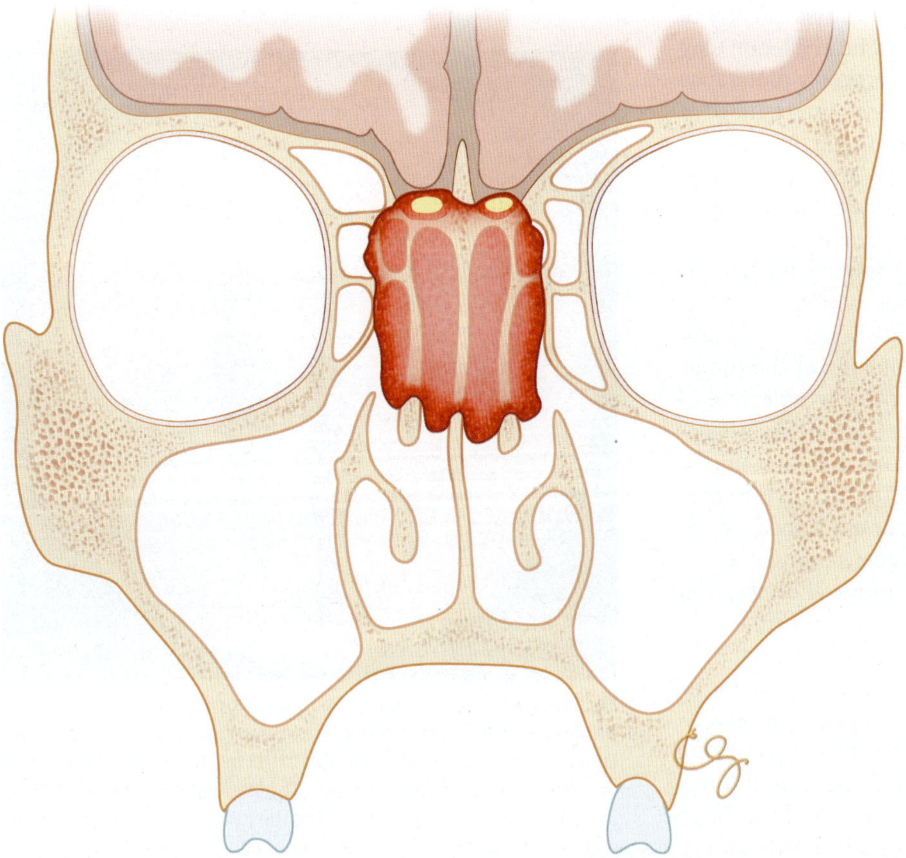

Fig. 45.10 Illustration depicting the extent of resection for bilateral endoscopic anterior skull base resections in the coronal plane.

it is often difficult to harvest a large nasoseptal flap that can be used for reconstruction of large anterior skull base defects. If this graft is used in malignant cases, frozen section analysis of its edges is necessary to eliminate possible tumor involvement.

If lyophilized dura is used, the surgeon should ascertain that the manufacturer has been approved by the U.S. Food and Drug Administration, and the donors were appropriately tested for potentially communicable diseases. For large defects extending the full length of the anterior skull base (~2 × 3 cm), the lyophilized dura or acellular dermal graft is tucked at least 1 cm circumferentially between the remaining dura and the orbital roof (**Fig. 45.11**). A pedicled nasoseptal flap or contralateral inferior turbinate-free mucosal graft may be used in conjunction, although it is not often necessary for anterior skull base reconstruction. Smaller defects are typically less challenging and may be closed using a variety of reconstructive techniques. After proper graft positioning, a layer of moist absorbable gelatin sponge (Gelfoam; Pfizer; New York, NY), fibrin matrix (Tisseel; Baxter, IL), or polymerized hydrogel (DuraSeal; Confluent Surgical, Waltham, MA) is placed against the graft, and a nasal tampon (Merocel Corp; Mystic, CT) is used for packing.

Endoscopic anterior skull base resection without craniotomy is not currently appropriate for large tumors with dermal involvement, marked intracranial extension with significant brain parenchyma involvement, orbital penetration, lateral extension over the orbit, and extensive frontal or infratemporal fossa involvement. In these cases, an endoscopically assisted anterior craniofacial resection or an external anterior craniofacial resection is more appropriate.

Complications

With the exception of external wound infections and skin necrosis, the possible complication profile is similar whether an open or endoscopic approach is undertaken during anterior skull base resection. This is inherent to the location of the tumor and the defect created after its removal. However, the relative incidence of these complications varies with the approach used. Significant complications include postoperative cerebrospinal (CSF) leakage with concurrent meningitis, pneumocephalus, seizures, strokes, intracranial hematoma, intracranial abscess, orbital hematoma, and death.

Postoperative CSF leak is common to both open and endoscopic anterior skull base resections and depends on the quality of the repair. Traditionally, it was believed that

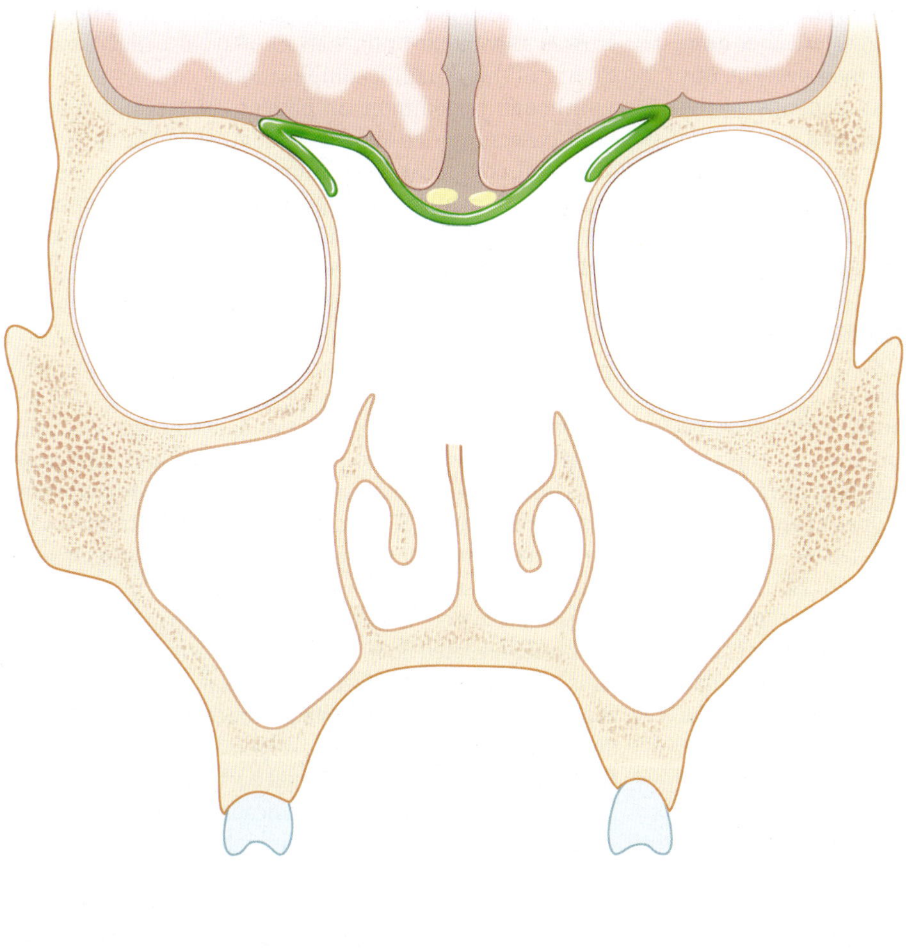

Fig. 45.11 A coronal depiction of the anterior skull base defect reconstructed with acellular dermal allograft. Note the proper watertight positioning (intracranial and extradural) of the graft for adequate support and minimization of postoperative displacement, cerebrospinal fluid leakage, or pneumocephalus.

large anterior skull base repair could only be successfully performed with a pericranial flap, adjacent temporalis muscle transfer, or free tissue transfer. However, recently many endoscopic skull base surgeons have shown the feasibility and efficacy of endoscopic repair for large skull base defects with acellular dermal allografts, septal cartilage, and or mucoperichondrial/mucoperiosteal vascularized rotational flaps.[13,29,30]

The most important factor in decreasing postoperative CSF leak during anterior skull base defect repair is obtaining a watertight dural closure. The use of a lumbar drain in this situation is still controversial. Although some authors believe that its usage decreases intracranial pressure and reduces pressure on the repair, thereby preventing a leak, others believe CSF drainage through the lumbar spine lifts the brain off the anterior skull base, thus pulling the closure inward.[15] Supporters of the latter theory also claim that downward pressure of the frontal lobe will theoretically assist in sealing the closure, and that possible air aspiration via an anterior cranial defect may predispose patients to pneumocephalus and subsequent herniation. Nevertheless, both groups agree a lumbar drain is beneficial in patients with known high intracranial pressure or sleep apnea whereby significant increases in intracranial pressure can lead to flap prolapse and CSF leakage.

As with any craniotomy, a small degree of intracranial air is expected and acceptable after an anterior skull base resection. Tension pneumocephalus usually occurs as a result of a ball-valve effect from a small defect in the repair coupled with improper lumbar drain usage. Judicious lumbar drain usage and meticulous repair may prevent this life-threatening complication. Treatment depends on the patient's neurologic status. Patients without neurologic changes may be treated by clamping the lumbar drain, intravenous antibiotics, frequent neurologic evaluation, and serial head CT scanning. In patients with acute neurologic changes, immediate decompression is warranted in addition to those previously listed.

Although previously common during intracranial tumor resection, the current widespread use of perioperative and postoperative prophylactic anticonvulsants in most neurosurgical procedures has tremendously decreased the occurrence of seizures after these surgeries. In the rare event when this occurs, treatment consists of intravenous administration of one of the different types of anticonvulsants and airway protection in the acute setting.

Strokes are usually a complication of ACFR and seldom occur in endoscopic transnasal anterior skull base resection. The mechanism of injury in ACFR involves the marked frontal lobe retraction necessary for adequate visualization. Prevention involves careful handling of the frontal lobes during ACFR and the avoidance of excessive retraction. Unfortunately, this may be difficult to achieve in tumors with significant posterior extent and may compromise surgical margins because of poor visualization.

Intracranial hematoma can occur in both endoscopic and open CFR. Avoidance of this complication may be achieved with meticulous hemostasis during and at the end of the procedure. The anterior cerebral arteries are within the field of dissection during the intracranial tumor resection segment of anterior skull base resection. Care should be taken to prevent excessive torsion or pulling on tumor adherent to these vessels because this may cause bleeding from its main trunks or branches. In revision cases with marked fibrosis and adhesion, if tumor separation from the vessels seems unsafe endoscopically, an open approach should be considered because this may decrease the chance of vascular injury. Because of adjacent neural tissue, monopolar cautery should be avoided for achieving hemostasis. If an intracranial hematoma is discovered postoperatively, treatment consists of drainage with control of hemorrhage (often no specific source is found) and prophylactic antibiotics to prevent meningitis or intracranial abscess.

Intracranial abscess can occur after all types of skull base procedures. A common source is CSF leak leading to meningitis and eventual abscess formation. Small intracranial hematomas may also remain unnoticed, becoming a culture media for bacterial overgrowth and empyema formation. Patients with pneumocephalus also tend to suction nasal flora intracranially, which may lead to intracranial contamination and abscess formation. Prevention requires adequate dural closure after anterior skull base surgery to prevent CSF leaks or pneumocephalus. Meticulous hemostasis can prevent residual hematoma. The use of a perioperative intravenous antibiotic that crosses the blood-brain barrier may also decrease the chance of this dreadful complication.

Although uncommon, all patients undergoing anterior skull base surgeries should be advised of the possibility of a fatal complication. Without timely recognition and appropriate medical or surgical management, any of the previously discussed complications can quickly evolve and lead to a preventable fatality.

Postoperative Care

Postoperatively, patients are extubated in the operating room with care taken to prevent bucking and sudden increases in intracranial pressure because this may cause graft displacement and CSF leak. Patients are then transferred to the recovery room or intensive care unit overnight for serial neurologic examination and blood pressure, urine output, and specific gravity monitoring. Patients are positioned with their head elevated at 30 degrees to prevent intracranial venous pooling and increased intracranial pressure. They are kept on bed rest for the first 48 postoperative hours. A stress dose of corticosteroid therapy is typically given intraoperatively, and patients are continued on a tapered dose 7 days postoperatively. Additional medications include subcutaneous heparin until patients are ambulatory, prophylactic antibiotics for 7 days or the duration of nasal packing, and anticonvulsants for 3 months. Although the latter use of anticonvulsants is commonly practiced, there are currently no accepted guidelines on their use in patients without prior history of seizures. MRI with gadolinium of the head, although not uniformly adopted, may be obtained on the second postoperative day to rule out perioperative intracranial complications, and at 3 months and annually thereafter to assess residual, persistent, or recurrent disease. Patients are usually transferred to a regular room on the second postoperative day and are encouraged to start ambulating at that time. In case a lumbar drain is used, it is clamped on the second or third postoperative day and removed one day later if patients show no signs of CSF leak.

Patients are routinely discharged home on the third or fourth postoperative day as long as they are neurologically intact, ambulate without difficulty, and tolerate a full diet. Nasal packing is removed on the fifth to seventh postoperative day, and the prophylactic antibiotic is usually discontinued thereafter. After removal of the nasal packing, the repair site is carefully examined endoscopically for evidence of CSF leak and proper graft positioning. It is paramount to avoid aggressive suctioning or debridement of the repair site at that time because this may cause dislodgement of the graft. The gelatin sponge overlying the grafted area is left undisturbed to fall off on its own. Nasal irrigation is not used until one month postoperatively. Most patients require adjunctive therapy (often radiotherapy), which can be started safely after three postoperative weeks.

Outcomes

Although the ACFR approach has been extensively studied over the past 50 years,[4–11] only limited retrospective datasets are currently available on endoscopic anterior skull base tumor resection.[2,16–26] A recent large international collaborative study showed that with the addition of adjuvant therapy, the 5-year overall, disease-specific, and recurrence-free survival rates for patients undergoing ACFR approximate 54%, 60%, and 53%, respectively. This study also indicated that histology of the primary tumor, its intracranial extent, and the status of surgical margins were independent predictors of overall, disease-specific, and recurrence-free survival on multivariate analysis.[10] Another large retrospective study found similar results after ACFR and reported that dural invasion, primary histologic diagnosis, and margin status had a significant impact on relapse-free and disease-specific survival.[7] However, both studies found similar rates of major complications and mortality (~40% and 5%, respectively) after ACFR.

An analysis of 19 patients (17 malignant and 2 benign lesions) by Casiano et al.[25] who underwent endoscopic anterior craniofacial resection without craniotomy or external incision showed a local control rate of 95% for all neoplasms and 94% for malignant tumors. The major complication rate was 10% without any case of mortality. Unfortunately, the mean follow-up period in this study was only 34 months, and a large portion of the patients were at an early stage. Batra et al.[8] compared standard ACFR with endoscopic and endoscopic-assisted anterior skull base resection in a small retrospective study of 25 patients and found no difference in operative time, estimated blood loss, hospital stay, or recurrence. However, there was a moderate increase in major complications and mortality in the patients undergoing ACFR. The mean follow-up in this study was less than 3 years. A similar recent comparison at the University of Miami in 18 patients undergoing endoscopic anterior skull base resection and 48 patients who underwent ACFR for malignant tumors of the anterior skull base showed a decreased hospital stay and faster recovery favoring the transnasal endoscopic resection group.[31] No significant differences were found in survival, metastatic, and complication rates between the two groups. A lower local recurrence rate was observed in the transnasal endoscopic resection group, although it was not statistically significant. However, due to a significantly larger number of high-grade histologies and clinical stages in the ACFR group, no definite clinical conclusions could be drawn.

Conclusion

In the hand of experienced, skilled endoscopic skull base surgeons, most anterior skull base tumors (benign and malignant) can be safely and successfully treated with an endoscopic anterior skull base resection while maintaining proper oncologic principles. This technique allows better visualization for tumor removal and is associated with a faster recovery, decreased hospital stay, decreased major and minor complication rates, and potentially decreased local recurrence rates in properly selected cases when compared with external ACFR. Nonetheless, this technique does not currently represent the standard of care for malignant anterior skull base tumors and should be performed by trained endoscopic skull base surgeons. Endoscopic-assisted anterior craniofacial resection should be reserved for large tumors with marked intracranial, dermal, and orbital extension necessitating gross intracranial tumor resection, skin excision, and orbital exenteration, respectively. Due to the continuous advances in endoscopic skull base surgery, the external ACFR as described by Ketcham,[3] has fewer indications. ACFR remains essential for revision cases with significant fibrosis and extensive tumors with skin and orbital extension not amenable to a purely endoscopic approach. It should be assisted with endoscopic equipment when appropriate to provide better visualization during tumor extirpation. Surgeons performing endoscopic anterior skull base resection should be familiar and proficient in performing external ACFR in case complete tumor extirpation cannot be achieved endoscopically, thus necessitating conversion to an open approach for cure.

References

1. Dandy WE. Orbital Tumors: Results Following the Transcranial Attack. New York: Oskar Priest; 1941
2. Casiano RR, Numa WA, Falquez AM. Endoscopic resection of esthesioneuroblastoma. Am J Rhinol 2001;15(4):271–279
3. Ketcham AS, Wilkins RH, Vanburen JM, Smith RR. A combined intracranial facial approach to the paranasal sinuses. Am J Surg 1963;106:698–703
4. Kraus DH, Shah JP, Arbit E, Galicich JH, Strong EW. Complications of craniofacial resection for tumors involving the anterior skull base. Head Neck 1994;16(4):307–312
5. Bridger GP, Kwok B, Baldwin M, Williams JR, Smee RI. Craniofacial resection for paranasal sinus cancers. Head Neck 2000; 22(8):772–780
6. Shah JP, Bilsky MH, Patel SG. Malignant tumors of the skull base. Neurosurg Focus 2002;13(4):e6
7. Bentz BG, Bilsky MH, Shah JP, Kraus D. Anterior skull base surgery for malignant tumors: a multivariate analysis of 27 years of experience. Head Neck 2003;25(7):515–520
8. Batra PS, Citardi MJ, Worley S, Lee J, Lanza DC. Resection of anterior skull base tumors: comparison of combined traditional and endoscopic techniques. Am J Rhinol 2005;19(5):521–528
9. Ganly I, Patel SG, Singh B, et al. Complications of craniofacial resection for malignant tumors of the skull base: report of an International Collaborative Study. Head Neck 2005;27(6):445–451
10. Patel SG, Singh B, Polluri A, et al. Craniofacial surgery for malignant skull base tumors: report of an international collaborative study. Cancer 2003;98(6):1179–1187
11. Richtsmeier WJ, Briggs RJ, Koch WM, et al. Complications and early outcome of anterior craniofacial resection. Arch Otolaryngol Head Neck Surg 1992;118(9):913–917
12. Thaler ER, Kotapka M, Lanza DC, Kennedy DW. Endoscopically assisted anterior cranial skull base resection of sinonasal tumors. Am J Rhinol 1999;13(4):303–310
13. McCutcheon IE, Blacklock JB, Weber RS, et al. Anterior transcranial (craniofacial) resection of tumors of the paranasal sinuses: surgical technique and results. Neurosurgery 1996;38(3):471–479, discussion 479–480
14. Har-El G, Casiano RR. Endoscopic management of anterior skull base tumors. Otolaryngol Clin North Am 2005;38(1):133–144, ix
15. Anand VK, Schwartz TH. Surgical approaches to the anterior skull base. In: Anand VK, Schwartz TH, eds. Practical Endoscopic Skull Base Surgery. San Diego, CA: Plural Publishing, Inc; 2007: 71–88
16. Banhiran W, Casiano RR. Endoscopic sinus surgery for benign and malignant nasal and sinus neoplasm. Curr Opin Otolaryngol Head Neck Surg 2005;13(1):50–54
17. Yuen AP, Fung CF, Hung KN. Endoscopic cranionasal resection of anterior skull base tumor. Am J Otolaryngol 1997;18(6):431–433
18. Stammberger H, Anderhuber W, Walch C, Papaefthymiou G. Possibilities and limitations of endoscopic management of nasal and paranasal sinus malignancies. Acta Otorhinolaryngol Belg 1999;53(3):199–205
19. Walch C, Stammberger H, Anderhuber W, Unger F, Köle W, Feichtinger K. The minimally invasive approach to olfactory neuroblastoma: combined endoscopic and stereotactic treatment. Laryngoscope 2000;110(4):635–640
20. Unger F, Walch C, Stammberger H, Papaefthymiou G, Haselsberger K, Pendl G. Olfactory neuroblastoma (esthesioneuroblastoma): report of six cases treated by a novel combination of endoscopic surgery and radiosurgery. Minim Invasive Neurosurg 2001;44(2):79–84
21. Cakmak O, Ergin NT, Yilmazer C, Kayaselçuk F, Barutcu O. Endoscopic removal of esthesioneuroblastoma. Int J Pediatr Otorhinolaryngol 2002;64(3):233–238
22. Unger F, Haselsberger K, Walch C, Stammberger H, Papaefthymiou G. Combined endoscopic surgery and radiosurgery as treatment modality for olfactory neuroblastoma (esthesioneuroblastoma). Acta Neurochir (Wien) 2005;147(6):595–601, discussion 601–602
23. Roh HJ, Batra PS, Citardi MJ, Lee J, Bolger WE, Lanza DC. Endoscopic resection of sinonasal malignancies: a preliminary report. Am J Rhinol 2004;18(4):239–246
24. Casler JD, Doolittle AM, Mair EA. Endoscopic surgery of the anterior skull base. Laryngoscope 2005;115(1):16–24
25. Dave SP, Bared A, Casiano RR. Surgical outcomes and safety of transnasal endoscopic resection for anterior skull tumors. Otolaryngol Head Neck Surg 2007;136(6):920–927
26. Batra PS, Citardi MJ. Endoscopic management of sinonasal malignancy. Otolaryngol Clin North Am 2006;39(3):619–637, x–xi
27. Liu JK, O'Neill B, Orlandi RR, Moscatello AL, Jensen RL, Couldwell WT. Endoscopic-assisted craniofacial resection of esthesioneuroblastoma: minimizing facial incisions—technical note and report of 3 cases. Minim Invasive Neurosurg 2003;46(5):310–315
28. Yuen AP, Fan YW, Fung CF, Hung KN. Endoscopic-assisted cranionasal resection of olfactory neuroblastoma. Head Neck 2005;27(6):488–493
29. Germani RM, Vivero R, Herzallah IR, Casiano RR. Endoscopic reconstruction of large anterior skull base defects using acellular dermal allograft. Am J Rhinol 2007;21(5):615–618
30. Hadad G, Bassagasteguy L, Carrau RL, et al. A novel reconstructive technique after endoscopic expanded endonasal approaches: vascular pedicle nasoseptal flap. Laryngoscope 2006;116(10):1882–1886
31. Eloy JA, Vivero RJ, Hoang K, et al. Comparison of transnasal endoscopic and open craniofacial resection for malignant tumors of the anterior skull base. Laryngoscope 2009;119(5):834–840

46 Endoscopic Approaches to the Sella and Suprasellar Region

Anne E. Getz, Edward R. Laws, and Peter H. Hwang

The endoscopic approach to the sellar and suprasellar regions has evolved considerably from the classical sublabial transseptal transsphenoidal approach that originated in the early 20th century. The current methodology encompasses the advances of modern surgical technology to improve the procedure, its safety, and its outcomes. Three major conceptual changes in the 1970s influenced the extracranial transsphenoidal approach to the sellar region. The first was the identification of the microadenoma, which ushered in a conservational approach to tumor resection. Whereas pituitary surgery had historically been obliterative in nature, it was recognized that a small microadenoma could be removed with preservation of the normal pituitary gland. Second, the introduction of video fluoroscopy improved anatomic control of instrumentation and the approach. Finally, the introduction of the operating microscope allowed for excellent illumination, superb visualization, and the use of delicate microsurgical instruments in a confined space.

In the 1980s, the application of endoscopic techniques to sinus surgery emerged as an important new modality of surgery for rhinosinusitis. Adaptation of endoscopic approaches to the sella were described in the 1990s, with the first major series reported by Jho and Carrau in 1997.[1] In the words of de Divitiis, the emergence of the endoscope onto the contemporary neurosurgical landscape resulted in a "stone in the pond" effect, stimulating new indications and novel approaches to minimally invasive surgery of the skull base.[2]

Relevant Embryogenesis and Anatomy of the Sphenoid Sinus and Pituitary

The sphenoid sinus begins pneumatization around 10 months of age and is complete by 10 years of age. Pneumatization begins at the natural ostium and proceeds superiorly and posteriorly. Pneumatization of the posterior ethmoids progresses in an anterior to posterior direction from birth to 8 years. An Onodi cell is a posterior ethmoid cell that has pneumatized superior and posterior to the rostrum of the sphenoid sinus. When present, Onodi cells may encompass the optic and/or carotid canals, pituitary sella, and suprasellar regions, potentially compromising adequate surgical exposure if not recognized during sphenoidotomy.

The natural ostium of the sphenoid sinus lies medially and inferiorly along the rostrum of the sphenoid, typically located at a level approximately one-third of the distance from the inferior aspect of the superior turbinate to the skull base. The nasopalatine branch of the sphenopalatine artery travels from lateral to medial within the soft tissues covering the rostrum, and runs inferior to the ostium. Blunt elevation of this soft tissue prior to inferior widening of the sphenoidotomy can avoid bothersome epistaxis, both intra- and postoperatively. Furthermore, preservation of this arterial branch is necessary if a posterior septal mucosal flap is anticipated because it provides the primary vascular supply.

The pituitary gland develops from two discrete evaginations: Rathke's pouch, a dorsal outpouching of the stomodeum; and the infundibulum, a ventral outpouching of the diencephalon. The former becomes the anterior pituitary, or adenohypophysis, and the latter becomes the posterior pituitary, or neurohypophysis. A second dorsal evagination, the pouch of Sessel, contributes to the hypophysis in lower primates and rarely will persist in humans as a potential site of tumorigenesis. Rathke's pouch and the infundibulum fuse under the morphogenic influence of the anterior notochord around the second month of gestation to form the pituitary gland. The pars tuberalis, a superior extension of Rathke's pouch, and the stem of the infundibulum comprise the pituitary stalk.[3]

During the first trimester, the adenohypophysis begins secreting its hormones, which include corticotrophin, beta-endorphin, luteinizing hormone (LH), follicle-stimulating hormone (FSH), thyrotropin-releasing hormone (TRH), growth hormone (GH), and prolactin (PRL). The neurohypophysis begins secretion of oxytocin and vasopressin in late fetal life.

Surgical Anatomy of the Sphenoid Sinus, Sella Turcica, and Parasellar Regions

Sphenoid and Sellar Anatomy

The sella turcica is the bony depression in the middle cranial fossa that houses the pituitary gland. The sella turcica is bounded anterosuperiorly by the tuberculum sellae and posteriorly by the dorsum sellae. The chiasmatic groove, which houses the optic chiasm, can sometimes be visualized from within the sphenoid sinus as a transverse convexity just anterosuperior to the tuberculum sellae. The relationship between the floor of the sella and the roof of the sphenoid (planum sphenoidale) depends on the degree of pneumatization of the sinus. In a well pneumatized sphenoid sinus, the sellar floor is clearly delineated as a prominent midline surface landmark of the posterior sphenoid wall and has a well-demarcated junction with the planum sphenoidale. By contrast, in the hypo- or nonpneumatized sphenoid, the pituitary will be largely or totally encased by dense bone, and the sellar floor will not be readily visualized or surgically accessible without significant bony drilling. As the pneumatization pattern may vary greatly from one individual to the next, it is important to review sphenoid pneumatization during surgical planning. In a radiographic review of 296 patients undergoing transsphenoidal surgery, Hamid et al. found presellar pneumatization in 21%, sellar pneumatization in 54.7%, and postsellar pneumatization in 22.3%.[4]

Another important variation in sphenoid anatomy is the course and configuration of the intersinus septum or septae. In the same study by Hamid, 10% had no septum, 66% had a single, centrally located septum inserting in the midline, and 5% had a septum that inserted laterally onto the carotid canal.[4] When the intersinus septum inserts onto the bony carotid canal, particular care must be taken in surgical resection or manipulation of the bony septum. In up to 12% of the population, there may be a dehiscent or absent bony canal.[5,6] Another variable that may affect the surgical approach is the intercarotid distance, ranging from 12 to 30 mm (mean, 23 mm).[4]

Because bony sphenoid anatomy is highly variable, preoperative review of anatomic landmarks is essential to form a sound surgical plan and avoid potential disaster.

Parasellar Anatomy

Incomplete dural folds, known as the diaphragma sellae, envelop the superior and lateral aspects of the pituitary, and separate the anterior pituitary from the optic chiasm. The diaphragma extends laterally where it is continuous with the medial dural walls of the cavernous sinuses, one and the same with the lateral walls of the pituitary fossa. An opening of variable size in the superior midline aspect of the diaphragma transmits the pituitary stalk and the gland's blood supply. Congenital incompetence of the diaphragma or increased intracranial pressure (ICP) can lead to herniation of the arachnoid though the opening and filling of the sella with cerebrospinal fluid (CSF), also known as empty sella syndrome.[3]

The cavernous sinus houses venous sinusoids, the intercavernous internal carotid artery (ICA), and multiple nerves: the oculomotor nerve, the first two divisions of the trigeminal nerve, the trochlear and abducens nerves, as well as the ICA sympathetic nerve complex. The cavernous ICA courses anteriorly in a bony groove known as the carotid sulcus. Here it runs adjacent to the superolateral surface of the body of the sphenoid bone. It then turns superiorly to pierce the dura and enter the subarachnoid space. The bony carotid canals are inferior and lateral to the optic nerve canals, the space between which forms the opticocarotid recess—a bony groove usually visible within the well-pneumatized sphenoid, representing clinoid pneumatization.

Inferior to the sella and comprising the posterior inferior boundary of the sphenoid sinus is the clivus—the bony surface in the posterior cranial fossa that slopes posteroinferiorly from the dorsum sellae to the foramen magnum.

Sellar and Parasellar Masses

Pituitary adenomas are by far the most common sellar tumors. Nonadenomatous lesions, although much less common, may embody a wide range of pathologies. Pituitary adenomas, along with some of the more common nonadenomatous lesions, are highlighted in the following sections.

Pituitary Adenoma

An enlarged sella may indicate a pituitary neoplasm or pituitary hyperplasia, which can occur in the setting of pregnancy or long-standing primary thyroid or gonadal failure.[7] Pituitary adenomas comprise 10% of all primary neurologic neoplasms, and 90% of all sellar lesions. The reported prevalence of pituitary adenomas in the literature varies greatly: autopsy studies and CT/MRI studies have yielded estimates as high as 16.7%,[8] whereas epidemiologic studies of clinically diagnosed adenomas in the United Kingdom and Italy have yielded estimates of 19 to 28 cases per 100,000. A more recent intensive cross-sectional analysis of over 70,000 individuals showed the prevalence of clinically apparent adenomas to be much higher than previously published at 1 in ~1000 individuals.[9]

Clinical presentation of adenomas is highly variable depending on the size and functional status of the tumor. Large adenomas may present with hypopituitarism, headaches, or bitemporal hemianopsia due to compression of the optic chiasm. Functional microadenomas may present with subtle or gross systemic changes reflecting neuroendocrine hypersecretion.

A snowman- or dumbbell-shaped tumor on MRI with solid characteristics and homogeneous enhancement is suggestive of a pituitary adenoma. Regions of necrosis, cystic degeneration, and/or hemorrhage may alter these characteristics.[10]

Craniopharyngioma

These rare epithelial tumors arise from the craniopharyngeal duct, the canal that connects the ectoderm of the stomodeum with Rathke's pouch. Two pathogenic hypotheses exist: (1) neoplastic transformation of the involuted duct; and (2) metaplastic degradation of adenohypophyseal cells. The different theories may explain the bimodal incidence of these tumors in childhood and in the sixth to eighth decades.[11,12]

Craniopharyngiomas have a reported incidence of 0.13 cases per 100,000 person-years, and comprise 2 to 5% of all primary intracranial neoplasms. They are the most common tumor of the sellar/parasellar region in the pediatric population, accounting for 5 to 15% of intracranial tumors.[13]

Craniopharyngiomas tend to have a lobulated shape with a prominent suprasellar component. Radiologically, craniopharyngiomas have heterogeneous signal characteristics, reflecting their typical composition of both solid and cystic characteristics, with enhancement of the solid portion.[10]

Clinically, the cyst fluid, composed of desquamated squamous epithelial cells, is often described as "machinery oil." The tumor borders are typically irregular and elicit a reactive gliosis that often prevent safe complete surgical resection,[11,14,15] contributing to an overall poorer clinical response to surgery and higher likelihood of recurrence during long-term follow-up. For these reasons, treatment typically involves postoperative radiation therapy for residual tumor.

Rathke's Cleft Cyst

Rathke's cleft cysts develop from the remnant of Rathke's pouch and thus are situated between the pars anterior and the infundibulum. Although these lesions are quite common with an incidence of around 15%, they are frequently small and asymptomatic. Symptoms present when cyst growth results in compression of the pituitary gland, optic chiasm, or hypothalamus. Rathke's cleft cysts are benign epithelium-lined cysts with a fibrous wall and mucoid content. The epithelium may be cuboidal, columnar, ciliated, or nonciliated, and there may be areas of pseudostratification and squamous metaplasia. CT imaging characteristically demonstrates a hypodense, nonenhancing mass; however, the cyst wall may occasionally enhance. Sellar expansion is present in 80% of cases, with both intrasellar and suprasellar components in 70%.[16] MRI characteristics are more variable. The lesion will typically appear as an ovoid-shaped, low-volume mass. As expected, the lesions have cystic, nonenhancing qualities, with signal attenuation similar to CSF on T1 and T2 imaging. Enhancement of the cyst wall may be seen.[10]

Only 5% of Rathke's cleft cysts will enlarge to the point of producing symptoms. Surgical drainage and partial cyst wall removal is considered curative, and recurrence is rare.

Meningiomas

Meningiomas are extra-axial tumors that arise from the meningothelial cell of the arachnoid that forms the external lining of the brain, and typically attach to the dura. Meningiomas account for ~15 to 25% of all primary intracranial neoplasms.[17,18] Ten to 15% of meningiomas are located in the parasellar region, whereas those confined entirely within the sella are rare.[19,20] Although most are histologically benign, meningiomas can behave aggressively and invade surrounding structures, and may cause significant morbidity secondary to mass effect. Sellar meningiomas present most often with alterations to visual fields (bitemporal hemianopsia) and diminished visual acuity as a result of optic atrophy.[21] Risk factors for the development of meningioma include exposure to ionizing radiation and exogenous hormones.[17]

Magnetic resonance imaging demonstrates a mass hypo- or isointense to gray matter on both T1- and T2-weighted images.[20] Contrast enhancement is intense, homogeneous, and rapid. Adenomas, in contrast, tend to enhance less intensely and homogeneously. The classic sign of a meningioma is that of a dural tail, a flat, tapering enhancement of dura emanating from the tumor. This feature is present on MRI in 60 to 72% of meningiomas.[22]

Germ Cell Tumors

Anomalous migration of the totipotent germ cells to the cranial midline during embryogenesis can result in various tumors including germinoma, teratoma, embryonal cell carcinoma, choriocarcinoma, yolk sac tumor, and mixed germinal tumor. These rare malignant tumors account for 0.1 to 2% of primary brain neoplasms, of which germinomas represent two-thirds.

These are tumors of childhood and usually arise between the ages of 10 and 12, with the exception of pure germinomas, which may present later. Similar to all tumors in this region, signs and symptoms are related to mass effect and pituitary function. Mass effects may include hydrocephalus and visual symptoms, whereas the more common functional symptoms include diabetes insipidus, delayed sexual development, hypopituitarism, and isolated growth failure. Germ cell tumors may secrete either alpha-fetoprotein (AFP) or beta-human chorionic gonadotropin (BHCG). Levels can be measured in the serum or, once disseminated, in the CSF. Detection of either is pathognomonic for the diagnosis of a germ cell tumor.[19,23]

The MRI findings of germ cell tumors are nonspecific, and thus these tumors cannot be diagnosed from imaging alone. Typical features include an enhancing solid sellar mass with or without suprasellar extension; occasional cysts and/or calcifications may also be seen. Not surprisingly, MRI cannot reliably differentiate the different subtypes of germ cell tumors.

Most germ cell tumors are at least partially responsive to radiation therapy; however, it is generally accepted that surgery plays a role in tissue diagnosis, at least in the case of negative tumor markers. As these are generally tumors of childhood, the long-term effects of radiation to this region and secondary malignancies must also be considered. Chemotherapy may also be an important therapeutic option depending on the specific tumor subtype.[24]

Chordomas

Chordomas are rare primary bone tumors that arise from embryonic remnants of the notochord. Chordomas account for 0.1 to 0.2% of all intracranial tumors, and 1% of malignant bone tumors. In normal embryogenesis, the mature notochord obliterates centrally, leaving microscopic foci in the cranial and caudal positions. Thus, chordomas most frequently arise in the spheno-occipital region within the clivus (~30%) and the sacrococcygeal region (~30 to 50%). Spheno-occipital tumors usually demonstrate malignant transformation in the third to fourth decades of life, and somewhat later (fifth to sixth decades) in the case of sacrococcygeal tumors.[25,26]

Magnetic resonance T1 images demonstrate a homogeneous, hypo- to isointense signal, whereas T2 images characteristically demonstrate a hyperintense, heterogeneous signal. All chordomas enhance to some degree, with approximately half demonstrating intense enhancement.[27] Because chordomas have a proclivity for bony erosion, CT can provide important complementary data to MRI regarding the bony integrity of clival and paraclival structures. Nearly 100% of chordomas will have evidence of bone destruction, abnormal contour, and expansion. Sclerotic bony reaction is not seen.

The clinical presentation of chordoma is most often pain, with neurologic deficits unique to the extent of local tumor invasion. Approximately half of patients with chordomas will present with ocular symptoms of diplopia or visual impairment. Abducens nerve palsy and ipsilateral Horner syndrome may be manifestations of invasion of the posterior and inferior cavernous sinus, where the abducens nerve travels along with the intercavernous sympathetics. Impairment of the oculomotor and trochlear nerves is also not uncommon.

Although surgery is the mainstay of therapy for chordoma, adjunctive radiotherapy improves local control, particularly combined proton/photon beam radiotherapy.[26,28] In certain cases, complete resection may be precluded by tumor involvement in neighboring critical structures. Given that positive margins result in a high rate of recurrence on the order of 70%, the importance of adjuvant therapy is further highlighted.[29]

Metastases

Metastases to the pituitary gland and sella are rare, and represent only 1% of all sellar and parasellar tumors.[30] Breast and lung malignancies are most commonly known to metastasize to this region and, combined, account for roughly 60% of all sellar metastases.

A propensity exists for metastasis to the posterior lobe. A review of 201 cases reported involvement of the posterior lobe either alone or in combination with the anterior lobe in ~80% of cases, whereas sole anterior lobe involvement occurred in only 15%.[31] Given that metastatic spread is hematogenous, this discrepancy has been attributed to the lack of a direct arterial blood supply to the anterior lobe.

The most common symptom observed in patients with pituitary metastases is diabetes insipidus (DI), which occurs in 45 to 70% of cases, and is likely due to the predilection to posterior lobe involvement. Other signs and symptoms include those common to sellar masses, including visual field deficits, pituitary insufficiency, oculomotor palsies, and headache.[19,32]

Radiographic characteristics of sellar metastases are somewhat variable. In the absence of other brain lesions, differentiation from pituitary adenoma can be difficult. Sellar metastases tend to be hypo- or isointense with gray matter on T1, and may be hyperintense on T2-weighted imaging. Metastases enhance to varying degrees with contrast, and rim enhancement is not uncommon. Biopsy is necessary to establish the diagnosis; excisional biopsy may be a reasonable therapeutic option in surgically appropriate patients with significant symptoms of mass effect. However, surgical morbidity must be considered carefully against overall prognosis. Palliative treatment with radiation therapy may often be an appropriate option. DI, when present, is managed with vasopressin. Hormonal replacement is also warranted depending on the individual's functional status.

Clinical Presentation

Functional Versus Nonfunctional Adenomas

As 90% of sellar tumors are pituitary adenomas, a discussion of their specific presentation is warranted. Pituitary adenomas are classified by size as microadenomas (≤1.0 cm) or macroadenomas (>1.0 cm), and may be functional or nonfunctional. Any suspected adenoma warrants a complete laboratory and radiologic workup to determine whether it is secretory. When clinical features such as acromegaly or Cushing disease suggest overproduction of a particular hormone, diagnostic tests may be tailored. If no such features are apparent, a comprehensive laboratory screening should be performed (**Table 46.1**).

As mass effect is less of an issue in microadenomas, management is typically governed by functional status. Nonsecreting microadenomas, and select nonsecreting macroadenomas not causing mass effects, can typically be monitored for growth with serial MRI. Expectant management of macroadenomas must take into consideration the increased risk of apoplexy and mass effects, discussed later. Surgical resection is indicated for functional adenomas not adequately controlled medically, and for tumors causing mass effect, regardless of secretory status.

Table 46.1 Laboratory Screening for Patients with Pituitary Adenoma

Serum prolactin
Thyroid function tests • Thyroid stimulating hormone • Free thyroxine
Serum gonadotropins • Men: Testosterone • Women: Estradiol + progesterone
Insulin-like growth factor (IGF-1)
If considering acromegaly: oral glucose tolerance test (OGTT) with growth hormone obtained at 0, 30, and 60 minutes
If considering Cushing syndrome: 24-hour urinary free cortisol, dexamethasone (1.0 mg) suppression test

Source: Adapted with permission from Melmed S, Kleinberg D. Anterior pituitary. In: Melmed S, Polonsky KS, Larsen PR, Kronenberger HM. Williams Textbook of Endocrinology, 11th ed. Philadelphia: Elsevier; 2007; and Janus TJ, Yung WKA. Primary neurological tumors. In: Goetz CG. Textbook of Clinical Neurology, 3rd ed. Philadelphia: WB Saunders; 2007.

Cystic Pituitary Lesions

Cystic tumors of the pituitary may represent arachnoid cysts, craniopharyngiomas, or more commonly, Rathke's cleft cysts. Sanno et al. reported nearly 30% of incidentally diagnosed cystic tumors to be Rathke's cleft cysts in a series of over 500 patients.[33] Given that a significant proportion of cystic pituitary lesions may be incidentally diagnosed in the absence of significant signs or symptoms, careful workup and clinical discernment are necessary to avoid unnecessary alarm and needless intervention in the asymptomatic patient.[34]

Symptoms

All of the lesions listed previously have the potential to produce hormonal abnormalities and local tumor effects eliciting some or all of the following clinical signs and symptoms.

Visual Symptoms

The classic presentation of visual impingement by a sellar mass is bitemporal hemianopsia. Although the exact mechanism of this specific visual field defect is not completely understood, it may be due to increased susceptibility of the nasally oriented optic nerve fibers to pressure as compared with the temporal fibers,[35] or to a differential ability to sustain pressure due to the physical orientation of the fibers themselves.[36] In a multivariate analysis of 152 patients with sellar masses, Rambaldini et al. found self-reported visual field defects to be a significant independent clinical predictor of the presence of an advanced sellar mass.[37]

Oculomotor palsy and/or paralysis are uncommon symptoms of uncomplicated sellar and parasellar masses, and should heighten the suspicion of apoplexy (see the following) or malignancy. Several cases of paresis (typically, of cranial nerve III) with and without ophthalmoplegia, however, have been described.

Headache

Headache is a common complaint in the general population with a long list of possible etiologies. However, a newly presenting headache, or one that has changed in character, may raise clinical concern for the presence of an advanced sellar mass.

One large prospective study of 84 patients with pituitary tumors sought to classify headache characteristics and correlate these symptoms with tumor characteristics and response to therapy. Diagnoses consisted of prolactinoma, acromegaly, nonfunctioning adenomas, Cushing disease, and thyroid stimulating hormone-secreting adenoma in 37%, 33%, 24%, 5%, and 1%, respectively. Sixty-five percent were macroadenomas, whereas 35% were microadenomas. Cavernous sinus invasion was visible on MRI in 21% of cases. Headaches were most often classified as migraine type and most often localized to the orbit or retro-orbit (79%) and frontal (64%) regions.[38]

Of the patients who underwent surgery, nearly half experienced improvement (49%), whereas the other half noted no change (36%) or worsening (15%) in headache symptoms. The majority (58%) of patients treated with somatostatin analogues experienced improvement. Dopamine-agonists were much less likely to improve symptoms, and in a significant percentage, exacerbated headache.[38]

Although headache is a common symptom associated with pituitary tumors, the etiology of these headaches is not totally understood. Mechanical stretch of the dura and cavernous sinus invasion, as well as functional activity of the tumor have all been implicated. Inability to correlate tumor size or functional status to the presence and severity of headache, as well as wide variations in response to surgical and medical therapy, suggest multifactorial etiologies, some of which may not yet be fully understood.

Apoplexy

Pituitary apoplexy is neurologic impairment due to acute hemorrhage or infarction of the pituitary gland, most cases of which occur in the setting of a pituitary adenoma. Signs and symptoms suggestive of apoplexy include sudden onset of headache, vomiting, visual symptoms (including ocular paresis, reduction in visual fields and/or acuities), altered mental status, and hormonal dysfunction. Recognition and appropriate treatment, including surgical decompression, are critical in this potentially life-threatening condition. Once the apoplexy patient is medically stable, prompt surgical decompression is vital to prevent sequelae. Near-complete reversibility of ophthalmologic signs and symptoms is attainable when decompression is performed within 1 week of presentation.[39]

In contrast, recovery of endocrine function may not be as complete, with a higher likelihood of requiring subsequent long-term steroidal and hormonal therapy. In their series of 36 postsurgical patients, Bills et al. reported that greater than 80% of patients required long-term steroidal or thyroid hormone replacement, 11% required desmopressin, and 64% of males required testosterone replacement.[40]

Hemorrhagic Rathke's cleft cysts have also been described to cause apoplexy; however, these cases are exceedingly rare.

Preoperative Evaluation

The preoperative phase of the evaluation of patients for endoscopic transnasal skull base surgery involves a careful review of the patient's history, clinical findings, endocrine laboratory studies, and imaging studies. It is important to include evaluation of all of the pituitary hormones (see Clinical Presentation, previously), specifically looking for deficiencies in cortisol and thyroid function, along with low sex hormones (FSH and LH), which may lead to sexual dysfunction, low testosterone in men, and low estrogen in women. Men with low testosterone may also present with a comorbidity of anemia. Some patients with lesions in the region of the sella will present with DI, making their endocrine management more difficult.

Clinical and radiographic evaluation of the nasal structures and sinuses is important prior to surgery. All patients without contraindications should undergo an MRI of the brain with contrast. The MRI is examined to assess the location of the lesion and its extent, if any, outside of the sella into the parasellar structures or the suprasellar region. The positions of the normal pituitary gland, pituitary stalk, optic nerves, optic chiasm, and hypothalamus are determined. Note should be made of any evidence of cerebral atrophy or hydrocephalus. The paranasal sinus anatomy can typically be delineated adequately on coronal sections of the MRI. However, CT imaging can be useful in providing supplemental detail of the sinonasal anatomy and the bony integrity of the sella, parasellar, and clival regions. The presence of sphenoethmoidal (Onodi) cells and intrasinus septations within the sphenoid sinus are noted, with attention to their relationship to the sella itself and to the carotid and optic canals.

Nasal endoscopy is performed with special attention to evidence of prior nasal or sinus surgery and deviations of the nasal septum that may require correction for ease of instrumentation. With rare exceptions, it has been the authors' experience that most septal deviations can be worked around without the need for formal septoplasty.

Surgical Approach

The major advantage in transnasal approaches is the reduction in morbidity by virtue of the midline trajectory of resection. Lateral-to-medial approaches to the tuberculum sella, suprasellar, and parasellar regions' resection pose higher risks of retraction injuries such as edema, hemorrhage, and optic and olfactory nerve injury.[41] These riskier external approaches include the frontolateral, bifrontal, and pterional (frontotemporal) approaches.

Endonasal microsurgical approaches to this region are well documented and offer the advantages of excellent three-dimensional optics and depth of field. Access is obtained by identical means as in the case of endoscopic resection, via sublabial, rhinoseptal, or endonasal approaches. One major technical difference is the dependency of the microsurgical approach on significant retraction with a nasal speculum for exposure. The absence of a nasal speculum in the surgical field during the endoscopic approach allows for a greater range of motion in instrument handling and positioning.

The endoscope possesses several other advantages as compared with the operating microscope. The wide-angle view of the endoscope provides a more expansive field of view in all directions. In one study, the endoscopic volume of visualization was 1.75 times greater than with the microscope for the transcolumellar approach and four times greater for the sublabial approach.[42] Of note, this study employed only the 0-degree endoscope. Use of angled endoscopes further increases the visible surgical volume. The use of angled endoscopes also facilitates more complete tumor resection than possible with the operating microscope by better visualization of the periphery of the surgical dissection in all directions. In one study where flexible and rigid angled endoscopes were used to augment visualization with the microscope, 40% of patients had residual tumor identifiable on endoscopy that was not microscopically visualized.[43] By virtue of the endoscope's ability to be manipulated in a narrow surgical field, sinonasal tissue is also less traumatized, resulting in less subsequent pain and sinonasal dysfunction.[2,44]

As noted previously, there are several variations of the approach to the sella, namely the sublabial, rhinoseptal, and endonasal approaches. In the sublabial approach, an incision is made in the maxillary gingivobuccal sulcus from canine to canine, and the mucoperiosteum is elevated superiorly exposing the pyriform apertures of the nose. The nasal speculum is inserted in one side and a vertical incision through the posterior septum performed. The speculum is then used to disarticulate the nasal septum from the maxillary crest, displacing it laterally to expose the sphenoid rostrum. In the rhinoseptal or transcolumellar approach, an open rhinoplasty incision is made along the columella, retracting the medial crura of the lower lateral cartilages to expose the nasal septum. Again, the septum is disarticulated from the maxillary crest to allow insertion of the speculum.

In the endonasal approach, no incisions are used, and the septum is left attached to the maxillary crest. This method is favored for endoscopic approaches. The posterior exposure is achieved via turbinate outfracture and a limited posterior septectomy.

Initial Intraoperative Phase

The patient's nose is first decongested topically with oxymetazoline. Bilateral transoral greater palatine foramina injections are performed to decrease bleeding from the sphenopalatine arteries. A 25-gauge needle is bent at a 45-degree angle 2.5 cm from the tip. The needle is inserted into the foramina up to the bend in the needle to avoid infiltration into the inferior orbital fissure, decreasing the unlikely but dreaded complication of vasoconstrictive blindness. After aspiration to ensure that the needle is not intravascular, 1.5 mL of 1% lidocaine with 1:100,000 epinephrine is injected slowly into each side.

The abdomen is prepped in the subumbilical region for a possible incision to obtain a small fat graft in the event of an intraoperative CSF leak. A 2-cm curvilinear incision is usually made in the fold just below the umbilicus.

For some patients, a lumbar intrathecal drain will be inserted. This is not routinely done but may be indicated for patients who have large suprasellar extensions of tumor, or where a high-flow CSF leak may be anticipated. In the case of large suprasellar tumors, tumor dissection can be facilitated by injecting saline solution through the lumbar drain to displace the tumor downward. Lumbar drainage is occasionally useful for the intrathecal administration of fluorescein in very low concentrations to aid in identifying a cerebrospinal fluid leak (0.05 to 0.1 mL of 10% fluorescein diluted in 10 mL of either nonbacteriostatic [preservative-free] saline or the patient's own CSF).

The patient is carefully positioned with the head of the bed elevated 15 to 20 degrees, and the head is turned slightly to the patient's right. The elevation of the head and thorax is helpful for hemostasis, particularly in patients with elevated venous pressure, such as those with Cushing disease. Rigid fixation of the skull is optional because most image-guidance reference frames can be affixed securely to the scalp without pinning.

Nasal Phase

A 0-degree endoscope is used to examine the intranasal anatomy. Pledgets soaked in 1:1000 epinephrine are used for hemostasis and decongestion. In the majority of cases it is possible to work around septal deviations; however, in the rare case of severe deviation prohibiting easy admittance or adequate manipulation of instruments, an endoscopic septoplasty is initially performed. The inferior turbinates are outfractured with a Boies/Goldman elevator, followed by outfracture of the middle and superior turbinates with a Freer elevator. The ostia of the sphenoid sinuses are thus brought into view within the sphenoethmoidal recess.

If a pedicled septal flap is to be used for sellar reconstruction, it is elevated at this time. After harvest, the flap is then tucked out of the way into the nasopharynx during the subsequent tumor resection. (It is also possible to harvest the septal flap in a delayed fashion if its necessity is not certain. By preserving the inferior aspect of the posterior septum and the mucosa of the sphenoid rostrum during the approach, a viable pedicled flap can still be elevated at the conclusion of the tumor resection.)

After identification of the sphenoid ostia, bilateral sphenoidotomies are performed with through-cutting instruments (**Fig. 46.1**). Particular care must be taken to avoid injury to the posterior septal branch of the sphenopalatine artery, which runs in a transverse direction inferior to the sphenoid ostium. A posterior septectomy is then performed to connect the sphenoidotomies. Approximately 1.5 to 2 cm anterior to the rostrum, a through-and-through incision is made in the septum. Through-cutting instruments are used to remove the posterior septum. Carefully performed posterior septal resections should have minimal effect on ultimate nasal function; care should be taken to avoid high septal resections that may injure the olfactory neuroepithelium.

Resection of the inferior sphenoid rostrum is sometimes necessary to optimize exposure. The thicker inferior extent of the rostrum and vomer are resected with Kerrison rongeurs or drill. During this resection, it may be appropriate to identify, protect, and possibly clip or cauterize the septal branches of the sphenopalatine artery.

Communication between the neurosurgeon and the otorhinolaryngologist–head and neck surgeon is essential

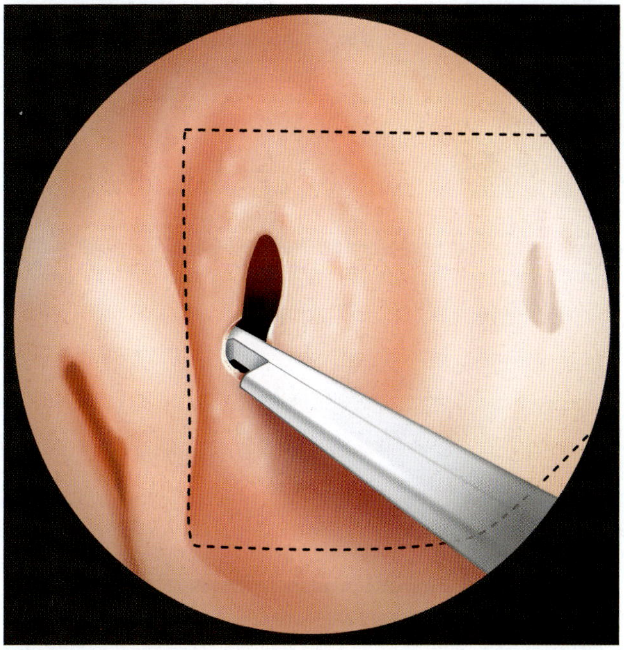

Fig. 46.1 Endoscopic view of right sphenoethmoid recess. The sphenoid ostium is identified after careful lateralization of the superior turbinate. A wide sphenoidotomy is then performed with the aim of mucosal preservation. The adjacent posterior septum will also be resected to allow the bilateral sphenoidotomies to be brought into continuity (area of resection outlined by *dotted line*). (Used with permission from Jackler RK. Atlas of Skull Base Surgery and Neurotology, 2nd ed. New York: Thieme; 2009: 157.)

to optimize the exposure for resection and ensure unencumbered movement of the endoscopes and instruments. Image-guidance navigation is often used at this point to confirm tumor extent and determine whether exposure is adequate. Wide exposure visualizing the carotid canals, the clival recess, the opticocarotid recesses, the planum sphenoidale, and the sphenoid floor is ideal. Broad exposure of the planum is particularly important in patients with suprasellar tumors because resection of a portion of the planum may be necessary to provide adequate exposure of the tumor (**Figs. 46.2 and 46.3**).

Sphenoid Phase

The sphenoid intersinus septum is then removed sharply until flush with the sella. Because the intersinus septum may insert laterally directly onto the carotid canal, foreknowledge of the patient's anatomy is essential to avoid potentially catastrophic injury. The sphenoid mucosa overlying the sella is then elevated laterally from the midline once the intersinus septum has been resected. The sphenoid mucosa should be preserved whenever possible.

The sella is then opened, either fracturing the thin floor or using a chisel or drill or a blunt nerve hook to expose the dura. Next, Kerrison punches are used to remove the sellar floor and expose the dura widely (**Fig. 46.4**). Lateral dissection is carefully performed until the bluish margin of the cavernous sinus is visible. Superior dissection should be performed with care as the dura is often adherent to the region of the tuberculum sellae. There may be an arachnoid diverticulum behind the dura at the upper margin of the sella, which, if disrupted, may result in CSF leakage.

The dura is then evaluated for the possibility of invasion or disruption by tumor, and for the venous channels that may occur in the dura, particularly the superior and inferior circular sinuses. The dura can be cauterized with bipolar cautery to secure hemostasis prior to the dural incision.

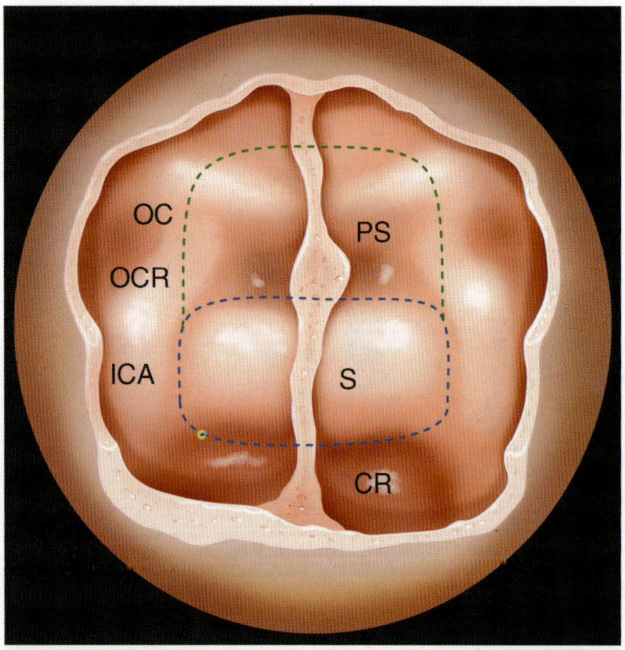

Fig. 46.2 Endoscopic view of bilateral sphenoid sinuses after bilateral sphenoidotomy and posterior septectomy. The *blue dotted line* demarcates the area of sellar (*S*) bone removal for intrasellar tumors; the *green dotted line* demarcates additional bone that needs to be removed from the planum sphenoidale (*PS*) for suprasellar approaches. Depending on the degree of sphenoid pneumatization, the optic canal (*OC*), opticocarotid recess (*OCR*), internal carotid artery (*ICA*), and clival recess (*CR*) may present as surface landmarks within the sphenoid sinus. (Used with permission from Jackler RK. Atlas of Skull Base Surgery and Neurotology, 2nd ed. New York: Thieme; 2009: 157.)

Sellar Phase

For the sellar phase, we use a 0-degree endoscope, and a two-surgeon binarial technique, where one surgeon manipulates the endoscope and the other uses two hands to perform the surgical resection (**Fig. 46.5**). A scope irrigator is particularly useful to wash blood and debris from the tip of the endoscope without needing to withdraw the scope from the field.

The sellar phase begins by coagulating and opening the dura. Fine-needle aspiration may be wise if there is any chance that the lesion could be an aneurysm or an empty sella. The dura is then opened with a shielded knife or a no. 10 scalpel. Usually, we use a rectangular excision of dura for large tumors (macroadenomas) and a cruciate incision for smaller tumors that do not invade the dura. A specimen of dura may be sent to pathology for evaluation of microscopic dural invasion.

The dural opening is then carefully extended, avoiding injury to the carotid and entry into the cavernous sinuses laterally. An initial helpful step is to establish a careful subdural plane using a blunt hook or a small curette. One can then identify and excise the lesion using an extracapsular dissection technique (**Fig. 46.6**). If not feasible, tumor dissection is performed by working outward from the center of the lesion and carefully dissecting it from surrounding structures. Every effort should be made to protect and preserve the normal anterior and posterior pituitary gland, and good visualization with careful hemostasis is critical in allowing this to occur.

Suprasellar extensions of tumor can be delivered by the injection of saline through a lumbar drain or by using a Valsalva maneuver or bilateral jugular compression. If exposure through the standard sellar exposure is not adequate for suprasellar tumor removal, the surgeon should be prepared to extend the dissection superiorly by resecting the tuberculum sella and planum sphenoidale. Hemostatic control of the superior intercavernous sinus is necessary before extending the dural opening superiorly.

Once the tumor has been removed, the endoscope is used to examine the periphery of the excision cavity and the underside of the diaphragm of the sella, including visualization of the cavernous sinus walls laterally and folds

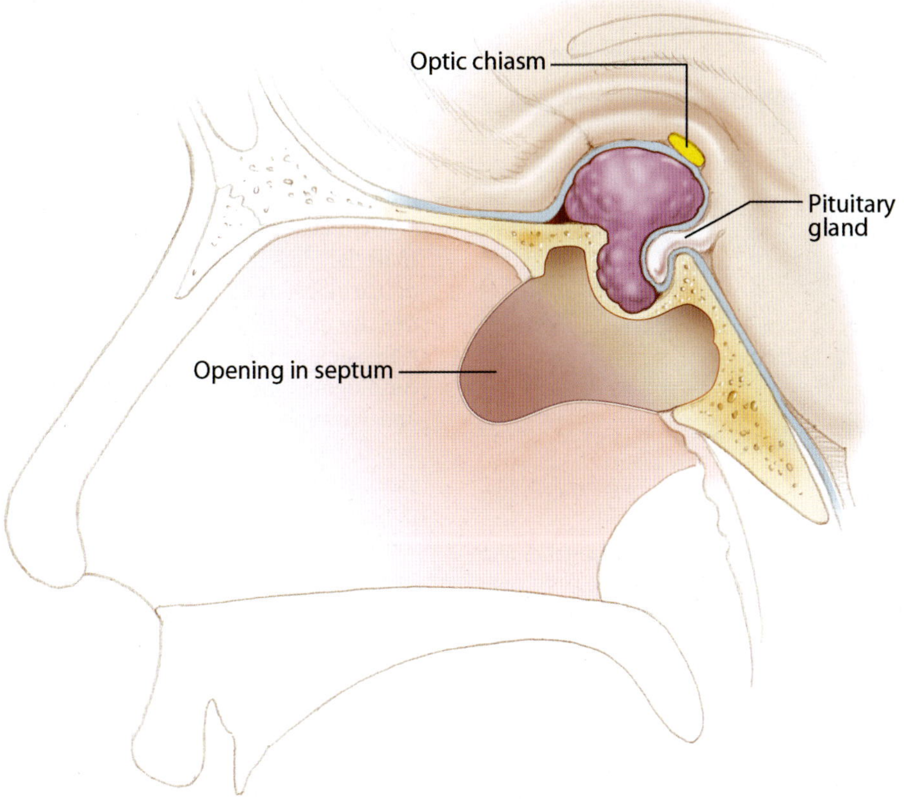

Fig. 46.3 A wide sphenoidotomy is desirable for optimal visualization and manipulation of parasellar structures, particularly when the tumor extends beyond the confines of the sella. Resection of the tuberculum sellae and planum sphenoidale may be required for exposure of suprasellar tumors.

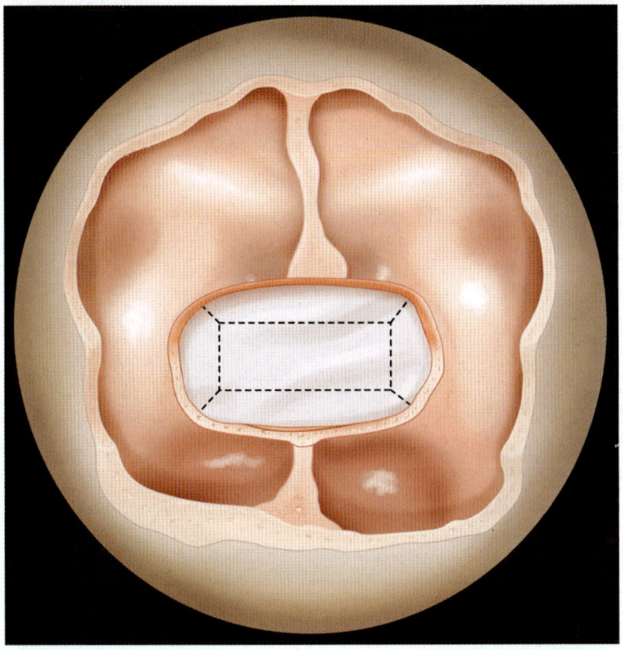

Fig. 46.4 Careful removal of sellar bone reveals the dura, which is incised sharply to access the tumor. (Used with permission from Jackler RK. Atlas of Skull Base Surgery and Neurotology, 2nd ed. New York: Thieme; 2009: 163.)

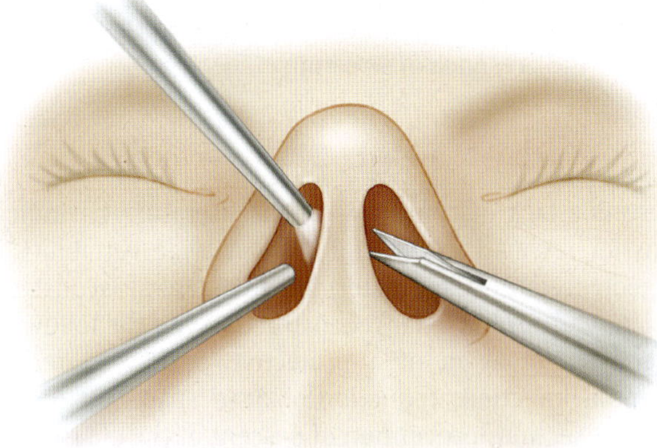

Fig. 46.5 Two-surgeon, binarial approach. The endoscope is placed at the superior aspect of the nasal vestibule with slight retraction, allowing room for passage of suction tips or instruments inferiorly. (Used with permission from Jackler RK. Atlas of Skull Base Surgery and Neurotology, 2nd ed. New York: Thieme; 2009: 156.)

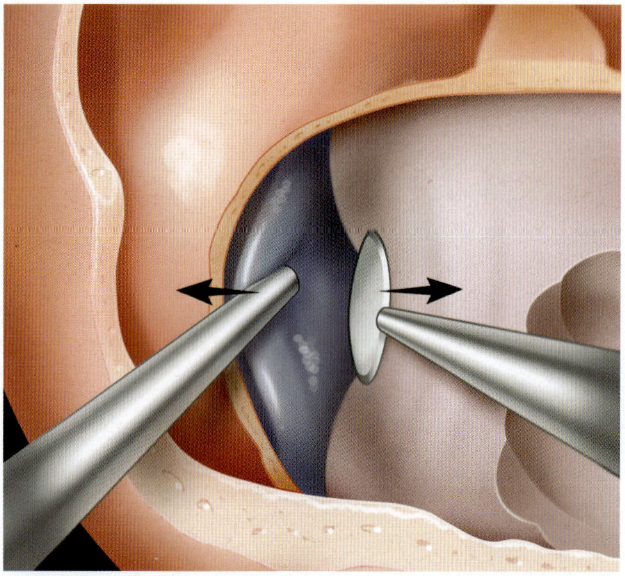

Fig. 46.6 Extracapsular dissection around the right lateral aspect of tumor bordering on the cavernous sinus. (Used with permission from Jackler RK. Atlas of Skull Base Surgery and Neurotology, 2nd ed. New York: Thieme; 2009: 165.)

of the diaphragm superiorly in the case of a large tumor. For this we use angled 30- to 45-degree endoscopes, when indicated.

At the conclusion of tumor resection, careful evaluation is made for hemostasis and possible CSF leak. Hemostasis is carefully achieved in the sellar region, with bipolar cautery for the dural margins and for vessels feeding the tumor, and oxidized cellulose packing for the cavernous sinuses and any areas of uncontrolled oozing. If hypotensive anesthesia has been administered, it is helpful to allow the blood pressure to normalize at this point to ensure hemostasis under normotensive conditions. Careful inspection of the diaphragm will usually reveal any CSF leaks, but administration of a Valsalva maneuver may be helpful to ensure complete assessment. The endoscopic finding of dark black "strings" or "tails" in the blood within the sella may indicate the presence of streaming CSF.

Reconstruction Phase and Closure of the Sella

There is a lack of consensus in the literature on indications for reconstruction, and there is wide variability in surgeon preference for materials and extent of reconstruction. Advocates for sellar reconstruction cite the following objectives: creation of a protective barrier to reduce potential infection; reduction of dead space left by the tumor resection; prevention of descent of the chiasm and other intracranial contents; and repair of CSF leak.[45]

Replacement of sellar volume may take the form of abdominal fat or an absorbable biomaterial, such as oxidized cellulose. However, the literature indicates that forgoing sellar packing may also be a viable option with no significant increased risk of postoperative complications in patients without sellar packing compared with those patients with sellar packing.[46] When a CSF leak is evident, sellar packing is typically indicated to facilitate leak closure and to avoid potentially serious complications including hemorrhage, infection, and tension pneumocephalus.[47] Careful attention must be paid to avoid overpacking the sella, which may result in deterioration of vision by mass effect, similar to that exerted by the original tumor.[46]

For reconstruction of the sellar floor, a wide variety of materials has been described, including autologous bone or cartilage, rigid biomaterial plates (e.g., porous high-density polyethylene), and pliable resorbable biomaterials such as gelatin foam and fibrin glue (**Fig. 46.7**).[48,49] Autologous materials carry the advantage of being inert and without cost, but can add additional operative time and donor site morbidity, and can possess limitations on size, shape, and malleability. Alternatively, alloplastic materials eliminate harvest time and can be fabricated to individualized reconstructive needs. However, alloplastic materials can add significant cost to the procedure, and their biocompatibility should be assessed carefully.

Cappabianca et al. examined their series of 170 transsphenoidal cases and found that only 28% of patients required sellar reconstruction.[46] No reconstruction or packing was performed in patients with microadenomas, macroadenomas without suprasellar extension, and macroadenomas with suprasellar extension, which

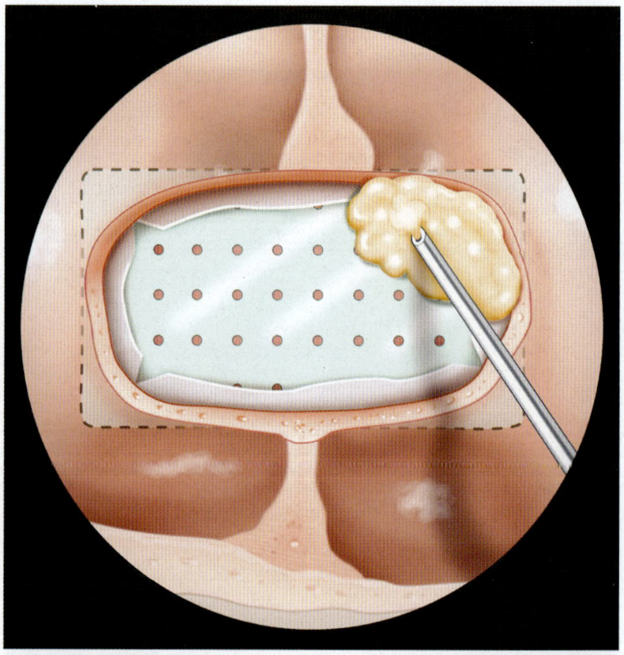

Fig. 46.7 Sellar reconstruction, when deemed necessary, can be performed with a wide range of autologous or alloplastic materials. Here, a bioabsorbable plate made of porous high-density polyethylene is seated in an underlay fashion intradurally. Application of fibrin glue is an optional additional step to secure the reconstruction. (Used with permission from Jackler RK. Atlas of Skull Base Surgery and Neurotology, 2nd ed. New York: Thieme; 2009: 163.)

were incompletely removed (to encourage descent of the residual lesion). Sellar packing and sellar floor reconstruction were performed in patients with prolapse of the suprasellar cistern toward the sellar floor; intraoperative CSF leak; bleeding from the medial wall of the cavernous sinus; or intracavernous carotid injury.

If a septal pedicled flap has been elevated, it can be rotated into the surgical field after the sellar dissection/reconstruction. Care must be taken to maintain the orientation of the flap with the mucosal side facing outward and to avoid kinking or twisting of the pedicle. The flap can be supported by a small amount of gelatin foam packing or fibrin glue. The sphenoid is otherwise left unpacked. In the case of extremely large defects, balloons or sponge packs may be required to provide additional bolstering of the closure. For additional information regarding closure of complex skull base defects, refer to Chapter 52 of this book.

Lumbar drainage is initiated intraoperatively when closure of a CSF leak is judged to not be watertight, as may occur in extended approaches, or postoperatively when a CSF leak is identified late during the convalescence period.[50]

Postoperative Care

The postoperative convalescence period requires careful monitoring for potential neurosurgical, neuroendocrine, and rhinologic complications. Neurosurgical complications may include headache, new visual loss, postoperative CSF leak, meningitis, and injury to the carotid artery with the possibility of a subsequent stroke. Neuroendocrine complications include diabetes insipidus, hyponatremia and syndrome of inappropriate antidiuretic hormone hypersecretion (SIADH), and new hypopituitarism. Complications related to the nasal and sinus aspects of the operation include delayed epistaxis, septal perforation, sinusitis, synechiae, and hyposmia. General complications may also include infection of the abdominal wound, deep venous thrombosis, and pulmonary emboli. Fortunately, these complications are rare and most can be dealt with successfully if recognized early and promptly corrected.

Postoperative sinonasal care is similar to that after standard endoscopic sinus surgery. The regimen includes frequent moisturization of the nasal cavity with saline nasal spray and saline irrigation. Serial nasal endoscopy with selective debridement is performed until complete remucosalization of the surgical field has been established.

Outcomes in Transsphenoidal Surgery

The transsphenoidal microsurgical approach to the sellar and parasellar region largely replaced transcranial approaches in the mid-20th century with the widespread use of the operating microscope. The endoscopic approach was first introduced to transsphenoidal surgery in the early 1990s, and has experienced steadily increasing use and acceptance since its inception. Published outcomes thus far have shown great promise for this approach as not only equal to the microsurgical approach, but superior in certain regards.[51–54]

It is generally accepted that transnasal approaches are less morbid and better tolerated than the transcranial approach. Furthermore, it stands to reason that the transseptal approach with septal dislocation and retractor placement may adversely affect nasal function postoperatively and be not as well tolerated than the endoscopic approach. Indeed, rhinology-specific outcomes as measured by the SNOT-22 questionnaire were improved in the endoscopic transsphenoidal approach as compared with the sublabial transseptal approach.[44] Local nasal complications including tears to the columella, septal perforation and deviation, and epistaxis are also significantly less common after endoscopic surgery.[55]

Mean hospital stay after endoscopic approach has been reported to be significantly shorter than for transseptal surgeries by an average of 2 days.[44,55,56] In an era of increasingly cost-conscious medicine, this too may be considered a significant outcome improvement.

Completeness of resection is certainly of greater importance than postoperative rhinologic function. For lesions extending beyond the sella, the endoscope has been shown to be superior in lowering the incidence of residual tumor volume,[51,55] likely attributable to the well-illuminated angulated views afforded by endoscopy. In a subsequent meta-analysis of nine endoscopic studies (821 patients), gross tumor removal was 78% and hormone resolution was 81 to 84% depending on tumor-secreting type.[55] In a comparison of 71 endoscopic and 122 sublabial transseptal microscopic surgeries, recurrence was more common in the sublabial cohort (28.4% versus 18.2%); however, this did not reach statistical significance.[44] Similar numbers have been reported for a transseptal series of 3093 patients followed for at least 10 years. Remission rates were found to be 84% for nonsecreting tumors; 88 and 65% for growth hormone micro- and macroadenomas; 87 and 56% for prolactin micro- and macroadenomas; and 91% and 65% for Cushing disease micro- and macroadenomas.[57]

Radiotherapy is used when indicated to address residual tumor. Murad et al. found that surgery coupled with radiotherapy in patients with residual nonsecreting pituitary adenomas significantly decreased recurrence.[58] Post-treatment sequelae from radiation, however, are not to be ignored. Evidence suggests that patients undergoing endoscopic surgery are statistically less likely to have radiation therapy due to increased completeness of resection.[55]

In patients with preoperative visual deficits, the majority experience improvement after surgery, regardless of approach. In a single series of over 3000 patients treated with a sublabial transsphenoidal approach, improvement of visual field deficit was seen in 87% of patients.[57] Incidence of visual improvement has been shown to be similar in studies assessing both endoscopic and transseptal approaches.[44,55,58]

Normalization of pituitary function following transseptal microsurgical surgery in a series of 3093 patients was 97% for growth hormone tumors, prolactinomas, and nonsecreting tumors.[57] In patients with normal preoperative pituitary function, the need for postoperative hormone therapy has been reported to be similar between endoscopic and transseptal groups. In a comparative series of endoscopic versus transseptal approaches, Graham et al. found that permanent DI was significantly more common in the transseptal microscopic group.[44] A meta-analysis of patients undergoing transsphenoidal (both endoscopic and transseptal) approaches reported an incidence of permanent DI of less than 5%.[58] Another meta-analysis of 481 endoscopic approaches reported permanent DI in only 1% of patients.[56]

Outcomes are also favorable with respect to other major complications. A meta-analysis of transsphenoidal (endoscopic and microsurgical) studies showed the rate of CSF leak, meningitis, and new visual field defects to be ≤5%.[58] Tabee et al. reported a 2% incidence of CSF leak in transsphenoidal approaches.[56] CSF leak was found to be significantly more common in the endoscopic group (10.6%) as compared with the transseptal group (2.5%) in a comparative series.[44] A similar incidence of CSF leak (19.7% intraoperative and 10.3% postoperative) was reported in Senior et al.'s series of 193 endoscopic procedures, and a similar trend was reported by Minet et al.[55,59] It has been proposed that increased rates of CSF leak may be a result of improved visualization owing to the more extensive resection of larger tumors. CSF leak may be an acceptable trade-off, however, for the sake of complete resection.

In a large meta-analysis of 51 studies pooling over 4000 patients with nonfunctioning pituitary adenomas, the relative risk ratio of death for transcranial versus transsphenoidal resection was 4.89.[58] Low mortality rates of 0 to 1% are reported in transsphenoidal series including sublabial, transseptal, and endoscopic approaches.[44,51,56,57,59]

The strength of the evidence on comparative outcomes of transsphenoidal surgical approaches is limited by the predominance of uncontrolled retrospective case series in the literature. As pituitary adenoma is the most common tumor in this region, most outcome data pertain to these patients and one must be mindful of this when considering the same approach for other pathologies. Long-term tumor control data are not yet available for the endoscopic approach; however, short-term data are favorable. Outcomes including mortality rate, perioperative complications, hormonal control, visual improvement, and extent of resection are available, and bode well for the endoscopic technique as a safe and effective approach to surgery of the sella and parasellar region.

Conclusion

The successful diagnosis and management of lesions of the sella require a multidisciplinary approach in both medical and surgical aspects. For lesions requiring surgery, evidence-based review of the literature indicates that lesions of the sella and suprasella can be safely and effectively approached with an endonasal endoscopic transsphenoidal approach. The rapid and increasingly broad acceptance of endoscopic surgical approaches since their inception foretells continued refinement and expansion of endoscopic techniques in years to come.

References

1. Jho HD, Carrau RL. Endoscopic endonasal transsphenoidal surgery: experience with 50 patients. J Neurosurg 1997;87(1):44–51
2. de Divitiis E. Endoscopic transsphenoidal surgery: stone-in-the-pond effect. Neurosurgery 2006;59(3):512–520, discussion 512–520
3. Amar AP, Weiss MH. Pituitary anatomy and physiology. Neurosurg Clin N Am 2003;14(1):11–23, v
4. Hamid O, El Fiky L, Hassan O, Kotb A, El Fiky S. Anatomic variations of the sphenoid sinus and their impact on trans-sphenoid pituitary surgery. Skull Base 2008;18(1):9–15
5. Unal B, Bademci G, Bilgili YK, Batay F, Avci E. Risky anatomic variations of sphenoid sinus for surgery. Surg Radiol Anat 2006;28(2):195–201
6. Nitinavakarn B, Thanaviratananich S, Sangsilp N. Anatomical variations of the lateral nasal wall and paranasal sinuses: a CT study for endoscopic sinus surgery (ESS) in Thai patients. J Med Assoc Thai 2005;88(6):763–768
7. Melmed S, Kleinberg D. Anterior Pituitary in Kronenberg: Williams Textbook of Endocrinology, 11th ed. Philadelphia: Saunders Elsevier; 2008
8. Ezzat S, Asa SL, Couldwell WT, et al. The prevalence of pituitary adenomas: a systematic review. Cancer 2004;101(3):613–619
9. Daly AF, Rixhon M, Adam C, Dempegioti A, Tichomirowa MA, Beckers A. High prevalence of pituitary adenomas: a cross-sectional study in the province of Liege, Belgium. J Clin Endocrinol Metab 2006;91(12):4769–4775
10. Choi SH, Kwon BJ, Na DG, Kim JH, Han MH, Chang KH. Pituitary adenoma, craniopharyngioma, and Rathke cleft cyst involving both intrasellar and suprasellar regions: differentiation using MRI. Clin Radiol 2007;62(5):453–462
11. Karavitaki N, Cudlip S, Adams CB, Wass JA. Craniopharyngiomas. Endocr Rev 2006;27(4):371–397
12. Garrè ML, Cama A. Craniopharyngioma: modern concepts in pathogenesis and treatment. Curr Opin Pediatr 2007;19(4):471–479
13. Kuratsu J, Ushio Y. Epidemiological study of primary intracranial tumors in childhood. A population-based survey in Kumamoto Prefecture, Japan. Pediatr Neurosurg 1996;25(5):240–246, discussion 247
14. Weiner HL, Wisoff JH, Rosenberg ME, et al. Craniopharyngiomas: a clinicopathological analysis of factors predictive of recurrence and functional outcome. Neurosurgery 1994;35(6):1001–1010, discussion 1010–1011
15. Miller DC. Pathology of craniopharyngiomas: clinical import of pathological findings. Pediatr Neurosurg 1994;21(Suppl 1):11–17
16. Voelker JL, Campbell RL, Muller J. Clinical, radiographic, and pathological features of symptomatic Rathke's cleft cysts. J Neurosurg 1991;74(4):535–544
17. Claus EB, Bondy ML, Schildkraut JM, Wiemels JL, Wrensch M, Black PM. Epidemiology of intracranial meningioma. Neurosurgery 2005;57(6):1088–1095, discussion 1088–1095

18. Larjavaara S, Haapasalo H, Sankila R, Helén P, Auvinen A. Is the incidence of meningiomas underestimated? A regional survey. Br J Cancer 2008;99(1):182–184
19. Huang BY, Castillo M. Nonadenomatous tumors of the pituitary and sella turcica. Top Magn Reson Imaging 2005;16(4):289–299
20. FitzPatrick M, Tartaglino LM, Hollander MD, Zimmerman RA, Flanders AE. Imaging of sellar and parasellar pathology. Radiol Clin North Am 1999;37(1):101–121, x
21. Laufer I, Anand VK, Schwartz TH. Endoscopic, endonasal extended transsphenoidal, transplanum transtuberculum approach for resection of suprasellar lesions. J Neurosurg 2007;106(3): 400–406
22. Tanaka A. Imaging diagnosis and fundamental knowledge of common brain tumors in adults. Radiat Med 2006;24(6):482–492
23. Packer RJ, Cohen BH, Cooney K. Intracranial germ cell tumors. Oncologist 2000;5(4):312–320
24. Kyritsis AP. Management of primary intracranial germ cell tumors. J Neurooncol 2010;96(2):143–149
25. McMaster ML, Goldstein AM, Bromley CM, Ishibe N, Parry DM. Chordoma: incidence and survival patterns in the United States, 1973-1995. Cancer Causes Control 2001;12(1):1–11
26. Chugh R, Tawbi H, Lucas DR, Biermann JS, Schuetze SM, Baker LH. Chordoma: the nonsarcoma primary bone tumor. Oncologist 2007;12(11):1344–1350
27. Pamir MN, Ozduman K. Analysis of radiological features relative to histopathology in 42 skull-base chordomas and chondrosarcomas. Eur J Radiol 2006;58(3):461–470
28. Mendenhall WM, Mendenhall CM, Lewis SB, Villaret DB, Mendenhall NP. Skull base chordoma. Head Neck 2005;27(2): 159–165
29. Boriani S, Bandiera S, Biagini R, et al. Chordoma of the mobile spine: fifty years of experience. Spine 2006;31(4):493–503
30. Fassett DR, Couldwell WT. Metastases to the pituitary gland. Neurosurg Focus 2004;16(4):E8
31. McCormick PC, Post KD, Kandji AD, Hays AP. Metastatic carcinoma to the pituitary gland. Br J Neurosurg 1989;3(1):71–79
32. Komninos J, Vlassopoulou V, Protopapa D, et al. Tumors metastatic to the pituitary gland: case report and literature review. J Clin Endocrinol Metab 2004;89(2):574–580
33. Sanno N, Oyama K, Tahara S, Teramoto A, Kato Y. A survey of pituitary incidentaloma in Japan. Eur J Endocrinol 2003;149(2): 123–127
34. Daly AF, Burlacu MC, Livadariu E, Beckers A. The epidemiology and management of pituitary incidentalomas. Horm Res 2007;68(Suppl 5):195–198
35. Kosmorsky GS, Dupps WJ Jr, Drake RL. Nonuniform pressure generation in the optic chiasm may explain bitemporal hemianopsia. Ophthalmology 2008;115(3):560–565
36. McIlwaine GG, Carrim ZI, Lueck CJ, Chrisp TM. A mechanical theory to account for bitemporal hemianopia from chiasmal compression. J Neuroophthalmol 2005;25(1):40–43
37. Rambaldini GM, Butalia S, Ezzat S, Kucharczyk W, Sawka AM. Clinical predictors of advanced sellar masses. Endocr Pract 2007;13(6):609–614
38. Levy MJ, Matharu MS, Meeran K, Powell M, Goadsby PJ. The clinical characteristics of headache in patients with pituitary tumours. Brain 2005;128(Pt 8):1921–1930
39. Muthukumar N, Rossette D, Soundaram M, Senthilbabu S, Badrinarayanan T. Blindness following pituitary apoplexy: timing of surgery and neuro-ophthalmic outcome. J Clin Neurosci 2008;15(8):873–879
40. Bills DC, Meyer FB, Laws ER Jr, et al. A retrospective analysis of pituitary apoplexy. Neurosurgery 1993;33(4):602–608, discussion 608–609
41. Fernandez-Miranda JC, Gardner PA, Snyderman CH, et al. Craniopharyngioma: A pathologic, clinical, and surgical review. Head Neck 2011 [Epub ahead of print]
42. Spencer WR, Das K, Nwagu C, et al. Approaches to the sellar and parasellar region: anatomic comparison of the microscope versus endoscope. Laryngoscope 1999;109(5):791–794
43. Helal MZ. Combined micro-endoscopic trans-sphenoid excisions of pituitary macroadenomas. Eur Arch Otorhinolaryngol 1995;252(3):186–189
44. Graham SM, Iseli TA, Karnell LH, Clinger JD, Hitchon PW, Greenlee JD. Endoscopic approach for pituitary surgery improves rhinologic outcomes. Ann Otol Rhinol Laryngol 2009;118(9):630–635
45. Cappabianca P, Cavallo LM, Esposito F, Valente V, De Divitiis E. Sellar repair in endoscopic endonasal transsphenoidal surgery: results of 170 cases. Neurosurgery 2002;51(6):1365–1371, discussion 1371–1372
46. Chen HC, Lee ST. Need for intrasellar packing in sellar reconstruction of transsphenoidal surgery: less is more? J Clin Neurosci 2006;13(4):423–427
47. Zieliński G, Podgórski JK, Koziarski A, Potakiewicz Z. [Reconstruction of the sellar floor in transsphenoidal surgery: our experience of 818 patients]. Neurol Neurochir Pol 2006;40(4):302–311, 312
48. Kaptain GJ, Vincent DA, Laws ER Jr. Cranial base reconstruction after transsphenoidal surgery with bioabsorbable implants. Neurosurgery 2001;48(1):232–233, discussion 233–234
49. Seiler RW, Mariani L. Sellar reconstruction with resorbable vicryl patches, gelatin foam, and fibrin glue in transsphenoidal surgery: a 10-year experience with 376 patients. J Neurosurg 2000;93(5):762–765
50. Sherman JH, Pouratian N, Okonkwo DO, Jane JA Jr, Laws ER. Reconstruction of the sellar dura in transsphenoidal surgery using an expanded polytetrafluoroethylene dural substitute. Surg Neurol 2008;69(1):73–76, discussion 76
51. Dehdashti AR, Ganna A, Karabatsou K, Gentili F. Pure endoscopic endonasal approach for pituitary adenomas: early surgical results in 200 patients and comparison with previous microsurgical series. Neurosurgery 2008;62(5):1006–1015, discussion 1015–1017
52. Frank G, Pasquini E, Farneti G, et al. The endoscopic versus the traditional approach in pituitary surgery. Neuroendocrinology 2006;83(3-4):240–248
53. Suberman TA, Zanation AM, Ewend MG, Senior BA, Ebert CS. Sinonasal quality-of-life before and after endoscopic, endonasal, minimally invasive pituitary surgery. Intl Forum Rhinol Allergy 2011;1(2):161–166
54. Messerer M, De Battista JC, Raverot G, et al. Evidence of improved surgical outcome following endoscopy for nonfunctioning pituitary adenoma removal. Neurosurg Focus 2011;30(4):E11
55. Minet WW, Sommer DD, Yousuf K, Midia M, Farrokhyar F, Reddy K. Retrospective comparison of an endoscopic assisted versus a purely endoscopic approach to sellar tumour resection. J Otolaryngol Head Neck Surg 2008;37(6):759–767
56. Tabaee A, Anand VK, Barrón Y, et al. Endoscopic pituitary surgery: a systematic review and meta-analysis. J Neurosurg 2009;111(3):545–554
57. Jane JA Jr, Laws ER Jr. The surgical management of pituitary adenomas in a series of 3,093 patients. J Am Coll Surg 2001;193(6):651–659
58. Murad MH, Fernández-Balsells MM, Barwise A, et al. Outcomes of surgical treatment for nonfunctioning pituitary adenomas: a systematic review and meta-analysis. Clin Endocrinol (Oxf) 2010;73(6):777–791
59. Senior BA, Ebert CS, Bednarski KK, et al. Minimally invasive pituitary surgery. Laryngoscope 2008;118(10):1842–1855

47 Endoscopic Approaches to the Petrous Apex and Cavernous Sinus

Paolo Castelnuovo, Andrea Pistochini, and Piero Nicolai

Endonasal endoscopic surgery, initially used for treatment of inflammatory diseases of the sinonasal tract,[1–5] has offered the possibility to access intracranial structures without violating the facial skeleton (transnasal neuroendoscopy). Transnasal endoscopic surgery is in accordance with the concept of minimally invasive surgery because it leaves anatomic structures intact and provides maximal control of the surgical target.[6–8] The validity of this new technique has been demonstrated by several surgical teams[9–20] that have shown the enormous potential of transnasal neuroendoscopy in properly selected patients, which leads to excellent results with less morbidity compared with conventional open procedures.[21–25] A common feature of all the established schools of endonasal neuroendoscopy is the continual collaboration between neurosurgeons and otorhinolaryngologists.

The development of transnasal neuroendoscopy was made possible due to improvements in surgical technique, such as four-handed endonasal techniques,[20] and dedicated surgical instrumentation. In fact, during the last decade, technological innovations have accompanied the evolution of the technique with corresponding improvements in its potential. Some of the major advances in instrumentation include rigid 45-degree endoscopes that are used in combination with double-angle instruments, and powered instruments such as intranasal drills, shavers, ultrasonic aspirators, and optic-cleaning systems that have reduced surgical times and allowed for the introduction of hydroscopy.[26] Other helpful tools are the diode laser, which provides the possibility of angled cutting, as well as Doppler surgical probes and neuronavigation systems based on optical or magnetic technology.

Using such instrumentation, it is possible to access the entire ventral skull base, from the crista galli to the odontoid process.[7] The nostrils and nasal fossae thus represent a natural port of surgical access to the skull base. Lesions located intracranially can be reached through an inverted cone-shaped "tunnel," constituted by the nasosphenoidal tract. This avoids violation of the facial skeleton, both anteriorly and laterally, and, in selected cases, permits preservation of important vascular and nervous structures. For surgical approaches involving the cavernous sinus and the petrous apex, anatomic and surgical knowledge of the sphenoid sinus is fundamental as it should be considered the main avenue to access the cranial base via a transnasal route.

Patient Selection/Indications

Preoperative workup includes assessment of respiratory and cardio-circulatory function in addition to routine blood and urine tests. To avoid excessive intraoperative bleeding, anticoagulants and nonsteroidal anti-inflammatory drugs (NSAIDs) should be discontinued. The former can be temporarily replaced with low molecular weight heparin (bridging therapy) and the latter substituted with paracetamol (acetaminophen) or codeine-based drugs. Concomitant rhinosinusitis should be treated before neuroendoscopic intervention. Patients should be informed about the risks associated with tumor excision, including vascular and neural injury, as well as of the possibility of duraplasty and the need to convert to an open procedure.

The type of approach depends on tumor location, histologic type, and relation with major vessels. In general, transnasal neuroendoscopic surgery is indicated when it is favorable to approach the lesion in a mediolateral direction and when neurovascular structures are on the periphery of the lesion. Tumors with limited vascular supply and/or that compress and devascularize the cavernous sinus are most favorable for endoscopic resection. Preoperative embolization of hypervascular skull base tumors can be useful.[27–29] Moreover, it is important to exclude invasion of the cavernous portion of the internal carotid artery (ICA), which would necessitate neuroradiologic treatment. The possibility of a minimally invasive access for biopsy procedures is particularly advantageous for lesions that are amenable to nonsurgical treatment (e.g., lymphomas, undifferentiated carcinomas, metastases). A minimally invasive approach is also indicated for the treatment of cerebrospinal fluid (CSF) leaks of the petroclival junction.[30]

Contraindications for excision include the encasement of vital vascular structures (ICA or perforating vessels) and the impossibility to remove the lesion by aspiration through the nasosphenoid tunnel due to its hard consistency and pial adherence. A purely endoscopic approach is also contraindicated in cases in which neurovascular surgery (shunting)[31,32] or orbital exenteration are needed. In these cases, a combined cranioendoscopic approach is favored.

A transnasal neuroendoscopic access to the cavernous sinus and the petrous apex allows for the treatment of several types of lesions[33,34] including pituitary macroadenomas, rare cases of petroclival meningioma tumors involving cranial nerves (CNs) III through VI (e.g., schwannomas),

CSF leak, meningoencephaloceles of the medial cranial fossa (e.g., Sternberg's canal) and the petroclival junction, benign lesions originating from the petrous apex and extending toward the clivus and the lateral recess of the sphenoid (e.g., cholesterol granulomas), and intra- or extradural malignant lesions involving the petroclival junction (e.g., chondrosarcomas, chordomas, lesions originating from the paranasal sinuses).[35]

Diagnostic Workup

Endoscopic and radiologic exams allow for evaluation of the location, size, and extent of lesions, and in some cases, can provide preoperative diagnosis (e.g., cholesterol granuloma) without resorting to biopsy. Computed tomography (CT) and magnetic resonance imaging (MRI) provide complementary information and their combined use can often lead to appropriate differential diagnosis,[36,37] permitting the identification of pseudolesions (e.g., presence of fat in the bone marrow in a unpneumatized petrous apex) that do not require surgical treatment. Preoperative endoscopic examination, together with CT, gives details on anatomic features (e.g., septal spur, concha bullosa, sphenoidal rostrum pneumatization, superior turbinate pneumatization), which can influence the choice of the ideal surgical corridor.

CT is extremely helpful in delineating the integrity of the bone and its variations in density: thickening as in the case of fibrous dysplasia; diffuse thickening combined with erosion as in chronic osteomyelitis; and thinning or various forms of erosion commonly associated with expansile lesions. The finding of bone remodeling or erosion on CT requires careful assessment of complementary soft tissue detail on MRI.

MRI with gadolinium (and angio-MRI) and angiography are particularly important to reveal the relationship between the lesion and adjacent vessels. MRI allows identification of intracavernous structures in extreme detail, perfectly highlighting the intracavernous portion of the cranial nerves. The boundaries of the cavernous sinus by MRI are well defined, and the dura and CSF are visible. At the level of the petrous apex and the middle cranial fossa, it is extremely important to identify the relation between the lesion and adjacent arteries and veins (especially if aneurysm or thrombosis is suspected). Therefore, MRI, angio-MRI, and angio-CT have a cardinal role.

In the case of lesions originating from the parasellar region and invading the middle cranial fossa, MR-cisternography should be performed to better delineate the cranial nerves at the levels of the root entry zone and cisternal-cavernous branches. The use of a contrast agent in both CT and MRI helps in characterizing the lesion and therefore the differential diagnosis. Positron emission tomography (PET)-CT is necessary for staging in malignant lesions prone to distant metastasis (**Tables 47.1 and 47.2**).[38,39]

Table 47.1 Differential Radiologic Diagnosis of Common Pathologies of the Cavernous Sinus

MRI	Additional Features	Diagnosis
⇒⇓T1, ⇑T2, enhancing	Typical dumbbell-shape, following the nerve from which they originate	Trigeminal schwannoma
⇒⇑T1, ⇒⇑T2, enhancing	⇑ age, progressive "filling in" after contrast administration	Cavernous hemangioma
⇓⇒T1, ⇓⇒T2, strongly enhancing	"Dural tail"	Meningioma
	Lateral growth (intracavernous ICA encasement: >30% of its diameter)	Pituitary adenoma
⇒T1, ⇒T2, strong inhomogeneous enhancing	Enhancing masses at orbital apex, ethmoid; presence of thrombosis and thickening of ICA walls	Fungal infection

Abbreviations: ⇒, intermediate signal; ⇓, decreased signal; ⇑, increased signal; ICA, internal carotid artery.
Sources: Data from Connor SE, Leung R, Natas S. Imaging of the petrous apex: a pictorial review. Br J Radiol 2008;81(965):427–435; and Jackler RK, Parker DA. Radiographic differential diagnosis of petrous apex lesions. Am J Otol 1992;13(6):561–574.

Surgical Anatomy

The cavernous sinuses are large venous spaces located laterally to the sphenoid body and interconnected by the intercavernous sinuses, almost forming a circular sinus (anterior coronary sinus, posterior and anterior to the foramen of Winslow) (**Fig. 47.1**). They contain the ICA with its intracavernous branches (meningohypophyseal trunk and the inferolateral trunk), the abducens nerve (cranial nerve VI), and sympathetic fibers that surround the ICA. The artery subdivides the cavernous sinus in a lateral and a medial portion (**Fig. 47.2**).[40] The oculomotor (CN III), trochlear nerve (CN IV), and ophthalmic branch (V1) and maxillary division (V2) of CN V run along the lateral wall in a dural sheath (**Fig. 47.3**).

The abducens nerve enters the cavernous sinus through Dorello's canal. This is an osteofibrous conduit between the petrous apex and the petro-sphenoidal ligament of Gruber. Above the petrous apex, it changes direction and reaches the ICA, and then folds forward to reach the superior orbital fissure. Inside Dorello's canal the nerve is strictly anchored to the endosteum and is in close contact with the meningeal dorsal artery in ~80% of individuals. Inside the cavernous sinus, the nerve runs along the lateral wall of the ICA, and sometimes divides into several branches.

The petrous apex is the portion of temporal bone located between the inner ear and the clivus. It may present with various degrees of pneumatization and varying quantities

Table 47.2 Differential Diagnosis of Primary Petrous Apex Lesions

CT	MRI	Additional Features	Diagnosis
Nonexpansile and nondestructive	⇑T1, ⇑T2		Diploic fatty marrow
	⇒⇓⇑T1, ⇑T2		Simple petrous apex diffusion (possible early cholesterol granuloma if ⇑T1)
	⇓T1, ⇑T2, ⇓T2 flair	From Meckel's cave	Cephalocele
Benign bony expansion	⇑T1, ⇑T2, nonenhancing		Cholesterol granuloma (consider aneurysm)
	⇒⇓T1, ⇑T2, nonenhancing	⇑ DWI	Cholesteatoma
		⇓ DWI	Mucocele or cyst
	⇒⇓T1, ⇑T2, enhancing		Rare benign tumors
Aggressive bony destruction	⇒⇓T1, ⇒⇑T2, enhancing	Infection, middle ear disease, diabetes immunodeficiency	Petrous apicitis or osteomyelitis
		⇑age	Metastasis, myeloma
		⇓age	Histiocytosis, sarcoma
	⇒⇓T1, ⇒⇑T2, enhancing with areas of ⇑T1	Along posterior petrous apex	Endolymphatic sac tumor

Abbreviations: ⇒, intermediate signal; ⇓, decreased signal; ⇑, increased signal; DWI, diffusion-weighted imaging; MRI, magnetic resonance imaging.
Sources: Data from Connor SE, Leung R, Natas S. Imaging of the petrous apex: a pictorial review. Br J Radiol 2008;81(965):427–435. Epub 2008 Jan 21; and Jackler RK, Parker DA. Radiographic differential diagnosis of petrous apex lesions. Am J Otol 1992;13(6):561–574.

of bone marrow. The internal acoustic meatus divides it into an anterior compartment that is larger and more frequently involved by pathologic processes, and a posterior compartment that borders the semicircular canals. The anterior compartment is crossed by the horizontal segment of the intrapetrous ICA and contains the fibrocartilaginous component of the foramen lacerum. The petrous apex adjoins the temporal lobe and cerebellum, cranial nerves, and large blood vessels. The superior border of the petrous apex encompasses the floor of the middle cranial fossa, the trigeminal nerve, and the dural wrapping of Meckel's cave. The petrous sinuses run posteriorly and inferiorly to the posterior margin, which is in relation with dura mater that covers the anterior portion of the pontocerebellar angle. Inferiorly, it adjoins with the infratemporal fossa; medially, with the clivus; and laterally, with the otic capsule.

A prerequisite of paramount importance in understanding this difficult anatomy is adequate experience in an anatomic laboratory, which can make the surgeon more familiar with the numerous anatomic variations. The main goal of cadaver dissection is to acquire a three-dimensional understanding of the anatomy to create a "patient-specific" navigation. In the live case, this experience leads the surgeon to safely identify anatomic landmarks and to select

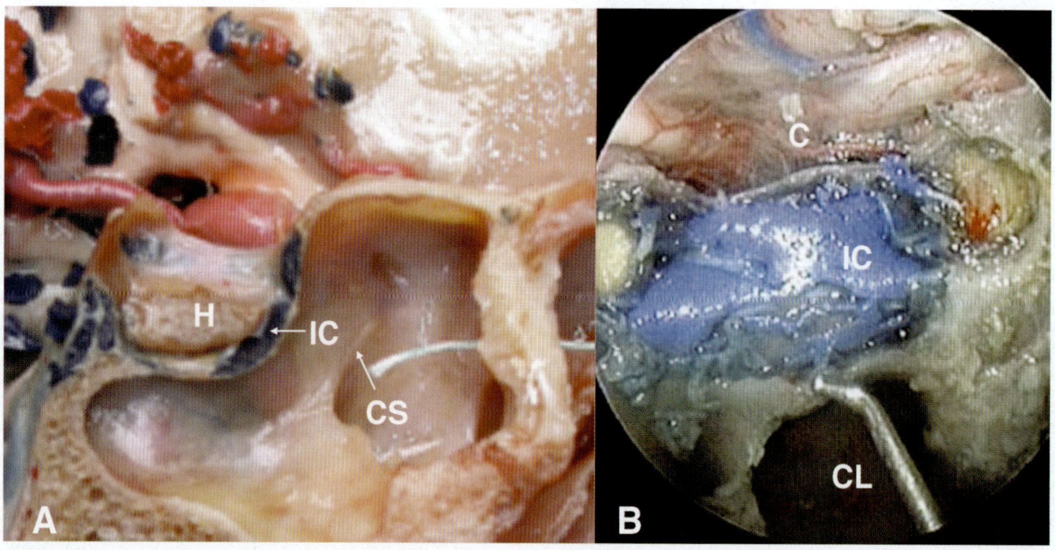

Fig. 47.1 (A) Cadaver specimen in sagittal section. The intercavernous sinus is visible anteroinferiorly to the hypophysis. *H*, hypophysis; *IC*, intercavernous sinus; *CS*, left cavernous sinus. **(B)** Endoscopic endonasal image with 0-degree, 4-mm endoscope. Cadaver dissection at the level of the sellar region. After removal of the osseous posterosuperior wall of the sphenoid, the sellar and suprasellar content is evident. The intercavernous sinus is located anteriorly to the sella (*IC*). *C*, chiasm; *CL*, clivus.

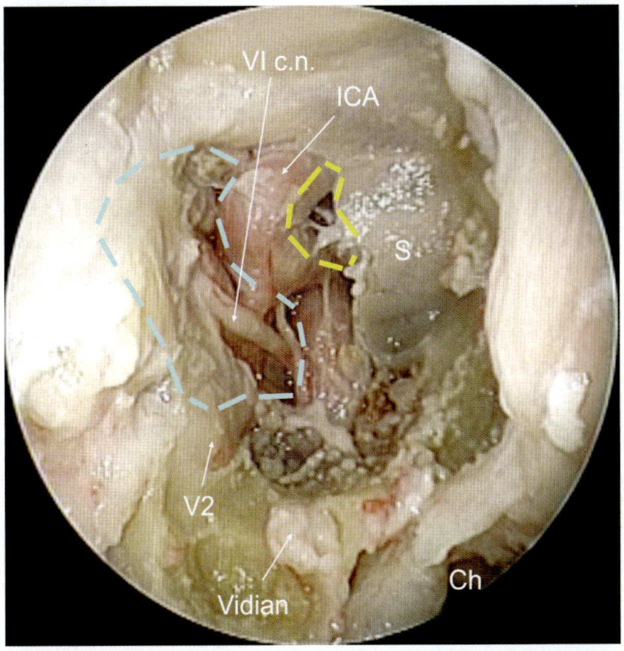

Fig. 47.2 Endoscopic endonasal image with 0-degree, 4-mm endoscope. Anatomic dissection. After a wide right sphenoethmoidectomy with drilling of the pterygoid bone, the bony wall covering the lateral parasellar region was removed. The course of the right internal carotid artery and cranial nerve VI, passing through the cavernous sinus, are evident. The lateral (*light blue*) and medial (*yellow*) component of the cavernous sinus are highlighted with different colors. *S*, sella; *ICA*, internal carotid artery; *V2*, second branch of cranial nerve V; *Ch*, choana.

the ideal surgical corridor for the specific pathology. In this regard, the classic neurosurgical subdivision of the cavernous sinus walls into subunits based on the different surgical approaches (anteromedial triangle, paramedial triangle, Parkinson triangle, oculomotor trigone, anterolateral triangle, lateral triangle, posterolateral triangle, and posteromedial triangle) is not particularly helpful in a transnasal endoscopic approach.[40]

The first step in a transnasal approach is the identification of the superior choanal border and the tail of the middle, superior, and supreme turbinates, before identifying the sphenoid floor and its natural ostium. The tails of the turbinates guide the surgeon toward the natural ostium and allow localization of the septal branch of the sphenopalatine artery (tail of the superior turbinate) (**Fig. 47.4**).

After removal of the anterior wall of the sphenoid sinus, the intrasphenoidal landmarks can be recognized as depressions and protrusions corresponding to the sellar floor, the paraclival and cavernous portions of ICA, V2, and the vidian canal (**Fig. 47.5**). These structures, which are the most important landmarks in surgery of the cavernous sinus and petrous apex, can be more or less evident depending on the extent of pneumatization of the sphenoid sinus. There are three basic patterns of sphenoid sinus pneumatization: sellar (complete pneumatization of the parasellar sphenoid with full exposure of the sellar bulge); presellar (partial pneumatization of the sphenoid but without extension to the sella); and conchal (nonpneumatized sphenoid). In the conchal variant, the lack of pneumatization makes it impossible to recognize the anatomic landmarks and thus requires special caution during surgical

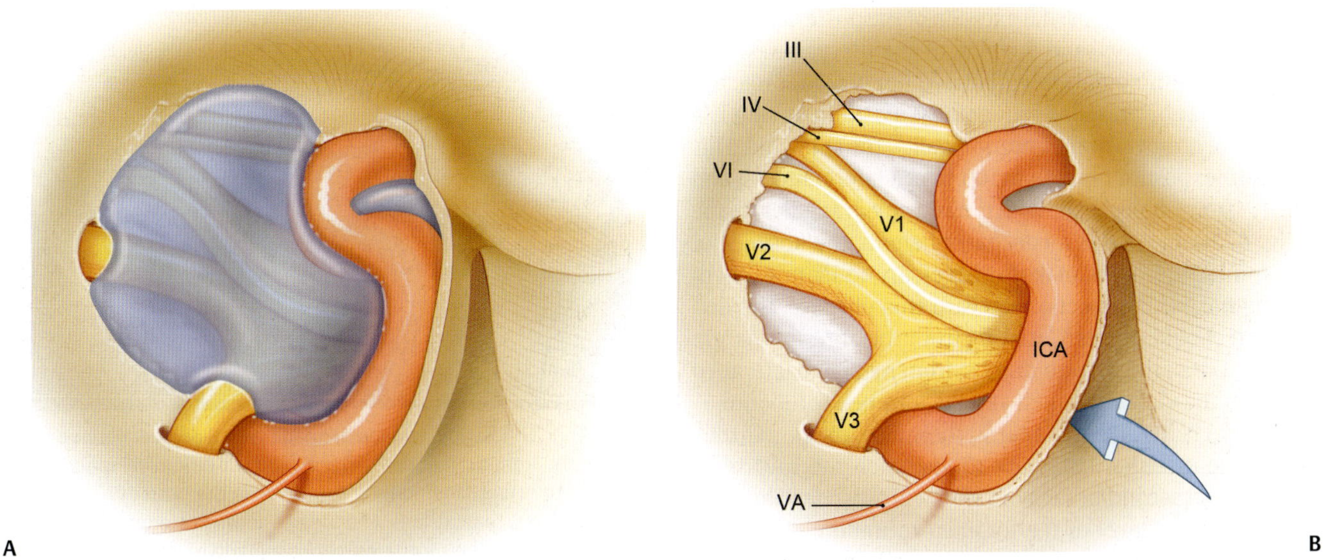

Fig. 47.3 **(A)** Illustration showing the right cavernous sinus after removal of the bony layer of the lateral sphenoidal wall. During dissection, the dural sheet below can be preserved. **(B)** The cavernous sinus contains the internal carotid artery, the abducens nerve (VI), the oculomotor nerve (III), the trochlear nerve (IV), and the branches of cranial nerve V (V1, V2, V3) running along the lateral wall in a dural sheath. The vidian artery (*VA*) originates from the internal carotid artery at the genu to its paraclival tract. The *light blue arrow* indicates the route to reach the petrous apex, which follows the VA inferomedially to avoid encountering the internal carotid artery.

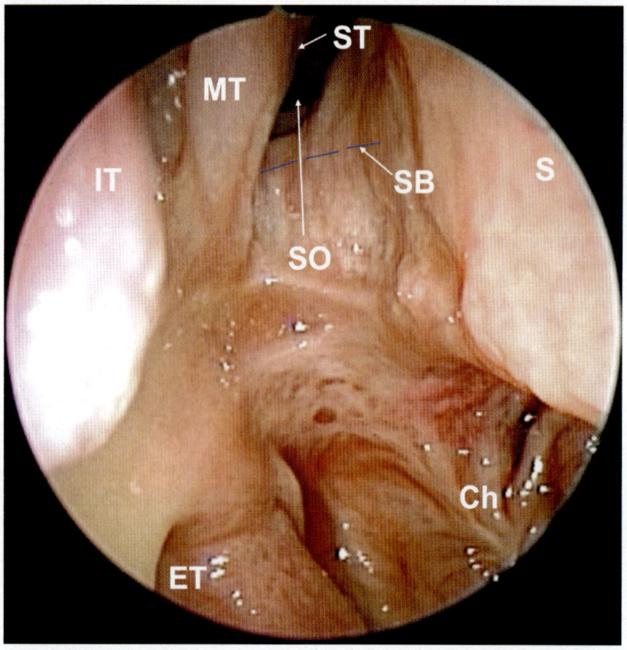

Fig. 47.4 Endoscopic endonasal image with 0-degree, 4-mm endoscope. After introducing the endoscope in the right nasal fossa along the nasal floor, at the level of the tail of the inferior turbinate (*IT*), it is possible to identify the sphenoid ostium (*SO*) by following the tails of the turbinates superiorly. At the level of the tail of superior turbinate (*ST*), the septal branch of the sphenopalatine artery (*SB*) crosses the superior choanal border. *Ch*, choana; *ET*, eustachian tube; *S*, nasal septum; *MT*, middle turbinate.

exposure. Surgical navigation may be a useful adjunct in these cases. Independent of the sphenoidal anatomy, the approach to lateral lesions of the cavernous sinus and petrous apex may also require creation of a surgical corridor via ethmoidectomy, partial excision of the posterior wall of the maxillary sinus, and opening of the pterygomaxillary fossa (transethmoidal-pterygoidal-sphenoidal approach).

In a sellar or presellar sphenoid sinus, the first step is a complete removal of the anterior wall of the sphenoid. This leads to exposure of its floor, up to the lateral recess, and of its lateral bony wall, which has a quadrangular shape (**Fig. 47.6**). In case of a conchal sphenoid, the absence of anatomic landmarks makes it necessary to identify them through careful dissection. Toward this purpose, the dissection should proceed, starting from the anterior margin of the floor of the sphenoid sinus, from medial to lateral, to identify the vidian foramen and the foramen rotundum.

Although the vidian canal is the guide to the petrous apex, the essential landmark to approach the cavernous sinus is the second branch of CN V, which is identified anteriorly at the level of the foramen rotundum. Following the protrusion of the lateral wall dorsally to the foramen, the lateral part of the cavernous sinus is reached.

To expose the medial portion of the cavernous sinus, the key anatomic landmarks are the sellar floor and the protrusion of the anterior arch of the cavernous ICA (carotid "C"). Complete removal of the sellar floor and the bone that covers the cavernous carotid exposes the region of the cavernous sinus that is delimited by the hypophyseal capsule medially and the cavernous ICA laterally and superiorly, whereas inferiorly, the boundary is the cranial portion of the paraclival ICA. At the level of the posterior genu between the paraclival and the cavernous ICA, the first branch of the meningohypophyseal trunk originates (tentorial artery of Bernasconi-Cassinari, which gives rise to the inferior hypophyseal arteries) (**Fig. 47.7**).[41]

Progressive drilling of the bony wall of the sphenoid sinus in a lateral direction from the interoptic-carotid recess to the orbital apex, with subsequent removal of the periosteal dural layer, allows access to the lateral portion of the cavernous sinus. If the dura is preserved and only the bony component is removed, it is possible to observe the venous plexus connecting the two cavernous sinuses. By excising the dural layer, the ICA can be observed along its entire paraclival and intracavernous course. Lateral to the vertical segment of the ICA, the abducens nerve can be seen entering the cavernous sinus, whereas medially, the sympathetic complex of the ICA is visible.

Moving laterally, it is possible to observe the imprints of the third and fourth cranial nerves that are contained within the dural portion of the lateral wall of the cavernous sinus. The nerve fibers that make up the first two branches

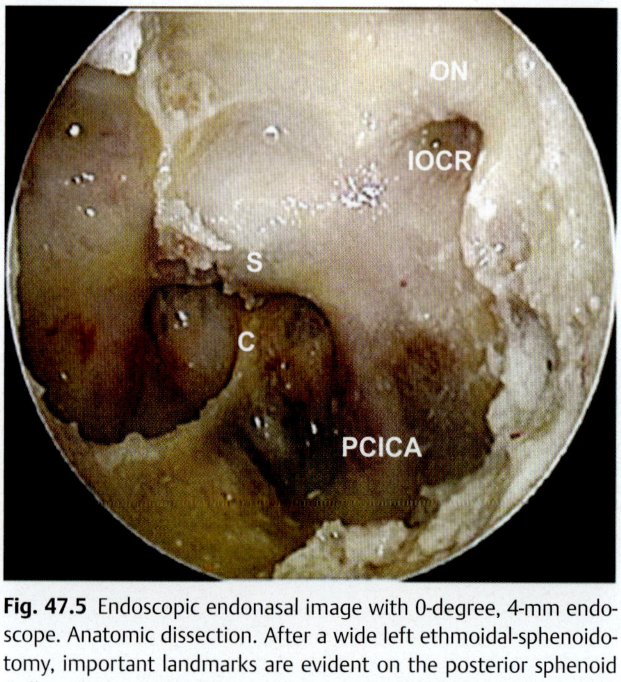

Fig. 47.5 Endoscopic endonasal image with 0-degree, 4-mm endoscope. Anatomic dissection. After a wide left ethmoidal-sphenoidotomy, important landmarks are evident on the posterior sphenoid wall as bony protrusions and depressions. Posteromedially, the depression and the protrusion corresponding to the sella floor can be seen. Superolaterally, the interoptic-carotid recess and the protrusion of the optic canal and cavernous portion of the internal carotid artery are visible. Inferiorly, the protrusion of the paraclival carotid is evident. *C*, Clivos; *S*, sella; *PCICA*, paraclival internal carotid artery; *IOCR*, interoptic-carotid recess; *ON*, optic nerve.

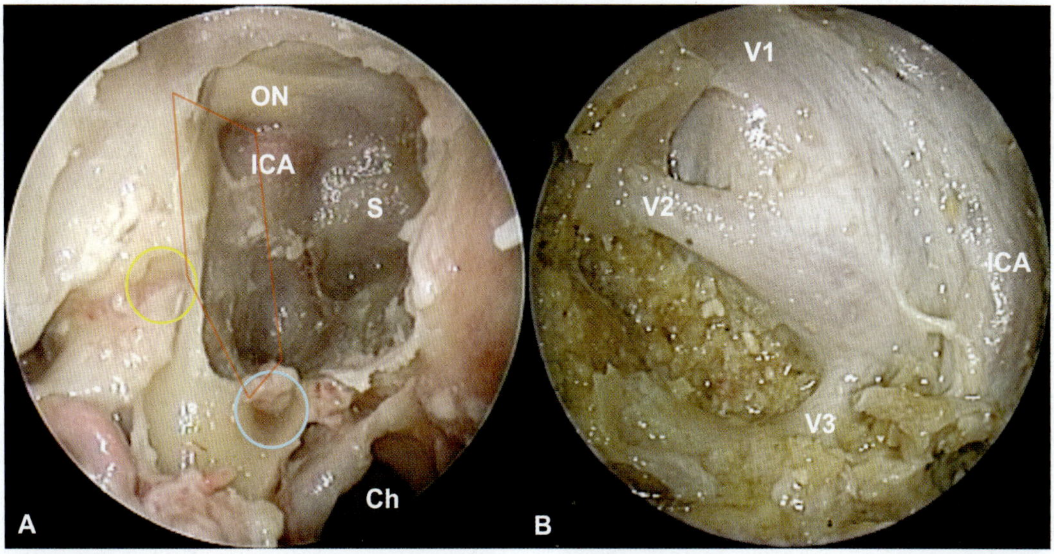

Fig. 47.6 (A) Endoscopic endonasal image with 0-degree, 4-mm endoscope. Anatomic dissection. After a wide right sphenoethmoidectomy, it is possible to identify at the level of the pterygoid base, the vidian canal (VC; *light blue circle*) and superolaterally to it, the foramen rotundum (*yellow circle*). The lateral sphenoidal wall has a quadrangular shape and is delimited by the following margins: *posteromedially*, the interoptic-carotid recess (with superiorly the optic canal and inferiorly the anterior curve of the cavernous portion of the internal carotid artery); *superolaterally*, the orbital apex with the initial portion of the optic canal; *medially*, the foramen rotundum with the longitudinal imprint of the second branch of cranial nerve V; and *inferiorly*, the lateral recess of the sphenoid with (at its medial border) the vidian canal within the sphenoid floor. *ON*, optic nerve; *S*, sella; *ICA*, internal carotid artery; *Ch*, choana. **(B)** Endoscopic endonasal image with 45-degree, 4-mm endoscope. Anatomic dissection. In the right part of the sphenoid sinus, after drilling the pterygoid, the use of an angled endoscope leads to identification of the whole cavernous sinus with the cranial nerve V branches.

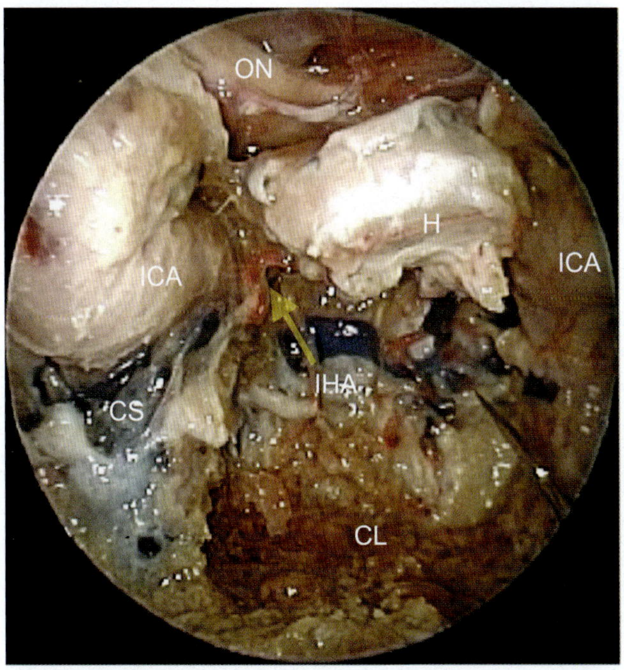

Fig. 47.7 Endoscopic endonasal image with 0-degree, 4-mm endoscope. Anatomic dissection. Exposure of the sellar and parasellar regions. The yellow arrow points at the inferior hypophyseal artery, a branch of the ICA, which originates at the junction between the paraclival and the cavernous portion of the internal carotid artery. *ICA*, internal carotid artery; *CL*, clivus; *IHA*, inferior hypophyseal artery; *ON*, optic nerve; *H*, hypophysis.

of CN V are more difficult to identify. At this point, drilling the basisphenoid and pterygoid root exposes the third branch of CN V.

To simplify a transnasal endoscopic approach to the cavernous sinus, surgical access can be gained through two routes[40]: one lateral to the carotid, which can be subdivided into four areas (posterosuperior triangle, corresponding to the anteromedial triangle for transcranial access and delimiting the parasellar region; anterosuperior triangle; superior quadrilateral; inferior quadrilateral), and one medial to the carotid "C," that allows the operator to expose the most proximal part of CNs III and IV (**Fig. 47.8**).

To reach the petrous apex, a ventrodorsal path along the vidian canal should be followed by skeletonizing the nerve to reach the angle between the vertical (paraclival) and horizontal portion (petrous) of the ICA at the end of its path, underneath which the petrous apex lies (**Fig. 47.9**). Whenever a conchal sphenoid is encountered, the vidian canal should be localized anteriorly at the level of the basisphenoid and followed posteriorly until the ICA is reached.

Following the same route, it is also possible to reach the petroclival region, which, to be exposed, generally requires removal of part of the petrous bone. In this case, the vidian canal is also a fundamental landmark. By following the vidian artery, in fact, it is possible to reach the anterior genu of the ICA. At this point, the bone of the petroclival region is removed until the underlying dura is exposed by

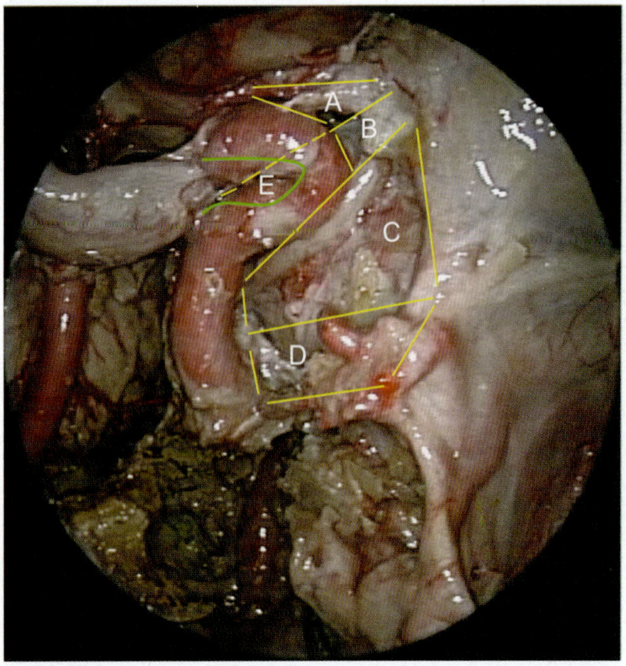

Fig. 47.8 (*A*) The posterosuperior triangle corresponds to the anteromedial triangle in transcranial access. (*B*) The anterosuperior triangle is bounded superiorly by cranial nerve (CN) III and inferiorly by CN IV; its base is the lateral loop of the internal carotid artery (ICA). The superior quadrangular area (*C*) is bounded superiorly by CN VI and inferiorly by V2; the bases are a segment of the ICA and the bony lateral wall of the sphenoid sinus. The inferior quadrangular area (*D*) is visible when the sphenoid is well pneumatized; its borders are superiorly, V2; inferiorly, the vidian nerve; posteriorly, the intrapetrous segment of the ICA; and anteriorly, the sphenoid bone between the foramen rotundum and the pterygoid or vidian canal. (Used with permission from Cavallo LM, Cappabianca P, Galzio R, Iaconetta G, de Divitiis E, Tschabitscher M. Endoscopic transnasal approach to the cavernous sinus versus transcranial route: anatomic study. Neurosurgery 2005;56(2 Suppl): 379–389; discussion 379–389.)

drilling medial to the genu of the ICA. The cavernous sinus and the middle cranial fossa represent the limits of superior and lateral dissection, respectively.

During anatomic dissection, after completing the drilling of the clival bone and opening of the prepontine dura, one can observe the basilar artery, posterior cerebral arteries, and the superior cerebellar artery. Lateral to the hypophysis and medial to the ICA, the posterior communicating arteries will be visible, and dorsally to the C1 tract of the intracavernous ICA, it is possible to observe the dural ring represented by Dorello's canal, where CN VI enters the cavernous sinus (**Fig. 47.10**).

In conclusion, the vidian canal is an important anatomic landmark: surgical access medial to it leads to the dura of the posterior fossa without encountering significant vascular or nervous structures. The end of the canal indicates the angle where the petrous segment of ICA joins the paraclival segment. Medial and inferior to this point of access, the orbital apex can be accessed safely (**Fig. 47.11**).

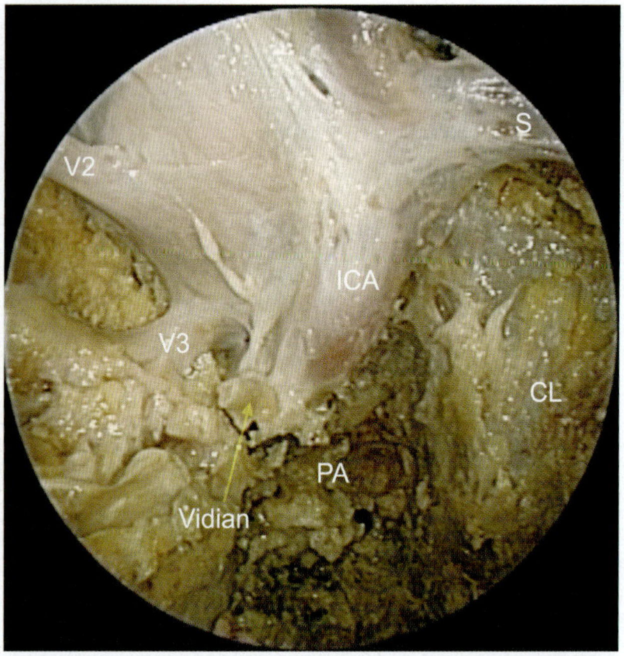

Fig. 47.9 Endoscopic endonasal image with 0-degree, 4-mm endoscope. Anatomic dissection. After exposure of the right cavernous sinus, by following the vidian canal, the junction between the petrous and the paraclival internal carotid artery can be identified. This is a safe landmark to approach the petrous apex (*PA*). *CL*, clivus; *ICA*, internal carotid artery; *S*, sella.

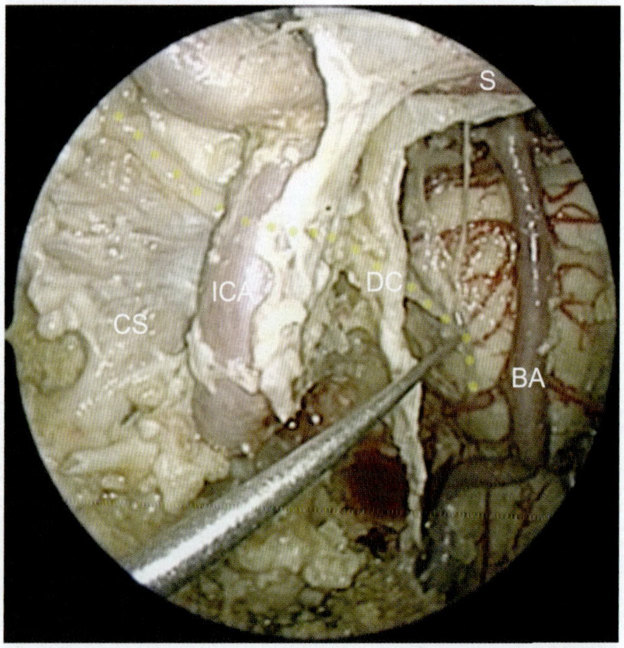

Fig. 47.10 Endoscopic endonasal image with 0-degree, 4-mm endoscope. Anatomic dissection. After removal of the bony wall covering the medial and posterior cranial fossa and after exposure of the right cavernous sinus and opening of the posterior cranial fossa dura, it is possible to follow the sixth cranial nerve from its origin to its intracavernous portion. *ICA*, internal carotid artery; *BA*, basilar artery; *DC*, Dorello's canal; *S*, sella; *CS*, cavernous sinus.

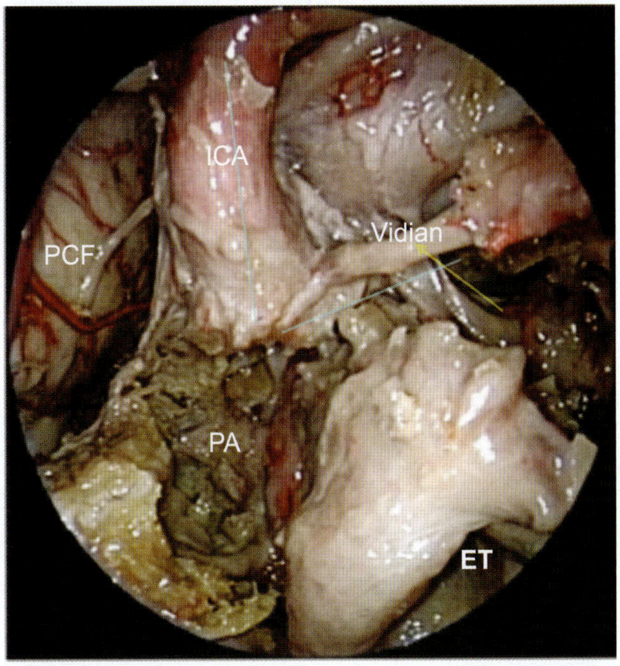

Fig. 47.11 Endoscopic endonasal image with 0-degree, 4-mm endoscope. Anatomic dissection. On the left side, the vidian nerve course leading to the internal carotid artery (*ICA*) can be seen. The petrous apex (*PA*) is inferomedial to the foramen lacerum. A curved seeker is introduced into the eustachian tube (*ET*). *PCF*, posterior cranial fossa.

Surgical Technique

As already mentioned, the approach to the sphenoid sinus and its complete exposure are the first steps in surgical treatment of the adjacent anatomic structures. The technique varies from a paraseptal to a transethmoidal-pterygoidal approach depending on the lateral extent of the lesion. In all cases, it is advisable to fully expose the sinus by creating a single cavity that is fully open anteriorly. The extension of the lesion will also determine the route of access beyond the sphenoid. The techniques used for extra- or intradural dissection of a mass under endoscopy require that initial debulking has already been performed. Techniques for debulking depend on the consistency of the lesion, but good choices include a suction aspirator and cutting or powered instruments (shaver, ultrasonic aspirator). Next, the tumor capsule is identified and, if present, is mobilized; the adjacent neurovascular structures should be dissected and protected, and the operator then proceeds with removal of the lesion by gentle use of bipolar coagulation (**Table 47.3**).

Bilateral Paraseptal Nasosphenoidal Surgical Approach: Petrous Apex

In surgery of the petrous apex, the target is located posteroinferiorly and then laterally to the genu between the vertical (paraclival) and horizontal segment (temporal) of the ICA (**Fig. 47.12**). The key landmark to reach this angle is the vidian canal.[42–44] The first surgical step is bilateral exposure of the sphenoid with removal of the intersinus septum, drilling of the sphenoid rostrum, and resection of the posterior portion of the vomer. Wide exposure in this manner allows the subsequent use of both nasal fossae for a four-handed technique, and it facilitates access to the lateral surgical field at the level of the petrous apex by allowing instruments to be passed through a contralateral nasal approach.

Table 47.3 Transsphenoidal Surgical Approaches

Four-Handed Transsphenoidal Surgical Approaches	Accessible Anatomic Regions
Bilateral paraseptal nasosphenoidal (transclival)	Sellar region and inferior parasellar region, petrous apex
Transethmoidal-sphenoidal	Superior and medial parasellar region (medial portion of the cavernous sinus)
Transethmoidal-pterygoidal-sphenoidal	Lateral parasellar region, middle cranial fossa

To reach the petrous apex, the medial pterygoid lamina is exposed anterosuperiorly to the eustachian tube, and the vidian canal is identified. Drilling the sphenoid floor and the required portion of the clivus is always performed following identification of the vidian canal.

Medial and inferior to the vidian canal there are no important vascular or nervous structures so that the dura of the posterior cranial fossa can be reached without any major risk. Laterally to the vidian canal, the other landmarks for lateral extension of the dissection are the cartilage of the eustachian tube and V3. Access to the petrous apex is sometimes facilitated by a medial and anterior growth of the lesion. In this case (e.g., cholesterol granuloma), it is sufficient to use a direct, bilateral paraseptal route with a wide medial opening of the sphenoidal sinus and marsupialization of the anterior wall of the granuloma at the level of the posteroinferior angle of the sphenoid sinus. (**Fig. 47.13**)

If inferior extension is needed (transclival), the surgical approach begins by elevating, with the help of a diode laser, an inferiorly based mucoperiosteal flap from the posterior wall of the nasopharynx, limited superiorly by the choanal border and laterally by the eustachian tube orifices, which are preserved. Next, the entire sphenoid floor and a portion of the clivus are drilled to widely expose the petrous apex. After marsupialization of a cholesterol granuloma, the key point is to keep the opening patent. This can be achieved by rotating into the cavity a septal mucosal flap based on the septal branch of the sphenopalatine artery (Hadad flap), which not only has the function of preventing closure of the cavity, but also favors the remucosalization of the cavity itself.[45]

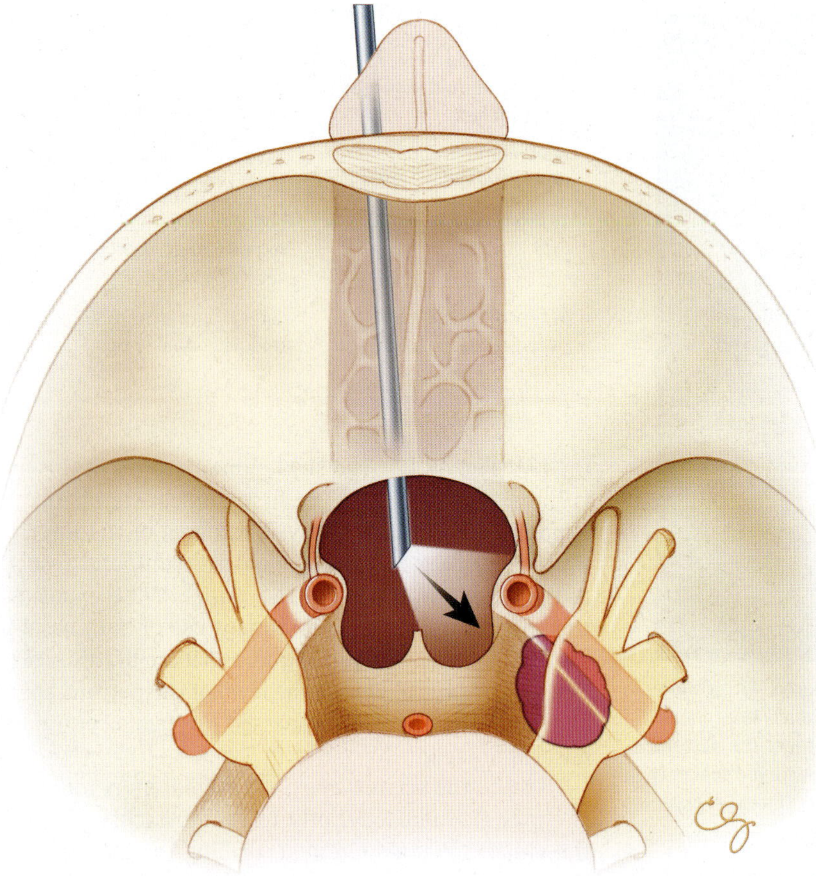

Fig. 47.12 The paraseptal bilateral approach allows one to reach lesions located at the petrous apex using the vidian artery as a landmark to preserve the internal carotid artery, thus avoiding major vascular complications. The illustration shows the use of angled scopes to illuminate and visualize the region; the resection of the posterior third of the nasal septum facilitates the four-hands technique at this level.

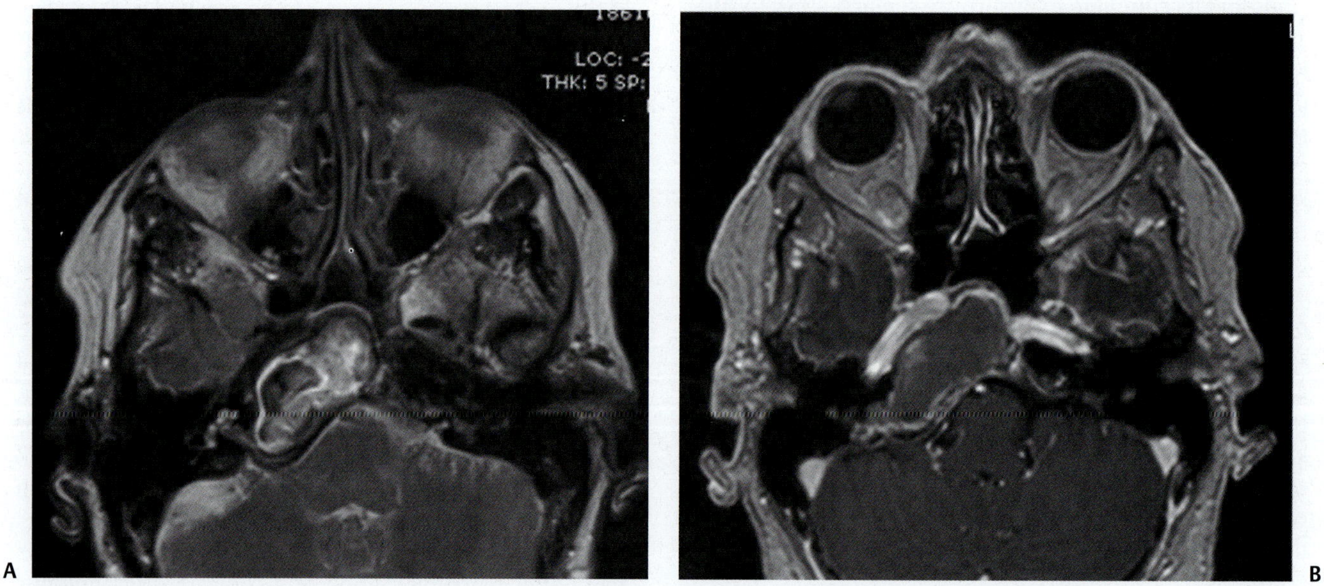

Fig. 47.13 Clinical case. **(A)** Preoperative magnetic resonance image (MRI) in the axial plane showing a cholesterol granuloma of the right petrous apex. In T2- but also in T1-weighted images the lesion is characterized by an increased signal. **(B)** Preoperative MRI after contrast medium administration. The lesion does not enhance, which is a typical feature suggesting the diagnosis of cholesterol granuloma. *(continued)*

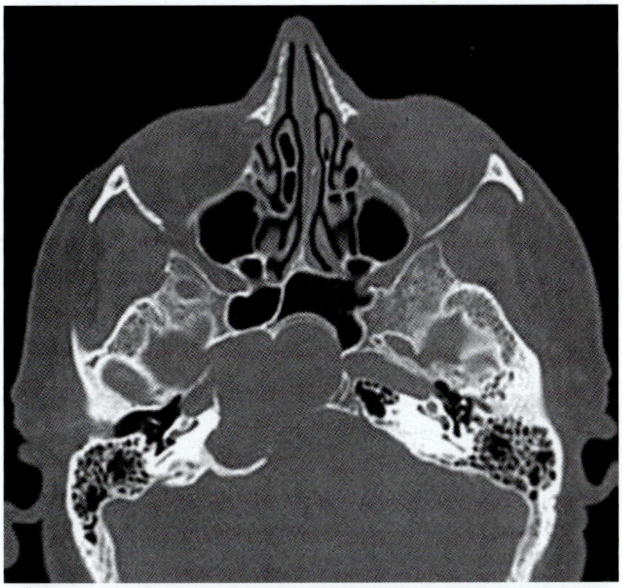

C

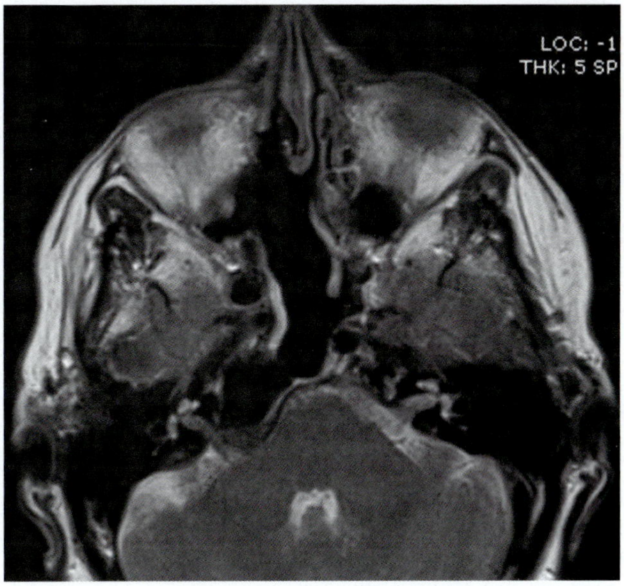

D

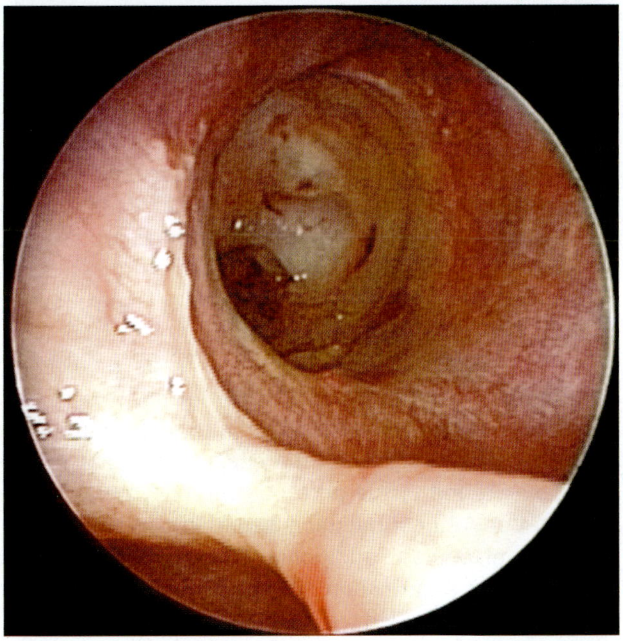

E

Fig. 47.13 *(continued)* **(C)** Preoperative computed tomography scan details the bony resorption caused by the lesion. **(D)** Postoperative (1 year) MRI shows a well-healed and aerated surgical cavity. **(E)** Endoscopic endonasal control with a 0-degree endoscope. The nasal mucosal flap used to cover the surgical cavity prevented stenosis and recurrence.

In cases in which the petrous apex is not pneumatized or the lesion does not extend far medially, the difficulty in the approach lies in moving inferiorly toward the clivus and laterally under the temporal portion of the ICA, which in some cases can also be lateralized. Depending on the need to extend laterally, transethmoidal-sphenoidal or a transethmoidal-pterygoidal-sphenoidal access can be used.

Transethmoidal-Sphenoidal Surgical Approach

This route of access is used for removal of lesions that involve the sellar region with extension to the medial parasellar region, to the lateral recess of the sphenoid, or to the posterolateral portion of the ethmoid. This approach is also suitable for endoscopic decompression of the optic nerve. With this route, it is easy to control the posterior ethmoid, the apex of the orbit, the lateral wall of the sphenoid (pterygoid recess), and, in particular, the medial component of the cavernous sinus. The inclination of surgical instruments is different in comparison to paraseptal access, offering more control over these anatomic structures.

Often, the extension of a sellar tumor to the cavernous sinus is through the space between the carotid siphon anteriorly and the clinoid process posteriorly, and the tumor can be accessed through this entry point. However, the complete exposure of the medial portion of the cavernous sinus requires, as described previously, removal of the bony wall that covers the cavernous ICA and of the lateral wall of the sphenoid up to the orbital apex. In sphenoids that are highly pneumatized, removal can involve the medial portion of the greater wing of the sphenoid. When the cavernous sinus is involved by an expansile process, venous bleeding is frequently minimal due to devascularization by compression of the lesion, whose removal is therefore made easier.

Transethmoidal-Pterygoidal Sphenoidal Surgical Approach

The indications for this surgical approach are the need for control of lateral structures of the anterior and medial skull base, such as the lateral portion of the cavernous sinus, the base of the middle cranial fossa (particularly in the case of pterygoidal-sphenoidal recesses that are highly pneumatized), and the infratemporal fossa. After removal of the posterior wall of the maxillary sinus and lateralization of the contents of the pterygomaxillary fossa, the vidian and the maxillary nerve are exposed and the vidian artery is cauterized. Drilling the base of the pterygoid and sphenoid sinus floor allows the surgeon to move laterally and to fully expose the vidian canal, which is an important safety landmark even for this type of approach. Superolaterally, in fact, at the level of V2, the base of the cavernous sinus can be identified. The possibility to access the lateral portion of the cavernous sinus is related, as mentioned, to devascularization due to tumor expansion.

Complications

Before planning removal of a lesion, it is important to consider the tumor's histology (to avoid unnecessary surgery), and the tumor's relation and possible adherence to vascular and nerve structures (to avoid iatrogenic injury). A complete understanding of anatomic relationships is a fundamental prerequisite. The basic extra- and intracranial landmarks must be constantly kept under control during surgery to guarantee safe access to deep structures.

When accessing the sphenoid sinus, the surgeon should keep in mind that he or she needs to identify the superior choanal border and the sphenoid rostrum. The removal of the sellar floor requires identification of the ICAs and, specifically, of the bulging of their cavernous portion. Opening the cavernous sinus is made after the exposure of the vidian canal and the foramen rotundum, recognizing that cranial nerve VI runs from lateral to medial. While accessing the petrous apex, the medial pterygoid lamina, the vidian canal, and the anterior genu of the ICA must be identified. This is necessary to avoid CSF leak from the posterior cranial fossa and to prevent severe vascular damage to the ICA or inferior hypophyseal artery. Hemorrhage of the ICA or major vessels can result in neurologic deficits or hemiparesis after ligation or can even lead to death.

The experience reported in the literature shows a significant reduction in CSF leak complications with the use of the Hadad flap[46] or, when this is not feasible, using a temporoparietal flap passed through the pterygopalatine fossa.[47] In the case that CSF leak does occur, a multilayer closure technique is preferred, with a tensor fascia lata free graft taken from the iliotibial tract as an intradural layer and a pedicled mucosal flap as an overlay.[48–50] It is not always straightforward to correctly place the intradural layer, such that alternative fixation techniques, such as the use of U-clips[51] or "gasket-seal" watertight closure,[52] have been recommended. Fibrin glue is placed only at the margins of the layers, and not between them because a dead space between layers can otherwise develop after glue resorption, placing the patient at risk for a recurrent CSF leak. The use of temporary lumbar-subarachnoid drainage during the postoperative period does not seem to decrease the rate of recurrence of CSF leak.[46] Generalized epilepsy possibly due to intraoperative massive CSF loss and consequent pneumocephalus has been observed.[53]

Cranial nerves can be damaged either directly or by injury to the vessels supplying them; temporary or permanent paralysis or sensory deficits are possible. We have also observed temporary paralysis of CN VI after lavage of the cavernous sinus to facilitate complete removal of a teratoma, in the absence of direct surgical trauma. Trauma to the optic nerve can lead to mono/binocular blindness.

Massive debulking of the hypophyseal gland can result in diabetes insipidus. Other complications are ascending bacterial meningitis, infections of the paranasal sinuses (i.e., sphenoid mycosis), postoperative epistaxis, and nasal airway difficulties due to scarring.[53]

A key aspect in surgical training is the acquisition of three-dimensional anatomic knowledge. This basic familiarity should allow the surgeon to achieve intraoperative orientation based on the integration of macroscopic, radiologic, and tactile perception to recreate a complete three-dimensional mental scheme. In this sense, neuronavigation offers an additional advantage to avoid complications, but its use should never substitute for anatomic and surgical knowledge.

As a final remark, transnasal neuroendoscopic surgery requires dedicated instrumentation. In recent years, significant innovations have been introduced such as intraoperative electromagnetic neuronavigation, intraoperative imaging systems, and extremely effective hemostatic materials. The wide availability of dedicated skull base instruments, together with the need for a more delicate and effective manipulation of anatomic structures, has contributed to the widespread use of the four-hand intranasal technique.[21] This has, in fact, offered the possibility for professional growth of otorhinolaryngologists and neurosurgeons, and requires dedicated cross-training in alternate roles during intervention.[54] The end result of interspecialist training is not only an increased knowledge of surgical technique, but also an important and valuable exchange of experience leading to better management of complications.

Postoperative Care

Lumbar drainage is not routinely indicated at the time of surgery unless the patient has clear signs of intracranial hypertension, but it can be helpful during the postoperative course for 5 to 6 days in case of suspicious CSF leak. In the case of preexisting endocranial hypertension, the possibility of positioning a ventriculoperitoneal shunt should be considered. Following intervention, the patient should not take nonsteroidal anti-inflammatory drugs (NSAIDs) for at least 20 days. Normally, a baseline CT or MRI should be obtained 24 hours after intervention to exclude hemorrhage, ischemia, or pneumocephalus.

Nasal packing is removed on the first or second postoperative day. Silicone sheets, which are placed paraseptally at the end of surgery to avoid synechiae and crust formation, are removed on days 15 to 20. Nasal washing and aerosols with mucolytics and saline solution allow for better cleansing of the nasal fossae. Patients should be kept under frequent endoscopic surveillance (monthly for the first 6 months, every 3 months for 2 years, and then at 6- to 12-month intervals in the absence of complications). During the first follow-up visit, at least 20 days after surgery, the surgical cavity should be cleansed of residual crusting, and the state of the flap should be examined. The presence of infection and macroscopic CSF leak are also ruled out. MRI is performed at 6, 12, and 24 months after intervention.

Outcomes

Transsphenoidal endonasal endoscopic approach for solid and cystic lesions of the petrous apex, in particular for cholesterol granulomas, is highly conservative and comparable to transtemporal/transcranial lateral approaches and avoids hearing and facial nerve risks,[55] also sparing cochlear and vestibular functions. Moreover, it allows for a larger and more natural drainage pathway into the sinuses and for effective endoscopic postoperative follow-up with easier transnasal management of recurrences.[56] Previous reports,[57,58] although on small patient cohorts, show that the approach can be used to completely remove the lesion with no or only minimal complications. In individual cases, recurrence has been reported to be related to stenosis caused by scarring at the site of surgery.

In contrast, extensive lesions involving the cavernous sinus, in particular pituitary adenomas, cannot always be completely removed by transnasal neuroendoscopic techniques. As a consequence, medical therapy and radiotherapy (stereotactic radiotherapy and radiosurgery) are still used as primary treatment for lesions of the cavernous sinus[59,60] and external intraextradural approaches still allow for the best surgical control in 1 to 4% of pituitary tumors, which extend to areas inaccessible by a purely endoscopic route.[61] In cases of large tumors with critical anatomic relationships, radiosurgery can be used after neuroendoscopic transnasal partial resection to provide long-term tumor control.[62]

There is good evidence in the literature that in pituitary adenomas invading the cavernous sinus, transnasal neuroendoscopic techniques yield good results in terms of tumor removal[63,64] with partial or total recovery of vision, when preoperatively compromised, and even provide good endocrine outcomes,[65] even though surgical resection cannot always be complete.[66]

Conclusion

The continual evolution of neuroendoscopic techniques, including hemostatic and reconstructive methods, in association with radiologic advances, will certainly lead to better outcomes in terms of resectability at the level of the cavernous sinus, even in intracranial areas at high neurovascular risk. However, radical resection of tumors that are firm, highly invasive to the cavernous sinus, or with multidirectional invasion remains a true challenge.[67,68]

References

1. Kennedy DW, Zinreich SJ, Rosenbaum AE, Johns ME. Functional endoscopic sinus surgery. Theory and diagnostic evaluation. Arch Otolaryngol 1985;111(9):576–582
2. Kennedy DW. Functional endoscopic sinus surgery. Technique. Arch Otolaryngol 1985;111(10):643–649
3. Kennedy DW, Kennedy EM. Endoscopic sinus surgery. AORN J 1985;42(6):932, 934, 936. No abstract available.
4. Stammberger H. [Endoscopic surgical treatment of mycoses of the paranasal sinuses]. Laryngol Rhinol Otol (Stuttg) 1984; 63(2):48–55 [German]
5. Stammberger H. Nasal and paranasal sinus endoscopy. A diagnostic and surgical approach to recurrent sinusitis. Endoscopy 1986;18(6):213–218
6. Stamm AM. Transnasal endoscopy-assisted skull base surgery. Ann Otol Rhinol Laryngol Suppl 2006;196:45–53 Review
7. Snyderman CH, Kassam AB. Endoscopic techniques for pathology of the anterior cranial fossa and ventral skull base. J Am Coll Surg 2006;202(3):563
8. Cappabianca P, Buonamassa S, Cavallo LM, Mariniello G, de Divitiis O. Neuroendoscopy: present and future applications. Clin Neurosurg 2004;51:186–190
9. Stammberger H, Anderhuber W, Walch C, Papaefthymiou G. Possibilities and limitations of endoscopic management of nasal and paranasal sinus malignancies. Acta Otorhinolaryngol Belg 1999;53(3):199–205
10. Walch C, Stammberger H, Unger F, Anderhuber W. [A new therapy concept in esthesioneuroblastoma]. Laryngorhinootologie 2000;79(12):743–748
11. Bockmühl U, Minovi A, Kratzsch B, Hendus J, Draf W. [Endonasal micro-endoscopic tumor surgery: state of the art]. Laryngorhinootologie 2005;84(12):884–891 [German]
12. Alfieri A, Jho HD. Endoscopic endonasal approaches to the cavernous sinus: surgical approaches. Neurosurgery 2001;49(2): 354–360, discussion 360–362
13. Mattox DE. Endoscopy-assisted surgery of the petrous apex. Otolaryngol Head Neck Surg 2004;130(2):229–241

14. Stammberger H, Anderhuber W, Walch C, Papaefthymiou G. Possibilities and limitations of endoscopic management of nasal and paranasal sinus malignancies. Acta Otorhinolaryngol Belg 1999;53(3):199–205
15. Unger F, Haselsberger K, Walch C, Stammberger H, Papaefthymiou G. Combined endoscopic surgery and radiosurgery as treatment modality for olfactory neuroblastoma (esthesioneuroblastoma). Acta Neurochir (Wien) 2005;147(6):595–601, discussion 601–602
16. Frank G, Sciarretta V, Calbucci F, Farneti G, Mazzatenta D, Pasquini E. The endoscopic transnasal transsphenoidal approach for the treatment of cranial base chordomas and chondrosarcomas. Neurosurgery 2006;59(1, Suppl 1):ONS50–ONS57, discussion ONS50–ONS57
17. de Divitiis E, Cavallo LM, Cappabianca P, Esposito F. Extended endoscopic endonasal transsphenoidal approach for the removal of suprasellar tumors: Part 2. Neurosurgery 2007;60(1):46–58, discussion 58–59
18. Schick B, Ibing R, Brors D, Draf W. Long-term study of endonasal duraplasty and review of the literature. Ann Otol Rhinol Laryngol 2001;110(2):142–147
19. Bockmühl U, Khalil HS, Draf W. Clinicoradiological and surgical considerations in the treatment of cholesterol granuloma of the petrous pyramid. Skull Base 2005;15(4):263–267, discussion 267–268
20. Castelnuovo P, Pistochini A, Locatelli D. Different surgical approaches to the sellar region: focusing on the "two nostrils four hands technique." Rhinology 2006;44(1):2–7
21. May M, Hoffmann DF, Sobol SM. Video endoscopic sinus surgery: a two-handed technique. Laryngoscope 1990;100(4):430–432
22. Briner HR, Simmen D, Jones N. Endoscopic sinus surgery: advantages of the bimanual technique. Am J Rhinol 2005;19(3):269–273
23. Hofmann T, Bernal-Sprekelsen M, Koele W, Reittner P, Klein E, Stammberger H. Endoscopic resection of juvenile angiofibromas—long term results. Rhinology 2005;43(4):282–289
24. Jho HD, Carrau RL. Endoscopic endonasal transsphenoidal surgery: experience with 50 patients. J Neurosurg 1997;87(1):44–51
25. Castelnuovo P, Battaglia P, Locatelli D, Delù G, Sberze F, Bignami M. Endonasal micro-endoscopic treatment of malignant tumors of the paranasal sinuses and anterior skull base. Oper Tech Otolaryngol—Head Neck Surg 2006;17(3):152–167
26. Senior BA, Dubin MG, Sonnenburg RE, Melroy CT, Ewend MG. Increased role of the otolaryngologist in endoscopic pituitary surgery: endoscopic hydroscopy of the sella. Am J Rhinol 2005;19(2):181–184
27. Gruber A, Bavinzski G, Killer M, Richling B. Preoperative embolization of hypervascular skull base tumors. Minim Invasive Neurosurg 2000;43(2):62–71
28. Rosen CL, Ammerman JM, Sekhar LN, Bank WO. Outcome analysis of preoperative embolization in cranial base surgery. Acta Neurochir (Wien) 2002;144(11):1157–1164
29. Oka H, Kurata A, Kawano N, et al. Preoperative superselective embolization of skull-base meningiomas: indications and limitations. J Neurooncol 1998;40(1):67–71
30. Castelnuovo P, Dallan I, Bignami M, Pistochini A, Battaglia P, Tschabitscher M. Endoscopic endonasal management of petroclival cerebrospinal fluid leaks: anatomical study and preliminary clinical experience. Minim Invasive Neurosurg 2008;51(6):336 –339
31. Scamoni C, Dario A, Castelli P, Caronno R, Picano M, Tomei G. Extracranial-intracranial bypass for giant aneurysms and complex vascular lesions: a clinical series of 10 patients. J Neurosurg Sci 2008;52(1):1–9, discussion 9–10
32. Liu JK, Couldwell WT. Interpositional carotid artery bypass strategies in the surgical management of aneurysms and tumors of the skull base. Neurosurg Focus 2003;14(3):e2
33. Kassam A, Snyderman CH, Mintz A, Gardner P, Carrau RL. Expanded endonasal approach: the rostrocaudal axis. Part II. Posterior clinoids to the foramen magnum. Neurosurg Focus 2005;19(1):E4
34. Kassam AB, Gardner P, Snyderman C, Mintz A, Carrau R. Expanded endonasal approach: fully endoscopic, completely transnasal approach to the middle third of the clivus, petrous bone, middle cranial fossa, and infratemporal fossa. Neurosurg Focus 2005;19(1):E6
35. Isaacson B, Kutz JW, Roland PS. Lesions of the petrous apex: diagnosis and management. Otolaryngol Clin North Am 2007;40(3):479–519, viii
36. Harnsberger HR, Glastonbury CM, Michel MA, et al. Diagnostic Imaging Head and Neck. Salt Lake City: Amirsys; 2004
37. Som PM, Curtin HD. Head and Neck Imaging. St. Louis: Mosby; 2003
38. Connor SE, Leung R, Natas S. Imaging of the petrous apex: a pictorial review. Br J Radiol 2008;81(965):427–435
39. Jackler RK, Parker DA. Radiographic differential diagnosis of petrous apex lesions. Am J Otol 1992;13(6):561–574
40. Cavallo LM, Cappabianca P, Galzio R, Iaconetta G, de Divitiis E, Tschabitscher M. Endoscopic transnasal approach to the cavernous sinus versus transcranial route: anatomic study. Neurosurgery 2005;56(2, Suppl):379–389, discussion 379–389
41. Reisch R, Vutskits L, Patonay L, Fries G. The meningohypophyseal trunk and its blood supply to different intracranial structures. An anatomical study. Minim Invasive Neurosurg 1996;39(3):78–81
42. Kassam AB, Vescan AD, Carrau RL, et al. Expanded endonasal approach: vidian canal as a landmark to the petrous internal carotid artery. J Neurosurg 2008;108(1):177–183
43. Osawa S, Rhoton AL Jr, Seker A, Shimizu S, Fujii K, Kassam AB. Microsurgical and endoscopic anatomy of the vidian canal. Neurosurgery 2009;64(5, Suppl 2):385–411, discussion 411–412
44. Vescan AD, Snyderman CH, Carrau RL, et al. Vidian canal: analysis and relationship to the internal carotid artery. Laryngoscope 2007;117(8):1338–1342
45. Hadad G, Bassagasteguy L, Carrau RL, et al. A novel reconstructive technique after endoscopic expanded endonasal approaches: vascular pedicle nasoseptal flap. Laryngoscope 2006;116(10):1882–1886
46. Snyderman CH, Kassam AB, Carrau R, Mintz A. Endoscopic reconstruction of cranial base defects following endonasal skull base surgery. Skull Base 2007;17(1):73–78
47. Fortes FS, Carrau RL, Snyderman CH, et al. Transpterygoid transposition of a temporoparietal fascia flap: a new method for skull base reconstruction after endoscopic expanded endonasal approaches. Laryngoscope 2007;117(6):970–976
48. Castelnuovo P, Locatelli D, Mauri S, De Bernardi F. Extended endoscopic approaches to the skull base, anterior cranial base CSF leaks. In: de Divitiis E, Cappabianca P, eds. Endoscopic Endonasal Transsphenoidal Surgery. New York: Springer Wien; 2003: 137–138
49. Locatelli D, Rampa F, Acchiardi I, Bignami M, De Bernardi F, Castelnuovo P. Endoscopic endonasal approaches for repair of cerebrospinal fluid leaks: nine-year experience. Neurosurgery 2006;58(4, Suppl 2):246–247
50. Castelnuovo PG, Delú G, Locatelli D, et al. Endonasal endoscopic duraplasty: our experience. Skull Base 2006;16(1):19–24
51. Gardner P, Kassam A, Snyderman C, Mintz A, Carrau R, Moossy JJ. Endoscopic endonasal suturing of dural reconstruction grafts: a novel application of the U-Clip technology. Technical note. J Neurosurg 2008;108(2):395–400

52. Leng LZ, Brown S, Anand VK, Schwartz TH. "Gasket-seal" watertight closure in minimal-access endoscopic cranial base surgery. Neurosurgery 2008;62(5, Suppl 2):E342–E343, discussion E343
53. Cappabianca P, Cavallo LM, Esposito F, De Divitiis O, Messina A, De Divitiis E. Extended endoscopic endonasal approach to the midline skull base: the evolving role of transsphenoidal surgery. Adv Tech Stand Neurosurg 2008;33:151–199
54. Snyderman CH, Kassam AB, Carrau RL, Mintz A, Gardner P, Prevedello DM. Acquisition of surgical skills for endonasal skull base surgery: a training program. Laryngoscope 2007;117(4):699–705
55. Zanation AM, Snyderman CH, Carrau RL, Gardner PA, Prevedello DM, Kassam AB. Endoscopic endonasal surgery for petrous apex lesions. Laryngoscope 2009;119(1):19–25
56. Presutti L, Villari D, Marchioni D. Petrous apex cholesterol granuloma: transsphenoid endoscopic approach. J Laryngol Otol 2006;120(6):e20
57. Georgalas C, Kania R, Guichard JP, Sauvaget E, Tran Ba Huy P, Herman P. Endoscopic transsphenoidal surgery for cholesterol granulomas involving the petrous apex. Clin Otolaryngol 2008;33(1):38–42
58. Mattox DE. Endoscopy-assisted surgery of the petrous apex. Otolaryngol Head Neck Surg 2004;130(2):229–241
59. Couldwell WT. Transsphenoidal and transcranial surgery for pituitary adenomas. J Neurooncol 2004;69(1-3):237–256
60. Kadashev BA, Kutin MA, Kalinin PL, Trunin IuK, Alekseev SN, Shkarubo AN. [Comparative assessment of the results of different surgical treatments in patients with pituitary adenomas infiltrating the cavernous sinus]. Vopr Neirokhir 2004;(3):14–17, discussion 17 [Russian]
61. Youssef AS, Agazzi S, van Loveren HR. Transcranial surgery for pituitary adenomas. Neurosurgery 2005;57(1, Suppl):168–175, discussion 168–175
62. Lunsford LD, Niranjan A, Martin JJ, et al. Radiosurgery for miscellaneous skull base tumors. Prog Neurol Surg 2007;20:192–205
63. Dehdashti AR, Ganna A, Karabatsou K, Gentili F. Pure endoscopic endonasal approach for pituitary adenomas: early surgical results in 200 patients and comparison with previous microsurgical series. Neurosurgery 2008;62(5):1006–1015, discussion 1015–1017
64. Kitano M, Taneda M, Shimono T, Nakao Y. Extended transsphenoidal approach for surgical management of pituitary adenomas invading the cavernous sinus. J Neurosurg 2008;108(1):26–36
65. Choe JH, Lee KS, Jeun SS, Cho JH, Hong YK. Endocrine outcome of endoscopic endonasal transsphenoidal surgery in functioning pituitary adenomas. J Korean Neurosurg Soc 2008;44(3):151–155
66. Frank G, Pasquini E. Endoscopic endonasal cavernous sinus surgery, with special reference to pituitary adenomas. Front Horm Res 2006;34:64–82
67. Zhao B, Wei YK, Li GL, et al. Extended transsphenoidal approach for pituitary adenomas invading the anterior cranial base, cavernous sinus, and clivus: a single-center experience with 126 consecutive cases. J Neurosurg 2010;112(1):108–117
68. Ceylan S, Koc K, Anik I. Endoscopic endonasal transsphenoidal approach for pituitary adenomas invading the cavernous sinus. J Neurosurg 2010;112(1):99–107

48 Endoscopic Approaches to the Clivus and Posterior Fossa

Aldo C. Stamm, Leonardo Balsalobre, and Larry Hilton Kalish

The treatment of lesions involving the clival area and the posterior fossa has changed dramatically through time. Before the introduction of endoscopic techniques, the management of lesions in these regions required extensive craniotomies resulting in significant morbidity to patients. Anterior approaches (transoral, transnasal, transfacial, transmaxillary) to the craniovertebral junction and the clivus, performed with microscopes, were originally proposed in the 1960s for the treatment of neoplasms and vertebrobasilar aneurysms.[1,2]

After the development and the dissemination of endoscopic technology and endoscopic surgical skills, particularly those involving the closure of dural defects, some authors have proposed several endoscopic approaches, seeking to optimize the exposure and minimize the risk of complications, avoiding nerve damage and excessive brain retraction. These endoscopic approaches were developed along two basic anterior midline routes, the transoral and the transnasal,[3–5] and they presented a lower rate of morbidity and complications when compared with the classic approaches.[6,7] However, even with the current use of technology of endoscopes, navigation systems, and powerful instrumentation, effective and safe treatment of lesions involving these regions is still a challenge.[8] Despite the lower morbidity and fewer complications, problems of infection, cerebrospinal fluid (CSF) leakage, difficulty controlling intradural bleeding, lack of experience, and appropriate surgical instruments still exist.[8] A thorough appreciation of the problems associated with endoscopic surgery is paramount to an informed discussion with the patient.

A multidisciplinary approach remains vital. Although the multidisciplinary team (MDT) has evolved only in the last few decades, improved survival and reduced complication rates in skull base surgery have been documented since its introduction.[9] The multidisciplinary team should include otorhinolaryngology–head and neck surgery, neurosurgery, intensive care, anesthesiology, pathology, endocrinology, and paramedical staff, including specialist nursing able to care for patients at risk of significant neurologic sequalae.[9–12]

A combination of a team approach, careful patient selection, a thorough understanding of the anatomy, appropriate expertise, and specialized equipment allows us to extend the transnasal approach to the clivus and posterior fossa and thus gives patients with previously surgically untreatable disease another option.

Patient Selection/Indications

There are a variety of indications for endoscopic approaches to the clivus and posterior fossa. Broadly, they include:

- The removal of disease
  - Clival lesions
    - Pituitary macroadenoma
    - Chordoma
    - Chondrosarcoma
    - Meningioma
    - Clival/sphenoid malignancy
    - Primary CFS leak
  - Petrous apex lesions
    - Cholesterol granuloma
    - Epidermoids
    - Mucoceles
    - Chordoma and chondrosarcoma
  - Craniocervical junction/odontoid lesions
    - Basilar invagination, secondary to rheumatoid arthritis
    - Exostosis
    - Osteoma
    - Foramen magnum meningiomas
    - Metastasis, specially of the odontoid process
- To minimize functional loss (decompression of cranial nerves with subtotal resection)
  - Optic nerve (vision)
  - Other cranial nerve integrity (CN III, IV, V, VI, IX, X, XI, XII)
  - Orbital contents
- To treat complications from previous surgery
  - CSF leaks
  - Mucoceles

Appropriate patient selection is vital to a successful outcome. Patient, disease, and surgeon factors must be considered, as follows:

- Patient factors include:
  - A suitable candidate for prolonged general anesthesia
  - No significant comorbidities (e.g., coagulopathy)

- An informed patient who is accepting of potential complications and resulting morbidity
- A patient who is motivated and compliant
- Disease factors include:
  - Benign pathology
  - Ability to surgically resect or decompress the disease
  - Favorable anatomy (e.g., internal carotids not obstructing field, well-pneumatized sphenoid for petrous apex approaches)
- Surgeon factors include:
  - Appropriate experience and expertise
  - Availability of equipment
  - Intensive care or closely monitored neurosurgical postoperative care

Contraindications

- Patient comorbidities precluding them from prolonged general anesthesia
- Unfavorable anatomy
- No multidisciplinary service
- Lack of specialized equipment/instruments

Diagnostic Evaluation

The effective and safe treatment of lesions involving the clivus and posterior fossa depends on several factors. These include a careful clinical history, preoperative evaluation with physical examination, and imaging studies and a well-developed surgical plan. A physician–patient informed discussion with frank conversations about the diagnosis, surgical plan, possible complications, and the roles of both the physician and the patient in the anticipated postoperative care plan is mandatory.

Physical Examination

The physical examination includes a gross neurologic assessment with special focus on cranial nerve function. Endoscopic assessment of the nasal cavity is recommended to visualize any nasal lesions and to document septal integrity, deviations, and other anatomic findings. An eye examination by an ophthalmologist is suggested if optic nerve or orbital integrity is compromised. A visual field examination is also recommended.

Imaging

Imaging is crucial in endoscopic approaches to the clivus and posterior fossa. This almost always includes both computed tomography (CT) and magnetic resonance imaging (MRI) modalities. A slice thickness of no more than 3 mm (and preferably less) and coronal, axial, and parasagittal CT images of the paranasal sinuses and skull base are essential in the preoperative assessment for surgery. CT permits assessment of anatomic information important during surgery, including:

- Presence and extent of erosions of the skull base
- Integrity of the medial orbital wall
- Position of the anterior skull base vessels
- Integrity and degree of aeration of the paranasal sinuses (particularly the sphenoid sinus)
- Location and presence of intersinus septae
- Position of the internal carotid arteries, optic nerves, and cavernous sinuses
- Relationships between the ethmoid sinuses, the orbits, and optic nerves
- Relationship between the roof of the ethmoid sinuses and the cribriform plate
- Presence of an Onodi cell

Especially for the clivus and posterior fossa approach, it is necessary to evaluate the size of the sphenoid sinus and the position of the internal carotid artery, particularly its paraclival portion, and the thickness of the clivus in a sagittal reconstruction. MRI is important to demonstrate the morphology of the soft tissues, but it is less helpful in assessing bony architecture. It can help to differentiate between either neoplastic or inflammatory tissue and retained secretions. MRI is especially valuable in excluding meningoencephaloceles when the CT reveals soft tissue densities adjacent to dehiscent bone in the skull base.

The evaluation of dehiscent areas becomes even more crucial when located in the lateral sphenoid. Iatrogenic injury to this region can result in bleeding, the formation of a carotid pseudoaneurysm, or optic nerve injury. Anatomic areas that pose greater challenges to resection should be carefully evaluated. These include the:

- Cavernous sinus
- Meckel's cave
- Jugular foramen
- Internal carotid artery (ICA)

Involvement of the carotid artery, vertebrobasilar system, or dural sinuses should also alert the surgeon to additional risk to the intracranial vasculature.[11]

Appropriate imaging sequences are necessary in order for correct interpretation of the MRI findings. T1-weighted images and fat suppression techniques before and after gadolinium enhancement will help reduce misdiagnosis, such as changes related to free fat grafts used in prior reconstructions. Often, scar and other high-signal tissues may not be discernible from recurrent disease, and changes on serial examinations, after an early postoperative baseline study, may be the only characteristic features of residual pathology.[11] Patients with complex skull base lesions may be candidates for fusion of CT and MR sequences for computerized intraoperative navigation. The navigation images can be variably blended to emphasize bone (CT) versus soft tissue (MRI) during different aspects of the skull base dissection.

CT angiography is a robust technology that allows simultaneous visualization of bony and vascular structures. Venous and arterial structures can be visualized separately in the venous and arterial phases, or seen together. CT angiography is especially useful in assessing the internal carotid and vertebrobasilar systems. Venous structures of particular interest include the cavernous sinus, the inferior aspect of the superior intercavernous sinuses, and the basilar venous plexus. This technology allows us to better plan surgical procedures.[13]

Magnetic resonance angiography (MRA) and/or CT angiography can assess the structure of medium to large arteries in patients with erosion of the sphenoid and clivus.[14] The relationship between the basilar and internal carotid arteries to pathology is crucial in this area. Venous structures are also visualized with these imaging modalities and particular interest should be given to the cavernous sinus, inferior end of the superior intercavernous sinuses, and the basilar venous plexus.

Although conventional angiography is not routinely performed, it can help to verify the functional integrity of the circle of Willis and the extent of any carotid artery compromise, and differentiate aneurysm from tumor.

Surgical Anatomy

All transnasal endoscopic surgical approaches to the clival region and posterior fossa involve the sphenoid sinus. We consider the sphenoid sinus "the hotel lobby," linked to almost all rooms in the building. For this reason, having a thorough knowledge of the sphenoid sinus anatomy is imperative. The other important anatomic structures related to this endoscopic approach include:

- The clivus
- The retroclival region (posterior fossa)
- The cavernous sinus and its contents

Sphenoid Sinus

The sphenoid sinus varies in shape and size and is often asymmetrically divided by an intersinus septum. When the sphenoid sinus is well developed, its thin lateral wall forms the medial wall of the cavernous sinus. The intracavernous portion of the internal carotid artery (ICA) is the most medial structure within the cavernous sinus and, in well developed sphenoid sinuses, it produces a bony projection in the lateral wall of the sinus called the carotid prominence.

The carotid prominence is divided into presellar, infrasellar, and retrosellar segments.[8] The presellar segment corresponds to the anterior vertical segment and the anterior bend of the intracavernous portion of the ICA.

The infrasellar segment corresponds to the short horizontal portion of the ICA, and the retrosellar segment reflects the posterior bend and posterior vertical segment.

The optic canal may be partially encompassed by the sphenoid sinus and creates a bony prominence in the superoanterior portion of its lateral wall. The bony depression between the optic canal and the presellar segment of the carotid prominence is called the opticocarotid recess.

The lateral sphenoid sinus wall over the internal carotid artery and the optic nerve is usually very thin and may be dehiscent in some areas.

The sella usually lies behind the posterior wall of the sphenoid sinus. Its prominence depends on the pneumatization of the sphenoid sinus. In a presellar ("conchal") configuration, the sella may not even feature as a prominence, whereas in the retrosellar configuration, the sellar prominence appears to be in the roof of the sinus. Between the two ICA prominences and above and below the sellar are numerous intercavernous vessels, which may result in nuisance bleeding in the transsellar approach.

Finally, one should always consider the presence of a sphenoethmoidal (Onodi) cell or posterosuperior pneumatization of the posterior ethmoid cells. These cells are easily mistaken for the sphenoid but may result in the surgeon being more superior than expected. They also may have a dehiscent optic nerve traveling through them.

Clivus

The clivus separates the nasopharynx from the posterior cranial fossa. It is composed of the posterior portion of the sphenoid body (basisphenoid) and the basilar part of the occipital bone (basiocciput) and it is further subdivided into upper, middle, and lower thirds. The upper third of the clivus is at the level of the sphenoid sinus and is formed by the basisphenoid bone including the dorsum sella. The middle clivus corresponds to the rostral part of the basiocciput and it is located above a line connecting the caudal ends of the petroclival fissures.[8]

The lower third of the clivus is formed by the caudal part of the basiocciput. The intracranial surface of the upper two-thirds of the clivus faces the pons and is concave from side to side.

The extracranial surface of the clivus gives rise to the pharyngeal tubercle at the junction of the middle and lower clivus. The upper clivus faces the roof of the nasopharynx that extends downward in the midline to the level of the pharyngeal tubercle.

The upper and middle clivus are separated from the petrous portion of the temporal bone on each side by the petroclival fissure. The basilar venous plexus is situated between the two layers of the dura of the upper clivus and is related to the dorsum sella and the posterior wall of the sphenoid sinus. It forms interconnecting venous channels between the inferior petrosal sinuses laterally, the cavernous sinuses superiorly, and the marginal sinus and epidural venous plexus inferiorly. The basilar sinus is the largest communicating channel between the paired cavernous sinuses.[8]

Retroclival Region (Posterior Fossa)

Although most of the structures of the suprasellar area, cavernous sinus, and clivus can be reached through the sphenoid sinus, the transnasal transclival endoscopic anatomy of the basal cisterns and posterior fossa through this approach remain unfamiliar to many surgeons.[8,15]

When all the bone of the posterior and lateral walls of the sphenoid sinus has been removed, only periosteum covers the underlying anatomy. The tectorial membrane protects the clival dura in the middle and lower clivus. When the external layer of the dura is opened, the basilar venous plexus and cranial nerve VI on each side can be seen.

After opening the inner layer of the clival dura, the view through the 0-degree endoscope reveals the vertebral arteries, basilar artery, and its branches (superior cerebellar arteries, anterior inferior cerebellar artery [AICA]), posterior cerebral arteries, brainstem, mammillary bodies, and the intradural pathway of cranial nerves III, IV, V, and VI. By introducing a 30- or 45-degree angled endoscope, it is also possible to view the cerebellopontine angle and CNs VII and VIII, as well as the lower cranial nerves and the retrosellar region.

Cavernous Sinus

The cavernous sinus is present bilaterally on each side of the sella turcica and body of the sphenoid bone. Each sinus has dural walls that surround a venous space through which a segment of the ICA with its branches, the abducens nerve (VI), and the sympathetic plexus course. Through the transnasal endoscopic surgical access, the ICA can be medially displaced, and CN VI is seen at the lateral surface. CN VI is the only intracavernous nerve, as the other cranial nerves III, IV, V_1, and V_2 are located between dural leaflets. Coming from the upper to the inferior part of the cavernous sinus, CNs III, IV, and the first division of the V are observed. The second division of CN V is seen inferiorly and laterally to the cavernous sinus.

Surgical Technique

Adequate instrumentation is essential for the endoscopic approach to the clivus and posterior fossa, and its lack is considered a contraindication to performing the procedure. The equipment includes (**Fig. 48.1**):

- High-quality endoscopes (0- and 45-degree)
- Video equipment (camera and monitor)
- Long endoscopic bipolar forceps, preferably suction bipolar
- Long and delicate high speed drills
- Long dissection instruments
- Hemostatic materials

In conjunction with Karl Storz, Inc., the lead author developed a 5-mm wide-angled 0-degree telescope for these procedures to increase the field of view and illumination.

The endoscopic surgical approach to the clivus and posterior fossa in primary surgery cases broadly follows the following sequence:

- Setup
  - Patient positioning
  - Topical vasoconstriction and infiltration
- Preparation
  - Combined transnasal/transseptal “binostril” approach[16]
  - Creation of pedicled nasal septal mucosal flaps (**Fig. 48.2**)
  - Wide opening of the sphenoid sinus
- Approaches
  - Transsphenoidal transclival
  - Petrous apex
  - Craniocervical junction/odontoid

Operative Setup

The surgery is performed under hypotensive general anesthesia with total intravenous anesthetic, using propofol and remifentanil as the preferred approach. The patient is placed in a supine position on the operating table, head elevated 30 degrees, neck slightly flexed, and head extended and turned toward the surgeon.

Neuropatties soaked in adrenaline 1:1000 are placed in the nasal cavity for 10 minutes before the surgical procedure begins. The septum is infiltrated with lidocaine with adrenaline 1:100,000.

Preparation

The access initiates with the combined transnasal/transseptal binostril approach,[16] which is described as follows.

After a standard anterior septoplasty incision, mucoperichondrial/mucoperiosteal flaps are created bilaterally. Most of the septal cartilage and bone are removed, preserving an L-shaped cartilage strut to support the nasal dorsum and tip. The cartilage harvested is preserved in normal saline solution. The sphenoid rostrum and anterior wall of the sphenoid sinus are exposed. The mucosal flaps are lifted until both natural sphenoid ostia are in view. The next step is the creation of sphenopalatine artery-based nasal septal mucosal flaps (**Fig. 48.2**).

Three incisions are made in the septal mucosa to create a rectangular flap; these include an anterior vertical

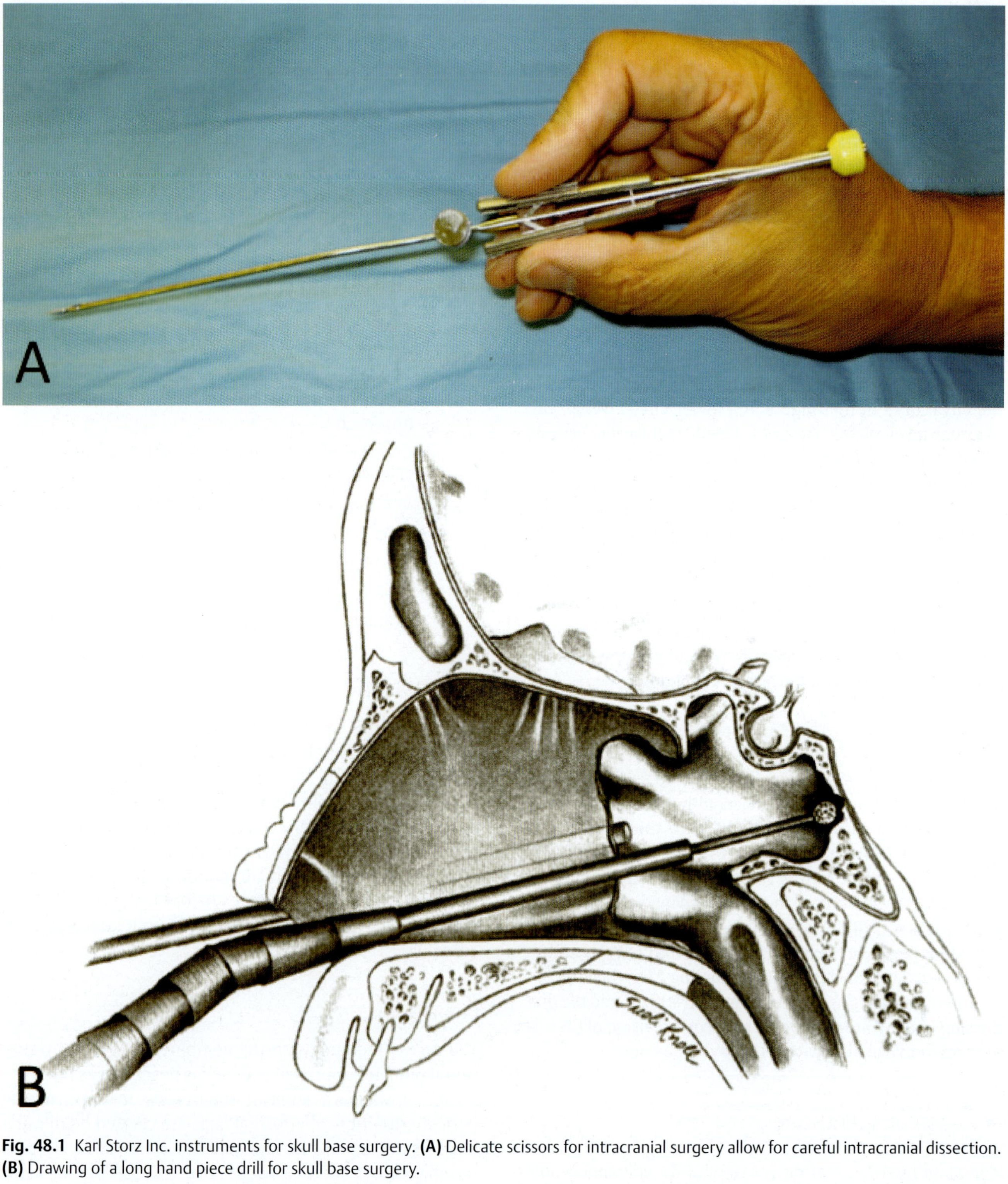

Fig. 48.1 Karl Storz Inc. instruments for skull base surgery. **(A)** Delicate scissors for intracranial surgery allow for careful intracranial dissection. **(B)** Drawing of a long hand piece drill for skull base surgery.

incision, and then superior and inferior horizontal incisions, contralaterally to the hemitransfixion incision made for the septoplasty. The vertical incision can be made as anterior as necessary because it will define the length of the flap. The superior horizontal incision is made 1 cm above the roof of the nasal cavity, and a parallel inferior incision borders the superior edge of the choana and, if continued, in an imaginary line heads toward to the sphenopalatine foramen. These horizontal incisions define the width of the flap.

The resulting mucosal flaps can be rotated and placed on the nasal floor back toward the choana or safely

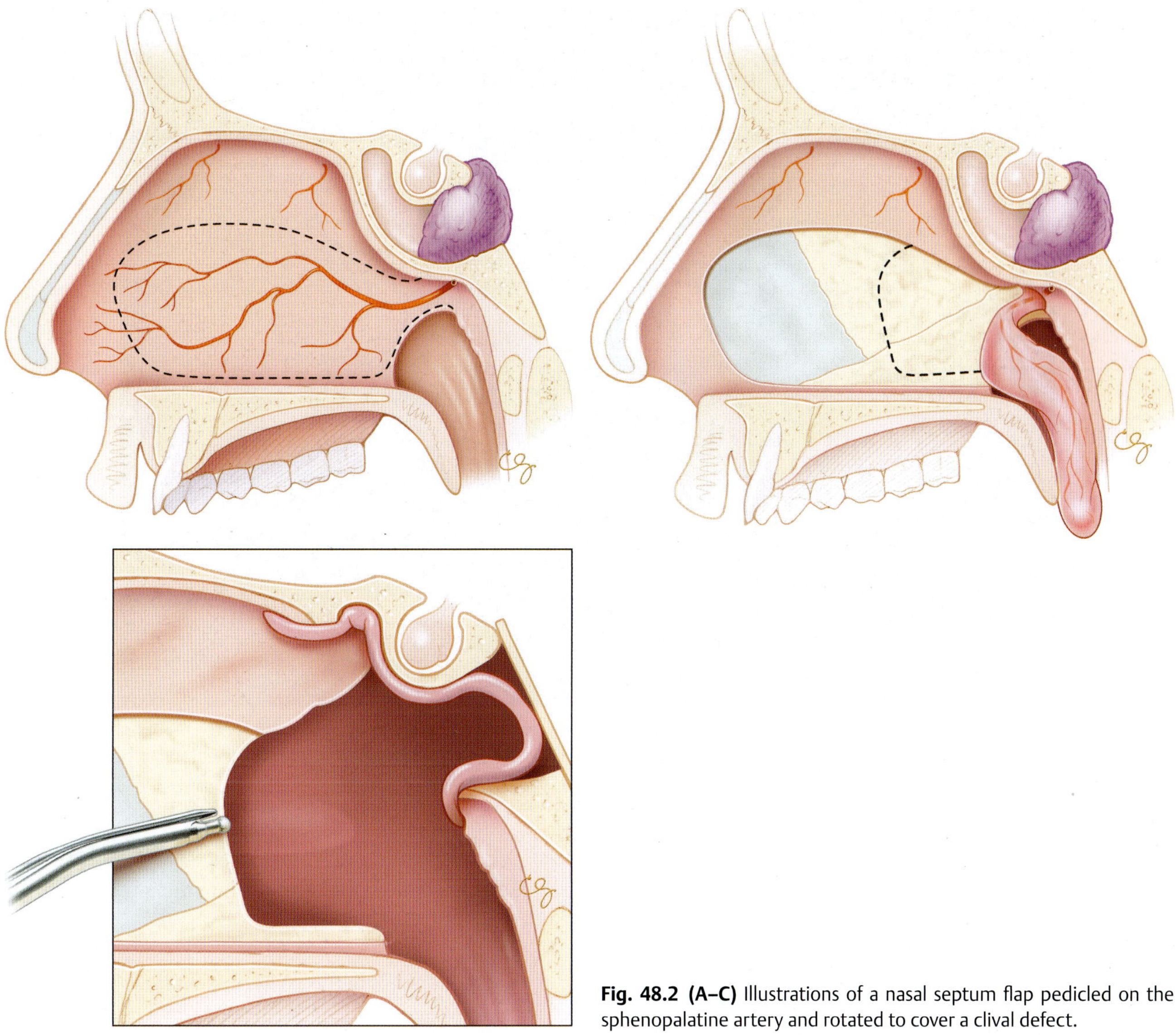

Fig. 48.2 (A–C) Illustrations of a nasal septum flap pedicled on the sphenopalatine artery and rotated to cover a clival defect.

placed into the maxillary sinus cavity through a large middle meatal antrostomy. This maneuver prevents the flaps from obstructing the surgical field or being accidentally injured.

This nasal septal flap preserves the posterolateral neurovascular pedicle (sphenopalatine artery). Multiple modifications regarding length and width are possible, and the flap should be created according to the size and shape of the planned defect.[17]

A wide opening of the anterior sphenoid sinus wall is created with a micro-Kerrison punch, and a drill is used to lower the sphenoid rostrum. The floor of the sella, the two carotid protuberances, the medial aspect of the optic canals, and the upper clivus should all be easily visualized. The sinus mucosa that lines the clival area is reflected carefully, exposing the clival bone. Care is usually taken to preserve this mucosa if possible to aid with closure.

This approach allows two surgeons to simultaneously manipulate surgical instruments using both nostrils. It incorporates a very robust vascularized flap to help in the closure of skull base defects. Furthermore, it preserves the nasal septal mucosa of one side, thus avoiding nasal septal perforation.

The approach can be expanded as required by removing the middle and superior turbinates and opening the maxillary and ethmoid sinuses.

Approaches

Transsphenoidal Transclival Approach

The transsphenoidal transclival approach is used for lesions involving the clivus or retroclival region (posterior fossa). The most common lesions indicated for this access are clival chordomas (**Fig. 48.3**) and

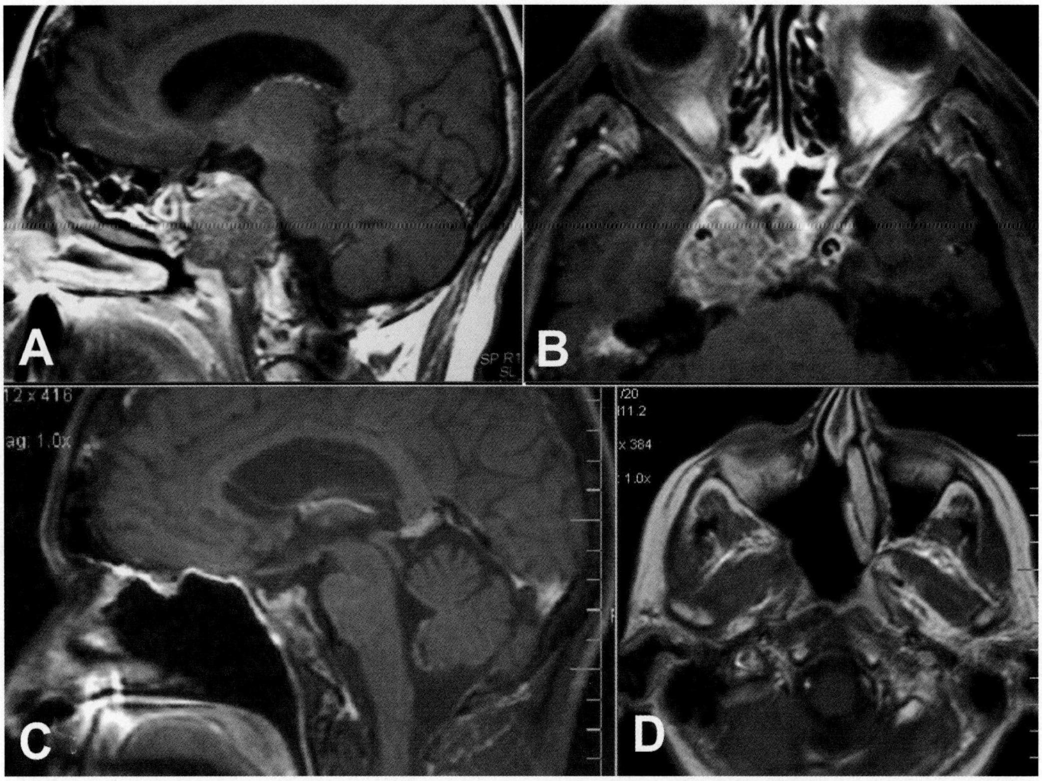

Fig. 48.3 **(A)** Parasagittal and **(B)** axial T1-weighted magnetic resonance images with gadolinium of a clivus chordoma preoperatively, and **(C)** parasagittal and **(D)** axial views postendoscopic resection. Skull base reconstruction was performed with a nasal septal flap pedicled on the sphenopalatine artery.

chondrosarcomas, followed by cholesterol granulomas and mucoceles.

The clival bone is fully exposed and its removal is initiated with a diamond burr drill and continued carefully with a micro-Kerrison punch if necessary. The limits of the clival bone removal include:

- Superiorly: Floor of the sella
- Inferiorly: Foramen magnum
- Laterally: Internal carotid arteries and occipital condyles

To create an intradural exposure, the external layer of the dura is first incised, and the basilar venous plexus and CN VI are encountered. Bleeding in the plexus cannot be cauterized safely but is usually controlled with packing using pieces of Surgicel. Large lesions often encroach on and obliterate much of the plexus, but if the lesion is not large or if the plexus is not completely compressed, profuse and intense bleeding can occur. Judicious packing, time, patience, and experience are required to control it.[13]

The opening of the internal layer of the dura at the level of the middle and superior clivus must be accomplished with great care to avoid injury to the underlying basilar artery. Once the dura is opened, minor bleeding is stopped by bipolar coagulation, and it is finally possible to introduce the 0-degree endoscope carefully into the intradural space and to identify the following:

- Major vessels of the posterior fossa
  - Basilar artery and branches
  - Anterior inferior cerebellar arteries
  - Vertebral arteries
  - Superior cerebellar artery
  - Posterior cerebral arteries
- Intradural course of cranial nerves
  - CNs III, IV, V, and VI
- Brainstem
  - Mammillary bodies

With angled endoscopes, it is also possible to visualize the following:

- Cerebellopontine angle
- Cranial nerves
  - CNs VII, VIII, IX, X, XI, and XII
- Retrosellar regions[13]

Once the anatomy is appreciated, meticulous dissection is required to remove the pathology. To optimize the surgeon's view, persistent hemostasis of the tissues of the nasal cavity and sphenoid needs to be maintained to minimize soiling of the endoscopes. A four-handed technique can be used. Frequent irrigation and suction with neurosurgical tip-protected low suction is used to maintain good vision. Once meticulous dissection and removal of the lesion is completed, the surgeon can proceed to repair the surgical site.

Dural repair in the region of the clivus is difficult. If the defect is large, we first occlude it with abdominal fat and then cover the defect with grafts of fascia lata or a synthetic material such as Duragen (Integra Life Sciences Corporation; Plainsboro, NJ) and/or Duraform (Codman; Raynham, MA). These grafts are covered by the sphenopalatine-based pedicled nasal septal flap(s), as described previously. Fibrin glue is not typically necessary but may be used to hold the graft and flap in position. Spongostan powder (Ethicon; Somerville, NJ) and Gelfoam (Pfizer; New York, NY) is layered directly over the flap and followed by gauze packing soaked in antibiotic paste. A silastic splint is inserted into the nose on the side from which the graft was taken to promote reepithelialization. The packing is supported by a RapidRhino 900 (Arthrocare; Austin, TX) or similar pack. With pedicled flaps, fibrin glue is not usually necessary. Broad-spectrum antibiotics are used for 10 days or as long as necessary.[8]

The main advantages of the transsphenoidal transclival approach include the ability to avoid any cerebral retraction and to decrease the incidence of injury to the lower cranial nerves. In addition, the approach is direct and does not require any external incisions. It is also relatively quick and preserves anatomic structures.

Even though endoscopes do not allow a three-dimensional perspective, they do provide a close view of the operative field from different angles. However, endoscopes only allow for a narrow operative field, which is surrounded by critical neurovascular structures, thus making the risks of major intradural bleeding, CSF leakage, and neural damage still possible.

Petrous Apex Approach

This type of surgical access can be useful for biopsy and drainage purposes. It can be particularly helpful in selected cases of cholesterol granuloma of the petrous apex (**Fig. 48.4**) when complete excision is unnecessary.

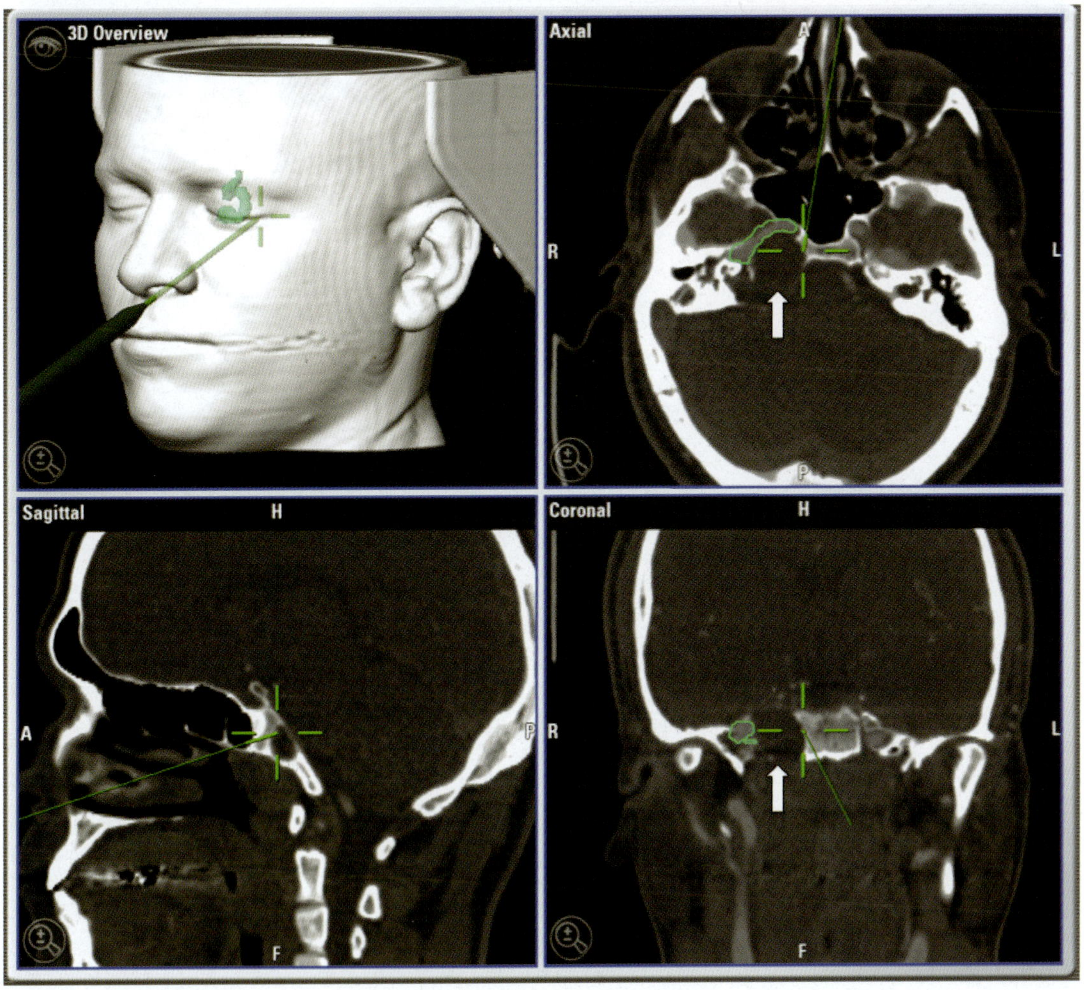

Fig. 48.4 Intraoperative screenshot of the image guidance system displaying the endoscopic petrous apex approach for cholesterol granuloma in situ (*arrow*).

Although surgical drainage is usually accomplished through the temporal bone, the transsphenoidal endoscopic approach may be indicated when the lesion abuts against the posterior and lateral wall of the sphenoid sinus. In these cases, the use of image guidance can be very helpful to precisely identify the internal carotid artery, optic nerve, and the lesion.

The clival region is completely exposed, and both ICA canals are identified. When the anatomy is clearly apparent, these canals are easily recognized. If the canals are difficult to identify, diamond burrs with suction irrigation can be useful to identify the vertical segment, particularly at the junction of the cavernous and petrous portions of the ICA.[18]

Craniocervical Junction/Odontoid Approach (Fig. 48.5)

The most common indication for this access is an extradural compressive lesion such as basilar invagination secondary to rheumatoid arthritis. Other indications for this access are exostosis, osteoma, foramen magnum meningiomas, clivus chordomas with inferior extension, and metastasis (especially in the odontoid process). The surgeon should follow the following sequence:

- General exposure
- Osseous exposure
- Removal of lesions
- Reconstruction

The surgery is usually performed through both nostrils by two surgeons to permit using multiple surgical instruments including suctions, drills, and a navigation system. The drill system must be thin, delicate, and long enough to allow its passage through the nose, but without interfering with the endoscopic vision. The image guidance system is very helpful in these cases.

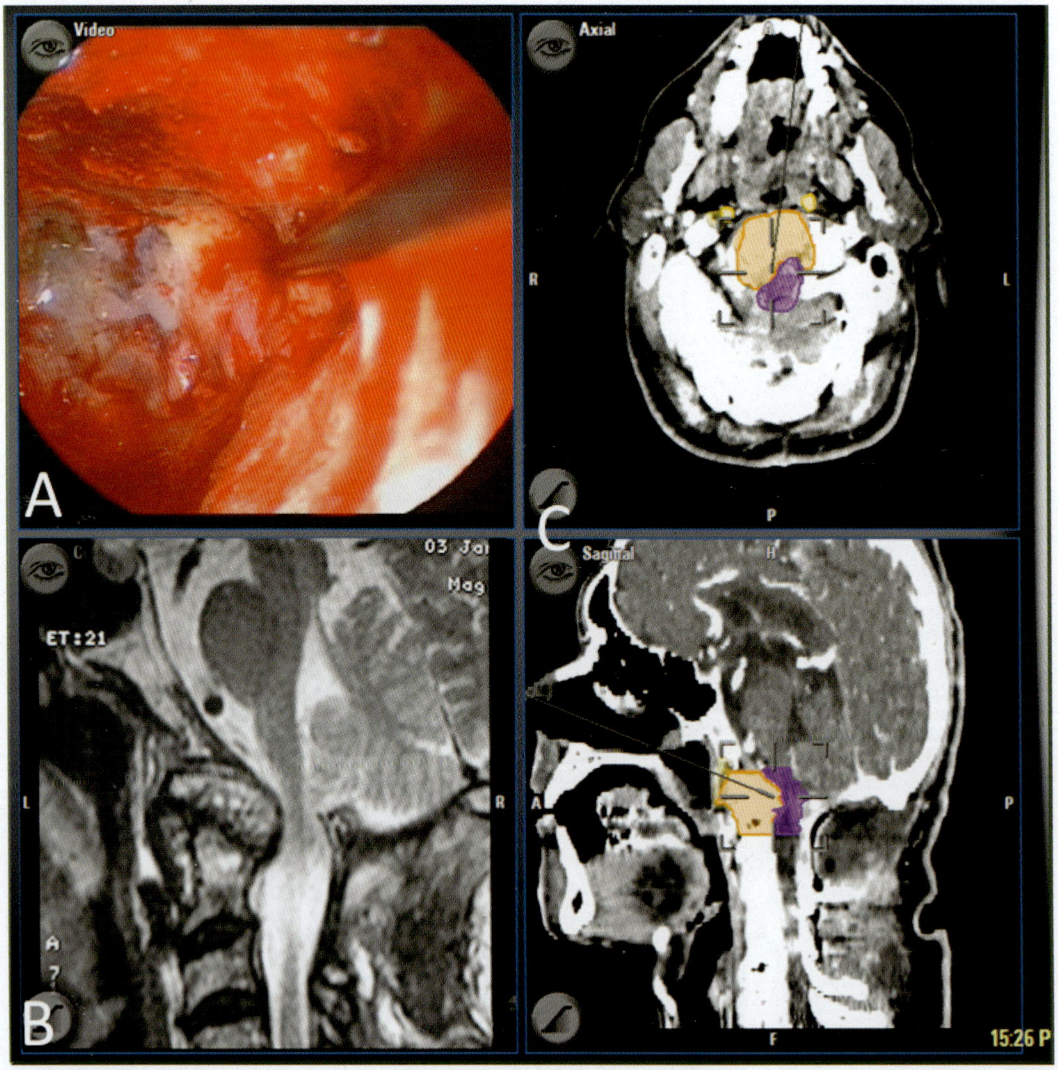

Fig. 48.5 Screenshots of the image guidance system displaying **(A)** the intraoperative endoscopic craniocervical approach, and **(B)** T2-weighted magnetic resonance image (MRI) demonstrating the compressive lesion–osteoma at the craniocervical junction. **(C)** Intraoperative view of the computed tomography–MRI fusion.

A panclival exposure creates a single cavity that extends from the sphenoid sinus to the level of the fossa of Rosenmüller. To expose the odontoid and the foramen magnum, additional soft tissue removal is required. The nasopharyngeal mucosa is cauterized with monopolar electrocautery and then resected from the sphenoclival junction to the level of the soft palate. The longus capitis and longus colli muscles are exposed and partially resected to expose the ring of C1. Care should be taken to stay medial to the eustachian tubes, especially when using electrocautery, because the parapharyngeal portion of the internal carotid artery is directly posterolateral to the eustachian tube. After finishing the procedure, the nasopharyngeal tissues do not need reapproximation and the surgical defect is covered with fibrin glue. The nasal passages are cleared of blood, and silastic septal splints are inserted to minimize the risk of postoperative synechiae.

Complications

The complications can be classified according to severity as minor or major and according to time of appearance as immediate or delayed. Minor complications present little morbidity and do not compromise the patient's life, although they may be annoying and troublesome. Most of the minor complications will resolve with time and conservative treatment.[8]

However, major complications present significant morbidity and the possibility of mortality. Most orbital complications stem from direct injury to the optic nerve or the extraocular muscles or from arterial or venous bleeding within the rigid bony orbit. These injuries can result in diplopia, hematoma, proptosis, and decreased visual acuity or blindness (which can be temporary or permanent). Direct or indirect damage to the optic nerve usually occurs at the superolateral sphenoid sinus wall or in the posterior ethmoid cells.

Intracranial complications can result from direct injury to brain, cranial nerves, meninges, blood vessels, or venous sinuses. The resulting deficits can include the following:

- Loss of function of the surgically damaged structures (brain and/or cranial nerves)
- Loss of vascular supply to critical areas
- Mass compressive effects (hematoma, others)

Also, CSF leakage can cause symptoms directly, as well as predispose the patient to meningitis and pneumocephalus, which can cause mass effect symptoms.

Bleeding is a risk in any surgical procedure, but seldom are so many important vessels susceptible to injury. The transnasal approaches outlined previously visualize and put the following vessels at risk:

- Anterior and posterior ethmoid arteries
- Sphenopalatine and maxillary arteries, and their branches
- Internal carotid artery
- Anterior cerebral artery
- Basilar and vertebral arteries, and their branches
- Venous sinuses of the skull base:
  - Cavernous sinus
  - Basilar venous plexus
  - Anterior intercavernous sinus

Immediate complications can occur during surgery. The most frequent of these are CSF leakage, intraoperative bleeding, orbital hematoma, and injuries to the brain and CNs III and VI. Delayed complications include progressive loss of vision, meningitis, bleeding, synechia, and infection.[8]

Postoperative Care

A satisfactory postoperative result depends on both appropriate operative technique and meticulous postoperative care. Wide-spectrum antibiotics are given during the operation and for 10 days postoperatively or until the nasal packing is removed.

Adequate postoperative care of the operative site requires appropriate instrumentation, including 4-mm 0- and 45-degree endoscopes, straight and curved atraumatic aspirators, and straight and curved microforceps for outpatient debridement and follow-up.

The anterior pack is removed after 5 to 7 days. The ribbon gauze is removed after 10 to 14 days. Vigilance is required in the postoperative period for CSF leaks and the risk of infections.

After the removal of the packing, the operative cavity is carefully suctioned and any residual bony fragments are removed. The patient is instructed to perform frequent nasal irrigations with buffered 0.9% saline solution.

After any dural repairs, it is recommended to avoid physical activities, nose blowing, and sneezing with a closed mouth for a period of ~30 days. All patients are prescribed stool softeners.

Follow-up takes place at least every 2 weeks or more frequently if there are any concerns. At each visit the operated nasal cavity is cleaned of crusts, granulation tissue, clots, and secretions. Imaging is only performed after the cavity has satisfactorily healed.

Outcomes

From 1996 to 2007, 22 patients with chordomas and chondrosarcomas were referred to our institution. Six patients had been treated previously by several surgical procedures, including craniotomies. After all preoperative care, they were submitted to endoscopic transnasal transclival approach for the resection of the tumor.

In 10 patients, a gross-total resection was achieved. Six patients had subtotal resection and 6 patients had partial resection.

Some authors believe that the main limits of the endoscopic technique are represented by extensive dural invasion of the tumor and the tumor centered on the inferior clivus.[19] Our study reports 7 cases with posterior fossa extension, all of which were treated with transnasal transclival endoscopic-assisted approach, which in four patients gross-total resection was achieved.

In our opinion, this procedure is feasible even for those cases of dural invasion. The greatest concern with regard to the technique is the extensive dural resection and resulting high-volume CSF leak that can be difficult to control. For this, the authors have found that the septal mucosal flap, pedicled at the sphenopalatine bundle, acts as a robust vascularized tissue and has enhanced our ability to close these defects.

Based on outcomes from our patients, we believe that the endoscopic-assisted transnasal surgery is an alternative way to treat these cases and, in expert hands, this technique can obtain good results. The extent of resection was better in patients having primary surgeries than in revision surgical cases. Posterior fossa invasion was not an impediment to obtaining a gross-total resection.

Conclusion

Surgical approaches for the clivus and posterior fossa require input from both neurosurgical and otorhinolaryngologic services. The ability of the surgical team to access these regions endoscopically greatly benefits patients with a variety of benign and malignant pathologies. Comfort and expertise with endoscopic techniques to control intracranial bleeding, reconstruct skull base defects, and manage intradural structures are all prerequisites for the operative team. These skills, combined with a detailed knowledge of the endoscopic anatomy of the region and its distortion from disease, serve as a foundation for addressing this complex pathology.

References

1. Mullan S, Naunton R, Hekmat-Panah J, Vailati G. The use of an anterior approach to ventrally placed tumors in the foramen magnum and vertebral column. J Neurosurg 1966;24(2):536–543
2. Sano K, Jinbo M, Saito I. Vertebro-basilar aneurysms, with special reference to the transpharyngeal approach to basilar artery aneurysm. No To Shinkei 1966;18(12):1197–1203
3. Crockard HA. The transoral approach to the base of the brain and upper cervical cord. Ann R Coll Surg Engl 1985;67(5):321–325
4. Draf W, Weber R, Keerl R. Endonasale chirurgie von tumoren der nasennebenhohlen und rhinobasis. Med Bild 1995;2:13–17
5. Harsh GR IV, Joseph MP, Swearingen B, Ojemann RG. Anterior midline approaches to the central skull base. Clin Neurosurg 1996; 43:15–43
6. Alfieri A, Jho HD. Endoscopic endonasal approaches to the cavernous sinus: surgical approaches. Neurosurgery 2001;49(2): 354–360, discussion 360–362
7. Jho HD. The expanding role of endoscopy in skull-base surgery. Indications and instruments. Clin Neurosurg 2001;48:287–305
8. Stamm AC, Pignatari SSN. Transnasal endoscopic-assisted surgery of the skull base. In: Cummings CW, Flint PW, Harker LA, eds. Otolaryngology Head Neck Surgery. 4th ed. Philadelphia: Elsevier Mosby; 2005; 3855–3876
9. Beals SP, Joganic EF, Holcombe TC, Spetzler RF. Secondary craniofacial problems following skull base surgery. Clin Plast Surg 1997;24(3):565–581
10. Kaylie DM, Wittkopf JE, Coppit G, Warren FM III, Netterville JL, Jackson CG. Revision lateral skull base surgery. Otol Neurotol 2006;27(2):225–233
11. Nguyen-Huynh A, Blevins NH, Jackler RK. The challenges of revision skull base surgery. Otolaryngol Clin North Am 2006;39(4): 783–799, viii
12. Pieper DR, LaRouere M, Jackson IT. Operative management of skull base malignancies: choosing the appropriate approach. Neurosurg Focus 2002;12(5):e6
13. Stamm AC, Pignatari SS, Vellutini E. Transnasal endoscopic surgical approaches to the clivus. Otolaryngol Clin North Am 2006;39(3):639–656, xi
14. Leong JL, Batra PS, Citardi MJ. Three-dimensional computed tomography angiography of the internal carotid artery for preoperative evaluation of sinonasal lesions and intraoperative surgical navigation. Laryngoscope 2005;115(9):1618–1623
15. Fakhri S, Citardi MJ, Wolfe S, Batra PS, Prayson RA, Lanza DC. Challenges in the management of sphenoid inverted papilloma. Am J Rhinol 2005;19(2):207–213
16. Stamm AC, Pignatari S, Vellutini E, Harvey RJ, Nogueira JF Jr. A novel approach allowing binostril work to the sphenoid sinus. Otolaryngol Head Neck Surg 2008;138(4):531–532
17. Hadad G, Bassagasteguy L, Carrau RL, et al. A novel reconstructive technique after endoscopic expanded endonasal approaches: vascular pedicle nasoseptal flap. Laryngoscope 2006;116(10):1882–1886
18. Stamm AC, Pignatari SN. Transnasal endoscopic surgical approaches to the posterior fossa. In: Anand VK, Schwartz TH, eds. Practical Endoscopic Skull Base Surgery. San Diego: Plural Publishing; 2007
19. Crockard HA, Cheeseman A, Steel T, et al. A multidisciplinary team approach to skull base chondrosarcomas. J Neurosurg 2001; 95(2):184–189

49 Endoscopic Approaches to the Pterygopalatine and Infratemporal Fossae

Ameet Singh, Vijay K. Anand, and Theodore H. Schwartz

Endoscopic approaches to the pterygopalatine and infratemporal fossae demonstrate the lateral infraorbital extent of the endonasal approach. The deep and lateral location of the complex anterolateral skull base renders this approach more challenging than midline approaches. Furthermore, the complexity of the anatomy and the high density of neurovascular structures in these two fossae challenge the surgeon to address the pathology without compromising function (**Fig. 49.1**).[1–8] Recent advances in endoscope technology, instrumentation, and image guidance have enhanced the endoscopic approach to these inaccessible skull base regions. Furthermore, the expanding knowledge of endoscopic lateral skull base anatomy as well as collaborative efforts between subspecialties has led to successful outcomes in addressing pathology of the pterygopalatine and infratemporal fossae.[8–15]

Traditionally, open surgical techniques have involved anteriorly based transmaxillary approaches to the pterygopalatine fossa (PPF) and laterally based preauricular approaches to the infratemporal fossa (ITF). Risks of the anteriorly based approaches include facial edema, pain, hypesthesia, oroantral fistulas, sinusitis, and vascular or dental injuries. Open surgical access to these regions is limited laterally by the parotid gland, mandible, facial nerve, and masticator muscles. Endoscopic surgical management of these lesions can provide direct access to these regions with superior visualization and magnification. Furthermore, early identification and preservation of neurovascular structures results in less functional and cosmetic morbidity than the external approaches.

The endoscopic transpterygoid approach is considered the workhorse for addressing lesions of the PPF, ITF, petrous

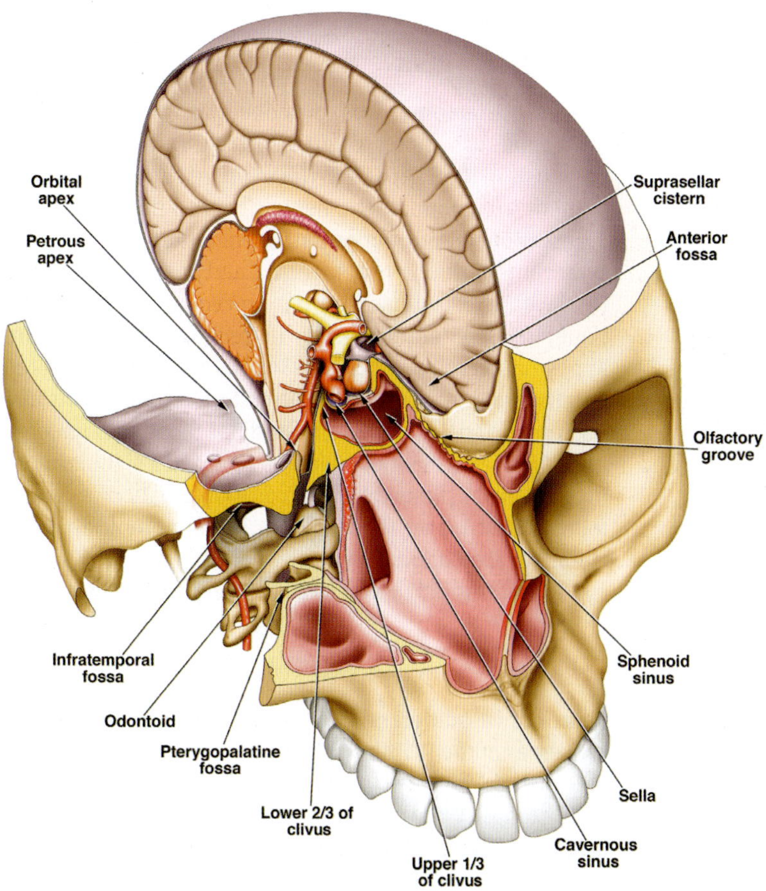

Fig. 49.1 Location of the pterygopalatine fossa and infratemporal fossa in relation to other intracranial and extracranial structures. (Used with permission from Schwartz TH, Fraser JF, Brown S, Tabaee A, Kacker A, Anand VK. Endoscopic cranial base surgery: classification of operative approaches. Neurosurgery 2008;62(5):991–1002; discussion 1002–1005.)

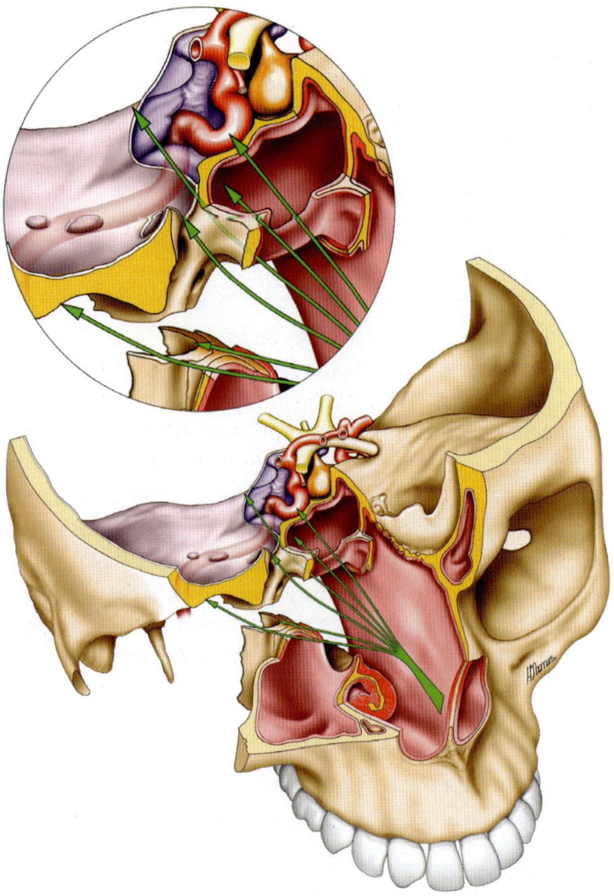

Fig. 49.2 The transpterygoid approach to the lateral sphenoid sinus, pterygopalatine fossa, infratemporal fossa, petrous apex, Meckel's cave, orbital apex, and lateral cavernous sinus. (Used with permission from Schwartz TH, Fraser JF, Brown S, Tabaee A, Kacker A, Anand VK. Endoscopic cranial base surgery: classification of operative approaches. Neurosurgery 2008;62(5):991–1002; discussion 1002–1005.)

apex, petroclival junction, and lateral sphenoid sinus. In select cases, this approach may be used to address pathology of the lateral cavernous sinus, Meckel's cave, and medial middle cranial fossa. In general, lesions medial and inferior to the petrous portion of the internal carotid artery (ICA) are more amenable to the endoscopic approach. The key corridor for this approach is the maxillary sinus, which can be entered and expanded endonasally to provide superior exposure and visualization (**Fig. 49.2**).[2,8,11,12,15,16]

Patient Selection/Indications

A variety of infectious, vascular, benign, and malignant pathologies are encountered in the PPF and ITF. Although primary tumors rarely originate from the PPF, this region can be secondarily involved by locally aggressive lesions of the nose and skull base. Secondary involvement occurs via the multiple foramina and canals that connect the PPF to the middle cranial fossa, orbit, nasal cavity, oral cavity, and ITF.

Advances in endoscopic techniques and instrumentation have broadened the indications for approaches to the PPF and ITF without altering functional morbidity. These include control of epistaxis by ligation of branches of the internal maxillary artery, vidian neurectomy for vasomotor rhinitis, and resection of benign and malignant tumors.[8–10,13,14,17–20] In addition, the transpterygoid approach is often used to provide exposure for resection of a lateral sphenoid sinus encephalocele.[11] Given the historically high recurrence rates, this approach is infrequently used for resection of the pterygopalatine ganglion for intractable facial pain or transection of the maxillary nerve for tic douloureux.

Posterior Epistaxis

Traditionally, open approaches to the PPF for surgical treatment of posterior epistaxis were difficult and potentially morbid. The emergence of interventional angiography to visualize and embolize branches of the internal maxillary artery greatly reduced the need for open surgical intervention. Endoscopic approaches to the sphenopalatine artery and other branches of the internal maxillary artery have reintroduced surgery as a safe, efficient, and successful method of controlling posterior epistaxis, perhaps even preferable to interventional techniques. Successful long-term (9 to 12 months) control of epistaxis after endoscopic sphenopalatine artery ligation has been reported to be over 90% in multiple publications.[17,20]

Vidian Neurectomy

Vidian neurectomy was described as a treatment for intractable vasomotor rhinitis, allergic rhinitis, and nasal polyposis in the 1960s. The vidian nerve supplies parasympathetic and sympathetic nerve fibers to the nasal cavity. Transection of the nerve has been reported to improve symptoms of rhinorrhea, sneezing, and postnasal discharge. However, the usefulness of the procedure has been questioned in the literature given the recurrence of symptoms in postneurectomy patients, as well as concerns over potential dry eye morbidity. Nevertheless, successful results have been reported, including one study of 9 patients undergoing 14 procedures where patients reported a significant improvement in rhinorrhea and nasal obstruction at a mean follow-up of longer than 2 years. Minor complications included exacerbation of sneezing postoperatively (33%), dry eye symptoms (35%), and nasal crusting (28%).[8]

Benign and Malignant Tumors

There is a vast differential for primary benign and infectious processes of the PPF and ITF. Common benign lesions of the PPF include inverted papillomas (IPs), juvenile nasal angiofibromas (JNAs), lipomas, schwannomas, and neuromas (**Fig. 49.3**). Successful endoscopic management with good long-term results has been reported for these lesions in the

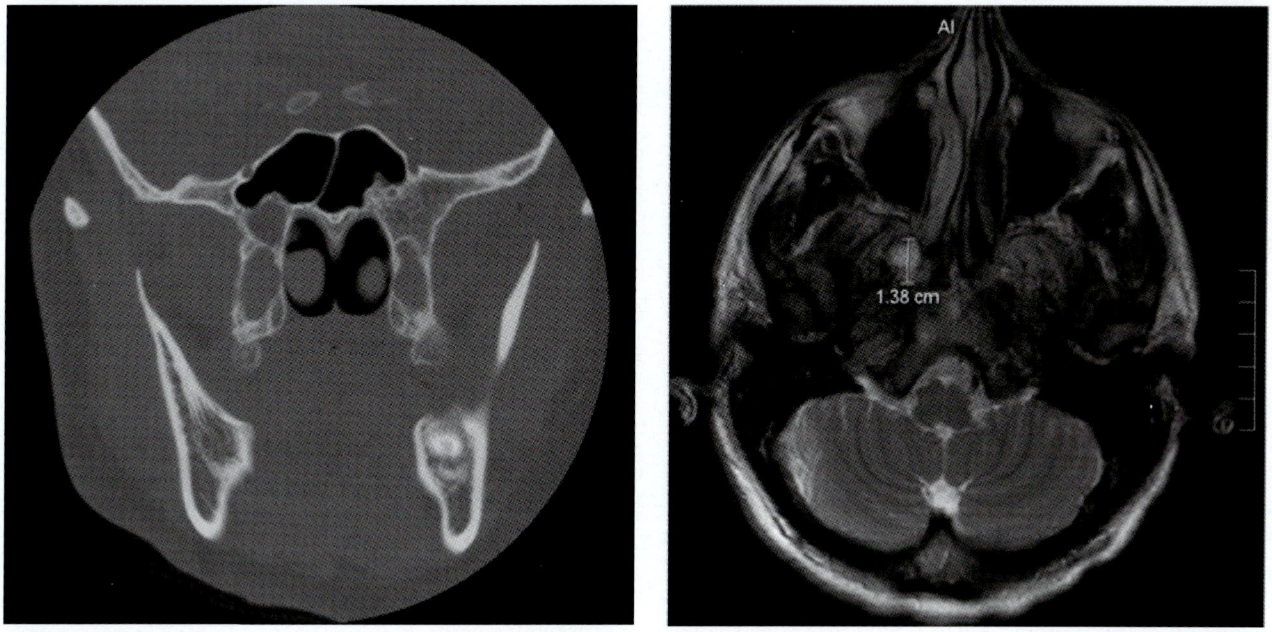

A B

Fig. 49.3 (A) Coronal computed tomography and **(B)** axial magnetic resonance image of a right primary lipoma involving the pterygopalatine fossa and pterygoid region.

literature.[8,10,11,14,18,21] For IPs, the recurrence rate for the endoscopic approach has been reported to be 12% compared with 18% for the open approach.[13] Similarly, successful endoscopic resections have been reported for JNAs. One study of 14 JNA patients, 8 of whom underwent an endoscopic medial maxillectomy for Radkowski stage IIC or IIIA, were disease-free with an average follow-up of 4.1 years.[8,18]

Malignant tumors with primary or secondary involvement of the PPF and ITF include tumors of epithelial origin such as squamous cell carcinoma, adenocarcinoma, and sinonasal undifferentiated carcinoma (SNUC); tumors of salivary gland origin such as mucoepidermoid and adenoid cystic carcinoma from parotid gland extension; lesions of neural origin such as gliomas and chordomas; tumors of mesenchymal origin such as rhabdomyosarcomas, neurofibrosarcomas, osteosarcomas, and chondrosarcomas; as well as melanomas, esthesioneuroblastomas, and lymphomas. Direct involvement of the PPF by malignant tumors may be secondary to direct extension, perineural invasion, lymphatic metastasis, or vascular seeding.

Endoscopic resection of malignant nasal and paranasal tumors is a controversial topic but reports are increasing in the literature. Arguments against endoscopic surgery emphasize the perceived difficulty in achieving the required negative margins and en bloc resection to achieve the optimal progression-free survival. However, it is not at all clear that en bloc resection is required to achieve a better outcome and studies exist to the contrary.[22,23] With regard to the need for negative margins, technically sophisticated endoscopic surgeons are able to achieve negative margins as readily as can be achieved transcranially, assuming there is no disease extending laterally over the orbits and no orbital exenteration is required. Likewise, in spite of aggressive attempts to achieve negative margins through the standard craniofacial approaches, recurrence rates approach 50%, indicating that this goal may be unachievable in a subset of patients regardless of the approach.[24] Hence, a less morbid and less invasive procedure may be preferable. Finally, palliative debulking may be better tolerated using an endonasal endoscopic approach.[25]

Nevertheless, although studies are ongoing, good long-term data are lacking to support endoscopic endonasal surgery as the sole method for resecting malignancies. Open surgical approaches remain the gold standard for sinonasal malignancies. Additionally, a cranioendonasal approach has been advocated, which provides suitable transcranial exposure without transfacial incision.[26] Previously described contraindications for endoscopic resection of nasal and sinonasal malignancies have included bony erosion of the skull base, lamina papyracea, and nasal floor; involvement of brain parenchyma or orbit; extension into the PPF or ITF; and involvement of the frontal sinus or lacrimal pathway.[9,19] However, these are relative contraindications based on the technical abilities of the endoscopic surgeon. Preoperative imaging on CT (for bony erosion) and MRI (for orbital or intracranial invasion) are critical for assessing the surgical candidacy of a patient with a sinonasal malignancy.

Diagnostic Workup

A thorough history and physical exam—in particular, assessing the patient's vision, extraocular movements, facial sensation, and all the cranial nerves—is essential. Patients with primary PPF lesions may present with a diverse and seemingly unrelated constellation of symptoms. Typical symptoms or signs may include unilateral midface hypesthesia, dental complaints, diplopia, proptosis, pain, and nasal congestion. A thorough nasal endoscopic evaluation of the tumor is also prudent to identify the origin and plan the surgical approach. Biopsy should be deferred for JNAs or other vascular tumors given the risk of bleeding. In this instance, diagnosis should rely on clinical and radiologic findings. Preoperative laboratory evaluation should include a complete blood count, metabolic evaluation, and a blood typing and cross-matching.[2,9]

Preoperative imaging is necessary to adequately define lesions of the PPF and ITF. CT imaging is important for elucidating the bony anatomy of the region, whereas MRI is critical for soft tissue detail and extension of lesions into the orbit or intracranial cavity. Critical evaluation of preoperative imaging is particularly important for tumors deeply invading into the ITF abutting the orbital apex, middle cranial fossa, cavernous sinus, or carotid artery. Close inspection of infraorbital fissure, which separates the PPF and ITF, orbital apex, cavernous sinus, and supra- and infrapetrous carotid artery, is important prior to the surgical approach. In addition, widening of foramina such as the foramen rotundum, foramen ovale, and sphenopalatine foramen, as well as passages such as the vidian, pterygomaxillary fissure, palatovaginal, and greater palatine must be noted on preoperative imaging. This is particularly true for JNAs that can invade multiple foramina and result in an incomplete resection and recurrence (**Fig. 49.4**).

Careful evaluation of preoperative imaging is critical to determine the difficulty of the resection, the risk of recurrence, or whether the lesion should be treated endoscopically. Absolute contraindication for the endoscopic approach includes significant orbital or skin involvement. Finally, image guidance is an important surgical adjunct for lesions of the PPF and ITF. This technology can not only help during resection of tumors, but also guide tissue biopsies for primary, secondary, or metastatic lesions of the PPF and ITF. As always, image guidance should never substitute or override the anatomic knowledge of a skull base surgeon.

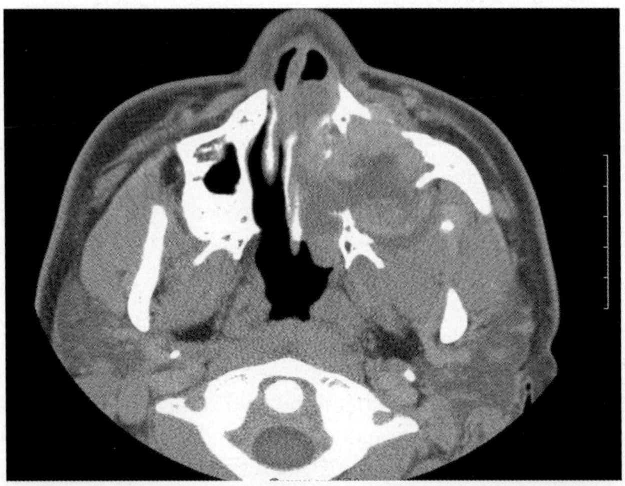

A

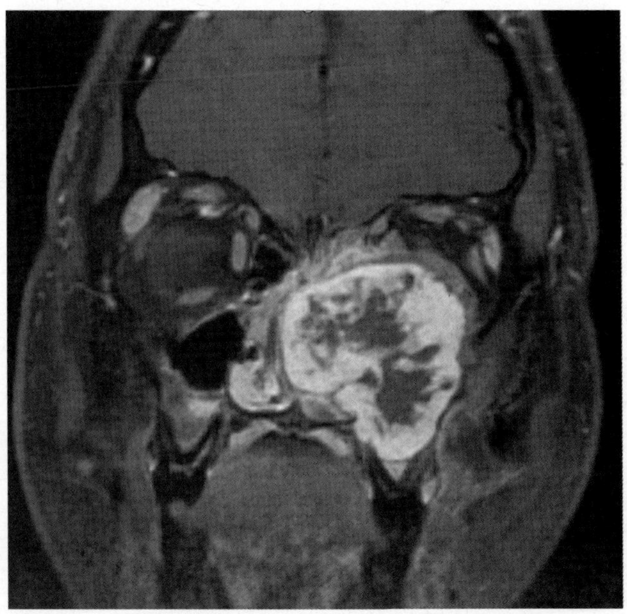

B

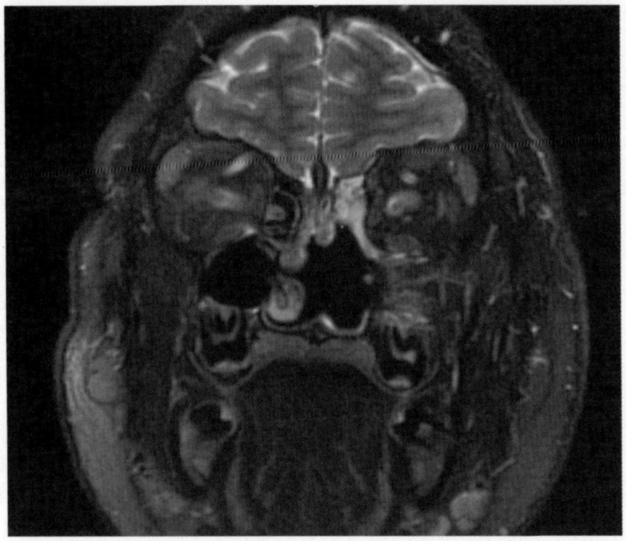

C

Fig. 49.4 **(A)** Axial computed tomography and **(B)** coronal magnetic resonance image of left juvenile nasal angiofibroma involving the nasal cavity, pterygopalatine fossa, medial infratemporal fossa, vidian canal, and pterygoid region. **(C)** Postoperative resection cavity.

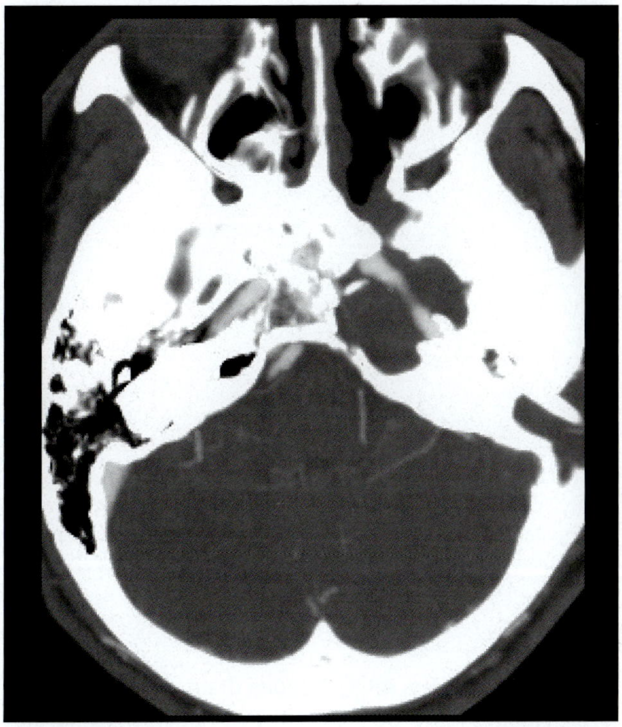

Fig. 49.5 Computed tomographic angiogram demonstrating a dehiscent horizontal petrous carotid artery within a multiple recurrent left petrous apex cholesterol granuloma.

Angiography may also be useful to not only visualize the ICA and its branches, but also to embolize tumors such as JNAs, which are prone to heavy bleeding during surgical resection. However, CT angiography may often be adequate to define the vascular anatomy if embolization is not required. CT angiography may also be helpful to plan a surgical approach when a lesion is intimately associated with a major arterial vessel (**Fig. 49.5**). Finally, if there is significant risk of surgical injury to the carotid artery, a balloon occlusion test should be performed to assess collateral flow, and strong consideration should be given to the open approach.

Gross Surgical Anatomy

Pterygopalatine (Pterygomaxillary) Fossa

The pterygopalatine (pterygomaxillary) fossa is a small inverted pyramidal space bounded by the posterior wall of the maxilla anterolaterally, the pterygoid plates of sphenoid bone posteriorly, the perpendicular plate of the palatine bone medially, the pterygomaxillary fissure laterally, the greater wing of the sphenoid bone superiorly, and the pyramidal process of the palatine bone inferiorly (**Fig. 49.1**).[1–4] Cadaveric anatomic measurements demonstrate a height of 2 cm, width of 1.5 cm, and depth of less than 1 cm. One anatomic study demonstrated an average height of 27 mm, a width of 23 mm, and depth of 7.3 mm. The PPF is widest superiorly and narrowest inferiorly.[6] Major neurovascular structures in the PPF include the internal maxillary artery and its branches, the maxillary nerve (V2) and its branches, the pterygopalatine ganglion, and vidian nerve.

Eight different openings transmit neurovascular structures in and out of the PPF. The inferior orbital fissure communicates with the orbit anteriorly and laterally, transmitting the infraorbital nerve, the zygomatic nerve, infraorbital vessels, veins to pterygoid plexus, and the ophthalmic vein. Laterally, the pterygomaxillary fissure opens up into the ITF, transmitting the maxillary vessels. The sphenopalatine foramen communicates with the nasal cavity medially, transmitting the sphenopalatine vessels and nerves to the nose. Inferiorly, the greater and lesser pterygopalatine canals, forming the bottom of the inverted cone, transmit the greater and lesser palatine nerves and vessels to supply the palate.

Three of the eight openings are present posteriorly in the PPF, which include the foramen rotundum, the vidian (pterygoid) canal, and the pharyngeal (palatovaginal) canal. The maxillary nerve exits the foramen rotundum and traverses the superior PPF on its way to the inferior orbital fissure. The vidian canal, located medially and inferiorly and separated from the foramen rotundum by a 7 to 10 mm vertical crest of bone, transmits the vidian nerve to the pterygopalatine (sphenopalatine) ganglion. The pharyngeal canal opens into the lateral part of the posterior choanae and sends branches of the internal maxillary artery into the nasopharynx (**Fig. 49.6**).

The PPF contains a high density of neurovascular structures. Arteries include the pterygopalatine (third) portion of the internal maxillary artery and its numerous branches. These vessels include the posterior superior alveolar artery, the infraorbital artery, the descending palatine artery, pharyngeal artery, artery of the pterygoid canal, and the sphenopalatine artery. The posterior superior alveolar

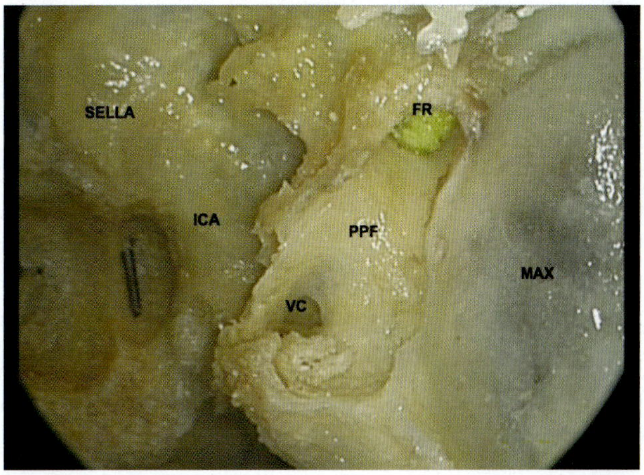

Fig. 49.6 Endoscopic view of posterior wall of the left pterygopalatine fossa. *FR*, foramen rotundum; *VC*, vidian canal; *MAX*, maxillary sinus (posterior wall); *ICA*, internal carotid artery.

artery initially runs over the posterior surface of the maxillary tuberosity, branches into small feeding vessels, and runs with the posterior superior alveolar nerve to supply the maxillary sinus, molar and premolar teeth, and gums. The infraorbital artery runs anteriorly into the infraorbital groove and canal and exits at the infraorbital foramen and branches extensively to supply the extraocular muscles, lacrimal gland, teeth, and maxillary sinus. The descending palatine artery gives rise to two arteries: the greater palatine artery, which exits the greater palatine foramen and supplies the roof of the mouth, palatine glands, and gums, and the lesser palatine artery, which exits the lesser palatine foramen and supplies the oral surface of the soft palate and palatine tonsils. The artery of the pterygoid canal, or vidian artery, accompanies the vidian nerve to provide blood supply to the eustachian tube and sphenoid sinus (**Fig. 49.7**).

The sphenopalatine artery, the terminal branch of the internal maxillary artery, enters the nasal cavity at the superior meatus adjacent to the pterygopalatine ganglion and divides into the posterolateral nasal and posterior septal branch after exiting the sphenopalatine foramen. The posterior lateral nasal branches supply the nasal turbinates and the paranasal sinuses, whereas the posterior septal branch traverses the anterior inferior portion of the sphenoid sinus and anastomoses with the anterior and posterior ethmoidal arteries to supply the posterior nasal septum. These terminal branches supply a range of pedicled intranasal flaps for skull base reconstruction, including the nasoseptal flap (**Fig. 49.8**). Venous drainage from the PPF is provided by the pterygoid venous plexus, which lies between the masticator, temporal, and the internal and external pterygoid muscles. This plexus of veins connects to an expansive network of veins, which include the inferior alveolar, middle meningeal, deep temporal, masseteric, buccal, posterior superior alveolar, pharyngeal, descending palatine, infraorbital, and sphenopalatine veins.

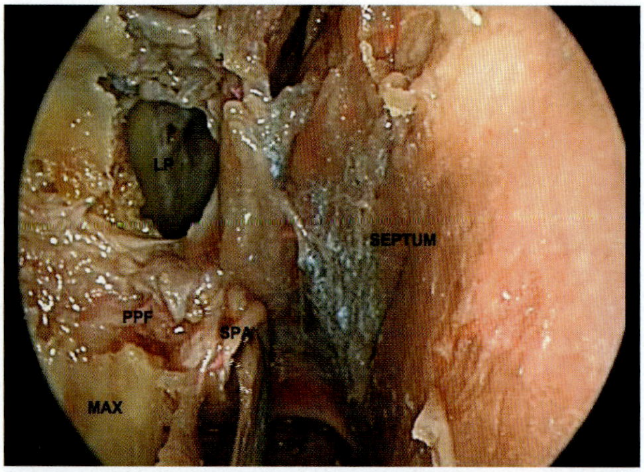

Fig. 49.8 Cadaveric dissection of the right pterygopalatine fossa demonstrates the sphenopalatine artery (SPA) emerging from the pterygopalatine fossa (PPF) to supply the nasal cavity, including the posterior septum for a vascularized pedicled flap. *LP*, lamina papyracea; *MAX*, maxillary sinus; *PC*, choana

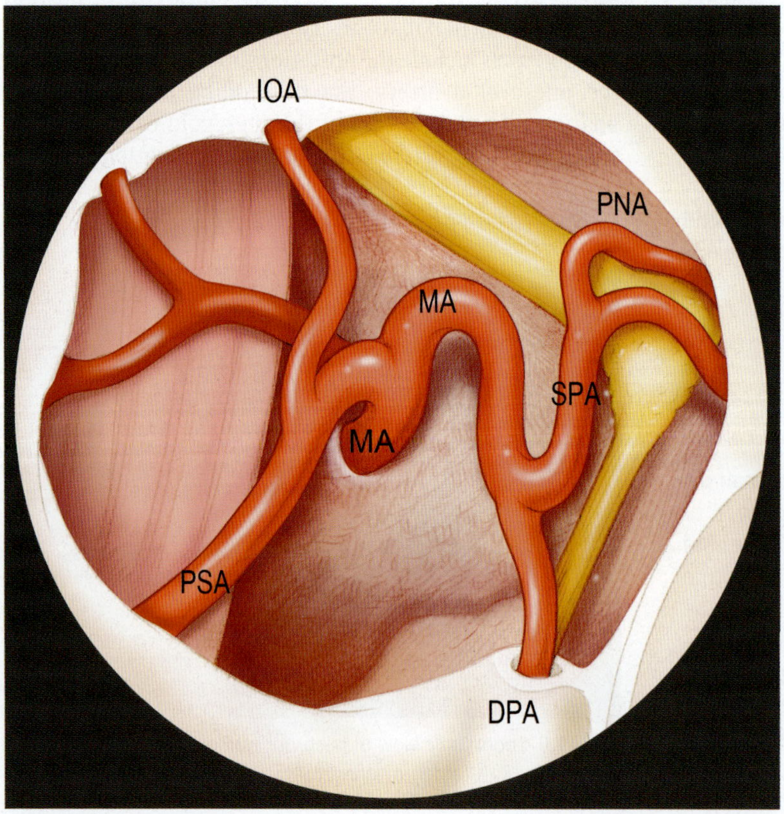

Fig. 49.7 Vascular anatomy of the pterygopalatine fossa and infratemporal fossa: *IOA*, infraorbital artery; *PSA*, posterior superior alveolar artery; *MA*, maxillary artery; *PNA*, posterior nasal artery; *SPA*, sphenopalatine artery; *DPA*, descending palatine artery.

The sphenopalatine ganglion (or pterygopalatine ganglion), one of four parasympathetic ganglions in the head and neck, rests in the PPF. It contains sympathetic and parasympathetic fibers from the vidian nerve. The maxillary nerve exits the foramen rotundum and enters the pterygomaxillary fossa where it branches into the zygomatic nerve, which supplies the orbit through the inferior orbital fissure, and ganglionic branches to the sphenopalatine ganglion. The maxillary nerve continues as the infraorbital nerve, which denotes an important division between the PPF (medial) and the ITF (lateral). Other nerves associated with the ganglion may be divided into ascending (to the orbit), posterior (to the pharynx), internal (to the nose), and inferior (to the palate). These nerves include the vidian nerve, pharyngeal nerve, descending palatine nerves, nasopalatine nerves, and posterior superior nasal nerve (**Fig. 49.9**).[4,27]

Infratemporal Fossa

The ITF is a large irregular space located above the parapharyngeal space, which is bound medially by the lateral pterygoid plate, the pyramidal process of palatine bone, and squamous portion of the temporal bone; laterally by the zygomatic arch and mandible; superiorly by the greater wing of the sphenoid; inferiorly by the alveolar processes; anteriorly by the posterior surface of the maxilla; and posteriorly by the auricular tubercle of the temporal bone and spine of the sphenoid bone (**Fig. 49.1**).

The ITF communicates superiorly with the temporalis fossa transmitting the temporalis muscle, nerve, and vessels. It also accepts the mandibular division of the trigeminal nerve, traveling through the foramen ovale and the middle meningeal vessels from the foramen spinosum. Anteriorly, it communicates with the orbital cavity via the infraorbital fissure, which is located between the greater wing of the sphenoid and maxilla; and medially with the PPF via the pterygomaxillary fissure, which sends through the terminal branches of the internal maxillary artery.

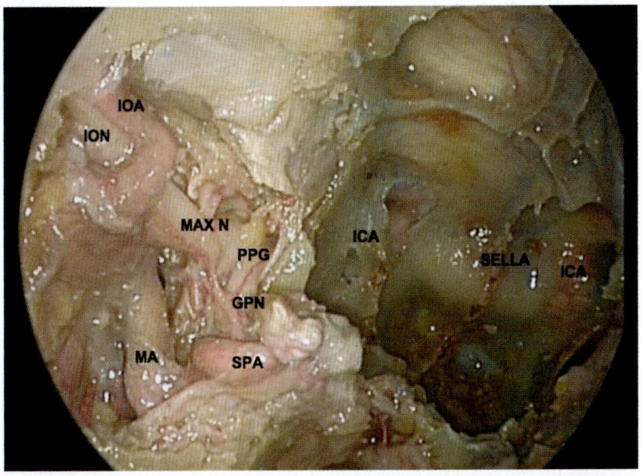

Fig. 49.9 Neural anatomy of the pterygopalatine fossa and infratemporal fossa. *MAX N*, maxillary nerve; *PPG*, pterygopalatine ganglion; *GPN*, greater palatine nerve; *SPA*, sphenopalatine artery; *MA*, maxillary artery; *ION/IOA*, infraorbital nerve and artery; *ICA*, internal carotid artery.

The fossa contains several structures that are bound by fatty fibroconnective tissues, which include the medial and lateral pterygoid muscles, the sphenomandibular ligament, the mandibular division of the trigeminal nerve, the chorda tympani nerve, the internal maxillary artery and branches of its mandibular and pterygoid divisions, the middle meningeal artery, and the pterygoid venous plexus.

External Approaches

Traditional approaches to the PPF and ITF have included anterior as well as lateral-based approaches. The most common anterior facial approach to the PPF is the transantral maxillectomy. This entails gaining access to the fossa through the anterior and posterior walls of the maxillary sinus. The technique involves making a gingivobuccal incision, a wide anterior maxillary wall antrostomy inferior to the infraorbital nerve, transgression through the maxillary sinus to the posterior wall, and removal of the bony wall medially and laterally to expose the pterygomaxillary and anterior ITF, respectively. Dissection within the PPF and ITF is then performed under microscopic guidance. Other approaches include midfacial degloving, lateral rhinotomy, and extended maxillectomy approaches. The risks of anterior-based approaches include facial edema and pain, infraorbital nerve injury, hypesthesia, lacrimal dysfunction, dental injuries (alveolar necrosis, dental granuloma, tooth loss, oroantral fistula), and chronic maxillary sinusitis.

Lateral approaches include temporal approach to the PPF as well as preauricular and facial translocation approaches to the ITF.[28,29] Postauricular approaches were described by Fisch who divided these approaches into type A, B, and C dissections. Type A entails a radical mastoidectomy, anterior transposition of the facial nerve, and cervical dissection allowing exposure to the posterior ITF, jugular bulb, and vertical petrous carotid artery. Type B dissection explores the petrous apex, clivus, and superior ITF. The type C approach permits exposure of the nasopharynx, rostral clivus, parasellar area, PPF, and anterosuperior ITF.[28] The preauricular approaches described by Sekhar expose the same anatomic regions accessed by the postauricular type B and C approaches from a pure lateral vector rather than an anteromedial vector. All the ITF approaches have been well described in the literature and are useful for extracranial lesions with or without intracranial extension. However, extensive soft tissue dissection and removal of bone result in complications that include masticatory difficulties, dental malocclusion, trigeminal nerve deficits, facial dysfunction, cosmetic deformities, conductive hearing loss, and potential intracranial complications such as seizures with extended temporal lobe retraction. Combined endoscopic transmaxillary-transantral approaches to the pterygoid region, lateral sphenoid sinus, and orbital apex have been reported, extolling the benefits of enhanced surgeon comfort and instrument maneuverability.[26] However, these approaches still risk the complications inherent in the open approaches.

Endoscopic Anatomy, Approach, and Technique

The endoscopic surgical approach to the PPF and ITF is influenced by the pathology being addressed. A tissue biopsy of a well-circumscribed schwannoma in the PPF requires a different set of surgical steps compared to the resection of a JNA that invades the PPF and ITF. For the purposes of describing the complex bony, vascular, and neural relationships of this region, a normal PPF and ITF will be assumed. This will be followed by a brief discussion of surgical modifications required with different pathologies.

Nasal Preparation

The nasal cavity is decongested with 4% cocaine-soaked pledgets placed in the middle meatus and floor of the nasal cavity. The pledgets are kept in place for 10 minutes or less to decrease absorption and avoid any risk of cardiac toxicity. The patient is routinely given cefazolin (2 g IV), dexamethasone (10 mg IV), and diphenhydramine (50 mg IV).[30] The two latter drugs are given as premedication for administration of intrathecal fluorescein to decrease the risk of seizures. A Foley catheter and an arterial line are placed for fluid monitoring. A lumbar puncture is performed and 0.25 mL (25 mg) of 10% fluorescein (AK-Fluor; Akron, IL) is mixed with 10 mL of withdrawn cerebrospinal fluid (CSF) and injected back slowly intrathecally. Although this agent is not U.S. Food and Drug Administration (FDA) approved for use intrathecally, we have published on its safety and use in detecting small CSF leaks during the operation.[31] Intrathecal fluorescein may also be used to stratify and direct the complexity of skull base closure.[32] The patient's head is placed in a horseshoe, elevated above the heart, slightly extended, and turned to the right (15 degrees). The headset for neuronavigation is placed and the patient is registered with the preoperative CT or MRI. Neuronavigation is routinely used throughout the procedure for surgical planning, confirmation of critical neurovascular structures, and determining the limits of dissection.

Using a rigid 0-degree endoscope, the sphenopalatine foramen is located and infiltrated with 1% lidocaine with 1:100,000 epinephrine to vasoconstrict the terminal branches of the sphenopalatine artery. This maneuver significantly reduces intraoperative bleeding.[8] The uncinate process, root, and anterior face of the middle turbinate and bilateral mucoperichondrial septal flaps are also infiltrated with local anesthesia.

Septoplasty

Although the transpterygoid approach is usually unilateral, the procedure is sometimes begun with a posterior septectomy to use the endoscope and surgical instruments through both nostrils. Removal of the posterior septum allows for a wider surgical exposure and greater maneuverability for surgical instrumentation.[1,6,10] However, a unilateral approach may be used for tissue biopsies of well-circumscribed PPF lesions, small lateral sphenoid sinus encephaloceles, or pathologies with limited involvement of the PPF. A septoplasty is performed to harvest the perpendicular plate of the ethmoid and vomeric bone to provide autologous tissue for skull base reconstruction.

Transpterygoid Approach

Although the transpterygoid approach primarily uses the transmaxillary corridor, the procedure requires a total ethmoidectomy and sphenoidotomy to widely expose the lateral nasal wall. The majority of the procedure is performed with a 0-degree endoscope. However, 30- and 45-degree endoscopes are often used to visualize and dissect the far lateral anatomic structures. The transpterygoid approach is begun with an uncinectomy, widening of the maxillary sinus ostium, a total ethmoidectomy, and a sphenoidotomy. The sphenoid sinus is entered through a transethmoidal approach, and the natural ostium is widely enlarged. This is particularly important when the transpterygoid approach, is performed to provide exposure to resect a lateral sphenoid sinus encephalocele.

Next, the maxillary sinus ostium is enlarged by removing the orbital process of the palatine bone (crista ethmoidalis) and the posteromedial wall of the maxillary sinus. This is accomplished by elevating the mucosa over the vertical palatine bone and removing the bone with a variety of instruments (Kerrison rongeurs, Grünwald forceps, drill with a diamond burr). The sphenopalatine foramen is identified, sitting between the articulation of the orbital and sphenoid processes of the palatine bone. The orbital process attaches to the orbital surface of the maxillary bone and inferior surface of the sphenoid bone. The sphenoid process articulates with the medial pterygoid plate posteriorly (**Fig. 49.10**).

Branches of the sphenopalatine artery usually include the posterior lateral nasal artery coursing superiorly and medially, and the posterior septal artery heading inferiorly and laterally toward the anterior face of the sphenoid. These branches are cauterized with bipolar forceps, ball tip cautery, or controlled with clips and sectioned. The sphenoid process of the palatine bone is then removed posteriorly, exposing the medial pterygoid plate and floor of the sphenoid sinus. The middle turbinate is preserved under most circumstances in a unilateral approach to the PPF. However, in cases that involve pathology of the lateral ITF, a binostril approach may necessitate resection of the inferior

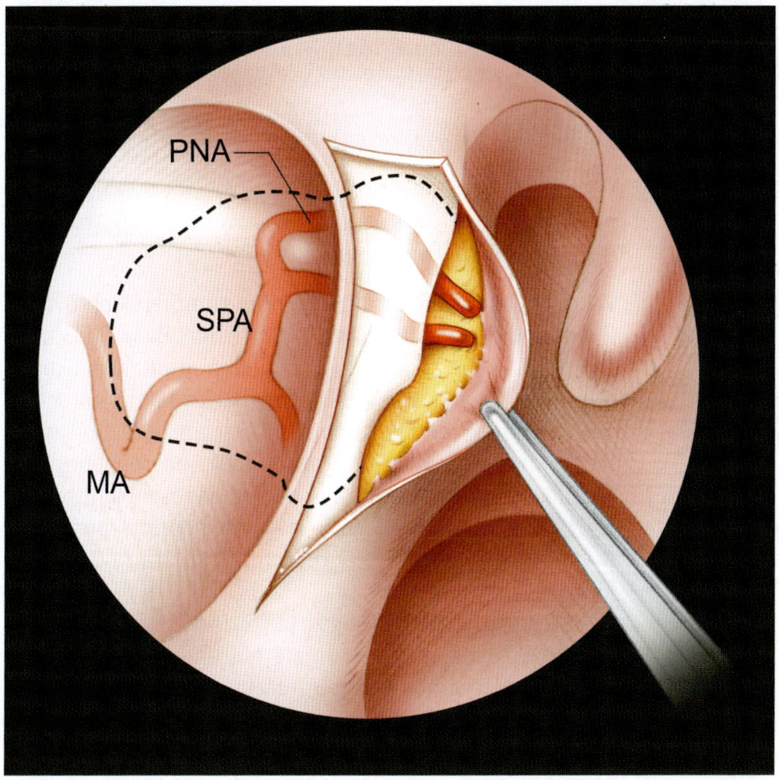

Fig. 49.10 Primary surgical steps in the approach to the pterygopalatine fossa. *SPA*, sphenopalatine artery; *PNA*, posterior nasal artery; *MA*, maxillary artery.

one-third of the middle turbinate. In extensive tumors of the nasal cavity extending to the PPF and ITF or malignant pathologies, the middle turbinate is obviously sacrificed.

Pterygopalatine Fossa Dissection

To expose the anterior face of the PPF, the posterior wall of the maxillary sinus is removed in a medial to lateral direction, superiorly to the roof, and inferiorly to the floor of the maxillary sinus. The thin fascia covering the PPF is removed, exposing the fat in the fossa. The PPF can be largely divided into an anterior and posterior compartment. The anterior compartment contains fat and blood vessels, whereas the posterior compartment contains neural elements.[8,10,16] Gentle dissection of the fat reveals the vascular anatomy of the fossa. Bipolar cauterization of small vessels is important to preserve a bloodless surgical field. Distal branches of the internal maxillary artery are often encountered before the main artery is identified. The most commonly described anatomic pattern of these vessels places the posterior superior alveolar artery and infraorbital artery proximally in the PPF, followed distally by the descending palatine, pharyngeal artery, artery of the pterygoid canal, and sphenopalatine artery.[27] This, however, does not always hold true, especially if the anatomy is distorted by the pathologic process. In addition, it is important to understand that if the approach to the pterygopalatine ganglion is from a medial to lateral direction, branches of the sphenopalatine and descending palatine are encountered before any of the other structures.

The internal maxillary artery is identified as it emerges from the lateral and inferior portion of the fossa along the anterior margin of the lateral pterygoid muscle. The posterior superior alveolar artery heads to the anterior inferior margin of the fossa to enter the maxillary bone. The infraorbital artery originates from the maxillary artery but is often seen originating from the posterior alveolar artery. This artery courses superiorly and laterally and is joined by the inferior orbital nerve to exit the inferior orbital fissure. The descending palatine artery and vidian artery often arise from the posterior portion of the maxillary artery, and therefore are not seen initially during the dissection. The descending palatine artery travels with the greater palatine nerve, and is in close association with the surface of the palatine bone. Precise identification of the maxillary artery and its branches is sometimes challenging given their tortuosity and the surrounding adipose tissue.[1,5] As a terminal branch of the internal maxillary artery, the sphenopalatine artery can often be followed retrograde into the fossa to help identify other branches. This retrograde approach is sometimes difficult if the artery courses through the tumor (**Fig. 49.11**).

Deep to the vascular structures lies the neural structures of the PPF. The maxillary nerve is seen at the superior margin of the fossa traveling laterally and superiorly toward the inferior orbital fissure. When traced posteriorly, this nerve can be used to identify the foramen rotundum. Minor nerve branches from the maxillary nerve can be identified traveling inferiorly to the PPF ganglion. The terminal branch of the maxillary nerve is the infraorbital

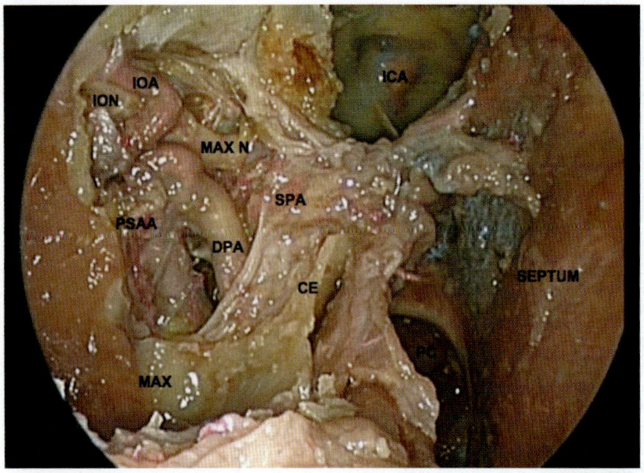

Fig. 49.11 Vascular anatomy of the pterygopalatine fossa and infratemporal fossa. *MAX*, maxilla; *CE*, crista ethmoidalis; *SPA*, sphenopalatine artery; *DPA*, descending palatine artery; *PSAA*, posterior superficial alveolar artery; *IOA/ION*, infraorbital artery and nerve; *ICA*, internal carotid artery.

nerve, which divides the PPF from the ITF. The vidian nerve is usually identified inferior and medial to the maxillary nerve and is formed by the parasympathetic fibers of facial nerve (greater petrosal nerve) and sympathetic fibers (deep petrosal nerve) of the superior cervical ganglion. The vidian nerve passes through the middle cranial fossa and foramen lacerum, enters the PPF through the pterygoid canal, and ends at the pterygopalatine ganglion. The triangular-shaped pterygopalatine ganglion lies anterior to the pterygoid canal, superior to the greater palatine foramen, and posterior to the branches of the sphenopalatine vessels. The principal branches of the ganglion include the vidian nerve superomedially, the maxillary nerve superolaterally, and the greater and lesser palatine nerves inferiorly.[6,10] Other neural branches include the sphenopalatine and pharyngeal branches coming from the medial surface of the pterygopalatine ganglion, and the orbital branch originating from its superior surface.[27]

The vidian nerve deserves additional discussion, particularly because of its relationship with the anterior genu of the ICA. In a radiologic study of 44 triplanar CT scans, the carotid artery was consistently found superior and medial to the vidian canal. Given this anatomic relationship, safe identification of the carotid artery is done and inadvertent injury is avoided by initially drilling on the inferior medial and lateral surfaces of the vidian canal. Also, in a majority of cases, the vidian canal runs in a medial-to-lateral direction when drilling in a superior-to-inferior direction. This anatomic relationship can aid in identifying the nerve during the transpterygoid approach. The mean length of the vidian canal in this study was 18 mm, the average distance from the origin of the medial pterygoid plate to the vidian canal was 9.3 mm, and the mean distance from the vidian canal to foramen rotundum was 5.5 mm. In addition, the vidian canal was found to lie medial to the medial pterygoid plate in majority of cases. These anatomic relationships are critical for not only identifying the vidian nerve, but also providing a road map for the skull base surgeon. A simple method to identify the vidian nerve is to explore the junction of the medial pterygoid plate with the floor of the sphenoid sinus (**Fig. 49.12**).[7]

Infratemporal Fossa Dissection

Wide exposure of the ITF requires complete removal of the posterior and lateral walls of the maxillary sinus from the floor to the roof of the maxillary sinus. This usually thin bone is removed from a medial-to-lateral direction with a variety of instruments. These include the endoscopic drill with diamond burrs, Kerrison rongeurs, and extended-length straight and angled endoscopic through-cutting instruments. Occasionally, the superior portion of the inferior turbinate is also removed to improve the exposure.

Tracing the maxillary nerve posteriorly from the PPF reveals the orbital apex superolaterally and lateral sphenoid sinus superomedially. The infraorbital fissure and maxillary nerve are important anatomic landmarks that separate the PPF (medial) from the ITF (lateral). Removal of bone around the maxillary nerve and floor of the sphenoid sinus provides access to the space that lies between the lateral wall of the sphenoid sinus and medial wall of the middle cranial fossa. Progressive removal of bone contributing to the floor and lateral wall of the sphenoid sinus initially exposes the floor of the middle cranial fossa, and with a deeper dissection, the cavernous sinus and carotid artery. Drilling away bone with a diamond burr to identify the maxillary and vidian nerves aids in the identification of these deeper structures. As mentioned previously, drilling around the inferior half of the vidian nerve before the superior portion helps to establish the depth and location

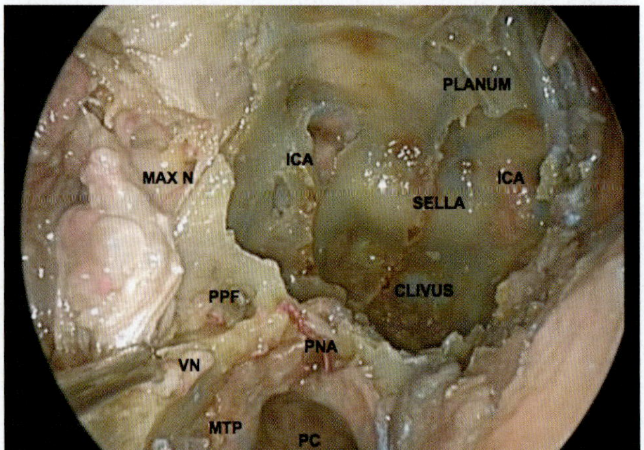

Fig. 49.12 Anatomy of the vidian nerve (*VN*) in relationship to the pterygopalatine fossa and internal carotid artery. *PC*, posterior choanae; *MTP*, medial pterygoid plate; *MAX N*, maxillary nerve; *PNA*, posterior nasal artery.

of the carotid artery.[7] Tumors from the PPF and ITF can spread around the infraorbital fissure, above and below the maxillary nerve, and then further posteriorly to the cavernous sinus and carotid artery.[8]

Removal of bone along the lateral wall of the sphenoid sinus exposes the pterygoid plates of the sphenoid bone. Removal of these plates to the maxillary nerve reveals the upper head of the lateral pterygoid muscle that lies in the superior part of the ITF under the floor of the middle cranial fossa. Medial to this muscle but lateral and anterior to the carotid artery lies the mandibular branch of the trigeminal nerve exiting the foramen ovale (**Fig. 49.13**). Superior to the foramen ovale lies the cavernous sinus, which in turn lies inferior to the orbital apex, which transmits the optic nerve to the chiasm. Lateral removal of bone around the middle temporal fossa reveals the middle fossa and cavernous sinus dura. The presence of multiple thin-walled venous plexi in this region can make dissection particularly tedious in this region.

Surgical Modification for Specific Pathologies

Although our philosophy to the PPF and ITF involves a graded medial-to-lateral endoscopic endonasal approach, other directed approaches have been described in the literature. These include the medial transpalatine approach for exposure of the medial PPF, the middle meatal transantral approach for a more lateral exposure of the PPF where the infraorbital nerve is the first landmark to be identified, and the inferior turbinectomy transantral approach, which provides the widest exposure to the PPF and ITF.[1] Techniques to improve exposure and the reach of instruments laterally include a canine fossa puncture and a staggered septal window. The canine trephine can be used as an additional port for the endoscope or dissecting instruments to address pathology of the maxillary sinus, PPF, or ITF. Similarly, a staggered transseptal window can serve the same purpose for lesions that involve the anterior maxillary wall or extend laterally into the ITF.[8,14]

The most common pathologies that require endoscopic approaches to the PPF and ITF include IPs and JNAs. Small IPs and JNAs originating from the nasal cavity with minimal extension into the PPF can be easily addressed by a simple endoscopic resection. This often requires removing the intranasal component of the tumor and then addressing the extension. An IP involving the lateral nasal wall requires an endoscopic medial maxillectomy. In addition, given their tendency to invaginate into bone, it is crucial that bone at the site of origin be drilled with a diamond burr to prevent recurrence.[9,13,21] Large JNAs and most smaller JNAs require preoperative embolization within 24 hours of surgery to reduce their vascularity. The two-surgeon approach, use of

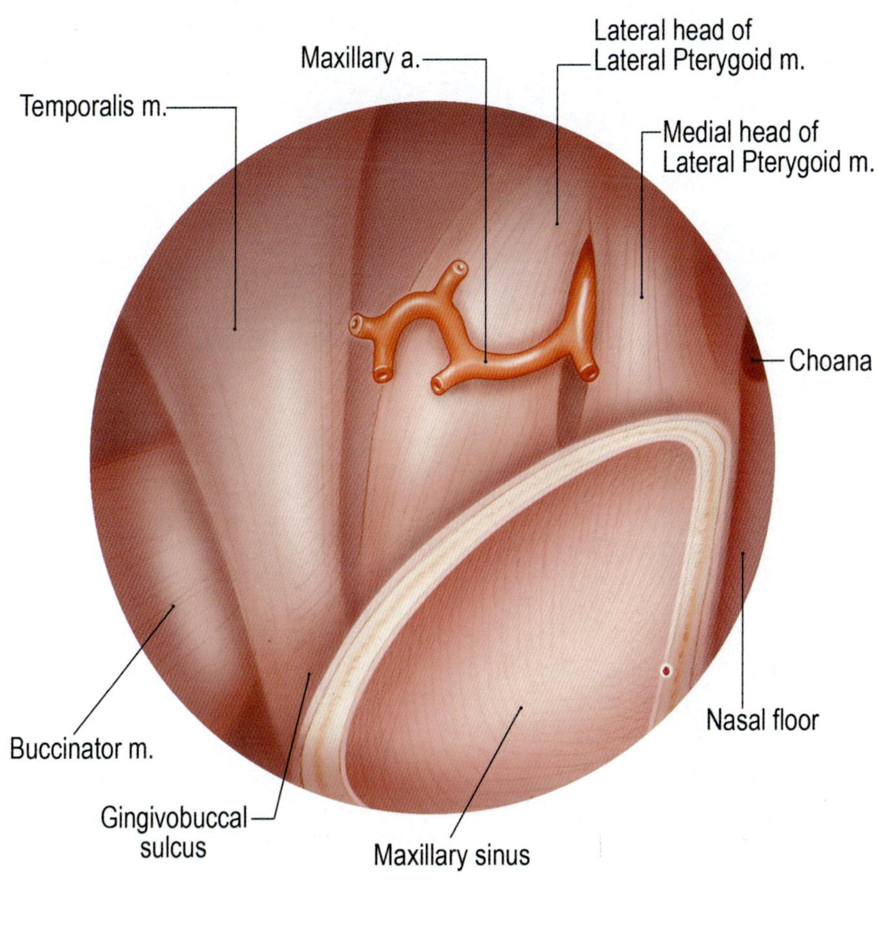

Fig. 49.13 Infratemporal fossa.

high volume suction, and traction techniques are useful for JNAs that extend around the infraorbital nerve far lateral into the ITF.[8] Finally, for exposure and resection of a lateral sphenoid sinus encephalocele, a complete dissection of the PPF is often unnecessary. Enlargement of the maxillary sinus, elimination of its posteromedial wall, removal of the vertical palatine bone, and drilling down of the medial pterygoid plate is usually all that is required (**Fig. 49.14**).[11,15]

On a cautionary note, although the endoscopes provide unsurpassed views of the surgical field, the diffuse presence of fat, anatomic rearrangement secondary to inflammatory or neoplastic processes, and engorged venous plexus may complicate the correct identification of structures during surgery. This is especially true in the ITF where the expansion of tumors pushes muscles and vessels away, and makes the vasculature difficult to identify and control. The endoscopic surgical team seeking to gain experience in this area should begin with lesions that are medial and inferior to critical neurovascular structures prior to embarking on more lateral approaches into the ITF. Finally, a solid knowledge of the anatomy, including anatomic variations, is necessary to successfully address the intraoperative and postoperative challenges encountered with these approaches.

Endoscopic Skull Base Reconstruction

Skull base reconstruction is individualized for patients based on the pathology, extent of dissection, location, and presence or absence of an intraoperative CSF leak. Transpterygoid approaches for PPF or ITF pathology may result in large, laterally placed defects that may be challenging to access and reconstruct. This is particularly true

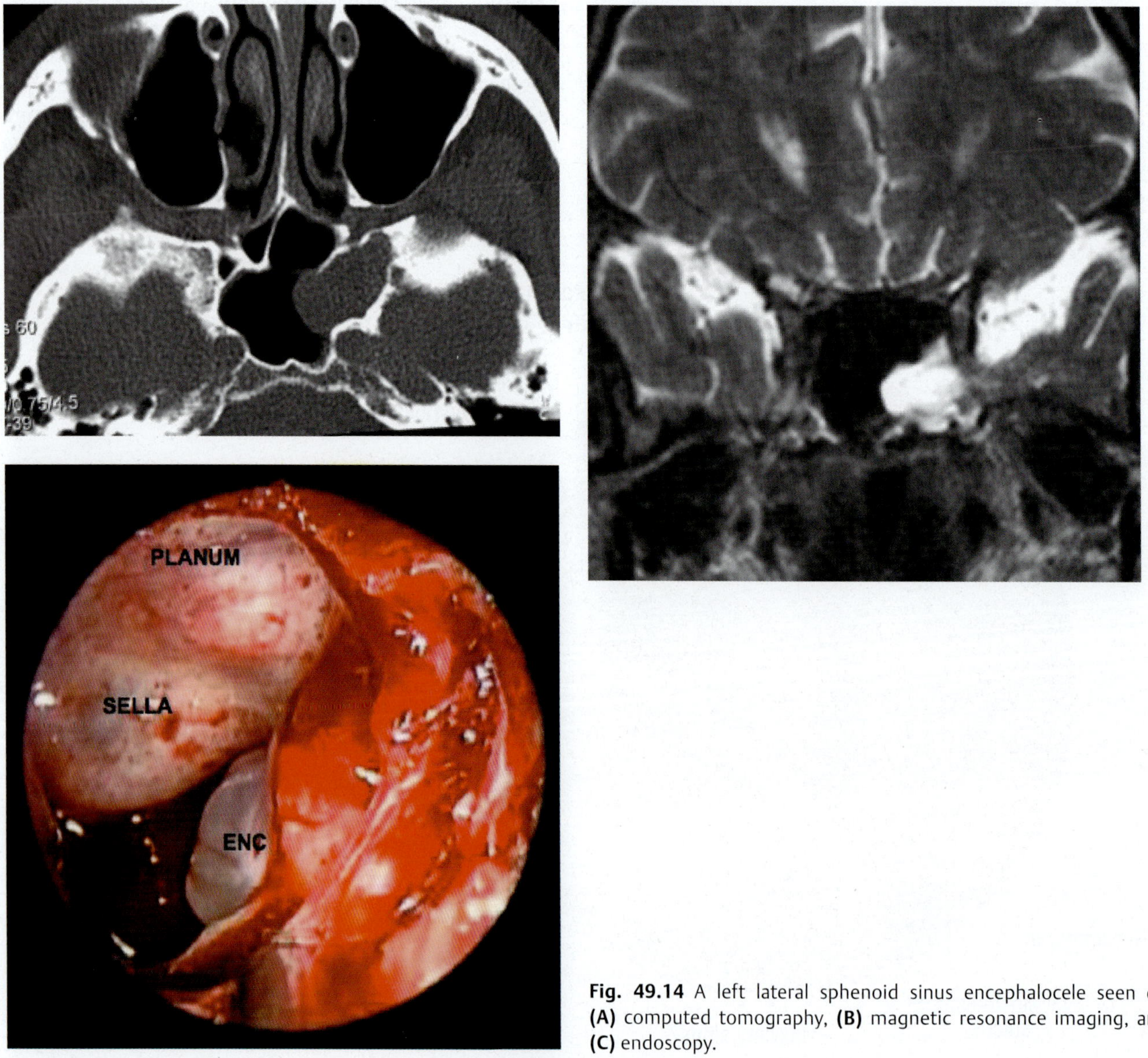

A B C

Fig. 49.14 A left lateral sphenoid sinus encephalocele seen on **(A)** computed tomography, **(B)** magnetic resonance imaging, and **(C)** endoscopy.

after resecting encephaloceles of the middle cranial fossa using a transpterygoid approach. Akin to midline skull base defects, endoscopic closure of transpterygoid defects with multilayered free tissue grafts represents the mainstay of reconstruction. In general, given the lack of extensive intradural dissection for transpterygoid approaches, the postoperative rate of CSF leaks is lower than midline approaches.

Our approach usually involves a multilayered closure based on the size, volume, and location of the CSF leak. Small defects with a small CSF leak and favorable patient factors may be closed with a small amount of Gelfoam or autologous fat, followed by a rigid buttress (quadrangular cartilage, vomer, ethmoidal plate, titanium miniplate, or synthetic graft), and overlayed with a tissue sealant (Tisseel, Baxter Healthcare Corp., Deerfield, IL; or DuraSeal, Confluent Surgical Inc., Waltham, MA) (**Fig. 49.15**). Larger defects require fat, an inlay fascial graft (fascia lata or temporalis fascia), a rigid buttress, and a tissue sealant. A rigid buttress is particularly important for reconstruction after resection of a Sternberg canal encephalocele. Occasionally, an additional onlay graft (fascia, dural substitute, or mucosa) is necessary for an additional layer of security in a large defect with high-flow CSF leak and unfavorable patient factors.[11,32] Other reconstructive materials may be used such as a collagen matrix or acellular dermal graft as underlay or onlay grafts. The authors have recently described a technique for closure called the "gasket seal," in which a fascia lata onlay graft is countersunk into the cavity with the use of a rigid buttress to achieve a watertight closure.[33] Finally, although long segments of carotid artery exposure are rare, the exposed carotid can be covered with fat or acellular dermis bolstered with tissue glue or sealant. Another option is the nasoseptal flap, a vascularized mucosal flap pedicled on the posterior nasal artery that can be harvested at the beginning of a case and then immobilized.[34] This is particularly useful for patients who have previously had or who require radiation therapy. Balloon stents may be used to bolster the reconstruction, especially if circumferential margins are not available for retention of the skull base reconstruction.

Surgical adjuncts such as a lumbar drain, fluorescein, and image guidance are often important for performing a reliable skull base reconstruction. Lumbar drainage is used in cases of a high-volume preoperative CSF leak, extended skull base defects, large body habitus, concern regarding the closure, or for a small persistent leak after skull base reconstruction. Although some authors recommend avoiding lumbar drainage for fear of pneumocephalus, we have not found this to be a problem as long as a good multilayer closure is performed and limited drainage is used (5 mL per hour). Fluorescein is a bright yellow compound that stains CSF and may be used to identify subtle CSF leaks in the presence of blood and mucus. A lumbar tap is performed and 10 mL of CSF is withdrawn, mixed with 25 mg of injectable fluorescein (0.25 mL of 10% solution), and reintroduced into the intrathecal space. The patient is premedicated with 10 mg of intravenous dexamethasone and 50 mg of intravenous diphenhydramine to reduce the risk of seizures, meningismus, and radicular symptoms. The risk of intrathecal fluorescein is dose dependent, and its safety has been well established in a series of patients.[31] Introduction and refinement of CT, MRI, and CT-MRI fusion image guidance is beneficial not only for tumor extirpation, but also skull base reconstruction, particularly in cases of previous skull base surgery or trauma.

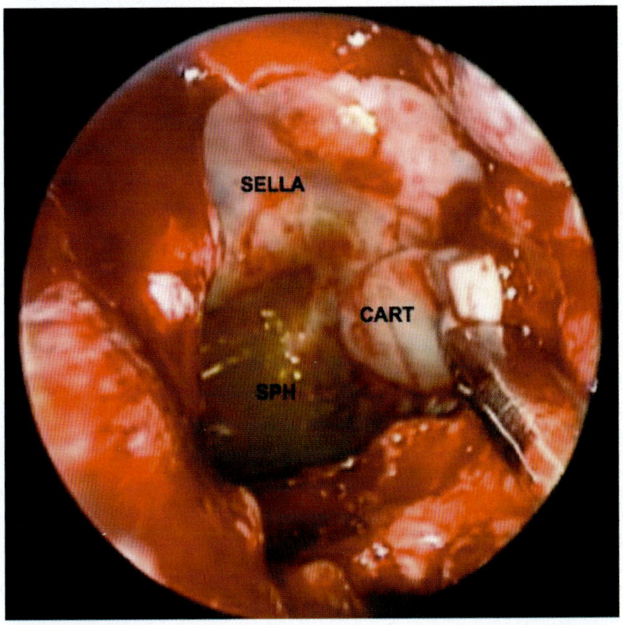

Fig. 49.15 Reconstruction of skull base defect with cartilage (*CART*) in the sphenoid (*SPH*).

Complications

Complications of endoscopic approaches to the PPF and ITF are similar to those encountered in open skull base approaches. These include bleeding, infections, orbital injury, cerebral injury, CSF leaks, tension pneumocephalus, and stroke. Injury to vascular structures, such as branches of the internal maxillary artery, are usually easily controlled without any morbidity. Damage to the internal maxillary artery or carotid artery are devastating vascular injuries that can result in significant morbidity or mortality. Complications can vary from minor (anemia, hypotension, and necrosis) to major (stroke and death). Bleeding from the pterygoid plexus or cavernous sinus can usually be controlled with pressure and hemostatic agents without incident. Injury to the maxillary nerve, mandibular nerve, vidian nerve, or rami from the pterygopalatine ganglion may result in hypesthesia, pain secondary to neuromas, decreased lacrimation, keratoconjunctivitis, and a variety of nasal complaints from loss of parasympathetic tone. Extensive lesions involving the sella or suprasellar region may result in endocrine dysfunction as seen after resection of pituitary adenomas. Minor nasal complications include sinusitis, crusting, and synechiae.

Given the high density of vascular structures in the PPF and ITF, perioperative bleeding presents one of the complications for endoscopic surgery in this region. The internal maxillary artery, ICA, smaller caliber arterial vasculature, as well as a multitude of venous plexi can contribute to significant perioperative bleeding. Several hemostatic strategies have been developed to counteract this difficulty during an endoscopic dissection. Minor bleeding from the venous plexus and small caliber vessels is easily controlled with Gelfoam soaked in thrombin and epinephrine applied to the bleeding area. This is often followed with a pledget placed over the Gelfoam to suction the excess blood and fluid. The Gelfoam is often left in place to continue to provide hemostasis as long as it does not compromise the surgical view. FloSeal, a hemostatic agent (Baxter Healthcare Corp.), may also be used for minor-to-moderate bleeding. More brisk arterial bleeding can often be controlled with ball tip cautery or endoscopic hand grip bipolar cautery if it lies in the vicinity of dura or brain. If the cut lumen of an arterial bleeder can be clearly identified, it may also be clipped. Severe arterial hemorrhage in cases of internal carotid or internal maxillary artery injury are best prevented by careful evaluation of all preoperative imaging, judicious use of image guidance technology, and recognizable and established endoscopic landmarks. Injury to a major vessel, such as the carotid artery, requires immediate control of the hemorrhage with packing material as well as placement of an intranasal Foley catheter to temporalize the bleeding. Angiography and embolization of the vessel is usually considered the safest and most expeditious method of controlling the bleeding. If no arterial defect is discovered, repeat angiography should be performed in 1 to 2 weeks to rule out a pseudoaneurysm.

CSF leaks may be encountered early or late in the postoperative period. Transpterygoid approaches to the PPF and ITF may be used for lesions abutting the dura of the medial wall of the middle temporal fossa. Lateral sphenoid sinus encephaloceles may present with a CSF leak, necessitating a transpterygoid approach to address this pathology. Postoperative CSF leaks may be the result of a multitude of factors. These include reconstruction failures, which include inadequate closure of a CSF leak, graft displacement, or inadequate recognition of a CSF leak. Patient factors such as hydrocephalus or obesity, as well as the nature of the surgical defect may also contribute to a higher leak rate.[32] The lateral or oblique orientation of some of these defects, as opposed to midline defects, may also pose reconstruction challenges for the surgeon. For low volume CSF leaks, conservative measures may be initiated such as bed rest, head of bed elevation, stool softeners, and/or lumbar drain. If these measures fail after a period, the wound must be reexplored. Our experience suggests that the majority of low-volume leaks will resolve with conservative measures. Other authors report that these leaks rarely resolve with conservative measures and must be reexplored immediately.[35] The etiology of these leaks frequently involve graft displacement or migration. Closure of leaks may involve minor revision with autologous grafts such as fat, fascia lata, or polymers such as Medpor and, very rarely, titanium plates.

Postoperative Care

Postoperative care for patients is appropriately tailored based on the pathology, extent of the approach, dural involvement, reconstructive strategy, and lumbar drain use. Postoperative care begins in the operating room with an understanding with our anesthesiology colleagues on the importance of a deep extubation to preserve the integrity of the skull base reconstruction and prevent CSF leaks and any increase in pneumocephalus. Dural or intracranial dissection with use of a lumbar drain necessitates monitoring in the intensive care unit (ICU) with frequent neurologic checks, lumbar drain monitoring, and close observation for CSF leaks. The nature of the reconstruction and packing also dictates postoperative management. In most cases, our skull base reconstruction does not require any specific postoperative care. Our nasal dressing consists of FloSeal for hemostasis and Telfa packs to wick minor bleeding.

Routine monitoring for CSF leaks in transpterygoid approaches is performed postoperatively. This includes sitting the patient up and leaning his or her torso forward for a few minutes to elicit any clear or serosanguinous rhinorrhea. In subtle cases, the patient is asked to perform a gentle Valsalva maneuver. In the event that rhinorrhea is elicited or the patient complains of continuous rhinorrhea or a salty taste in his or her mouth, this fluid is collected and evaluated for CSF-specific biochemical markers, such as beta-2-transferrin (most common), prostaglandin-D-synthase, and transthyretin. Diagnosis of a subtle CSF leak is sometimes difficult given the anticipated drainage of blood and breakdown products used for skull base reconstruction. In our experience, the majority of postoperative CSF fistulas are diagnosed clinically without waiting for biochemical confirmation.[2]

Diagnosis of a CSF leak mandates a nonenhanced CT scan to evaluate the possibility of clinically significant pneumocephalus. Expanding pneumocephalus or worsening neurologic status mandates an immediate endoscopic or open exploration to correct the pneumocephalus and seal the defect. Anticipated or minimal pneumocephalus may be managed with conservative measures such as a trial of bed rest, head of bed elevation, stool softeners, and lumbar drainage. Lumbar drainage is routinely used in cases of a preoperative CSF leak, extended skull base defects, patient large body habitus, concern regarding the closure, or for a small persistent leak after skull base reconstruction. If a lumbar drain is used, monitoring in the intensive care unit or step-down unit is necessary to monitor for pneumocephalus because continuous CSF drainage can promote a pressure gradient that can produce increasing pneumocephalus through a fistula.

Disorders of the hypothalamic-pituitary-adrenal axis with approaches to the PPF and ITF are rare. However, extensive skull base lesions that involve the sellar and suprasellar region, cavernous sinus, orbital apex, PPF, and ITF may cause hypopituitarism. This is managed with postoperative serum sodium and osmolality, urine sodium, and specific gravity, as well as cortisol levels. Perioperative antibiotics are continued for 24 hours after the surgical procedure and discontinued. Nasal Telfa pads are typically removed on the first or second postoperative day and an MRI is performed to assess the surgical bed, extent of tumor resection, integrity of skull base reconstruction, and clinically significant pneumocephalus. The patient is discharged after ensuring the absence of a CSF leak, a normal hypothalamic-pituitary-adrenal axis and electrolyte status, resolution of postoperative pain, and a normal neurologic exam.

Patients are typically followed by the rhinologist 1 week, 4 weeks, and 3 months after discharge from the hospital. At the first postoperative visit, gentle debridement of old blood, crusting, and breakdown products of FloSeal and DuraSeal is performed. In addition, patients are placed on gentamicin nasal spray three times a day to provide nasal hygiene and improve nasal ciliary function. Patients are instructed to refrain from nose blowing and to avoid strenuous activity for 10 to 14 days. Patients are evaluated for clinically significant rhinosinusitis and placed on antibiotics if necessary. At the 4-four week visit, the patient undergoes additional debridement of crusting and gentle lysis of synechiae if present. Some patients suffer from long-term crusting due to incomplete mucociliary clearance. This is treated with repeated debridements and nasal irrigations. Careful examination of the skull base reconstruction is also performed, and any signs or symptoms of meningismus are elicited. Any complaint of unilateral rhinorrhea must be evaluated for CSF rhinorrhea, as previously described. The 3-month visit usually entails endoscopic evaluation of the nasal cavity, skull base reconstruction, lysis of synechiae, and careful evaluation of the postoperative MRI.

Conclusion

The transpterygoid approach through the transmaxillary corridor is the primary endoscopic approach to the PPF and ITF. The anatomic complexity of these regions represents a challenge for the endoscopic surgeon addressing pathology in these areas. A solid knowledge of the anatomy and variations is critical for successful surgical management. Advances in endoscopic technology, instrumentation, and anatomic knowledge have enabled surgeons to achieve successful outcomes for diseases of the pterygopalatine and infratemporal fossae.

References

1. Alfieri A, Jho HD, Schettino R, Tschabitscher M. Endoscopic endonasal approach to the pterygopalatine fossa: anatomic study. Neurosurgery 2003;52(2):374–378, discussion 378–380
2. Anand VK, Schwartz TH. Practical Endoscopic Skull Base Surgery. San Diego, CA: Plural Publishing; 2007
3. Cavallo LM, Messina A, Gardner P, et al. Extended endoscopic endonasal approach to the pterygopalatine fossa: anatomical study and clinical considerations. Neurosurg Focus 2005;19(1):E5
4. Janfaza P. Surgical Anatomy of the Head and Neck. Philadelphia, PA: Lippincott Williams & Wilkins; 2001
5. Morton AL, Khan A. Internal maxillary artery variability in the pterygopalatine fossa. Otolaryngol Head Neck Surg 1991; 104(2):204–209
6. Solari D, Magro F, Cappabianca P, et al. Anatomical study of the pterygopalatine fossa using an endoscopic endonasal approach: spatial relations and distances between surgical landmarks. J Neurosurg 2007;106(1):157–163
7. Vescan AD, Snyderman CH, Carrau RL, et al. Vidian canal: analysis and relationship to the internal carotid artery. Laryngoscope 2007;117(8):1338–1342
8. Wormald PJ. Endoscopic Sinus Surgery: Anatomy, Three-Dimensional Reconstruction, and Surgical Technique. 2nd ed. New York: Thieme; 2008
9. Batra PS, Citardi MJ. Endoscopic management of sinonasal malignancy. Otolaryngol Clin North Am 2006;39(3):619–637, x–xi
10. DelGaudio JM. Endoscopic transnasal approach to the pterygopalatine fossa. Arch Otolaryngol Head Neck Surg 2003;129(4): 441–446
11. Hofstetter CP, Singh A, Anand VK, Kacker A, Schwartz TH. The endoscopic, endonasal, transmaxillary transpterygoid approach to the pterygopalatine fossa, infratemporal fossa, petrous apex, and the Meckel cave. J Neurosurg 2010;113(5):967–974
12. Kassam AB, Gardner P, Snyderman C, Mintz A, Carrau R. Expanded endonasal approach: fully endoscopic, completely transnasal approach to the middle third of the clivus, petrous bone, middle cranial fossa, and infratemporal fossa. Neurosurg Focus 2005;19(1):E6
13. Melroy CT, Senior BA. Benign sinonasal neoplasms: a focus on inverting papilloma. Otolaryngol Clin North Am 2006;39(3): 601–617, x
14. Robinson S, Patel N, Wormald PJ. Endoscopic management of benign tumors extending into the infratemporal fossa: a two-surgeon transnasal approach. Laryngoscope 2005;115(10):1818–1822
15. Schwartz TH, Fraser JF, Brown S, Tabaee A, Kacker A, Anand VK. Endoscopic cranial base surgery: classification of operative approaches. Neurosurgery 2008;62(5):991–1002, discussion 1002–1005
16. Fortes FS, Sennes LU, Carrau RL, et al. Endoscopic anatomy of the pterygopalatine fossa and the transpterygoid approach: development of a surgical instruction model. Laryngoscope 2008;118(1):44–49
17. Abdelkader M, Leong SC, White PS. Endoscopic control of the sphenopalatine artery for epistaxis: long-term results. J Laryngol Otol 2007;121(8):759–762
18. Douglas R, Wormald PJ. Endoscopic surgery for juvenile nasopharyngeal angiofibroma: where are the limits? Curr Opin Otolaryngol Head Neck Surg 2006;14(1):1–5

19. Nicolai P, Battaglia P, Bignami M, et al. Endoscopic surgery for malignant tumors of the sinonasal tract and adjacent skull base: a 10-year experience. Am J Rhinol 2008;22(3):308–316
20. Wormald P-J, Wee DT, van Hasselt CA. Endoscopic ligation of the sphenopalatine artery for refractory posterior epistaxis. Am J Rhinol 2000;14(4):261–264
21. Schlosser RJ, Mason JC, Gross CW. Aggressive endoscopic resection of inverted papilloma: an update. Otolaryngol Head Neck Surg 2001;125(1):49–53
22. McCutcheon IE, Blacklock JB, Weber RS, et al. Anterior transcranial (craniofacial) resection of tumors of the paranasal sinuses: surgical technique and results. Neurosurgery 1996;38(3): 471–479, discussion 479–480
23. Steiner W, Vogt P, Ambrosch P, Kron M. Transoral carbon dioxide laser microsurgery for recurrent glottic carcinoma after radiotherapy. Head Neck 2004;26(6):477–484
24. Patel SG, Singh B, Polluri A, et al. Craniofacial surgery for malignant skull base tumors: report of an international collaborative study. Cancer 2003;98(6):1179–1187
25. Tabaee A, Nyquist GG, Anand VK, Singh A, Kacker A, Schwartz TH. Palliative endoscopic surgery in advanced sinonasal and anterior skull base neoplasms. Otolaryngol Head Neck Surg 2010;142(1):126–128
26. Har-El G. Combined endoscopic transmaxillary-transnasal approach to the pterygoid region, lateral sphenoid sinus, and retrobulbar orbit. Ann Otol Rhinol Laryngol 2005;114(6):439–442
27. Roberti F, Boari N, Mortini P, Caputy AJ. The pterygopalatine fossa: an anatomic report. J Craniofac Surg 2007;18(3):586–590
28. Fisch U, Fagan P, Valavanis A. The infratemporal fossa approach for the lateral skull base. Otolaryngol Clin North Am 1984;17(3):513–552
29. Janecka IP. Classification of facial translocation approach to the skull base. Otolaryngol Head Neck Surg 1995;112(4):579–585
30. Brown SM, Anand VK, Tabaee A, Schwartz TH. Role of perioperative antibiotics in endoscopic skull base surgery. Laryngoscope 2007;117(9):1528–1532
31. Placantonakis DG, Tabaee A, Anand VK, Hiltzik D, Schwartz TH. Safety of low-dose intrathecal fluorescein in endoscopic cranial base surgery. Neurosurgery 2007; 61(3, Suppl)161–165, discussion 165–166
32. Tabaee A, Anand VK, Brown SM, Lin JW, Schwartz TH. Algorithm for reconstruction after endoscopic pituitary and skull base surgery. Laryngoscope 2007;117(7):1133–1137
33. Leng LZ, Brown S, Anand VK, Schwartz TH. "Gasket-seal" watertight closure in minimal-access endoscopic cranial base surgery. Neurosurgery 2008; 62(5, Suppl 2)E342–E343, discussion E343
34. Hadad G, Bassagasteguy L, Carrau RL, et al. A novel reconstructive technique after endoscopic expanded endonasal approaches: vascular pedicle nasoseptal flap. Laryngoscope 2006;116(10):1882–1886
35. Kassam A, Carrau RL, Snyderman CH, Gardner P, Mintz A. Evolution of reconstructive techniques following endoscopic expanded endonasal approaches. Neurosurg Focus 2005;19(1):E8

50 Transnasal Endoscopic Approach to the Craniocervical Junction

Jayakar V. Nayak and Stefan A. Mindea

Midline lesions of the craniocervical junction are rare pathologic entities that can cause significant neurologic compromise by way of secondary brainstem and spinal cord compression. The standard avenue for achieving brainstem decompression in these challenging patients is through either a transoral or, more rarely, a lateral cervical approach, both of which have been well described elsewhere.[1,2] Despite its use, the transoral approach has been associated with varying challenges, including the ease of surgical exposure, wound healing difficulties, postoperative pain, dental trauma, soft palate edema, and airway compromise. In light of these concerns, interest in an endonasal approach to the upper cervical spine, in which the surgeon can capitalize on the natural anatomic surgical corridors conferred by the nasal cavity, has flourished in recent years. Coupled with advances in endoscopic technology and instrumentation, and burgeoning collaborative efforts between neurosurgery and otorhinolaryngology–head and neck surgery, the transnasal endoscopic approach has now gained considerable traction as an acceptable alternative method to decompressing the spinal cord at the craniocervical junction.[3]

This chapter covers three principal topics: (1) preoperative considerations to guide judicious patient selection; (2) operative technique and technical nuances to the procedure based on our experience; and (3) complication avoidance and management. We also discuss the limited outcomes data that exist for this procedure.

Pathophysiology

The most common cause of extradural pathology in this location is pannus formation from rheumatoid arthritis, which promotes myxoid tissue deposition into, and displacement of, the atlantoaxial joint space.[4] Other entities that arise at this site include other benign processes such as degenerative fibroconnective tissue disease (also termed degenerative pseudotumor) (**Fig. 50.1A**); infection/osteomyelitis of the foramen magnum and anterior cervical skull base (**Fig. 50.1B**); and benign neoplasms such as meningioma. Unfortunately, malignant disease at this site can also manifest, including chordoma or distant metastasis to the C1/C2 vertebral bodies (**Fig. 50.1C**). Each of these diverse processes shares the common property of creating a nonreducible lesion of osteitic and/or devitalized bone admixed with soft tissue that creates spinal cord compression with progressive neurologic decline.

Clinical Presentation

Patients with anterior spinal cord compression or basilar invagination at the craniocervical junction may demonstrate signs of progressive myelopathy and upper motor neuron disease and may present with symptoms of motor incoordination, imbalance, dysarthria, dysphagia, and neck pain despite stabilizing cervical collars. Because of concurrent spinal degenerative joint disease, complex neurologic findings may exist, often prompting the appropriate referrals to colleagues in neurology, pain medicine, physiatry, and psychiatry for selected patients. In severe cases of medulla and upper cord compression, patients may develop respiratory decline. On the other hand, patients do not complain of new nasal obstruction, sinusitis, or postnasal discharge.

The physical exam in this setting is often challenging because patients frequently present in a debilitated state with ongoing weight loss from poor nutritional intake. Patients may also be emotionally taxed, in part from the progressive loss of personal independence. Objective neurologic findings include upper and lower limb paresis, gait ataxia, and lower cranial nerve palsies affecting both speech and swallowing control. Nasal endoscopy does not typically reveal any regional asymmetries to the region of the posterior nasopharynx, eustachian tubes, or posterior oropharynx. If severe septal deviation or turbinate hypertrophy is noted, the patient should be counseled about the possibility of septoplasty or turbinate outfracture for unobstructed access through the nares at the time of transnasal skull base surgery.

After appropriate diagnostic workup (see next section), indications for surgery in this setting include a definitive tissue biopsy and resection of devitalized tissue and, more importantly, mechanical decompression of the brainstem and cervical spinal cord.[4,5]

Diagnostic Workup

Imaging and Planning for Navigation

The use of both magnetic resonance imaging (MRI) and computed tomography (CT) is the most critical diagnostic element in the preoperative assessment of craniocervical junction pathology. Many patients present to the neurosurgeon or otorhinolaryngologist with a battery of both baseline cervical spine CT and MRI imaging, which enables an initial diagnosis consistent with basilar invagination

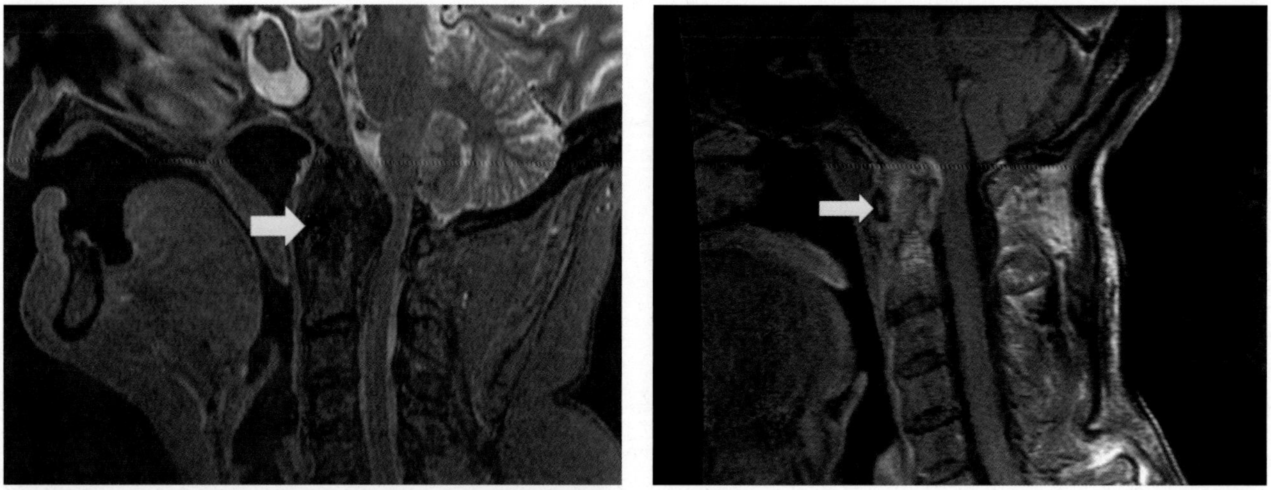

A B

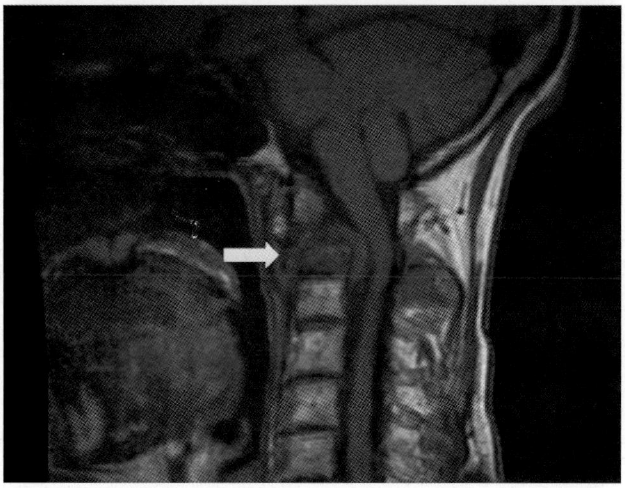

C

Fig. 50.1 **(A)** Skull base lesion at the craniocervical junction in a patient presenting with myelopathic symptoms and unilateral tongue paralysis. Surgical pathology showed degenerative fibroconnective tissue, also termed degenerative pseudotumor. **(B)** *Staphylococcus aureus* osteomyelitis of the odontoid process causing dural enhancement and compression at the medulla/C1 spinal column. **(C)** Metastatic neuroendocrine carcinoma from a lung primary producing painful myelopathic symptoms. The *arrow* in each image indicates the C1/C2 lesion producing basilar invagination.

(**Fig. 50.2**). Review of radiologic studies is critical in determining if the lesion can be successfully approached and resected endoscopically. Each lesion requires judicious assessment, including breadth both rostrocaudally and mediolaterally, localization both extradural versus intradural, extension both above the foramen magnum and below C2, and proximity to the vertebrobasilar arterial system. Accurate measurements of the surgical trajectories and the extent of the surgical approach required for access in the rostral-caudal and medial-lateral dimensions can be readily determined from these modalities. *Ultimately, the principal feature that determines the feasibility of the transnasal approach to the craniocervical junction is whether the position and plane of the hard palate, when projected posteriorly, allows unrestricted access to the anterior spinal pathology in a given patient.*

If surgery is indicated, stereotactic imaging for intraoperative navigation is typically mandated. It is helpful to develop imaging protocols that incorporate as many surface facial landmarks as possible, which are often truncated on selective cranial imaging protocols. Enhanced surface anatomic details facilitate rapid intraoperative registration and accurate intraoperative merging, or overlaying, of disparate CT and MRIs. To this end, we have developed fine-cut sinus and cervical CT scan protocols to clearly delineate the hard palate and the sphenoid, clivus, and atlantoaxial bony anatomy in candidate patients. Our stereotactic MRI sequences typically include the entire skull base, paranasal sinuses, brain parenchyma up to the ventricular horns, and brainstem. We also specifically incorporate the forehead and nasal tip to assist with registration in image guidance, foregoing imaging of the cerebellum and occiput. Finally, for select cases, CT angiogram technology can be implemented to determine the course of the extradural vasculature proximal to the ventral cranial base. If used, we recommend fine-cut (0.625 cm) sequences, which allow for the incorporation of these images for intraoperative navigation. We typically reserve the CT angiogram as the final study prior to transnasal endoscopic surgery. The CT angiogram is typically performed after the patient's initial posterior cervical fusion (see later text), thereby providing updated imaging of subtle changes in the anatomy of the cervical vertebrae and

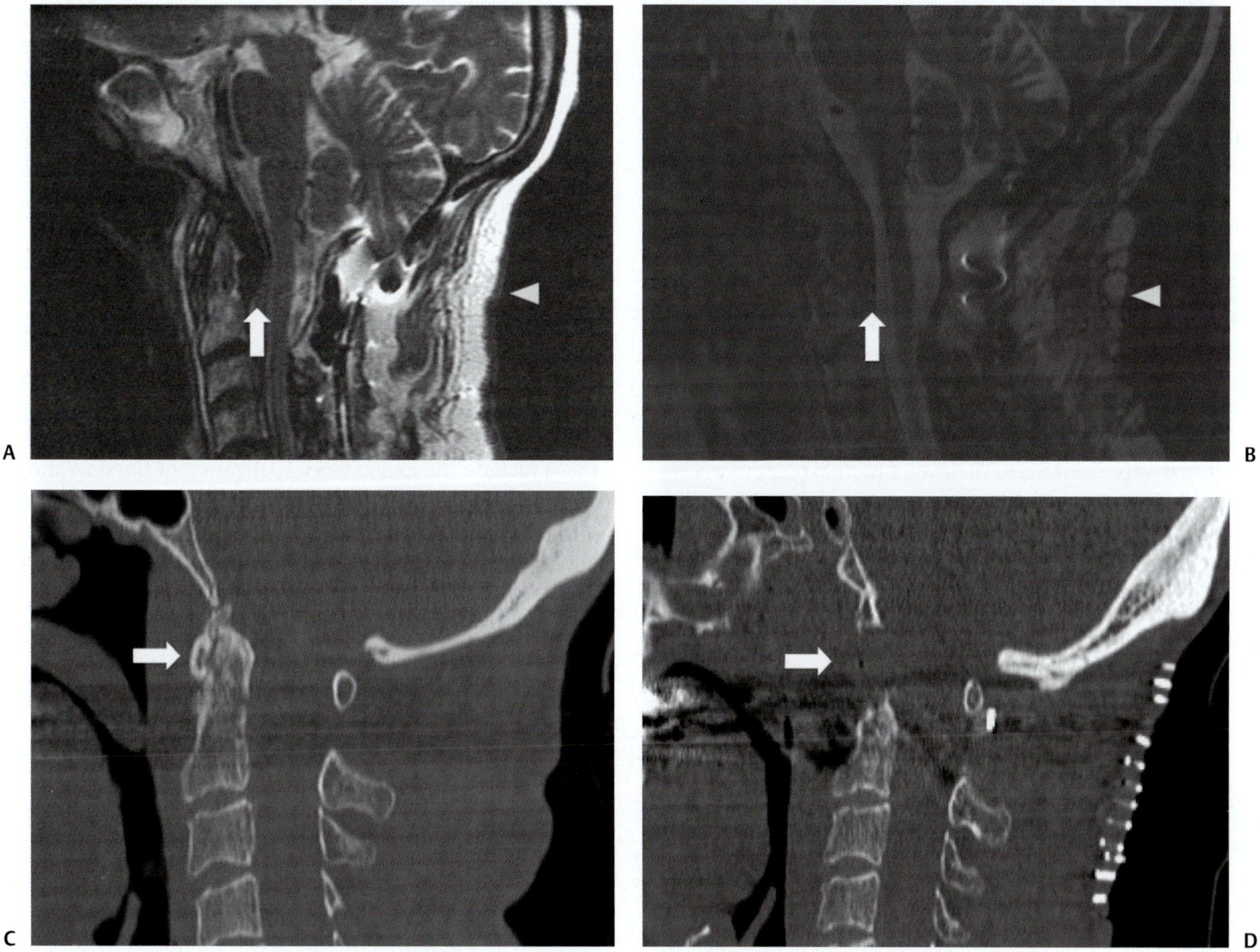

Fig. 50.2 Preoperative and postoperative imaging of craniocervical junction lesions. **(A)** T2-weighted sagittal magnetic resonance image (MRI) demonstrating cervical cord compression in preoperative imaging of a benign skull base lesion. The *arrow* demonstrates compressed cord with restricted CSF fluid signal. The *arrowhead* shows the site of anticipated occipital cervical fusion. **(B)** Six-weeks postoperative T2-sagittal MRI of the patient in **(A)** showing restored cerebrospinal fluid compartment (*arrow*) and absence of brainstem decompression. The *arrowhead* shows slight soft tissue remodeling after posterior fusion. **(C)** Preoperative cervical spine computed tomography (CT) scan demonstrating osteitic changes of C1 and odontoid process (*arrow*) in the setting of isolated skull base osteomyelitis. **(D)** Three days following transnasal decompression, postoperative cervical spine CT in the same patient as **(C)** shows C1 resection with complete odontoidectomy (*arrow*) to improve neurologic function.

spinal column that may have transpired after posterior decompression and stabilization screw placement. These most current images also allow for greater accuracy in intraoperative navigation.

Vasculature

Careful evaluation of the vertebral artery anatomy, especially in the setting of substantial bony disruption, rotatory subluxation, or tumor encasement of the vessel, is essential in avoiding vertebral artery injury (**Fig. 50.3A**). In most cases, the vertebral arteries are displaced posterolaterally by the lesion located in the craniocervical junction. Preoperative balloon test occlusion (BTO) of the vertebral artery may be helpful if this vessel is either felt to be at higher risk for injury or encased in tumor. The results of BTO can be helpful in discussing preoperative risks with the patient.

Stability of the Craniocervical Junction

In patients with lesions of the craniocervical junction, our practice has been to proceed with posterior spinal instrumentation and stabilization with either an occipit-C4 or C1-C4 posterior arthrodesis prior to endonasal decompression. However, there is debate regarding the true level of postoperative instability and potential for subluxation after anterior surgical decompression in this subsite. Determination of spinal stabilization is based on the degree of bony destruction and ligamentous injury associated with the disease process and the extent of bone removal required to achieve sufficient brainstem decompression.

This is in large part due to the fact that the two primary ligaments stabilizing the occipitocervical junction—the alar ligament connecting the occipital condyles to the dens and the transverse ligament stabilizing the dens to the atlas—are either degenerated by disease or will be compromised by the surgical resection at the level of C2.

In support of this, classic studies using the transoral approach by Dickman et al. found that patients with rheumatoid arthritis required posterior spinal arthrodesis given their propensity for spinal instability secondary to inflammatory pannus, ligamentous destruction, and extensive bone softening associated with this disease process.[6] Craniovertebral junction decompression tends to destabilize even previously stable patients, again suggesting the need for antecedent posterior spinal stabilization.[6] Alternatively, patients with developmental osseous anomalies, having a normal ligament and bone structure with abnormal configurations, still tend to maintain stability after transoral decompression, thus obviating the need for posterior stabilization. Although not rigorously studied, the need for spinal fusion appears to be predicated on the degree and quality of normal bone and ligament preservation prior to, and subsequent to, surgical extirpation.

Treatment

Advantages and Drawbacks of the Endonasal Approach

Endoscopic endonasal decompression of the craniocervical junction can confer several potential benefits compared with a transoral approach. For the surgical team, these include the expanded visualization of the operating field using fiberoptic endoscopy, improved instrumentation for safely accessing and deftly decompressing the cervical spine, coordinated use of intraoperative stereotactic

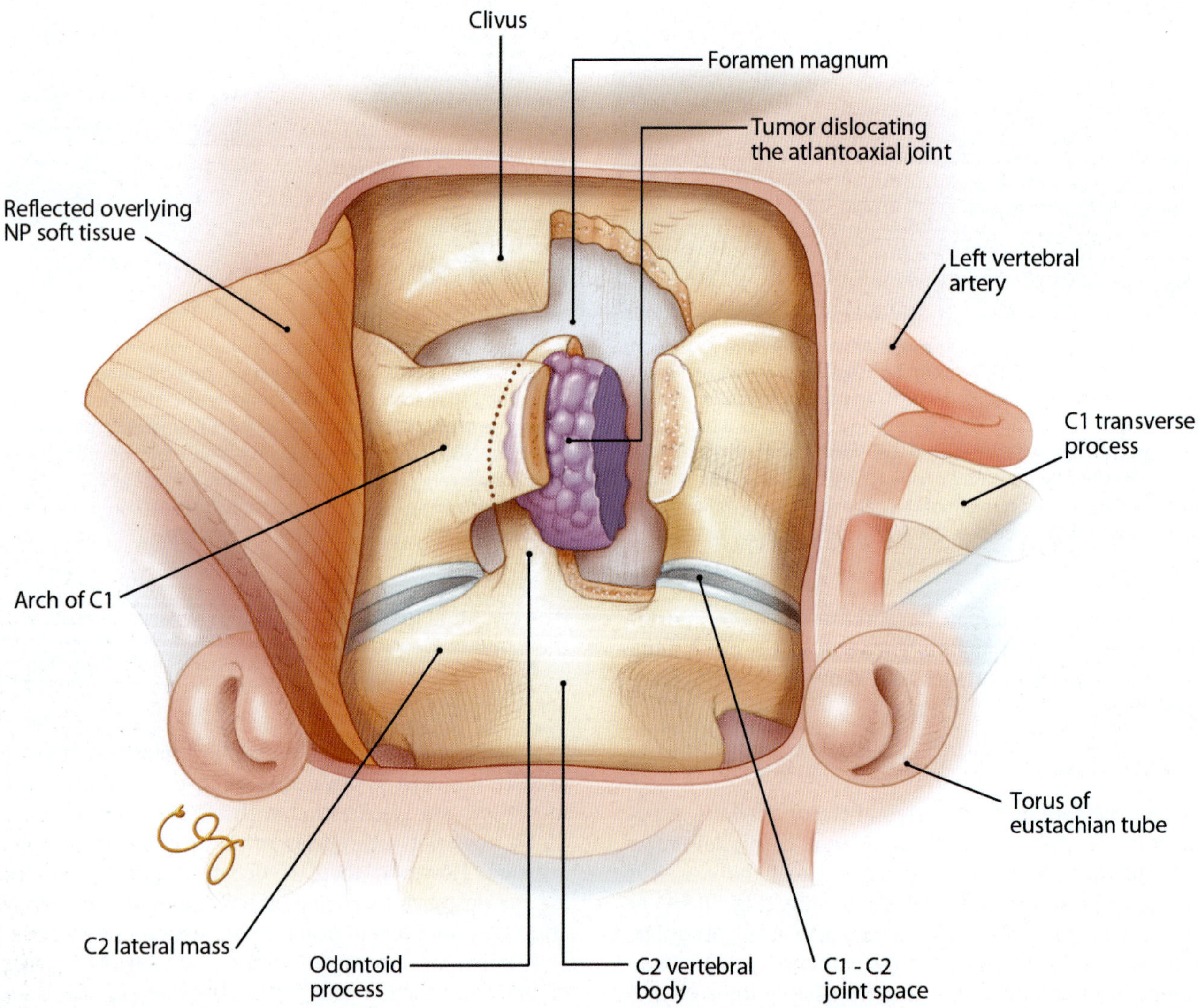

Fig. 50.3 (A) Coronal illustration of critical intraoperative landmarks and vasculature, most notably the vertebral arteries in their sinuous course in this region. *(continued)*

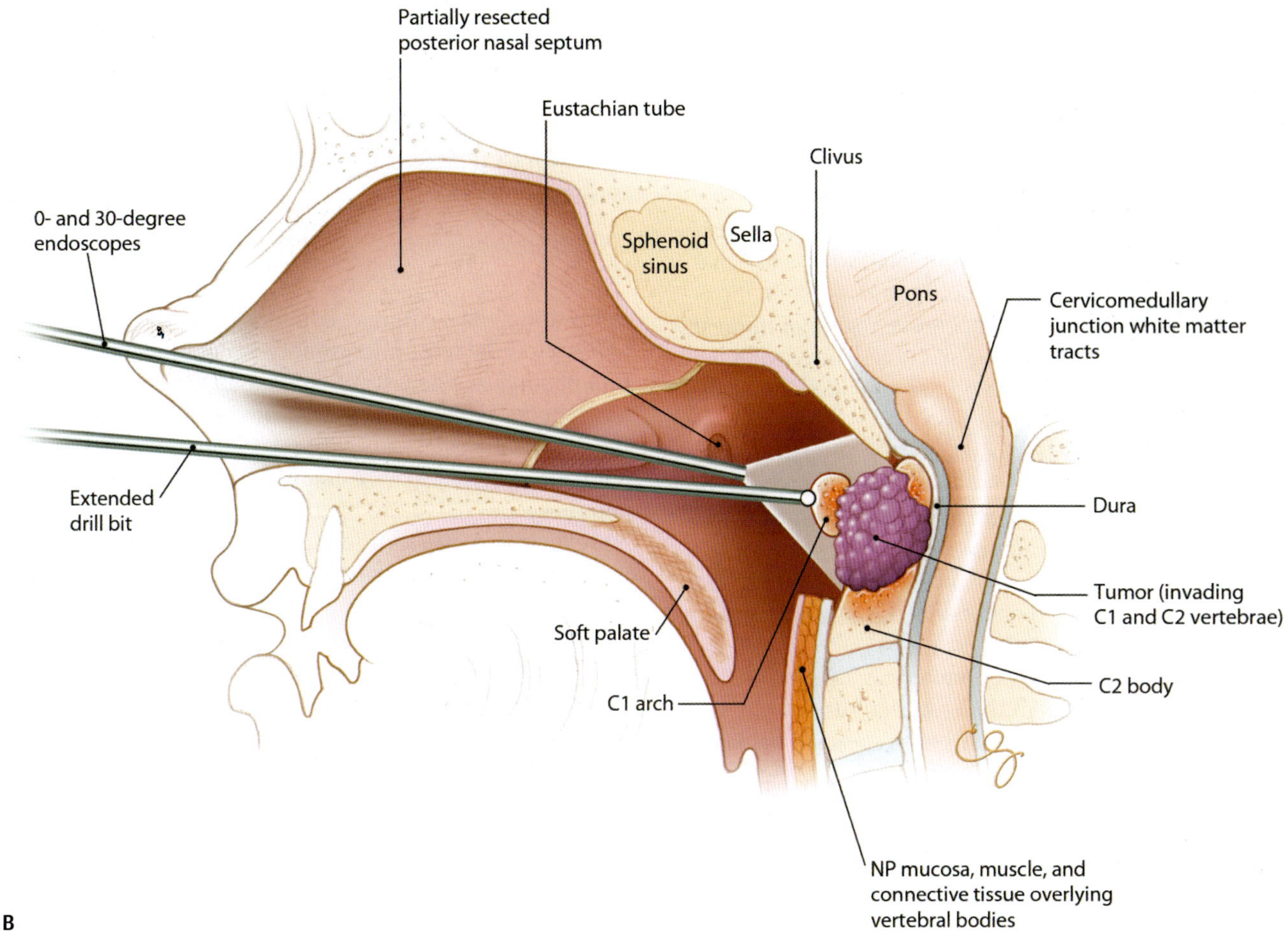

B

Fig. 50.3 *(continued)* **(B)** Illustration in sagittal plane of transnasal odontoidectomy approach, and some of the extended instrumentation required to resect a lesion at this site.

navigation, and the refined ability to recognize and manage cerebrospinal fluid (CSF) leaks when present (**Fig. 50.3B**). For the patient, advantages include reduced wound morbidity and incisional pain, limited velum and pharyngeal swelling, earlier oral nutritional advancement, and decreased pulmonary-associated complications. The major disadvantage of the transnasal approach is topographic: the anatomic constraint in the craniocaudal plane from the underlying nasal floor and hard palate. The latter structures confine surgical access primarily to the foramen magnum, and anterior and lateral arches of the C1 and C2 vertebral bodies. Pathology that produces myelopathy at C3 or lower vertebrae would therefore necessitate a transoral or transcervical surgical approach.

Additionally, both the otorhinolaryngologist–head and neck surgeon and the neurosurgeon require expertise with the use of endoscopic instrumentation, and a collaborative, experienced working relationship is necessary to effectively assist one another throughout this type of challenging case. The authors hope to provide a meaningful protocol for optimizing surgical results with this procedure.

Staging of Surgical Procedures

We have found that staging the posterior arthrodesis and the endonasal odontoidectomy is quite beneficial for numerous reasons. Intraoperatively, patients have a reduced duration of exposure to both a single anesthetic and immobilization on the operating room table. It is also less cumbersome to stage procedures, rather than convert from a prone position with padding and endotracheal tube stabilization for posterior fusion into a supine position for a transnasal approach and risk cord instability. Additionally, dividing the procedure into two stages allows sufficient time for the patient to recover from a posterior fusion procedure in preparation for the endoscopic approach. It perhaps goes without saying that the surgical teams also benefit from staging in avoiding surgeon fatigue, which may adversely affect a long, complex case. The planned staging of the endonasal portion of the procedure has resulted in a limited duration of hospital admission after an endonasal odontoidectomy, with an average stay of 72 to 96 hours after surgery.

Transnasal Odontoid Instrumentation and Equipment Planning

Specialized equipment is required to successfully and reliably perform the endoscopic approach to the craniocervical junction. Several considerations are discussed here.

1. Intraoperative stereotactic navigation is exceedingly helpful, and numerous platforms exist that each promote accurate computer-assisted localization. Given that the operative region of interest is 12 to 14 cm from the nasal alar rim, extended length image guidance probes and suction instrumentation are required.
2. Standard microdebrider and reverse-facing ("adenoid") blades provide for rapid resection of excess nasopharyngeal soft tissue. Some blades include bipolar cautery in their design, allowing for perhaps more hemostatic tissue resection and for others to register effectively within image guidance platforms.
3. Monopolar and bipolar cautery is needed at distinct points through the case, and disposable, extended length attachments are especially valuable for this surgery.
4. High-speed drills that accommodate extended-length fluted and diamond drill bits allow for precision bone removal without heating of the handpiece, which can possibly burn the alar vestibule skin.
5. Ultrasonic soft tissue and bone aspirators can be advocated for the removal of admixed soft tissue and deformed vertebral cortex in this area. These instruments typically limit heat transmission to the surrounding tissues, which is attractive when proximal to the dural lining.
6. Currently available biosealants, hemostatic agents, and tissue adhesives can save time in controlling minor sites of venous hemorrhage and in reconstruction of the final skull base defect.

Patient Positioning and Setup

The transnasal approach to the craniocervical skull base mandates careful attention to positioning. Where possible, our practice has been to position the patient and fiberoptically intubate while awake, both of which ensure that no undue neurologic sequelae occur with head extension. Mayfield pinning for head positioning is advocated, despite the antecedent occipital cervical fusion, to maintain head and cervical spine fixation through the case.

Preoperative antibiotics, such as third-generation cephalosporins, are routinely administered given their excellent penetration into the CSF. Dexamethasone is additionally administered to minimize neural and airway edema. A preferred dose of 8 to 10 mg has been sufficient. Our practice has been to implement neural monitoring via somatosensory-evoked potentials and motor-evoked potentials as well as brainstem auditory-evoked potentials. Electrophysiologic monitoring can be helpful in the event of progressive cord edema, where the surgeon can alter the degree of head extension to optimize canal diameter and minimize spinal cord compression.

Description of Operative Approach

Delineating the anatomic boundaries of the transnasal approach is the most important consideration in anticipation of surgery. The critical landmarks to respect are the basisphenoid and anterior arch of the clivus superiorly, the bilateral eustachian tubes laterally, and the nasal floor inferiorly, which is comprised of the hard palate anteriorly and curvature of the soft palate posteriorly. In our experience, the corridor created within these borders is both necessary and sufficient to access the C1/C2 spinal cord, compared with previous reports (**Fig. 50.3B**).[2,7,8]

After unobstructed access to the posterior nasal cavity is conferred and appropriate landmarks identified, a posterior, inferior septectomy is first performed, removing 2 cm of vomer bone as it intercalates with the hard palate (**Fig. 50.4**). This is accomplished with the use of microdebrider attachments and back-biter hand instruments, and allows for more fluid binarial instrumentation throughout the surgery. In contrast to previous reports,[3] our team rarely performs sphenoidotomies at the outset of the case, favoring the base of the anterior arch of the clivus as the superior limit of dissection. The nasopharyngeal mucosa and longus colli musculature, with its origin at the C1 tubercle, is then resected as a single large

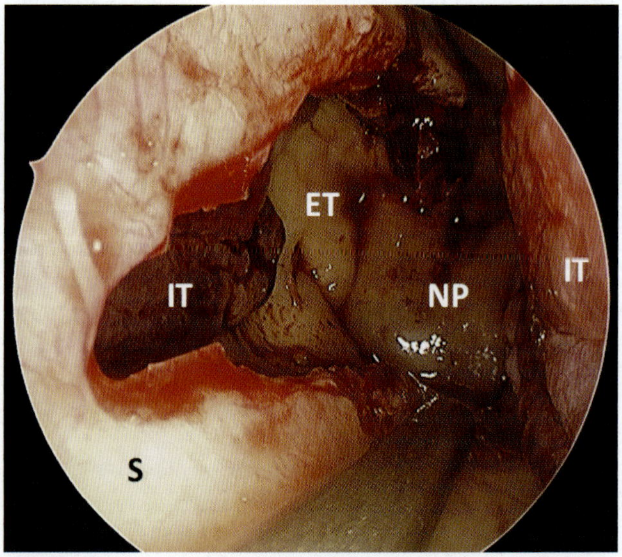

Fig. 50.4 Intraoperative highlights from a transnasal endoscopic odontoidectomy dissection, beginning with the posterior septectomy. *S*, nasal septum; *IT*, inferior turbinate; *ET*, eustachian tube; *NP*, nasopharynx.

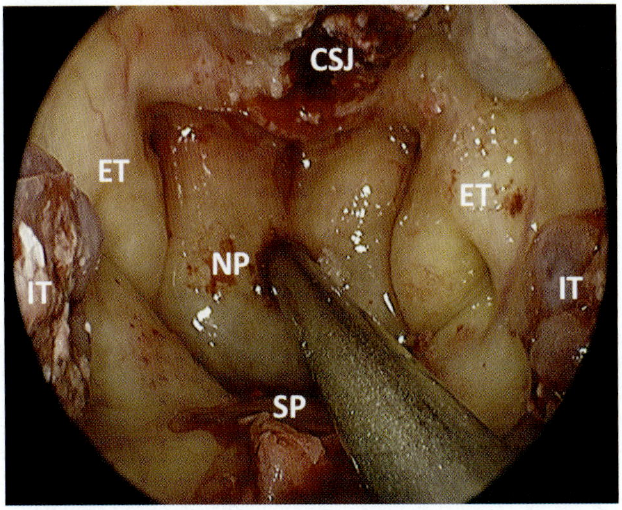

Fig. 50.5 Nasopharynx primary surgical access site with dissection borders. *SP*, soft palate; *CSJ*, clivus/septum junction.

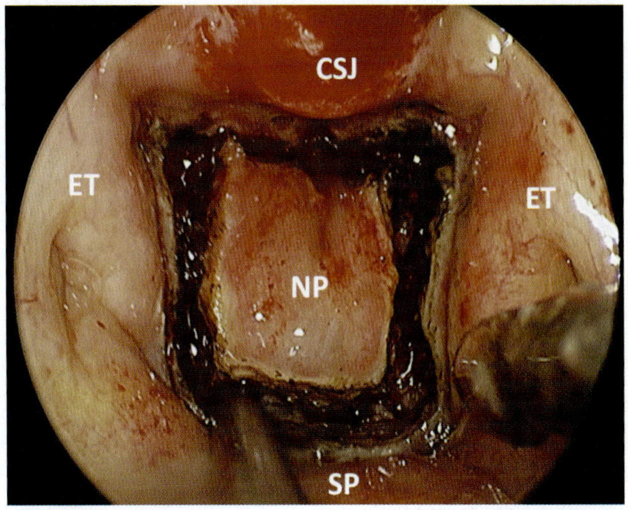

Fig. 50.6 Borders of nasopharynx flap outlined prior to soft tissue resection. Note absence of mucosal injury to lateral eustachian tube orifices and inferior soft palate tissues.

block specimen through the use of extended needle-tip electrocautery (**Figs. 50.5 and 50.6**). This tissue removal is achieved using a four-handed approach for control of the endoscope, cautery device, extended suction tip, and transnasal tissue retractor. There is debate about whether to preserve a tissue flap of nasopharyngeal mucosa at this step, but we have not found it to be especially critical in this setting. Additional submucosal soft tissue is resected via angled microdebrider, ultrasonic aspirator, and/or suction cautery (**Fig. 50.7**).

These coordinated procedures lead to wide exposure of the body and arch of C1 and C2 (**Fig. 50.8**). For the otorhinolaryngologist, a brief anatomic review may be helpful. The central C1 tubercle can serve as a midline bony landmark for the ventral craniovertebral junction. The tubercle prominence is generally equidistant to the tubercles of the C1 lateral masses and vertebral arteries bilaterally. It should be noted, however, that the integrity and orientation of the tubercle may be altered in settings of rotatory subluxation and lateral mass destruction by rheumatoid arthritis or neoplastic processes.

In terms of critical vasculature, at the level of the C1 tubercle, the vertebral artery is located 24 mm laterally, whereas more inferiorly at the C2/3 junction, the vertebral artery tapers medially and is approximately only 11 mm lateral to the midline. At the craniocervical junction, therefore, the vertebral artery is usually sufficiently lateral and essentially protected from injury by the walls of the

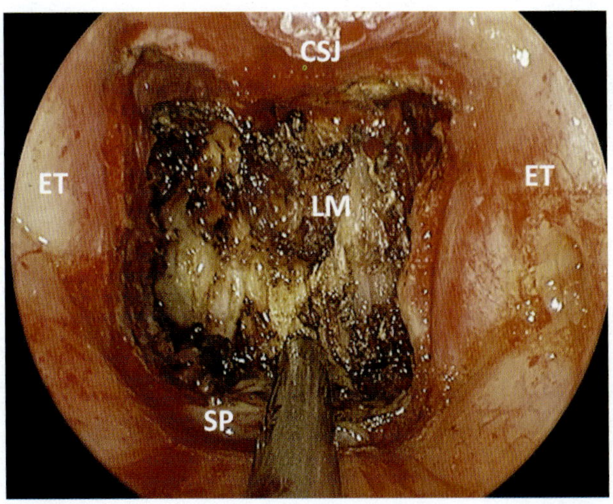

Fig. 50.7 Ligamentous and muscular soft tissue deep to nasopharyngeal flap that requires meticulous clearance. *LM*, submucosal ligaments and musculature.

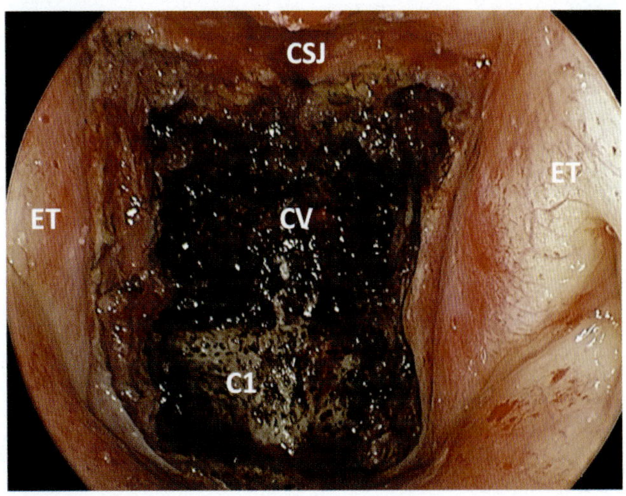

Fig. 50.8 Exposed bony anatomy of the craniovertebral junction and anterior arch of C1. *C1*, anterior arch of C1 vertebral body; *CV*, clivus.

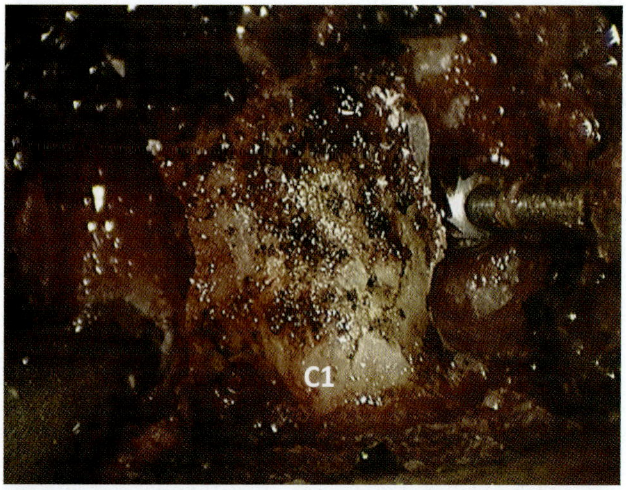

Fig. 50.9 Endoscopic drilling of osteitic C1 using extended drill bits and suction instrumentation.

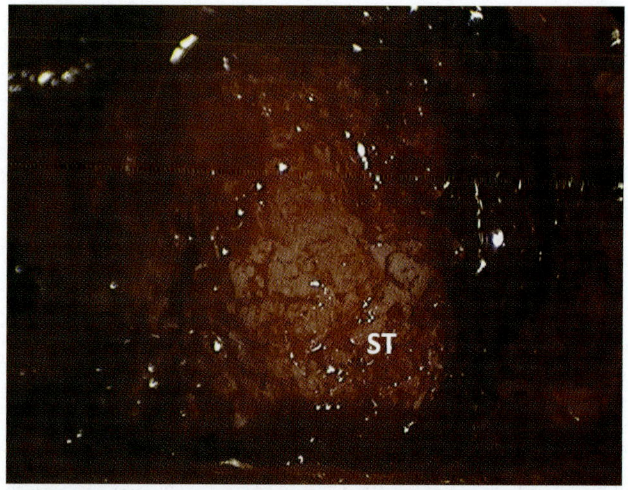

Fig. 50.10 Upon C1 removal, abnormal deposits of soft tissue such as rheumatoid pannus or inflammatory granulation tissue, can be encountered and resected. *ST*, soft tissue.

C1 lateral masses bilaterally. As noted previously, in the setting of C1 tubercle subluxation from midline, one of the displaced tubercles of the C1 lateral mass may inadvertently be interpreted as the midline C1 tubercle, leading to potential vertebral artery injury.

Finally, two venous plexi are noteworthy at this skull base site. At the inferior margin of the clivus, the midline is devoid of major vascular structures, although bleeding from the diploic channels in communication with the clival-dural venous complex may be treacherous. Similarly, at the occipitoatlantal junction, small venous tributaries from the jugal venous complex will commonly be encountered.

The C1 arch is taken down and resected using extended-length endoscopic drill bits and Kerrison rongeurs (**Fig. 50.9**). The ultrasonic aspirator can be used at the lateral extents of the exposure to resect remnant bone and soft tissue in an atraumatic fashion. At this time, if there is pathology affecting and expanding the atlantoaxial joint space, such as rheumatoid pannus, it will become apparent (**Fig. 50.10**). Lesions or degenerated tissue at this site should be readily resected to reveal the odontoid process of C2. Consideration should be given to sending this tissue for pathologic analysis and culture, depending on the contributing disease mechanism. The dens can then be addressed by precision drilling of its base (**Fig. 50.11**). This directed action will allow the tip of the odontoid to collapse anteriorly into the surgical field, which can then be removed with extended hand instruments to decompress the brainstem (**Fig. 50.12**).

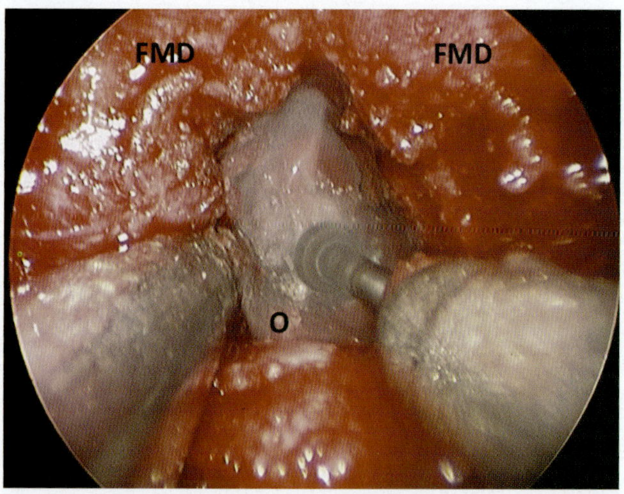

Fig. 50.11 Continuing more posteriorly, the odontoid process can be mottled and retrodisplaced onto the brainstem dura, making the surrounding dura of the foramen magnum billow out around this site of basilar invagination, as seen here. Drill out of the dens base is typically required to achieve the most effective decompression. *O*, odontoid process; *FMD*, foramen magnum dura.

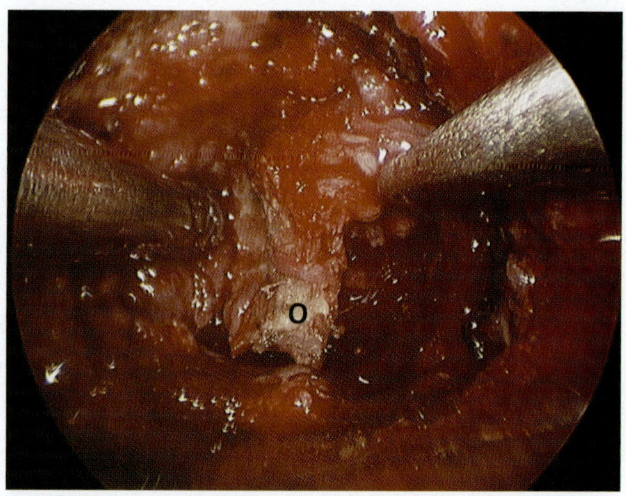

Fig. 50.12 Meticulous resection of the irregular odontoid process away from the spinal canal using appropriate-length hand instruments, picks, and suctions.

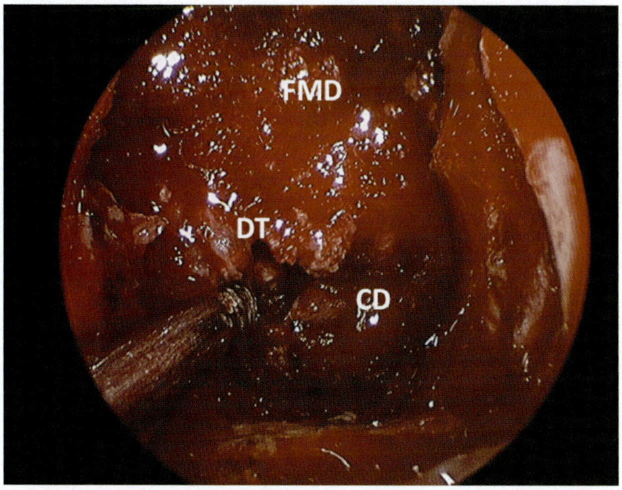

Fig. 50.13 After odontoidectomy is completed with restoration of brainstem pulsations, in select cases, a dural tear is created leading to cerebrospinal fluid leak. *DT*, dural tear; *CD*, cervical spine dura after decompression.

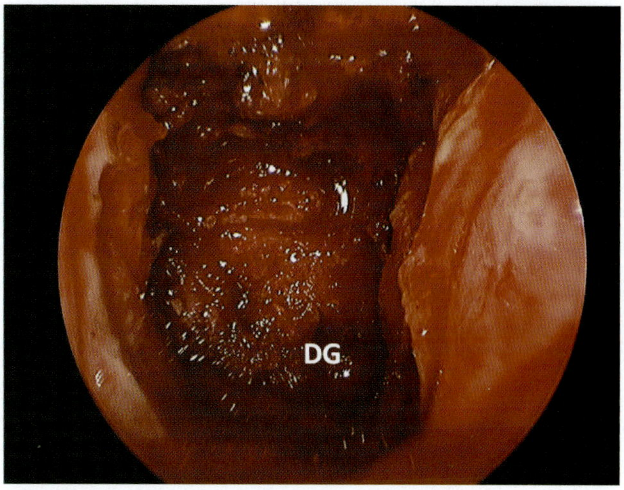

Fig. 50.14 Multilayered reconstruction of dural tear and cerebrospinal fluid leak using a Duragen matrix graft as first layer. *DG*, Duragen onlay graft.

Depending on the location of the pathologic process, the dens itself can be adherent to dura, making a CSF leak likely upon odontoid resection (**Fig. 50.13**). In other cases, the extradural disease process resides at the craniocervical junction between the dens and dura. Following dens resection, the lesion in this space can be meticulously dissected for tissue biopsy and resected partially or completely as exposure and neurologic parameters allow, with the principal goal of decompressing the brainstem and cervical spine. The latter is demonstrated by the renewed transmission of arterial pulsations through the meningeal membranes, which are typically devoid at the inception of the surgery.

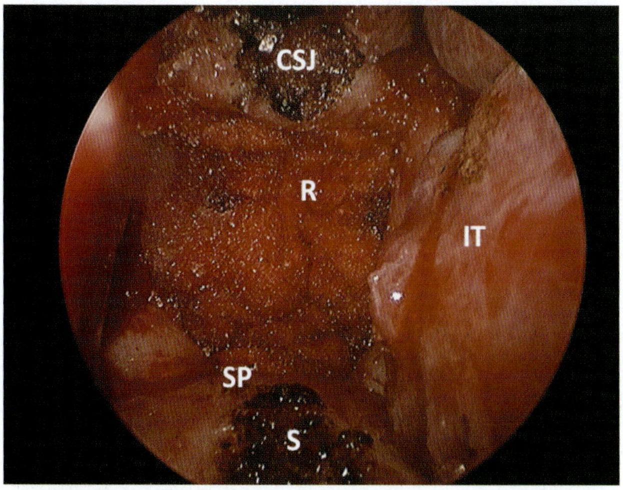

Fig. 50.15 Final view of intraoperative nasopharynx reconstruction access site after layered placement of abdominal fat, tissue adhesives, and squares of Gelfoam matrix. A pedicled septal flap was not felt to be required for reconstruction in this patient. *R*, final reconstruction.

Reconstruction can range from limited to extensive. Simple reconstruction in the absence of CSF leak can be achieved with absorbable gelatin sponges and tissue sealants alone. The leakage of CSF through a cervical dural tear can be repaired through a multilayered closure using a synthetic dural substitute (**Fig. 50.14**), abdominal fat, and bioresorbable layers of gelatin sponges (**Fig. 50.15**). A regional, pedicled nasoseptal flap, described elsewhere, can also be harvested and rotated into this defect for tissue coverage.

Patients are typically kept in house for several days to closely monitor hemodynamics, counteract pain, assess the ability to perform the activities of daily living, and achieve safe postoperative swallowing function. Intravenous antibiotics with effective central nervous system (CNS) penetration are maintained for 1 to 2 days postoperatively, and saline irrigations are initiated on the first postoperative day. Upon discharge, the otorhinolaryngologist typically oversees each patient's progress and healing during routine office debridements of the nasal cavity 2 weeks and then 2 months postoperatively (**Fig. 50.16**). Depending on surgical team preferences, immediate postoperative imaging, such as CT of the cervical spine, may be undertaken, although our team favors a single comprehensive skull base and cervical spine MRI sequence 2 to 3 months after surgery when most of the anticipated changes from swelling and tissue ingrowth have subsided.

Complications

The primary potential complication from the transnasal approach to the craniocervical junction is inadequate brainstem decompression due to a subtotal resection of the odontoid and extradural lesion. A persistent CSF leak can be anticipated in this location given the

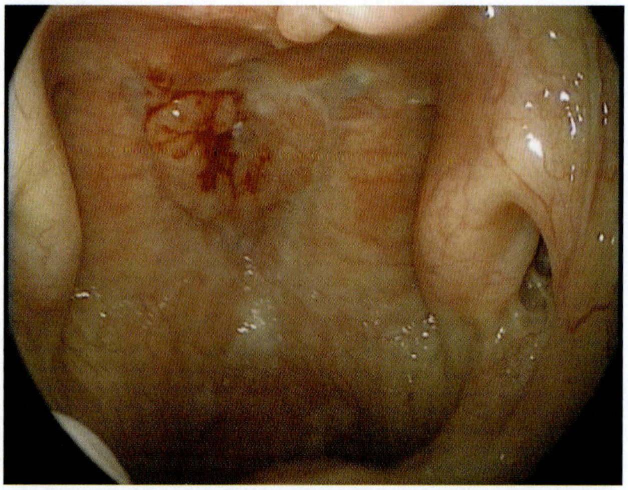

Fig. 50.16 Favorable healing of nasopharynx surgical corridor at 2-month postoperative time point in same patient. Slight blood seen here only noted after debridement of minute overlying crust at this site. This patient experienced no postoperative eustachian tube dysfunction, velopharyngeal insufficiency, or postnasal drip, with uneventful closure of cerebrospinal fluid leak and complete resolution of preoperative neck pain and myelopathic symptoms.

difficulty in placing a reinforced bolster, but dural closure can usually be achieved using a multilayered reconstruction. Vertebral artery injury can be avoided in most cases through careful preoperative assessment of imaging sequences and the use of stereotactic intraoperative navigation in the lateral aspects of the surgical field. However, a vascular injury of this magnitude can be difficult to manage. Attempts at clamping the offending vessel using hand instruments, vascular clip application, and bipolar cautery should be considered, although pressure tamponade of the affected vessels with emergent neurointerventional embolization of the offending vessel would likely be required.

Outcomes

Several case reports are now available that describe successful outcomes with the transnasal approach to the odontoid and craniocervical junction for various pathologies.[3,9,10] Two current reports describe surgical patient series with the endoscopic approach.[4,5] Both articles demonstrate quite favorable outcomes with regard to complete odontoid resection, cervical decompression, and an improvement in preoperative symptomatology. In one study, there was one death (of a 96-year-old patient) that was attributed to perioperative sequelae such as pulmonary embolus,[4] but the remainder of the patients in this retrospective group with atlantoaxial rheumatoid pannus had dramatic improvements in myelopathic symptoms and preoperative dysphagia. Of note, perioperative velopharyngeal insufficiency and respiratory issues resolved or improved measurably in all patients studied.

Conclusion

Although decompression of the craniocervical junction can be performed using an open transoral approach, anterior decompression of the spinal cord at the craniocervical junction through a transnasal approach is an attractive alternative for this challenging skull base subsite. We present our experiences and considerations herein with the endonasal endoscopic approach and outline the surgical strategies that may facilitate performance of this procedure and minimize operative pitfalls and complications. The transnasal approach can be a technically demanding procedure for the combined neurosurgery and otorhinolaryngology–head and neck surgery teams, but offers demonstrable advantages in terms of improved surgical visualization and reduced perioperative morbidity for the properly selected patient.

References

1. Costagliola C, Di Lorenzo N. Extreme lateral-transatlas approach. J Neurosurg 2003;98(1, Suppl):115–116, author reply 116–117
2. Kingdom TT, Nockels RP, Kaplan MJ. Transoral-transpharyngeal approach to the craniocervical junction. Otolaryngol Head Neck Surg 1995;113(4):393–400
3. Kassam AB, Snyderman C, Gardner P, Carrau R, Spiro R. The expanded endonasal approach: a fully endoscopic transnasal approach and resection of the odontoid process: technical case report. Neurosurgery 2005;57(1, Suppl):E213, discussion E213
4. Nayak JV, Gardner PA, Vescan AD, Carrau RL, Kassam AB, Snyderman CH. Experience with the expanded endonasal approach for resection of the odontoid process in rheumatoid disease. Am J Rhinol 2007;21(5):601–606
5. Gempt J, Lehmberg J, Grams AE, Berends L, Meyer B, Stoffel M. Endoscopic transnasal resection of the odontoid: case series and clinical course. Eur Spine J 2011;20(4):661–666
6. Dickman CA, Locantro J, Fessler RG. The influence of transoral odontoid resection on stability of the craniovertebral junction. J Neurosurg 1992;77(4):525–530
7. Cavallo LM, Cappabianca P, Messina A, et al. The extended endoscopic endonasal approach to the clivus and cranio-vertebral junction: anatomical study. Childs Nerv Syst 2007;23(6): 665–671
8. Seker A, Inoue K, Osawa S, Akakin A, Kilic T, Rhoton AL Jr. Comparison of endoscopic transnasal and transoral approaches to the craniovertebral junction. World Neurosurg 2010;74(6):583–602
9. Gempt J, Lehmberg J, Meyer B, Stoffel M. Endoscopic transnasal resection of the odontoid in a patient with severe brainstem compression. Acta Neurochir (Wien) 2010;152(3):559–560
10. Leng LZ, Anand VK, Hartl R, Schwartz TH. Endonasal endoscopic resection of an os odontoideum to decompress the cervicomedullary junction: a minimal access surgical technique. Spine (Phila Pa 1976) 2009;34(4):E139–E143

51 Extended Applications of Endoscopic Skull Base Surgery

Carl H. Snyderman, Paul A. Gardner, and Daniel M. Prevedello

Since the introduction of the endoscope, there has been an evolution of surgical techniques in all of the surgical disciplines from *maximally* invasive open approaches to *minimally* invasive endoscopic approaches. Cranial base surgery is the latest surgical specialty to embrace endoscopic techniques and it is revolutionizing the practice of skull base surgery.[1] Endoscopic techniques have increased access to complex anatomic areas and enabled more invasive surgery with less morbidity. It is important to realize, however, that endonasal endoscopic skull base surgery is maximally invasive; it has extended the limits of cranial base surgery. The major concept of endonasal surgery is not the use of the endoscope but the choice of a nasal corridor for ventral skull base pathology. The endoscope is simply a tool that allows the modern skull base surgeon to choose the best approach for the patient's pathology.

Table 51.1 Classification of Endonasal Approaches to the Ventral Skull Base

Sagittal Plane
Transfrontal
Transcribriform
Transplanum (suprasellar/subchiasmatic)
Transsellar
Transclival
Superior: Posterior clinoid
Middle: Midclivus
Inferior: Foramen magnum
Transodontoid
Coronal Plane
Superior (anterior cranial fossa)
Supraorbital
Transorbital
Middle (middle cranial fossa)
Transpterygoid
Transcavernous
Medial petrous apex
Suprapetrous (middle fossa)
Infratemporal skull base
Inferior (posterior cranial fossa)
Infrapetrous
Transcondylar
Parapharyngeal space
Medial (jugular foramen) Lateral

The classification of endonasal approaches to the ventral skull base is based on anatomic relationships and orientation in radiologic planes (**Table 51.1**).[2–4] The sphenoid sinus is the starting point for most surgical modules because of its important anatomic relationships (internal carotid artery [ICA], optic nerves). The sagittal plane extends from the frontal sinus to the second cervical vertebra (**Fig. 51.1**). The coronal plane is divided into three planes corresponding to the anterior, middle, and posterior cranial fossae (**Fig. 51.2**). The superior (anterior) coronal plane extends to the midorbital roof; the middle coronal plane extends across the floor of the middle cranial fossa superior to the petrous ICA; and the inferior (posterior) coronal plane extends across the occipital condyle to the jugular bulb and parapharyngeal space. Suprapetrous (middle coronal plane) and infrapetrous (inferior coronal plane) approaches are defined relative to their relationship to the petrous segment of the ICA (**Fig. 51.3**). Individual surgical modules vary greatly in anatomic complexity, technical difficulty, and potential risk to neurovascular structures. To address these issues, we have devised a training program that classifies endonasal surgical modules into five levels that are incremental and modular (**Table 51.2**).[5] Mastery of each level is necessary before proceeding to the next.

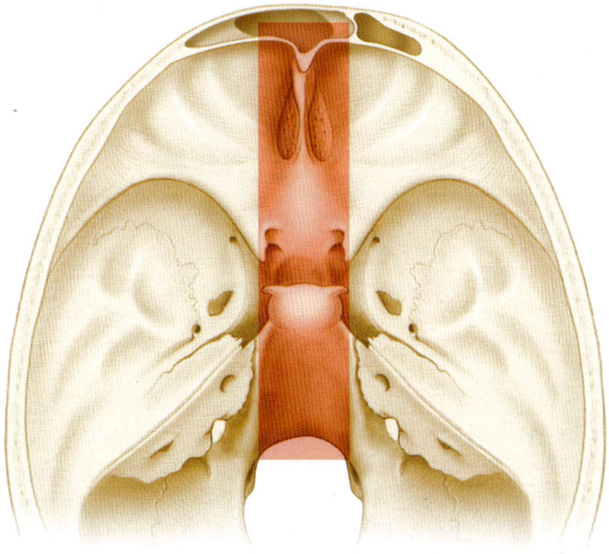

Fig. 51.1 In the sagittal plane, surgical modules extend from the frontal sinus to the second cervical vertebra in the midline.

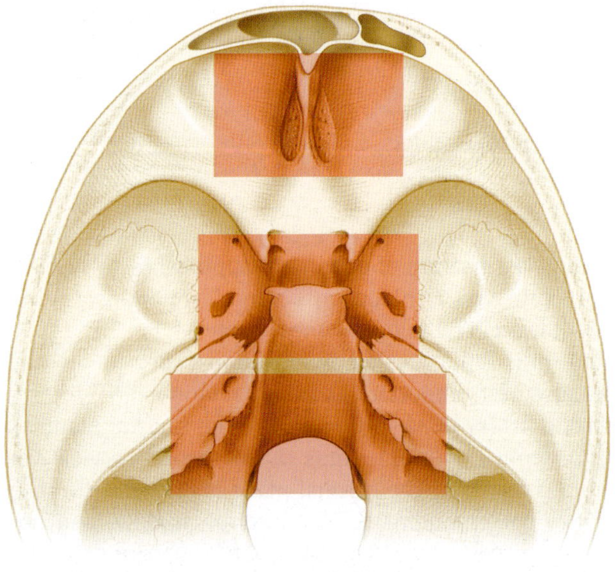

Fig. 51.2 Superior (anterior), middle, and inferior (posterior) coronal planes extend laterally from the midline corridor and correspond to the respective cranial fossae.

Table 51.2 Training Levels for Endonasal Skull Base Surgery

Level I:
Sinus surgery
Level II:
Advanced sinus surgery
Cerebrospinal fluid leaks
Sella/pituitary (intrasellar)
Level III:
Sella/pituitary (extrasellar)
Optic nerve decompression
Extradural skull base surgery
Level IV:
A. With cortical cuff
Transplanum
Transcribriform
Type I craniopharyngiomas
B. Lack of cortical cuff
Type II/III craniopharyngiomas
Transclival intradural
Level V:
Coronal plane (carotid dissection)
Vascular surgery

Endoscopic treatment of pituitary tumors is quickly becoming the new standard. Endonasal endoscopic approaches have been applied to the treatment of extrasellar pituitary tumors, sinonasal neoplasms, clival tumors, expansile lesions of the petrous apex, aneurysms, and even the upper cervical spine.[6–13] What, then, are *extended* applications? The greatest challenges of endonasal skull base surgery are found with level IV and V procedures (**Table 51.2**). These involve intradural dissection of tumors from cerebral vessels and dissection in the coronal plane along the course of the ICA. It has been said that skull base surgery "is all about the carotid." Familiarity with the course of the ICA and its branches and the ability to deal with hemorrhage (both venous and arterial) is necessary to perform these more complex procedures. Surgical approaches to the ICA (suprapetrous and infrapetrous) are the focus of this chapter.

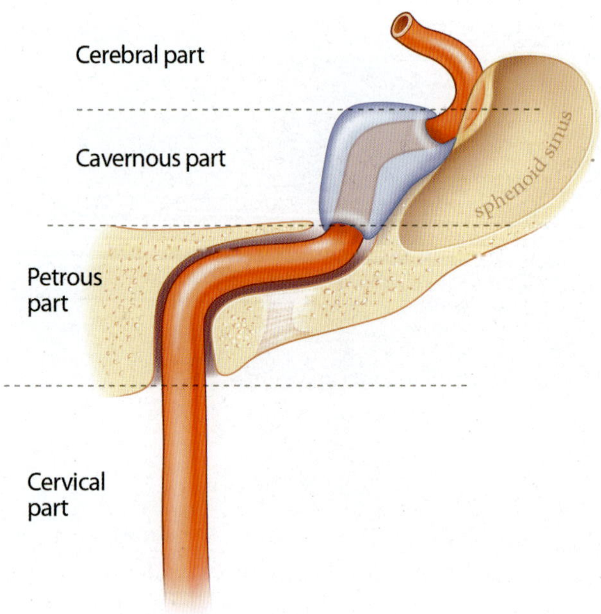

Fig. 51.3 Supapetrous and infrapetrous approaches are defined relative to the petrous segment of the ICA.

Patient Selection/Indications

The selection of a surgical approach is predicated on multiple factors: diagnosis, sites of involvement, extent of disease, prior treatment, medical comorbidities, surgical expertise, reconstruction, tumor vascularity and consistency, and patient preference. There must exist a dedicated surgical team (otolaryngology and neurosurgery) with adequate surgical expertise and resources (equipment, staff) to perform extended endonasal procedures. The surgical team needs to understand endonasal skull base anatomy and have mastery of hemostatic and reconstructive techniques. The choice of an endonasal approach may be limited by the ability to perform a complete resection and the ability to deal with potential complications (vascular injury), reconstructive needs (dural reconstruction), and the duration of the surgery (impact on the patient and surgeon).

The guiding principle of endonasal skull base surgery is to minimize displacement of normal neural and vascular structures. Tumors such as olfactory groove meningiomas

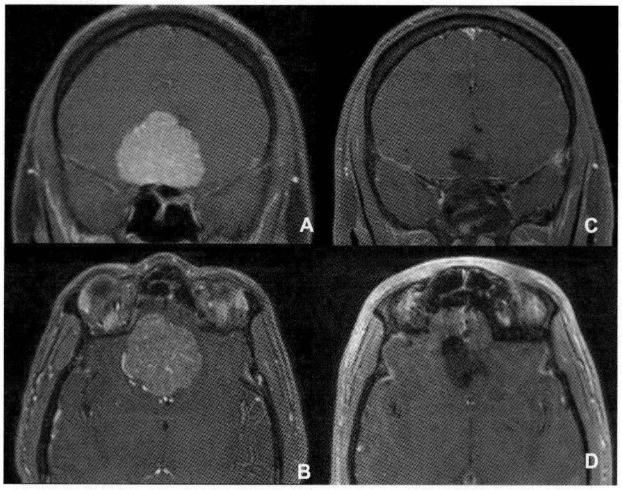

Fig. 51.4 The endonasal corridor provides direct access to an olfactory groove meningioma and avoids any retraction of the frontal lobes: preoperative **(A,B)** and postoperative **(C,D)** coronal and axial views.

and chordomas that originate from the ventral skull base are ideally suited to an endonasal approach (**Fig. 51.4**). The key anatomic structures of the skull base are the cranial nerves (optic nerves) and major blood vessels (ICA and vertebrobasilar arteries). Tumors that are situated superolateral to the optic nerves or require transposition of a major vessel are examples of situations in which a different surgical corridor or the use of multiple corridors must be considered. Tumors that are located posterior to the pituitary stalk may be accessed using a pituitary transposition with preservation of pituitary function.[7]

When there is encasement of the ICA by tumor (**Fig. 51.5**), the goals of surgery may be limited. For high-grade malignancies, nonoperative therapy is usually selected although there may be a role for palliative debulking of bulky tumors or limited resection of residual tumor following radiochemotherapy. En bloc excision of the ICA is no longer performed due to the limited oncologic benefit and potential morbidity. Benign tumors can usually be dissected free with preservation of the ICA.

The suprapetrous approach to the middle cranial fossa is used to access tumors that arise within Meckel's cave (neurilemomas), petroclival tumors that involve the floor of the middle cranial fossa (meningiomas), benign tumors that arise extracranially and extend through the

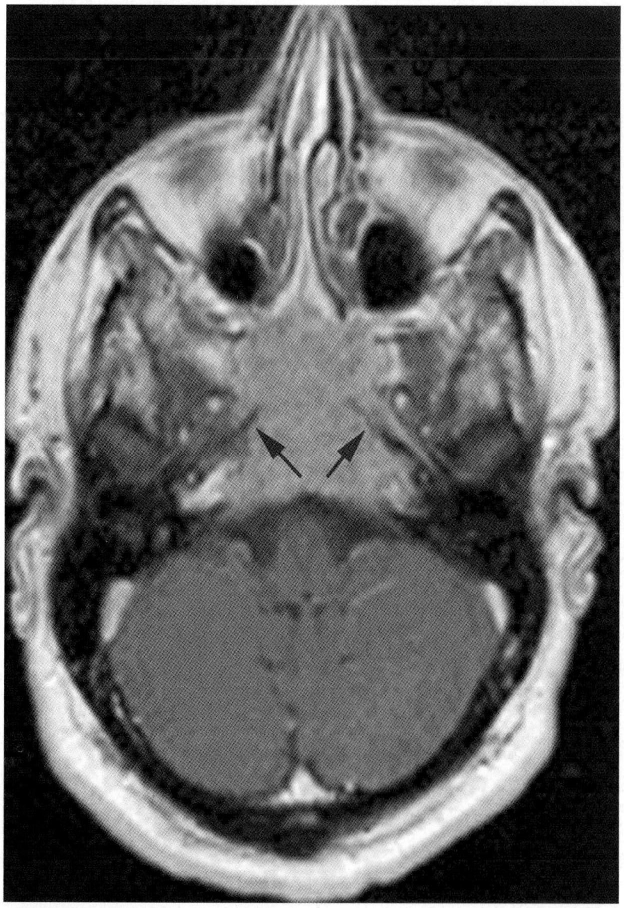

Fig. 51.5 Surgery has a limited role in the treatment of high-grade neoplasms with carotid involvement (*arrows*). This patient had a keratinizing nasopharyngeal carcinoma (Type 1) and underwent endoscopic debulking of the neoplasm to relieve a sixth cranial nerve palsy prior to radiochemotherapy.

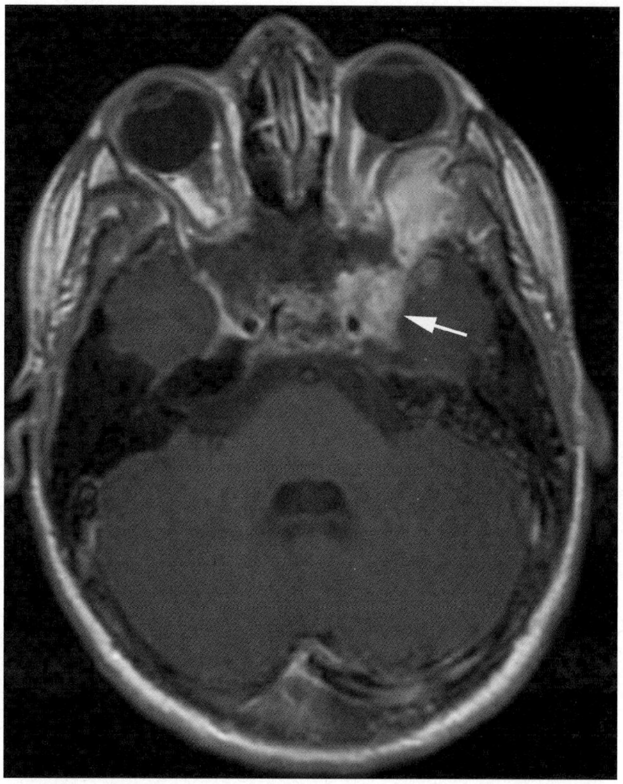

Fig. 51.6 Residual juvenile nasopharyngeal angiofibroma following an endonasal excision of the extracranial portion of the tumor. Tumor in the left middle cranial fossa (Meckel's cave [*arrow*]) is removed using a suprapetrous approach superior to the petrous ICA and lateral to the paraclival ICA.

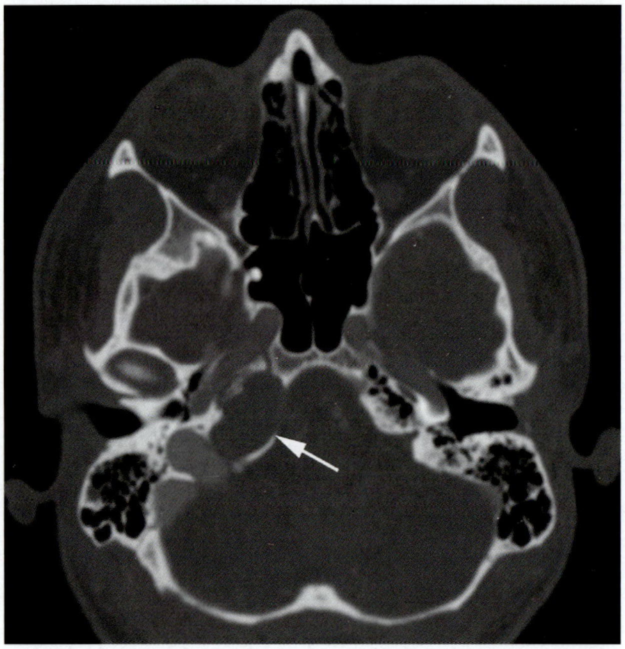

Fig. 51.7 An expansile cystic lesion (cholesterol granuloma) of the right petrous apex (*arrow*) requires an infrapetrous approach when it does not expand medially into the sphenoid sinus and it is deep or inferior to the petrous internal carotid artery.

skull base foramina (angiofibromas), and malignant sinonasal neoplasms with perineural extension along the infraorbital nerve (squamous cell carcinoma, adenoid cystic carcinoma) (**Fig. 51.6**). An infrapetrous approach provides access to the petrous apex and region of the petroclival synchondrosis. Expansile petrous apex lesions that do not extend medial to the paraclival ICA into the sphenoid sinus cannot be approached through the sphenoid sinus and require an infrapetrous approach, and include petrous apicitis, cholesterol granulomas (**Fig. 51.7**), epidermoids, metastases. Neoplasms that occur at the petroclival synchondrosis include chondrosarcomas and chordomas and are typical indications for infrapetrous approaches.

Diagnostic Workup

A definitive diagnosis should be ascertained prior to surgery whenever possible. In most cases, a diagnosis can be established (or limited) from radiologic imaging. Computed tomography (CT) and magnetic resonance imaging (MRI) provide complementary information. CT provides superior visualization of bony anatomy, such as normal anatomic landmarks and extent of bone destruction. MRI helps differentiate tumor from obstructed secretions in the sinuses and provides superior visualization of the tumor-brain interface. It is also helpful in delineating tumor extension along vascular and neural structures. Although sinonasal neoplasms are frequently amenable to biopsy in the outpatient setting, biopsy may be deferred due to concerns about hemorrhage. When a definitive diagnosis is not apparent from imaging and the treatment plan may be altered (e.g., plasmacytoma), a surgical biopsy may be warranted. For sinonasal neoplasms with skull base or orbital involvement, the ability to provide informed consent to the patient and the choice of primary therapy (surgery versus radiochemotherapy) is dependent on the grade of the neoplasm. In such cases, an extradural/extraorbital resection of the tumor is performed to obtain tissue for diagnosis, palliate symptoms, and avoid a complication (cerebrospinal fluid [CSF] leak) without compromising subsequent treatment. For deeply situated tumors (middle cranial fossa), an endonasal approach provides the least invasive approach for diagnosis, and the extent of tumor resection will depend on a frozen histologic section.

In preparation for surgery, the preoperative imaging is obtained using an image-guidance protocol. An intraoperative navigational system is routinely used in all endonasal surgeries to help identify key anatomic landmarks and the limits of resection. For tumors with minimal intracranial extension, CT angiography provides important bony details for drilling and visualization of the ICA throughout its course. For pure intracranial tumors with minimal vascular involvement such as pituitary adenomas, MRI can be used independently for image guidance. For tumors with skull base involvement and intracranial extension or a heterogeneous composition (solid and cystic components), CT and MRIs are fused for surgical navigation.

Preoperative angiography is reserved for vascular tumors in proximity to the ICA. Large juvenile nasopharyngeal angiofibromas (JNAs) invariably derive some blood supply from the ICA, but only the contribution from the external carotid artery is embolized to minimize the risk of secondary brain infarct. However, the extent and location of ICA contributions is important in the planning of surgery; early isolation is performed to minimize blood loss. When extensive dissection of the ICA is anticipated and there is an increased risk of vascular injury, preoperative balloon-occlusion testing of the ICA is performed to assess collateral cerebral blood flow and predict the consequences of a vascular sacrifice. If the patient fails a balloon occlusion, the goals of surgery may be restricted; if the patient passes, a carotid sacrifice is an option in the event of injury.

Surgical Anatomy

The ICA is the main structure that defines the surgical modules of the ventral skull base. It is helpful to divide the course of the ICA into several segments: parapharyngeal, petrous, paraclival, cavernous, and supraclinoid (**Fig. 51.8**). The most important anatomic relationships are found in the environs of the sphenoid sinus. Within the sphenoid sinus, it is important to remember that lateral septations of the sphenoid sinus customarily attach

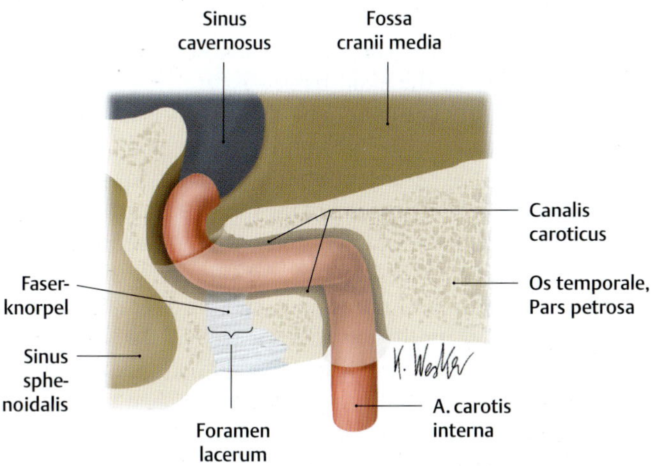

Fig. 51.8 For the endonasal surgeon, it is helpful to divide the internal carotid artery into parapharyngeal, petrous, paraclival, cavernous, and supraclinoidal (cerebral) segments *A* artery.

to the carotid canal. Aggressive removal of septations can result in injury to the artery. The cavernous ICA is often dehiscent or covered by a thin shell of bone and is susceptible to direct trauma from a sharp instrument such as a drilled suction tip. The cavernous and paraclival segments are readily apparent in a well pneumatized sphenoid sinus. The cavernous segment defines the lateral margin of the sella and curves medially at its junction with the optic nerve. This junction is formed by a triangular piece of bone that projects between the ICA and optic nerve and represents the lateral portion of the tuberculum sella. This is also a site for potential carotid injuries with opening of the sella. Laterally, the pneumatization of the anterior clinoid through the optic strut forms the optic-carotid recess. The paraclival ICA forms the lateral margins of the clival recess. The bone deep to the paraclival ICA is the petrous apex and the sixth cranial nerve courses across its surface through Dorello's canal. The abducens nerve has an oblique trajectory and its more medial aspect is found posterior to the paraclival ICA just above its junction with the sphenoid floor; drilling of bone deep to the ICA at this level may injure the nerve. In acromegalic patients, the ICA is often tortuous and elongated and the distance between the arteries can be narrowed.

The petrous ICA extends from its first genu at the entrance of the carotid canal to the second genu at the foramen lacerum in a lateral-to-medial and posterior-to-anterior direction. Because the second genu is the most anterior projection of the petrous ICA, it is an important site for initial exposure of the artery. The key landmark for the second genu is the pterygoid canal that transmits the vidian artery and nerve (**Fig. 51.9**).[14] The pterygoid canal is inferolateral to the lateral recess of the sphenoid sinus in the base of the pterygoid plates and courses posterolaterally in the axial plane. The vidian artery joins the ICA at the genu and the vidian nerve originates over the petrous ICA where the greater superficial petrosal nerve joins the deep petrosal nerve.

The posterior edge of the lateral pterygoid plate can be followed directly to the foramen ovale and the third division of the trigeminal nerve. The mandibular nerve crosses over the petrous ICA laterally and the petrous ICA can be approached medial to the nerve with a transpterygoid

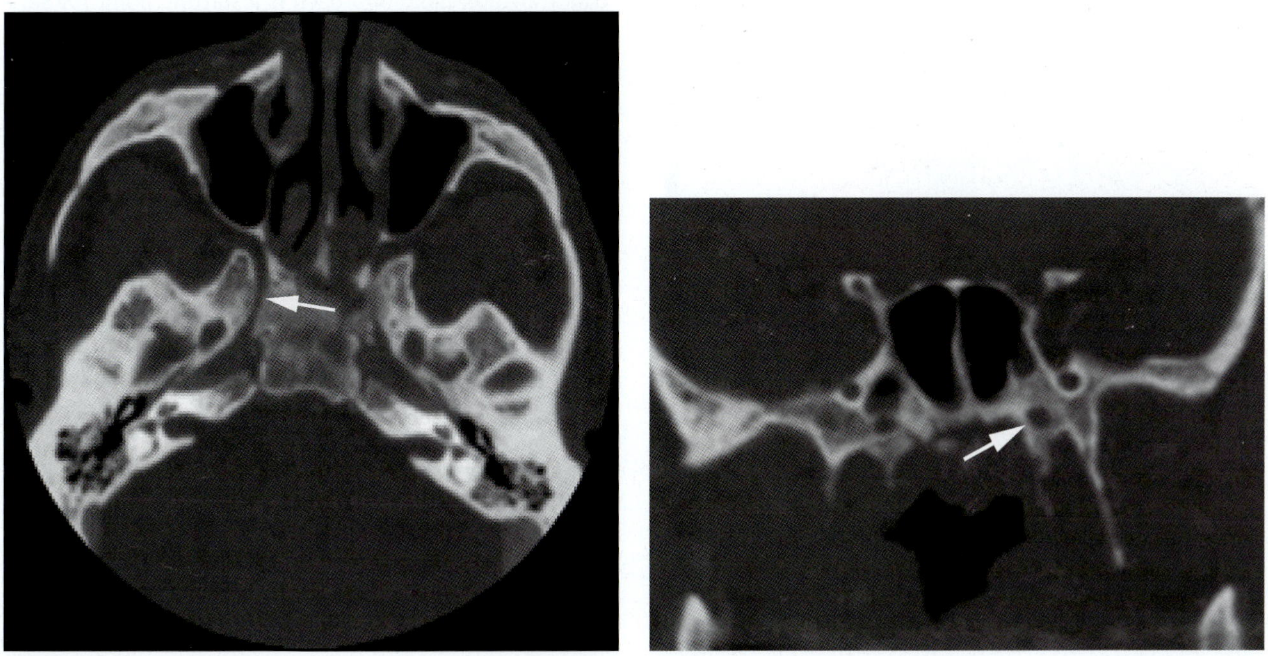

A B

Fig. 51.9 (A) Axial and **(B)** coronal views of the pterygoid canal (*arrows*), which transmits the vidian artery and nerve, is a useful landmark for exposure of the second genu of the internal carotid artery at the junction of the petrous and paraclival segments.

approach. The eustachian tube is also superficial and lateral to the petrous ICA and the cartilaginous portion must be resected to gain access to the parapharyngeal ICA. The parapharyngeal ICA enters the carotid canal posterior to the mandibular nerve and foramen ovale.

Surgical Technique

The patient is positioned at right angles to the anesthesia team with surgical access to the right side of the patient. The patient's head is fixed in a Mayfield clamp and the head is rotated slightly to the right with no significant flexion or extension. Following registration of the image guidance system, needle electrodes are placed for neuromonitoring of somatosensory-evoked potentials (cortical function). Electromyographic (EMG) monitoring of extraocular muscles is performed if dissection in proximity to the cavernous sinus or petrous apex (abducens nerve) is anticipated. Monitoring of brainstem function with brainstem-evoked responses is performed when there is significant brainstem compression or dissection of the vertebrobasilar vessels. The nasal cavity is decongested with 0.5% oxymetazoline solution on pledgets and systemic antibiotic prophylaxis is administered.

Septal Mucosal Flap[15]

Reconstruction of the surgical defect must be considered at the beginning of the operation so that the vascular pedicle of the septal flap is preserved. A septal mucosal flap is elevated on the side of the nasal septum opposite the side requiring the greatest exposure (**Fig. 51.10**). The sphenoid os is visualized and mucosal incisions are made with a needle-tip electrode. The superior incision extends from the os parallel to the skull base ~1 cm below the nasal vault and cribriform plate. The inferior incision extends from the bottom of the sphenoid rostrum along the posterior edge of the nasal septum to the nasal floor and runs anteriorly along the junction of the nasal septum and nasal floor. An anterior vertical incision ~1 cm posterior to the columella connects the superior and inferior incisions. The septal flap is then elevated in a submucoperichondrial/subperiosteal plane to the anterior face of the sphenoid sinus. The pedicle is mobilized laterally with preservation of the posterior septal artery. The flap is then displaced into the nasopharynx or maxillary sinus until it is needed for reconstruction.

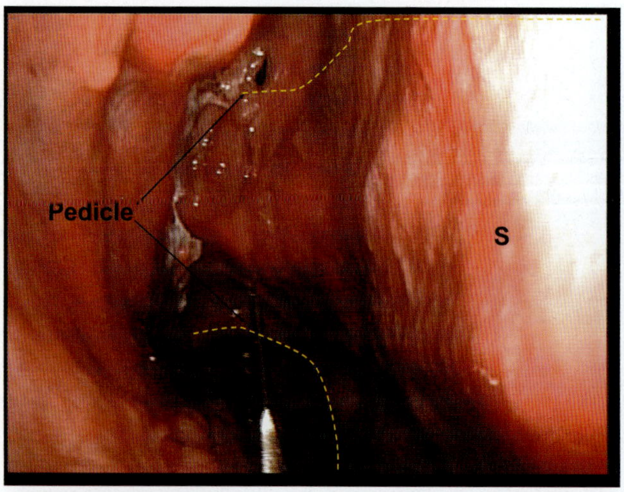

Fig. 51.10 The septal mucosal flap is pedicled on the posterior nasal artery, which is a distal branch of the sphenopalatine artery. The vascular pedicle is between the sphenoid ostium and the posterior choana. The flap can incorporate the entire mucoperichondrium/mucoperiosteum of the ipsilateral septal surface (S).

Bilateral Sphenoidotomy

Once the septal mucosal flap has been elevated, the posterior septum is disarticulated from the rostrum of the sphenoid bone. The bone of the rostrum is removed with a rongeur or drill to create an opening into the sphenoid sinus bilaterally. The sphenoidotomy is maximally enlarged to the margins of the sinus with Kerrison rongeurs so that all walls of the sinus are visible. Intrasinus septations are removed, with the realization that lateral septations lead to the carotid canal and the cavernous ICA may be dehiscent. Landmarks within the sinus are identified to provide orientation: sella, clival recess, paraclival ICA, cavernous ICA, optic canals, and lateral opticocarotid recesses.

Transpterygoid Approach[16,17]

The transpterygoid approach is a starting point for surgical approaches in the coronal plane of the ICA. A maxillary antrostomy is performed with removal of the uncinate process. The antrostomy is enlarged posteriorly and inferiorly. The lateral nasal wall is dissected in a subperiosteal plane posterior to the antrostomy, and the sphenopalatine foramen is identified posterosuperior to the crista ethmoidalis. The bone overlying the pterygopalatine space is then removed with a 1-mm angle Kerrison rongeur to expose the contents of the space. The sphenopalatine and posterior nasal arteries are transected and the contents of the pterygopalatine space are elevated from the underlying bone (base of the pterygoid plates) in a medial to lateral direction. This exposes the pterygoid canal containing the vidian artery and nerve. If a more lateral dissection is necessary, the vidian artery and nerve are cauterized and transected and additional subperiosteal dissection is performed laterally. The infraorbital nerve can be traced posteriorly from the roof of the maxillary sinus and the foramen rotundum is identified superolateral to the lateral recess of the sphenoid sinus. Additional bone can be removed from the lateral recess of the sphenoid sinus to maximize the exposure.

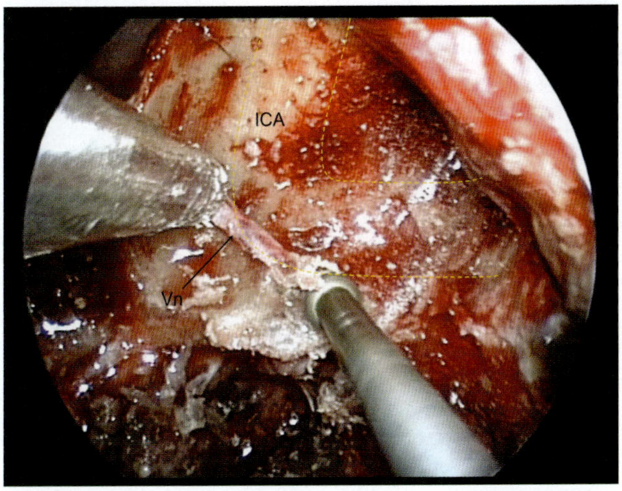

Fig. 51.11 A left transpterygoid approach with drilling of bone circumferentially around the vidian nerve (*Vn*). The course of the left internal carotid artery is outlined.

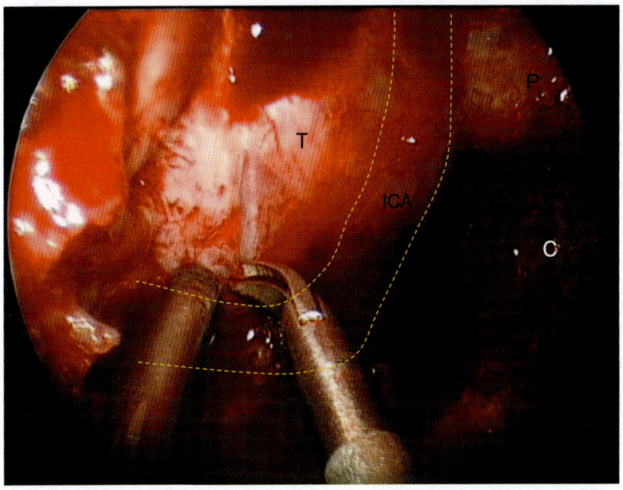

Fig. 51.12 Right suprapetrous approach with exposure of the dura overlying tumor (*T*) in the middle cranial fossa (Meckel's cave). The course of the right internal carotid artery is outlined. *P*, pituitary; *C*, clival recess.

Suprapetrous Approach

The bone surrounding the pterygoid canal is drilled with a 3-mm hybrid diamond bit to establish the depth of the second genu of the ICA (**Fig. 51.11**). The bone between the foramen rotundum and pterygoid canal is thinned with the drill to expose the dura of the middle cranial fossa. As one approaches the middle cranial fossa, the distance between the pterygoid canal and foramen rotundum narrows. The dura is now exposed superior to the petrous ICA and is lateral to the paraclival ICA (**Fig. 51.12**). These structures form the inferior and medial borders of the quadrangular space (Meckel's cave), respectively. The superior border is the abducens nerve and lateral portion of the cavernous sinus. The mandibular nerve is the lateral border. The dura is incised to access this space and the trigeminal nerve (**Fig. 51.13**).

Infrapetrous Approach

Following a bilateral sphenoidotomy, the mucosa and underlying longus capitis muscle are cauterized and resected to expose the clival bone inferior to the sphenoidotomy. Resection of soft tissue continues into the fossa of Rosenmüller on the side of the lesion. The position of the parapharyngeal ICA is visualized with image guidance; a tortuous ICA can deviate medially into the nasopharynx and be at risk for injury. The mucoperiosteum is elevated from the medial "wedge" of the medial pterygoid plate, and the anterior surface of the pterygoid plates is exposed. The genu of the petrous ICA is identified via a transpterygoid approach. The stump of the vidian artery marks the superior limit of the dissection. The base of the pterygoid plates is further drilled to expose the medial pterygoid muscle. The cartilaginous portion of the eustachian tube

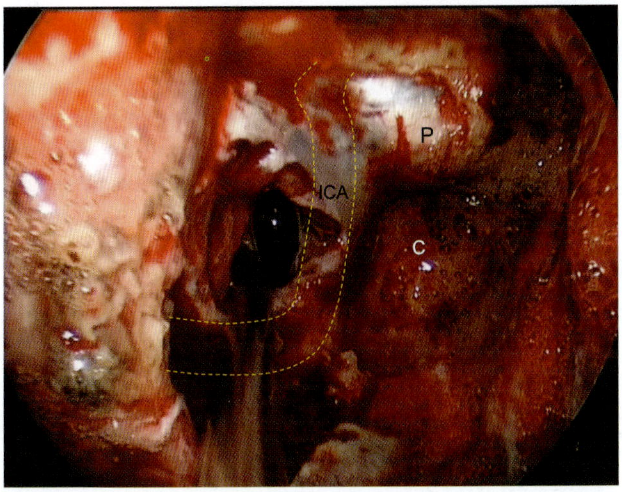

Fig. 51.13 Right suprapetrous approach with surgical defect in the middle cranial fossa (Meckel's cave). The course of the right internal carotid artery is outlined. *P*, pituitary; *C*, clival recess.

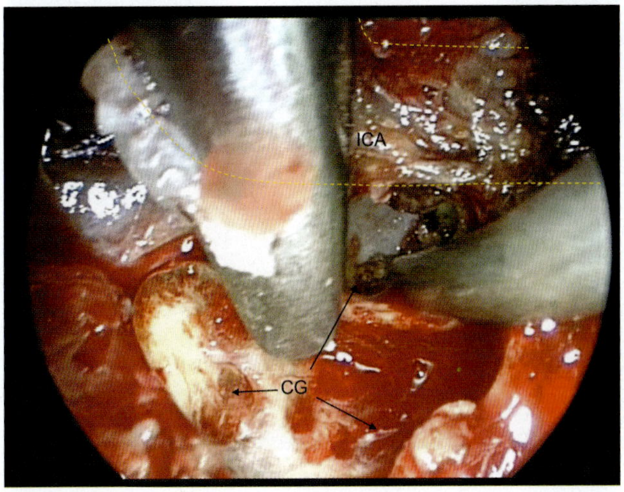

Fig. 51.14 Left infrapetrous approach with evacuation of cholesterol granuloma (*CG*). The course of the internal carotid artery is outlined.

is then resected, taking care to avoid deep scissor cuts that could injure the parapharyngeal ICA lateral to the fossa of Rosenmüller. At this point, the inferior surface of the petrous bone is exposed lateral to the clivus, inferior to the petrous ICA, and medial to the parapharyngeal ICA (**Fig. 51.14**). Image guidance is used to confirm the location of the petrous apex, and careful drilling deep to the petrous ICA allows entry into the air cells.

Reconstruction

If the dura is intact, surrounding bone edges are smoothed with the drill and the septal mucosal flap is transposed to cover the exposed dura and ICA (**Fig. 51.15**). The entire flap should be in contact with bone or soft tissue to avoid contracture and delayed healing. If there is a dural defect, it is first repaired with inlay and onlay fascial grafts, and the septal flap is transposed. The edges of the septal flap are covered with oxycellulose, and a synthetic glue or fibrin glue is applied. This is followed by a layer of absorbable hemostatic material and packing with expandable tampons or a balloon catheter to provide external support for 2 to 7 days. The exposed septal cartilage from the flap donor site is covered with a Silastic stent for 3 weeks.

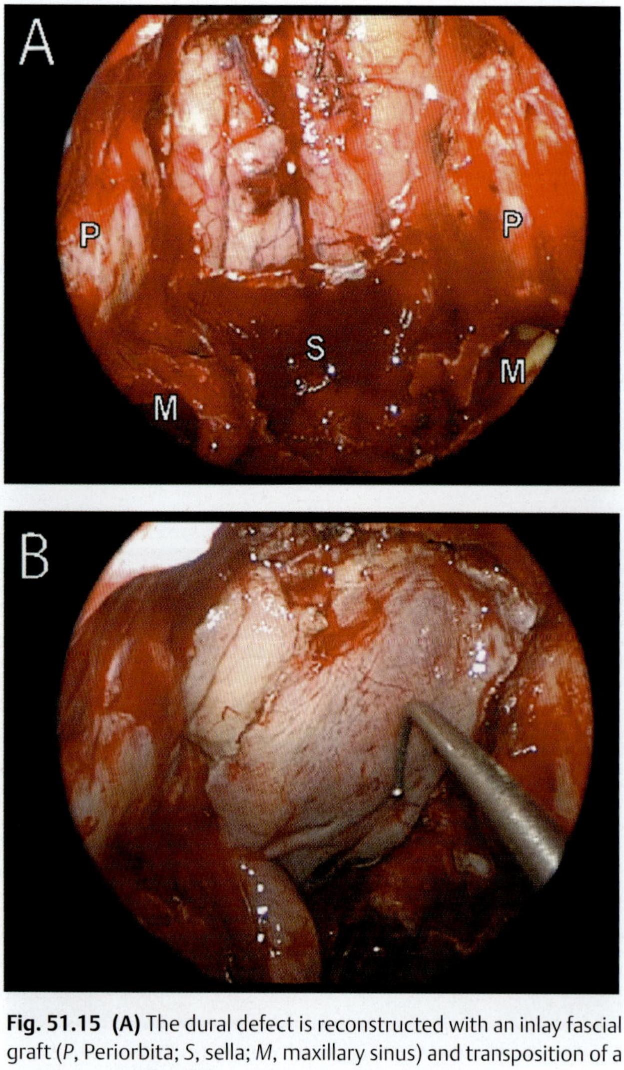

Fig. 51.15 (A) The dural defect is reconstructed with an inlay fascial graft (*P*, Periorbita; *S*, sella; *M*, maxillary sinus) and transposition of a septal mucosal flap **(B)**.

Complications

Complications that are not unique to the suprapetrous and infrapetrous approaches include CSF leaks and meningitis. The transpterygoid approach results in sacrifice of the sympathetic and parasympathetic nerves within the pterygopalatine space. Loss of the vidian nerve is usually not noticed but patients may admit to decreased tearing of the ipsilateral eye with emotional crying or windy conditions. Baseline tearing is usually not affected but could be a concern in patients who are elderly or already have dry eyes. Exposure of the pterygoid muscles and surrounding soft tissues increases the risk of postoperative cellulitis, and patients may develop significant pain and trismus that persists for weeks following surgery. Injury to sensory branches of the trigeminal nerve may result in palatal or facial numbness. Resection of the eustachian tube will result in a serous middle ear effusion that can be treated with a tympanostomy tube if there is no CSF leak.

Whenever there is extensive drilling and removal of bone around the paraclival ICA, there is a risk of injury to the abducens nerve in Dorello's canal posteromedially. During suprapetrous approaches, the sixth cranial nerve can also be injured if dissection is performed above the level of V2 where the abducens nerve runs parallel to V1 inside the cavernous sinus to enter the superior orbital fissure.

The hypoglossal nerve is at risk with inferior extensions during infrapetrous approaches. The hypoglossal canal is located superolateral to the occipital condyle. Intraoperative EMG monitoring can be very helpful in identifying the nerve before injury occurs. Cranial nerves IX and X are also susceptible to injury with posterolateral extension of the infrapetrous approach to the region of the jugular foramen.

The greatest concern with the suprapetrous and infrapetrous approaches is injury to the ICA. This can be avoided with secure knowledge of the anatomic relationships, use of image guidance, proper dissection technique, and realistic surgical goals. Wide exposure of the skull base is necessary to visualize the anatomic landmarks and to have unimpeded access to instruments. It is especially important to have good tactile feedback from the drill bit when drilling around the carotid canal. Drilling should always follow the course of the ICA and should be done with a diamond bit. In the event of a vascular injury, a wide exposure provides the room necessary to deal with the hemorrhage. In the event of a vascular injury, the goal should be to control the bleeding with a focal pack at the site of the injury and then evaluate the patient with angiography. It is helpful to direct the blood up the tip of the suction so that it does not squirt onto the tip of the endoscope, obscuring the view. Surrounding bone can be removed to better visualize the injury. Direct suture repair of a laceration is technically feasible but is unlikely to be successful. A very small hole can often be "welded" shut with bipolar electrocautery but should be reinforced with a fascial graft. Hemostatic materials applied to the wall of the artery may be helpful but will require additional packing. If preoperative testing has determined that a sacrifice of the ICA will be tolerated, aneurysm clips can be placed on both sides of the injury. Blood pressure should be maintained throughout the surgery and in the postoperative period to prevent cerebral ischemia from decreased cerebral blood flow. If an angiography demonstrates a pseudoaneurysm, treatment options include endovascular stenting or sacrifice of the ICA.

Postoperative Care

Patients are monitored in an intensive care unit or intermediate unit for at least 24 hours in case of a neurologic complication. A postoperative CT scan of the head without contrast is obtained within 12 hours to rule out intracranial hemorrhage or significant pneumocephalus. If tumor resection is subtotal, an early MRI is helpful in quantifying the amount of residual tumor. A lumbar spinal drain to lower CSF pressures is not routinely used.

In the absence of an intraoperative CSF leak, nasal packing is removed in 1 to 2 days. In the presence of a CSF leak, packing is removed in 5 to 7 days. Patients receive antibiotic prophylaxis until the packing is removed. Once nasal packing is removed, gentle use of a nasal saline spray is instituted. Patients are instructed to avoid activities that increase CSF pressure such as nose blowing, heavy lifting, bending over, and stifling a sneeze. Patients are seen 1 to 2 weeks after surgery, and minimal debridement of the nasal cavity is performed. More aggressive irrigations of the nasal cavity with a saline flush are instituted several weeks after surgery. Septal splints are removed 3 weeks after surgery and patients are instructed to apply ointment to the healing septum. Periodic visits at monthly intervals allow for the endoscopic debridement of nasal crusts until healing is complete (3 to 4 months). Postoperative trismus can be treated with anti-inflammatory medication or a

Table 51.3 Intraoperative Complications After Endoscopic Endonasal Surgeries in 800 Patients

Category	Consequence	• Type of Lesion and/ or Deficit
Vascular (0.9%)	Death (0%)	• ∅
	Transient deficit (0.1%)	• P1 perforator
	Permanent deficit (0.4%)	• Pontine bleed (quadriplegic) • IMA laceration (hemiplegic) • Frontopolar avulsion (R lower limb paresis)
	No deficit (0.4%)	• One ophthalmic (already blind) • Two ICA lacerations
Neural Injury (2.2%)	Transient deficit (1.5%)	• III nerve (2 cases) • V3 motor (1 case) • VI nerve (4 cases) • IX, X (1 case) • Hemiparesis (4 cases)
	Permanent deficit (0.7%)	• II -vision deterioration (2 cases) • IX, X, XII (1 case) • IX, X (1 case) • VI (2 cases)

Abbreviations: IMA, internal maxillary artery; ICA, internal carotid artery; R, right.

Table 51.4 Postoperative Complications After Endoscopic Endonasal Surgeries in 800 Patients*

Category	Consequence	Type of Complication
Infection (1.4%)	Death (0.1%)	• Meningitis + status epilepticus (1 case)
	Successfully treated (1.1%)	• Intradural abscess (1 case) • Extradural abscess (1 case) • Meningitis (7 cases)
	Deficit (0.1%)	• Intradural abscess – incapacitated (1 case)
Systemic (2.8%)	Death (0.7%)	• PE <30d (2 case) • PE >30d (2 cases) • Pneumonia + MI <30d (1 case) • Multiorgan failure > 30 days (1 case)
	Successfully treated (2.1%)	• Acute renal failure transfusion (1 case) • Respiratory failure (7 cases) • PE <30d (5 case) • MI (3 cases) • Immediate postop asystole (1 case)
Delayed Deficit* (1.6%)	Permanent deficit (0.4%)	• Unilateral blindness (late hypotension) 1 case • Hemiplegia (postoperative) 1 case • Visual deficit (hematoma) 1 case
	Transient deficit (1.2%)	• Visual deficit (encephalocele) 1 case • Visual deficit (hematoma) 4 cases • Visual deficit (nasal balloon) 2 cases • III nerve (hematoma) 1 case • Proptosis (retrobulbar hematoma) 1 case • Ataxia (orogastric tube complication) 1 case

Abbreviations: PE, pulmonary embolism; MI, myocardium infarct; d, days.
*There were 5 patients who had seizures during the postoperative period with no sequelae.

Therabite appliance if severe. Patients who complain of a dry eye are evaluated by an ophthalmologist.

Outcomes

Over the last decade, the authors have performed more than 1500 completely endonasal skull base procedures. During the first 4 to 5 years of our experience, the majority of cases were level II and III procedures: CSF leaks, pituitary tumors with minimal extrasellar extension, and extradural skull base procedures. Increased comfort with hemostatic[18] and reconstructive techniques,[19,20] an improved understanding of endonasal skull base anatomy, and the development of endonasal instruments enabled progression to more demanding level IV and V procedures with intradural dissection and exposure of the ICA in the coronal plane. Due to the diverse types of pathologies encountered in the skull base, it is difficult to provide outcomes data on large series of individual tumor types at this time.

Two tumor types that usually involve significant coronal plane exposure and dissection are schwannomas and chordomas. Between 2003 and 2009, 17 nonvestibular schwannomas underwent resection via endoscopic endonasal approach (EEA; three combined with open approaches) at our institution.[21] Eighty percent of patients underwent near ($n = 3$) or gross total ($n = 9$) resection. There were no postoperative CSF leaks in this series. Sixty patients underwent EEA for chordoma between 2003 and 2011. Eighty-three percent of primary tumors underwent gross total resection (GTR) (67% overall). Lower lateral clival extension (coronal plane) was a significant factor that adversely influenced GTR. In addition, GTR rates improved over time, demonstrating a learning curve with this tumor. There was a 20% CSF leak rate in this series.

Major complications have been remarkably rare considering the potential risks of surgery (**Tables 51.3 and 51.4**). The incidence of postoperative CSF leaks in our last 150 prospective endonasal surgeries reconstructed with a septal mucosal flap is 4%.[22] The incidence of bacterial meningitis is less than 2%.[23] We have observed six ICA injuries (0.4%) in our cumulative experience: two pituitary adenomas, three chondroid tumors, and one adenoid cystic carcinoma. Four patients had their ICA sacrificed either intraoperatively or postoperatively without neurologic sequelae. Two ICAs were preserved. All bleeding was controlled intraoperatively. There was one postoperative death due to cardiac ischemia. Other major vascular injuries are noted in **Table 51.3**.

Conclusion

Extended applications of endoscopic endonasal skull base surgery provide access to the entire ventral skull base and can be organized along sagittal and coronal planes. In the coronal plane, surgical approaches are categorized based on their relationship to the ICA. A strong foundation in endoscopic surgical anatomy and proper surgical technique allow safe dissection in this plane. Clinical series have demonstrated the safety and oncologic efficacy of extended applications of endoscopic endonasal surgery for multiple skull base pathologies. Proper training in endoscopic endonasal techniques using an incremental training program is essential for success.

References

1. Mehta RP, Cueva RA, Brown JD, et al. What's new in skull base medicine and surgery? Skull Base Committee Report. Otolaryngol Head Neck Surg 2006;135(4):620–630
2. Kassam AB, Snyderman CH, Mintz A, Gardner PA, Carrau RL. Expanded endonasal approach: the rostrocaudal axis. Part I. Crista galli to the sella turcica. Neurosurg Focus 2005;19(1):E3 http://www.aans.org/education/journal/neurosurgical/July05/19-1-3.pdf
3. Kassam AB, Snyderman CH, Mintz A, Gardner PA, Carrau RL. Expanded endonasal approach: the rostrocaudal axis. Part II. Posterior clinoids to the foramen magnum. Neurosurg Focus 2005;19(1):E4 http://www.aans.org/education/journal/neurosurgical/July05/19-1-4.pdf
4. Kassam AB, Gardner PA, Snyderman CH, Mintz A, Carrau RL. Expanded endonasal approach: fully endoscopic, completely transnasal approach to the middle third of the clivus, petrous bone, middle cranial fossa, and infratemporal fossa. Neurosurg Focus 2005;19(1):E6 http://www.aans.org/education/journal/neurosurgical/July05/19-1-6.pdf
5. Snyderman CH, Kassam A, Carrau R, Mintz A, Gardner P, Prevedello DM. Acquisition of surgical skills for endonasal skull base surgery: a training program. Laryngoscope 2007;117(4):699–705
6. Bhatki A, Pant H, Snyderman C, et al. The expanded endonasal approach for the treatment of anterior skull base tumors. Otolaryngol Head Neck Surg 2010;21(1):66–73
7. Kassam AB, Prevedello DM, Thomas A, et al. Endoscopic endonasal pituitary transposition for a transdorsum sellae approach to the interpeduncular cistern. Neurosurgery 2008;62(3, Suppl 1): 57–72, discussion 72–74
8. Gardner PA, Prevedello DM, Kassam AB, Snyderman CH, Carrau RL, Mintz AH. The evolution of the endonasal approach for craniopharyngiomas. J Neurosurg 2008;108(5):1043–1047
9. Snyderman CH, Kassam AB, Carrau RL, Mintz A. Endoscopic approaches to the petrous apex. Otolaryngol Head Neck Surg 2006;17(3):168–173
10. Kassam AB, Gardner PA, Snyderman C, et al. Endoscopic, expanded endonasal approach to the jugular foramen. Otolaryngol Head Neck Surg 2005;8(Issue 1):35–41
11. Gardner PA, Kassam AB, Spiro R, et al. Endoscopic endonasal approach to the odontoid. In: Mummaneni P, Kanter A, Wang M, Haid R, eds. Cervical Spine Surgery: Current Trends and Challenges. St. Louis: Quality Medical Publishing; 2009
12. Kassam AB, Mintz AH, Gardner PA, Horowitz MB, Carrau RL, Snyderman CH. The expanded endonasal approach for an endoscopic transnasal clipping and aneurysmorrhaphy of a large vertebral artery aneurysm: technical case report. Neurosurgery 2006; 59(1, Suppl 1):E162–E165, discussion E162–E165
13. Kassam AB, Thomas AJ, Zimmer LA, et al. Expanded endonasal approach: a fully endoscopic completely transnasal resection of a skull base arteriovenous malformation. Childs Nerv Syst 2007;23(5):491–498

14. Vescan AD, Snyderman CH, Carrau RL, et al. Vidian canal: analysis and relationship to the internal carotid artery. Laryngoscope 2007;117(8):1338–1342
15. Hadad G, Bassagasteguy L, Carrau RL, et al. A novel reconstructive technique after endoscopic expanded endonasal approaches: vascular pedicle nasoseptal flap. Laryngoscope 2006;116(10): 1882–1886
16. Fortes FS, Sennes LU, Carrau RL, et al. Endoscopic anatomy of the pterygopalatine fossa and the transpterygoid approach: development of a surgical instruction model. Laryngoscope 2008; 118(1):44–49
17. Gardner PA, Kassam AB, Carrau RL, Snyderman CH, Mintz A. The endoscopic, endonasal transpterygoid approach. In: Practical Endoscopic Skull Base Surgery. San Diego, CA: Plural Publishing; 2007: 163–174
18. Kassam AB, Snyderman CH, Carrau RL, Gardner PA, Mintz A. Endoneurosurgical hemostasis techniques: lessons learned from 400 cases. Neurosurg Focus 2005;19(1):E7
19. Bhatki A, Pant H, Snyderman C, et al. Reconstruction of the cranial base after endonasal skull base surgery: local tissue flaps. Otolaryngol Head Neck Surg 2010;21(1):74–82
20. Bhatki A, Pant H, Snyderman C, et al. Reconstruction of the cranial base following endonasal skull base surgery: regional tissue flaps. Otolaryngol Head Neck Surg 2010;21(1):83–90
21. Shin SS, Gardner PA, Stefko ST, Madhok R, Fernandez-Miranda JC, Snyderman CH. Expanded endoscopic endonasal approach for non-vestibular schwannomas. Neurosurgery [accepted for publication March 2011]
22. Zanation AM, Carrau RL, Snyderman CH, et al. Nasoseptal flap reconstruction of high flow intraoperative cerebral spinal fluid leaks during endoscopic skull base surgery. Am J Rhinol Allergy 2009;23(5):518–521
23. Kono Y, Prevedello DM, Snyderman CH, et al. One thousand endoscopic skull base surgical procedures demystifying the infection potential: incidence and description of postoperative meningitis and brain abscesses. Infect Control Hosp Epidemiol 2011;32(1):77–83

52 Endoscopic Skull Base Reconstruction

Adam M. Zanation, Mihir R. Patel, Ricardo L. Carrau, and Daniel M. Prevedello

Over the past 10 years, significant anatomic, technical, and instrumentation advances have facilitated the exposure and resection of intradural lesions via a fully endoscopic expanded endonasal approach (EEA). This chapter describes our sequential learning from our initial free tissue grafting reconstructive techniques, advancing to our current vascularized flaps. Outcomes and limitations of the current endoscopic reconstructive techniques are discussed. This chapter does not discuss idiopathic cerebrospinal fluid (CSF) leaks because those are covered in Chapter 44.

The goals of reconstructing defects produced by the EEA are identical to those of reconstructing conventional external approaches: to completely separate the cranial cavity from the sinonasal tract, eliminate dead space, and preserve neurovascular and ocular function.[1] The underlying principle of multilayered reconstruction to reestablish tissue barriers is also the same as traditional open techniques. Using endonasal pedicled vascular flaps and a reconstruction based on the aforementioned principles, we have been able to reduce our postoperative CSF leak rates below 5%, which is comparable with that reported for open cranial base reconstructive techniques.

■ Endoscopic Reconstruction with Free Tissue Grafts

Prior to the adoption of the vascularized tissue flaps as our primary reconstructive technique (see later text) skull base reconstruction after EEA (i.e., large skull base defects) was limited to the use of free tissue grafts. These techniques were adapted from experience accumulated with the endoscopic repair of CSF leaks associated with endoscopic sinus surgery and trauma,[2] and then expanded to repair larger dural defects as well as high-flow CSF leaks. A monolayer free tissue graft, placed onlay or inlay, results in a successful repair of a small CSF fistula in over 95% of the cases. However, when this technique was applied to larger defects, such as those created during endoscopic skull base surgery, we encountered a significant increase in postoperative CSF leaks. After experimenting with different variations of the technique, we deemed that a multilayer approach seemed advantageous for a successful endoscopic dural reconstruction of large defects.

First, a subdural inlay graft (between the brain and the dura) of collagen matrix is placed; this helps to obliterate the intradural dead space and helps to contain the flow of CSF. Its pliability and texture allows for its safe manipulation around neurovascular structures. Ideally, this subdural graft should extend 5 to 10 mm beyond the dural margins in all directions. A subsequent inlay graft of acellular dermis or fascia is placed in the epidural space (between the dura and the skull base). Occasionally, the bony ledges are not adequate to support an inlay graft; therefore, the acellular dermal graft is placed extracranially (at the nasal side of the defect) as an onlay graft. It is of utmost importance that all the periphery of the defect is denuded of mucosa to allow for the revascularization of the graft (i.e., take) and to avoid mucocele formation. Alternatively, this graft can be sutured to the dura with nitinol U-clips (Medtronic, Minneapolis, MN); however, their use is technically challenging and requires an adequate dural cuff to anchor the graft. U-clips prevent migration of the graft, yet they do not result in a watertight suture line.

Although this is an off-label indication for the acellular dermal graft, we found that its handling characteristics, its availability (no need for skin graft harvesting), and ingrowth of the patient's own tissue with rapid epithelialization are advantages that outweigh its cost in many patients. It is important to use a single graft with dimensions that will extend beyond the defect margins in all directions, and that the graft is adequately hydrated in normal saline solution prior to its insertion. In our experience, a thinner graft offers the best take, although it is somewhat difficult to manipulate endonasally.

Once both grafts are in place, the edges of the acellular dermal graft are bolstered intranasally with oxidized cellulose (absorbable hemostatic dressing), a biologic or synthetic glue is sprayed or applied over the edges, and absorbable gelatin sponge squares are used to further bolster the reconstruction. These layers of absorbable packing accomplish three goals. First, they fix the free tissue grafts in place and protect them from changes in airflow and pressure within the nose. Second, they serve as "filler" to flatten the concavities and convexities of the skull base; therefore, allowing an even distribution of the pressure applied by a removable packing (expandable sponges, gauze strip, or Foley catheter balloon). Third, the last layer of gelatin sponges is nonadherent; thus, it prevents traction or sliding of the grafts during removal of the packing 3 to 5 days postoperatively. Most frequently, the authors use the balloon of a 12-French Foley catheter or 10-cm expandable sponge packing to stabilize and bolster the inlay/onlay grafts, and to prevent early brain herniation. It should be noted that this only occurs during the early postoperative period when there may be a brain edema or if the patient develops high ventricular pressure, which will push the brain parenchyma through a bony defect; therefore, a permanent bolster, such a bone, cartilage, or titanium mesh seem unnecessary.

Placement of the packing and inflation of the catheter balloon is also performed under endoscopic vision. Overinflation of the balloon may result in compressive effects over neurovascular structures. If the optic nerves or chiasm are exposed during the dissection, then a balloon packing is avoided as it may exert excessive pressure on these structures. Under these circumstances, the authors advocate the use of an expandable sponge packing in lieu of the balloon. Any nasal packing or balloon is removed 3 to 5 days after the EEA.

For small- to moderate-sized skull base defects, the authors have also used an onlay free mucosal graft harvested from the resected middle turbinate instead of fascia or an acellular dermal graft. The remainder of the reconstructive procedure is as described previously. The take of free mucoperiosteal grafts is excellent; however, they are limited by their surface area and by the fact that they can only be placed as an onlay. Lastly, abdominal free fat is used mainly as a bolster or biologic dressing to the multilayered reconstruction. Fat is also used to obliterate spaces such as the clival recess or the nasopharyngeal defect after a transnasal approach to the anterior spine. Harvesting abdominal fat has the added morbidity of an abdominal incision, scar, and the potential for infection, hematoma, or seroma formation.

Endoscopic reconstructions with multilayered free tissue grafts for larger dural defects during skull base tumor cases resulted in postoperative CSF leak rates of 20 to 30%.[3] These leaks were usually managed with further endoscopic bolstering of the reconstruction, additional free fat grafting, and some required CSF diversion with a lumbar spinal drain for 3 to 5 days (see later for further details). Endoscopic revisions made evident that the vast majority of postoperative CSF leaks were due to graft migration or CSF fistula formation in the most dependent area of the flap. It is important to note that almost all postoperative fistulas were managed endoscopically and resulted in no permanent sequelae or ascending meningitis. Only one of our first 400 EEA patients had to undergo an open reconstruction for a persistent CSF leak. This patient had undergone chemoradiotherapy for a sinonasal malignancy, and the remaining blood supply to the nose was inadequate to sustain the take of the grafts. The overall incidence of meningitis in the first 400 EEAs was less than 3%, which is on par with the incidence associated with open skull base techniques. However, we deemed that a CSF leak rate of 20 to 30% was unacceptable, therefore propelling us to assess vascularized tissue options.

Endoscopic Reconstruction with Vascular Pedicled Flaps

Nasoseptal Flap (Hadad-Bassagasteguy Flap)

During the past 5 years, a vascular pedicle flap has become our preferred reconstructive technique for defects resulting from endoscopic skull base surgery. Most commonly, we use a vascular flap of the nasal septum mucoperiosteum and mucoperichondrium pedicled on the nasoseptal artery, a branch of the posterior septal artery, which is one of the terminal branches of the internal maxillary artery.[3]

The nasal cavity is decongested with oxymetazoline 0.05% on pledgets and the anterior nasal septum is infiltrated with lidocaine 0.5 to 1% with epinephrine 1:100,000 to 1:200,000. The inferior and middle turbinates are out-fractured to allow for visualization of the entire height of the nasal septum from the olfactory sulcus to the nasal floor. To facilitate a bimanual technique during the EEA, we usually remove the right middle turbinate. In addition, resection of the middle turbinate facilitates the visualization of the nasoseptal flap (NSF) vascular pedicle and ipsilateral elevation of the septal flap. The side of the flap harvesting (right or left) is determined by several factors. First, if the lesion requires dissection of the lateral pterygoid recess or the pterygomaxillary fossa, the vascular supply of the flap will be compromised; thus, the flap is harvested from the opposite side. Similarly, lesions that invade the rostrum of the sphenoid or the septal mucoperiosteum will mandate harvesting an NSF on the contralateral side. If the lesion is median, and no significant lateral dissection is required, then sharp or large septal spurs (placing a risk for laceration of the flap during dissection) may dictate the side from which the flap is harvested. Lastly, the right side is usually an easier dissection for the right-handed surgeon, especially in the setting of removal of the right middle turbinate. The flap may be designed according to the size and shape of the anticipated defect. It is best, however, to harvest the largest possible flap, then trim it if needed (rarely necessary). Two parallel incisions are performed following the sagittal plane of the septum, one over the maxillary crest and the other 1 to 2 cm below the most superior aspect of the septum (this preserves the olfactory epithelium) (**Figs. 52.1, 52.2, and 52.3A,B**).

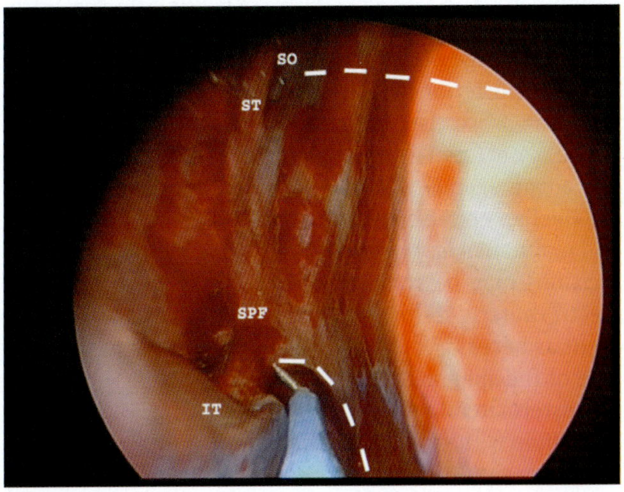

Fig. 52.1 Planned incisions around the pedicle of the nasoseptal flap. *IT*, inferior turbinate; *ST*, superior turbinate; *SO*, sphenoid ostium; *SPF*, mucosa over the sphenopalatine foramen.

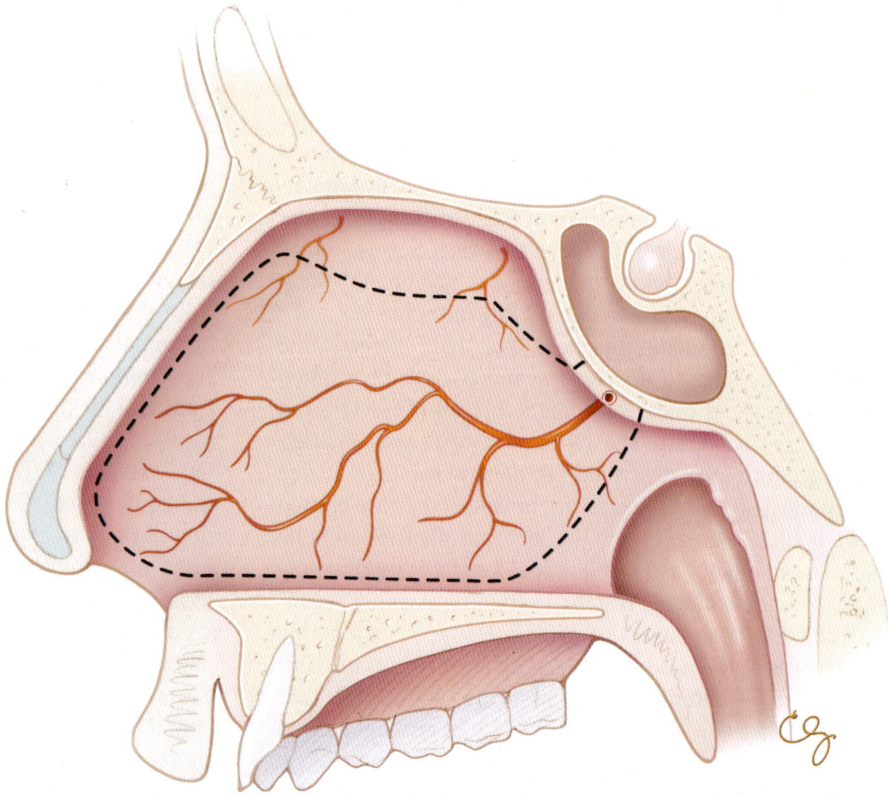

Fig. 52.2 Nasoseptal flap incisions: superiorly from the natural ostium of the sphenoid sinus and inferiorly along the choana to the nasal floor. The flap is supplied by the posterior nasal artery as shown.

These incisions are joined anteriorly by a vertical incision at a level that is always anterior to the anterior head of the inferior turbinate (**Fig. 52.3C**). To harvest the largest possible area, this incision is placed at the mucocutaneous junction of the columella. These incisions may be modified to account for the specific area of reconstruction or to allow for adequate oncologic margins. Posteriorly, the superior incision is extended laterally with an inferior slant and crosses the rostrum of the sphenoid sinus horizontally at the level of the natural ostium (**Fig. 52.1**). The inferior incision is extended superiorly parallel to the posterior free edge of the nasal septum and then laterally to cross the posterior choana toward the lateral nasal wall. Its elevation proceeds in an anteroposterior direction using a Cottle dissector or a small suction dissector (**Fig. 52.3D,E**). It is advantageous to complete all incisions before elevating the flap because it may be difficult to orient the tissue and maintain it at tension once it has been elevated. Septal incisions may be completed with a needle-tip insulated electrocautery, scalpel, scissors, or any other sharp instrument as necessary. Elevation of the flap from the anterior face of the sphenoid sinus is completed while preserving its posterolateral neurovascular pedicle (**Fig. 52.3F**).

The flap is then placed in the nasopharynx or inside the maxillary sinus until it is needed for reconstruction at the end of the resection. Multiple modifications of the flap regarding length and width are possible. The entire ipsilateral mucoperiosteum and mucoperichondrium may be harvested to cover anterior skull base defects as extensive as those that include the area from the posterior wall of the frontal sinus to the sella turcica and from orbit to orbit. A wider flap may be harvested by extending the incision to include the mucoperiosteum of the floor of the nose. A radioanatomic study of the nasoseptal flap compared the relative size of the anterior skull base to the size of the potential nasoseptal flaps, and demonstrated that most anterior skull base defects can be completely covered with the nasoseptal flap (**Fig. 52.4**).[4,5]

Additional considerations must be taken into account when reconstructing pediatric skull base defects with the NSF. It is clear that before the age of 10, the NSF area is significantly smaller than the area of large, age corresponding skull base defects (such as a transcribiform defect). Between the ages of 10 and 14 years, the NSF area approaches, but is not larger than, the size of the defect.[5] This is due to the fact that cranial growth occurs earlier in life, and septal growth does not occur until around puberty when midface growth accelerates.[5] Bilateral flaps are conceptually possible; however, they are rarely used. During surgery, it is important to be careful with bone removal lateral to the pterygoid canal so that the vascular pedicle is not injured.

Once the extirpative portion of the procedure is complete (**Fig. 52.5A**), a multilayer cranial base repair is performed. An inlay collagen matrix is placed as previously described (**Fig. 52.5B**). The NSF is then placed as an onlay

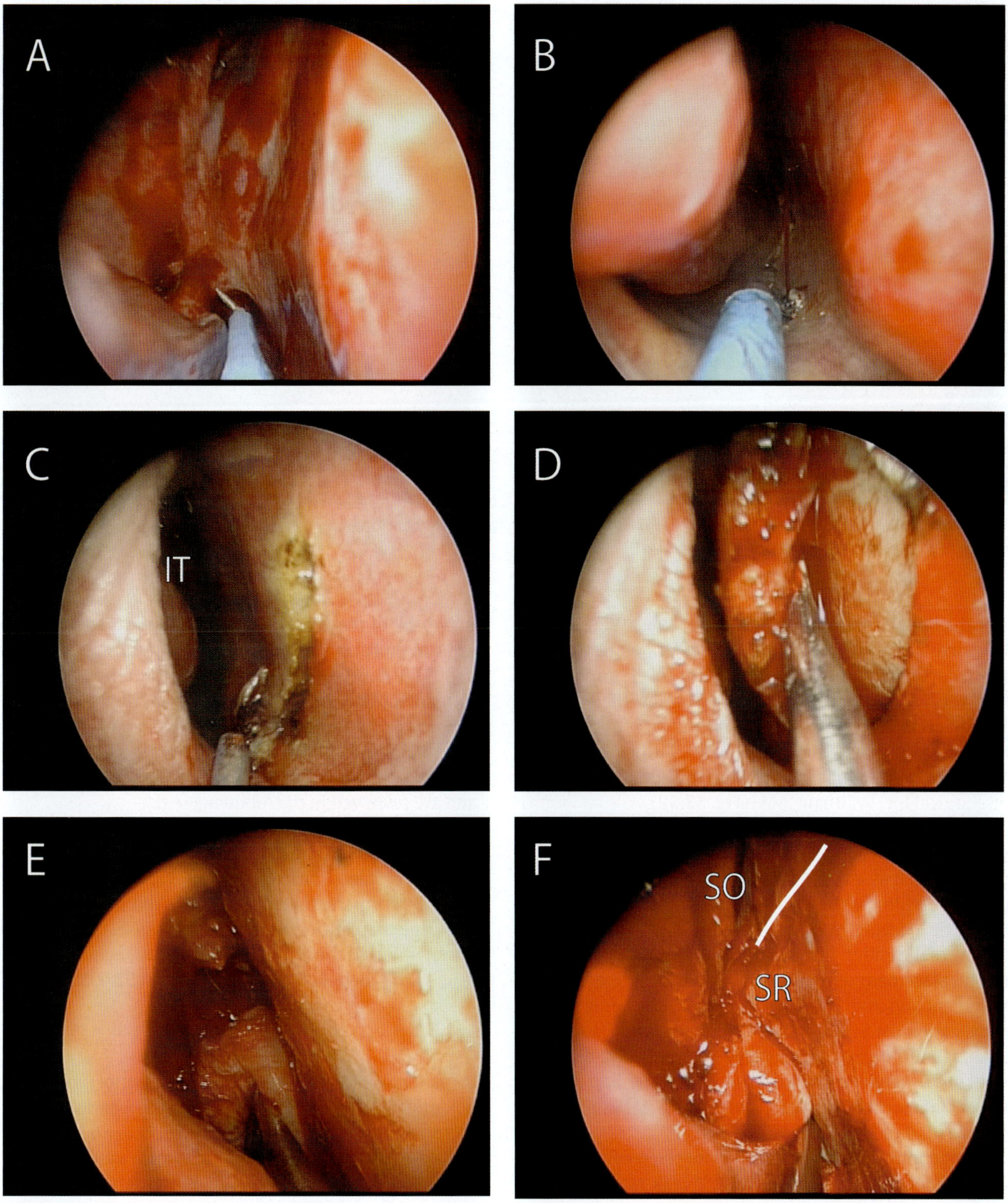

Fig. 52.3 Intraoperative dissection of nasoseptal flap (aka Hadad-Bassagasteguy flap). **(A)** Starting the incision crossing the posterior choana. **(B)** Continuing the inferior incision along the nasal floor. **(C)** Connecting the inferior and superior incisions via a vertical incision anterior to the inferior turbinate *(IT)*. **(D)** Starting to dissect the anterior nasoseptal flap. **(E)** Continuing to dissect the nasoseptal flap from the underlying septal cartilage. **(F)** Final posterior dissection of the flap along the area of the pedicle over the sphenoid rostrum (*SR*). The *white line* represents the area of the superior incision as it continues right below the sphenoid ostium (*SO*).

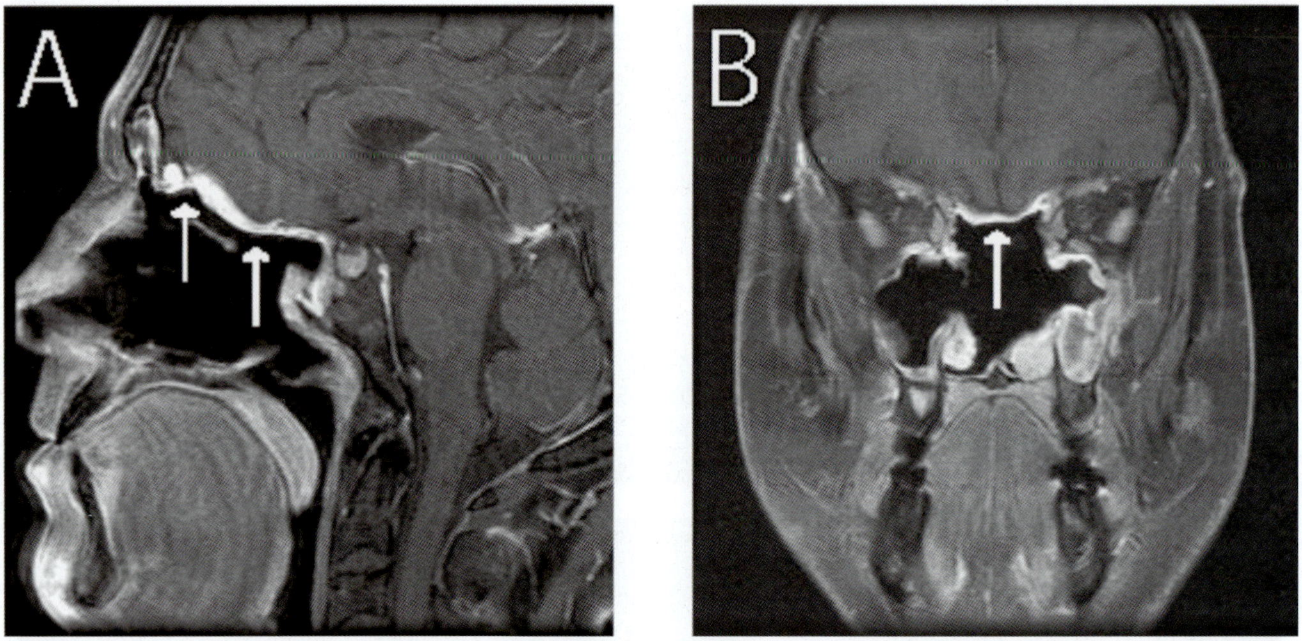

Fig. 52.4 Postoperative sagittal **(A)** and coronal **(B)** T1 with contrast magnetic resonance image; an anterior transcribriform skull base resection with excellent nasoseptal flap reconstruction (*arrows*).

over the bony edges of the cranial base defect (**Fig. 52.5C**). All mucosa is removed around the defect before the flap is placed to prevent nonhealing or mucocele formation. After the collagen graft and flap are in place, the edges of the flap are bolstered intranasally with oxidized cellulose absorbable packing (**Fig. 52.5D**) and further stabilized with a synthetic or biologic glue, such as DuraSeal (Confluent Surgical Inc, Waltham, MA) (**Fig. 52.5E**).

As previously mentioned, it is critical to separate the grafts from the packing using some type of nonadherent material, such as an absorbable gelatin sponge or absorbable gelatin film, as this will prevent traction on the grafts when the packing is removed (**Fig. 52.5F**). In addition, shifting of the underlying inlay/onlay grafts may occur during the placement of the packing; thus, the surgeon must be vigilant and insert the packing under direct endoscopic visualization. Packing consists of either a Foley balloon or expandable sponges as previously described. Sealants are never used between the grafts or under the flap as this prevents direct tissue contact and healing. Packing is kept in place for 3 to 5 days.

After adopting the nasoseptal flap for the reconstruction of EEA defects, our postoperative CSF leak rates dropped to less than 5% for all endonasal defects, a rate that compares with the those of traditional open techniques.[3,6] In a prospective series of 70 NSF skull base reconstructions for high-flow leaks with large dural defects (either cisterns or a ventricle was widely opened into the nasal cavity during the dissection), the postoperative leak rate was 5.7% (4/70).[7] Advantages of the NSF as a reconstructive option include that a second approach or incision is not necessary and that the flap can be harvested endoscopically. A major drawback of the NSF is that its need must be anticipated prior to embarking on the resection because the vascular pedicle of this flap is frequently compromised during the sphenoidotomy and posterior septectomy. In addition, if a revision procedure is necessary, the flap may have been used previously or the pedicle previously damaged; therefore, other endonasal pedicled flaps have been described and are reviewed in the following text.

In select revision cases, the NSF can be dissected from the defect and reused. In a series of 20 NSF takedowns and reuses for staged procedures or recurrence, only one of 20 (5%) reconstructions leaked.[8] We did not encounter a nonviable flap during takedown and reuse. Healing of the intranasal dissection and nasoseptal flap reconstruction is usually complete in 6 to 12 weeks (**Figs. 52.4, 52.6**).

Posterior Pedicled Inferior Turbinate Flap

In patients with prior septectomy or prior wide sphenoidotomies, the NSF blood supply has been interrupted; therefore, this option is not available. Other options, such as free grafting or other local or regional vascular pedicle flaps, have to be considered. The posterior pedicle inferior turbinate flap (PPITF) is based on the inferior turbinate artery, a terminal branch of the posterior lateral nasal artery (PLNA), which arises from the sphenopalatine artery (SPA).[9] Its design and harvesting requires the understanding of the anatomic course of the PLNA.[9] The PLNA runs in a descending vertical or anteroinferior course over the perpendicular plate of the ascending process of the palatine bone, giving a branch medially to supply the middle turbinate. As the artery courses inferiorly, it enters the

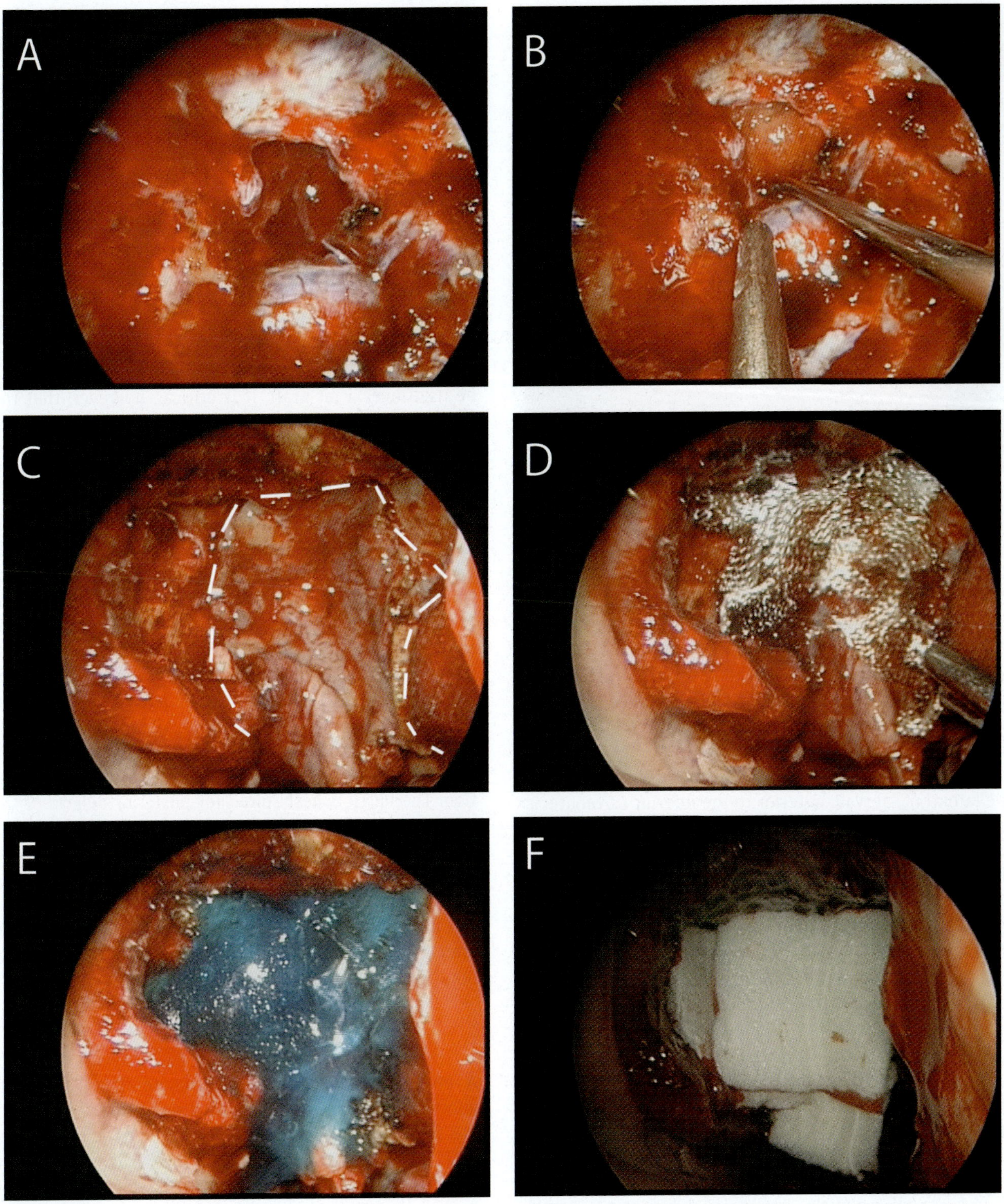

Fig. 52.5 Placement of nasoseptal flap (aka a Hadad-Bassagasteguy flap). **(A)** A transsellar and transplanar skull base defect over the area of the suprasellar cistern. **(B)** A collagen matrix inlay graft. **(C)** Placement of the nasoseptal flap over the entire defect and over the denuded surrounding bone. **(D)** The edges of the flap are bolstered intranasally with oxidized cellulose absorbable packing. **(E)** DuraSeal placement. **(F)** Absorbable gelatin sponge is placed. This will prevent traction on the repair when the nonabsorbable packing is removed.

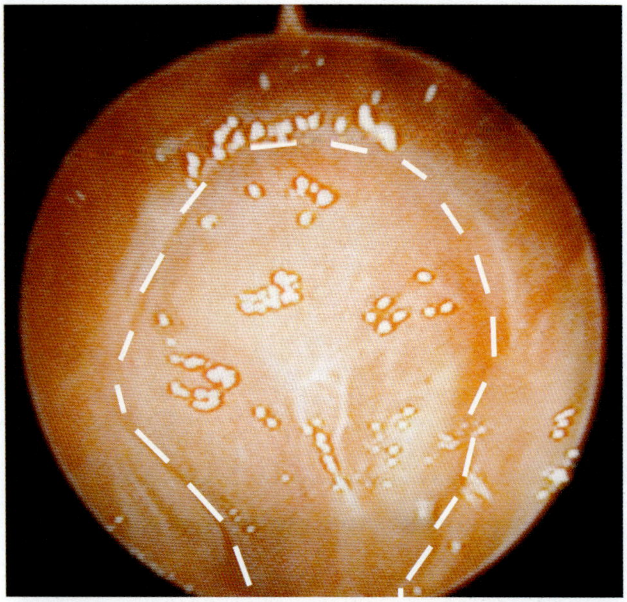

Fig. 52.6 Healed nasoseptal flap over a transsellar and transclival defect.

inferior turbinate on the superior aspect of its lateral attachment, 1.0 to 1.5 cm from its posterior tip.[10] Some have found that the artery may lie within the bone (50%) or within the soft tissue (14%), or may follow a mixed pattern (36%).[11] The artery runs for some distance (mean of 1.2 cm) before piercing the bone and soft tissue and splitting off into two to six branches.[11]

To harvest the PPITF, the nasal cavity is decongested and the lateral nasal wall, anterior to the inferior turbinate, is injected with a solution of lidocaine 1% with epinephrine 1:100,000. We harvest the PPITF after the completion of the EEA ipsilateral to the approach whenever possible to minimize the distance of the pedicle to the defect. Initially, the inferior turbinate is gently medialized to better expose the entire medial surface of the inferior turbinate. Given that this flap is substantially smaller than the NSF, it is best to harvest the entire turbinate mucoperiosteum to ensure adequate coverage (**Figs. 52.7, 52.8, 52.9A**).

A wider flap may be harvested by transposing the lower incision laterally to include the lateral mucoperiosteum of the turbinate and even the mucoperiosteum of the lateral wall of the middle meatus. The first step is to identify the SPA as it exits the sphenopalatine foramen and follow it distally to identify the PLNA. The flap will be based solely on this vascular pedicle. Two parallel incisions are performed endoscopically following the sagittal plane of the inferior turbinate, the superior one just above the inferior turbinate, and the inferior one following the caudal margin of the turbinate or, as previously described, its lateral aspect (**Fig. 52.9A**).

A vertical incision, placed over the anterior head of the inferior turbinate, connects the two previous incisions (**Figs. 52.8, 52.9B**). Its mucoperiosteum is elevated, starting at the anterior aspect of the inferior turbinate. A variable amount of bone may be elevated also, depending on the ease of dissecting the mucoperiosteum from the underlying bone. Care must be taken to avoid injuring the vascular pedicle as it enters at the superior aspect of its lateral attachment ~1.0 and 1.5 cm from its posterior tip. In addition, it is important to preserve the lateral nasal artery as it descends vertically over the ascending process of the palatine bone. It may course anteriorly to the posterior wall of the maxillary sinus; therefore, this should be considered when extending the maxillary antrostomy posteriorly.

Once harvested, the flap is gently unrolled and mobilized to cover the skull base defect (**Fig. 52.9C**). The PPITF can be applied directly to dura or denuded bone or may be used over a fat graft. It is critical, however, that the vascularized flap be in direct contact with the margins of the defect and to remove any nonvascularized tissue or foreign body between the margins of the defect and the flap. A sealant is applied over the flap, absorbable gelatin sponges are placed, and sponge nasal packing or the balloon of a 12-French Foley catheter is inserted to gently press the PPITF against the defect. Silicone nasal splints are used to protect the denuded lateral wall and are left in place for ~10 to 21 days. According to an anatomic analysis of the anteriorly based inferior turbinate flap, the mucosal surface area of this flap is ~4.97 cm^2 (2.8 × 1.7 cm).[12] Bilateral flaps can be harvested to cover larger defects.

The limitations of this flap are that, in comparison to the NSF, it has a smaller surface area and a limited arc of rotation. The PPITF is best suited for posterior defects of the sella, or parasellar and midclival areas. The flap size limits its use for anterior skull base reconstruction. Another disadvantage of using the PPITF is the formation of crusting over the inferior turbinate bone remnant in the postoperative period. Mucosalization of the donor site was observed after a period of 3 to 4 weeks (removal of the turbinate bone hastens healing) (**Fig. 52.9D**).[5]

Posterior Pedicled Middle Turbinate Flap

A posterior pedicle middle turbinate flap (PPMTF) is another option for the reconstruction of small- to moderate-size anterior skull base defects. The middle turbinate (MT) attaches to the lateral nasal wall at its anterior and posterior segments. Its midportion attaches to the skull base at the vertical lamella of the cribriform plate. The anatomic description of the vasculature around the lateral nasal wall has been described previously. Cadaver studies showed that the MT draws its blood supply from a branch of the sphenopalatine artery coursing through its posterior attachment.[13] It is this artery that serves as the pedicle for the PPMTF.

The flap is harvested by first making a vertical incision along the anterior face of the MT head (**Fig. 52.7**). A second

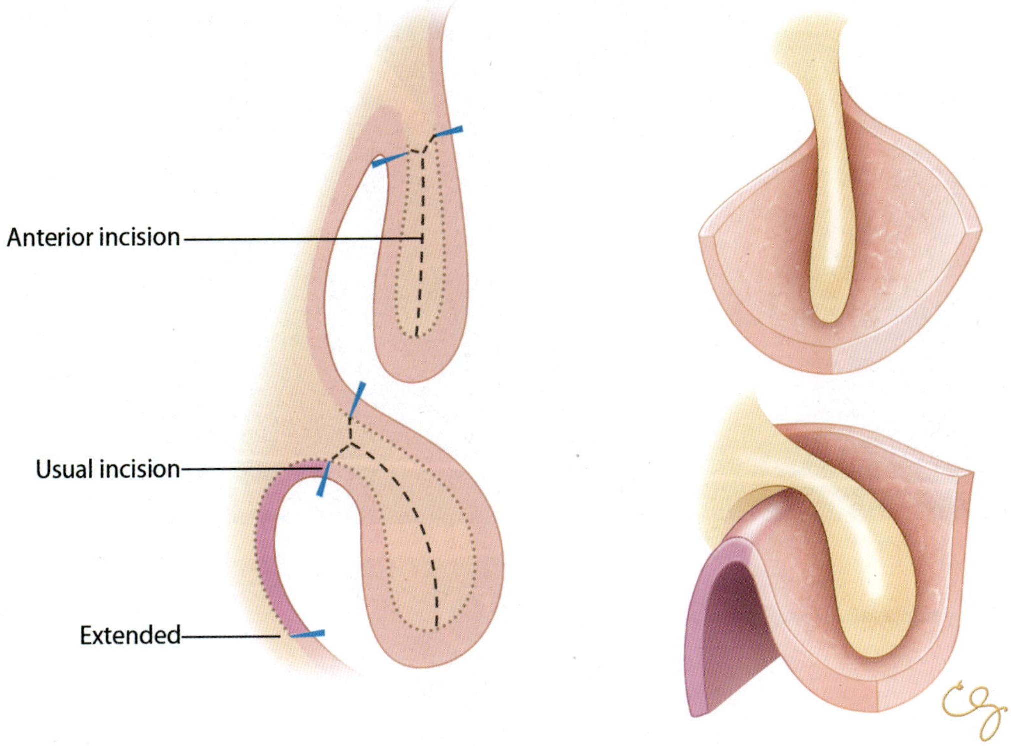

Fig. 52.7 Middle turbinate and inferior turbinate posteriorly pedicled flap incisions based off the corresponding branches from the sphenopalatine artery.

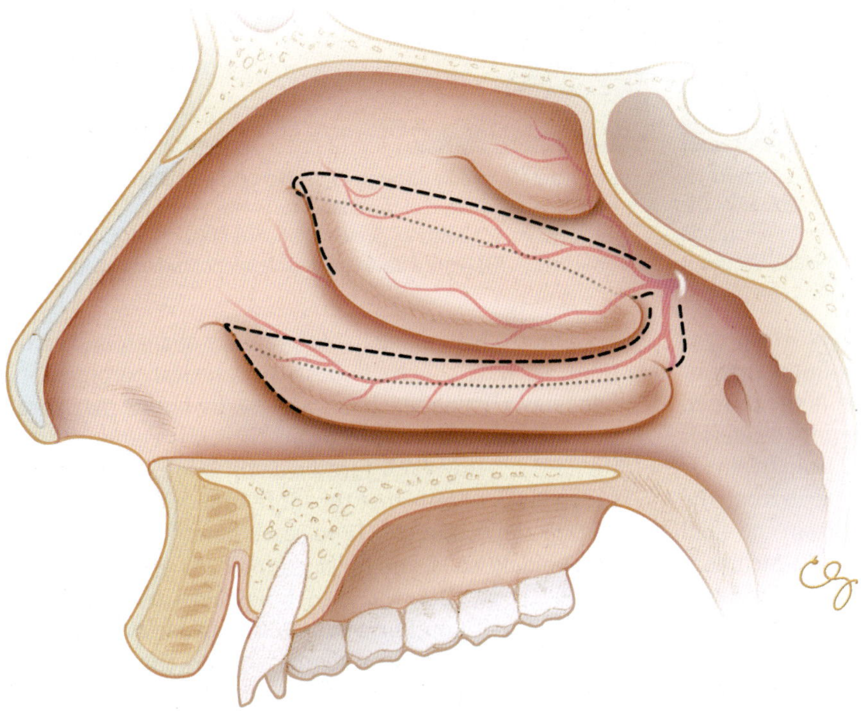

Fig. 52.8 Cross section of middle turbinate and inferior turbinate flap incisions. The inferior turbinate flap can have an extension onto the nasal floor for added width if needed.

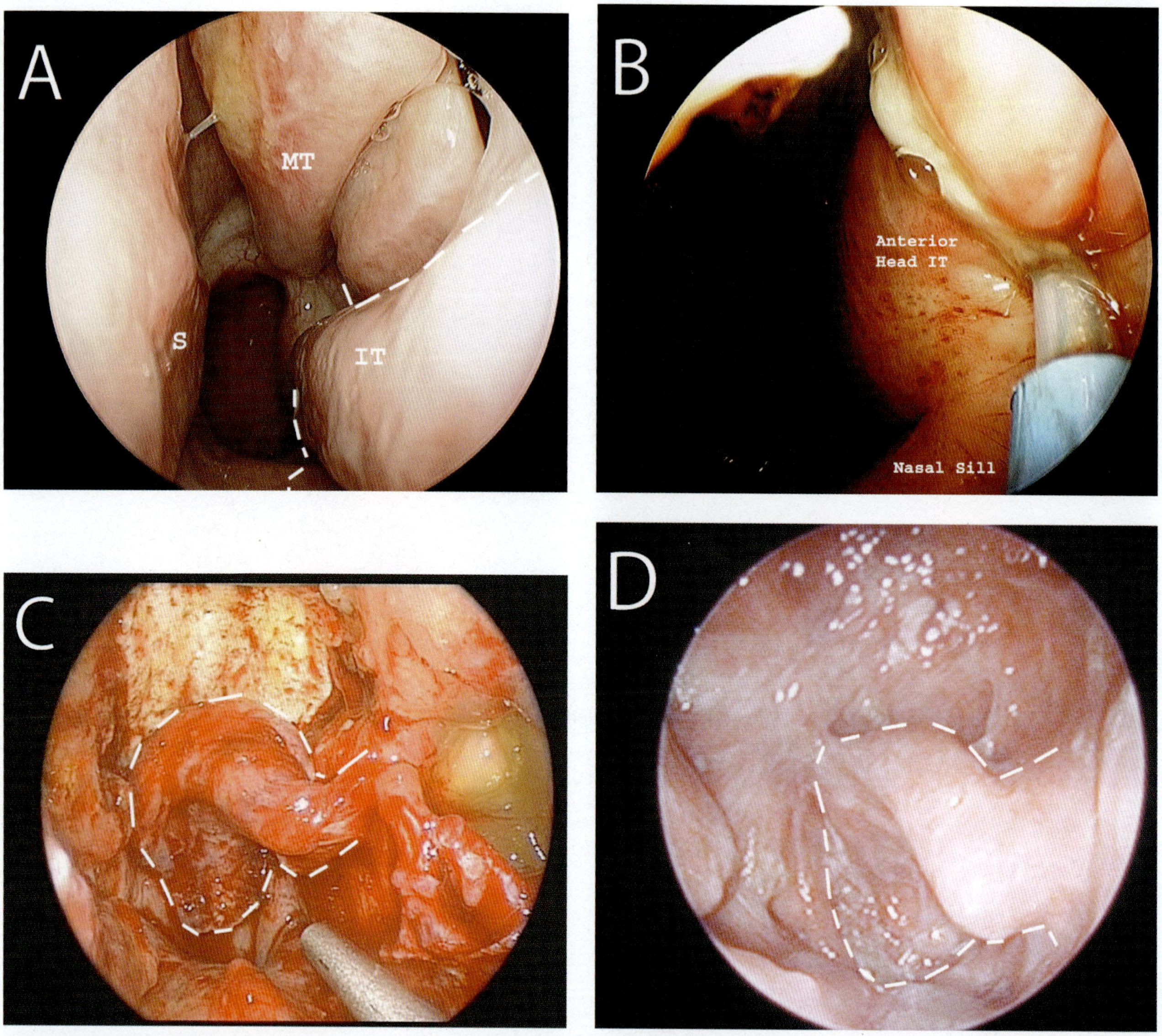

Fig. 52.9 Posterior pedicle inferior turbinate flap. **(A)** Two parallel incisions are performed endoscopically following the sagittal plane of the inferior turbinate: the superior one just above the inferior turbinate and the inferior one following the caudal margin of the turbinate. *IT*, inferior turbinate; *MT*, middle turbinate; *S*, septum. **(B)** A vertical incision, placed over the anterior head of the inferior turbinate, connects the two previous incisions. **(C)** Posterior pedicle inferior turbinate flap is placed over a clival defect. **(D)** Healed posterior pedicle inferior turbinate flap.

incision is made horizontally along the vertical attachment of the turbinate just below the skull base, in an anterior to posterior direction. Its mucoperiosteum is then raised from the medial aspect of the MT in a superior-to-inferior direction. Its thin bone is carefully removed from the inner aspect of the flap, concomitantly dissecting it from the lateral mucoperiosteum and transecting it from the skull base. Once the bone is removed, the lateral attachment of the flap to the skull base is sharply released (**Fig. 52.8**). Further elevation of the flap posteriorly and removal of the basal lamella yields a posteriorly pedicled flap. The pedicle is further dissected to improve its arc of rotation and to extend its reach.

One of the limitations of the PPMTF is the technical difficulty associated with elevating the flap. It becomes even more challenging in the presence of anatomic variations, such as concha bullosa, paradoxical turbinate, or hypoplasia. Its dimensions vary greatly but its mean area is somewhat limited at 5.6 cm^2, which is comparable to the PPITF.[13] However, further comparison of the PPMTF to the PPITF reveals that the more superior position of its pedicle allows the PPMTF to reach defects of the planum sphenoidale, sella, and fovea ethmoidalis area better than the PPITF. To date, the PPMTF has been used sparingly as a secondary option when an NSF is not available and the defect is of small to moderate size. The middle turbinate flap is most useful for reconstruction of small- to moderate-size defects of the planum sphenoidale, cribriform plate, or sella, but can be used to reconstruct the defects of the clivus.

Endoscopic-Assisted Pericranial Flap

The pericranial flap has been one of the most commonly used reconstruction options for traditional open anterior cranial base resection. It is an axial flap based on the supraorbital and supratrochlear arteries, which yields large, durable vascularized tissue that can cover the entire skull base (**Fig. 52.10A**). However, the use of the pericranial flap became limited with the advent of endoscopic skull base techniques due to inability to incorporate the externally harvested flap into the nasal cavity. By developing a technique that transposes the flap through a bony window at the nasion, the pericranial flap was reintroduced into the reconstructive arsenal after endoscopic skull base surgery.[14]

This flap may be harvested using a traditional coronal incision (preferred) or an endoscopic-assisted technique via "port" scalp incisions. A 2-cm midline incision and a 1-cm lateral port incision are made along the coronal plane of the scalp (**Fig. 52.10A**). The supraorbital and supratrochlear arteries are located by Doppler ultrasound, around which a 3-cm-wide flap pedicle is marked at the level of the supraorbital rim. A subgaleal plane dissection is performed through the vertex incisions, extending it to the vascular pedicle. The pericranium is incised using an extended insulated needle-tip electrocautery to the desired surface area. The pericranial flap is then elevated from the underlying bone down to the pedicle.

A 1-cm transverse glabellar incision is made and it is dissected down to the periosteum of the nasion. A subperiosteal plane is developed, communicating it with the subperiosteal plane of the flap dissection. Then the bone over the nasion is drilled to form a horizontal channel that enters into the nasal cavity. The pericranial flap is transposed through the glabellar incision (**Fig. 52.10B**) and then into the endonasal surgical field via a bony window at the nasion. Care must be taken not to twist the flap as it passes through the glabellar incision and the bony window. The flap should be applied to the skull base defect as it would in an open approach; the superficial surface of the flap should be in contact with the dural defect (**Fig. 52.10C,D**).

The flap is then bolstered into place as described previously for the nasoseptal flap reconstruction. A PCF, however, is most commonly harvested via a coronal incision as its design and dissection is more reliable and faster; the nasion bony window can be completed without a glabellar incision.

A pericranial flap is ideal for endoscopic reconstruction of the anterior cranial base given its pedicle location; it is well suited for reconstruction of cribriform and planar defects and can be extended to cover defects of the clivus. The length of the flap can be extended by placing the incisions further posterior on the scalp or by dissecting posterior to the incisions.

From April 2008 (when the first endoscopic PCF was performed) until December 2008, ten cases of endonasal skull base reconstruction with the pericranial flap have been performed at our institutions without a postoperative leak. The pericranial flap healed without any complication in three patients who had previous radiation treatment. In addition, the PCF withstood postoperative irradiation in five patients who required this treatment.

Temporoparietal Fascial Flap

The temporoparietal fascial flap (TPFF) has been used extensively for reconstruction of defects resulting after various head and neck extirpative procedures and its anatomy is well described. This section describes the use of the TPFF in endoscopic skull base reconstruction.[15] This flap is used when no viable endonasal options are available for reconstruction of large clival and parasellar defects.

The temporoparietal fascia (TPF) is a strong fascial layer that is connected to the overlying fibrous septae of the subcutaneous tissue. The blood supply of the TPF comes from the superficial temporal artery (STA), one of the terminal branches of the external carotid artery. It courses through the retromandibular parotid gland, crosses the posterior root of the zygomatic process, and becomes incorporated into the temporal fascia at the level of the zygomatic arch. The average diameter of the vessel is 2.73 mm over the zygomatic arch, and the mean distance between the STA and the tragus is 16.68 mm.[10] In most patients, the STA divides into an anterior frontal and a posterior parietal branch at the level of the zygomatic arch (61 to 88%); however, the bifurcation point can be superior to the arch (4 to 26%) or inferior to the arch (7 to 12%).[16,17] One or two veins accompany the STA, which lies just deep to them.[10] The frontal branch of the facial nerve courses just under the TPF after it crosses the superficial surface of the zygomatic arch.[18] The TPF is 2 to 3 mm in thickness over the parietal region and extends in a fanlike manner from the preauricular region, comprising a surface area as large as 17×14 cm.[19]

Harvesting and transposition of the TPFF to the nasal cavity is performed after the EEA dissection is complete so the defect size is known. It may be harvested from either side of the scalp, but we most commonly use the side that is ipsilateral to the defect. Previous incisions over the area of the flap may alter the laterality of the harvesting.

If not performed previously as a part of the EEA, an anterior and posterior ethmoidectomy and a large maxillary antrostomy are performed. Then, the SPA and posterior nasal artery are clipped at the level of the sphenopalatine foramen. A retrograde dissection of the SPA serves to remove the posterior wall of the maxillary sinus, thus exposing the pterygopalatine fossa (PPF). In addition, a portion of the lateral wall of the maxillary sinus is removed to open a wide communication with the infratemporal fossa (ITF). The descending palatine artery is identified in

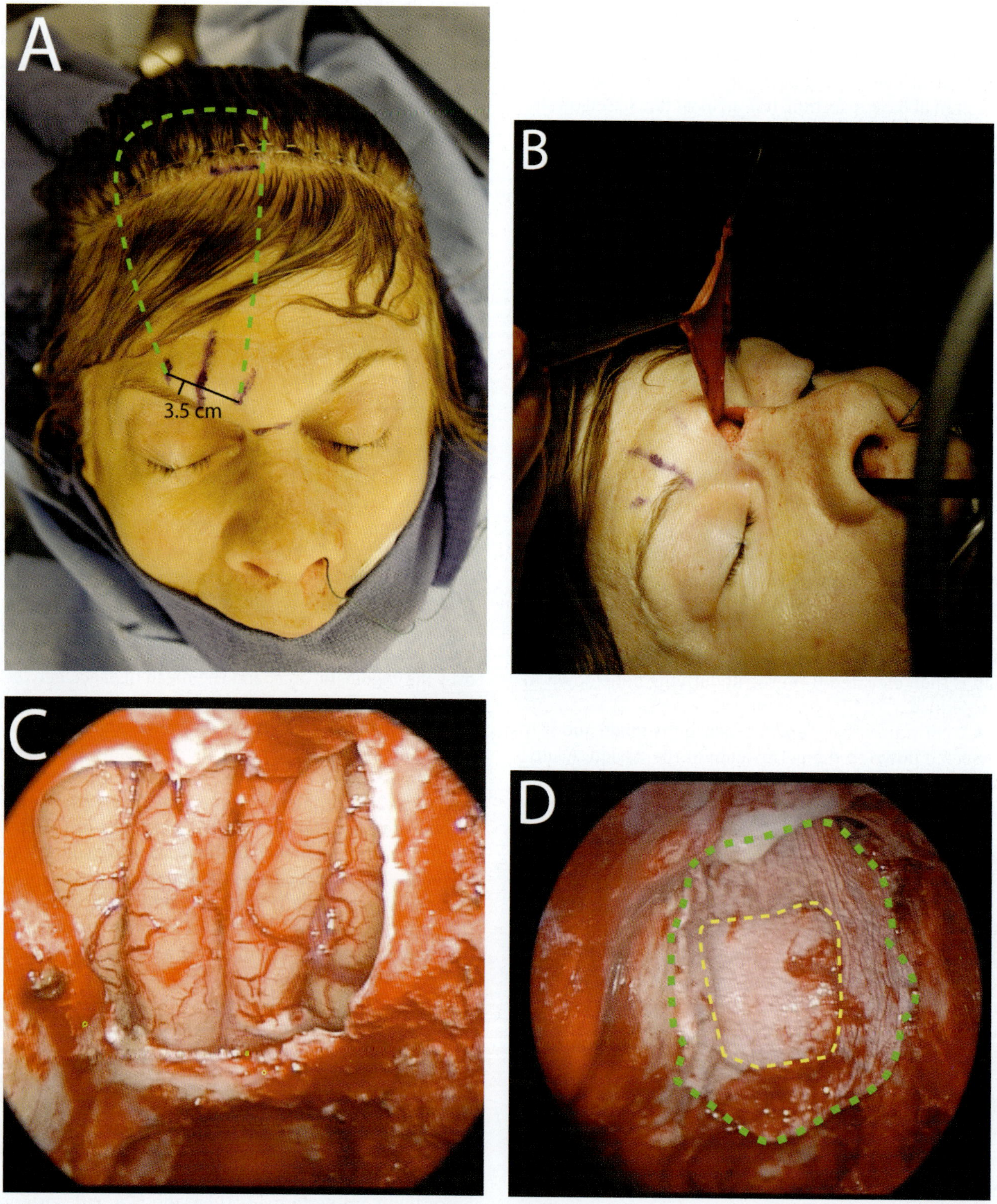

Fig. 52.10 Minimally invasive pericranial flap. **(A)** Planned endoscopic pericranial flap incisions from a unilateral 3-cm pedicle. **(B)** Pericranial flap rotated from beneath the scalp out a 1-cm glabellar incision. **(C)** Transcribriform defect from esthesioneuroblastoma. **(D)** Reconstruction of the defect with significant overlay of the defect in **(C)**.

its inferior vertical trajectory from the internal maxillary artery (IMA) and is dissected from its canal. This allows the inferior and lateral displacement of the contents of the upper PPF, therefore exposing the pterygoid plates. The pterygopalatine ganglion may be preserved, but the vidian nerve has to be divided to allow for the displacement of the ganglion. Then, the anterior aspect of the pterygoid plates is reduced with a high-speed drill to enlarge the space for transposition of the TPFF. At this point, one should have full access into the ITF and the IMA should be completely mobile at the pterygomaxillary fissure.

A TPFF is harvested from the ipsilateral side using a conventional technique. A hemicoronal incision is carried down to the level of the hair follicles. Care must be taken to avoid injuring the pedicle during the hemicoronal incision because the STA lies directly under the skin within the subcutaneous tissue. Dissection of the TPF from the subcutaneous tissue effectively elevates the flap. Once enough surface area is exposed, the fascia is incised at its lateral margins and elevated from the cranium and deep temporal fascia down to its pedicle. The superficial layer of the deep temporal fascia is incised vertically, and the fascia is separated from the muscle following this plane of dissection inferiorly to elevate the periosteum from the surface of the zygomatic arch. This creates a wide tunnel beneath the superficial layer of the deep temporalis fascia that will accept the passage of the pedicle without compression.

To help the transposition of the TPFF, a lateral canthotomy incision may be used to expose and separate the temporalis muscle from the lateral orbital wall and from the pterygomaxillary fissure. This creates a tunnel that communicates the temporal, the infratemporal fossa, and the endoscopic transpterygoid approach. This soft tissue tunnel is sequentially dilated, advancing percutaneous tracheotomy dilators over a guidewire. After an adequate tunnel is created, the dilators are removed, and the flap is tied to the external end of the guidewire. As the nasal end of the guidewire is pulled out through the nostril, it pulls the flap through the tunnel into the nasal cavity. The mobilization of the flap through the tunnel is assisted with external manipulation, keeping in mind to avoid a rotation of the flap because this may compromise its blood supply. The external incisions are closed with a running absorbable suture after insertion of a suction drain. The reconstruction of the skull base begins with the placement of an inlay graft of a collagen matrix. The edges of the defect are refreshed, and the TPFF is placed over the defect. A sealant may be used after the flap is in position. The flap is then covered with absorbable gelatin sponges, and a sponge packing is placed to stabilize the flap. The packing is removed 3 to 5 days later.

Advantages of the TPFF include a large surface area, a pliable flap with sufficient thickness, and tissue that is outside the boundaries of customary therapeutic fields in the setting of prior sinonasal or skull base radiotherapy. Disadvantages of this technique include the need for an external approach and a surgical scar, risk of alopecia, risk to the frontal branch of the facial nerve, and the need for a corridor from the nose to the infratemporal fossa.

Oliver Pedicled Palatal Flap

We have described a pedicled flap based on the descending palatine artery, which, like the previously described endonasal flaps pedicles, also arises from the internal maxillary artery. The pedicled palatal flap can be used in skull base reconstruction by transposing the vascularized mucoperiosteal tissue of the hard palate into the nasal cavity through the enlarged greater palatine foramen.[20] This flap is considered a last resort if other tissue options are not available due to the potential associated morbidity, the introduction of oral flora into the surgical field, and clinical inexperience at this time.

High-Risk Factors for a Postoperative Cerebrospinal Fluid Leak

High-risk factors for a postoperative CSF leak include the following:

1. Body habitus of the patient. Large body mass is associated with high ventricular pressure.
2. Pathology, especially lesions involving the cisterns and craniopharyngiomas.
3. Entry into arachnoid cisterns or ventricles.
4. Site and size of the defect. Defects in the anterior cranial base are much more likely to leak than clival defects.
5. Cushing disease patients, due to poor tissue healing.
6. Patients with no vascularized tissue reconstructive options due to prior surgery or chemoradiation therapy.

Lumbar Cerebrospinal Fluid Drainage

Lumbar spinal drains are not routinely used in the postoperative period after EEA except in the cases that had a significant intraoperative high-flow CSF leak or patients suspected to have high ventricular pressure. Any patient with a postoperative leak is taken back to the operating room for endoscopic exploration and repair. If, at this time, the patient is noted to have a high-flow leak, a spinal lumbar drain is considered. CSF diversion is usually continued for 3 to 5 days, using intermittent drainage of 50 mL of CSF every 8 hours. This is preferable to leaving the lumbar drain open to gravity, because excessive CSF drainage may occur with changes in patient position.

Table 52.1 Intranasal and Regional Vascular Flaps Available for Skull Base Reconstruction

Location	Vascular Tissue Flap	Pedicle	Comments/ Limitations
Intranasal Vascular Tissue Flap	NSF	Sphenopalatine artery	• All skull base defects (two adjacent anatomic modules)
	ITF	Inferior turbinate artery*	• Small clival defects • Cannot reach ACF or sella
	MTF	Middle turbinate artery*	• Small ACF or sellar defects • Small size • Thin mucosa • Difficult to elevate
Regional Vascular Tissue Flap	PCF	Supraorbital and supratrochlear artery	• Hearty flap with versatile dimensions • ACF to sella • Requires frontal sinusotomy and total ethmoidectomy • Poor choice for posterior skull base
	TPFF	Superficial temporal artery	• Clival or parasellar defects • 90-degree pedicle rotation limits reconstruction of ACF
	PF	Greater palatine artery	• Reaches all areas of skull base • 3 cm pedicle, but difficult to harvest • Limited experience

*Terminal branch of posterior lateral nasal artery of the sphenopalatine artery
Abbreviations: ACF, anterior cranial fossa; NSF, nasoseptal flap; ITF, inferior turbinate flap; MTF, middle turbinate flap; PCF, pericranial flap; TPFF, temporoparietal fascia flap; PF, palatal flap.

Rarely, patients have CSF leaks that persist even after endoscopic reexploration and repair and spinal lumbar drain. In these situations, the CSF pressure is measured, and if a high-pressure hydrocephalus is noted, permanent CSF shunting is considered.

Skull Base Reconstructive Algorithm

Clearly, there are various free graft and vascularized tissue options for the reconstruction of large skull base defects. We offer here a brief description of an algorithm that guides the surgeon through the preferable options.[21]

First, if there is an intraoperative CSF leak, the flow intensity of the leak must be determined. If the leak is a low-flow leak, then the defect site and size will determine the vascular tissue flap needed. If the leak is a high-flow leak, then the defect site alone guides the choice of the reconstructive technique.

Advantages of each vascular tissue flap based on the size and site are discussed later and outlined in **Table 52.1**. The NSF may be applied to any skull base defect and size. The PPITF excels in the reconstruction of small clival defects. Due to limitations in pedicle length, the PPITF cannot reach the anterior cranial fossa or sella area. The PCF has an extended pedicle that supports the reconstruction of defects that extend from the anterior cranial fossa to the sella. The need for a frontal sinusotomy (endoscopic Lothrop or Draf III) and a total ethmoidectomy makes the PCF a less optimal flap for the reconstruction of posterior skull base defects. The TPFF is ideal for large clival, middle cranial fossa, and parasellar defects. The TPFF is a poor choice for anterior skull base defects due to limitations in the arc of rotation necessary to tunnel the pedicle through the pterygopalatine fossa. The remaining two vascular tissue flaps are more difficult to harvest and have specific indications. The PPMTF is small, difficult to elevate, and is comprised of a thin mucosa layer. Nevertheless, the flap is good for reconstruction of small and small-to-moderate anterior cranial fossa (planum and cribriform plate) defects. In theory, the palatal flap can reach all areas of the skull base given its 3-cm-long pedicle; however, the dissection of the vascular pedicle from the descending palatine canal is difficult. This flap is usually a last resort due to the previously mentioned morbidity.

Conclusion

Advancements in endoscopic skull base reconstruction must match the ever increasing size and complexity of the defects produced by endoscopic resections. The principles of multilayer reconstructions and the routine use of vascularized flaps in expanded endonasal surgery have reduced the incidence of postoperative CSF leak to less than 5%. Future advances will help us to understand and manage patients with a high risk for a postoperative CSF leak, especially those patients who have been previously irradiated and patients that require revision surgery.

References

1. Neligan PC, Mulholland S, Irish J, et al. Flap selection in cranial base reconstruction. Plast Reconstr Surg 1996;98(7):1159–1166, discussion 1167–1168
2. Hegazy HM, Carrau RL, Snyderman CH, Kassam A, Zweig J. Transnasal endoscopic repair of cerebrospinal fluid rhinorrhea: a meta-analysis. Laryngoscope 2000;110(7):1166–1172
3. Hadad G, Bassagasteguy L, Carrau RL, et al. A novel reconstructive technique after endoscopic expanded endonasal approaches: vascular pedicle nasoseptal flap. Laryngoscope 2006;116(10): 1882–1886
4. Pinheiro-Neto CD, Prevedello DM, Carrau RL, et al. Improving the design of the pedicled nasoseptal flap for skull base reconstruction: a radioanatomic study. Laryngoscope 2007; 117(9):1560–1569
5. Shah RN, Surowitz JB, Patel MR, et al. Endoscopic pedicled nasoseptal flap reconstruction for pediatric skull base defects. Laryngoscope 2009;119(6):1067–1075
6. Kassam AB, Thomas A, Carrau RL, et al. Endoscopic reconstruction of the cranial base using a pedicled nasoseptal flap. Neurosurgery 2008;63(1, Suppl 1):ONS44–ONS52, discussion ONS52–ONS53
7. Zanation AM, Carrau RL, Snyderman CH, et al. Nasoseptal flap reconstruction of high flow intraoperative cerebral spinal fluid leaks during endoscopic skull base surgery. Am J Rhinol Allergy 2009;23(5):518–521
8. Zanation AM, Carrau RL, Snyderman CH, Gardner PA, Prevedello DM, Kassam AB. Nasoseptal flap takedown during endoscopic skull base surgery. Neurosurgery 2009; In press
9. Fortes FS, Carrau RL, Snyderman CH, et al. The posterior pedicle inferior turbinate flap: a new vascularized flap for skull base reconstruction. Laryngoscope 2007;117(8):1329–1332
10. Padgham N, Vaughan-Jones R. Cadaver studies of the anatomy of arterial supply to the inferior turbinates. J R Soc Med 1991;84(12):728–730
11. Hadar T, Ophir D, Yaniv E, Berger G. Inferior turbinate arterial supply: histologic analysis and clinical implications. J Otolaryngol 2005;34(1):46–50
12. Murakami CS, Kriet JD, Ierokomos AP. Nasal reconstruction using the inferior turbinate mucosal flap. Arch Facial Plast Surg 1999;1(2):97–100
13. Prevedello DM, Barges-Coll J, Fernandez-Miranda JC, et al. Middle turbinate flap for skull base reconstruction: cadaveric feasibility study. Laryngoscope 2009;119(11):2094–2098
14. Zanation AM, Snyderman CH, Carrau RL, Kassam AB, Gardner PA, Prevedello DM. Minimally invasive endoscopic pericranial flap: a new method for endonasal skull base reconstruction. Laryngoscope 2009;119(1):13–18
15. Fortes FS, Carrau RL, Snyderman CH, et al. Transpterygoid transposition of a temporoparietal fascia flap: a new method for skull base reconstruction after endoscopic expanded endonasal approaches. Laryngoscope 2007;117(6):970–976
16. Moore KL, Dalley AF. Clinically Oriented Anatomy, 5th ed. Baltimore: Lippincott Williams and Wilkins; 2006: 788–798
17. Pinar YA, Govsa F. Anatomy of the superficial temporal artery and its branches: its importance for surgery. Surg Radiol Anat 2006;28(3):248–253
18. Casoli V, Dauphin N, Taki C, et al. Anatomy and blood supply of the subgaleal fascia flap. Clin Anat 2004;17(5):392–399
19. David SK, Cheney ML. An anatomic study of the temporoparietal fascial flap. Arch Otolaryngol Head Neck Surg 1995;121(10): 1153–1156
20. Oliver CL, Hackman TG, Carrau RL, et al. Palatal flap modifications allow pedicled reconstruction of the skull base. Laryngoscope 2008;118(12):2102–2106
21. Patel UA, Keni SP. Pectoralis myofascial flap during salvage laryngectomy prevents pharyngocutaneous fistula. Otolaryngol Head Neck Surg 2009;141(2):190–195

53 Complications of Endoscopic Skull Base Surgery

Ernesto Pasquini and Giorgio Frank

Over the last decade, the advent of extended endoscopic approaches has expanded the indications for endoscopic endonasal surgery from strictly sellar pathology to a broad array of skull base tumors.[1] To take advantage of this new technique, training is required to become familiar with two-dimensional (2D) vision, with endoscopic anatomy, with the surgical approaches in general, and with the new instrumentation.[2] In this chapter the most frequent complications occurring during endoscopic skull base surgery are described along with suggestions regarding how to prevent and treat them using endoscopic technique. The first step in avoiding complications is to perform only operations for which the surgeon is highly trained. A training program, such as that initially suggested by the Pittsburgh group,[2] may be a useful instrument for assisting the surgeon in handling incremental and modular surgical difficulties. Complications of skull base resection and repair may be classified as vascular, neurologic, and infectious.

Vascular Complications

Vascular complications may be related to the approach phase and/or to vascular dissection during tumor resection; these may be categorized into arterial or venous hemorrhages.

Vascular Complications in the Approach Phase

Arterial Hemorrhages

The most frequent arterial hemorrhage during endoscopic skull base surgery occurs as a result of bleeding from branches of the external carotid artery, namely the sphenopalatine artery and the maxillary artery. Only rarely is there bleeding from the internal carotid artery (occurring in 1% of the procedures).[3,4]

The primary sources of bleeding are frequently either the main trunk of the sphenopalatine artery or its branches (the septal branch and the posterior nasal or external branch; **Fig. 53.1**). When using a midline transsphenoidal approach, the septal branch may accidentally be lacerated during the enlargement of the sphenoid ostium inferiorly, and the external nasal branch may be interrupted at the posterior end of the middle turbinate when performing a middle turbinectomy.[5] Conversely, interruption of the main trunk of the sphenopalatine artery is planned when performing a transpterygoid approach.[6] The sphenopalatine artery reaches the nasal cavity through the sphenopalatine foramen, which is located laterally to the attachment of the middle turbinate at the posterosuperior corner of the maxillary sinus. To

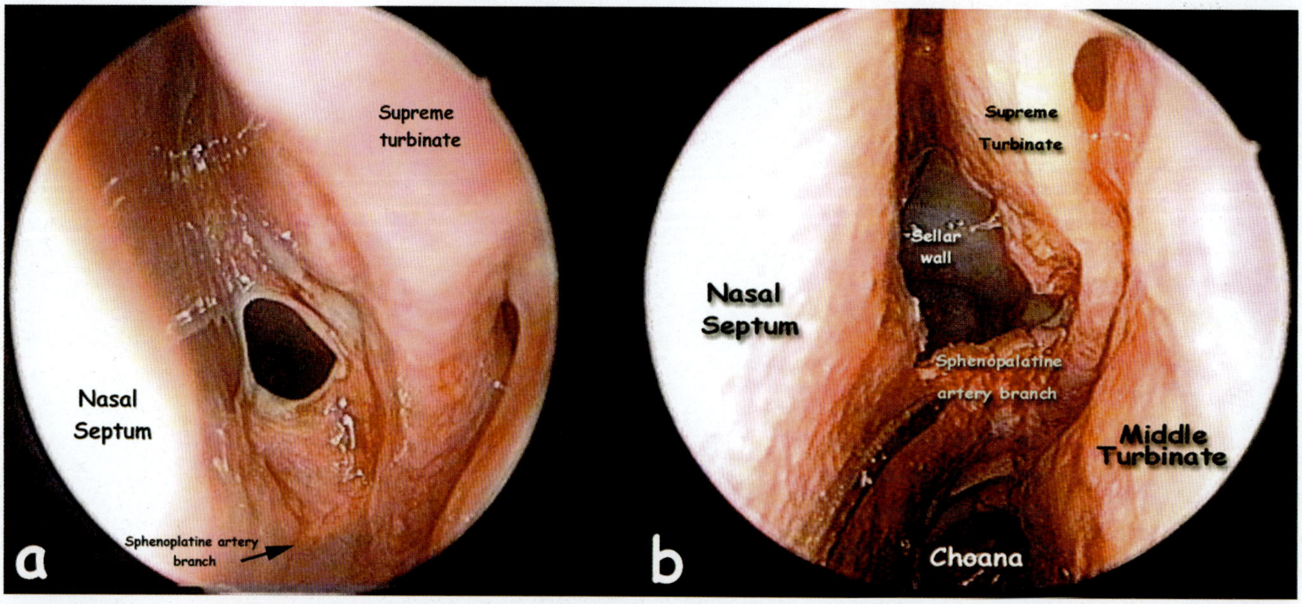

Fig. 53.1 (A,B) The sphenopalatine artery reaches the nasal cavity through the sphenopalatine foramen. It has two branches, the medial or septal branch and the lateral or external branch, which vascularizes the turbinates. The artery traverses in a submucosal plane, and careful elevation of the mucosa from the bone helps to prevent vascular damage.

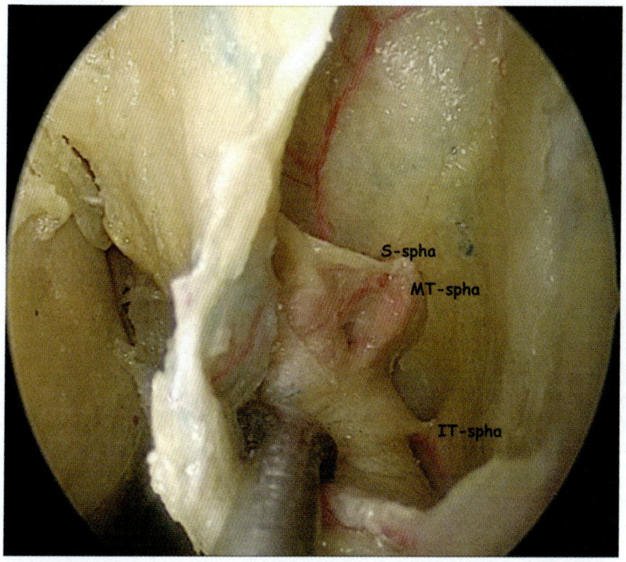

Fig. 53.2 In this specimen, the left sphenopalatine artery is exposed at the sphenopalatine foramen located laterally to the attachment of middle turbinate at the posterosuperior corner of maxillary sinus. *S-spha*, septal sphenopalatine artery; *MT-spha*, middle turbinate sphenopalatine artery; *IT-spha*, inferior turbinate sphenopalatine artery.

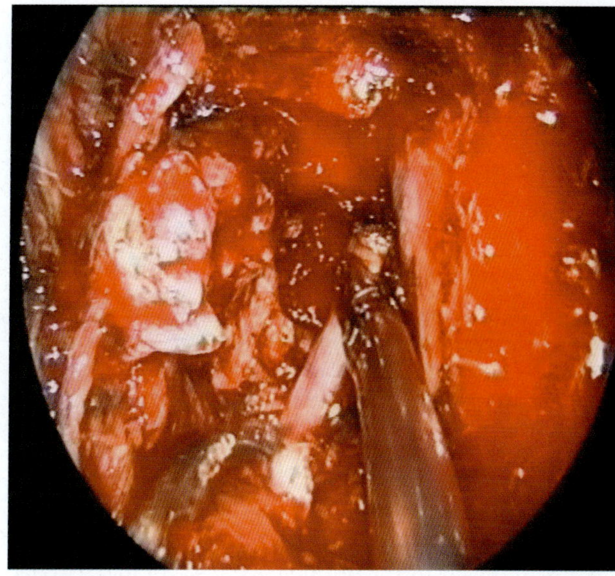

Fig. 53.3 Clipping the maxillary artery during endoscopic approach of a juvenile angiofibroma growing in the right infratemporal fossa.

expose the main trunk of the sphenopalatine artery, the foramen should be opened using a rongeur, after which it should be cauterized or clipped before its transection (**Fig. 53.2**). In all cases, bleeding of the main trunk or of the branches of the sphenopalatine artery requires the meticulous coagulation of the vessel, not only to stop the blood loss but also to prevent possible delayed epistaxis.

The main trunk or branches of the maxillary artery are involved during endoscopic approaches to the pterygopalatine or infratemporal fossae, such as during the removal of a juvenile angiofibroma. In fact, during this procedure, the identification, coagulation, and interruption of the maxillary artery should anticipate the tumor removal either to prevent hemorrhage from its laceration or to reduce the blood supply to the tumor. To control the maxillary artery, simple coagulation may not be sufficient and the clipping of the vessel trunk may be preferred (**Fig. 53.3**).

Hemorrhage from the Internal Carotid Artery

Hemorrhage from the internal carotid artery (ICA) is a rare complication of transsphenoidal surgery.[4] The incidence of arterial lesions during transsphenoidal surgery varies between 0.4% for expert surgeons to 1.4% for less experienced surgeons.[3] Raymond pointed out an incidence of 1% bleeding during or after transsphenoidal pituitary surgery with a morbidity of 24% and a mortality of 14% of these cases.[7] Some anatomic variations may favor this grave complication. The most important anatomic variants are[8] (1) bulging of the ICA within the sphenoidal sinus at the level of the parasellar tract where, in 4% or more of cases, the bony wall may be lacking;

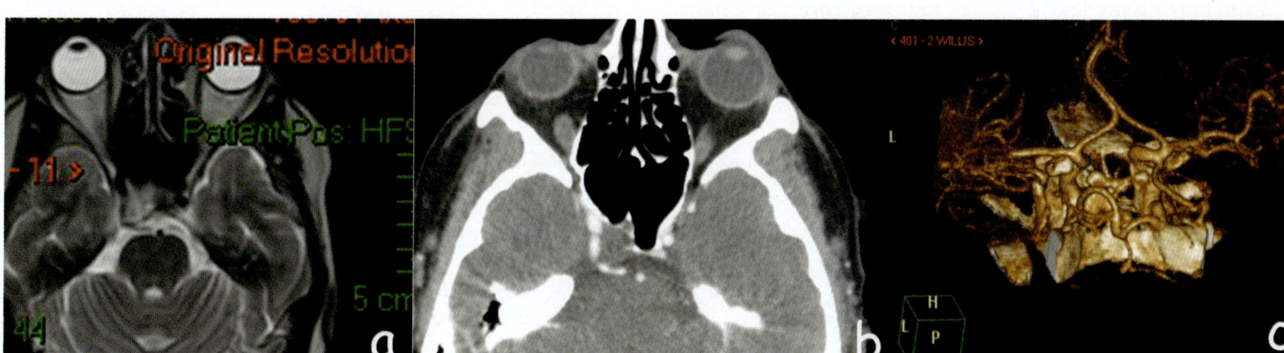

Fig. 53.4 **(A)** Magnetic resonance image, **(B)** computed tomographic angiogram, and **(C)** computed tomographic angiogram three-dimensional reconstruction showing a persistent right-sided trigeminal artery, thus complicating the procedure to remove a pituitary macroadenoma involving the right cavernous sinus.

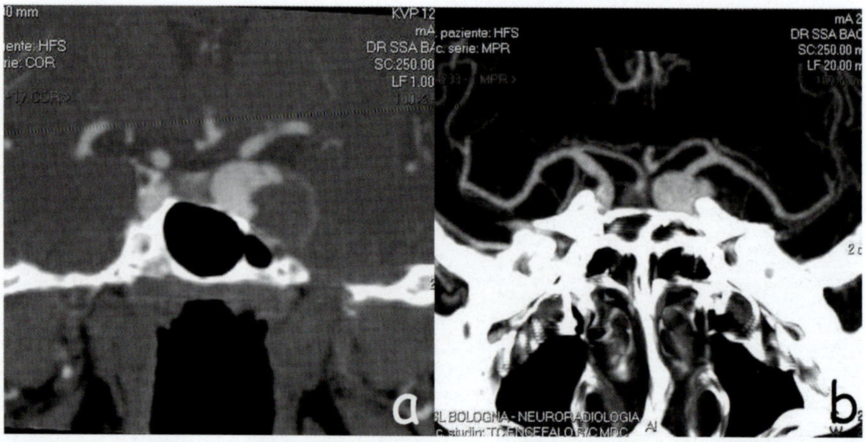

Fig. 53.5 (A,B) Computed tomography angiograms showing a giant aneurysm, which are partially thrombosed and which are arising from the medial wall of the left internal carotid artery.

(2) sphenoidal septa inserting on the prominence of the ICA; (3) reduced intercarotid space; (4) the persistence of the trigeminal artery, which consists of a connection between the carotid-vertebral system (**Fig. 53.4**) or the presence of vascular malformations, such as an aneurysm (**Fig. 53.5**).

Other factors that may favor these arterial hemorrhages are carcinomas encroaching on the wall of the arteries and the presence of scar tissue derived from previous surgical procedures or from radiotherapy.

Although the possibility of injuring the carotid artery through a transsphenoidal route is remote, the same thing cannot be said for cases of extended surgical approaches requiring an anatomic dissection in the proximity and along the pathway of the internal carotid artery. The surgical routes or corridors used to gain access to the ventral skull base were described and identified by Kassam and colleagues[9–11] according to their relationship to the four main segments of the ICA (ascending parapharyngeal segment, horizontal petrous segment, vertical paraclival/parasellar segment, paraclinoid segment).

In carrying out these approaches, knowledge of the course of the ICA and its landmarks is of paramount importance to avoid vascular complications. The main landmark is the medial aspect of the anterior clinoid process for the identification of the paraclinoid segment of the artery, the vidian canal for the junction between the horizontal petrous portion of the carotid and its ascending paraclival portion, and the eustachian tube for the parapharyngeal arterial segment (**Fig. 53.6**).

Some devices, such as the neuronavigator (**Fig. 53.7**)[12] and the Doppler (**Fig. 53.8A**)[13] are useful aids for the early identification of the vessel. When the anatomy is normal, they simply confirm previous anatomic identification but, in the presence of anatomic variants, such as in the case of an anomalous course of the vessel, they are of paramount importance in selecting the safest approach and identifying the vessel in an unexpected location. However, if a carotid injury occurs, the surgeon should be able to control the bleeding immediately. In such dramatic circumstances, working as a team with the second surgeon is of great importance. The second surgeon must hold the endoscope at a specific distance from the source of the bleeding while trying to maintain clear vision and using a suction device to eliminate the blood from the field. On the other hand, the first surgeon should control the bleeding by compressing the vessel with pledgets. Then, moving the pledget aside, the edges of the bleeding site are cauterized using bipolar coagulation.[14]

If cauterization fails and/or when the bleeding source is extradural and the dura is intact, packing should be considered. Conversely, packing in a surgical field with opened dura should be avoided because the bleeding could become intradural. The contribution of the anesthesiologist during these maneuvers is crucial. In fact, the

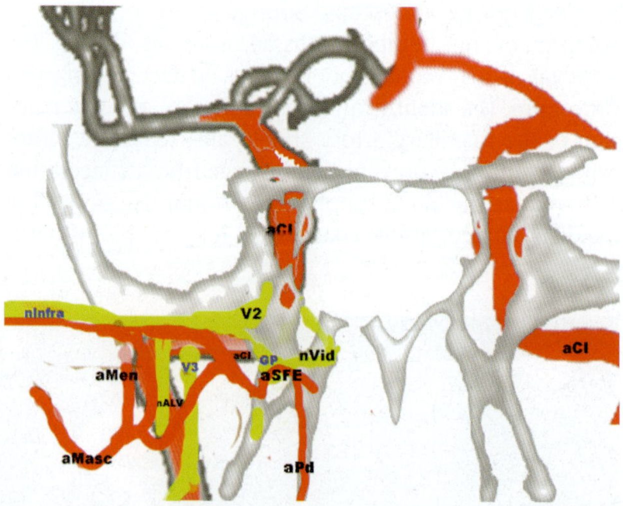

Fig. 53.6 Schematic drawing over a bone window computed tomography scan showing the course of the internal carotid artery and the maxillary branch of the external carotid artery. The complex relationship between vessels and nerves is depicted. *aCI*, internal carotid artery; *aMasc*, maxillary artery; *aMen*, middle meningeal artery; *aPd*, palatine artery; *aSFE*, sphenopalatine artery; *GP*, palatine ganglion; *nALV*, alveolar nerve; *ninfra*, infraorbital nerve; *nVId*, vidian nerve; *V2*, maxillary branch of trigeminal nerve; *V3*, mandibular branch of trigeminal nerve.

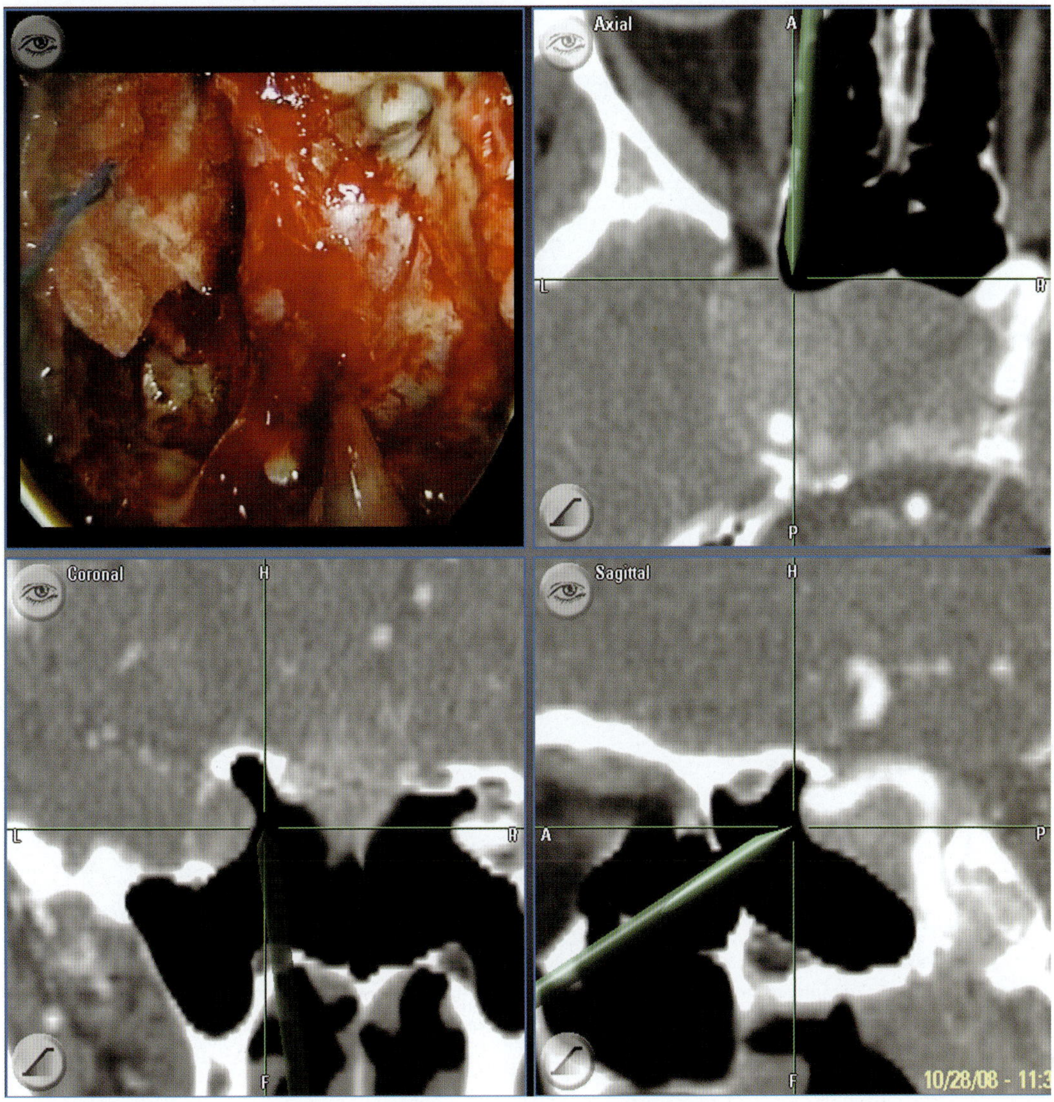

Fig. 53.7 Intraoperative endoscopic view and corresponding neuronavigator imaging (axial, coronal, and sagittal computed tomography angiogram) before the opening of the left cavernous sinus invaded by a pituitary adenoma. This control allows identification of the safest entry point.

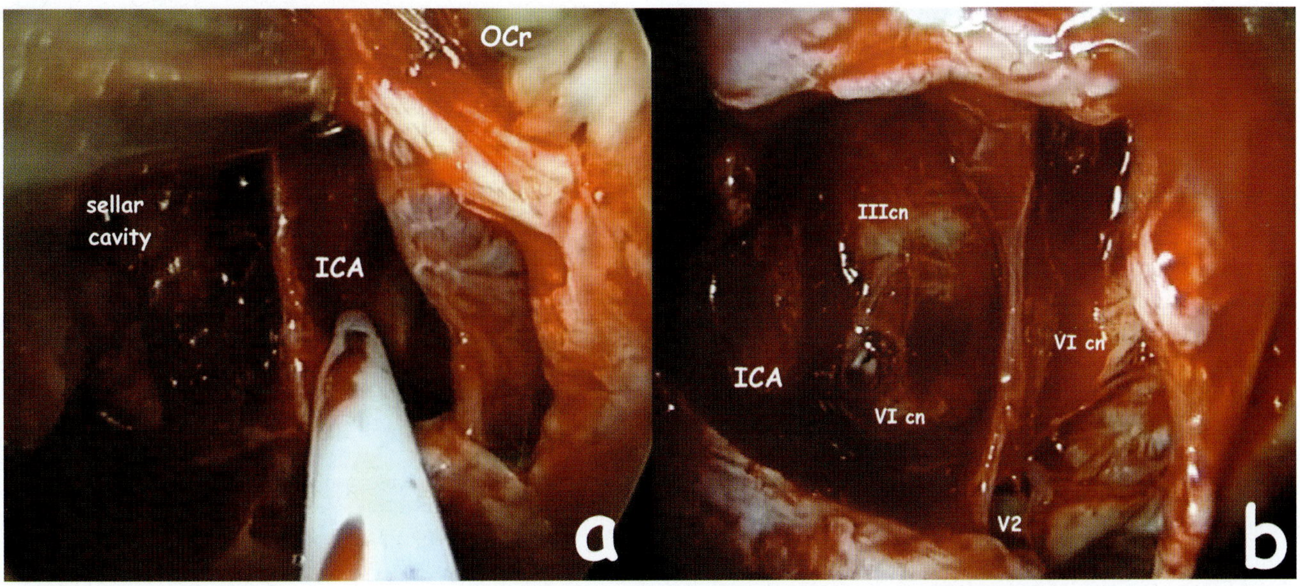

Fig. 53.8 **(A)** Operative image showing the use of the Doppler to check the intracavernous internal carotid artery. **(B)** After tumor removal from the cavernous sinus, the internal carotid artery is highly visible as is the oculomotor nerve, which is embedded in the lateral wall of the cavernous sinus. The sixth nerve course runs free in the cavernous sinus having a superolateral direction toward the superior orbital fissure.

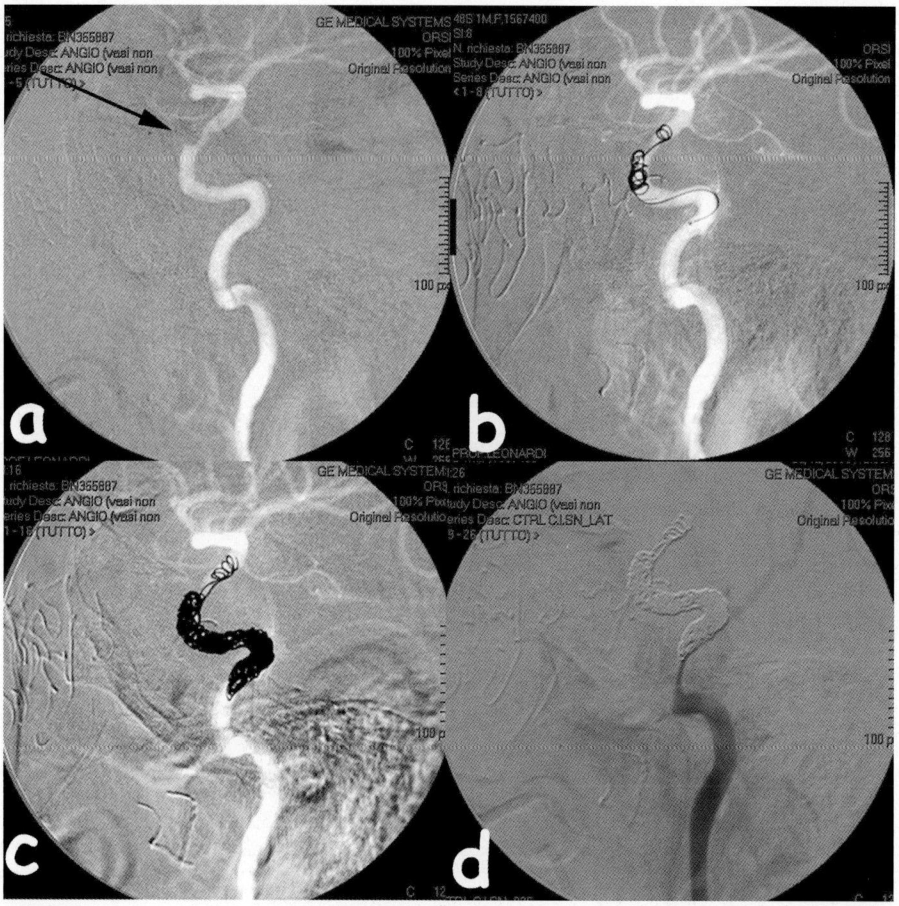

Fig. 53.9 Emergency carotid angiography performed after injury of the left internal carotid artery, which occurred during an endonasal transsphenoidal procedure. **(A)** The *black arrow* points out the laceration of the vessel appearing as a defect of the wall. **(B)** First coils at the injured site. **(C)** Completed occlusion of the vessel by coils. **(D)** Final image.

anesthesiologist should maintain the blood pressure and vascular volume, thus ensuring adequate cerebral perfusion. With the same aim, if the patient is in a semisitting position and/or with the head elevated, the surgeon should restore the supine position with the head at heart level.

After the bleeding is controlled, angiography should be performed to confirm the presence of either a pseudoaneurysm at the site of the vascular injury or of the effectiveness of the collateral circulation.[7] The first therapeutic choice could be to repair the vessel through the endovascular placement of a stent, thus occluding the tear in the vessel wall and maintaining blood flow.[15] The second therapeutic choice[7] is an endovascular permanent occlusion of the ICA, including at the site of bleeding (**Fig. 53.9**). This option should only be considered if adequate collateral circulation exists. Otherwise, a bypass should be performed before there is occlusion of the vessel (**Fig. 53.10**). There is still disagreement regarding the value of routinely performing a preoperative balloon occlusion test.[16] Due to the potential procedure complications, a balloon occlusion test is advisable only in selected cases where the risk of carotid injury is greater than that of the test.

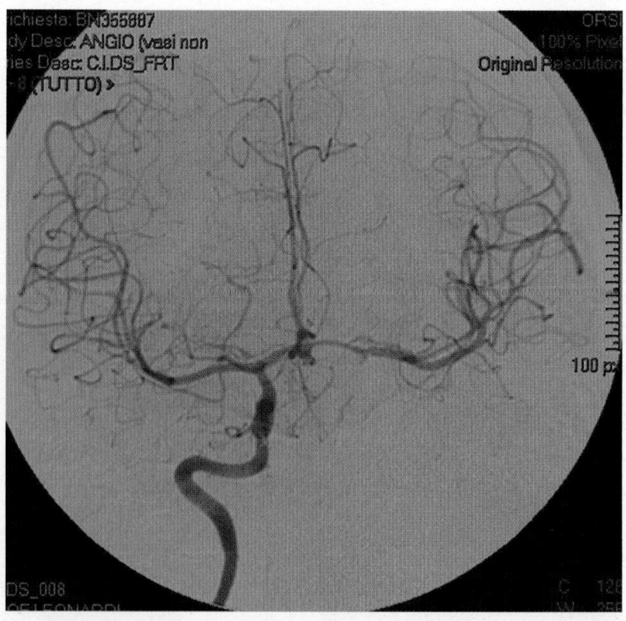

Fig. 53.10 The same case as shown in Fig. 53.9. Balloon occlusion test is performed before the left-side carotid artery embolization. With this test, the effectiveness of the collateral circulation coming from the right side is checked.

Venous Hemorrhages

During skull base surgery, some venous hemorrhages, although foreseeable, are unavoidable due to the presence of venous structures in the approach pathway.[8] One example of this is during a midline transsphenoidal approach in the presence of a wide intercavernous connection from which bleeding may be unavoidable during the opening of the sellar meningeal layer. Similarly, there are venous sinuses that have to be transected during some extended transsphenoidal approaches. For example, in the supradiaphragmatic approach to gain access to the diaphragma and expose the pituitary stalk, transection of the superior intercavernous sinus is anticipated (**Fig. 53.11**)[17]; in the transclival approach, to open the dura and gain access to the intradural space, the basilar venous plexus has to be transected. Bipolar coagulation is generally effective, particularly after the dura is opened. Otherwise, several hemostatic materials may contribute to controlling venous bleeding (e.g., FloSeal, Avitene, Gelfoam).

Some venous hemorrhages are not foreseeable or avoidable. Such an example is when the cavernous sinus (CS) is erroneously opened as a result of an inappropriate surgical trajectory. To prevent such a complication, it is necessary to open the dura in the midline, keeping in mind the anatomic landmarks (sphenoidal septa, parasellar carotid protuberances, and opticocarotid recesses) and/or using devices such as the neuronavigator. To control the bleeding from the CS, bipolar coagulation may be harmful, thus increasing the diameter of the tear due to the retraction of the cauterized margins. In such a situation, the use of hemostatic agents (e.g., FloSeal, Avitene, Gelfoam) is preferable. Some of those agents (FloSeal and Avitene) have the advantage of being removable by washing without interfering with the visual control of the surgical field.

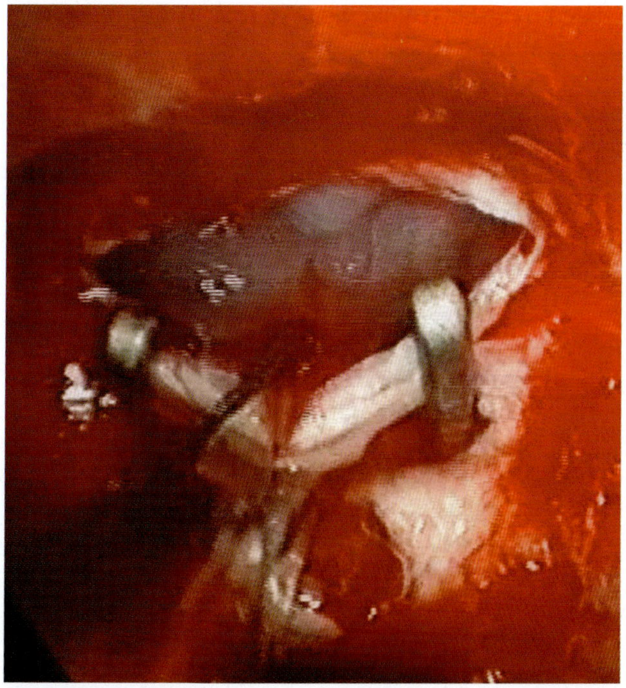

Fig. 53.11 Operative view. During a supradiaphragmatic approach, coagulation and/or clipping of the superior intercavernous sinus should anticipate the sinus transection.

Vascular Complications in the Dissecting Phase

The rules of microsurgery do not change with endoneurosurgery.[14,18] The surgeon operates using both hands, one for suction and the other for dissection; tumor debulking anticipates sharp extracapsular dissection and, only after this step, can the tumor be removed. Unfortunately, even respecting such rules, bleeding may occur and significant attention must be applied to hemostasis. The management of extradural arterial or venous bleeding is identical to the approach phase. However, the management of intradural bleeding is more intuitive, being a compromise between what we can do and what is more convenient. The hemostatic techniques used are simple packing and irrigation with warm water (effective for venous oozing); the use of hemostatic agents (effective for venous bleeding and also for mild arterial bleeding); and the use of bipolar cauterization (especially necessary for arterial bleeding). The experience of the surgeon guides the choice of the technique because each technique has advantages and disadvantages. The packing-waiting-washing technique is time-consuming and is mainly effective in stopping minor oozing of blood. On the other hand, the use of hemostatic agents is effective for venous bleeding, but some nonremovable agents may hide the presence of retrograde bleeding toward the brain. Focal bipolar cauterization is the technique of choice for arterial bleeding, but its use is limited by the functional role of the bleeding vessel.

In spite of the meticulous hemostatic technique, the absolute avoidance of postoperative hematoma seems to be impossible.[4] Asymptomatic hematomas in the surgical field incidentally discovered at routine postoperative neuroradiologic controls (computed tomography [CT] scan or magnetic resonance imaging [MRI]) are not infrequent and do not require treatment, but are to be monitored until their disappearance. Conversely, symptomatic hematomas are to be promptly treated; an endonasal reintervention may be sufficient, but sometimes a craniotomy procedure is necessary, particularly when the surgeon suspects that the bleeding source is a major arterial vessel (**Fig. 53.12**).

Neurologic Complications

Neurologic complications may be the consequence of vascular damage or may be due to direct injury of the nervous tissue (e.g., the curettes, which pierce the diaphragma sellae and penetrate the nervous tissue) and nerves. It is assumed that endoscopic skull base surgery is more

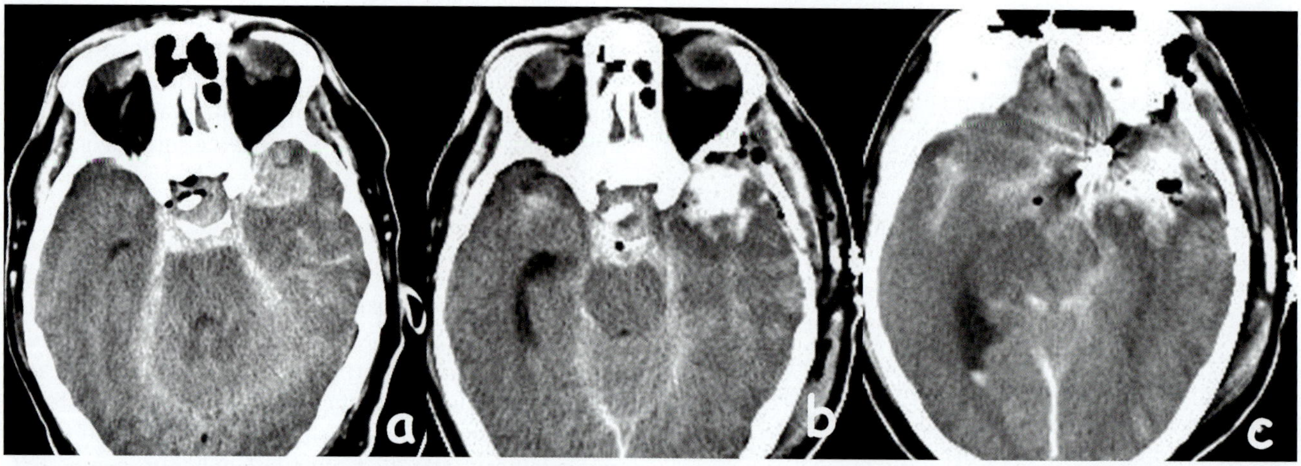

Fig. 53.12 Computed tomography scans performed at different times after the operation. **(A)** Immediately after surgery, a temporopolar hemorrhage and a subarachnoid hemorrhage are visible. **(B)** Six hours later, the patient was worse and the temporal herniation was increasing. **(C)** An emergency craniotomy was performed to control the bleeding due to a patent vessel of the internal carotid artery, and the computed tomography scan shows the artifact due to the clip on the bleeding vessel.

conservative in respect to craniotomic microsurgery and this is generally correct. Craniotomy approaches to the ventral skull base require brain manipulation even if an incremental demolition of the bone of the skull base allows this to be minimized. Furthermore, craniotomy approaches follow a lateral-to-medial direction, and access to midline lesions requires the dissection of the neurovascular structures displaced at the periphery of the expanding mass. Conversely, endoscopic skull base approaches allow for an extracerebral direct access to the ventral skull base, avoiding brain manipulation and neurovascular dissection. These are the reasons why endoscopic approaches are well tolerated and why they are generally considered minimally invasive.

The following section will describe the cranial nerves that are most frequently involved in endoscopic approaches and specify the most frequent points of risk.

Olfactory Nerve Injury

Anosmia is the clinical consequence of bilateral damage to the olfactory nerves and/or of the resection of the neurosensorial olfactory mucosa. Bilateral olfactory nerve damage is rarely due to the approach, being more frequently due to the involvement of the olfactory pathways by the tumor itself, which frequently has anosmia as a presenting symptom. The unilateral sacrifice of the olfactory nerve is generally without functional consequences, but the olfactory mucosa should be maintained to preserve the olfaction.

Optic Nerve and Chiasm Injury

The sellar and suprasellar regions are bracketed superolaterally and posteriorly by the optic nerve and the chiasm. When using an endoscopic approach, the zone at maximum risk for the optic nerve is the optic canal. The optic nerve may be damaged by direct and indirect trauma, and its recovery ability is very low. Therefore, utmost care should be taken not only to avoid direct injury to the nerve, but also to avoid indirect damage, such as that which can be induced by excessive heating during the drilling of the optic canal. When using a transethmoidal approach to the sella, the surgeon should be aware of the presence of the Onodi variants of the posterior ethmoidal cells because this anatomic variant increases the risk of direct optic nerve injury in the ethmoid sinus. In an extended transtuberculum sellae approach, the optic canals represent the lateral limit of the opening and, being well identified in this approach, must be preserved.[17] Furthermore, in a transtuberculum approach intended to open the dura of the suprasellar area, the surgeon should be aware of the displacement of the chiasm, which may be pushed immediately behind the dura and thereby be at risk of damage during this phase of the procedure.[17]

Oculomotor, Trochlear, and Abducens Nerve Injuries

Lesions to these nerves induce ophthalmoplegia. The zone at risk for damage is mainly the CS.[13] The third and fourth cranial nerves course across the lateral wall of the cavernous sinus, where they are embedded and protected between the endosteal and meningeal layers, which make up the lateral wall. The sixth nerve runs free in the cavernous sinus having a medial to lateral ascending course as it moves toward the superior orbital fissure (**Fig. 53.8B**). The abducens nerve is also at risk of damage during the opening of the clival dura. Accordingly, the opening should be in the midline and, if possible, it should start in the lower part of the clival dura where the nerve can more easily be identified at the level of vertebro-basilar junction where it emerges a few millimeters above the latter junction.

Trigeminal Nerve Injury

Lesions to the branches of the trigeminal nerve induce neuralgia, anesthesia, or both (painful anesthesia). There are different zones at risk regarding damage to the branches of the trigeminal nerve. The first branch of the trigeminal nerve, the ophthalmic branch, may be injured in the parasellar area where it courses in the lateral wall of the CS; by avoiding transection of the lateral wall, the nerve is preserved. The second and the third branches of the trigeminal nerve, the maxillary branch and the mandibular branch, respectively, are at risk of damage mainly during the transmaxillary approach to the pterygopalatine and infratemporal fossae.[19] In this approach, the course of the infraorbital nerve indicates the lateral limit of the resection of the posterior wall of the maxillary sinus. The infraorbital nerve is a branch of the maxillary branch of the trigeminal nerve. The maxillary nerve is reached by following the infraorbital nerve backward. It emerges from the cranium through the foramen rotundum and courses in the region of the lateral wall of the sphenoid sinus where it is covered by a bony prominence called the trigeminal prominence. The mandibular branch of the trigeminal nerve emerges from the cranium through the foramen ovale and it courses along the infratemporal fossa. It is generally exposed during the approach to the infratemporal fossa.

Vidian Nerve Injury

The vidian nerve derives from the union of the greater petrosal nerve, which arises from the facial nerve at the geniculate ganglion, and the deep petrosal nerve, which originates from the carotid sympathetic plexus (**Fig. 53.13**). Although it is frequently electively resected, the vidian nerve plays an important role in maintaining normal lacrimation and nasopharyngeal physiology. Damage to the vidian nerve can lead to a loss of lacrimation with desiccation of the cornea and dry nose due to damage to the parasympathetic fibers. The vidian nerve runs in the vidian or pterygoid canal together with the vidian artery. The vidian canal is located in the floor of the sphenoid sinus where, in well pneumatized sinuses, it is visible as a prominence. However, in the presellar and conchal variants of the sphenoid sinus, this prominence is not visible and, therefore, its exposure should start at the level of the pterygoid process. In a subperiosteal approach performed along the face of the pterygoid process, the vidian canal is located 5 to 6 mm laterally to the sphenopalatine foramen. The posterior end of the vidian canal delimits the genu between the petrous carotid artery and the paraclival artery. This is an important landmark for the carotid artery and, indirectly, for the trigeminal Meckel's ganglion, which is located in a space bounded by the horizontal and paraclival carotid arteries medially and inferiorly, by the maxillary branch laterally, and the abducens nerve superiorly. Kassam recommended drilling the vidian canal in its ventral surface, between 3 and 9 o'clock, to avoid injuring the carotid artery with the drill.[20]

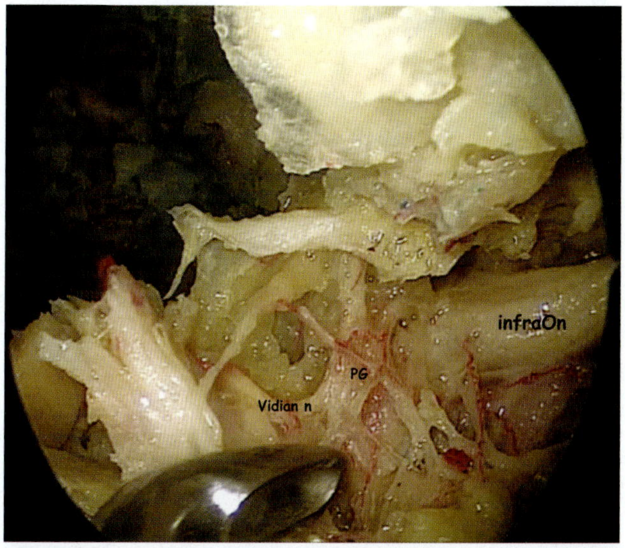

Fig. 53.13 Anatomic specimen: the vidian nerve entering the pterygoid channel is exposed in a view from maxillary sinus at level of pterygoid process. The sphenopalatine ganglion or pterygoid ganglion, which receives otho/parasympathetic bundles from vidian nerve and sensitive somatic fibers from maxillary nerve, is also shown. The infraorbital nerve is well visualized, which is the terminal branch of maxillary nerve. *Vidian n*, vidian nerve; *PG*, pterygoid ganglion or sphenopalatine ganglion; *InfraOn*, infraorbital branch of maxillary nerve.

Other Nerves

The facial nerve and the vestibulocochlear nerves are too lateral to be involved during endoscopic endonasal approaches even if, exceptionally, the internal auditory canal can be reached following the tumor along its direction of growth.

The glossopharyngeal, vagus, and the hypoglossal nerves are also distant from the surgical corridors normally used in the endoscopic endonasal approach. The surgeon should keep them in mind when carrying out an approach to the jugular foramen or to the foramen magnum. In the latter circumstance (i.e., during an approach to the foramen magnum), the posterior half of the occipital condyle should be preserved to avoid hypoglossal nerve injury.[10]

Cerebrospinal Fluid Leak

Leakage of cerebrospinal fluid (CSF) from the subarachnoid space into the paranasal sinuses and, finally, into the nasal cavities may produce disastrous intracranial complications such as meningitis and pneumocephalus. Accordingly, this is the reason why the repair of such leaks is mandatory. Generally, the incidence of a CSF leak after pituitary surgery is ~2 to 3%, but a higher incidence is reported after extended transsphenoidal approaches.[21]

A CSF leak may occur intraoperatively or postoperatively. An intraoperative CSF leak appears as the flow of clear fluid from the suprasellar cisterns. Sometimes a tear in the cisterns is not evident and the CSF oozes through a macroscopically

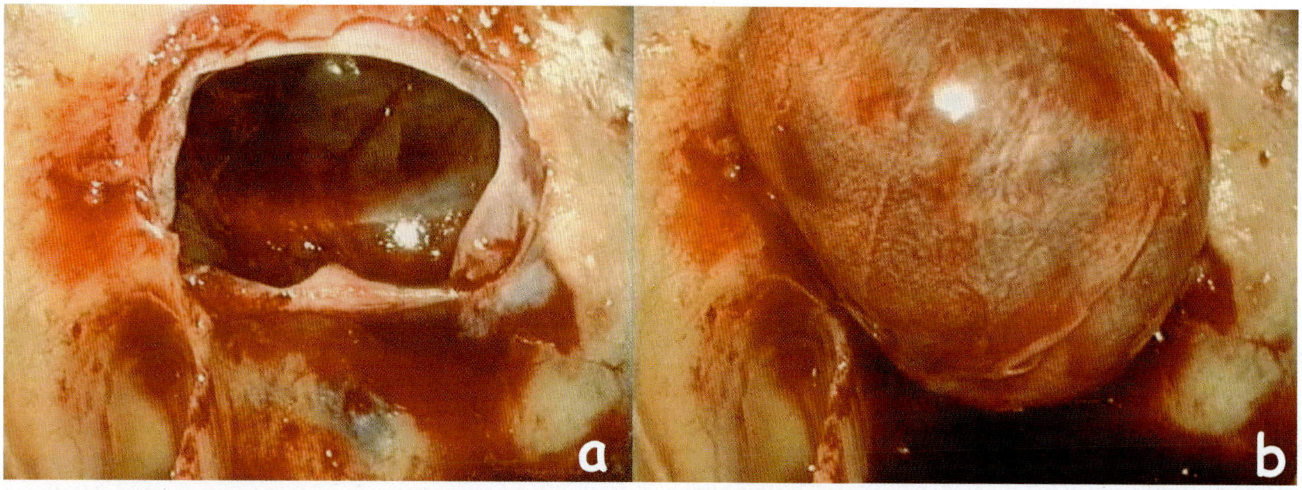

Fig. 53.14 Operative views. **(A)** The sellar empty cavity after a tumor removal is highly visible. **(B)** During the Valsalva maneuver, the suprasellar cistern is pushed outside the sella and no defects or cerebrospinal fluid leaks are detectable.

intact arachnoid membrane; a Valsalva maneuver is always suggested to confirm its presence (**Fig. 53.14**). A postoperative CSF leak normally occurs within a few days following surgery. The main reasons for a delayed CSF leak lie primarily in the tearing of previously intact suprasellar membranes or in displacement of a graft. The features favoring such a complication are mostly uncontrollable expiratory reflexes, such as sneezing, coughing, or vomiting. A smooth emergence from anesthesia as well as preoperative instructions regarding activity restrictions are useful expedients in preventing such events.

In postoperative CSF leaks, different algorithms are proposed to confirm the diagnosis. The suspicion that clear fluid leaking from the nose is CSF may be increased significantly using the tilt test (head flexed). However, the certainty that the fluid is CSF may be reached only by the beta-2-transferrin test or the beta-trace protein test.[22] Unfortunately, these two highly sensitive tests, based on a specific marker of CSF, are not always available. A further key point in the management of a CSF leak consists in the localization of the dural defect.

High-resolution CT, combining fine slices in two planes, is the primary and often the only imaging modality for the localization of defects.[23] It may show the bone defect and the opacification of contiguous sinuses or air cells. MR cisternography[24] is another noninvasive imaging method used in the evaluation of a patient with CSF rhinorrhea; a continuous T2-weighted high signal extending from the subarachnoid space into the paranasal sinuses is a sign of a CSF leak. Furthermore, the use of intrathecal fluorescein is strongly suggested as a guide during surgery to indicate the sites of the leak and to confirm the effectiveness of the repair.[25]

Management of a Skull Base Defect

According to the Esposito-Dusik classification,[26] the authors believe that the repair should be tailored to the grade of the CSF leak: grade 0 no leak (no repair); grade 1, small leak without an obvious diaphragmatic defect (simple reinforcement with fat and/or mucoperiosteum from the middle turbinate or septum may be sufficient); grade 2, a moderate leak with a definite diaphragmatic defect (a multilayer repair [fat + fascia lata + mucoperiosteum] is suggested); grade 3, a large diaphragmatic/dural defect (multilayer repair or a pedicled flap is required) (**Fig. 53.15**).[27] The material available for a tissue repair may be heterologous or autologous. At present, the authors prefer to use only autologous material because it allows stable healing with viable material. A debate still exists regarding the advisability of the use of lumbar drainage. Such conservative management is used by the

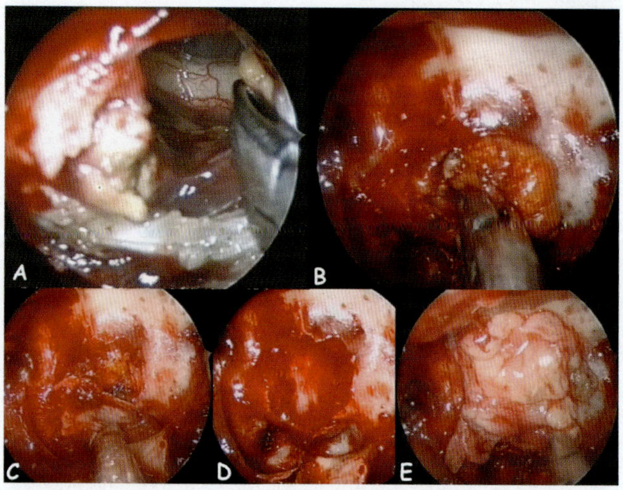

Fig. 53.15 Operative views of a multilayer plastic repair of the sella. **(A)** A wide defect of the diaphragma/suprasellar cisterns makes visible the intracranial content (chiasm). **(B)** Abdominal fat is introduced in the sellar space, being careful to avoid an overpacking. **(C,D)** A piece of bone is introduced extradural to support the fat graft. **(E)** Mucoperiosteum of the middle turbinate or of the septum is applied overlay.

authors in only two circumstances: (1) recurrent small leakage after a previous tissue repair; and (2) the presence of CSF hypertension suggesting the use of lumbar drainage to support a tissue repair because it reduces the pressure on the graft.

It should be kept in mind that lumbar drainage may precipitate a rare and severe complication of CSF leak: tension pneumocephalus. Pneumocephalus normally occurs in conjunction with a CSF leak, and may be considered an indirect sign of this complication due to the fact that there is a CSF outflow from the intracranial spaces and an air inflow at the same time. Typically, pneumocephalus is asymptomatic, but the potential concern is tension pneumocephalus. There are a few reports stating that lumbar drainage may increase the volume of the penetrating air, thus inducing intracranial hypertension and a clinical deterioration of the patient. In this rare condition, it is mandatory to remove the lumbar drainage, evacuate the air, and repair the fistula directly at the site of origin.[28]

Infections

Two main types of infection may occur: systemic infections (urogenital, pulmonary, and cardiac infections) and local infections. The former depends on the operative time, the recovery time, and bed rest, and on factors related to the general health conditions of the patient; they are not affected by antibiotic prophylaxis.[29] Their management is part of the general health care and is not treated in the present chapter.

Conversely, local infection at the surgical site (rhinosinusitis, meningitis) is related to the surgical procedure. Endonasal skull base surgery is clean contaminated surgery.[30] A direct connection between the nasal cavity and the intracranial cavity and multiple passages with the surgical instruments through a contaminated field occur systematically during endonasal surgery. Despite the theoretical high risk of intracranial contamination with sinus nasal flora, present experience shows a relatively low incidence of central nervous system infections arising from rhinosinusitis.

Factors influencing the reduction of infections of the surgical field include antibiotic prophylaxis, sealed closure of the dural defect and prompt management of the postoperative CSF leak, and operative and postoperative management of the sinonasal cavity.

1. Antibiotic prophylaxis[29] is highly recommended. It helps to prevent infection by reducing the "infectious load" in the presence of the clean contaminated surgery inherent in transnasal skull base surgery. A standardized regimen of antibiotic prophylaxis maintains a low incidence of postoperative infection, decreasing the risk of infection resulting from resistant organisms, allergic reactions and side effects, and antibiotic-related complications such as *Clostridium difficile* enterocolitis and thrombophlebitis from intravenous lines. Multiple factors influence the choice of antibiotic prophylaxis, at the forefront of which are patient demographics and the nature of the surgical procedure.

   The authors' antibiotic prophylaxis scheme is short-term prophylaxis with cephazolin (an initial dose of 2 g and then 1 g 6 hours postoperatively). In patients allergic to penicillin, either gentamicin or vancomycin is used at the discretion of the surgeon. In the case of infection, antibiotic therapy is mandatory.
2. The dural defect is sealed closed and the CSF leak is managed postoperatively. Anytime there is a suspicion or evidence of a CSF leak, a meticulous waterproof closure of the exposed dural plane is mandatory. In the case of an evident or persistent leak, we recommend carrying out revision duraplastic surgery as soon as possible to reduce the time of exposure involving the sinus flora and the intracranial cavity. In our experience, all cases of postoperative meningitis have occurred in patients with a postoperative CSF leak.[5,13]
3. The sinonasal tract is managed operatively and postoperatively. All surgical injury of the mucosa reduces mucociliary transport in the nose and sinus cavities. Moreover, if the sinus mucosa is removed, the new epithelium is not ciliated and subsequent mucus clearance may be impaired. If the natural ostial patency of the sinus is not respected, it may possibly lead to acute or, more frequently, chronic sinusitis and, over the long term, a postsurgical mucocele. Therefore, to prevent acute or chronic alterations of the sinuses and nasal cavity functioning and/or infection and/or postsurgical mucocele, it is important to avoid unnecessary stripping of mucosa, to preserve sinus patency, and to correct any tendency toward lateralization of the middle turbinate. In the postoperative period, we suggest frequent nasal cleaning with saline solution and a transnasal endoscopic examination 3 to 4 weeks after the surgical procedure. An earlier examination should be performed in the case of an extended approach or in the case of disturbing sinus symptoms, such as rhinorrhea, a foul smell, and/or nasal obstruction.

Conclusion

Endoscopic skull base surgery is the most recent development of endoscopic transsphenoidal surgery and is based on the use of expanded endonasal approaches. The key for its widespread acceptance results from the direct extracerebral access to the ventral skull base and the avoidance of brain manipulation and neurovascular dissection. In other respects, endoscopic approaches follow the same rules as for microsurgery. It is a technique that can give great results, but that may pose many pitfalls for the surgeon. Safety may be preserved following some golden rules: (1) perform only operations for which the surgeon is highly trained; (2) prevent complications by strictly following the technical rules; and (3) be prepared to treat complications that unfortunately occur even when the surgery is performed in the best hands using careful and cautious management. The latter statement implies that such procedures have to be performed only by surgeons or in centers where all competencies are present—namely, the possibility of switching to open surgery, having rapid access to endovascular treatment, and having an experienced intensive care unit.

References

1. Cappabianca P, Cavallo LM, Esposito F, De Divitiis O, Messina A, De Divitiis E. Extended endoscopic endonasal approach to the midline skull base: the evolving role of transsphenoidal surgery. Adv Tech Stand Neurosurg 2008;33:151–199
2. Snyderman C, Kassam A, Carrau R, Mintz A, Gardner P, Prevedello DM. Acquisition of surgical skills for endonasal skull base surgery: a training program. Laryngoscope 2007;117(4):699–705
3. Ciric I, Ragin A, Baumgartner C, Pierce D. Complications of transsphenoidal surgery: results of a national survey, review of the literature, and personal experience. Neurosurgery 1997;40(2): 225–236, discussion 236–237
4. Laws ER Jr. Vascular complications of transsphenoidal surgery. Pituitary 1999;2(2):163–170
5. Frank G, Pasquini E, Farneti G, et al. The endoscopic versus the traditional approach in pituitary surgery. Neuroendocrinology 2006;83(3-4):240–248
6. Pasquini E, Sciarretta V, Farneti G, Mazzatenta D, Modugno GC, Frank G. Endoscopic treatment of encephaloceles of the lateral wall of the sphenoid sinus. Minim Invasive Neurosurg 2004;47(4):209–213
7. Raymond J, Hardy J, Czepko R, Roy D. Arterial injuries in transsphenoidal surgery for pituitary adenoma; the role of angiography and endovascular treatment. AJNR Am J Neuroradiol 1997;18(4):655–665
8. Snyderman C, Kassam A, Carrau R, Mintz A, Gardner P, Prevedello DM. Acquisition of surgical skills for endonasal skull base surgery: a training program. Laryngoscope 2007;117(4):699–705
9. Kassam A, Snyderman CH, Mintz A, Gardner P, Carrau RL. Expanded endonasal approach: the rostrocaudal axis. Part I. Crista galli to the sella turcica. Neurosurg Focus 2005;19(1):E3
10. Kassam A, Snyderman CH, Mintz A, Gardner P, Carrau RL. Expanded endonasal approach: the rostrocaudal axis. Part II. Posterior clinoids to the foramen magnum. Neurosurg Focus 2005;19(1):E4
11. Kassam AB, Gardner P, Snyderman C, Mintz A, Carrau R. Expanded endonasal approach: fully endoscopic, completely transnasal approach to the middle third of the clivus, petrous bone, middle cranial fossa, and infratemporal fossa. Neurosurg Focus 2005;19(1):E6
12. Lasio G, Ferroli P, Felisati G, Broggi G. Image-guided endoscopic transnasal removal of recurrent pituitary adenomas. Neurosurgery 2002;51(1):132–136, discussion 136–137
13. Frank G, Pasquini E. Endoscopic endonasal cavernous sinus surgery, with special reference to pituitary adenomas. Front Horm Res 2006;34:64–82
14. Kassam A, Snyderman CH, Carrau RL, Gardner P, Mintz A. Endoneurosurgical hemostasis techniques: lessons learned from 400 cases. Neurosurg Focus 2005;19(1):E7
15. Archondakis E, Pero G, Valvassori L, Boccardi E, Scialfa G. Angiographic follow-up of traumatic carotid cavernous fistulas treated with endovascular stent graft placement. AJNR Am J Neuroradiol 2007;28(2):342–347
16. Sorteberg A, Bakke SJ, Boysen M, Sorteberg W. Angiographic balloon test occlusion and therapeutic sacrifice of major arteries to the brain. Neurosurgery 2008;63(4):651–661
17. Frank G, Pasquini E, Doglietto F, et al. The endoscopic extended transsphenoidal approach for craniopharyngiomas. Neurosurgery 2006;59(1, Suppl 1):ONS75–ONS83, discussion ONS75–ONS83
18. Snyderman CH, Carrau RL, Kassam AB, et al. Endoscopic skull base surgery: principles of endonasal oncological surgery. J Surg Oncol 2008;97(8):658–664
19. Pasquini E, Sciarretta V, Farneti G, Ippolito A, Mazzatenta D, Frank G. Endoscopic endonasal approach for the treatment of benign schwannoma of the sinonasal tract and pterygopalatine fossa. Am J Rhinol 2002;16(2):113–118
20. Kassam AB, Vescan AD, Carrau RL, et al. Expanded endonasal approach: vidian canal as a landmark to the petrous internal carotid artery. J Neurosurg 2008;108(1):177–183
21. Cappabianca P, Cavallo LM, Esposito F, Valente V, De Divitiis E. Sellar repair in endoscopic endonasal transsphenoidal surgery: results of 170 cases. Neurosurgery 2002;51(6):1365–1371, discussion 1371–1372
22. Bachmann-Harildstad G. Diagnostic values of beta-2 transferrin and beta-trace protein as markers for cerebrospinal fluid fistula. Rhinology 2008;46(2):82–85
23. Lloyd KM, DelGaudio JM, Hudgins PA. Imaging of skull base cerebrospinal fluid leaks in adults. Radiology 2008;248(3): 725–736
24. El Gammal T, Sobol W, Wadlington VR, et al. Cerebrospinal fluid fistula: detection with MR cisternography. AJNR Am J Neuroradiol 1998;19(4):627–631
25. Stammberger H, Greistorfer K, Wolf G, Luxenberger W. Surgical occlusion of cerebrospinal fistulas of the anterior skull base using intrathecal sodium fluorescein. Laryngorhinootologie 1997;76(10):595–607
26. Esposito F, Dusick JR, Fatemi N, Kelly DF. Graded repair of cranial base defects and cerebrospinal fluid leaks in transsphenoidal surgery. Neurosurgery 2007;60(4, Suppl 2):295–303, discussion 303–304
27. Kassam AB, Thomas A, Carrau RL, et al. Endoscopic reconstruction of the cranial base using a pedicled nasoseptal flap. Neurosurgery 2008;63(1, Suppl 1):ONS44–ONS52, discussion ONS52–ONS53
28. Candrina R, Galli G, Bollati AJ. Subdural and intraventricular tension pneumocephalus after transsphenoidal operation. J Neurol Neurosurg Psychiatry 1988;51(7):1005–1006
29. Carrau RL, Snyderman C, Janecka IP, Sekhar L, Sen C, D'Amico F. Antibiotic prophylaxis in cranial base surgery. Head Neck 1991;13(4):311–317
30. Brown SM, Anand VK, Tabaee A, Schwartz TH. Role of perioperative antibiotics in endoscopic skull base surgery. Laryngoscope 2007;117(9):1528–1532

54 Cranial and Combined Approaches

Michael J. Kaplan, Nancy J. Fischbein, and Griffith R. Harsh IV

This last chapter focuses on indications for and techniques of transcranial approaches to pathology at the intersection of the cranial and sinonasal (or rhinal) spaces. It emphasizes the value of multidisciplinary cooperation in choosing among management options, procedures, and patient follow-up. This includes: (1) using high-resolution skull base imaging to assess the extent of disease; (2) appreciating the efficacy of alternatives or adjuncts of surgery such as chemotherapy and conformal radiotherapy (e.g., IMRT and stereotactic radiosurgery); and (3) exploiting the complementarity of cranial and rhinal approaches to achieve maximal resection of neoplastic or infectious pathology or repair of developmental or traumatic defects with minimal morbidity.

Surgical approaches to the anterior skull base have evolved since an initial paper in 1954 by Smith[1] described resection of a frontal sinus tumor. Prior to Smith's report, two papers appeared in which an orbital tumor had been resected via a craniotomy[2] or a craniotomy-transorbital[3] approach. Between 1963 and 1973, Ketcham[4,5] demonstrated clearly that surgery in this area, although associated with significant morbidity, improved the likelihood of cure of malignant tumors. Since that time, numerous surgical techniques have been introduced to extend or improve anatomic access for resection or reconstruction, and/or to reduce functional or aesthetic morbidity. Small transfacial incisions that supplement a bicoronal craniotomy incision are widely used[6] and, increasingly, endoscopic and endoscopic-assisted approaches are being perfected for selected cases, as reviewed by Har-El.[7] Today, anterior skull base surgery by experienced multidisciplinary teams is performed and accepted internationally. Compared with a generation ago, improved local control and survival rates have been documented, and the incidence of severe morbidity and mortality has been reduced to much lower than 5%.[8]

This evolution demonstrates a shift from cranial to rhinal approaches as the default choice in an attempt to reduce the risk of brain injury. Thus, a purely rhinal and often endoscopic approach is preferred unless this would significantly limit the extent of tumor resection or preclude adequate repair of the anterior skull base. Identification of such limitations of a rhinal approach requires familiarity with surgical anatomy, the natural history of neoplastic diseases of the area, and the efficacy of adjuvant therapies.

Indications

Although extensive bacterial or fungal infections of the anterior or lateral skull base occasionally require combined transcranial and rhinal approaches, tumors far more frequently require these combined approaches and are the focus of this review. Tumors that may require anterior skull base resection include selected malignant tumors of the paranasal sinuses that extend superiorly through the cribriform plate, ethmoid roof, and planum sphenoidale or posteriorly through the posterior wall of the frontal sinus; benign and malignant meningiomas that involve the same areas; and selected benign tumors or tumorlike lesions such as orbital apex schwannomas, large nasal tumors such as juvenile angiofibromas and inverted papillomas, and occasional encephaloceles and mucoceles.

The goals of anterior skull base surgery for tumors have remained constant throughout the continuing evolution of surgical and radiation oncology techniques. These goals include the following:

1. Resection of tumor with negative margins
2. Preservation of neurologic function, including vision and olfaction
3. Reduction of operative complications via:
   a. Minimal brain retraction
   b. Cerebrospinal fluid (CSF) leak repair; dural repair and/or flaps (myogenous, fascial, or mucosal)
   c. Segregation of intracranial contents from the contaminated paranasal sinuses, reducing the incidence of meningitis
4. Improved aesthetic outcome

Contraindications to aggressive surgical resection include tumor extension that precludes resection of tumor with negative margins (e.g., tumor in the cavernous sinus lateral to the internal carotid artery); tumor surrounding the optic chiasm; and/or perineural spread to Meckel's cave or the cavernous sinus. Involvement of the internal carotid artery is often deemed unresectable. Additional contraindications include distant metastatic disease unlikely to respond to chemotherapy and patient medical fragility.

Specific indications for craniotomy or a combined procedure over a rhinal approach alone include the following:

1. Tumor involvement superior to the orbit (and lateral to the ethmoid roof) in cases in which preservation of the orbit is anticipated (**Fig. 54.1**)

A B C D

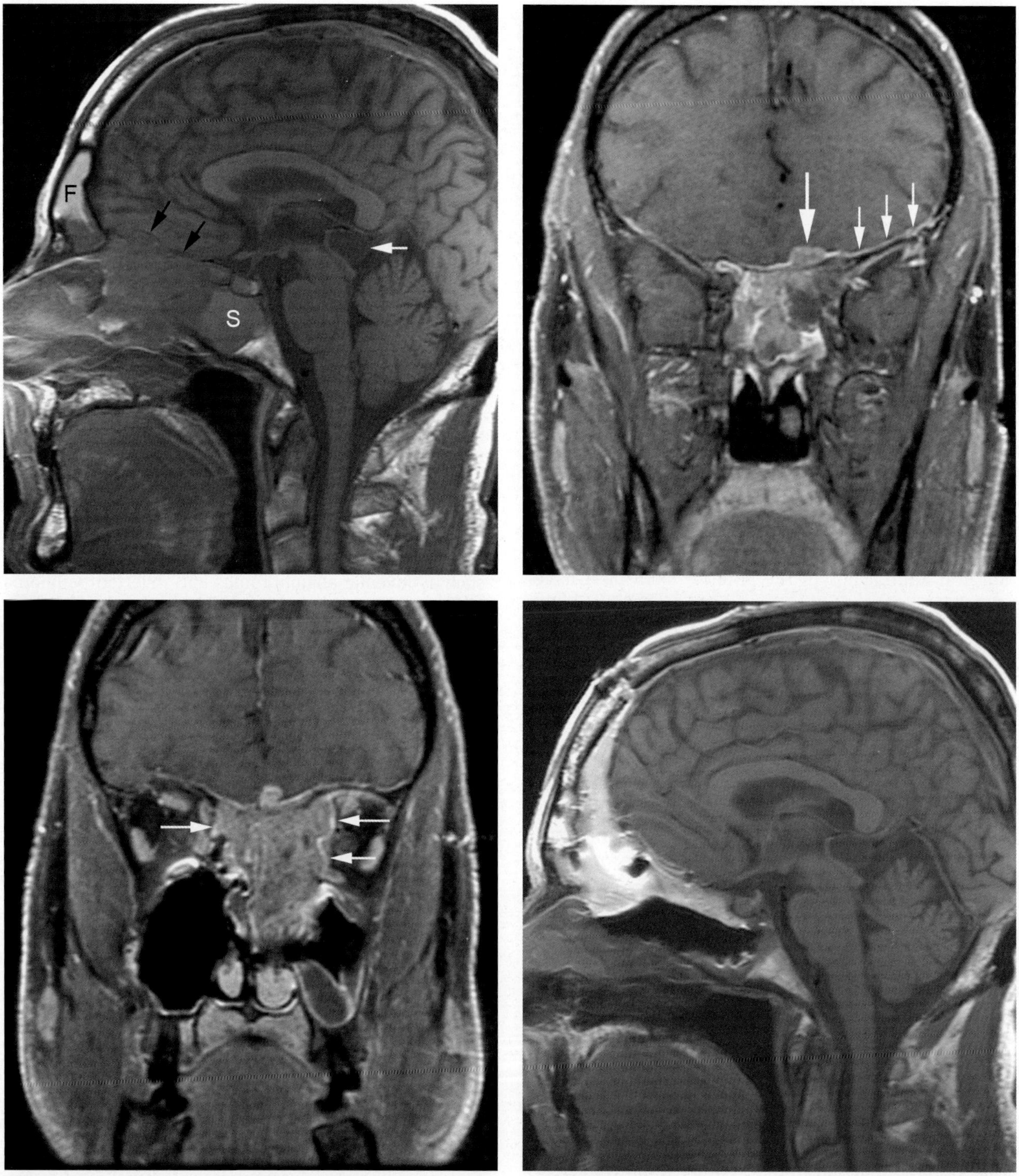

Fig. 54.1 A 57-year-old man with poorly differentiated squamous cell carcinoma. **(A)** Sagittal T1-weighted image demonstrates a soft tissue mass extending from the nasal cavity and ethmoid sinus into the anterior cranial fossa through the ethmoid roof *(black arrows)* and also into the anterior sphenoid sinus. Obstructive proteinaceous secretions are present in the sphenoid (*S*) and frontal (*F*) sinuses. Incidental pineal cyst (*white arrow*). **(B)** Coronal T1-weighted postgadolinium image with fat saturation demonstrates enhancing tumor extending superiorly through the planum sphenoidale to infiltrate the dura in a nodular (*large white arrow*) and linear fashion but without brain involvement. Dural enhancement extends laterally (*small white arrows*), beyond the reach of an endoscopic approach. **(C)** A more anterior coronal T1-weighted postgadolinium image with fat saturation again demonstrates nodular dural involvement as well as linear dural enhancement superior to the orbits bilaterally, mandating craniotomy. In addition, bilateral left-greater-than-right extension of tumor into the orbit is seen (*white arrows*). The lamina papyracea and orbital periosteum were involved. As anticipated because of the full extraocular motility, the medial rectus and inferior rectus muscles were not involved, and the orbits were preserved. **(D)** Sagittal T1-weighted image shows typical appearance following bifrontal orbital-cranial approach to tumor resection, followed by reconstruction of the anterior skull base with a pericranial galeal flap. Blood products are present in the anterior cranial fossa and paranasal sinuses. *(continued)*

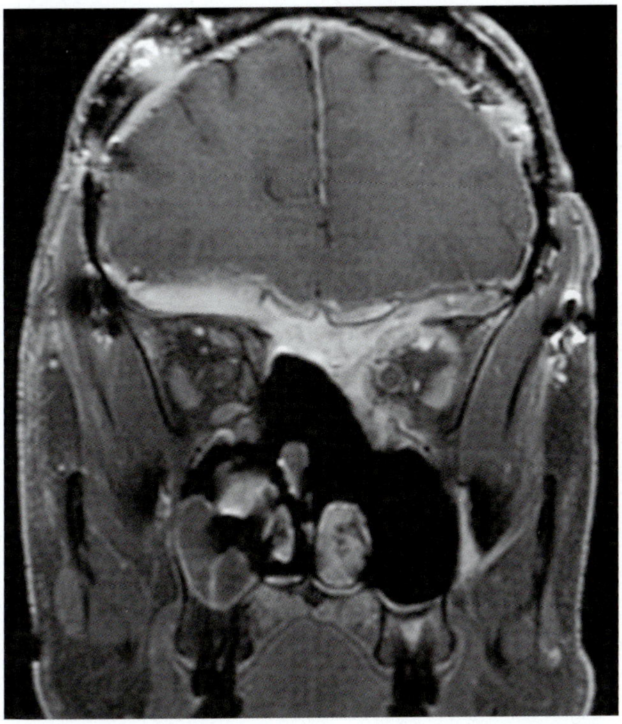

E

Fig. 54.1 *(continued)* **(E)** Postoperative coronal T1-weighetd postgadolinium image with fat saturation also shows evidence of the bifrontal craniotomy, extensive surgery of the paranasal sinuses and orbits, and reconstruction with a pericranial-galeal flap. Negative margins were achieved.

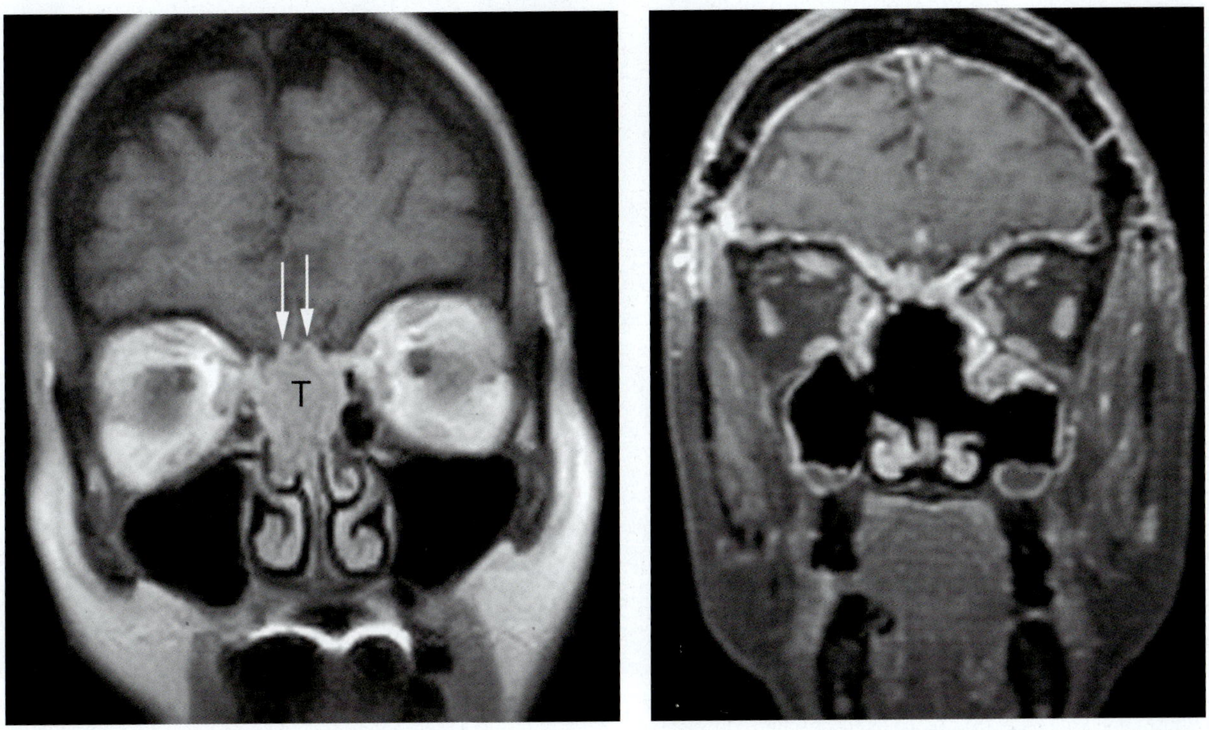

A B

Fig. 54.2 A 66-year-old woman with poorly differentiated squamous cell carcinoma of the superior nasal septum and ethmoid sinuses penetrating the anterior skull base. **(A)** Coronal T1-weighted postgadolinium image demonstrates enhancing tumor (*T*) involving the nasal septum and ethmoid labyrinth, with superior extension to the anterior skull base and extension intracranially (*white arrows*) to involve dura. Some might have resected this lesion endoscopically, but the site of tumor precluded the use of a robust regional mucosal flap.[46] A bifrontal craniotomy facilitates both excellent dural margins and definitive cerebrospinal fluid leak repair via a pericranial-galeal flap. **(B)** Coronal T1-weighted postgadolinium image with fat saturation shows expected postoperative appearance following bifrontal craniotomy, anterior skull base resection, pericranial-galeal flap reconstruction, and paranasal sinus and nasal septal resection. A rim of enhancing nonspecific soft tissue is expected around the periphery of the operative bed.

2. Resectable tumor attached to the dorsal or lateral aspects of the optic nerve, optic chiasm, or the intracranial internal carotid artery and its branches
3. Tumor widely involving subfrontal dura, especially over the orbital roofs, such that watertight closure is precluded (**Fig. 54.1**)
4. Tumor involvement precluding septal mucosal flap for repair of CSF fistula (**Fig. 54.2**)

Orbital Tumor and Preservation of the Orbit

There remains some controversy regarding how much of the orbit can be resected while still retaining adequate functional integrity. Some feel that involvement of the lamina papyracea demands orbital exenteration. Many feel, as do we, that the orbit can be functionally preserved in an oncologically sound fashion if there is no significant involvement of the orbital fat, even if the orbital periosteum is involved with the tumor. The thin fascial layer that surrounds the orbital fat just inside the orbital periosteum[9] probably accounts for orbital integrity after the resection of significant periosteum. In our experience, when the patient has full extraocular motility on preoperative clinical examination, one can usually preserve the orbit. If there is diplopia solely because of mass effect leading to proptosis and interference with extraocular muscle function but without radiologically evident extension of tumor into orbital fat, then the orbit also is likely to be able to be preserved. Extension of tumor superiorly through the orbital roof limits tumor resection from below, mandating craniotomy. The exception to mandated craniotomy is tumor involvement of the orbit sufficiently extensive to warrant exenteration, in which case tumor that is superior to the orbit can be removed transorbitally (**Fig. 54.3**). Compare **Fig. 54.3** with **Figs. 54.4** and **54.5**; an orbital exenteration was required in the former but, despite bilateral medial orbital periosteal involvement in the latter two cases, both orbits were preserved. Although magnetic resonance imaging (MRI) is extremely helpful in evaluating the orbit, the final decision with regard to orbit preservation may

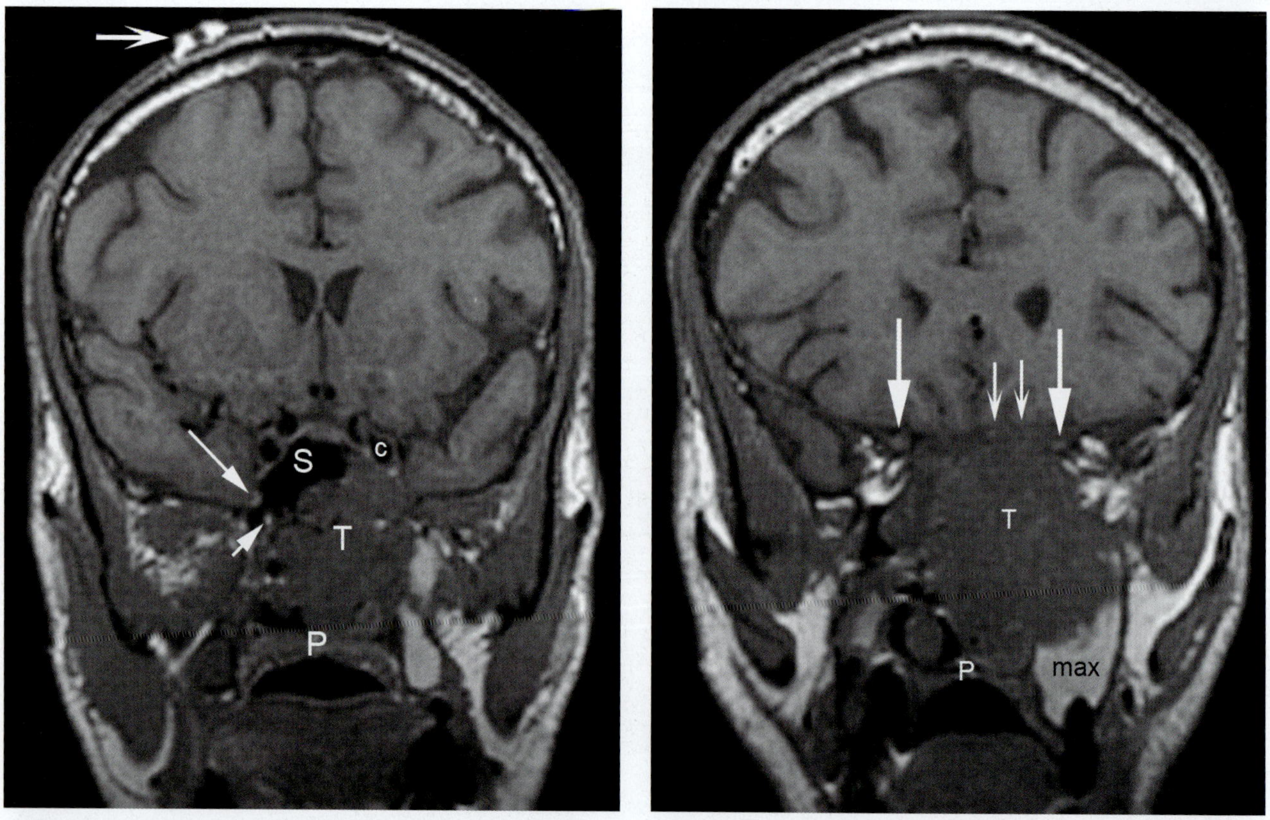

A

B

Fig. 54.3 A 60-year-old man with adenoid cystic carcinoma of the paranasal sinuses and skull base. **(A)** Coronal pregadolinium T1-weighted image from a preoperative stereotactic scan done for intraoperative navigation (note fiducial marker on the scalp, *concave white arrow*) demonstrates a large tumor mass (*T*) involving the sinonasal cavity and skull base. The tumor rests on the uninvolved hard palate (*P*) inferiorly and extends superiorly into the sphenoid sinus (*S*), eroding its floor. Foramen rotundum (*long white arrow*) and the vidian canal (*short white arrow*) are normal on the right, but are involved by tumor and poorly defined on the left. Tumor abuts the left cavernous internal carotid artery, (*c*). **(B)** A more anterior coronal pregadolinium T1-weighted image again demonstrates the large tumor mass (*T*) extending from the hard palate (*P*) through the nasal cavity to involve the anterior skull base superiorly (*concave arrows*). Tumor extends into and obstructs the maxillary sinus (*max*), with T1 bright proteinaceous secretions seen in the sinus. This image includes the posterior orbits, with the optic nerves (*large white arrows*) demonstrated. The right optic nerve is normal; the left optic nerve is involved and compressed by tumor. *(continued)*

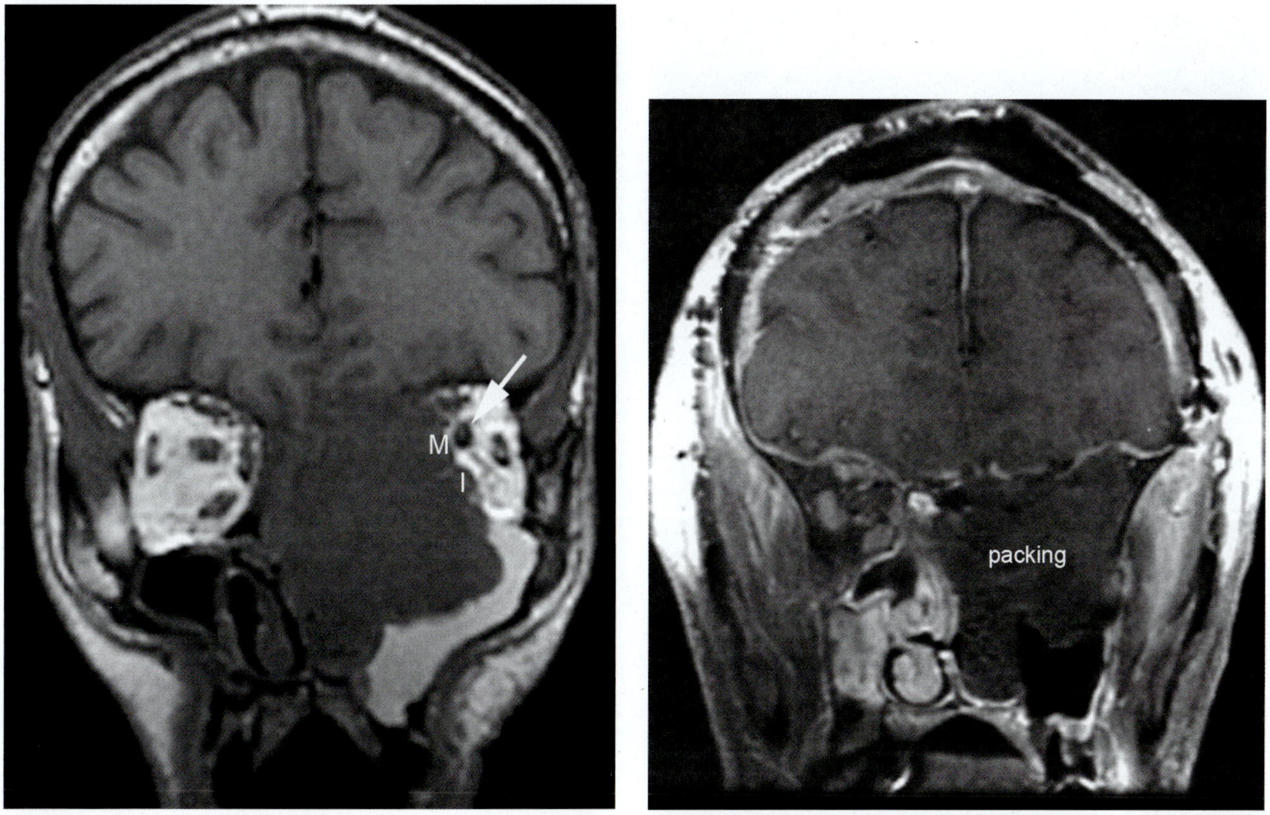

C D

Fig. 54.3 *(continued)* **(C)** More anteriorly, another coronal pregadolinium T1-weighted image through the midorbit level demonstrates tumor extension into the maxillary sinus, anterior skull base, and left orbit. The inferior (*I*) and medial (*M*) rectus muscles are involved by tumor. The optic nerve-sheath complex (*white arrow*) is not involved at this level. Involvement of the inferolateral sphenoid sinus and foramen rotundum is well managed endoscopically, but involvement of the orbit posterosuperiorly mandates a craniotomy approach for effective cerebrospinal fluid leak repair. In addition, optic nerve involvement and rectus muscle involvement (with diplopia) requires orbital exenteration. **(D)** Coronal postgadolinium T1-weighted image with fat suppression acquired following resection. Tumor was removed largely through the orbital exenteration cavity, including resection of the anterior cranial fossa and nasopharynx, maxillectomy, ethmoidectomy, sphenoidectomy, and a craniectomy for tumor within the frontal bone (not shown). No frontal lobe elevation was required. A pericranial-galeal flap was used both to resurface the skull base and line the orbital defect. Gross total resection of tumor was achieved, although with microscopically positive posterior margins, as expected due to the perineural spread common in adenoid cystic carcinoma. A large Merocel sponge (*packing*) is seen inferior to the pericranial flap. The patient received intensity-modulated radiation thereapy postoperatively and has remained free of disease at the primary site, though discontinuous dural metastases subsequently developed.

have to be made intraoperatively, and should be discussed in advance with the patient and family.

Preservation of Vision and Protection of the Internal Carotid Artery

The optic nerve and the internal carotid artery (ICA) are usually covered by bone in the superolateral aspect of the sphenoid sinus, though the bone is occasionally dehiscent. The optic nerve lies just superior to the ICA. Tumor and tumor-infiltrated bone can be removed transsphenoidally from these structures unless tumor invades the optic nerve sheath or the arterial adventitia, in which case tumor should be left behind lest the artery or nerve be injured. The ophthalmic artery arises from the ICA superiorly or superomedially near the cranial end of the optic canal and then courses through the optic canal along the optic nerve. It typically runs on the lateral surface of the nerve in the anterior optic canal. Thus, dissection of the anterior optic chiasm and the medial optic canal is generally safe.

When tumor is attached to the dorsal or lateral surfaces of the optic nerve, optic chiasm, or the intracranial internal carotid artery and its branches, and particularly when it surrounds these structures, then the risk of dissection from below is substantial and a craniotomy is indicated if it is the judgment of the team that tumor resection is appropriate at all. Tumor within the cavernous sinus, particularly if it surrounds the internal carotid artery, usually cannot be removed safely by even a transcranial approach.

Lateral Dural Extension and Preservation of Smell

Although areas of dura infiltrated or penetrated by tumor can be resected and the resultant defect repaired

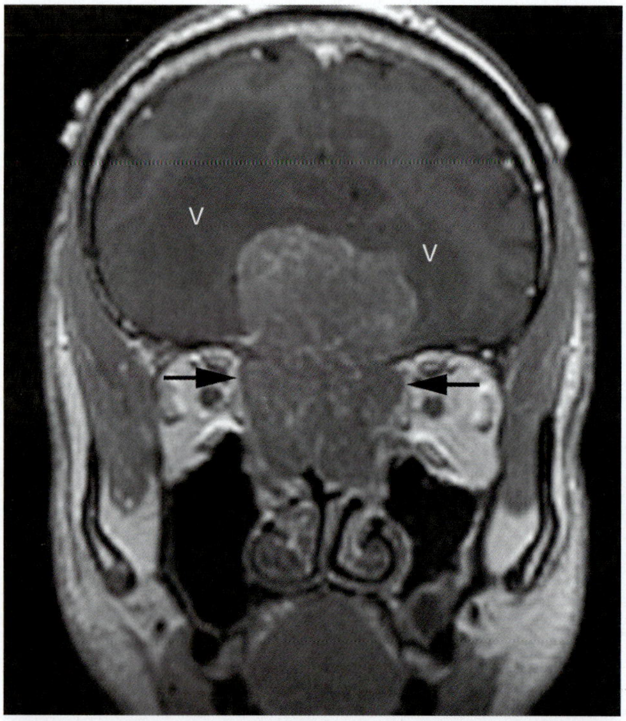

A

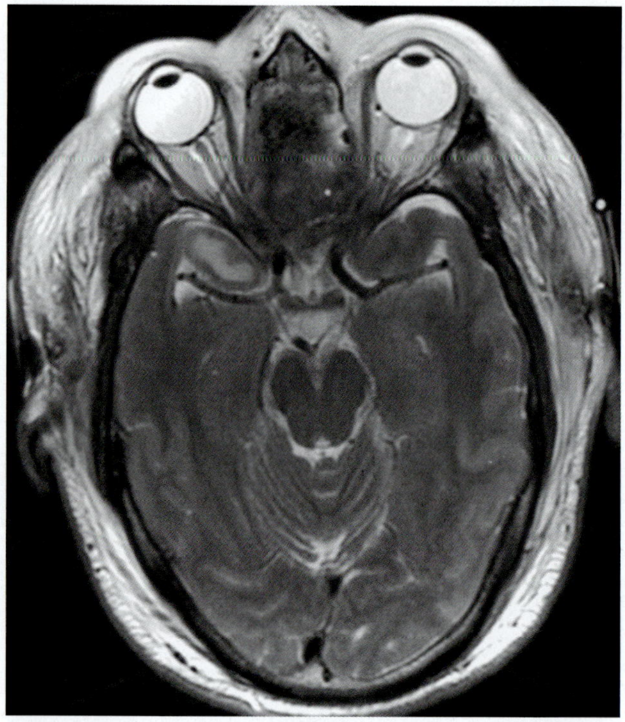

B

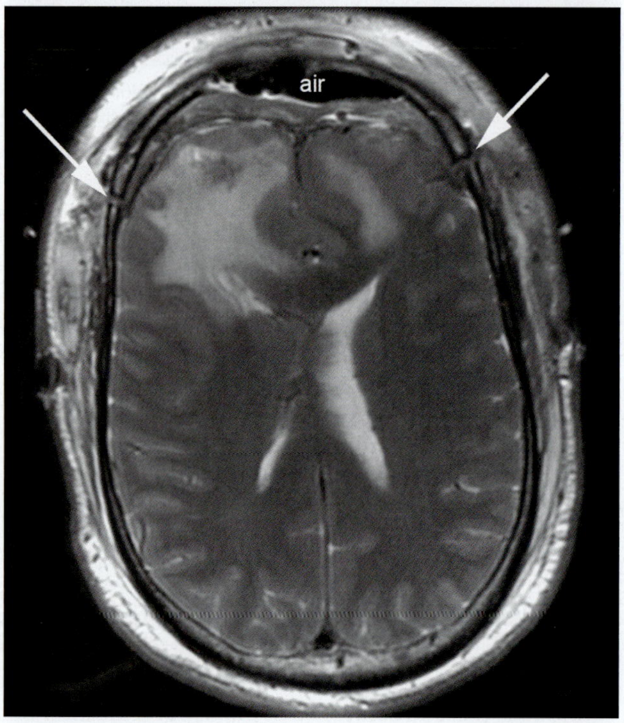

C

Fig. 54.4 A 53-year-old man with sinonasal undifferentiated carcinoma of the paranasal sinuses and skull base, with normal extraocular motility (*EOM*). **(A)** A coronal postgadolinium T1-weighted image from a preoperative stereotactic scan (note fiducial markers on the scalp) demonstrates a large tumor mass involving the nasal cavity, the ethmoid sinuses, anterior skull base, and orbits bilaterally (*black arrows*). A large component of tumor extends into the anterior cranial fossa, displacing the bilateral frontal lobes and causing vasogenic edema (V) in them. **(B)** An axial T2-weighted image from a postoperative day 3 scan demonstrates gross total resection of tumor in the sinonasal cavity and orbits. The orbital periosteum was involved bilaterally, but no orbital fat was involved. The orbits were preserved, and the patient maintained normal extraocular motility postoperatively. **(C)** A more superior axial T2-weighted image from the postoperative scan demonstrates the bifrontal craniotomy (*white arrows*), as well as extra-axial air and hemorrhage. Residual bifrontal vasogenic edema is present.

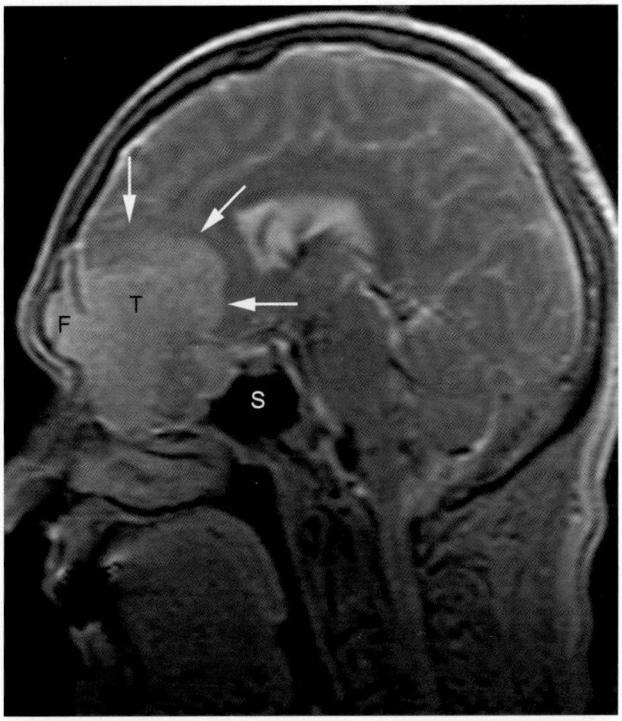

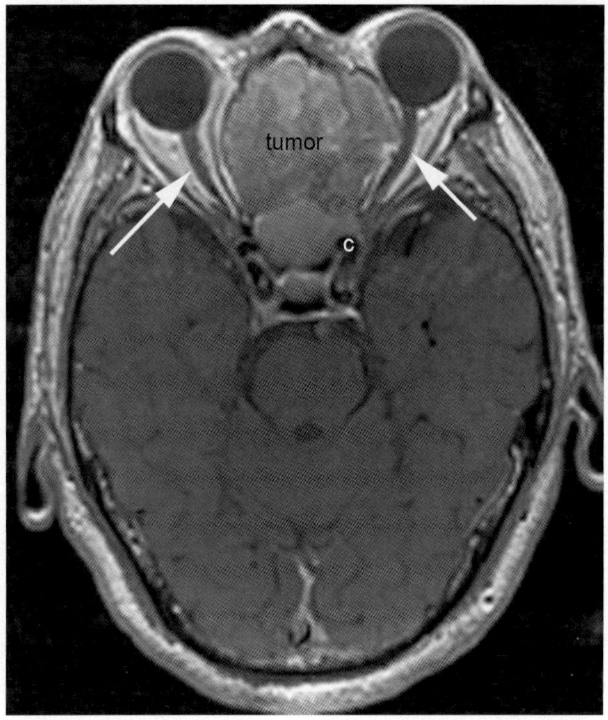

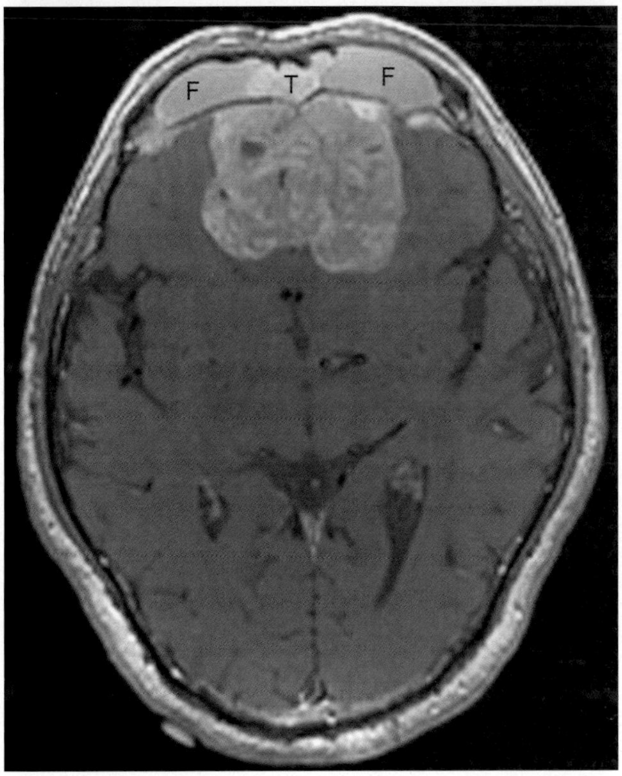

Fig. 54.5 A 61-year-old man with adenoid cystic carcinoma of the sinonasal cavity and anterior skull base. **(A)** Sagittal T2-weighted low resolution scout image from a stereotactic preoperative magnetic resonance examination demonstrates a large tumor (*T*) involving the nasal cavity, nasal septum, and ethmoid sinuses, extending into the frontal sinus (*F*). A large component in the anterior cranial fossa (*white arrows*) displaces the frontal lobes and corpus callosum, but no brain edema is seen. The anterosuperior aspect of the sphenoid sinus (*S*) is involved, but not the sella. **(B)** An axial postgadolinium T1-weighted image from the same preoperative stereotactic study demonstrates the large tumor mass extending into the orbits bilaterally. There is mass effect on the optic nerves (*white arrows*) and globes, but the patient had normal bilateral extraocular motility. Tumor approaches the cavernous internal carotid arteries (*c*) bilaterally, but inspissated secretions are present between the tumor and internal carotid artery. **(C)** A more superior axial postgadolinium T1-weighted image demonstrates bulky tumor in the anterior cranial fossa, but no evidence for transdural extension. The upper aspect of tumor (*T*) within the frontal sinus is indicated, as are obstructive proteinaceous secretions laterally in the frontal sinuses (*F*). The patient underwent bifrontal craniotomy and anterior skull base resection, including bilateral orbitotomy, frontal sinusectomy, and reconstruction with a pericranial-galeal flap. Gross total resection of tumor was achieved, followed by intensity-modulated radiation therapy. *(continued)*

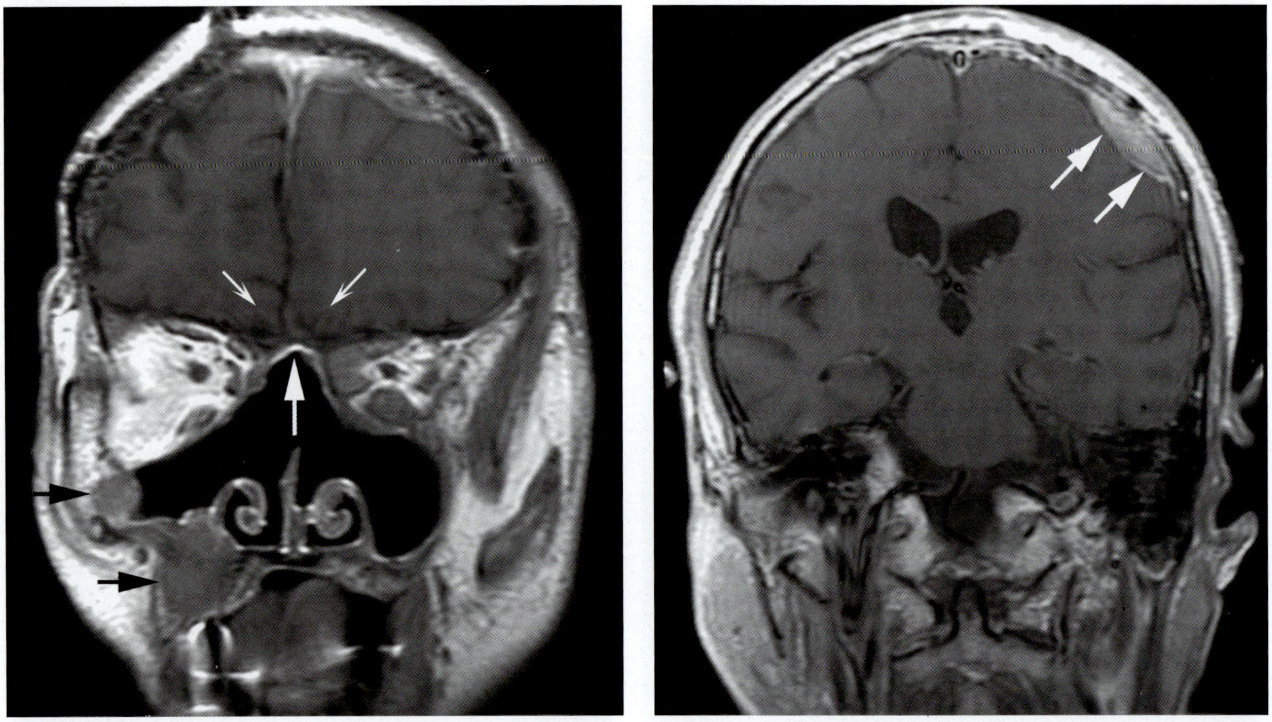

D E

Fig. 54.5 (D) *(continued)* A coronal postgadolinium T1-weighted image from an magnetic resonance scan performed 21 months after the initial surgery demonstrates expected postcraniotomy changes (including subtle bifrontal encephalomalacia, *small concave arrows*) and no evidence of recurrence at the sinonasal/anterior skull base, which was the original site of disease (*white straight arrow*). Recurrence is noted in the right lateral maxilla, however (*straight black arrows*). In addition, the left extraocular muscles are swollen due to an orbital apex metastasis (not shown). The patient also had developed extensive pulmonary metastases (not shown), as occurs in ~20% of patients with adenoid cystic carcinoma. **(E)** A more posterior coronal postgadolinium T1-weighted image demonstrates a plaquelike dural metastasis (*arrows*) that was not contiguous with the initial primary site.

endoscopically, durotomies much larger than several square centimeters are more challenging to repair with high reliability; this is a particular problem if tumor involves the septum from which a flap might be obtained or when there has been prior irradiation. In the absence of viable nasal septum, an endoscopically harvested and rotated pericranial flap offers a reconstructive alternative, but with very large defects, a craniotomy may be warranted. This is particularly true when the dura involved extends lateral to the cribriform plate and planum sphenoidale and dorsal to the orbital roofs (**Fig. 54.1**).

The olfactory rootlets penetrate the cribriform plate, which lies just medial and usually slightly inferior to the ethmoid roof. Dura is much more tightly adherent to bone at the cribriform plate than at the ethmoid roof. A thin-section (≤1 mm) coronal computed tomography (CT) scan is useful for assessing the bony integrity of the cribriform plate and ethmoid roof. This area can also be assessed with MRI, which better depicts the dural and parenchymal extension of tumor. Thin-section coronal fast-spin echo T2-weighted images are often most useful for assessing the presence or absence of subtle anterior skull base penetration (**Fig. 54.6**), whereas coronal postgadolinium T1-weighted images with fat saturation will most sensitively demonstrate or exclude dural, leptomeningeal, and brain parenchymal extension.

If the olfactory apparatus is involved only minimally and unilaterally by, for example, a small esthesioneuroblastoma, then preservation of the contralateral olfactory apparatus by a unilateral approach may be possible. Such a patient would be first evaluated for the feasibility of an endoscopic conservational approach. If the patient is not deemed to be an endoscopic candidate, then a unilateral frontal craniotomy could be considered. The exposure from a limited craniotomy could be augmented as necessary by endoscopic or external ethmoidectomy to enable complete tumor resection.

Cerebrospinal Fluid Fistula

Anticipation of creating a large fistula by removing a tumor with substantial transcranial and transdural extension warrants strong consideration of a cranial approach. Craniotomy provides wide exposure and is conducive to placing an inlay dural graft beneath an elevated frontal lobe (which has the advantage of peripheral buttressing of the graft against downward CSF pulsation). It also allows direct suture repair of dural rents and circumferential suturing of dural grafts, both of which are more difficult to accomplish using a transnasal endoscope. Paramedian or lateral fistulas are also more readily repaired from above

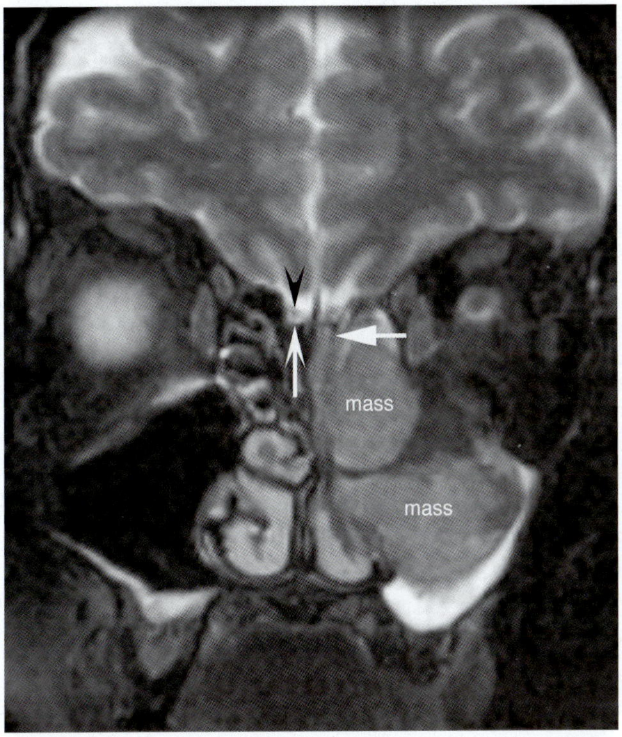

Fig. 54.6 A 55-year-old woman with squamous cell carcinoma of the maxillary and ethmoid sinuses and nasal cavity. Coronal fast spin echo T2-weighted image with fat saturation demonstrates a lobulated mass in the left maxillary and ethmoid sinuses, with tumor extending superiorly in the olfactory recess (*straight white arrow*) toward the anterior cranial fossa. The normal right cribriform plate (*concave white arrow*) and right olfactory bulb (*concave black arrowhead*) are shown. Although tumor abuts the left cribriform plate, the left olfactory apparatus is well seen and there is no evidence of tumor penetration of the anterior cranial fossa. The orbit is intact.

than from below. The advantages of improved exposure are of course mitigated by the need for brain retraction and by the increased difficulty of maintaining the integrity of the contralateral olfactory tract in unilateral disease.

Other Limits of Resectability

Poor clinical prognostic indicators include dural and, especially, brain involvement. Orbital involvement and extension of tumor to the pterygoid plates, infratemporal fossa, and/or nasopharynx are also indicators of poor prognosis. Although tumor involvement of these areas portends a worse prognosis, however, it is not an absolute contraindication for surgery, and proceeding with surgery may be worthwhile. Fee[10,11] and To[12,13] have demonstrated, for example, that resection of the soft tissue and cartilage of the nasopharynx can be accomplished effectively in selected cases of recurrent nasopharyngeal carcinoma. The authors and others have resected tumors that extend to the infratemporal fossa and greater wing of the sphenoid with acceptable morbidity and with long-term results dependent largely on the underlying histology. Malignant tumors that envelop the cavernous or petrous internal carotid artery, however, are usually regarded as unresectable. Although tumor abutting the anterior or inferior optic chiasm can be successfully resected, most surgeons feel that more extensive involvement of the optic chiasm by a malignancy is an absolute contraindication for surgery because of the likely resultant complete bilateral blindness.

Preoperative Clinical and Radiologic Assessment

Medical history and general physical examination with special attention to rhinologic and neurologic symptoms and signs are mandatory. The patient's current sense of smell should be noted and possibly documented with scent testing, and the patient should be fully informed regarding its vulnerability to surgery. Nasal endoscopy should establish the inferior boundaries and attachments of the mass. It is usually wise to have obtained a biopsy of accessible tumor, but in a few cases, notably juvenile angiofibroma, the history, clinical findings, and radiologic findings are essentially pathognomonic (**Fig. 54.7**); operative management (discussed in detail later) is indicated, and a preoperative biopsy is unnecessary, if not contraindicated. In other cases where surgery is indicated regardless of the histology, then histologic confirmation may be deferred to an early frozen section at the time of surgery.

Prior to planning a surgical approach to a tumor of the anterior skull base, it is important to have considered those histologies for which surgical resection may not be indicated. Primary lymphomas of the skull base and paranasal sinuses comprise one important category of nonoperative skull base lesions. Because lymphomas are common enough to be considered in the differential diagnosis of many aggressive lesions of the anterior skull base, biopsy may be indicated to exclude lymphoma.

Establishing that a mass is a metastasis from a prior malignancy should lead to further metastatic evaluation. If additional metastases are found, then a palliative approach with chemotherapy may be preferable to skull base surgery. On the other hand, there are times that surgical resection might be indicated even for a metastasis to the skull base or for an anterior skull base primary tumor with distant metastases. Examples of surgical indications where curative tumor resection is not expected include repair of an existing or imminent CSF leak or amelioration of mass effect and more effective palliation.

Radiologic imaging facilitates both preoperative planning and subsequent clinical follow-up. A high-quality MRI is almost always indicated as the imaging examination of choice, sometimes supplemented with coronal CT for assessment of the cribriform plate. CT scans are, however, particularly useful if the primary pathology is a fibro-osseous lesion of the skull base (**Fig. 54.8**). In addition

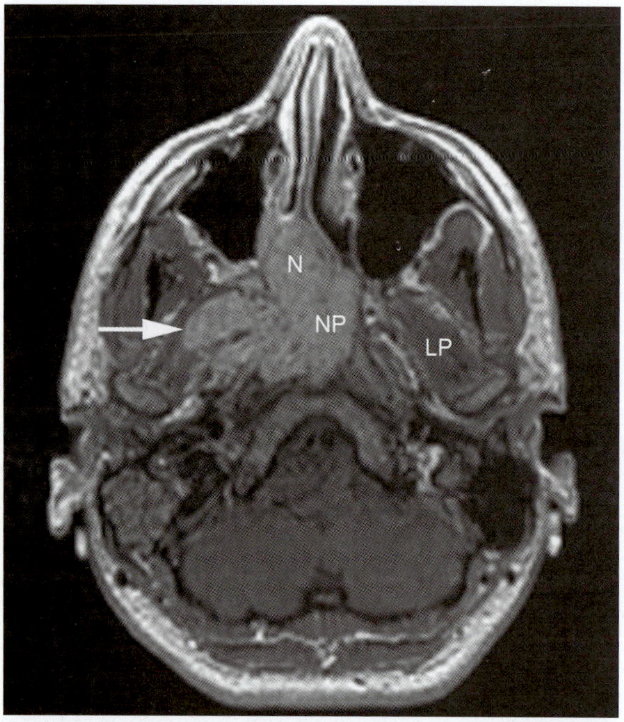

A

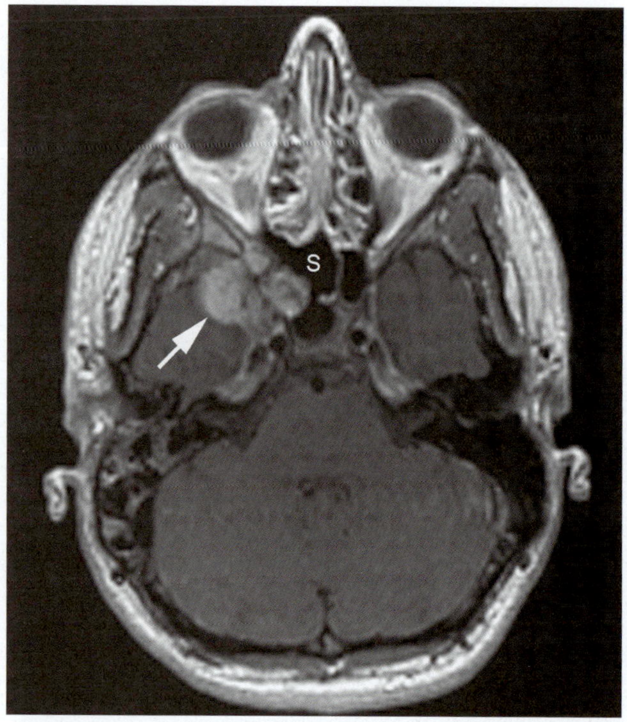

B

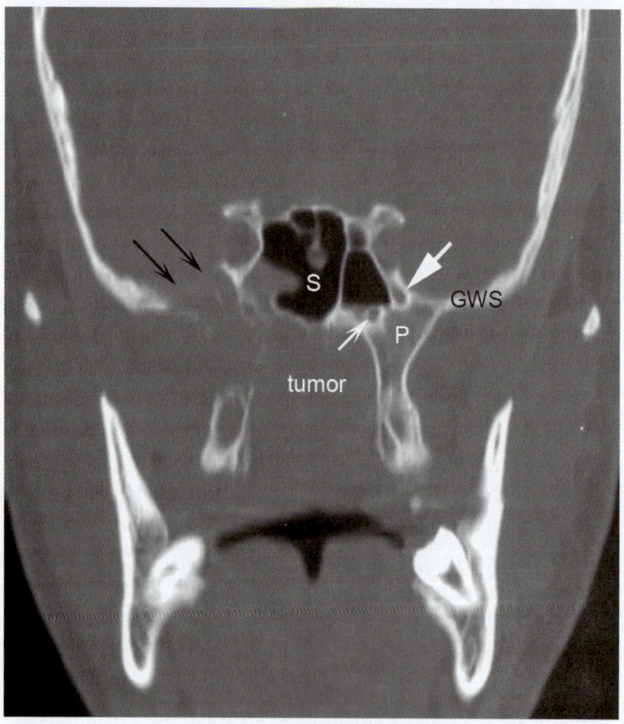

C

Fig. 54.7 A 19-year-old man with an extensive juvenile angiofibroma. **(A)** An axial postgadolinium T1-weighted image from a preoperative stereotactic magnetic resonance image demonstrates a lobulated, intensely enhancing sinonasal mass; internal foci of low signal intensity are consistent with the flow voids that characterize this highly vascular neoplasm. The nasal cavity (*N*) and nasopharyngeal (*NP*) components of the mass are indicated. In addition, the mass extends deep and laterally (*white arrow*) into the right infratemporal fossa, where it erodes the pterygoid plates and encroaches on the lateral pterygoid muscle (left lateral pterygoid, *LP*; shown for comparison). **(B)** A more superior axial postgadolinium T1-weighted image demonstrates enhancing tumor in the right lateral aspect of the sphenoid sinus (*S*), as well as extension of tumor into the right middle cranial fossa (*white arrow*), where it displaces but does not invade the right temporal lobe. **(C)** A preoperative coronal computed tomography directly demonstrates some of the areas where tumor has eroded bone. On the right, the tumor has eroded the pterygoid process of the sphenoid bone as well as the greater wing of the sphenoid (*black arrows*) to extend into the right middle cranial fossa. Tumor also involves the sphenoid sinus (*S*) and foramen rotundum and vidian canal. The normal structures are shown on the left for comparison. *P*, pterygoid process; *GWS*, greater wing of sphenoid; *straight white arrow*, foramen rotundum; *concave white arrow*, vidian canal. *(continued)*

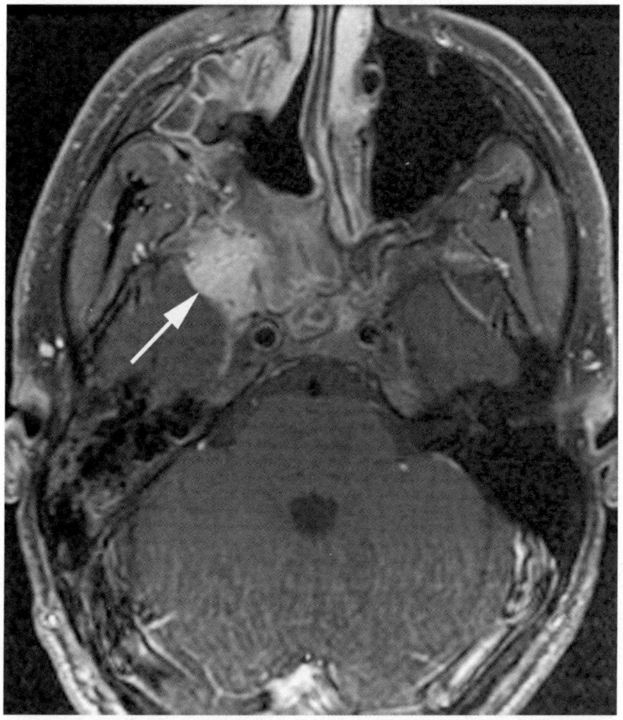

D

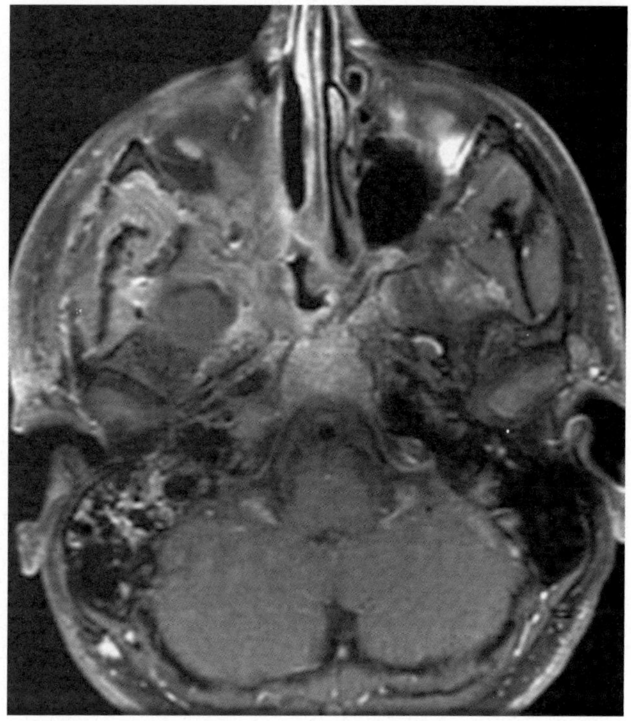

E

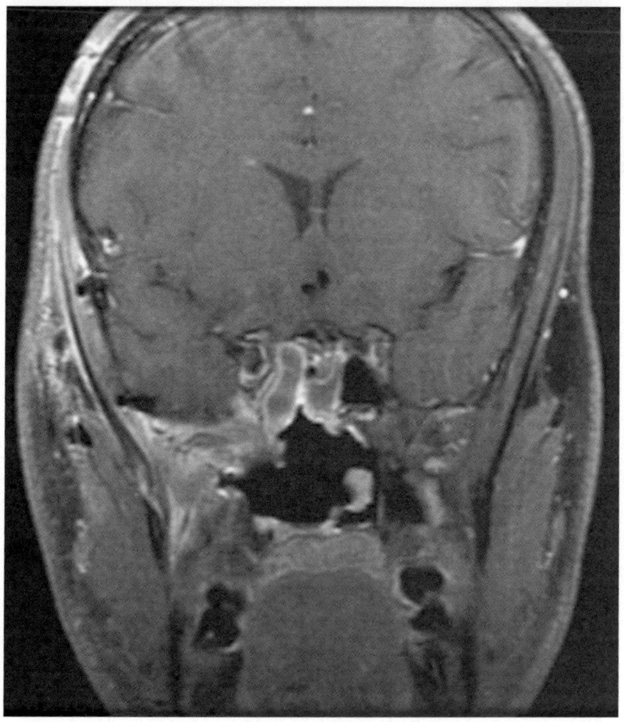

F

Fig. 54.7 *(continued)* **(D)** The tumor was resected in two stages following preoperative embolization. This axial postgadolinium T1-weighted image with fat suppression was acquired following the first stage: a right transsphenoethmoidal approach to the skull base, with medial maxillectomy, ethmoidectomy, sphenoidotomy, dissection in the pterygomaxillary space, and exposure of dura at the middle fossa but no dural entry. A 2-cm external ethmoidectomy facial incision facilitated access to all of the nasal, nasopharyngeal, and infratemporal fossa components of tumor, with wider exposure than an endoscopic approach would have afforded. On the postoperative magnetic resonance scan, expected postsurgical changes are seen in the paranasal sinuses and skull base without any residual tumor. A nodule of tumor remains in the middle cranial fossa (*white arrow*). **(E)** A subsequent middle cranial fossa approach was used to remove the residual tumor in the middle cranial fossa. An axial postgadolinium T1-weighted image with fat suppression shows expected changes after this operative approach, and no residual tumor. **(F)** The lack of any residual is demonstrated on a coronal postgadolinium T1-weighted image with fat suppression, and the patient has remained disease free in follow-up.

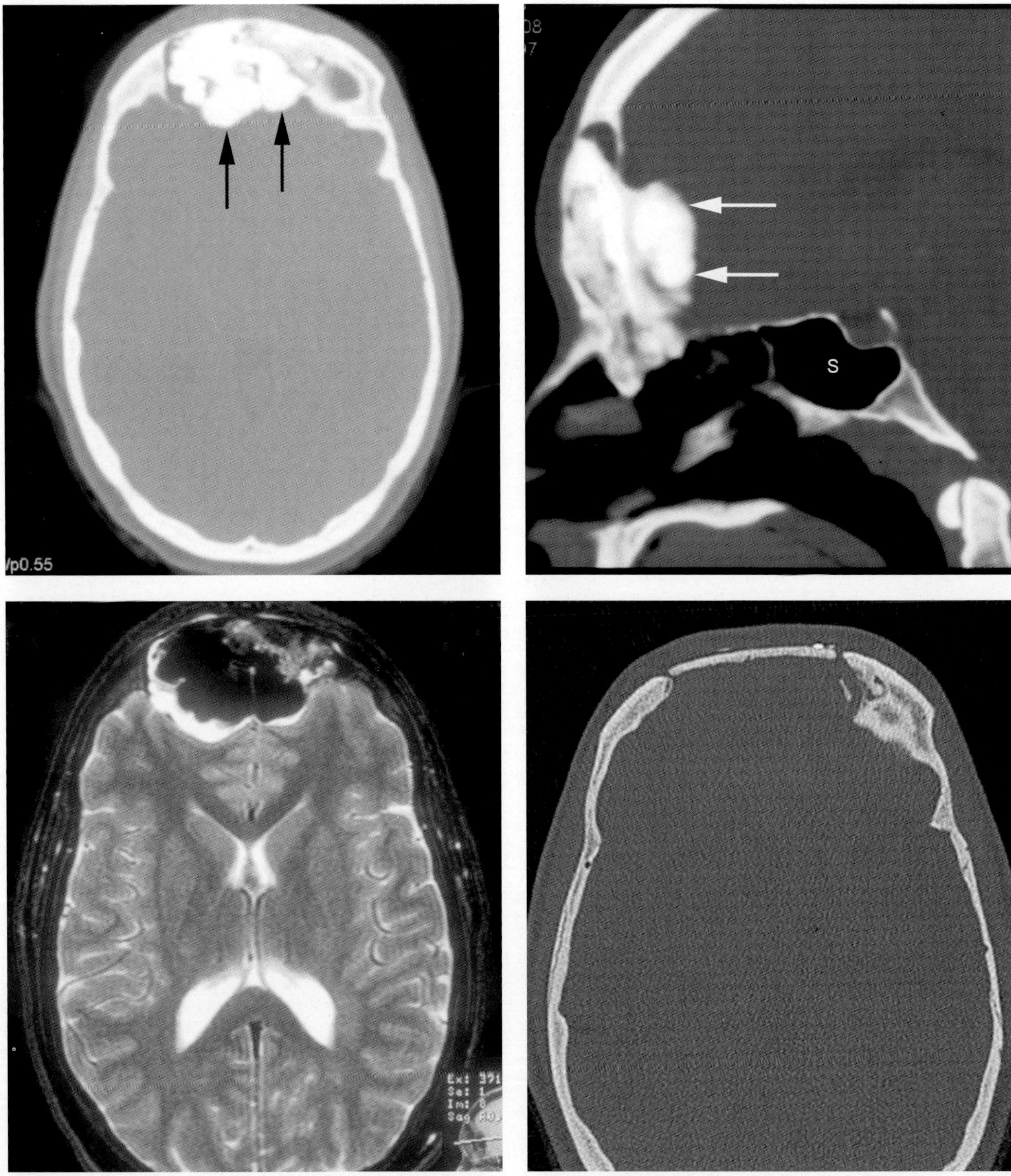

A B C D

Fig. 54.8 A 29-year-old woman with a sino-orbital osteoma with osteoblastomalike areas. **(A)** An axial computed tomography (CT) scan demonstrates a large lobulated mass (*black arrows*) involving the frontal sinuses and frontal bone. The mass is very dense, consistent with an osseous tumor. **(B)** A sagittal CT scan demonstrates the dense lobulated mass involving frontal sinus and frontal bone, with posterior extension into the anterior cranial fossa (*white arrows*). *S*, sphenoid sinus. **(C)** On an axial T2-weighted magnetic resonance image, the mass is very low in signal intensity given its bony nature. Although there is mass effect on the frontal lobes, no brain edema is present, and the lesion is benign appearing. **(D)** Postoperative axial CT image shows resection of the mass and reconstruction with a split calvarial graft. The tumor was resected via a combined endoscopic and external approach, with negative margins. The patient has remained disease free.

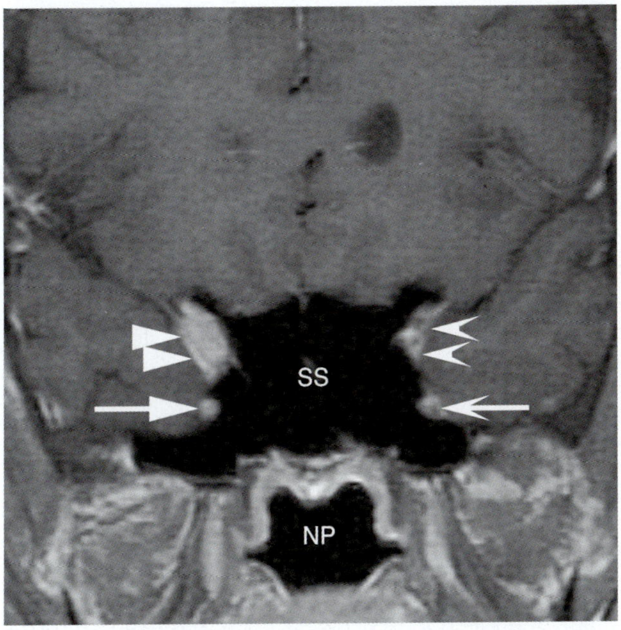

Fig. 54.9 A 66-year-old man with squamous cell carcinoma of the skin of the forehead and numbness of the right forehead and cheek. A coronal postgadolinium T1-weighted image with fat saturation demonstrates abnormal enhancing soft tissue in the right superior orbital fissure (*straight arrowheads*), consistent with perineural extension of the tumor along V_1, as well as enlargement and enhancement of V_2 (*straight arrow*) secondary to perineural spread of tumor. The normal left superior orbital fissure (*concave arrowheads*) and left V_2 in foramen rotundum (*concave arrow*) are shown for comparison.

to providing the surgeon with critical information regarding the extent of tumor and its relationships to important nerves and arteries, the MRI also allows for assessment of potential perineural spread of tumor along branches of the trigeminal nerve (**Fig. 54.9**). As mentioned earlier, MRI may also suggest specific histologies, such as primary lymphoma or angiofibroma. For many histologies in which neck metastases are common, a baseline assessment of the neck is helpful for accurate tumor staging, current treatment planning, and future tumor surveillance. Furthermore, preoperative angiography and embolization for radiologically highly vascular tumors should be considered, as reducing the blood supply from branches of the internal maxillary artery is likely to reduce the need for intraoperative transfusion. Preoperative catheter angiography is not warranted if the tumor blood supply is likely to be largely from the anterior and posterior ethmoidal arteries, however, because these branches of the ophthalmic artery cannot be safely embolized unless vision has already been lost.

Careful review of the preoperative MRI is essential to understand the anatomic relationships in a particular patient. Intraoperative navigation, usually with MR-based systems but at times with a CT-based system instead, is often helpful to the surgeon, depending on the surgical approach planned and whether the tumor has obscured important surgical landmarks. Current navigation software also allows merging of CT and MRI to allow blending of modalities, taking advantage of the better bone detail of CT and better soft tissue detail of MRI. Navigation is also important if the tumor is to be resected via an approach with a narrow vista (such as endoscopic approaches) or when critical structures will be immediately distal to tumor or an eroded landmark. Dissection near the internal carotid artery and optic chiasm, for instance, is often aided by intraoperative navigation.

If fludeoxyglucose (FDG) position emission tomography (PET)-CT imaging is to be considered as part of long-term surveillance, then it may be helpful to obtain a baseline FDG PET-CT preoperatively so that any areas that demonstrate unexpected increased activity can be evaluated; this also confirms whether a particular tumor is FDG-avid, a fact that is useful in ongoing tumor surveillance. A PET-CT should also be considered if unexpected metastases would lead to a reassessment of the indications for surgery. In other words, if surgery with curative intent is futile, then the question becomes: do the potential palliative benefits of surgery still outweigh its risks, or should the patient be managed with nonsurgical palliative methods?

Surgical Anatomy

The anterior skull base includes the posterior frontal sinus, cribriform plate, and roofs of the orbits and ethmoid sinuses. More posteriorly, it includes the planum sphenoidale and lesser wing of the sphenoid bone. Details of this anatomy are reviewed in Chapter 41 of this book and in previous works by Lang and Jho.[14,15]

Assessment of the skull base anatomy and pathology by high-resolution imaging is critical to development of a differential diagnosis, design of a therapeutic plan, execution of surgery or irradiation, and subsequent assessment of intervention.

Surgical Approaches: Details of Technique

At each institution performing skull base surgery, the accumulated experience of the individual surgeons will shape the decision as to what approach is most appropriate for a particular tumor in a particular patient. This judgment will be affected by the known or suspected histology and whether there has been prior irradiation or surgical intervention, as well as by the patient's preferences regarding risks and alternatives. Key anatomic issues that will affect this decision include adequate access for tumor resection with negative margins, the angle of approach so as to minimize brain retraction, the extent of dural or intradural involvement, and the need for access to difficult sites such as the optic chiasm, lateral sphenoid sinus recess, nasopharynx, lesser wing of the sphenoid, and/or craniocervical junction. When possible, anatomic circumscription of the tumor in three dimensions prior to its actual excision, with control of margins by frozen section, will usually afford the best chance of complete resection. At times, some piecemeal endoscopic or nonendoscopic resection is strategically planned and accepted as part of the resection; careful notation of tumor attachments allows selective piecemeal resection without compromising margins or overall oncologic effectiveness.

Bifrontal Craniotomy Approach

The anterior skull base has classically been approached via a bifrontal craniotomy with elevation of the frontal lobe or lobes. This craniotomy provides excellent exposure from the frontal sinuses to the perichiasmal region including the cribriform plate, planum sphenoidale, tuberculum sella, sella, central clivus to the spheno-occipital junction, orbital roof, medial and inferior orbits, ethmoid sinuses, sphenoid sinus, and nasopharynx. Pathologies accessed by this approach include meningiomas of the cribriform plate, planum sphenoidale, tuberculum sella, and diaphragm sella; esthesioneuroblastomas and paranasal carcinomas of mucosal or minor salivary gland origin; and melanoma (see also Chapter 42). Intraoperative magnification and navigation, microscopic dissection, modern high-speed drills, and, when needed, preoperative tumor embolization have significantly improved operative capability.

Position and Incision

The patient is placed supine with the head neutral, and cranial pin fixation is applied. Marked neck extension to promote frontal lobe elevation by gravity is unnecessary and can cause any remnant orbitonasal bar to obscure the view of posterior pathology if the orbital roofs are tilted beyond vertical. Stereotactic fiducial markers or facial surface contours are registered in anticipation of stereotactic guidance.

The bicoronal incision preserves pericranium vascularized by supraorbital arterial branches, exposes the undersurface of the orbital rims for osteotomies, avoids injury to zygomatic branches of the facial nerve, and promotes cosmesis. It begins 1 cm anterior to the tragus just above the root of the zygoma and passes superiorly, just posterior to the midline hairline across to the opposite pretragal area (**Fig. 54.10A**).

Ventriculostomy

Where ventriculostomy is required, a small trephination is drilled in the midpupillary parasagittal line of the nondominant side, 1 cm anterior to the coronal suture. The frontal horn of the lateral ventricle is then cannulated, and CSF is withdrawn to facilitate frontal lobe elevation (~40 mL throughout the case, then is replaced during closure). Placement of a lumbar subarachnoid drain, which also may be electively continued postoperatively for ~4 days, is an alternative preferred by some.

Soft Tissue Dissection

The incision is carried through skin and galea but not temporal fascia. The posterior margin of the incision is elevated and pericranium is incised by a coronal cut several centimeters posteriorly (as needed, depending on the posterior subfrontal extension of tumor disruption of the anterior skull base). The resulting soft tissue flap comprised of skin and pericranium is elevated anteriorly toward the orbital rims and nasion. The supraorbital branches of the frontal nerve may need to be freed from their foramina to facilitate this elevation. Anterolaterally on both sides, 1 to 2 cm posterior to the lateral orbital rims, superficial fascia is incised to allow the plane of dissection to progress deep to the lateral retro-orbital fat pad containing distal branches of the facial nerve. Anterior elevation is then continued over the nasion and superior orbital rims bilaterally, with care to preserve the thin periorbita, and the flap is wrapped in a moist pad until closure. The temporal fascia is incised at the anterior end of the superior temporal line to expose the external orbital angle, taking care to leave a cuff of tissue for closure.

Craniotomy

Three trephinations, one in each external orbital angle and one in the midline just behind the hairline at the top of the forehead (with care to avoid injury to the superior sagittal sinus), are used to elevate a free bone flap that traverses the orbital rims, nasion, and frontal sinuses (**Fig. 54.10B**). Inclusion of the superior orbital rims but not much of the orbital roofs provides a low trajectory to the undersurface of the frontal lobe while minimizing the risk of disruption of the periorbita (whose integrity may help preserve orbital shape, especially if tumor involvement necessitates removal of substantial lamina papyracea or medial orbital roof). Any frontal sinus component included in the bone plate is exenterated of mucosa and the posterior bone cortex is removed; the bone plate is kept moist, often in an antibiotic-soaked pad, until closure. Epidural tack-up sutures are placed superiorly and any dural tears are repaired.

Subfrontal Exposure

The posterior wall of the remaining frontal air sinus and the crista galli are removed, and the sinus is exenterated of its mucosa. Using microscopic illumination and magnification and self-retaining retractors, the subfrontal dura is elevated from the cribriform plate and orbital roofs back

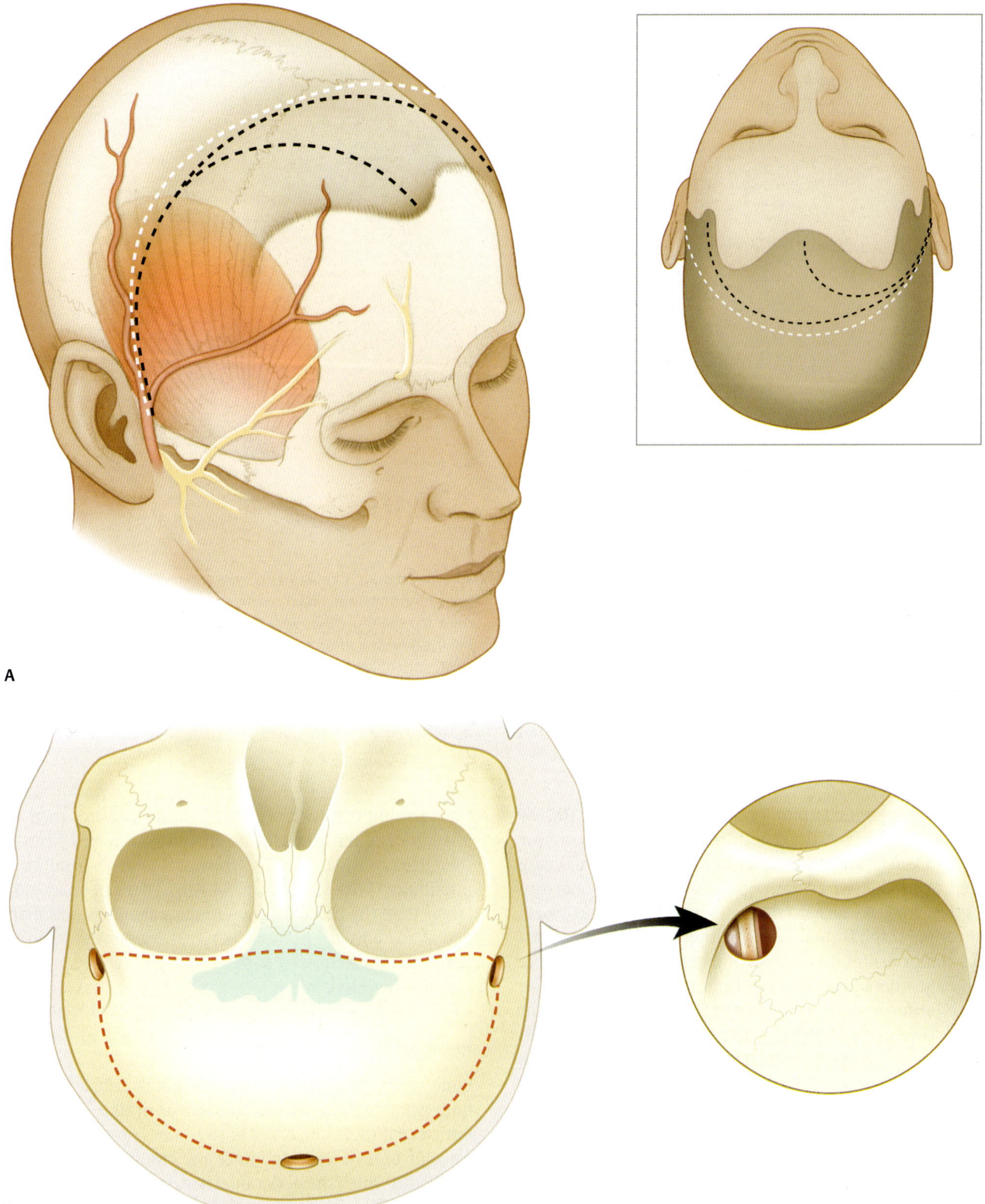

Fig. 54.10 Bifrontal cranio-orbital approach. **(A)** With the supine head held in a neutral position, a bicoronal incision is used (*dotted yellow line*). Each supraorbital nerve is freed from its notch/foramen and the zygomatic and temporal branches of the facial nerve are preserved (nerves in *solid yellow*). The scalp flap, including pericranium extending posterior to the incision, is carried forward and reflected over the nasion and superior orbital rims. **(B)** Craniotomy. Three trephinations, one in each external orbital angle and one in the midline just behind the hairline at the top of the forehead (with care to avoid injury to the superior sagittal sinus), are used to elevate a free bone flap that traverses the orbital rims, nasion, and frontal air sinuses. *(continued)*

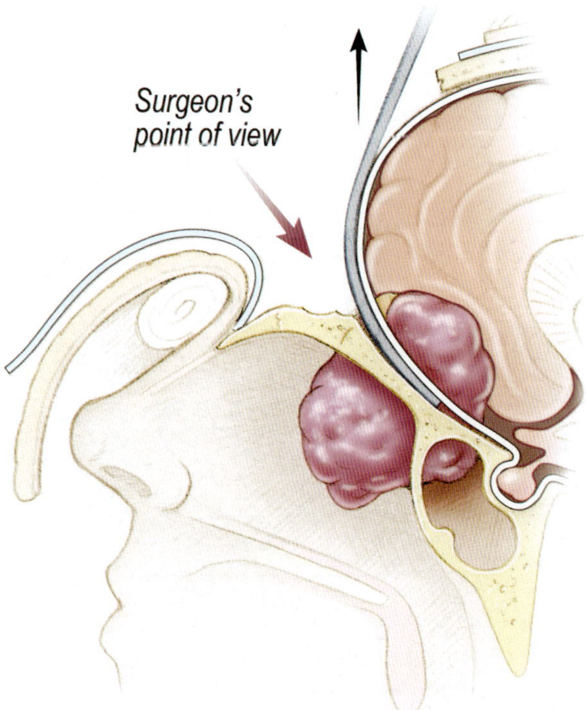

C

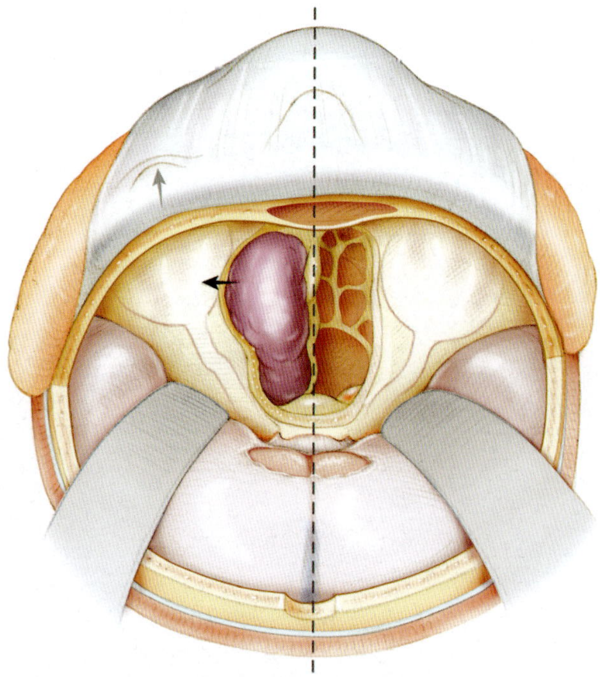

D

Fig. 54.10 *(continued)* **(C)** Subfrontal exposure (lateral view). The subfrontal dura is elevated by paramedian self-retaining retractors from the cribriform plate and orbital roofs back to the level at which tumor breaches bone or dural attachments to the cribriform plate restrict posterior access. Tumor protruding through the cribriform plate is amputated at its dural attachment and is compressed inferiorly until intracranial tumor can be resected and the dura repaired. **(D)** Removal of tumor (superior view). The subfrontal dura is incised circumferentially about any tumor, any intradural tumor is dissected from brain and removed, and the dura is repaired (*red*). Resection of anterior cranial fossa floor involved with tumor provides wide access to tumor (*T*) of the sella, sphenoid (*SS*) and ethmoid sinuses, medial orbits and inferomedial optical canals, portions of the petrous and cavernous internal carotid artery (ICA), nasal septum and cavity, and medial maxillary sinuses. *(continued)*

to the level at which tumor breaches bone (**Fig. 54.10C**) or dural attachments to the cribriform plate restrict posterior access. Even if tumor does not traverse dura, the dura may need to be incised at the cribriform plate and olfactory rootlets may be sacrificed to allow sufficient extradural elevation of the frontal lobe to either access more posterior tumor or to provide a favorable angle of exposure of tumor in the sinuses below. Tumor protruding through the cribriform plate is amputated at its dural attachment and is compressed inferiorly until intracranial tumor can be resected and the dura repaired. Clean instruments are then substituted.

Removal of Intracranial and Intradural Tumor, and Dural Repair

The subfrontal dura is then incised circumferentially around any regions involved with the tumor, and any intradural tumor is dissected from brain and removed (**Fig. 54.10D**, brain). After hemostasis is obtained, the dura is repaired. Primary dural closure is performed with 6-0 synthetic sutures, using a patch of dural substitute as needed. If the location or the size of the defect or attenuation of the surrounding dura precludes suture closure, then an inlay graft of dural substitute should be inserted deep to the edges of the defect and the dural edges partially approximated with suture (**Fig. 54.10E**). Then, an onlay graft larger than the defect is sewn to dura about its periphery and is coated with tissue adhesive. Exposed dura and its repair are then covered with a moist pad while sinonasal tumor is resected.

Removal of Sinonasal Tumor

Bone of the anterior cranial fossa floor—cribriform, planum sphenoidale, tuberculum sella, orbital roofs, and optic canal roofs—involved with tumor is resected with a rongeur or drill (leaving intact any uninvolved bone as a shelf onto which the pericranial flap can be wedged during closure). This both removes tumor and facilitates surgical exposure to tumor of the sella, sphenoid and ethmoid sinuses, medial orbits and inferomedial optic canals, nasal septum and nasal cavity, and medial maxillary sinuses (**Fig. 54.10D**). Tumor is removed under direct inspection. Transnasal endoscopy may be helpful to guide mucosal incisions or tumor removal from below or, in certain

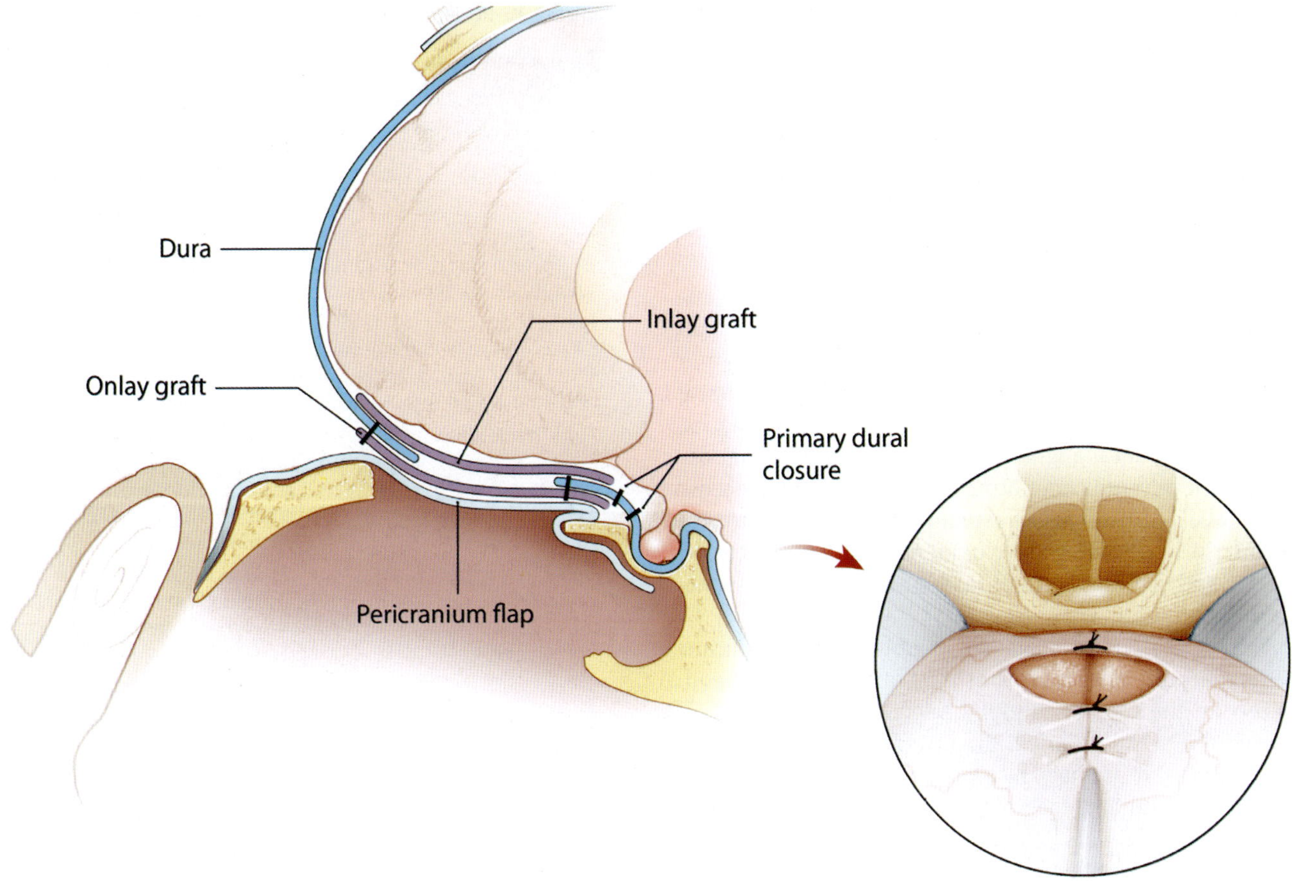

Fig. 54.10 *(continued)* **(E)** Closure (sagittal view; *insert*). Dura is closed with primary suture (detail, superior view), inlay graft (purple), and onlay graft (purple). The pericranial flap is turned posteriorly to reconstitute the medial anterior cranial fossa floor. Its distal portion is tucked between the posterior subfrontal dura (posterior to the dural repair) and any remaining planum sphenoidale and turned inferiorly into the sella.

cases, even from above.[16–18] An endoscope is particularly valuable for lesions located anterosuperiorly in the nose, for example. Endoscopic-assisted approaches can provide complementary access to the pterygopalatine fossa/infratemporal fossa[19,20] and the lateral recess of the sphenoid sinus.[21] Dissection of tumor extensions in the area of the optic nerve, cavernous sinus, and internal carotid artery can be facilitated by stereotactic computer-assisted navigation. Negative margins should be confirmed by intraoperative pathologic analysis of frozen specimens.

Closure

Repair of the anterior cranial fossa floor, even after extensive removal of the lamina papyracea, does not require orbital reconstruction with bone or metal plates. A broad-based pericranial or pericranial-galeal flap provides a supple, well vascularized barrier that is ideal for preventing CSF leakage and segregating the brain from the paranasal sinuses (**Figs. 54.2B, 54.3D, and 54.10E**). Dissection of the pericranial flap from the frontal bone should be carried to the orbital rims to avoid furrowing the skin above the eyebrows that may occur when retained attached muscle is reflected and advanced across the skull base defect. The pedicled flap is reflected posteriorly over the orbital roofs and wedged between subfrontal dura and any remaining ledge of planum sphenoidale or tuberculum sella. The flap separates the dura from the ethmoid and sphenoid sinuses. After positioning, the pericranial-galeal flap is covered with a layer of absorbable gelatin foam to protect the flap from disruption during removal of transnasally placed nonabsorbable sponge packs (**Fig. 54.10E**). If there is no shelf of bone posteriorly, then the pericranial flap will extend into the posterior sphenoid sinus (which has been carefully stripped of all mucosa) and will be held there by the absorbable and nonabsorbable packing.

After the ventricles are reexpanded by fluid infusion through the ventriculostomy, then additional epidural tack-up sutures are placed and the cranial plate is fixed with titanium miniplates. A subgaleal drain is placed, and it and the ventricular catheter are brought through the skin and connected to collecting reservoirs. Temporalis fascia, galea, and skin are then closed. The drain, which evacuates subgaleal and intracranial air as well as extradural fluid, should exert minimal negative pressure (which might challenge the dural repair) and should be removed when mass effect from air and/or blood has been alleviated. The ventriculostomy is removed thereafter, following confirmation of the absence of rhinorrhea (usually on postoperative day 3).

Advantages and Disadvantages

The major advantage of the external craniofacial approach is superb exposure and familiarity to most skull base surgeons because it incorporates the key access and anatomy of a common surgical external ethmoidectomy approach to the paranasal sinuses, albeit from a superior rather than frontal angle of view, along with familiar aspects of a bifrontal craniotomy. It also facilitates access to uninvolved orbital periosteum either anteromedially or inferiorly, allowing development of a plane between tumor and the involved periosteum if orbital preservation is planned.

This approach does have two potentially significant disadvantages: retraction of at least one frontal lobe and, except in the case of carefully selected anterior tumors, loss of the sense of smell. Brain retraction can be minimized with CSF drainage by a ventriculostomy or a lumbar subarachnoid drain, each of which carries its own attendant risks. For tumors extending posteriorly along the planum sphenoidale, the removal of the superior orbital rims and nasion affords an angle of exposure that reduces the amount of frontal lobe retraction needed.

Complications

Complications (and means of avoidance) include the following (**Table 54.1**):

1. Injury to the zygomatic and temporal branches of the facial nerve at the zygomatic arch or in the anterior temporal fat pad, resulting in frontalis muscle weakness (incision should traverse the zygomatic arch in its posterior half, and dissection about the lateral orbital rim should be just superficial to deep fascia and beneath the temporal fat pad)[22]
2. Injury to orbital contents causing intraorbital hematoma, enophthalmos, diplopia, and visual loss (careful dissection)
3. CSF rhinorrhea through the frontal sinus or anterior cranial fossa floor (repair of dura and anterior cranial fossa floor, as described previously)
4. Injury to the optic nerves during tumor dissection (careful dissection and minimizing inferior dissection along the optic nerve anterior to the chiasm [where the ophthalmic artery originates from the ICA], and use of irrigation during coagulation to minimize heat injury to nerve)
5. Injury to the ICA causing hemorrhage or stroke during tumor dissection (suspicion of artery displacement by tumor; insonation with the microvascular Doppler can supplement stereotactic image guidance by intraoperatively locating the artery)
6. Injury to the frontal temporal lobes from retraction or tumor dissection (gentle use of retractors and careful tumor dissection)
7. Poor aesthetic result (attention to proper realignment of the cranial plate and soft tissue layers, and dissection to the superior orbital ridge when creating the pericranial-galeal flap)

Table 54.1 Potential Complications of Anterior Approaches

Complication	Prevention
VII injury (temporalis and zygomatic branches)	Incision traverses the zygomatic arch posteriorly, and lateral orbital rim dissection is just superficial to deep fascia beneath the temporal fat pad
Intraorbital injury: hematoma, enophthalmos, diplopia	Maintain periorbital integrity where possible, extraconal dissection, hemostasis
Cerebrospinal fluid rhinorrhea into frontal sinus, or sphenoid and ethmoid sinuses	Dural repair, pericranial-galeal flap
Optic nerve injury	Irrigation during coagulation to minimize heat injury to nerve, careful dissection mindful of location of origin of ophthalmic artery
Injury to internal carotid artery (ICA)	(1) Preoperative imaging through the displacement of the ICA by tumor (2) Microvascular Doppler to assist in localization of ICA
Frontal lobe injury	Gentle retraction, precise tumor dissection
Aesthetic defects	Realign cranial plate precisely; the pericranial flap dissection should continue to superior orbital ridge

Modifications and Alternatives

Subcranial Approach

Raveh popularized the subcranial approach via a bicoronal incision that was initially described for trauma but was subsequently extended to tumor resection.[23] This approach removes the nasal bone and medial orbital walls. The major advantage of this low craniotomy is the minimization of brain retraction, similar to adding a temporary removal of the orbital rim to the classic bifrontal craniotomy. A potential disadvantage of the subcranial approach, when it is used in resection of malignant tumors, is osteomyelitis and/or osteoradionecrosis of the disconnected and replaced bone that includes the medial orbital rim, glabella, and part of the nasal bone. The aesthetic deformity that may result from subsequent removal of infected or radionecrotic bone is greater than with a more superior craniotomy. If this region of bone is involved by tumor such that its resection is required, then the subcranial approach is ideal. Otherwise, it does not offer significant advantage. Repair of the dura is similar to that in a bifrontal craniotomy.

At times, the frontal sinus is the primary site of pathology, which then extends posteriorly toward the frontal lobes. When this occurs, resection of the frontal sinus-containing frontal bone will afford the intracranial access needed. Reconstruction is accomplished with a pericranial-galeal flap if the skull base requires repair and by the split calvarial bone to reconstitute the anterior bony contour (**Fig. 54.8**).

Complementary Transfacial Exposure

The anterior skull base has classically been approached via a bifrontal craniotomy with elevation of the frontal lobe or lobes, combined with a transfacial approach to supplement the paranasal sinus exposure. A limited external ethmoidectomy incision that extends inferiorly along the nose to the axial plane of the inferior nasal bone provides adequate exposure for most procedures. There is rarely a need for a lateral rhinotomy or a Weber-Ferguson approach that splits the upper lip. If the hard palate requires extirpation, then a supplementary intraoral approach is added. This combined craniotomy and transsphenoethmoid approach provides excellent exposure from the optic chiasm to the spheno-occipital junction, including the planum sphenoidale, orbital roof, frontal sinuses, ethmoid sinuses, sphenoid sinus, and nasopharynx. The medial, superior, and inferior orbital areas are well exposed, as are the maxilla and nose. The transsphenoethmoid component also provides access to the pterygomaxillary fissure and pterygopalatine fossa, pterygoid plates, and nasopharynx. Using complementary endoscopic approaches, surgeons have learned that paranasal exposure is often adequate without a supplemental facial incision.[24] In fact, at most institutions, endoscopic techniques are replacing external incisions as the approach of choice for transfacial access to tumors.

Supplemental Midfacial Degloving Intraoral Incision (± LeFort I Osteotomy or Maxillotomy)

Some patients are adverse to any facial scar, even the small and well camouflaged one that results from an external ethmoidectomy incision. A midfacial degloving approach is a well recognized approach to the paranasal sinuses that avoids a facial incision. It can supplement either a bifrontal craniotomy or a subcranial approach. A LeFort I osteotomy may be added, especially if one is approaching the craniocervical junction. A unilateral maxillotomy[25] approach can also be used, which mobilizes the inferior maxilla while keeping it attached to the soft palate. Some find this useful if access to the central skull base is needed.

Endoscopic Approach Without Craniotomy

As detailed in other chapters of this book, selected tumors of the anterior skull base can be resected solely via an endoscopic approach by highly experienced endoscopic surgeons. With an esthesioneuroblastoma,[26] for example, such an approach takes advantage of intraoperative image-guided navigation, specialized equipment, acquired surgical skill, and effective endoscopic repair of CSF leaks using pedicled or free mucosal grafts. Extended endoscopic exploration beyond the paranasal sinuses may allow resection of tumor involving the dura and (adjacent to the optic nerve) cavernous sinus and ICA.

Orbitozygomatic Approach

Access to the superior parapharyngeal space as well as access along the floor of the middle cranial fossa can be gained by a temporary and often en bloc removal of the zygomatic arch, lateral orbit, and part of the zygomatic body. This may at times be needed to supplement an anterior cranial base approach to provide superolateral access to the foramina rotundum and ovale, posterolateral maxillary antrum, pterygomaxillary space, lateral orbit, greater wing of the sphenoid, and floor of the middle cranial fossa. Pathologies possibly requiring this approach include: V_3 schwannomas, meningiomas extending from above, sarcomas extending from below, salivary gland tumors, or lateral extension of more anteriorly originating squamous cell carcinomas. Occasionally, this approach is also used in uncommon settings such as skull base extension of invasive fungal infection requiring aggressive debridement (**Fig. 54.11**).

Position and Incision

The patient is placed supine and the ipsilateral shoulder is elevated to permit turning the head into the lateral position. A Mayfield headholder is placed and the head is rotated 20 degrees contralaterally and tilted down 20 degrees to bring the pterion uppermost. The incision is designed to expose the temporalis muscle while preserving the posterior branch of the superficial temporal artery and the temporal and zygomatic branches of the facial nerve. It begins in the pretragal crease just below the root of the zygoma and passes superiorly across the superior temporal line behind the coronal suture before arcing anteriorly to the midline hairline. A receding hairline may require a full bicoronal incision (**Fig. 54.10A**).

Soft Tissue Dissection

The incision is carried through skin, galea, and pericranium but not temporalis fascia. The resulting scalp flap is elevated anteriorly, leaving the temporal fascia intact except far anteriorly, just posterior to the lateral orbital rim. Here, superficial temporal fascia is incised to expose a fat

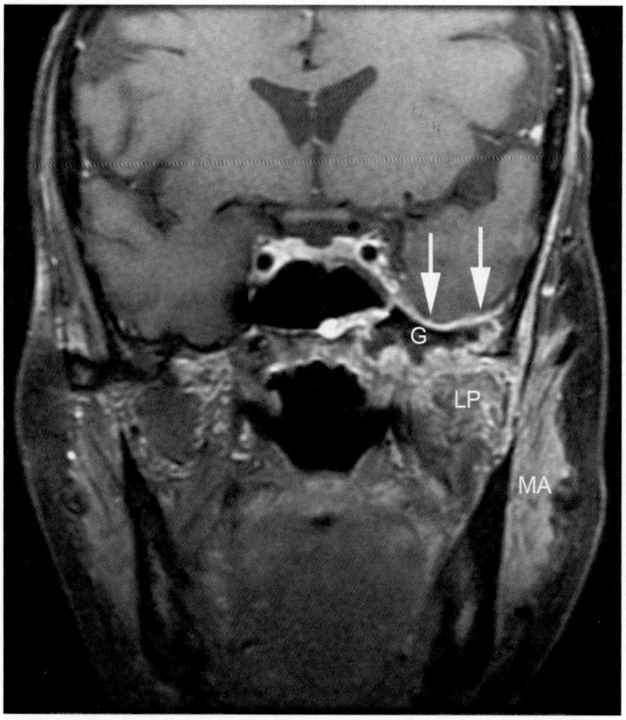

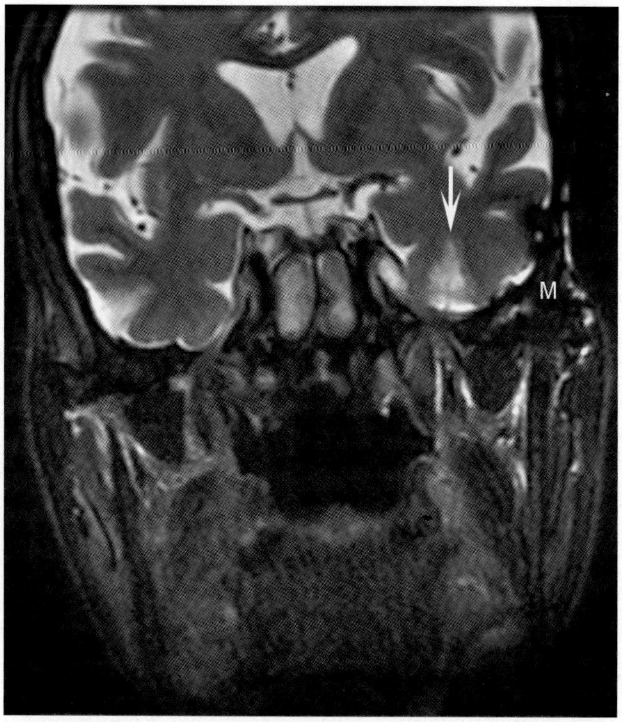

Fig. 54.11 A 47-year-old man with chronic myelogenous leukemia in remission following a recent bone marrow transplant, with *Rhizopus* infection of the paranasal sinuses. The patient had already undergone several endoscopic debridements of necrotic tissue as well as antifungal therapy. **(A)** A coronal postgadolinium T1-weighted image with fat saturation demonstrates swelling and enhancement of the left lateral pterygoid (*LP*) and masseter (*MA*) muscles. In addition, there is irregular erosion of the greater wing of the sphenoid bone (*G*) and diffuse dural enhancement along the floor of the left middle cranial fossa (*large white arrows*). The patient was taken to the operating room for a zygomaticotemporal craniectomy with an osteotomy of the zygomatic arch, debridement (near complete resection) of the greater wing of the sphenoid, infratemporal fossa dissection, and inferolateral sphenoid sinusotomy. The dura was debrided, and no cerebrospinal fluid leak occurred. **(B)** The patient improved postoperatively and continued an additional 6-week course of antifungal agents. A follow-up magnetic resonance scan was obtained 1 year later, without gadolinium because the patient had developed renal insufficiency associated with antifungal treatment. A coronal fast spin echo T2-weighted image with fat suppression demonstrated a metal artifact (*M*) at the site of the prior surgery, as well as a gliosis/encephalomalacia in the left temporal lobe (*white arrow*).

pad that lies superficial to the deeper temporal fascia and contains distal temporal and zygomatic branches of the facial nerve. The fat pad and nerves are elevated along with the scalp and pericranium over the lateral orbital rim. The dissection is continued to expose the superior orbital rim (where the supraorbital branch of the frontal nerve may need to be freed from its foramen) and inferiorly to expose the zygomatic arch back to its root. The temporal fascia is incised at its superior and posterior margins, leaving a cuff to which to sew at closing. The muscle is then mobilized from its fossa with a dissection from inferior to superior along its deep surface (**Fig. 54.12A**).

Frontotemporal Craniotomy With Orbitozygomatic Osteotomy

A low unilateral frontal and anterior and middle temporal craniotomy is performed using four burr holes: (1) external orbital angle, entering both the anterior cranial fossa and the orbit; (2) anterior inferior lateral frontal; (3) superior posterior temporal; and (4) anterior inferior temporal. The last three are connected with a craniotome, the cut of which is extended anteriorly into the supraorbital notch (**Fig. 54.12A**). A more anterior elevation of the pericranium and the superolateral orbital periosteum to which it transitions permits three osteotomies in the orbital roof and lateral wall. The first, from within the orbit across the orbital roof, connects the supraorbital notch to the orbital portion of the burr hole in the external orbital angle (long horizontal dotted line). The second, from within the anterior temporal fossa through the lateral orbital wall, connects the orbital portion of this burr hole with the lateral end of the inferior orbital fissure (long vertical dotted line). The third, from within the orbit, connects the lateral end of the inferior orbital fissure with the superior limb of the cut through the zygomatic body to be made later (short horizontal dotted line). Retraction of the scalp flap inferiorly permits osteotomies across the frontal process of the maxilla (angled dashed line) and the posterior end of the zygomatic arch (short vertical dashed line).

The greater wing of the sphenoid bone is then divided by connecting the cranial portion of the external orbital angle burr hole with the anterior inferior lateral temporal burr hole and the lateral end of the inferior orbital fissure (vertical groove and horizontal short dashed lines). This frees the craniotomy plate, superior orbital rim, lateral orbital rim, frontal and zygomatic processes of the zygoma, and zygomatic arch, all of which are removed as a single construct (or, if necessary, in two pieces as the lateral orbit and the maxilla-zygomatic arch). The temporalis muscle is then retracted inferiorly through the gap in the zygomatic arch so as to expose the inferior lateral wall, the anterior lateral wall, and the lateral floor of the middle cranial fossa.

This craniotomy and these osteotomies thus remove the lateral frontal and the anterior and middle aspects of the lateral temporal cranial bone, as well as the lateral portions of both lesser and greater wings of the sphenoid bone, superior and lateral orbital rims, frontal and zygomatic processes of the zygoma, and the zygomatic arch (**Fig. 54.12B**: axial view from above, dark green, 1). The approach facilitates access to more medial frontal, temporal, and sphenoid bones of the skull base.

Exposure of the Central Skull Base

Progressively greater exposure of the central skull base can then be achieved. Bones of the lateral frontal fossa floor (orbital roof back to the optic canal), the lateral middle

A

B

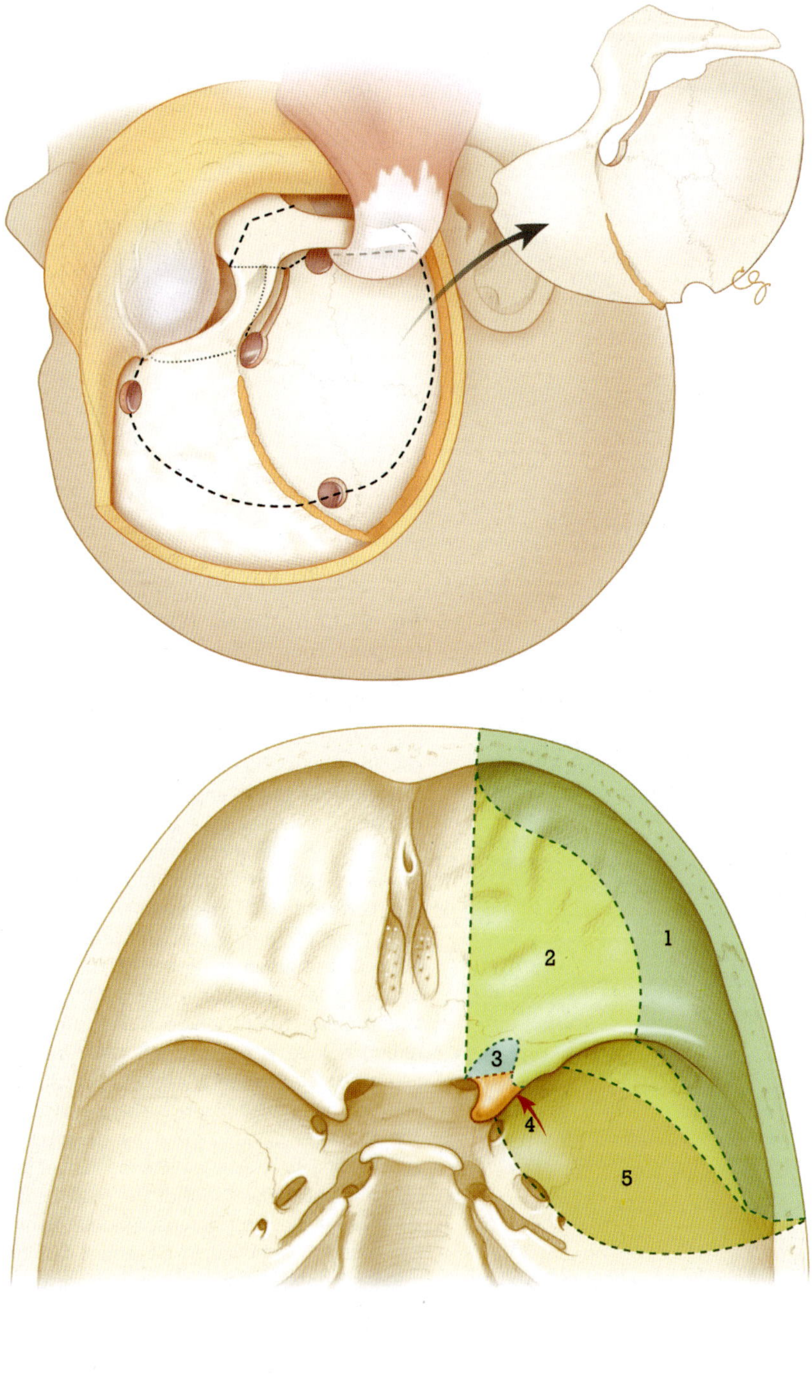

Fig. 54.12 Orbitozygomatic craniotomy. **(A)** Incision, soft tissue dissection, and craniotomy (superior view). With the head rotated 20 degrees contralaterally and tilted down 20 degrees to bring the pterion uppermost, the incision extends from the pretragal crease superiorly, anteriorly, and contralaterally as needed given the hairline (Fig. 54.1, *black dashed lines*). The scalp flap is elevated anteriorly. The temporal muscle is mobilized from its fossa and four trephinations are placed: (1) external orbital angle, entering both the anterior cranial fossa and the orbit; (2) anterior inferior lateral frontal; (3) superior posterior temporal; and (4) anterior inferior temporal. The last three are connected with a craniotome, the cut is extended anteriorly into the supraorbital notch. Three osteotomies in the orbital roof and lateral wall connect the supraorbital notch to the orbital portion of the burr hole in the external orbital angle (*dotted line*), the orbital portion of this burr hole with the lateral end of the inferior orbital fissure (*dashed line*), and the lateral end of the inferior orbital fissure with the superior limb of the cut through the zygomatic body to be made later (*single dash*). Osteotomies across the frontal process of the zygoma and the posterior end of the zygomatic arch and division of the greater wing of the sphenoid bone frees the craniotomy plate, superior orbital rim, lateral orbital rim, frontal and zygomatic processes of the zygoma, and zygomatic arch, all of which are removed as a single construct. The temporalis muscle is then retracted inferiorly. **(B)** Removal of bone for an approach to parasellar and subtemporal tumors (superior view). An approach to the parasellar region involves removal of frontotemporal cranial bone, lateral portions of both lesser and greater wings of the sphenoid bone, superior and lateral orbital rims, frontal and zygomatic processes of the zygoma, and zygomatic arch by an orbitozygomatic craniotomy (*dark green*); rongeuring off the orbital roof and medial portions of the lesser and greater sphenoid wings forming the middle cranial fossa (*light green*); and drilling away the anterior clinoid process (*light brown*), the roof of the optic canal (*blue*), and the optic strut (*purple*). *(continued)*

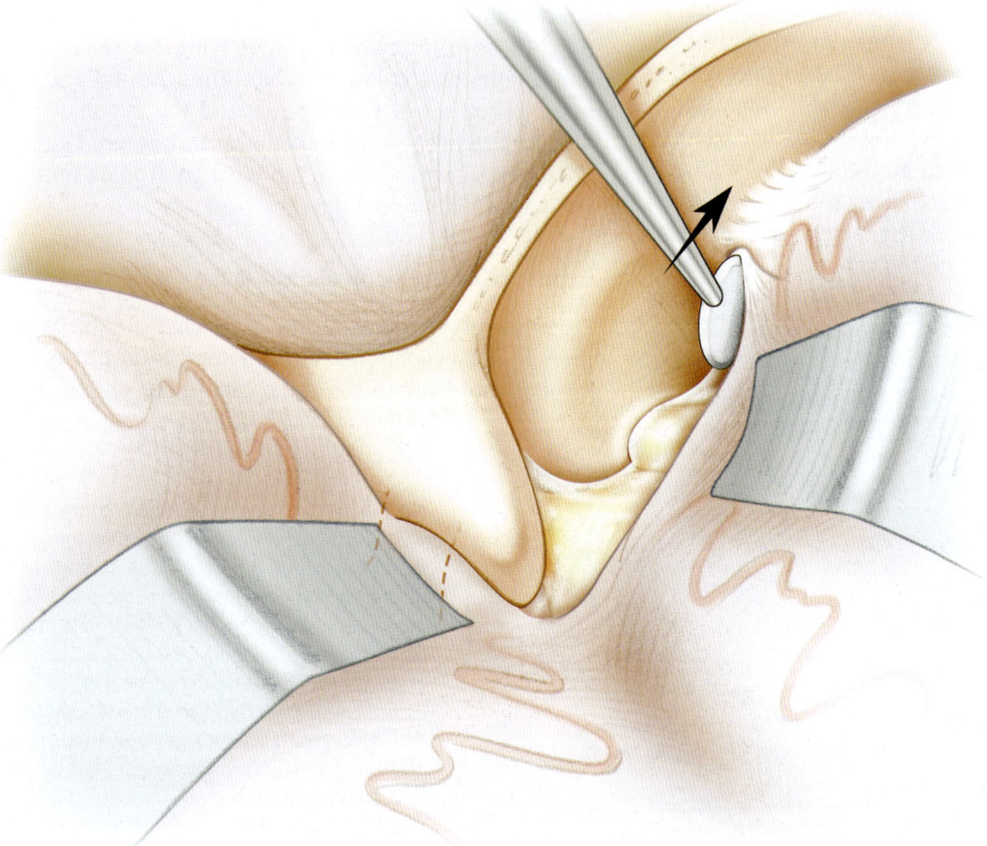

C

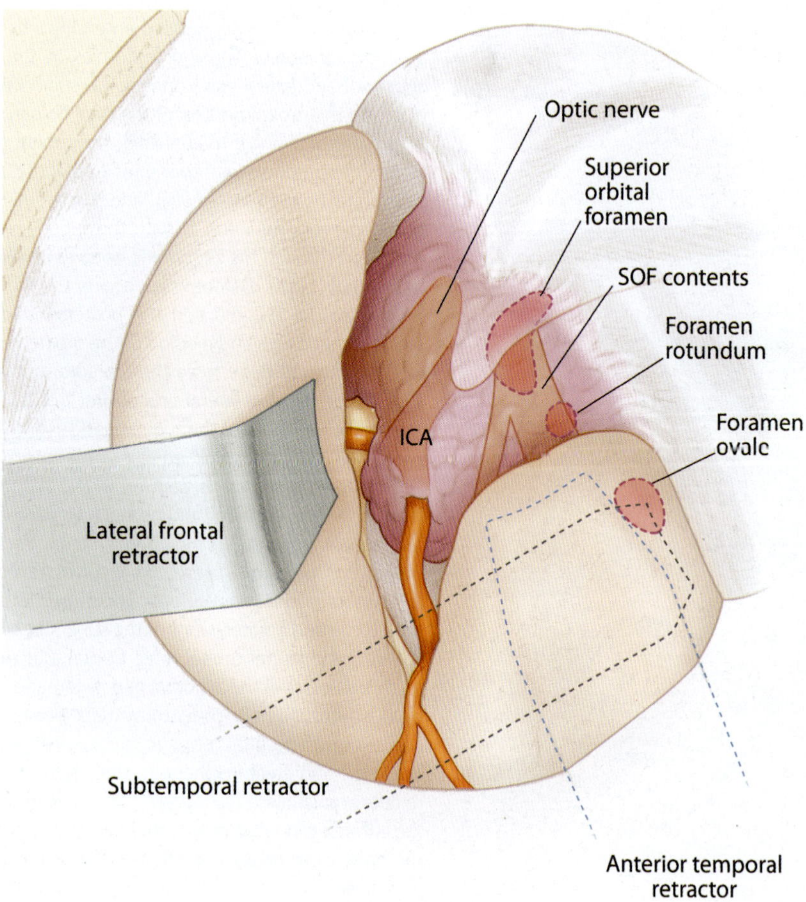

D

Fig. 54.12 *(continued)* **(C)** Exposure of the temporal floor. Self-retaining retractors are placed extradurally to separate the frontal and temporal lobes and reveal the most medial lesser wing of the sphenoid wing and anterior clinoid process. The anterior temporal lobe is elevated from the anterior wall and floor of the middle cranial fossa by extradural dissection. This exposes the lateral wall of the cavernous sinus and its transition into the superior orbital fissure (*SOF*), the foramen rotundum, and, more posteriorly (not shown), foramen ovale and foramen spinosum. **(D)** Resection of a clinoidal meningioma. The dura over the lateral inferior frontal lobe, Sylvian fissure, and temporal lobe is opened and the resulting flap is retracted anteriorly, and the arachnoid bridging the Sylvian fissure is sharply divided. The tumor is devascularized by coagulating and dividing its attachments to the dura of the planum sphenoidale, roof of the optic canal, anterior clinoid, and anterior middle cranial fossa, and is removed in piecemeal fashion using arachnoidal planes about major arteries as a guide to dissection.

cranial fossa floor, and intervening medial portions of the lesser and greater sphenoid wings are removed by rongeur (**Fig. 54.12B**, light green, 2).

To expose the parasellar region, self-retaining retractors are placed to separate the frontal and temporal lobes and reveal the most medial lesser wing of the sphenoid wing and the anterior clinoid process. The anterior temporal lobe is elevated from the anterior wall and floor of the middle cranial fossa by extradural dissection (**Fig. 54.12C**). This exposes the lateral wall of the cavernous sinus and its transition into the superior orbital fissure, the foramen rotundum, and, more posteriorly (not shown), foramen ovale and foramen spinosum.

Using microscopic illumination and magnification, a superior parasellar perioptic or paraclinoidal lesion is exposed by removing the anterior clinoid process (light brown), the roof of the optic canal (blue, 3), and the optic strut (purple, 4) as needed to access the optic nerve and the clinoidal segment of the internal carotid artery. A fine diamond drill under continuous irrigation is used to remove the roof of the optic canal and the anterior clinoid process. This exposes the dura of the superior orbital fissure and reveals the optic strut forming the inferolateral wall of the intracranial end of the optic canal. This too can be drilled away to widen access to the paraclinoidal internal carotid artery as needed to expose tumor.

An inferior parasellar and subtemporal lesion is exposed by removing bone from the medial middle cranial fossa floor (**Fig. 54.12B**, *olive*, 5). Self-retaining retractors are placed extradurally in a more lateral-to-medial orientation. Bone is rongeured away until the foramina rotundum and ovale are approached, after which a high-speed drill is used. Care must be taken to avoid injury to the horizontal petrous segment of the internal carotid artery, the canal roof may be deficient.

Tumor Removal

If the tumor is predominantly extradural, then it is removed without opening the dura. Any dura suspicious for tumor invasion should be biopsied and specimens sent for frozen section analysis to ensure that surgical margins are free of tumor. Any penetrating tumor is followed intradurally, separated from brain, and removed. If the tumor is predominantly intradural (as in the case of a clinoidal meningioma; **Figs. 54.12D, 54.13**), then after extradural removal of bone, the dura over the lateral inferior frontal lobe, Sylvian fissure, and temporal lobe is opened and the resulting flap is retracted anteriorly. After application of gentle retraction to separate the two lobes, the arachnoid bridging the Sylvian fissure is sharply divided. Care is taken to avoid injury to underlying vessels within the fissure. The dural attachments of the tumor are coagulated and divided so as to devascularize the tumor of any dural blood supply prior to

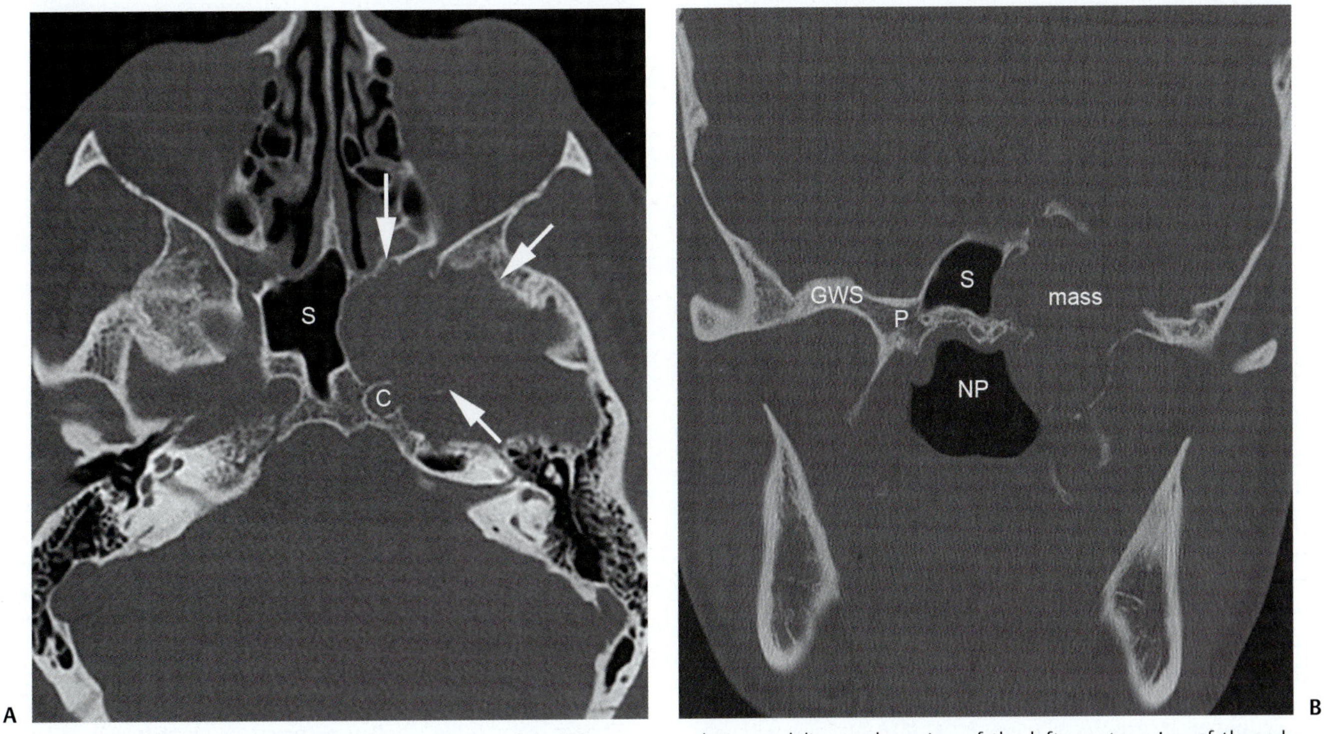

Fig. 54.13 A 65-year-old woman with a meningioma of the left cavernous sinus and middle cranial fossa. **(A)** An axial computed tomography (CT) scan demonstrates erosion and remodeling of the left sphenoid bone by a mass lesion (*arrows*). *C*, cavernous internal carotid artery; *S*, sphenoid sinus. **(B)** A coronal CT demonstrates again the remodeling and erosion of the left greater wing of the sphenoid, pterygoid process, and left lateral wall of the sphenoid sinus (*S*) by the meningioma. The normal right pterygoid process (*P*) and greater wing (*GWS*) are shown for comparison. *NP*, nasopharynx. *(continued)*

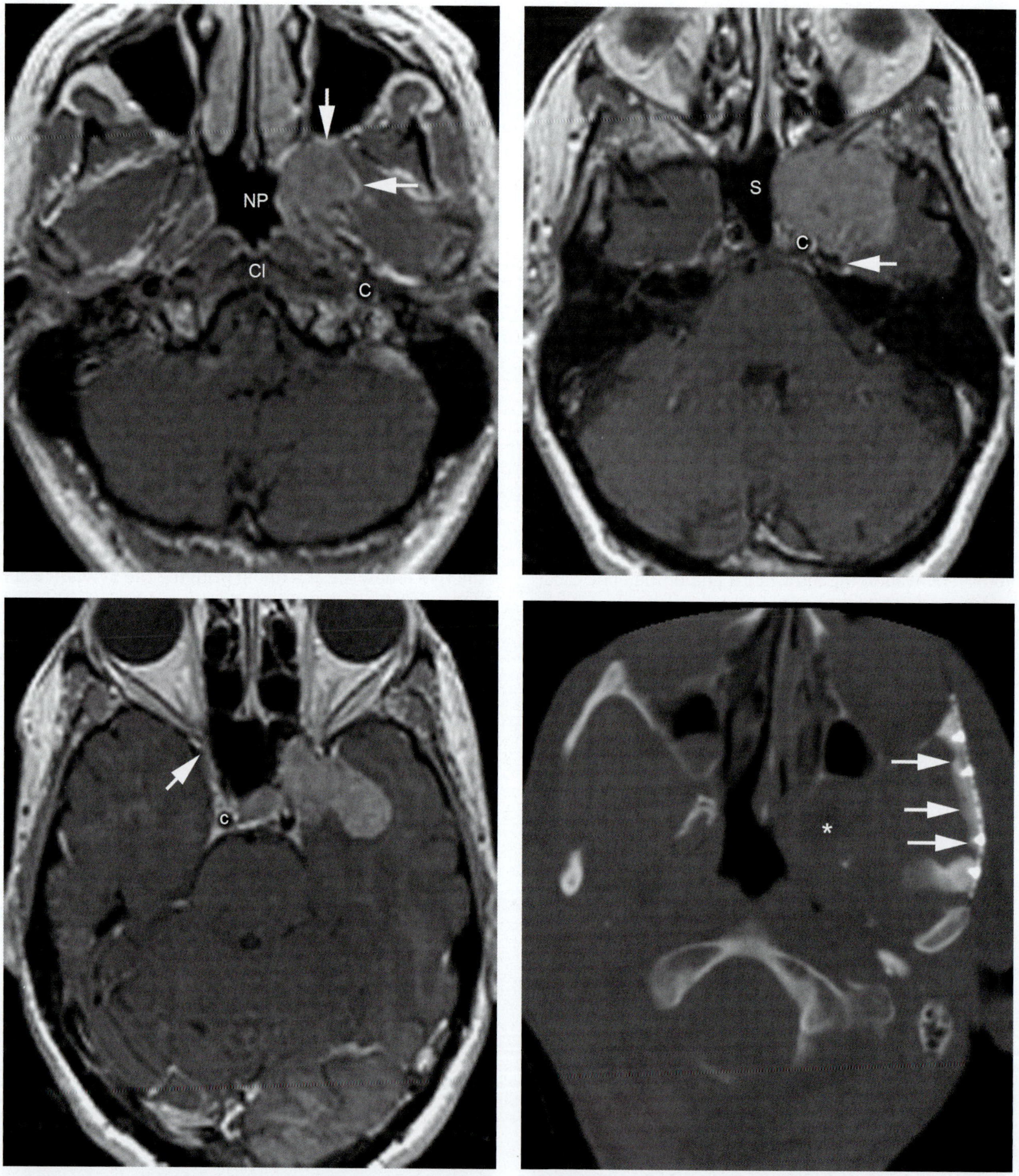

C D E F

Fig. 54.13 *(continued)* **(C)** An axial T1 postgadolinium image from a preoperative stereotactic magnetic resonance scan demonstrates the enhancing tumor involving the left pterygoid process (*arrows*). *NP*, nasopharynx; *C*, internal carotid artery; *Cl*, clivus. **(D)** A more superior image demonstrates the large enhancing tumor mass in the left middle cranial fossa. The left internal carotid artery (*C*) is contacted and displaced posteriorly, as is Meckel's cave (*arrow*). **(E)** A more superior image demonstrates tumor at the level of the superior orbital fissure and the cavernous sinus, as well as a lobule of tumor that is deeply impressing upon the left temporal lobe. The normal right superior orbital fissure is indicated (*arrow*), as is the right cavernous carotid artery (*C*). **(F)** An axial CT scan following orbitozygomatic approach to the tumor. Plating of the left zygoma is seen (*arrows*), as well as Gelfoam and packing material in the region of the left pterygoid process (*asterisk*). *(continued)*

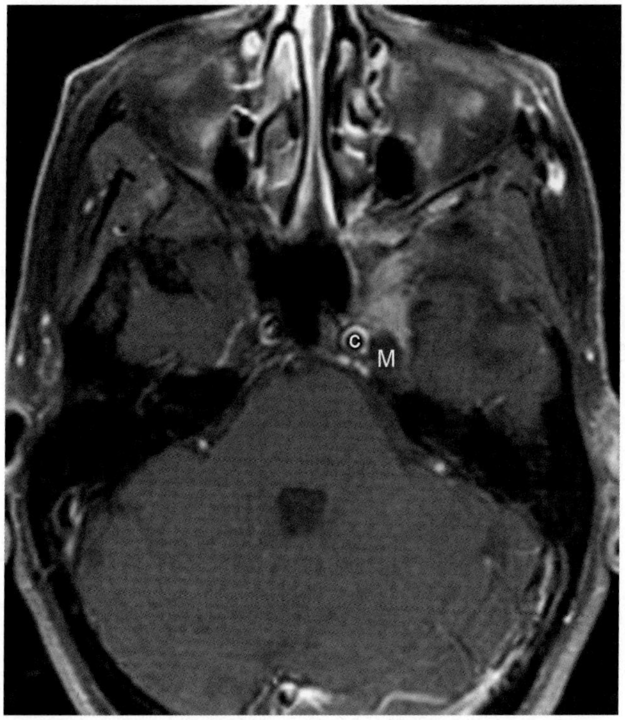

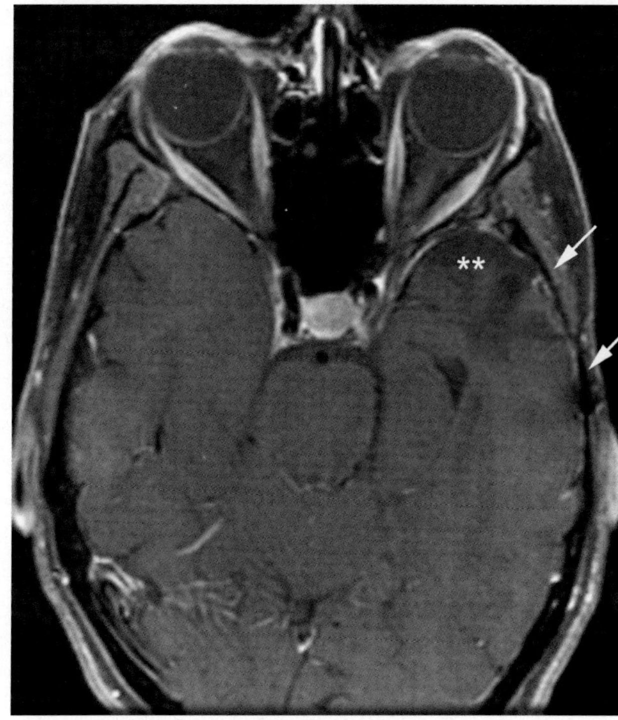

Fig. 54.13 *(continued)* **(G)** An axial postgadolinium T1-weighted image with fat saturation demonstrates a residual enhancing tumor in the medial aspect of the left middle cranial fossa, anterior to Meckel's cave (*M*) and the cavernous carotid artery (*c*). This tumor could not be resected without great risk to the neurovascular structures. **(H)** A more superior axial postgadolinium T1-weighted image with fat saturation demonstrates complete resection of the component of tumor that had been compressing the left temporal lobe. Encephalomalacia of the left temporal tip (*double asterisk*) is present. Metal artifact from craniotomy (*arrows*).

microdissection of tumor from the brain, cranial nerves, and cerebral arteries (**Fig. 54.12D**); branches of the middle cerebral artery emerging from the tumor are a good guide to more proximal vessels.

Closure

Watertight dural closure, achieved as described previously, is important, especially if the sphenoid sinus has been entered or if previously irradiated superficial soft tissues are compromised. Titanium miniplates are used to repair osteotomies and fix the cranial plate, and a subgaleal drain is placed. Soft tissue and skin are closed in an anatomically correct, cosmetically acceptable manner.

Advantages and Disadvantages

The orbitozygomatic approach affords excellent near-field exposure of tumors of the parasellar and subtemporal skull base with minimal brain retraction, which has the advantage of reducing the risk of contusion or venous infarction of frontal and temporal lobes (**Fig. 54.13**). It also affords excellent exposure of tumors that involve the floor of the middle cranial fossa and lateral orbit (**Figs. 54.14 and 54.15**).

This approach involves extensive dissection of soft tissue about the orbit and temporal area. There is a risk of disruption of the periorbita and consequent loss of intraorbital fat, followed by enophthalmos. Aesthetic deformity about the lateral orbital rim may also result if the osteotomies are not accurately realigned. Finally, if the temporalis muscle is reflected into the skull base to assist in CSF leak repair, then replacing its anterior half in its anatomically normal position avoids a deep lateral skull soft tissue depression above the zygomatic arch.

Complications

Complications (and means of avoidance) include the following (**Table 54.2**):

1. Injury to the zygomatic and temporal branches of the facial nerve during traverse of the zygomatic arch or in the anterior temporal fat pad, resulting in frontalis muscle weakness (incision should traverse the zygomatic arch in its posterior half and the dissection about the lateral orbital rim should be just superficial to deep fascia, beneath the temporal fat pad)[22]
2. Injury to orbital contents causing intraorbital hematoma, enophthalmos, diplopia, and visual loss (careful dissection)
3. CSF rhinorrhea through the sphenoid sinus (avoid opening into the sinus unless required for tumor removal), and repair of any opening with anterior

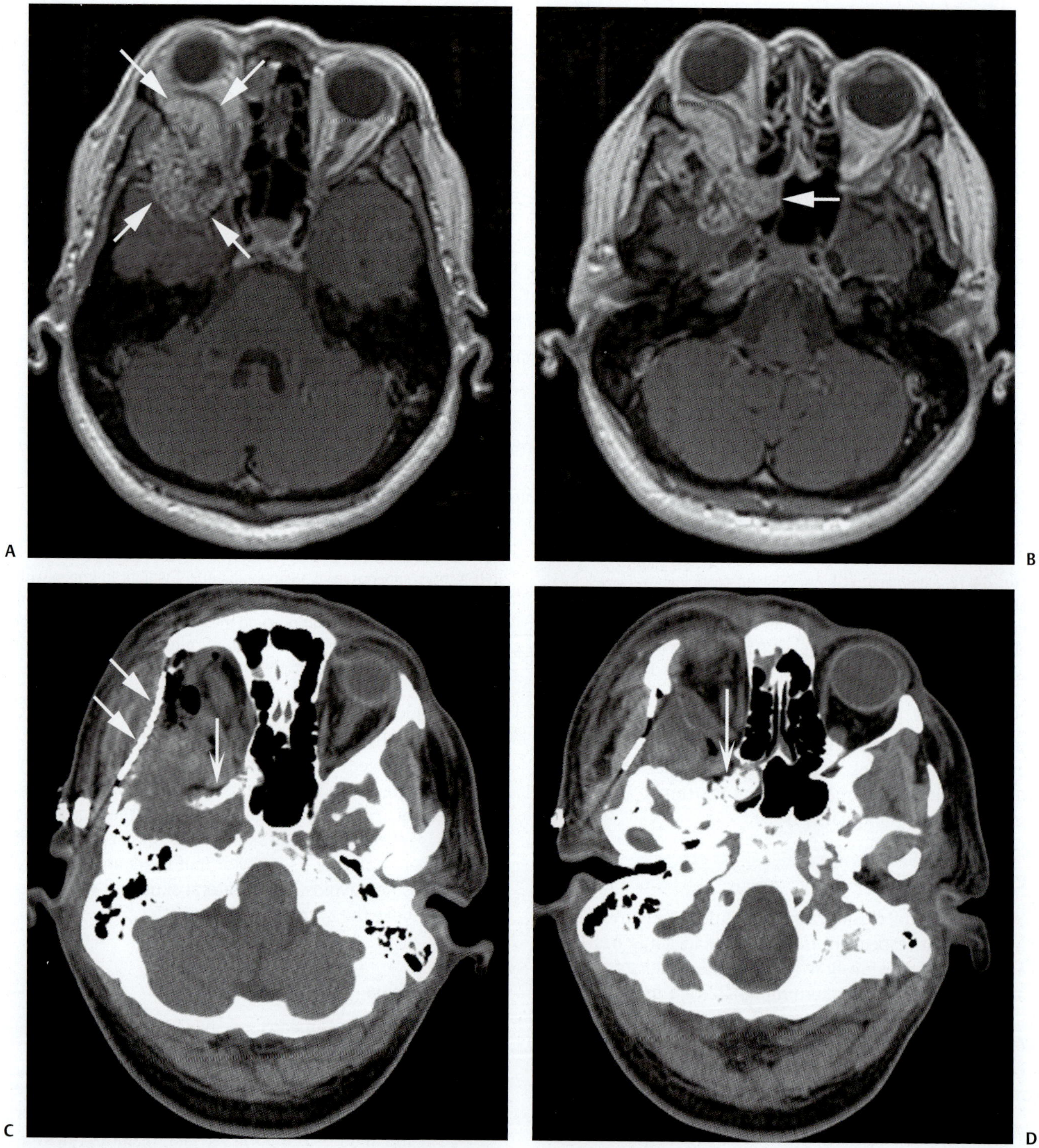

Fig. 54.14 A 53-year-old woman with a rare epithelioid hemangioma of bone. **(A)** An axial postgadolinium T1-weighted image from a preoperative stereotactic magnetic resonance image demonstrates an enhancing mass centered on and destroying the right greater wing of sphenoid, sphenotemporal buttress, and posterior aspect of the right lateral orbital wall. The mass extends into the orbit, but it displaces the lateral rectus muscle and does not appear to cross the orbital periosteum. There is mass effect on the right temporal lobe, but no evidence of transdural extension or brain edema. **(B)** A more inferior axial postgadolinium T1-weighted image demonstrates extension of enhancing tumor into the right sphenoid sinus (*white arrow*). **(C)** Axial noncontrast head computed tomography (CT) following orbitozygomatic approach to the middle cranial fossa and sphenoid sinus, as well as lateral orbitotomy, pericranial flap, and reconstruction with titanium mesh (*straight white arrows*). A small piece of residual hyperostotic bone remains (*concave white arrow*). **(D)** An axial noncontrast CT image at a slightly more inferior level again demonstrates the expected postoperative changes and residual hyperostotic bone medially (*white arrow*); otherwise a gross total resection of tumor was achieved and the orbit was preserved.

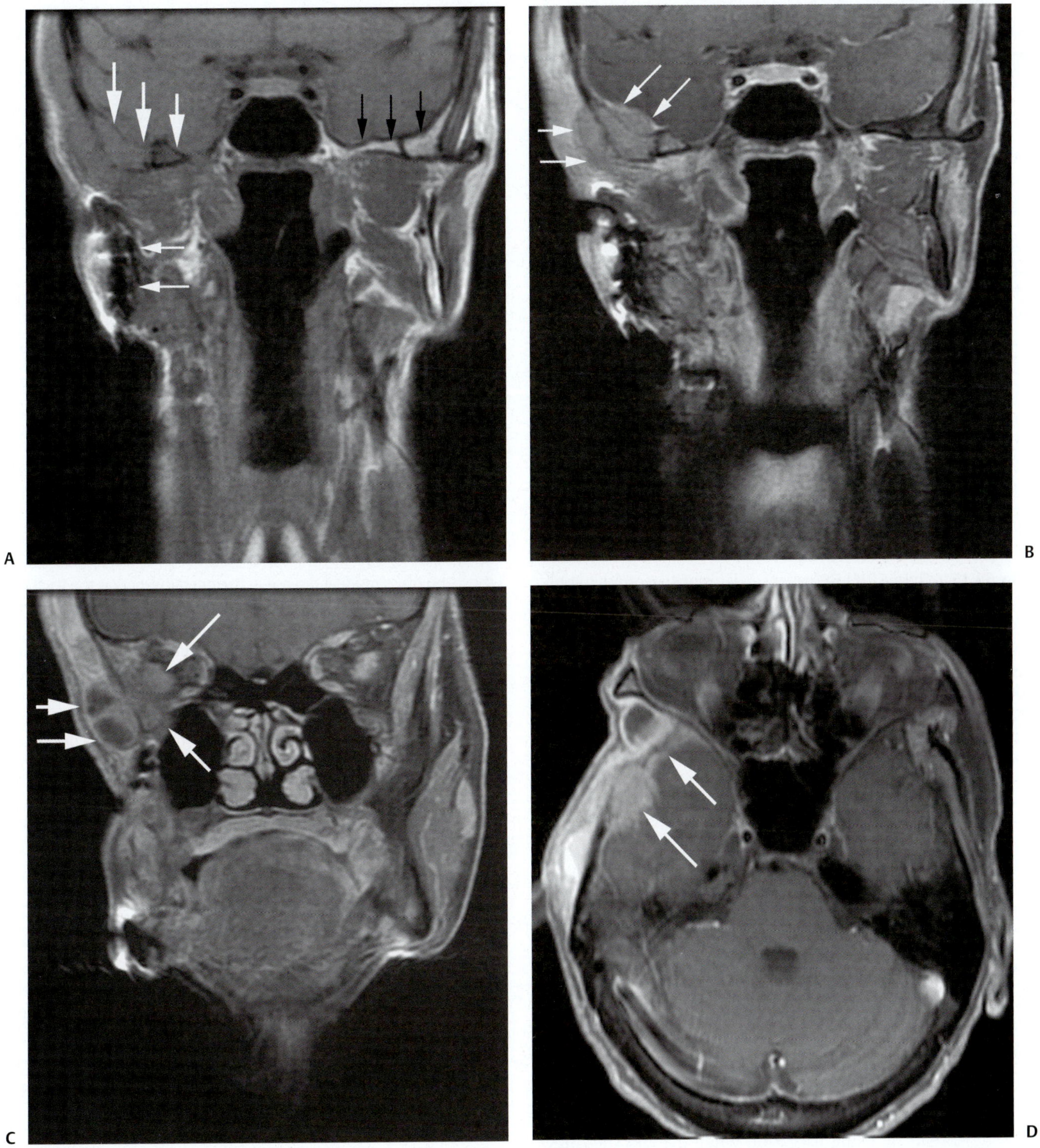

Fig. 54.15 A 56-year-old woman with recurrent poorly differentiated squamous cell carcinoma, status post prior surgery and chemoradiation. **(A)** The patient had previously undergone extensive surgery, including mandibulectomy and mandibular reconstruction, for a retromolar trigone squamous cell carcinoma. This coronal T1-weighted image demonstrates recurrent tumor extensively involving the greater wing of the sphenoid/floor of the right middle cranial fossa (*large white arrows*). The normal bone is shown on the left for comparison (*black arrows*). There is metal artifact from the mandibular reconstruction (*small white arrows*). **(B)** A coronal postgadolinium T1-weighted image with fat saturation at the same level demonstrates the lobulated enhancing recurrence (*white arrows*) centered on the greater wing of the sphenoid and sphenotemporal buttress with involvement of the dura but no evidence of transdural tumor extension. **(C)** A more anterior coronal postgadolinium T1-weighted image with fat saturation demonstrates recurrent tumor (*white arrows*) involving the lateral orbital wall as well as adjacent superficial soft tissues. **(D)** An axial postgadolinium T1-weighted image with fat saturation again demonstrates the irregular nodular infiltration of the dura overlying the right temporal lobe. After considerable discussion, a decision was made that significant palliation for this highly functional patient would more likely be achieved surgically than via chemotherapy and/or reirradiation. The patient's eye was working and she had severe unremitting pain despite maximal pain management efforts. *(continued)*

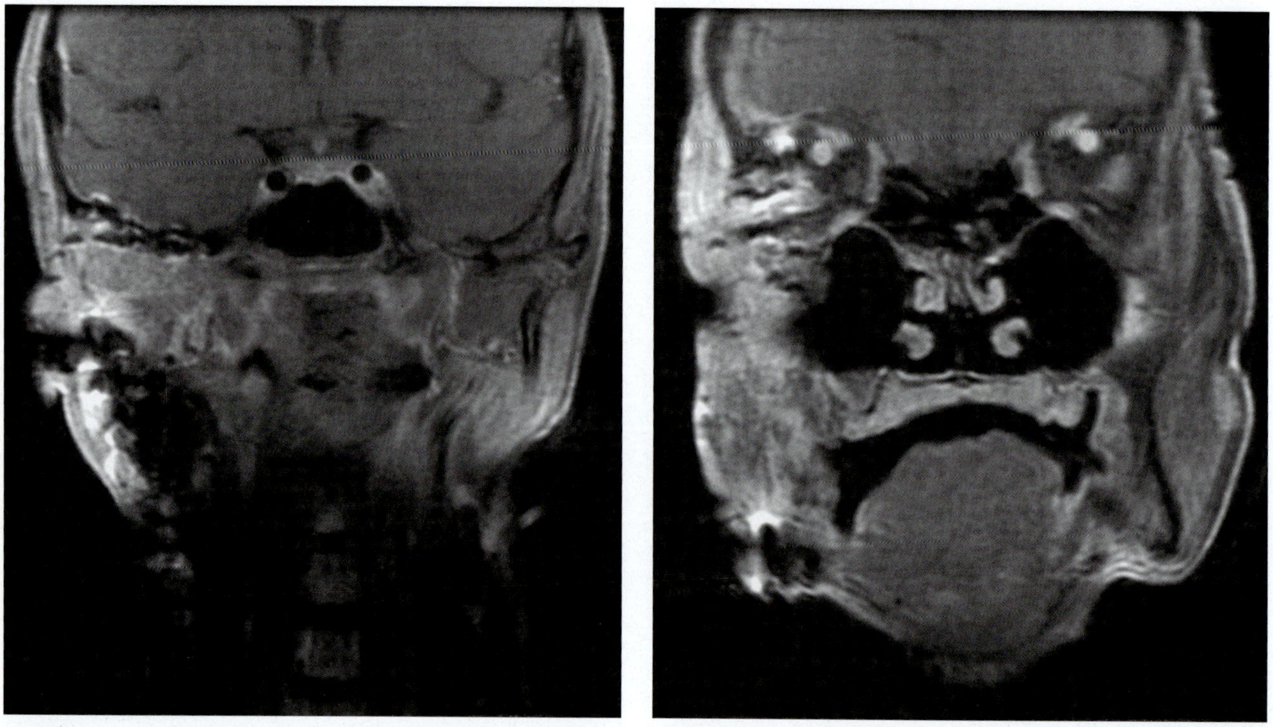

E F

Fig. 54.15 *(continued)* **(E)** The patient underwent a lateral orbitotomy and orbitozygomatic approach to resect the middle cranial fossa component of tumor. A parotidectomy and completion mandibulectomy with temporomandibular joint resection were also performed, and intraoperative radiation therapy (IORT) was administered. The dura was repaired with bovine dura, and the uninvolved temporalis muscle was reflected beneath the middle cranial fossa floor. No sphenoid sinus or maxillary antrum entry was made. A postoperative coronal postgadolinium T1-weighted image with fat saturation shows no gross residual disease in the operative bed at the level of the middle cranial fossa. **(F)** A more anterior coronal postgadolinium T1-weighted image with fat saturation shows resection of the orbital component of tumor. Given the recurrent nature of her tumor, the close margins at the dura, the functional eye, and the palliative intent of the surgery, the patient's orbit was not exenterated. The patient received an additional 30 Gy of external beam radiation therapy and she achieved significant palliation for 22 months and was pain free and fully functional before her tumor eventually recurred.

and inferior rotation of a portion of the temporalis muscle

4. Injury to the branches of the trigeminal nerve in the temporal floor or lateral cavernous sinus wall causing facial sensory loss or pain (identify and preserve these nerves when drilling the floor of the middle cranial fossa from lateral to medial)
5. Injury to the oculomotor, trochlear, or abducens nerves in the cavernous sinus or orbit causing diplopia (avoid excessive surgical traction or heat spread during coagulation)
6. Injury to the optic nerve during the opening of the optic canal resulting in blindness (minimize heat spread by using irrigation when drilling the optic canal, anterior clinoid process, and optic strut)
7. Injury to the internal carotid artery causing hemorrhage or stroke during subtemporal exposure or parasellar dissection (assess preoperative images for evidence of a dehiscent horizontal petrous canal or artery displacement by tumor; insonation with the microvascular Doppler can help to locate the artery)
8. Injury to the frontal and temporal lobes from traction or tumor dissection (gently use retractors and careful tumor dissection)
9. Poor aesthetic result (attention to proper realignment of the osteotomy fragments and soft tissue layers)

Areas of Controversy

Given the low incidence of anterior skull base tumors, it is difficult to accrue patients for randomized controlled studies of various therapeutic approaches. Hence, there remain aspects of surgical management that are handled differently by individual surgeons based on their own and their institutional experience. Some of these areas are discussed briefly.

1. Can the contralateral olfactory apparatus be preserved when an esthesioneuroblastoma appears to involve only the ipsilateral olfactory bulb at the cribriform plate?

This is difficult to do, and should be considered only in highly selected patients. Good quality, thin-section coronal MRIs, notably high-resolution fast spin echo (FSE)

Table 54.2 Potential Complications of Orbitozygomatic Approach

Complication	Prevention
VII injury (temporalis and zygomatic branches)	Incision traverses the zygomatic arch posteriorly, and lateral orbital rim dissection is just superficial to deep fascia, beneath the temporal fat pad
Intraorbital injury: hematoma, enophthalmos, diplopia	Maintain periorbital integrity to extent possible, hemostasis, extraconal dissection
Cerebrospinal fluid rhinorrhea into sphenoid sinus	Open into sphenoid sinus only if needed; repair dura and use temporalis flap to segregate opened sinus from dura
V2 numbness	Avoid infraorbital foramen when making zygomatic body osteotomies; at middle cranial fossa floor, respect foramen rotundum
Injury to cranial nerves III, IV, VI	Avoid excessive traction and coagulation heat at cavernous sinus and annulus of posterior orbit; maintain periorbital integrity
Optic nerve injury	Irrigate when using drill or bipolar electrocautery when opening optic canal or operating near adjacent structures such as the anterior clinoid or optic strut
Injury to internal carotid artery (ICA)	(1) Preoperative imaging evaluation for dehiscent horizontal petrous canal or displacement of ICA by tumor (2) Microvascular Doppler to assist in locating the ICA
Frontal lobe edema	Minimize retraction, gentle tumor dissection
Aesthetic defects	Align osteotomies at closure; replace anterior half of temporalis muscle to its usual location

T2-weighted images, are very helpful in determining whether the opposite cranial nerve (CN) I can be spared. The issues are that the opposite CN I is quite fragile and may be damaged anyway, and the space to repair a CSF leak becomes narrow when one preserves the crista galli. The surgical margin will also be closer in these cases. Given the relatively good response of these tumors to the combination of surgery and postoperative radiation therapy, and given that there are some who advocate a nonsurgical treatment option involving only radiation and chemotherapy, some patients might opt to accept a closer surgical margin rather than necessarily sacrifice olfaction. The authors' own experience is that in highly selected patients, we have occasionally successfully preserved the opposite CN I while obtaining both clean surgical margins and an effective CSF leak repair using a pericranial flap. The chance of contralateral olfactory preservation is greatly enhanced if the tumor can be resected by an entirely endoscopic approach.

2. Orbit preservation: How much of the medial orbit can be involved to still achieve both an oncologically sound resection and useful eye function?

This is controversial, and was discussed earlier. Some feel that involvement of the lamina papyracea is an indication for orbital exenteration. More feel that bone involvement per se does not require exenteration but that orbital periosteal involvement does. One can, however, remove considerable periosteum and still maintain conjugate vision without diplopia if the medial and lateral canthal ligaments are preserved and there is no orbital fat involvement by the tumor. An MRI is very helpful in assessing the orbit, but one cannot always definitely establish the presence or absence of fat involvement by radiologic criteria, and careful intraoperative evaluation is essential. Preoperative full extraocular motility correlates well with the likelihood of preserving orbit function, but this criterion is also not perfect. To further complicate the matter, there may be times when tumor does extend intraorbitally to focally involve orbital fat, but orbit preservation remains a viable option. This is an individual judgment decision by the surgeon, in conjunction with the radiation oncologist and the patient. If a close decision (such as a concerning margin elsewhere) is anticipated, then it is often best to make this decision late in the surgical procedure, after an assessment by frozen sections of other key potential margins such as dura, lateral sphenoid sinus, and posterior orbital periosteum. If close or microscopically positive margins are inevitable at other locations and the eye was functional preoperatively, then the surgeon must decide whether exenteration would either (1) materially improve the prognosis or (2) significantly facilitate postoperative radiation treatment.

3. How should the frontal sinus be managed?

The best way to prevent a possible late complication of a frontal sinus mucocele is to ensure that all areas of the frontal sinus can drain into the ethmoid sinuses. If the frontal sinus is entered as part of the frontal craniotomy and a pericranial galeal flap is used, then it will be necessary to remove the mucosa from the now segregated superior portion of the frontal sinus, and also to burr away 1 to 2 mm of the surface as one would as part of a frontal sinus obliteration. Fat obliteration or removal of the posterior table may at times be indicated to prevent a mucocele or to facilitate prevention of a CSF leak.

Occasionally, epidural air may fill the frontal fossa postoperatively, particularly if a dehydrated, CSF-depleted brain does not fully reexpand. Excessive drainage of lumbar CSF can also contribute to this. If a CSF leak has been excluded as the etiology of the air, then it is likely that the source of the extradural air is nasally inspired air accessing the extradural space via the superior ethmoid and/or frontal sinus surgical defect. Intubation and maintenance of an inflated endotracheal cuff for several days usually facilitates resolution of the problem. If the air persists, then a tracheotomy may be indicated, as well as careful reassessment to be sure there is not an occult CSF leak.

4. When is supplemental bony reconstruction of the anterior skull base indicated?

Smith and Ducic[27] nicely reviewed the anatomy and versatility of extended pericranial flaps for closure of the anterior skull base. Pericranial or pericranial-galeal flaps, usually anteriorly based but sometimes lateral based, are vascularized pieces of tissue positioned and sealed in a watertight manner so that they prevent CSF leakage and so they segregate the brain from the contaminated paranasal sinus flora. They also eliminate dead space and serve as a sling to support the brain, thus preventing frontal lobe herniation.

In some cases, however, reconstruction of large anterior skull base defects may benefit from adding split calvarial bone from the inner table of the craniotomy flap to further support the brain, thus preventing herniation as well as oscillopsia or pulsatile exophthalmos if the orbital roof has been removed, or if the frontal sinus required resection (**Fig. 54.6**). Large defects are defects greater than 3 to 4 cm both in anteroposterior and transverse dimensions; they typically include the orbital roof and part of the planum sphenoidale.[28] The split calvarial bone is placed superior to the pericranial flap, and then the distal part of the soft tissue flap is reflected back over the bone to fully enclose it within soft tissue.

5. Should drainage of cerebrospinal fluid be performed, by what means, and for how long?

Drainage of CSF can decompress the brain, thus reducing both the amount of brain that needs to be retracted and the retractor pressure needed to accomplish the needed elevation. Use of a ventricular catheter rather than a lumbar subarachnoid drain to remove CSF has the advantage of facile reexpansion of the ventricles by the infusion of fluid at the end of the case. Return of the frontal lobe to its original position occupies extra-axial space that might otherwise fill with air, fluid, or blood and may help secure the tissues repairing the anterior cranial fossa floor. Ventricular puncture creates a hole at the top of the CSF column and may thus be less likely to cause gravity-dependent overdrainage of CSF with the risks of pneumocephalus and downward brain herniation inherent in lumbar drainage. Postoperative drainage of CSF also increases the possibility of bacterial contamination of the CSF. If a ventricular catheter is left in place, it is clamped unless there is CSF rhinorrhea. While substantial nasal packing remains, it may be difficult to assess for CSF rhinorrhea. Hence, some maintain the ventricular drain in place until 24 hours after any nasal packs are removed (usually by postoperative day three).

Complications: Frequency, Avoidance, and Management

Complications have become less frequent as more experience with anterior skull base surgery has been gained. Although the rate of all complications, major and minor, is ~35%, the rate of complications with long-term consequences is less than 5% in most series. Operative mortality is well under 1%; we have had no operative deaths in over a decade. The incidence of CSF leaks is less than 2%, as is the incidence of meningitis or brain abscess. CSF leaks have been addressed with re-repair (and the rare ventriculoperitoneal shunt). Infectious complications have resolved with antibiotics and/or surgical drainage. Serious central nervous system injuries (including cerebrovascular accidents, unanticipated blindness, postinfection deficits, and autonomic dysfunction) have occurred in only 2 to 3% of patients. Intracranial bleeding and venous infarction can be devastating, and meticulous dissection and hemostasis is a must. Loss of the anterior bone flap secondary to osteomyelitis, once a serious problem in anterior skull base surgery, is now rare. Pericranial-galeal flaps and, for larger defects and for those patients who have undergone prior irradiation, microvascular free flaps[29] have contributed greatly to the reduced incidence of postoperative CSF leaks and wound or bone infections. It is also our impression that we have seen less postoperative frontal lobe encephalomalacia as we have tailored approaches to minimize the need for brain retraction. Finally, medical complications such as pneumonias, arrhythmias, and (rare) myocardial infarctions have been steady at ~10%, sometimes extending hospitalizations but rarely fatal.

Outcome of Transcranial Skull Base Surgery Plus Adjuvant Therapy

Radiation Therapy[30–33]

A major impetus to the development of anterior cranial base surgery was the disappointing results of radiation with or without the surgery of the time for tumors that extended to the skull base. Numerous series showed no better than 50% survival (and in most series 25 to 35%) for the more common malignancies. Planning radiation fields near the brain, optic nerves, and optic chiasm[34] is challenging. The ocular lens can tolerate ~50 Gy. Above this, cataracts develop, but they are treatable. Regarding the optic nerve and chiasm, there is a 10% incidence of optic neuritis if the dose received is 50 to 55 Gy, whereas the incidence increases to 20% above 65 Gy. Minor radionecrosis of the inferior portions of the frontal lobe is often tolerated with few if any long-term symptoms, but this is not always the case. Radionecrosis of the brain may lead to severe cerebral edema, brain herniation, and death. Although there is variation in the literature regarding what dose of radiation should be given to the gross tumor volume, most centers aim for a minimum of 60 Gy, with many centers advocating a minimum of 65 Gy or more.

Prior to the development of intensity-modulated radiation therapy (IMRT), charged particles were often used when radiating the anterior skull base. The rapid falloff in dose afforded by protons permitted, for example, a dose of 60 to 80 Gy to be administered to clival chordomas without undue risk to the optic nerves and chiasm. Proton beam radiation therapy is available at only a few centers, however, severely limiting its usefulness. Preliminary experience does suggest that proton IMRT may offer even tighter fields than conventional IMRT, allowing more of a tumor to receive adequate doses safely. Stereotactic radiosurgery directed at small regions of residual or recurrent tumor is also being used to supplement IMRT, and the increasingly widespread availability of stereotactic radiosurgical systems is likely to result in it being used more frequently in the future.

Chemotherapy

Concomitant postoperative chemotherapy and radiation therapy is indicated for squamous cell carcinoma (SCC) of the paranasal sinuses that extends through the skull base. For lymphomas, chemotherapy is usually the mainstay of treatment depending on the specific histologic type of lymphoma and the stage of disease. For esthesioneuroblastoma, the role of chemotherapy is controversial; some recommend it for all Kadish C lesions, whereas others reserve it for only the most extensive tumors. For high-grade neuroendocrine carcinomas and sinonasal undifferentiated carcinomas, chemotherapy in conjunction with irradiation and surgery is generally considered. Specific regimens directed toward a particular tumor histology will depend on the overall health and tolerance of the patient.

Many series[35–44] from different centers, including our own, have documented encouraging local control rates compared with historical results that do not include skull base resection for several malignant histologies (including esthesioneuroblastoma, adenoid cystic carcinoma [ACC], adenocarcinoma, and SCC). These are summarized in **Table 54.3** and also discussed in Chapter 42. Esthesioneuroblastomas and adenocarcinomas generally respond best, with 5-year survival rates approaching or exceeding 80%. Several tumors are in the middle, with 5-year survival rates on the order of 50 to 60%. Melanoma and sinonasal undifferentiated tumors do much more poorly, and treatment strategies for patients with these two histologies should stress functional preservation and the need for multicenter trials to attempt to elucidate how best to incorporate chemotherapy and IMRT or possibly proton IMRT into the management of these patients.

Table 54.3 Prognosis by Histology

Histology	Five-Year Survival (%)
Esthesioneuroblastoma	62–95 (most: 80–95)
Adenocarcinoma	78 (meta-analysis)
Adenoid cystic carcinoma	40–60 (additional 15–20% alive with disease)
Sarcomas	50–60 (additional 20% alive with disease)
Squamous cell carcinoma, including skin extending into paranasal sinuses via perineural spread	60 (meta-analysis)
Melanoma	23 (meta-analysis)
Sinonasal undifferentiated sarcoma	<10–15

Recurrent Disease and Its Treatment

Local Recurrence

Treatment of paranasal sinus malignancies that recur locally is usually limited by prior radiation and prior surgery. In addition, a tumor that has recurred may be relatively resistant to irradiation and chemotherapy. Depending on the histology, there may be chemotherapy protocols or combined chemotherapy and reirradiation protocols that are of some value. Depending on current symptoms and extent of recurrence, there may also be a role for palliative surgery.

Perineural Extension to Meckel's Cave and the Cavernous Sinus

Perineural extension, generally along V_2 or in some cases V_1, is particularly common in SCC and ACC, but is seen with many other histologies as well. New dysesthesia or hypesthesia, with or without pain, along the lateral nose and maxillary alveolar ridge (V_2) or above the eye (V_1) warrants an MRI. The MRI must be done with meticulous attention to the skull base and cavernous sinuses, as imaging findings of perineural extension may be subtle and are often overlooked by inexperienced interpreters. Spread from CN V to VII may occur via several routes, notably the auriculotemporal nerve or the greater superficial petrosal nerve, and this possibility should be carefully assessed in any patient with a history of paranasal sinus malignancy and a new facial palsy. Radiosurgery has been used in perineural extension of tumor both to control pain and to retard tumor growth, with pain relief often occurring ~6 months and with a 40% rate of clinical and radiologic 5-year durable response in controlling tumor progression.

Cervical Nodal Metastases

Cervical nodal metastases occur in ~30% of cases of SCC of the paranasal sinuses and in ~10% of esthesioneuroblastomas, but may occur with any malignant neoplasm of the paranasal sinuses. If the primary site is controlled, then a neck dissection is indicated, with postoperative irradiation performed if not already done. When there has been prior neck radiation, then there may be a role for intraoperative radiation therapy at the time of the neck dissection.[45]

Conclusion

Cranial and combined approaches to the anterior skull base, parasellar area, and subtemporal region have evolved significantly over the past 50 years, moving from early experimental procedures with dismal control rates and a high risk of life-threatening complications, to a well accepted multidisciplinary subspecialty with much improved results. Further reductions in perioperative side effects, decreased length of hospital stay, and improved aesthetic results are ongoing goals of the discipline. Modified surgical approaches are constantly under development and review. The standard against which these modifications will be judged remains a bifrontal craniotomy with or without a supraorbital rim approach, and with or without a well camouflaged transfacial extended external ethmoidectomy incision without a lateral rhinotomy. For an increasing number of cases, endoscopic-assisted approaches provide the visualization that allows foregoing a facial incision, and endoscopic techniques will continue to evolve and disseminate. Selected highly experienced centers are exploring the increased use of endoscopic resections without a craniotomy, demonstrating that this approach is feasible for highly selected tumors. A subfrontal approach with minimal brain retraction is occasionally ideal when the frontal bone and nasal bone necessarily need to be removed because of tumor involvement.

Effective skull base surgery requires a multidisciplinary team that involves otorhinolaryngologists–head and neck surgeons, neurosurgeons, plastic surgeons, neuroradiologists, medical oncologists, radiation oncologists, and prosthodontists, as well as other supporting physicians and allied health professionals. Guided by local experience and influenced by a variety of patient and physician factors, this group should cooperatively choose which set(s) of approaches and their variations appear most appropriate for each individual patient.

References

1. Smith RR, Klopp CT, Williams JM. Surgical treatment of cancer of the frontal sinus and adjacent areas. Cancer 1954;7(5):991–994
2. Dandy WE. Orbital Tumor: Results Following the Transcranial Operative Attack. New York: Oskar Priest; 1941
3. Rae BS, McLean JM. Combined intracranial and orbital operation for retinoblastoma. Arch Ophthal 1943;30:437–445
4. Ketcham AS, Wilkins RH, Vanburen JM, Smith RR. A combined intracranial approach to the paranasal sinuses. Am J Surg 1963;106:698–703
5. Van Buren JM, Ommaya AK, Ketcham AS. Ten years' experience with radical combined craniofacial resection of malignant tumors of the paranasal sinuses. J Neurosurg 1968;28(4):341–350
6. Kaplan MJ, McDermott M, Gutin P, et al. Transcutaneous transfacial approaches to the anterior skull base. Oper Tech Neurosurg 2000;3:53–56
7. Har-El G. Anterior craniofacial resection without facial skin incisions—a review. Otolaryngol Head Neck Surg 2004;130(6):780–787
8. Patel SG, Singh B, Polluri A, et al. Craniofacial surgery for malignant skull base tumors: report of an international collaborative study. Cancer 2003;98(6):1179–1187
9. Tiwari R, van der Wal J, van der Waal I, Snow G. Studies of the anatomy and pathology of the orbit in carcinoma of the maxillary sinus and their impact on preservation of the eye in maxillectomy. Head Neck 1998;20(3):193–196
10. Fee WE Jr, Moir MS, Choi EC, Goffinet D. Nasopharyngectomy for recurrent nasopharyngeal cancer: a 2- to 17-year follow-up. Arch Otolaryngol Head Neck Surg 2002;128(3):280–284
11. Ibrahim HZ, Moir MS, Fee WW. Nasopharyngectomy after failure of 2 courses of radiation therapy. Arch Otolaryngol Head Neck Surg 2002;128(10):1196–1197
12. To EW, Yuen EH, Tsang WM, et al. The use of stereotactic navigation guidance in minimally invasive transnasal nasopharyngectomy: a comparison with the conventional open transfacial approach. Br J Radiol 2002;75(892):345–350
13. To EW, Lai EC, Cheng JH, Pang PC, Williams MD, Teo PM. Nasopharyngectomy for recurrent nasopharyngeal carcinoma: a review of 31 patients and prognostic factors. Laryngoscope 2002;112(10):1877–1882
14. Jho HD, Ha HG. Endoscopic endonasal skull base surgery: Part 1—The midline anterior fossa skull base. Minim Invasive Neurosurg 2004;47(1):1–8
15. Lang J. The anterior and middle cranial fossae including the cavernous sinus and orbit. In: Sekhar LN, Janecka IP, eds. Surgery of Cranial Base Tumors. New York: Raven Press; 1993: 99–121
16. Thaler ER, Kotapka M, Lanza DC, Kennedy DW. Endoscopically assisted anterior cranial skull base resection of sinonasal tumors. Am J Rhinol 1999;13(4):303–310
17. Yuen APW, Fung CF, Hung KN. Endoscopic cranionasal resection of anterior skull base tumor. Am J Otolaryngol 1997;18(6):431–433
18. Har-El G, Todor R. Anterior craniofacial resection without facial skin incisions—a review. Otolaryngol Head Neck Surg 2004; 130(6):780–787
19. Fagan JJ, Snyderman CH, Carrau RL, Janecka IP. Nasopharyngeal angiofibromas: selecting a surgical approach. Head Neck 1997;19(5):391–399
20. Carrau RL, Snyderman CH, Kassam AB, Jungreis CA. Endoscopic and endoscopic-assisted surgery for juvenile angiofibroma. Laryngoscope 2001;111(3):483–487
21. Al-Nashar IS, Carrau RL, Herrera A, Snyderman CH. Endoscopic transnasal transpterygopalatine fossa approach to the lateral recess of the sphenoid sinus. Laryngoscope 2004;114(3):528–532
22. Stuzin JM, Wagstrom L, Kawamoto HK, Wolfe SA. Anatomy of the frontal branch of the facial nerve: the significance of the temporal fat pad. Plast Reconstr Surg 1989;83(2):265–271
23. Raveh J, Laedrach K, Speiser M, et al. The subcranial approach for fronto-orbital and antero-posterior skull base tumors. Arch Otolaryngol Head Neck Surg 1993;119:382–393

24. Har-El G. Anterior craniofacial resection without facial skin incisions–a review. Otolaryngol Head Neck Surg 2004;103:780–787
25. Cocke EW, Robertson JH. Extended unilateral maxillotomy approach. In: Donald PJ, ed. Surgery of the Skull Base. Philadelphia: Lippincott-Raven; 1998: 207–237
26. Casiano RR, Numa WA, Falquez AM. Endoscopic resection of esthesioneuroblastoma. Am J Rhinol 2001;15(4):271–279
27. Smith JE, Ducic Y. The versatile extended pericranial flap for closure of skull base defects. Otolaryngol Head Neck Surg 2004;130(6):704–711
28. Rodrigues M, O'Malley BW Jr, Staecker H, Tamargo R. Extended pericranial flap and bone graft reconstruction in anterior skull base surgery. Otolaryngol Head Neck Surg 2004;131(1):69–76
29. Clayman GL, DeMonte F, Jaffe DM, et al. Outcome and complications of extended cranial-base resection requiring microvascular free-tissue transfer. Arch Otolaryngol Head Neck Surg 1995;121(11):1253–1257
30. Adams EJ, Nutting CM, Convery DJ, et al. Potential role of intensity-modulated radiotherapy in the treatment of tumors of the maxillary sinus. Int J Radiat Oncol Biol Phys 2001;51(3):579–588
31. Claus F, De Gersem W, De Wagter C, et al. An implementation strategy for IMRT of ethmoid sinus cancer with bilateral sparing of the optic pathways. Int J Radiat Oncol Biol Phys 2001;51(2): 318–331
32. Waldron JN, O'Sullivan B, Gullane P, et al. Carcinoma of the maxillary antrum: a retrospective analysis of 110 cases. Radiother Oncol 2000;57(2):167–173
33. Waldron JN, O'Sullivan B, Gullane P, et al. Carcinoma of the maxillary antrum: a retrospective analysis of 110 cases. Radiother Oncol 2000;57(2):167–173
34. Rasch C, Eisbruch A, Remeijer P, et al. Irradiation of paranasal sinus tumors, a delineation and dose comparison study. Int J Radiat Oncol Biol Phys 2002;52(1):120–127
35. Janecka IP, Sen C, Sekhar LN, et al. Cranial base surgery: results in 183 patients. Otolaryngol Head Neck Surg 1994;110(6):539–546
36. Janecka IP, Sen C, Sekhar L, Curtin H. Treatment of paranasal sinus cancer with cranial base surgery: results. Laryngoscope 1994;104(5 Pt 1):553–555
37. Irish JC, Gullane PJ, Gentili F, et al. Tumors of the skull base: outcome and survival analysis of 77 cases. Head Neck 1994; 16(1):3–10
38. O'Malley BW Jr, Janecka IP. Evolution of outcomes in cranial base surgery. Semin Surg Oncol 1995;11(3):221–227
39. McCaffrey TV, Olsen KD, Yohanan JM, Lewis JE, Ebersold MJ, Piepgras DG. Factors affecting survival of patients with tumors of the anterior skull base. Laryngoscope 1994;104(8 Pt 1): 940–945
40. Boyle JO, Shah KC, Shah JP. Craniofacial resection for malignant neoplasms of the skull base: an overview. J Surg Oncol 1998;69(4):275–284
41. Shah JP, Kraus DH, Arbit E, Galicich JH, Strong EW. Craniofacial resection for tumors involving the anterior skull base. Otolaryngol Head Neck Surg 1992;106(4):387–393
42. Harbo G, Grau C, Bundgaard T, et al. Cancer of the nasal cavity and paranasal sinuses. A clinico-pathological study of 277 patients. Acta Oncol 1997;36(1):45–50
43. Lund VJ, Howard DJ, Wei WI, Cheesman AD. Craniofacial resection for tumors of the nasal cavity and paranasal sinuses—a 17-year experience. Head Neck 1998;20(2):97–105
44. Dulguerov P, Jacobsen MS, Allal AS, Lehmann W, Calcaterra T. Nasal and paranasal sinus carcinoma: are we making progress? A series of 220 patients and a systematic review. Cancer 2001;92(12):3012–3029
45. Coleman CW, Roach M III, Ling SM, et al. Adjuvant electron-beam IORT in high-risk head and neck cancer patients. Front Radiat Ther Oncol 1997;31:105–111
46. Harvey RJ, Nogueira JF, Schlosser RJ, Patel SJ, Vellutini E, Stamm AC. Closure of large skull base defects after endoscopic transnasal craniotomy. Clinical article. J Neurosurg 2009;111(2): 371–379

Index

Note: Page numbers in *italic* indicate figures.

N

O

P

Q

R

MENU FOR THE ACCOMPANYING DVD

Video 1: Anatomy of the Paranasal Sinuses
Richard R. Orlandi

Video 2: Endoscopic Septoplasty
Parul Goyal

Video 3: Inferior Turbinate Submucosal Resection
Parul Goyal

Video 4: Maxillary Antrostomy
Eric H. Holbrook

Video 5: Total Ethmoidectomy
Amin R. Javer and Carl Philpott

Video 6: Sphenoidotomy
John Lee

Video 7: Frontal: Draf Types 1 and 2A
Joseph K. Han

Video 8: Endoscopic Draf Type 3 Procedure (Modified Lothrop Procedure)
Alexander G. Chiu and Jayakar V. Nayak

Video 9: Endoscopic Resection of Inverting Papilloma
Rakesh K. Chandra and Andrew J. Fishman

Video 10: Sphenopalatine Artery Ligation
Amin R. Javer and Carl Philpott

Video 11: Cerebrospinal Fluid Leak Repair/Encephalocele
Rodney J. Schlosser and Richard J. Harvey

Video 12: Dacryocystorhinostomy
Todd T. Kingdom and Vikram Durairaj

Video 13: Orbital Decompression
Winston Vaughan and Roy F. Thomas

Video 14: Esthesioneuroblastoma
Belachew Tessema, Jean Anderson Eloy, and Roy R. Casiano

Video 15: Endoscopic Resection of a Juvenile Angiofibroma
Peter-John Wormald

Video 16: Endoscopic Approach to the Odontoid
Carl H. Snyderman, Amin B. Kassam, Ricardo L. Carrau, Daniel M. Prevedello, Juan C. Fernandez-Miranda, and Paul A. Gardner

Video 17: Sublabial Trans-Septal Endoscopic Repair of Bilateral Choanal Atresia
Peter J. Koltai

Video 18: Endoscopic Resection of Pituitary Adenoma
Brent A. Senior

Video 19: Endoscopic Approach to the Clivus and Posterior Fossa
Aldo C. Stamm, João Flávio Nogueira, and Larry Hilton Kalish

Video 20: Free Graft Skull Base Reconstruction after Endoscopic Skull Base Surgery
Pete S. Batra

Video 21: Septal Sphenopalatine Flap for Skull Base Reconstruction
Aldo C. Stamm and João Flávio Nogueira